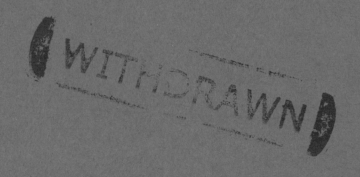

HEALTH ASSESSMENT
Across the Life Span

HEALTH ASSESSMENT
Across the Life Span

Dorothy A. Jones, R.N., C., M.S.N., F.A.A.N.
Editor-in-Chief
Associate Professor
Boston College School of Nursing

Mary Kolassa Lepley, R.N., M.S.N., P.N.P.
Assistant Professor
University of Colorado Health Sciences Center
School of Nursing

Bette A. Baker, R.N., M.S.N., J.D.
Formerly Instructor
University of Texas Health Science Center
School of Nursing

Consulting Editor　　Jerome T. Glickman, Ed.D. Candidate (Boston University)
Director, Educational Media Support Center
Assistant Professor
Boston University School of Medicine

Consulting Editor and　Marcia L. Williams, M.S.M.I.
Visual Coordinator　　Art Staff Coordinator
Educational Media Support Center
Boston University School of Medicine

Photography　　Fred W. Delorey, B.S., M.Ed.
Assistant to the Director for Production
Educational Media Support Center
Boston University School of Medicine

McGraw-Hill Book Company
New York St. Louis San Francisco Auckland Bogotá Hamburg
Johannesburg London Madrid Mexico Montreal New Delhi
Panama Paris São Paulo Singapore Sydney Tokyo Toronto

HEALTH ASSESSMENT ACROSS THE LIFE SPAN

234567890   VNHVNH   8987654

ISBN 0-07-032805-6

This book was set in Century Schoolbook by York Graphic Services, Inc.
The editors were Karol M. Carstensen and Stephen Wagley;
the designer was Merrill Haber;
the production supervisor was Charles Hess.
The drawings were done by Boston University Medical Center.
Von Hoffmann Press, Inc., was printer and binder.

NOTICE

As new medical and nursing research and clinical experience broaden our knowledge, changes in treatment and drug therapy are required. The editors and the publisher of this work have made every effort to ensure that the drug dosage schedules herein are accurate and in accord with the standards accepted at the time of publication. Readers are advised, however, to check the product information sheet included in the package of each drug they plan to administer to be certain that changes have not been made in the recommended dose or in the contraindications for administration. This recommendation is of particular importance in regard to new or infrequently used drugs.

Library of Congress Cataloging in Publication Data

Jones, Dorothy A.
    Health assessment across the life span.

    Includes indexes.
    1. Physical diagnosis. 2. Nursing. I. Lepley,
Mary Kolassa. II. Baker, Bette A. (Bette Ann)
III. Title. [DNLM: 1. Nursing process. WY 100 H4335]
RT48.J66   1984   616.07'54   83-9846
ISBN 0-07-032805-6

CONTENTS

LIST OF CONTRIBUTORS · vii

PREFACE · ix

1 HOLISTIC HEALTH AND NURSING PRACTICE · 1
Bette A. Baker and Dorothy A. Jones

2 BEHAVIORAL DEVELOPMENT · 31
Joan McParland, Karen A. Szymanski, and Mary Kolassa Lepley

3 ESTABLISHING A DATA BASE: THE HEALTH HISTORY · 69
Mary Kolassa Lepley, with contributions by Dorothy A. Jones

4 PHYSICAL EXAMINATION · 117
Dorothy A. Jones, with contributions by Carol Bowen, Meredith Censullo,
Lynne Colby, Maureen Jane Guarino McRae, Mary Ellen Maguire,
Margaret Allen Murphy, Geralyn R. Spollett

5 THE NEONATE · 351
Phyllis A. Autotte and Mary Kolassa Lepley

6 THE INFANT · 413
Arlene Misklow Sperhac

7 THE TODDLER · 467
Cheryl A. Olson and Mary Kolassa Lepley

8 THE PRESCHOOLER · 509
Nancy Kay Olson Hester and Mary Kolassa Lepley

9 THE SCHOOL-AGED CHILD · 559
Gladys M. Scipien, Marilyn A. Chard, and Dorothy A. Jones

10 ADOLESCENCE · 597
Karen L. Miller

11 THE YOUNG ADULT · 637
Lynne E. Johnson Phillips

12 PREGNANCY · 669
Maureen Jane Guarino McRae and Mary Kolassa Lepley

13 THE MIDDLE ADULT · 725
Mary P. Cadogan

14 AGING · 757
Nancy J. Kehrli and Marian G. Spencer

APPENDIXES · 801

INDEXES · 839
Author and Title Index
Subject Index

LIST OF CONTRIBUTORS

Phyllis A. Autotte, R.N., M.P.H., C.P.N.P.
Consultant in Maternal Child Health
Pan American Health Organization
World Health Organization
Tegucigalpa, Honduras

Formerly Clinical Instructor
University Graduate Division
University of Wisconsin School of Nursing
Madison, Wisconsin

Bette A. Baker, R.N., M.S.N., J.D.
Formerly Instructor
University of Texas Health Science Center
School of Nursing
San Antonio, Texas

Carol Bowen, R.N., C., M.S.N.
Clinical Specialist, Primary Care
Lemuel Shattuck Hospital
Boston, Massachusetts

Mary P. Cadogan, R.N.M.N.
Assistant Clinical Professor
Department of Family Medicine
School of Medicine
University of California, San Diego
San Diego, California

Meredith Censullo, R.N., M.S.,
    Doctoral Candidate (Boston College)
Assistant Professor
Massachusetts General Institute
Boston, Massachusetts

Marilyn A. Chard, R.N., B.S., Ed.M., M.S., Ed.D.
Faculty/Clinical Specialist
Department of Pediatrics
School of Nursing and School of Medicine
University of Kansas College
Lawrence, Kansas

Lynne Colby, R.N.C., M.S.
Clinical Specialist—Primary Care
Family Health Services
Sommerville Hospital
Sommerville, Massachusetts

Nancy Kay Olson Hester, R.N., Ph.D.
Assistant Professor
University of Colorado Health Sciences Center
School of Nursing
Denver, Colorado

Dorothy A. Jones, R.N., C., M.S.N., F.A.A.N.,
    Ed.D. Candidate (Boston University)
Associate Professor
Graduate Medical Surgical Nursing
Project Director, Primary Care
Boston College School of Nursing
Chestnut Hill, Massachusetts

Nancy J. Kehrli, R.N., M.S.
Assistant Professor, Primary Care Nursing
    Program
Boston University School of Nursing
Boston, Massachusetts

Mary Kolassa Lepley, R.N., M.S.N., P.N.P.
Assistant Professor
University of Colorado Health Sciences Center
School of Nursing
Denver, Colorado

Mary Ellen McGuire, R.N., C., M.S.
Nurse Practitioner–Clinical Specialist,
    Primary Care
Leonard Morse Occupational Services, Inc.
Natick, Massachusetts

Joan McParland, R.N., M.S.
Assistant Chief of Nursing Service for Education
Bedford Veterans Medical Center
Bedford, Massachusetts

Maureen Jane Guarino McRae, R.N., M.S.N.
Maternity Clinical Specialist
Beth Israel Hospital
Boston, Massachusetts

Karen L. Miller, R.N., M.S.
Director of Nursing Education
Lutheran Medical Center
Wheatridge, Colorado

Formerly Assistant Professor
University of Colorado Health Sciences Center
School of Nursing
Denver, Colorado

Margaret Allen Murphy, R.N., C., M.A.
Assistant Professor
Boston College School of Nursing
Chestnut Hill, Massachusetts

Cheryl A. Olson, R.N., M.S., C.F.D.P.
Educational Director
Montana State University (Missoula Campus)
Bozeman, Montana

Lynne E. Johnson Phillips, R.N., M.S.N.
Manager of Patient Services
Home Health Care of America, Inc.
Denver, Colorado

Formerly Assistant Professor
University of Colorado Health Sciences Center
School of Nursing
Denver, Colorado

Gladys M. Scipien, R.N., M.S., F.A.A.N.
Associate Professor
Boston University School of Nursing
Boston, Massachusetts

Marion G. Spencer, R.N., M.S., C.A.G.S.
Associate Professor
Gerontological Nursing Program
Boston University School of Nursing
Boston, Massachusetts

Arlene Misklow Sperhac, R.N., P.N.P., Ph.D.
Assistant Professor
Institute for Health Professions
Massachusetts General Hospital
Boston, Massachusetts

Geralyn R. Spollett, R.N., S., M.S.N.
Occupational Health Nurse Practitioner
McLean Hospital
Belmont, Massachusetts

Karen A. Szymanski, R.N., M.S., M.B.A.
Management Consultant
Value Management Inc.
Wheaton, Illinois

PREFACE

During the last few decades, the growth of professional nursing has been significant. Many social, political, economic, and educational trends, such as the women's movement, cost containment and economic constraints, increased technology, national health insurance, the nurse practitioner movement of the 1970s, the open classroom, and the computer age, have made a profound impact on the direction of professional nursing today. Evidence of growth in context, theory, and process abounds, not only in curriculum development, but in research and practice as well. During the past ten years alone, the number of textbooks written on nursing theory has greatly increased, reflecting the continued evolution of the science of nursing.

The art of nursing, the creative application of nursing science to practice, has also changed. At all levels of professional education, there is a demand for nurses to articulate and teach that domain of knowledge called nursing. Therefore, increased attention has been paid to those activities engaged in by the professional nurse in the delivery of nursing care.

One significant result of this development has been to place increased emphasis upon the decision making process and how it determines nursing action. Central to this process is the acquisition, processing, and interpretation of data collected from individuals, families, or groups.

Early interpretation of this process relied heavily on the medical model of assessment and emphasized the medical history and physical assessment skills. However, as nurses further defined their profession, it became apparent that a comprehensive system of data collection oriented to professional nursing activities was needed. This system would enable nurses to assess, diagnose, treat, and evaluate clients' responses to actual or potential health problems.

Health Assessment Across the Life Span presents such an approach to data collection. This book takes a holistic approach to assessing human beings and their response to the life process. It focuses upon organizing data collection around a nursing model. Human beings are viewed as dynamic, changing individuals, interacting continuously with their environment. Their responses to the life process are complex, highly integrated, and very individualized. Growth and development, along with past experiences, sociocultural backgrounds, and economic forces, constitute additional variables which affect data collection and influence data analysis.

Health Assessment Across the Life Span does not define what is normal in relation to abnormalities or diseases. Instead, it describes in elaborate detail a range of expected responses which the nurse can then evaluate in light of such variables as the client's age, developmental process, and present health status. The purpose of this textbook is to provide the professional nurse with a method of data collection that yields information to guide nursing decisions.

The text is designed to present an overall framework for data collection in the first four chapters and then to apply this framework to various age groups in the remaining ten chapters.

Chapter 1 presents a historical overview of the concept of holistic health and incorporates it into a nursing framework. In addition, various frameworks of practice proposed by current nursing theorists are discussed along with an overview of the nursing process. Because of the importance of human responses to health and illness, Chapter 2 emphasizes components of behavioral development. Within the chapter, a variety of developmental theories is presented along with a description of associated behaviors for a variety of ages and stages of growth. The reader should also refer to specific developmental chapters for discussions of theories more specific to that age group.

Chapter 3 integrates the holistic philosophy presented in Chapter 1 with Gordon's functional pattern typology of human responses as a framework for data collection.* Specific functional patterns, for example, Nutritional Pattern, Elimination Pattern, Exercise-Activity Pattern, are discussed in terms of normal dimensions. In addition, discussion of each pattern is followed by a listing of suggested questions that can be used to elicit data. This format is used in describing findings unique to each age group discussed throughout the remainder of the book.

The format for presenting physical assessment information in Chapter 4 has been specifically created to fit the holistic framework of this book. In addition, text and illustrations interact to facilitate learning. The chapter incorporates a head-to-toe approach to the examination and presents the techniques used to collect data in each body component. Also included is a discussion of the nurse's approach to the client and a section on equipment used to collect data. It should be noted that the young adult is used as the model for Chapter 4 since it is at this period that optimal physical growth should be achieved.

Chapters 5 through 14 present normal assessment for each age group across the life span: neonate, infant, toddler, preschooler, schoolage child, adolescent, young adult, middle adult, and older adult. Of particular interest is Chapter 12, which discusses pregnancy throughout each trimester, and illustrates and identifies the normal changes that accompany pregnancy. In addition, there is a parallel discussion of the development of the fetus for each month of pregnancy and its effect on the mother's physical state.

Health Assessment Across the Life Span incorporates a multiplicity of features that will offer professional nursing an approach to collect data and diagnose health problems for which they are accountable. We hope that the consistant format along with the illustrated physical assessment sections will have an impact, not only on the student of nursing, but on the profession as a whole.

ACKNOWLEDGMENTS

The production of *Health Assessment Across the Life Span* has been a monumental task made possible through the efforts of many people. To acknowledge everyone's efforts would not be possible; however, there are several people who should be recognized:

To Jerry Glickman, our thanks for your friendship, sensitivity to goals of the book, and continued efforts in helping us translate into visual form what we were able to describe in words

---

*Marjory Gordon, *Nursing Diagnosis: Process and Application,* McGraw-Hill, New York, 1982.

To Marcia Williams, our deepest appreciation for your loyalty, talent, patience, and dedication beyond the call of duty

To Fred DeLorey, our deepest gratitude for your wit, your energy, your willingness to adapt to our schedule, and, above all, your photographic skill and ability

Special thanks are also extended to the secretarial and support staff of Boston University Educational Media Support Center: Stacey Farratti, graphic design assistant; Jo Ellen Murphy, biomedical illustrator; Mark Lefkowitz, medical illustrator; Kathleen Cote, medical photographer; Jim Grochecki, senior photographer; William J. Tocci, Jr., medical illustrator; Diane Glickman, senior typographer; and Ginney Halliday, typographer.

Recognition is given to John Sanders, Jr., of Forsyth Dental Center, Boston, Massachusetts, for photography of the mouth found in Chapter 4; Newton Wellesley Hospital, Newton, Massachusetts, for permitting us to photograph pictures of the newborn found in Chapter 5; William K. Frankenburg, Arnold D. Goldstein, and John Barker, University of Colorado Medical Center, for permission to reproduce the Denver Eye Screening Test; William K. Frankenburg and J. B. Dodds, University of Colorado Medical Center, for permission to reproduce the Denver Developmental Screening Test; Amelia F. Drumwright, University of Colorado School of Nursing, for permission to reproduce the Denver Articulation Screening Exam; and Ross Laboratories for permission to reproduce the growth percentile charts.

Thanks must also be given to the personnel at McGraw-Hill who supported this endeavor: Orville Haberman, Laura Dysart Marcy, Dave Carroll, Karol Carstensen, and Stephen Wagley.

A special thank-you is extended to the undergraduate and graduate faculty of the University of Colorado School of Nursing for providing an atmosphere of educational excellence and encouragement and support in making this text a reality, and to the graduate students and faculty in the primary care curriculum of Boston College for participating in this project as authors, models, consultants, and resource persons.

Finally, our deepest thanks must be extended to our families and friends who have supported us throughout this endeavor:

To Dorothy and Thomas Jones, for creating a loving environment that allowed for development while nurturing personal growth

To Thomas, Lorraine, Roy, Thomas, and Christopher, for always being interested and loving generously

To Bill, Diane, and Pamela, for bringing a new joy to life; for being there and caring

To Charles R. and Charles H. Lepley, who provided support, encouragement, love, understanding, and inspiration for a sometimes tedious and yet gratifying effort and accomplishment

To Vivian and Jerome Kolassa and Margaret and Hollie Lepley, for being such loving, caring, and supportive parents throughout this lengthy endeavor

To Isabelle and Kenneth C. Baker, Mary M. Baker, Kenneth Baker, Deborah Baker, and Kristina Baker for their support and love throughout all the challenges and changes.

To all of the numerous nurses and nursing students who over the years have challenged our ways of teaching and inspired us to strive for excellence in education

Dorothy A. Jones
Mary Kolassa Lepley
Bette A. Baker

HOLISTIC HEALTH AND NURSING PRACTICE

CHAPTER ONE

Bette Baker and Dorothy A. Jones

INTRODUCTION

In our complex society, an individual's search for optimal health seems to be limited by the fact that human beings are not viewed in their entirety. Historically, health providers have tended to isolate certain portions of the mind or body for study. In many instances examination of the "whole" person—that is, study of the mind, body, and spirit, beyond the sum of all the parts of an individual—has been put aside for study of the intricacies of one system or organ.

Holism (sometimes spelled *wholism*) is a concept that accepts as its basic premise an individual as a total being, composed of a continuously interacting body, mind, and spirit in harmony with itself and the environment.

It is difficult to attain and maintain health if the essential aspects of health—namely, the physical, spiritual, and psychological perspectives—are not addressed. The information contained throughout the text is presented from the perspective of a holistic framework, so as to emphasize the totality of clients interacting with the self and others to promote health.

Holism views human beings as a total interaction of mind, body, and spirit.

Definition of Health

"Health" is a term familiar to everyone. Yet, despite the universality of the concept of health, there is little agreement on its definition. Many groups at various times have attempted to define health; however, their definitions often seemed vague and unclear.

Despite the elusiveness of a definition of health, nurses and other health care providers are charged with the responsibility of promoting the health of a large number of people. If health is to be successfully promoted, a health standard must be established. This standard should specify clear criteria by which the health provider can measure attainment of the optimal health for a particular individual or group of individuals. Over the years a number of health descriptions have been developed. These definitions reflect the gamut of interpretations given to the term by both traditional medicine and the promoters of a holistic perspective. These definitions include the absence of disease concept, the World Health Organization (WHO) definition, Dunn's levels of wellness, an adaptation model, Cannon's homeostasis, the freedom from pain model, holism, and Travis's concept of wellness.

Definitions of health have been proposed by many groups, but there is no agreement on one definition.

Model definitions of health include:
1. Absence of disease
2. WHO definition
3. Dunn's levels of wellness
4. Adaptation model
5. Cannon's homeostasis
6. Freedom from pain
7. Holistic health
8. Travis's concept of wellness

Absence of Disease Concept

Traditional medicine has defined health as merely the "absence of disease." However, much evidence has accumulated to show that the health state involves more than the lack of detectable pathogens in the body. Despite this information, the basic stance of traditional medicine concerning the attainment of health has not changed. Frequently, medical schools promulgate this traditional orientation by teaching that diagno-

Traditional medicine views health as the absence of disease.

sis and treatment of pathological disease is the major path toward health. Although some health care programs now include holistic medicine, the detection and removal of actual or potential pathogens is still an important component of health care practices today.

WHO Definition of Health

In 1946 WHO medical experts recognized the dilemma in delineating the nature of health. Members of this group tried to sharpen and expand the definition of health by affirming that health implies not only the absence of disease, but also a generally positive attitude toward life. The introductory paragraph of the WHO statement reads: "Health is a state of complete physical, mental, and social well-being and is not merely the absence of disease or infirmity."[1]

Dunn's Levels of Wellness

Halpert L. Dunn (1959) went further in his explorations of health. He argued that there are different levels of the health states which were later described as *levels of wellness*. Some levels are depicted as states of passive adaptability to the environment and others, as a dynamic process in which the objective is the attainment of one's optimal potential. Dunn's concept saw the absence of disease as only a beginning step toward health. He used the term "high-level wellness" to describe a dynamic state where the individual moved toward a more optimal state of wellness. Concepts related to prevention were also incorporated into this definition.

Adaptation

In the nineteenth century the renowned French physiologist Claude Bernard promoted the concept of adaptation. He believed that health depended on one's ability to maintain a stable internal environment despite changes in the external environment through use of regulatory mechanisms within oneself. The same theme was advanced in the 1930s by the American physiologist Walter B. Cannon, who referred to the adaptation process as *homeostasis*. Cannon suggested that when an organism was unable to maintain homeostasis, it was out of balance and thus could not be called healthy. Critics of the term "homeostasis" suggest that the term implies a static rather than a more dynamic state of being.

Others viewed health as a continuous process, involving adaptation to the environment. According to a proponent of George Engle (1962):

> When the organism is successfully adjusting to the environment and is able to maintain this state free of undue excitation, capable of growth, development, and activity in an integrated and effective sense . . . then an active dynamic process is taking place in the face of an ever-changing environment. There is a continued need for adjustment and adaptation to maintain this state in face of tasks imposed from the outside or from within the organism itself.[3]

Health as Freedom from Pain

Before scientific technology pervaded our lives, people from different civilizations recognized that to be healed meant to be "whole." All available records suggest that many ideas on treatment of illness and promotion of health were developed long before the advent of modern medicine. René Dubos, a public health microbiologist and philosopher, recognized this heritage when he suggested that "the nearest approach to health is a physical and mental state fairly free of discomfort and pain . . . a state of adaptness which permits the person concerned to function as effectively

World Health Organization defines health as "a state of complete physical, mental and social well being and not merely the absence of disease or infirmity."

Dunn defines health according to *levels of wellness*. High-level wellness is an all-encompassing term focusing on a dynamic process toward optimal functioning of an individual, family, and community.

The adaptation model suggests that health depends on the organism's ability to adapt to the internal and external environment.

Homeostasis is the maintenance of a balance of conditions within a system. Originally the term applied to only physiological concepts but today has been expanded to include mental and social aspects as well. Homeostasis can be regarded as the maintenance of:

1 body balance, sometimes within very fine ranges;
2 psychologic and emotional balances;
3 cultural, social and political balances; and
4 spiritual and philosophic balances.[2]

as long as possible in the environment where chance or choice has placed him."[4]

Holistic Health

The holistic health movement began in the nineteenth century and has brought with it a different yet surprisingly similar definition of health and wellness. Holistic health is based on the idea that the "body-mind-spirit trinity has the inherent capacity to heal and that the environment—air, food, water, and space—have more influence on humans than anything else."[5]

The word "holistic" is derived from the Greek word *holos,* meaning whole. The word "health" is derived from the Anglo-Saxon term *hal,* also meaning whole. The terms "holistic" and "wholistic" are used interchangeably. Arthur Koestler (1967) used the word "holon" to mean a self-contained whole.[6]

In 1926 a South African philosopher, Jan Christiaan Smuts, introduced the concept of holism in a text entitled *Holism and Evolution.* His work views a human being as an organized whole greater than the sum of its parts and constantly interacting with its environment.

Work completed by D. C. Phillips expands the efforts of Smuts. While supporting the belief that the whole is greater than the sum of its parts, Phillips suggests that the whole also determines the nature of its parts and that the parts cannot be analyzed in isolation from the whole and are dynamically interrelated and interdependent.[7]

The term "holism" also refers to the beliefs that all parts of a living organism work together to determine the health of the entire person. This interdependence of body, mind, and spirit in dynamic interaction with the environment is being recognized as fundamental to health promotion efforts.

The holistic health movement further proposes that health problems result from a complex interaction of many factors that arise from within the individual person as well as the external environment. Because the causation of disease is viewed as multifaceted, development of solutions to deal with these problems must also be as complex. For these reasons the holistic health movement seeks to combine the efforts of traditional and nontraditional health care practices to promote health.

Concept of Wellness

The concept of wellness has been more recently expressed by a leading figure in the holistic health movement, Dr. John Travis. He suggests that

> Wellness is not a static state. It results when a person begins to see themself as a growing, changing person. High level wellness means giving good care to your physical self, using your mind constructively, expressing your emotions effectively, being creatively involved with those around you, being concerned about your physical and psychological environment, and becoming aware of other levels of consciousness.[8]

Another proponent of the wellness concept (Hettler) states that "wellness can also be defined as an active process through which the individual becomes aware of and/or makes choices toward a more successful existence." He further states that one's daily life is constantly changing "in the reflection of his or her intellectual, emotional, physical, social, occupational, and spiritual dimensions."[9]

Don Ardell describes high-level wellness as a life-style-focused approach which allows the individual to personally design a way to achieve

Holistic health is based on the interdependence of the body, mind, and spirit.

The work completed by Smuts suggests that the organism is greater than the sum of its parts.

Wellness is a dynamic state, reflecting growth and change physically, emotionally, and socially.

Wellness is an active process through which an individual makes choices which result in a more successful existence.

optimal wellness within the limits of his or her own capacity. Life style is an integrated, ever changing state which focuses on self responsibility, nutritional awareness, physical fitness, stress management and environmental sensitivity as critical components of optimal wellness.

Disease

When unsuccessful attempts to attain or maintain health occur, the individual lapses into a state of disease (spelled *dis-ease* by many holistically oriented people). The unique spelling of the word "dis-ease" connotes that the lack of health brought on by a general disharmonious state of dis-ease extend beyond the idea that microbial pathogens alone are the causative factor in illness.

Dis-ease: all deviations from health. Dis-ease is not limited to problems resulting from microbial pathogens; it can be a result of a variety of factors, many of which are discussed in this text.

Summary

Definitions of health have followed a path of broadening perspectives from the rather limited idea of "absence of disease" to a dynamic state of interaction of the total being's interaction (mind, body, and spirit) with the surrounding environment. Throughout the text, reference is made to the definitions of holism and wellness as they serve as the philosophical basis for assessing the client across the life span.

INFLUENCES ON HEALTH AND HOLISM

The philosophy of holistic health requires abandonment of the belief that health care should look only to traditional western medicine for answers and solutions to health care delivery. Proponents of holism take a broader view of the world and study other cultures and times to discover what has been useful and healthful. The following discussion looks more closely at some of the many cultural practices that have influenced health care practices throughout the United States and the world. They include the Oriental and Greek influences; the effects of the Middle Ages, the microbial era, and popular health movements.

Asian Influence

The Chinese and Japanese promoted holistic health practices for many thousands of years before the birth of Christ. "Traditional Oriental medicine does not conceive of the body in parts, it considers an organ a part of the whole and disease a deterioration of the entire body system. Its highest practitioners reflect constantly upon the role of man in this world and the role of disease in this life."[10]

Unlike modern Americans, the ancient Asians viewed health care as an extension of one's approach to life and not as a separate entity. The way one lived, worked, ate, and interacted with the environment was all part of the harmony of life that determined health. Nutrition and peace of mind were considered as much a part of health as physical endowment.

Confucian and Taoist beliefs also impacted on the Chinese attitudes toward health. Confucius shared his commonsense approach to life with his believers, supporting the use of practical knowledge as a way of achieving good health.

Taoism, on the other hand, supported the notion of trusting in one's instincts and judgments and acting on impulse and following the natural order of things to achieve harmony.[11]

Asians view health care as an extension of one's approach to life.

The Asian philosophy supports the notion that the physician is the promoter of health and the individual responsible for maintaining harmony or balance with the internal and external environment.

The Chinese called this harmony a *balance of yin and yang*; yin represented negative forces in the environment and yang positive. The struggle was to keep these dynamic forces in harmony with the environment and avoid disharmony. Today, disharmony would be equated with illness. It is interesting to note that the philosophy affected health practices. For example, a Chinese physician was paid only when a client remained well; no payment was received when the individual was ill.

Greek Influence

The ancient Greeks also fused medicine and philosophy into a way of life. The Greek physician viewed the wholeness of things, helping nature to heal by restoring the balance that was disturbed by disease, rather than by interfering with nature.[12] The Greek physician focused on educating healthy people about diet and exercise in order to keep individuals in a state of health through a balanced internal environment. More time was spent in attempts to maintain balance of mind and body than in the detection of disease.

The influence of the external environment was also considered when the Greeks assessed health. Such things as geography, tides, climate, and lunar cycles were studied in relation to the general health state of a population. Hippocrates was regarded as the best of the Greek physicians. His treatise, which was a compilation of many people's efforts, was derived in part from Egyptian sources. Hippocrates' view of health is well expressed within a holistic framework: "Health means a healthy mind in a healthy body and can be achieved only by governing daily life in accordance with the natural laws, which ensures an equilibrium between the different forces of the organism and those of the environment."[13]

Influence of the Middle Ages

The classical theory of the separation of humans into body, mind, and spirit was continued in the Middle Ages. The appeal of this differentiation seems related to the increasing societal divisions that were becoming more pronounced during that time. One influence occurred in medieval Europe, where the mind was considered to be within the realm of "occult" sciences, such as *magic* and *alchemy*. The spirit, however, was considered within the strict provinces of orthodox religions. The division of mind and body in medieval health practices can still be observed in current health care practices. Today health care is still segmented, with physicians giving care to the body, psychiatrists and psychologists to the mind, and the clergy responding to spiritual matters.

Yet, despite segmented care by health professionals, holistic practices continued to surface even in the Middle Ages. Unfortunately, the lay people, who relied on holistic practices, felt a split with the professional groups, who rejected holistic ideas in favor of the more "modern" notion of viewing people in defined parts. The differing perspectives between professionals and lay groups created a schism that has remained to present times.

The Age of Reason

The attitudes toward health established in the Middle Ages continued to flourish into the seventeenth century. Holistic practices were questioned with renewed interest during the so-called age of reason. René Descartes and others held the theory that the mind and matter were separate entities.

Their ideas negated much of what was useful knowledge of health care learned from previous generations and civilizations. The *rationalists* embraced a school of thought termed *allopathy.* This approach was opposite to that of *homeopathy,* an approach promoted in this country in the eighteenth century by Samuel Hahnemann. Today, the use of live virus immunizations is perhaps the closest example of a homeopathic approach.

The Microbial Era

With the discovery of the microbial diseases in the nineteenth century, the *specific* or *single-agent theory* of disease emerged and was embraced by allopathists. Louis Pasteur and other scientists demonstrated the presence of germs and connected that presence with the cause of disease. This discovery caused an ever-widening gap between holistic practices and the current approach to health care practices.

It is important to note, however, that even Pasteur recognized the need to consider other factors (e.g., emotions or environmental relationships) that caused disease. Unfortunately, the impact of the discovery of the *germ theory* caused science to look at the *invading organism* theory to the exclusion of other ideas. Development of the germ theory has become the single most powerful force in the development of medical care during the past century.

Popular Health Movements

Despite the movement within medical professional groups toward the specific-agent theory, popular health movements with a holistic basis continued to surface, reacting against orthodox medicine.

In the United States during the 1830s a health movement arose supported by farmers, artisans, and others from the working classes. Women were involved heavily in the movement and played a significant role in promoting health practices.[14] This group of health supporters developed alternatives to traditional medicine by first exchanging home remedies and then initiating their own techniques to gain knowledge.

"Ladies' physiological societies" were formed where women gathered in privacy to learn about female anatomy and functioning. From within these ranks, a Scottish-American reformer named Fanny Wright, an advocate of universal education, equal rights for women, and birth control, emerged as a spokesperson for the health movement. The effort of this group was directed toward freeing the working class from the professional aristocrats through knowledge. Wright's proposal of self-responsibility continues as a central tenet in the present-day holistic health movement.

Thomsonian Movement

While Fanny Wright was providing an impetus for those within the worker's health movement, a New Hampshire farmer, Samuel Thomson, was "reconstructing the folk medicine he had learned as a boy from a female lay healer and a midwife named Benton."[15] Thomson's system focused on the compilation of herbal remedies he had learned, many of which had been derived from native American healing lore.

Thomson's approach became very popular and encompassed more than merely a set of rote techniques and home remedies. His goal was to

Allopathy: a system of medicine characterized by the use of remedies that produced effects different from those of the disease under treatment.

Homeopathy: a system of medicine that utilizes remedies that produce a minimum of effects of the disease under treatment.

The single-agent theory is the unidimensional idea that disease results from one cause and is not the result of the interaction of many factors. The single-agent theorists tried to discover a single specific cause of each disease and supported the germ theorists in their pursuits.

Germ theory is the notion that all disease results from the invasion of the body by microbial pathogens. The germ theorists felt that if pathogens could be detected and eliminated, health could be restored.

Popular health movements were early advocates of self-responsibility for health.

The Thomsonian movement encouraged individual self-healing.

remove the control of health from the competitive market and encourage individual self-healing. Thomson felt this could be accomplished through increased consumer education which would lead to greater self-responsibility for health. His book, *New Guide to Health,* further emphasized this approach. By 1839, 100,000 copies of the text had been sold.

In the years following the publication of this book, Thomson founded hundreds of "Friendly Botanical Societies." Members met to share information and to study the Thomsonian system. Five Thomsonian journals were published, and at the height of its popularity, the Thomsonian movement claimed 4 million members of a potential 17 million population.

Hygienic Movement

Additional healing systems arose in the 1830s which were also opposed to the monopolism and elitism of the traditional medical care system of the period. Sylvester Graham headed one such movement. The *hygienic movement,* as it came to be known, proposed sweeping medical reforms, including the rejection of all types of drugs. Graham argued for a dramatic change in American living habits. He saw the eating of raw fruits and vegetables and the use of whole-grain breads and cereals as crucial to his proposed reforms of dietary habits. These ideas were considered quite outrageous in Graham's time, especially by the medical profession, who were advising people that ingestion of uncooked produce was injurious to health.

Nevertheless, people seemed to support Graham's ideas, and the movement proved popular. One Grahamian disciple described the movement by saying:

> Any system that teaches the sick that they can only get well through the exercise of the skill of someone else, and they remain alive only through the tender mercies of the privileged class, has no place in nature's scheme of things . . . .[16]

Unfortunately, the popular health movement was opposed by many traditional health care providers who saw it as a threat to the health care delivery system prevailing at the time. However, some advocates of traditional medicine were converted to this movement. One 19th century physician who had practiced traditionally and then embraced the hygienic movement wrote: "We cannot practice our system without educating the people . . . our patrons learn from our teachings, examples, and prescriptions [on] how to live and to avoid, (to a great extent), sickness of any kind."[17]

Summary

It is important to see that what is presently termed the *holistic health movement* has been influenced by many cultures and related health movements throughout recorded history. Historically, people have seen the value of a health care system that takes into account all the various factors that affect the healthy state. The impact of the discovery of microbes and development of the germ theory tended to overshadow and at times negate many of the holistic practices that existed within professional realms. Yet, despite this fact, popular health movements have continued to thrive, supporting health beliefs that stress optimization of health and maintenance of wellness.

Highlights

The hygienic movement proposed rejection of drugs and encouraged changes in living habits leading to positive health practices.

The present holistic health movement has been significantly influenced by the health care practices of other cultures and groups working to promote optimal health.

MODELS OF HEALTH CARE

Several models of health care are discussed in the following pages. These include the traditional *medical model,* the *holistic health* (incorporating self-care) *model,* and the *nursing model.* Each is presented in terms of its contributions to and limitations on health care delivery.

There are several health care models:
1 Medical model
2 Nursing model
3 Holistic model (including a self-care model)

The Traditional Medical Model of Health Care

Despite the popular health movements over the years, traditional health care providers have derived satisfaction and income from treating clients rather than assisting individuals in mobilizing personal resources to self-heal. This attitude of *treating the client* has increased dependency on health providers and created the need for health providers to continue to identify a cause for disease that they can isolate and control. Engel (1962) states that "physicians also find attractive ways of thinking, particularly if they see the 'cause' of disease as something which they can attack and destroy."[18]

Dr. David Hayes-Bautista, a medical sociologist, points out that the medical model places the ultimate origin of disease inside the individual on the microbiological level. Efforts to eradicate illness are, therefore, aimed at eliminating the problem. Our highly evolved medical technology is designed for the detection and treatment of disease processes whose etiologies are within the human body. Certainly this technology is very effective in the diagnosis and treatment of specific pathogen-caused diseases.

This same technology, with its focus on a microbial basis of illness, also supports a fragmented health care system. The fragmentation leads to a system where parts of an individual are considered while "the whole individual and the society in which he/she operates are lost in a welter of organs, tissues, cells, bacteria, and procedures."[19]

Response to the Medical Model

Irving Oyle, in his book *The Healing Mind,* states, "Of all patients who consult outpatient facilities in the United States, 70% are found to have no organic basis for their complaint."[20]

If indeed there is an absence of an organic etiology, what are the factors that lead these individuals to seek medical attention?

Despite the fact that only a small percentage of those who encounter the health care system have a health problem, there is still a resistance to exploring alternative ways of dealing with altered health status. One major reason for this resistance is the tenacious clinging to western scientific materialism. Another is a limited approach to dealing with a possible multifactorial analysis that needs to be done in order to affect health status.

Because of the limitations of and the frustrations generated by disease-oriented care, this approach has failed to meet the needs of the consumer. In the presence of today's rising health care costs, consumers still have limited alternatives to health care.

From 1965 to 1976 there was a 320 percent increase in personal consumption for medical care, hospital services, and physician services.[21] From 1967 to present there has been a 224 percent rise in the costs of other consumer goods and services.[22] Increases in health care costs outweigh other cost increases by a substantial margin.

Yet, despite dramatic cost increases in health care, America is not a nation of healthy people. For instance, at least 20 million people in the United States are afflicted with hypertension. Thirty million Americans

Table 1-1
Death Rates According to Sex and Cause 1976*

Cause	Male	Female
Diseases of the Heart	383.5	293.4
Malignant Neoplasms	196.6	156
Carebrovascular Accidents (Strokes)	77.1	98
Accidents	67.3	27.7
Pneumonia	31.1	26.6
Diabetes Mellitus	13.4	18.6
Cirrhosis of the Liver	19.8	9.8
Arteriosclerosis	11.3	15.9
Suicide	18.7	6.7
Early Infancy Diseases	13.6	9.6

*Rates per 100,000 population (all ages).

suffer from sleep-onset insomnia.[23] Over one-third of the deaths in the United States in 1970 were attributed to coronary heart disease.[24] Of 70 million alcohol users in the United States, it is estimated that 5 million are alcoholics.[25] Today, it is not uncommon for a friend or relative of a chronically ill person to be afflicted with one of the many stress-related diseases such as migraine headaches, heart disease, cancer, arthritis, or peptic ulcer.[26] (See Tables 1-1 and 1-2.)

In the United States, it would appear that the consumer is paying luxury medical prices for mediocre care. Much of the resulting disappointment and resentment on the part of the consumer often result from the widespread belief that physicians, whose primary task is the diagnosis and treatment of illness, should be experts on all other aspects of health. Failure to provide health care in all areas is not tolerated by the client. A client who is told that he or she is well but still does not feel well may feel that the physician is not providing adequate care. However, the problem may not be inadequate medical care but inadequate health care. Unrealistic expectations of medical treatment result in the single most common reason for the initiation of malpractice suits.[27] Pelletier argues that "If both patients and physicians clearly recognize that the doctor's function is simply to diagnose and treat disease, then the medical profession could once again receive the respect and dignity which their work deserves."[28]

The Holistic Model of Health Care

In contrast to the medical model, a holistic health model places the origin of disease outside the individual. The holistic model recognizes that microbiological factors affect illness, but also pays equal attention to other elements, such as "the political, economic, social, and psychological"[29] factors that affect the interactive nature of mind, body, and spirit. The proponents of holism do not ignore sophisticated technology but place it

The holistic model recognizes not only the microbial factors involved in illness, but other psychosocial, political, and economic factors as well.

Table 1-2
Persons with Activity Limitation by Selected Chronic Conditions*

Percent Limited by	Male	Female
Heart Conditions	16.7	14.8
Arthritis and Rheumatism	11.4	21.7
Visual Impairment	5.7	5.0
Hypertension	4.8	8.9
Marital and Nervous Disorders	4.4	5.4

*Total population affected 15.6 million.

in its proper perspective. Individuals are viewed not simply as vulnerable to wandering microbes, but capable of pulling together internal and external forces to resist illness. Holism recognizes that healing involves more than merely removing the overt manifestations of a disease process. Without treatment of the total person, interventions used may be limited in their overall effect. (See Fig. 1-1.)

Holistic Principles of Health

Although holistic practices encompass a variety of modalities, they share several basic assumptions about attitudes toward health.[30] These include some basic principles which are discussed in the pages to follow:

All states of health and disease have a psychological component. This assumption rests on the premise that the bodily state profoundly influences the mental state and vice versa. As a result, clients are seen as more than helpless victims of disease. Holistic health practitioners recognize the necessity of treating the *whole* person and explore the psychosociological as well as the biological causes of disease. In addition, holistic health practitioners view the individual (or self) as a regulator of health and carefully consider the extent to which a person can exert influence on states of health *and* illness.

Every person represents a complex but unique interaction of body, mind, and spirit. Holists define health as a harmonious balance among the body, mind, and spirit. Disease is viewed as a disturbance in the dynamic balance of this relationship. Within this framework, each individual responds differently, yet uniquely, to a set of factors that could potentially affect the health state. As a result, no two persons will respond in exactly the same way to a given set of circumstances. Health providers who claim to solve all problems through one approach, such as taking medicines as the only cure for a cold, are not holistic. The use of a single remedy does not take into account the multiple facets of an individual's life which can interact to cause illness or promote health. The holistic practitioner, therefore, must carefully consider the meaning and significance a particular problem has for each individual. In so doing, an individual's innate capacity to recognize the origins of a health problem can be utilized and healing resources stimulated.

The primary responsibility for health lies not with a health care provider, but with oneself. The tendency within the traditional model of care has been to force the client to seek the answers for problems from the health care providers and follow the directions without question or com-

All states of health and disease have a psychological component.

Health represents the complex but harmonious balance of mind, body, and spirit.

The responsibility for health lies with the client.

Figure 1-1 Holistic health model. (Adapted from John Travis, *Wellness Workbook,* Wellness Resource Center, Mill Valley, Cal., 1977.)

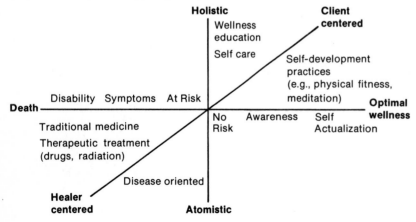

plaint. This parent-child relationship between health care providers and consumers can be detrimental to both groups.

Individuals need to be in control of and regulate their destiny. Clients need to acknowledge a primary responsibility for their personal health state. The holistic health model views individuals as capable of taking control of their lives and interactions with the world. Health care providers can *assist* individuals to optimize health by acting as health resources, but only the individual can ultimately determine his or her health state.

Holistic health care providers must determine to what extent the atmosphere of dependency is created within the context of helping roles. In other words, by fostering a relationship in which clients or patients are dependent, the question is asked as to whose needs are truly being met. Research by Williamson and Danaher suggests that individuals participate in self-health practices in relation to a variety of symptoms. Self-care "is a process whereby a lay person can function effectively on his or her own behalf in health promotion, decision making, disease prevention, detection and treatment at a level of the primary health resource in the Health Care System."[31] (See Fig. 1-2.)

Health care is not the exclusive province or responsibility of orthodox medicine or any other single system. Holistic health practitioners attempt to individualize care by assessing those factors in a client's lifestyle that make that person susceptible to disease. The client's inherent bodily defenses are strengthened to reduce or help to eliminate environmental stress that may impede health. Alternate traditional and nontraditional interventions are used to promote health. Conversely, medical practice has attempted to fit each individual into a generalized disease syndrome and offer an appropriate medical treatment for that disease. Since we are all uniquely different, the creation of one uniform program conducive to health maintenance and personal fulfillment may not always be appropriate. But the creation of a framework that allows the health provider to assess total health care needs of a client in the presence or absence of pathology helps to promote the attainment of health in the fullest sense of the word.

Illness is not necessarily "bad." Believers of the concept of holistic health take the position that illness is not bad. Rather, illness presents the client with an opportunity to learn more about the self and fundamental values and beliefs about the life process. Each state of altered health is an expression of some imbalance in an individual's life. Therefore, being ill may offer the person an opportunity to reflect on the self and factors that may be related to the imbalances. Confrontations with pain, chronic illness, and even the possibility of death provide the individual with opportunities for growth. A change in attitude toward an illness can cause marked changes in self-perception. To ask "What am I to learn from this?" rather than "Why me?" can cause a profound change in many people's attitudes toward life and death.

Positive wellness, and not just absence of disease, is the goal of holistic health. The conventional health care provider assesses a person as being "well" if there is an absence of physical or behavioral symptoms or if a series of diagnostic tests fall within normal limits. Yet this "well" person might smoke heavily, engage in no regular exercise program, eat irregularly, and be highly stressed at work. The holistic health model views the absence of disease as only the starting point. Individuals are encouraged to consider ways of assessing all the many life patterns that influence physical fitness and well-being and in so doing increase resistance to disease.

A study conducted by Lester Breslow, Dean of the University of Cali-

The provider (nurse) is a facilitator and a health resource for the client.

The holistic model encourages health care providers to examine their need to be depended on. Holistic providers place the responsibility for the success of any treatment or intervention ultimately on the person being treated. The health care provider can only give guidance, assistance, or support.

Interventions used to restore the health state of an individual should include both traditional and nontraditional treatments.

Illness may be an outward sign of an inner imbalance in the mind-body-spirit triad.

Positive wellness is the goal of holistic health.

Figure 1-2 What people do about their symptoms. (Adapted from J. D. Williamson and K. Danaher, "Self-care in Health," in A. C. Hastings, ed., Health for the Whole Person, Westview Press, Boulder, Col., 1980.)

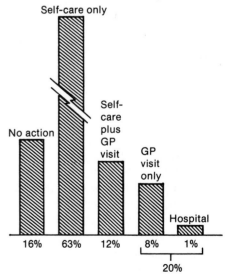

fornia at Los Angeles (UCLA) School of Public Health, explored the correlation between simple health habits and life expectancy. After studying 11,000 adults for $5\frac{1}{2}$ years, Breslow and his colleagues concluded that certain health habits are associated with a longer life. These health habits included three regular meals a day, with particular emphasis on a well-balanced breakfast; moderate exercise; 7 or 8 hours of sleep a night; no smoking; moderate weight; and moderate use of alcohol. According to Breslow's study, a 35-year-old man who practices three or fewer of these health habits has an average life expectancy of 67 years; whereas a man who practices six of them has an average life expectancy of 78 years.[32]

Practitioners of holism must come to know themselves as human beings. Before prompting optimal health in others, health providers must first be fully acquainted with personal strengths, weaknesses, conflicts, and general nature. The health provider must live and practice in the holistic mode, continuously exploring the self and related values and motivations. Nonjudgmental assistance of clients cannot be accomplished unless the provider engages in the process of exploring personal values and ideas.

Summary

The principles of holism provide a strong framework for health promotion and stimulate the pursuit of wellness. Although holistic health practices encourage different approaches to attaining health, all holistically oriented practitioners share these basic, underlying principles which encapsulate the essence of holism.

HOLISTIC HEALTH AND NURSING

Basic to the scientific body of nursing knowledge is the commitment to the "whole" person. By definition, holism implies a belief system which supposes an awareness of the total self, an attitude that encompasses a life-style which is open to change and sensitive to one's innate ability to heal and self-regulate. To accomplish this goal, the health provider must recognize the dynamic interaction that exists in each client, that is, the interdependence between mind, body, and spirit (see Fig. 1-3). This interaction is dynamic and changing in full communication with the environment.

Nursing has since its beginnings accepted this approach to the client as an essential part of its framework of practice. Its goal has been to prevent (maintain and promote health), nurture (care and comfort), and generate (foster healing) actions that stimulate the optimization of one's state of health.

Furthermore, it must be recognized that promotion of a holistic philosophy cannot occur in isolation. It occurs within three defined dimensions—intrapersonal space, interpersonal space, and community systems.[33]

Intrapersonal space involves interaction between the individual (life space) and the environment and those factors within its framework (e.g., nurse-client values and beliefs about health). Interpersonal space involves interaction between two or more groups, e.g., the family, the nurse, and the client.

The term "community systems" refers to the implementation of holistic principles of groups of individuals that have an organizational structure (base) and are interested in a common goal (e.g., health promotion). Today many wellness centers have successfully achieved this goal.

Highlights

Breslow's health habits include:
1 Three regular meals a day with an emphasis on a well-balanced breakfast
2 Moderate exercise
3 Seven to eight hours of sleep a night
4 No smoking
5 Weight within recommended limits for age, height, etc.
6 Moderate use of alcohol

Many practices advocated by holistic health are simple and can bring about marked changes in the client's health status.

The phenomenon of "self-care" must begin with the provider and then become an integral component of the client-provider relationship.

Holistic health principles:
1 All states of health and disease have a psychological component.
2 Every person represents a complex but unique interaction of body, mind, and spirit.
3 The primary responsibility for health lies not with a health care provider, but within oneself.
4 Health care is not the exclusive province or responsibility of orthodox medicine or any other single system.
5 Illness is not necessarily bad.
6 Positive wellness, not merely absence of disease, is the goal.
7 Practitioners of holism must come to know themselves as human beings.

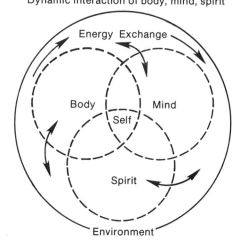

Figure 1-3 Interactive holistic health model.
Dynamic interaction of body, mind, spirit

Human beings are subject to a multiplicity of influences occurring outside the body structure. These influences include all those physical, biological, psychological, and social variables which may affect an individual's health status (patterns) at a given point. The milieu or external environment in which these factors exist is in a constant state of change, and the individual's balance within this environment influences the health state.

Theorists studying the relationship between humans and the environment have developed the concepts of *ecology* and *ecosystem*. These terms connote the dynamic, ever-changing state that exists between individuals and the environment. To achieve the role of provider within this holistic framework, the nurse takes responsibility for identifying not only biophysical factors affecting health, but those social, cultural, economic, psychological, maturational, and environmental factors which influence a person's wellness.

The holistic role of the nurse has become more openly promoted in the 1960s and 1970s, but historically nurses have always valued the idea of the consideration of the "whole" person. One needs only to glance through Florence Nightingale's *Notes on Nursing* to appreciate her consistently holistic approach to clients. Ms. Nightingale concerns herself with the impact of environment on health in various chapters, including those on ventilation and warming, housing sanitation, noise, light, and food.

A chapter entitled "Variety" is particularly holistic. Nightingale points out that "A patient can just as much move his leg when it is fractured as change his thoughts when no external help from variety is given him. This is, indeed, one of the main sufferings of sickness, just as the fixed posture is one of the main sufferings of a broken limb."[34] Nightingale's concern for the body is seen throughout the book in the form of specific therapeutic recommendations. She foretells what would become a major contemporary focus of nursing: "The same laws of health or of nursing, *for they are in reality the same,* obtain among the well as among the sick" (emphasis is present author's).[35]

Nursing Theory and Practice

As the science of nursing evolves, several theoretical frameworks have emerged to describe nursing and its interaction with clients to promote health. As these frameworks evolve, support for a holistic nursing framework seems to be most evident. For example, Myra Levine (1971) suggests that nursing intervention is directed toward a conservation of wholeness. She goes on to delineate four essential conservation measures that help to determine nursing practice; these include conservation of the individual's energy, structural integrity, personal integrity, and social integrity.

Martha Rogers's (1971) theoretical framework of nursing embraces holistic concepts by presenting a life process model of care. She states: "The life process of unitary man is a phenomena of wholeness, of continuity, of dynamic and creative change."[36] Within this change new patterns evolve and the individual's pattern and organization become more complex. According to Rogers, a human being is an energy field engaged in "mutual, simultaneous interaction" with the energy of the environment, requiring the open, active participation of both. The life process is the transaction between energy field and environment.

Furthermore, this theory emphasizes that human beings are interacting in a holistic way with the universe. She terms this wholeness as

Ecology: study of the interactions between organisms and their environment.
Ecosystem: composed of all the organisms (including humans) found in a particular place at a given time, together with their physical environment. The human organism is found in, is shaped by, and in turn shapes many kinds of ecosystems around the globe. Examples of these ecosystems are forests, deserts, and urban areas.

Emphasis of a holistic approach to nursing care is reflected by Florence Nightingale (*Notes on Nursing*).

Levine's conservation principles:
1 Conservation of energy
2 Conservation of structural integrity
3 Conservation of personal integrity
4 Conservation of social integrity

being *synergistic*—that is, humans are greater than the sum of their parts. Only where the individual is viewed totally rather than in components or parts does one's uniqueness (that which clearly describes each person from another) emerge.

Other nursing theorists have also described nursing within a holistic framework. Henderson (1960) described nursing as helping people to do things they would ordinarily do for themselves. Orem's (1971) model of a self-care agency parallels Henderson in several ways. Orem's model supports the principle of holism and stresses that individuals must take responsibility for their own health. Alterations in health result in self-care deficits which require assistance from the nurse until health is restored.

Johnson (1959) views the client as a complex, interrelated system. Each system has a pattern (e.g., behavioral patterns) which needs to be evaluated to determine insufficiency or discrepancy relative to a subsystems goal. She suggests that the role of nursing is to support clients physically and emotionally until their own resources enable them to deal with a particular situation.

Roy (1970), on the other hand, described an adaptation model in which nursing is concerned with the adjustments and adaptations that are necessary under the stress of change. Disease is viewed as an expression of a basic imbalance in human adaptation to the multiple physical and emotional stresses in the environment. She states that ineffective coping may be at the root of the problem and suggests that coping mechanisms *cognator* (e.g., learning) and *regulator* (endocrine) need to be affected to restore balance. These coping mechanisms manifest themselves by four modes of adaptive behavior (physiological, self-concept, role function, and interdependence modes) which form the basis for assessment and direct interventions.[37]

Orlando (1961) and Weidenbach (1964) pointed out the fact that the nurse must consider the person's needs and continuously validate perceived needs with the client. Their models emphasized the need for interaction between the nurse, the environment, and the client in order to promote health and prevent disease.

Mitchell (1973) summarizes holism in nursing as "a primary role in helping people to live with or avoid further disability or illness and in promoting wellness—living to one's fullest capacities."[38] She sees the nurse's role as independent as well as collaborative with other health care providers. As health care moves away from institutions and moves into the community, she suggests that the role of the nurse will continue to expand and impact on the consumer.

As nurses begin to define the clinical science of nursing, it is apparent that the goal of practice must reflect the needs of the total person. Traditionally, nurses' concerns have centered on persons who are ill and the environment surrounding them rather than the responses to disease itself.[39]

As nurses begin to evolve a theoretical base for the clinical science of nursing, attention must also be paid to the definition of nursing as presented by the American Nurses Association Congress for Nursing Practice (1980), in which nursing is defined as "the diagnosis and treatment of human responses to actual or potential health problems."[40] It suggests further that the practice of nursing can be characterized by four factors—phenomena, theory application, nursing action, and evaluation of the effects of such actions.[41]

The *phenomena* being described refer to the concern or attention nurses pay to those observable responses (signs and symptoms) that re-

Mutual, simultaneous interaction is a relationship between a person and the environment in which the interaction is so equally reciprocal that both entities are seen as one. The process of interacting is so balanced that one part cannot exist without the other.

Rogers's depiction of the constant interaction between humans and the environment takes the form of a helix. The interaction is seen as continuous unidirectional movement to increased complexity.

Cyclic spiral is used to represent Rogers's concept of change, reorganization, repatterning, and increased complexity.

Orem's self-care: helping people cope with those portions of their daily living patterns which are associated with actual or potential disease states or the treatment thereof. Daily living patterns include eating, moving, relating to others, etc.

Roy's model of adaptation suggests that a client's coping mechanisms (cognator and regulator) become imbalanced due to multiple physical and emotional stressors. Adaptation is the intervention used to restore balance through the four adaptive models.

"Nursing is the diagnosis and treatment of the human responses to actual or potential health problems."

The practice of nursing can be characterized by four factors—phenomena, theory application, nursing action, and evaluation.

flect human response to actual or potential health problems. For example, the nurse attends to the discomfort experienced by a client following a trauma or attempts to prevent the lack of information regarding health promotion activities by teaching the person about health promotion activities.

The use of *theory* provides the nurse with a set of comprehensive guiding principles and concepts which facilitate the practice of nursing. Today, there are many theoretical frameworks which have been set forth to serve this goal. These theories seem to reflect a model of nursing practice which helps to determine the nurse's actions in relation to the implementation of nursing process. These theories also help to serve as a foundational basis for researching the validity of nursing interventions.

Actions reflect those activities in which nursing engages to promote, maintain, restore, and optimize health. These actions occur within a highly developed technical yet interpersonal and scientific framework, emerge from the collection of a sound data base, determine the nursing diagnosis, and help to direct interventions.

The *effects* of nursing actions are those outcomes which occur as a result of nursing care. The evaluation of achievement of these outcomes (criteria or standards of performance) determine the accuracy of both the diagnosis and interventions and help to validate nursing practice.

Within this definition of nursing the scope of practice can be more clearly defined, boundaries determined, and intersections with other health providers more clearly established.

HOLISM AND THE NURSING PROCESS

The philosophy or conceptual framework of nursing, which evolves from a synthesis of values and beliefs about human nature, health, and nursing, provides a variety of evolving models which can be used to systematically order a set of related knowledges and principles. These include models such as problem solving, decision analysis and decision making, interaction, and maturational-developmental models. The models all seem to reflect a scientific approach to information gathering, diagnosis, analysis, and evaluation.

The standards of nursing practice established by the American Nurses Association advanced an approach to the process of nursing actions. These standards "provide a means for determining the quality of nursing which a client/patient receives" and "provide a systematic approach to nursing practice."[42]

This approach includes data collection (assessment), developing nursing diagnosis, establishment of the goals of care, planning interventions, and evaluating outcomes. The so-called nursing process provides the vehicle used to describe nursing practice.

Nursing Process

The nursing process is a scientific problem-solving process which focuses on the total health care needs of clients. In its most concise form, the nursing process consists of assessing the client's needs (physical, psychological, and spiritual), establishing nursing diagnosis, selecting appropriate nursing interventions, evaluating the client's response to the nursing action (outcomes), reassessing need, and reapplying the process in a cyclic pattern.[43] The utilization of the nursing process provides a system-

American Nurses Association standards of nursing practice (adapted)
1 Collection of data about the patient's health status
2 Nursing diagnosis derived from data
3 Formulation of goals for nursing care
4 Planning to achieve goals
5 Implementation of nursing plan
6 Evaluation of nursing care
7 Reassessment as a continuous process

The standards of care developed by the American Nurses Association's Council on Nursing Practice are used as the guiding framework for implementing the nursing process.

atic vehicle for critically analyzing care and implementing holistic health principles. Components of the nursing process are outlined in the list that follows:

Highlights

Nursing process includes

1. Assessment or data collection.
2. Nursing Diagnosis—through analysis of cue clusters.
3. Goal Setting—mutually set.
4. Intervention—individually selected.
5. Evaluation through established outcome criteria.

1 Assessment

  a. *Nursing history:* specific facts which are usually presented by the client with a particular health problem should be considered. Functional patterns (see Table 1-3) are used as the basis for this process.

  b. *Physical assessment:* specific changes that are commonly observed during a physical examination should be described (one-word lists should be avoided).

  c. *Diagnostic tests:* diagnostic tests relevant to the discussion should be defined, and changes associated with the problem being presented should be listed.

  d. *Problem list:* at the completion of the assessment, a problem list may be developed. This should include a list of nurse-oriented problems from which a nursing diagnosis can be made.

2 Nursing diagnosis. *"Nursing Diagnosis* describes health problems in which the responsibility for therapeutic decisions can be assumed by the professional nurse . . . these problems encompass *potential* or *actual* disturbances in life processes, functions, patterns, or development, including those occurring secondary to the disease" (Gordon). To identify a nursing diagnosis, the nurse must validate that the "etiology" of that diagnosis is carefully reflected in the assessment data.

3 Goal setting. Goals are clear realistic statements which describe, in measurable terms, intended client outcomes following the delivery of specific nursing care. Both short- and long-term goals can be identified; however, it is important to note that *time* and *individuality* of the client are determining factors in goal setting. For instance, if your goal was that in 20 weeks the client would lose 15.75 kilograms (kg) [35 pounds (lb)], this becomes a long-term goal. However, if you were planning to see the client on a bimonthly basis, you may plan short-term goals of a 0.45- to 0.9-kg (1- to 2-lb) weight loss at each interim visit. (When devel-

Table 1-3
Components of the Functional Assessment Tool: Functional Patterns

Health-Status–Health-Management (Including Values and Beliefs)
Life Pattern–Life-Style (Including Biological Rhythms, Sleep-Rest Pattern, and Elimination Pattern)
Role-Relationship Pattern
Self-Perception–Self-Concept Pattern
Cognitive-Perceptual Pattern
Sexuality-Reproductive Pattern
Nutritional-Metabolic Pattern
Activity-Exercise Pattern
Coping-Stress Pattern

Source: Adapted from M. Gordon, *Nursing Diagnosis: Process and Application,* McGraw-Hill, New York, 1982, p. 81.

oping goals, the nurse should reflect on nursing diagnosis stated to ensure that all issues are addressed.)

4 Intervention. Nursing intervention should be clearly stated and reflect an action(s) for each goal stated. The reader is reminded that while all nursing care is individualized to meet client needs, there are "standardized" or commonly accepted interventions unique to the health problem being discussed. If specific *medical* interventions are presented, the author should so indicate and list related nursing interventions as appropriate.

5 Evaluation. Evaluation should indicate the relative success or failure of nursing interventions; therefore, they should be stated in terms of achievement of outcome which will carefully delineate criteria against which goal attainment can be measured.

Use of an organized method for collecting data and classifying related health problems has resulted in a variety of assessment tools. These include Abdellah's "21 nursing problems" (1959) and Henderson's "14 basic needs classification system" (1966) as well as others, such as Johnson's "8 behavioral subsystems" or Roy's "4 adaptation modes" (1971).

In 1970 the First National Conference on the Classification of Nursing Diagnosis began to formulate a method for organizing information and classifying nursing diagnosis. From this work much information has evolved which carefully assesses the need for an organized mechanism for data collection.

COMPONENTS OF THE NURSING PROCESS

Assessment

Nursing assessment consists of data collection and analysis. Since data can be obtained from a variety of sources, the collection methods become vital to the process. Unless a systematic approach is used in the data collection phase, important needs will not be recognized and consequently nursing action will not adequately address these needs.[44]

Work by Gordon suggests that this can be accomplished through a *functional pattern assessment*. She defines patterns as a sequence of behaviors across time.[45] This suggests that the construction of a pattern requires not only current data (*current patterns*), but previous data (*previous patterns*) in order to make inferences as to the presence of actual or potential health problems.[46]

These patterns form a data base from which information can be viewed in its totality and decisions made about pattern disturbances on the basis of its impact on the total system. This clustering of data provides the nurse with an opportunity to analyze information and generate a list of characteristics which indicate an actual or potential nursing diagnosis.

For purposes of this text, the following patterns are addressed: health perception/health management, including values and beliefs; lifestyle and life patterns, including biological rhythms (e.g., sleep, rest, and elimination); roles and relationships; self-perception and conception patterns; cognitive perceptual patterns; sexuality reproductive patterns; nutritional patterns; exercise activity patterns; and coping patterns and stress tolerance.[47] (See Table 1-3.)

Data sources include client, family, friends or significant others, past hospital records, etc.

Patterns discussed throughout the text include all of Gordon's Functional Patterns; Sleep Rest patterns and elimination patterns are addressed under life style and life patterns.

Health Perception/Health Management

Health care perception focuses on the client's perception of the health care system. Evaluation of the person's current health, personal health habits followed to promote health and prevent illness, and previous health states are included in the discussion. Family history and a description of the client's values and beliefs and ethnic or racial influences on health care perception are incorporated into the assessment.

Some of the preventive measures that are more commonly accepted by society include (1) maintaining body awareness as reflected in a good diet, adequate sleep, routine exercise, recreation and relaxation, and caring for body functions, (2) engaging in periodic health screening (at least yearly) and seeking health care for acute conditions, (3) avoiding products known to contribute to unhealthy states, such as cigarettes, caffeine, alcohol, food additives, and environmental pollutants, and (4) learning the warning signals of illness and disease to facilitate early detection, diagnosis, and treatment.[48-52]

The late Dr. John Knowles, former president of the Rockefeller Foundation, summed up preventive care by saying:[53]

> Prevention of disease means forsaking the bad habits which many people enjoy—overeating, too much drinking, taking pills, staying up at night, engaging in promiscuous sex, driving too fast, and smoking cigarettes—or, put another way it means doing things which require special effort—exercising regularly, improving nutrition, going to the dentist, practicing contraception, ensuring harmonious family life, submitting to screening examinations.

Beliefs, attitudes, customs, behaviors, and practices must be assessed and evaluated in relation to the cultural meaning it holds for the individual. Racial influences must also be determined.

Race is defined as those characteristics that distinguish one particular group from another. Racial background can influence health care practices, family life, nutritional and other patterns, physical traits, and potential for specific health problems (e.g., prevalence of hypertension amongst black males 18 years of age and older).

Racial groups can contain many different ethnic groups. For example, the white racial group contains different ethnic groups who embrace different customs and traits despite a common racial background.

Ethnicity: refers to peoples and races and to their customs and traits.

As changes occur within cultures, the norms of the culture change. Societal norms of a group (status, position, money, power, as well as poverty, no power, etc.) can influence an individual's seeking out health care services. Because of the complexity of culture, the nurse may find it difficult to assess this component as it relates to health and illness.

Norm: a standard representing the average or typical.

Life-Style and Life Patterns

Assessment of these data provides the most comprehensive information about how individuals conduct their lives on a daily basis. Personal responses to season changes, age, birth, death, holidays, and vacations can be analyzed here. In addition, cultural norms and characteristics, growth and developmental patterns across the life span, behavioral development, and biological rhythms (including sleep, rest, and elimination patterns) are part of the discussion of this pattern area. At this time it is also important to consider the client's overall interaction with the environment so that economics, environmental factors, and community resources may be addressed.

Age may be defined as one's *chronological* age (birth to death) and *developmental* age (social and emotional development). Both chronological and developmental age should be reflected by the accomplishment of tasks as measured by specific standardized measures.

Information related to genetic endowment and heredity, familial traits, personal characteristics, and tendencies toward specific health problems should be identified. Such data will help to direct preventive care.

Growth and development of an individual represent the interaction between genetic endowment at birth and the environment in which these traits flourish. Growth and development normally proceed in an orderly fashion with each step or stage dependent on the one preceding. There is generally a positive correlation between physical growth and mental and emotional development.[54] Each individual progresses at his or her own rate of development.

Developmental screening tests (discussed throughout the text) are used to assess an individual's developmental progress [(e.g., Denver Developmental Screening Test (DDST)].

Biological rhythms regulate recurring life processes. There are several types of biological rhythm, generally differentiated according to extrinsic influences (e.g., time or length of day—circadian, ultradian, and infradian rhythms—and seasonal changes, viz., exogenous rhythms) and intrinsic factors (endogenous rhythms, synchrony, and desynchronization).

The environment is broadly defined as the external conditions which surround, act on, and influence an organism or its parts.[55] The external environmental factors to be assessed include the following:

1 Weather and climate. Extremes in heat and cold can affect health and metabolism. For instance, seasonal changes can affect health (e.g., increase allergic responses) and length and frequency of sunshine can affect one's mood and alter health perception and can also determine availability of food sources.

2 Water source. Water quality can be affected by chemicals and pollutants, and population density can increase potential for pollutants.

3 Air quality. Chemicals, automobile exhausts, metal compounds, sprays, etc. can contaminate the air source, exposure to harmful air sources must be evaluated in terms of its potential health risk.

4 Work environment. Safety factors and potential for harmful pollutants must be assessed; e.g., noise, contaminated air, and lack of activity increase stress. (Refer to Roles and Relationships below.)

5 Home environment. Potential for stress and social and intimate relationships must be assessed.

6 School environment. Potentials for stress and growth must be evaluated along with stressors that affect learning.

Individuals and family groups develop a life-style which includes use of and communication with community resources. Community resources include:

Acute-care facilities—services such as continuous close medical and nursing attention and use of complex equipment offered in a hospital for care of certain critically ill patients, with a view to restoring, when possible, normal life processes.

Highlights

Growth: the quantitative changes an individual undergoes.

Development: progressive increase in skill and capacity to function.

Maturation: development of genetic traits.

Circadian rhythm: corresponds to a 24-hour-period rhythm (e.g., day-night cycle).

Infradian rhythm: a rhythm that occurs in patterns of less than a day in length (e.g., body temperature).

Ultradian rhythms: rhythmic cycles that occur in patterns of longer than a day (e.g., menstrual cycle).

Endogeneous rhythms: patterns that develop within the organism and follow distinct cycles (the so-called internal clock; e.g., heart rate).

Exogenous rhythms: rhythms influenced by factors occurring outside the body (e.g., seasonal change).

Synchrony: event that occurs at the same time as another event or which depends on the other's coexistence (e.g., sleep-wakefulness).

Desynchronization: change in body rhythm that interrupts the internal clock, e.g., passing through time zones.

External environmental factors:
  1 Weather and climate
  2 Water source
  3 Air quality
  4 Work, home, and school environments

Medications are affected by rhythmic patterns.

There are four main types of community facility:
  1 Acute-care facilities
  2 Long-term care facilities
  3 Preventive health care facilities
  4 Walk-in clinics

Long-term care facilities—facilities providing symptomatic treatment or maintenance and rehabilitative services for clients of all ages in a variety of settings.

Preventive health care agencies—those functions performed by health professionals or health consumers for the purpose of avoiding illness or injury, including activities as immunizations, dietary control, and proper exercise.[55]

Walk-in clinics—clinics where clients are seen on a first-come, first-served basis to treat non-acute conditions.

Roles and Relationships

These patterns are explored to determine an individual's role as provider, head of household, child, parent, and so on, and the responsibility of that role and its impact on one's life and life-style are assessed. Interactions between family and community systems are analyzed, and these interactions are considered in terms of their impact on the individual members and group in both occupational and social relationships.

Roles and Relationship patterns focus on issues around role function and role perception.

Family structure roles and functions need to be assessed in terms of culture, society, occupation, mobility, and similar factors. The main tasks of families are to:

1 Provide for physical care of its members in areas such as food, clothing, shelter, safety, and health care

2 Determine roles and functions of each family member for the purpose of maintaining the household

3 Develop their capacities to socialize children through community relationships with church, schools, friends, and bureaucratic organizations and develop successful linkages with these nonfamily organizations

4 Facilitate development of a positive self-image and affectional responses in each member through open communication and supportive interaction

5 Encourage and enhance initiative, motivation, and ethical standards, rewarding achievement and adaptation to stressful life events through role modeling and transference of cultural values and beliefs

6 Create an atmosphere of love, satisfaction, and mental health essential to the well-being of a family

Changes in the role functions of each member of a family can be influenced by occupation. Today individuals can be employed at long distances from the home, which can affect relationships and increase separation of members. Increase in the numbers of women in the work force has influenced roles and relationships in the home and the workplace. Occupational stress should be explored in terms of its impact on the client's life-style.

Sexuality and Reproductive Patterns

Sexual patterns reflect an individual's interaction with others on a more intimate basis. Assessment of these patterns includes a discussion of satisfaction derived from the individual's own sexuality and sexual relationships with others. Female reproductive patterns, menstrual cycle, and male and female pre- and postmenopausal behavioral status can also be evaluated at this time. Since discussion of this area may be threaten-

Discussion of Sexuality and Reproductive Patterns may be uncomfortable for the client and the nurse.

ing, it is important that the client and provider have a sound relationship based on trust.

Sexuality involves one's complete personality development, including sexual identification, self-concept, self-esteem, and patterns of behavior. The sexuality of a person reflects attitudes towards one's body and one's sex and sexual role.

Sexual behavior is thought to be learned, not innate. Sexual expression will change with age, physical development, emotional maturity, social mores, and general health. The essence of sex has been described as the manner in which one relates to other people. Although sexual awareness develops early in an individual, there may be constraints (social, moral, and religious) on expression of that sexuality through intercourse prior to marriage.

Nutritional Patterns

Assessment of this area should include an attempt to determine an individual's nutritional status as determined by the metabolism (ingestion, digestion, and elimination) of food and water. Sociocultural variables, eating habits, food preferences, and impact of stress on eating are some of the areas explored under assessment of this pattern.

Nutritional requirements and related factors will vary from person to person. The *recommended daily allowances,* defined as the levels of intake of essential nutrients considered adequate to meet nutritional requirements of practically all healthy persons, can be used to assess intake.[57] It is essential to evaluate this component on an individual basis and in view of basic nutritional needs. In his book *Eating Right For You,* Dr. Carlton Fredricks promotes a holistic approach to diet assessment and counseling.

Exercise-Activity Patterns

Assessment of these patterns reflects on the client's ability to move around and carry out activities of daily living. In addition, the type, quality, and regularity in which exercise is engaged are assessed. Use of leisure time is evaluated, and the client's interaction with significant others whose company is shared at this time is addressed.

The *disuse phenomenon* is a description of individuals who do not exercise. It is simply stated as "use it or lose it." Disuse phenomena can be reversed through the development of a regular exercise program. Activity should be encouraged on a regular basis within the individual's financial and physical means.

Self-Perception–Self-Concept Patterns

An assessment of this area should include attempts to determine a person's attitude about himself or herself (self-image) in relation to personal appearance, cognitive style, and effective and psychomotor skills. In addition, the client's self-perception and sense of self-worth are evaluated in relation to the individual (self) and others. Personal goals, as well as accomplishments and future achievements, are also explored.

Cognitive and Perceptual Patterns

Evaluation of this pattern area should include an assessment of an individual's sensory competence (vision, hearing, taste, touch, and smell), cognitive abilities (e.g., language, intelligence, and memory), and the impact of these factors on the person's ability to attain and retain information. In addition, tolerance to pain or other noxious stimuli are addressed and the comfort measures used to promote rest and relaxation identified.

To assess the results of dietary practices, foods eaten must be explored, along with activity levels, health status, and related factors.

Nutritional assessment involves a critical look at the interaction between the individuals, the foods regularly eaten, and the impact on life-style of nutrition related factors (e.g. meals, time, planning, etc.).

Exercise and activity are central to one's life-style and overall health status.

Disuse phenomena occur due to a lack of activity and can be corrected with regular activity.

Intelligence is the "ability to perceive qualities and attributes of the objective world and to employ a means of the attainment of an end (goal).[58]

Intelligence is influenced by heridity, education, culture, health state, sensory capacity, etc.

Coping Patterns and Stress Tolerance

Evaluation of this pattern area reflects how an individual handles crisis, behavioral and physical responses to stress, and identification of actual or potential stress factors within the environment. In addition, modes of resolving conflicts are also determined.

Since life presents a constant series of stressors, it is important to differentiate between those which are normal and those that might lead to disease. In his book, *Mind as Healer, Mind as Slayer,* Kenneth Pelletier further elaborates on this distinction by saying:[59]

> Obviously, not all stress can or should be avoided. A normal adaptive stress reaction occurs when the source of stress is identifiable and clear. When this particular challenge is met, an individual returns to a level of normal functioning relatively quickly. However, when the source of stress is ambiguous, undefined, or prolonged, or when several sources exist simultaneously, the individual does not return to a normal mental and physiological baseline as rapidly. He or she continues to manifest a potentially damaging stress reaction.

Each client responds to a stressful event in an individual way, depending on the perceived threat of the experience.

When stressors are clearly identified, a normal adaptive stress reaction occurs.

Summary

The pattern areas described proved to be a framework for collecting and organizing data. Further delineation of these areas and related questions that can be used to elicit data are discussed in greater depth in Chapter 3.

Problem List

The problem list is a simple list which identifies actual or potential needs as noted by the client, the nurse, or both. These needs are listed according to priority of importance. The use of nursing diagnosis has replaced the problem list in most instances.

The problem list can include areas where specific nursing intervention is needed or where the services of other health professionals and other people in the community are required.

Nursing Diagnosis

Nursing diagnosis offers the nurse a way to conceptualize problems which can be positively changed by the client with the nurse's assistance. Those diagnoses for which the responsibility for therapeutic decisions is assumed by the nurse are included under the heading of "nursing diagnosis."

Nursing diagnosis can reflect the six dimensions of nursing practice. These nursing dimensions include:[60]

a) prevention of complications; b) the preservation of bodily defenses; c) the detection of changes in the body's regulatory systems; d) the re-establishment of the client with the outside world; e) the implementation of physician's prescribed diagnostic and therapeutic activity and f) the provision of comfort and safety. All of nursing actions designed to meet patient needs can be classified in one of the cited dimensions of nursing practice.

Diagnosis as defined by Gordon is "A concise term (phrase) representing a cluster of signs and symptoms (empirical indicators) describing an actual or potential health problem (pattern disturbance) which nurses by virtue of their education and experience are licensed to treat."[61]

A list of nursing diagnoses as accepted by the Fourth National Conference Group on the Classification on Nursing Diagnosis is presented in Table 1-4.

Since nursing diagnosis can be viewed as a statement of probability, it is important that the nurse try to minimize this uncertainty in clinical

Nursing diagnosis is "a concise term, representing a cluster of signs and symptoms describing an actual or potential health problem, which nurses by virtue of their education and experience are licensed to treat."

Nursing diagnosis is a statement of probability.

Table 1-4
List of Nursing Diagnoses Accepted at the Fourth National Conference*

Airway Clearance, Ineffective
Bowel Elimination, Alterations in: Constipation
Bowel Elimination, Alterations in: Diarrhea
Bowel Elimination, Alterations in: Incontinence
Breathing Patterns, Ineffective
Cardiac Output, Alterations in: Decreased
Comfort, Alterations in: Pain
Communication, Impaired Verbal
Coping, Ineffective Individual
Coping, Ineffective Family: Compromised
Coping, Ineffective Family: Disabling
Coping, Family: Potential for Growth
Diversional Activity, Deficit
Fear
Fluid Volume Deficit, Actual
Fluid Volume Deficit, Potential
Gas Exchange, Impaired
Grieving, Anticipatory
Grieving, Dysfunctional
Home Maintenance Management, Impaired
Injury, Potential for
Knowledge Deficit (Specify)
Mobility, Impaired Physical
Noncompliance (Specify)
Nutrition, Alterations in: Less than Body Requirements
Nutrition, Alterations in: More than Body Requirements
Nutrition, Alterations in: Potential for More than Body Requirements
Parenting, Alterations in: Actual
Parenting, Alterations in: Potential
Rape-Trauma Syndrome
Self-Care Deficit (Specify Level: Feeding, Bathing-Hygiene, Dressing-Grooming, Toileting)
Self-Concept, Disturbance in
Sensory Perceptual Alterations
Sexual Dysfunction
Skin Integrity, Impairment of: Actual
Skin Integrity, Impairment of: Potential
Sleep Pattern Disturbance
Spiritual Distress (Distress of the Human Spirit)
Thought Processes, Alterations in
Tissue Perfusion, Alteration in
Urinary Elimination, Alteration in Patterns
Violence, Potential for

Diagnoses "Accepted" without Defining Characteristics [Therefore, Unacceptable but to be
    Listed Separately, as Diagnoses to be Developed: (TBD)]
Cognitive Dissonance: TBD
Family Dynamics, Alterations in: TBD
Fluid Volume, Alterations in, Excess; Potential for: TBD
Memory Deficit: TBD
Rest-Activity Pattern, Ineffective: TBD
Role Disturbance: TBD
Social Isolation: TBD

*Refer to Table A-9 for additional diagnoses from the Fifth Conference.
Source: M. Gordon; *Nursing Diagnosis: Process and Application,* McGraw-Hill, New York, 1982, pp. 325–
326.

judgment. Collection of a comprehensive data base, correct interpretation of data and cues, knowledge on the part of the nurse, and commitment to the task at hand (i.e., correct interpretation and analysis of data)
are essential to the decision-making process.

The use of nursing diagnosis facilitates the validation of nursing
practice, can become the framework for clinical research, has been seen
as a mechanism for third party reimbursement, improves quality care
(care can be measured through outcomes), lends itself to the subjective-
objective assessment plan (SOAP) charting format, and carefully reflects
those nursing actions which fall within the nurse's scope of practice.

As work on the development and refinement of diagnostic categories
evolves, further uses will become more evident. But it is only through

Nursing diagnosis is used for:
1   Validation of practice
2   Third-party reimburse-
    ment
3   SOAP charting (see
    Chap. 2)
4   As a basis for clinical re-
    search
5   Quality assurance
6   Actualization of nursing
    practice

continued use and research in the area of nursing diagnosis that a classification system can be developed to its fullest potential.[62]

Planning

When the assessment phase is completed and an appropriate nursing diagnosis defined, the planning phase begins. The planning phase entails two parts which basically answer the questions of *what* nursing action to initiate and *when* that action should take place. An important part of planning is accomplished through setting goals.

Recently, it was discovered that the use of a contract or another form of a negotiated statement between the client and the provider can facilitate goal attainment. Contracts are viewed as a mechanism whereby an individual can actively participate in decisions related to therapy and thereby become more committed to the proposed health plan.[63] Figure 1-4 provides one sample of a contract that can be used to achieve a specific goal(s) of care.

Client-nurse contracts are currently being used to promote goal achievement.

Figure 1-4 Sample teaching-learning contract between client and nurse. (From D. Jones, et al., Medical-Surgical Nursing: A Conceptual Approach, McGraw-Hill, New York, 1982, p. 17. Used with permission.)

Contract

I, _____ agree to participate in the following contract

with _____ from _____, 19___ to _____, 19___,

for the purpose of achieving the goals listed below:

Goals: – to lose 30 pounds by _____;
  – to learn to control excessive weight gain through careful planning of well balanced meals;
  – to identify the times when my eating patterns change, recognize the precipitating behavioral changes and/or stress factors that accompany overeating, and learn to control the cause before it affects my eating habits.

I also agree to attend bimonthly meetings with _____ at the Primary Health Clinic to evaluate intermediate achievements toward accomplishing my goals.

Within one month from the date of this contract, I will reevaluate my goals and make necessary changes. If I am not satisfied with my progress, I may cancel this contract and future meetings. Should I intend to terminate this contract, I will inform _____ during our scheduled meeting time. I will also provide reasons for terminating the agreement.

At the completion of our scheduled meetings both _____ and myself will decide if additional meetings are needed.

I further agree that this contract can become part of my health record, accessible to both the nurse and physician only.

Date: _____

Name of the Client _____

Name of the Nurse _____

***A copy of this contract should be given to the client and reviewed as needed.**

Goals

Goals are clear, realistic statements of outcomes of client care. The establishment of goals should be mutually planned by both the client and the nurse. Goals are formulated on the basis of clients' aspirations and reflect an assessment of the client's capabilities. When goals are set, they should be listed in measurable terms with the outcomes expected and time frame for accomplishment clearly identified.

The specific activities that lead to meeting a goal must be individualized for the particular client. For example, setting the goal of running 1.6 kilometers (km) (1 mile) daily may be a long-term goal for a person who is not in good physical condition but could be a short-term goal for someone who has been exercising daily but wants to increase physical endurance by running.

Intervention

After goals have been mutually established, the next step is to plan nursing actions with the client and identify mechanisms for implementation. Interventions which have the greatest probability for success reflect a high level of knowledge as well as a sensitivity to the client's beliefs, attitudes, and perceptions.[64] The nurse may implement the actions directly, collaborate with the client, encourage the client to take responsibility for self-care, or utilize the services of other health care personnel. For example, a dietician may collaborate with the nurse to develop a diet appropriate for the client.

Within a holistic framework many types of intervention have been suggested for implementation by the nurse; these provide dimension and incorporate the use of a more creative approach to care. Table 1-5 provides a list of some suggested approaches to holistic health care. Careful exploration and attention to each of these approaches reflect on some of the basic precepts posited earlier in this chapter. They encourage clients to utilize their own self-healing potential in taking control of the life process to regain, maintain, and optimize health. In addition, they imply an interaction between the client and the environment and suggest the exchange of energy as a mechanism by which the nurse may facilitate the realization of optimal health by the client.

Activities such as *meditation, relaxation, visualization,* and *autogenic* training facilitate the self-regulation and self-generation of a client's own potential for self-healing by focusing introspectively on the self. In this way the flow of energy within the human system can be directed and controlled.

The use of *therapeutic touching,* for example, suggests that along with self-centering, one can transfer and exchange energy from one individual to another. In addition, through intentional assessment of the total system, imbalances in energy can be identified and energy transferred by the healer to the client in an attempt to restore a state of balance. Such actions support the concept that individuals are open systems, continually changing and exchanging and that symmetry or equal balance is needed on both sides of the body to restore its wholeness (yin and yang concepts mentioned earlier).

Many types of intervention which focus on stress reduction involve programs which also focus the individual on techniques that allow for further regulation and control of energy. *Biofeedback* and the use of sensory stimuli, including music, exercise, and light, have allowed clients to actively intervene in relieving the effects of a specific health problem and reducing its impact on their health status.

Goals should reflect mutual planning by the client and the nurse.

Example—long-term goal:
  1 Mr. S will lose a total of 18 kg (40 lb) within 4 months.

Example—short-term goal:
  1 Mr. S will have lost 2.25 kg (5 lb) by his next visit to the nurse in 3 weeks.

One should be as creative as possible in devising nursing actions, and there should be at least one nursing action for each goal stated.

Table 1-5
Nursing Interventions That Reflect Principles of Holism

Therapeutic Touching
Pressure (acupressure)
Guided Imagery
Stress Management
Autogenic Training
Biofeedback
Self-Health
Meditation
Nutrition
Music, Sound, Light, and Color Stimuli
Hypnosis
Herbs and Plants

Evaluation

Evaluation permits the nurse to validate the achievement of a particular outcome on the basis of objective criteria. Criteria for evaluating the effectiveness of a nursing action should be stated in specific outcome behaviors. Fundamental to goal-setting is the selection of criteria to measure the effectiveness of the intervention. If goals are clearly established, the evaluation becomes a simple process of looking at the success or failure of a nursing intervention in terms of the client's behavior.

Example—evaluation:
Mr. S returns in 3 weeks and has lost 2.25 kg (5 lb). How do you know it happened?
1 The client reports a 2.25-kg (5-lb) weight loss.
2 You weigh the client and note a 2.25-kg (5-lb) loss.

Evaluation: validates the client's achievements against clearly observable criteria.

Reassessment

Reassessment involves a reevaluation of the nursing process. It is implemented when specific goals are not met. There are many reasons why a goal may not be successfully achieved. These include:

1 More data are available which better define or change the problem

2 New problems appear or old ones are solved

3 One or more of the short-term goals are met, indicating the need to move on to long-term goals

4 The initially proposed action is not successful

5 The client or nurse modifies the goals

6 New resources become available or former resources are no longer available

Regardless of the feedback, new goals, interventions, and outcome criteria are then planned in view of the new data collected.

Summary

The nursing process is a mechanism whereby nursing practice is systematically organized. It allows for a more consistent approach to client care. In the succeeding chapters, much attention is paid to the assessment phase of the nursing process. Utilizing the conceptual framework of holistic health, an in-depth assessment format is developed in Chaps. 2 to 4 which will facilitate implementation of the remaining components of the nursing process.

See the list of steps in the nursing process earlier in this chapter.

THE CONSUMER AND HOLISM

When conducting the holistic health assessment, the nurse is not only aware of utilizing the principles of the nursing process to organize an approach, but is also putting into action the principles or assumptions of holism which were outlined earlier. One assumption that bears repetition is that the consumers of health care become active participants in the decision making regarding their own care. It is important to note that the use of the term "client" is supportive of this idea of self-responsibility.

Traditionally, we have referred to the consumer of health care as a "patient"—a term that often implies a more passive role on the part of the individual and connotes an illness rather than wellness orientation. It further suggests that the individual, as patient, relinquishes autonomy and self-direction. In addition, identification with the *illness role* allows the individual the freedom to reject personal responsibility for health care.

See the list of holistic health principles in the section on holistic health and nursing earlier in this chapter.

On the other hand, the term "client" implies that the individual is a consumer of health services and has the right to be involved in planning and deciding which type of care may be of optimal physical, social, or psychological benefit. This personal responsibility for health permits the client to freely choose health care services and become accountable for compliance or noncompliance to a recommended health regime. The term "client" broadens the scope of the individual's involvement in seeking, receiving, and responding to health care.

Summary

As the science of nursing continues to evolve, its focus on those concepts found within a holistic framework will be an integral part of any practitioner's theoretical framework. Therefore, it is important to study the constructs of holistic health care and its interrelated use in the data collection (assessment) process and the related judgments and actions that will be taken by the nurse to enhance quality care.

REFERENCES

1. World Health Organization, "The Constitution of the World Health Organization," *WHO Chron* 1:29 (1947).

2. R. French, *Dynamics of Health Care,* McGraw-Hill, New York, 1979, p. 3.

3. G. Engel, *Psychological Development in Health and Disease,* Saunders, Philadelphia, 1962, p. 46.

4. R. Dubos, *Man Adapting,* Yale University Press, New Haven, 1965, p. 9.

5. Valerie Harms, "What Is Holistic Health, Anyway?" *Ms.,* March 1978.

6. Barbara Blattner, *Holistic Nursing,* Prentice-Hall, Englewood Cliffs, N.J., 1981, p. 3.

7. Ibid., p. 5.

8. J. Travis, *Wellness Inventory,* Wellness Resource Center, Mill Valley, Cal., 1977.

9. B. Hettler, "Wellness Promotion on a University Campus," in M. Faber (ed.), *Family and Community Health,* vol. 3, no. 1, p. 77, (May 1980).

10. M. Abehsera (ed.), *Healing Ourselves,* Avon, New York, 1973, p. 4.

11. Blattner, *Holistic Nursing,* p. 8.

12. G. G. Luce, *Body Time,* Random House, New York, 1971, p. 27.

13. Ibid., p. 68.

14. B. Ehrenrich and D. English, "For Her Own Good," *Mother Jones,* August 1978, p. 23.

15. Ibid., p. 24.

16. Ibid., p. 28.

17. Ibid.

18. Engel, *Psychological Development,* p. 46.

19. D. Hayes-Bautista, "Holistic Health Care," *Social Policy,* March-April 1977, p. 8.

20. Irving Oyle, *The Healing Mind,* Celestial Arts, Millbrae, Cal., 1975, p. 29.

21. R. French, *Dynamics of Health Care,* p. 101.

22. J. Posner, "What Price Health?" *Newsweek,* December 10, 1979.

23. K. Pelletier, *Mind as Healer, Mind as Slayer,* Delta, New York, 1977, p. 7.

24. U.S. Bureau of the Census, *1970 Census of Population,* U.S. Government Printing Office, Washington, D.C., 1973.

25. Cheletz and Demone, *Alcoholism and Society,* Oxford University Press, New York, 1962, p. 9.

26. Pelletier, *Mind as Healer,* p. 7.

27. Ibid., p. 317.

28. Ibid.

29. D. Hayes-Bautista, "Holistic Health," p. 8.

30. G. Leonard, "Holistic Health Revolution," *New West,* May 10, 1976, p. 18.

31. J. D. Williamson and K. Danaher, *Self Care in Health,* Neale Watson, New York, 1978.

32. N. B. Bellock and L. Breslow, "Relationship of Physical Health Status and Health Practices," *Preventative Med* 1:409-421 (1972).

Highlights

The term "client" is used throughout this book to refer to an individual seeking health care services.

33. B. Blattner, *Holistic Nursing,* p. 23.

34. F. Nightingale, *Notes on Nursing,* Harrison, London, 1860, p. 34.

35. Ibid., p. 6.

36. M. Rogers, *Theoretical Foundations in Nursing,* F. A. Davis, Philadelphia, 1968.

37. M. Gordon, *Nursing Diagnosis: Process and Applications,* McGraw-Hill, New York, 1982, p. 67.

38. P. Mitchell, *Concepts Basic to Nursing,* McGraw-Hill, New York, 1971, pp. 15–22.

39. Dorothy Johnson, "Development of Theory: A Requisite to Nursing as a Primary Health Profession," in N. Chaska (ed.), *The Nursing Profession,* McGraw-Hill, New York, 1978, p. 211.

40. *Social Policy Statement on the Scope of Nursing,* ANA Congress on Nursing Practice, Kansas City, Mo., 1981, p. 9.

41. Ibid., p. 9.

42. *Standards of Practice,* ANA Congress for Nursing Practice, Kansas City, Mo., 1973, p. 1.

43. D. Brodt, "The Nursing Process," in N. Chaska (ed.), *The Nursing Profession,* McGraw-Hill, New York, 1978, p. 257.

44. D. Brodt, "The Nursing Process," p. 257.

45. M. Gordon, *Nursing Diagnosis,* p. 82.

46. Ibid., p. 83.

47. Ibid.

48. *Recommended Daily Allowances,* Food and Nutrition Board, National Academy of Sciences, Washington, D.C., 1974.

49. U.S. Bureau of the Census, 1977.

50. M. Byrne and L. Thompson, *Key Concepts for the Study and Practice of Nursing,* Mosby, St. Louis, 1972.

51. Gerald Beeson, "The Health-Illness Spectrum," *Amer J Pub Health* **11**:1901-1904 (1967).

52. R. Peters, H. Benson, and D. Porter, "Daily Relaxation Breaks in a Working Population, I: Effects on Self-Reported Measures of Health Performance and Well-Being," *Amer J Pub Health* **67**:946-953 (1977).

53. J. Knowles, excerpted from "Responsibility for Health," *Science* **198**:1106 (1977).

54. Robert Wilson, *The Sociology of Health, An Introduction,* Random House, New York, 1970.

55. D. Clark and B. MacMahon, *Preventive Medicine,* Little, Brown, Boston, 1967, pp. 4–8.

56. *McGraw-Hill Nursing Dictionary,* McGraw-Hill, New York, 1979, pp. 476, 538, 753.

57. *Recommended Daily Allowances.*

58. Sylvia Price and L. Wilson, *Pathophysiology, Clinical Concepts of Disease Processes,* McGraw-Hill, New York, 1982, pp. 9–10.

59. K. Pelletier, *Mind as Healer,* p. 42.

60. D. Brodt, "The Nursing Process," p. 256.

61. M. Gordon, *Nursing Diagnosis,* p. 2.

62. D. Jones, C. Dunbar, and M. Jirovec, *Medical-Surgical Nursing: A Conceptual Approach,* McGraw-Hill, New York, 1982, p. 33.

63. Ibid., p. 16.

64. P. Mitchell, *Concepts,* p. 166.

BIBLIOGRAPHY

Aamodt, A. M.: "Culture," in Clark, A. L., *Culture, Childbearing, Health Professionals,* F. A. Davis, Philadelphia, 1978.

Abehsera, M.: *Healing Ourselves,* Avon Books, New York, 1973.

Aiken, L. (ed.): *Health Policy and Nursing Practice,* McGraw-Hill, New York, 1981.

Battistella, R. M.: "The Right to Adequate Health Care," *Nurs Digest,* Jan.-Feb. 1976.

Becker, M. H.: "The Health Belief Model and Sick Role Behavior," *Health Educ Monogr,* **2**:409-19 (1974).

Bensen, H.: *The Mind Body Effect,* Simon and Schuster, New York, 1979.

Brink, Pamela J. (ed.): *Transcultural Nursing,* Prentice-Hall, Englewood Cliffs, N. J., 1976.

Burns, E. M.: "Critical Issues in Social Health Practice: Today and Tomorrow," *Man and Medicine,* **1**:205. (Spring 1976).

Chaska, Norma (ed.): *The Nursing Profession: Views through the Mist,* McGraw-Hill, New York, 1978.

Chin, P. (ed.): "Nursing Diagnosis," *Advances in Nurs Sci* **2** (October 1979).

————: "Holistic Health," *Advances in Nurs Sci* **2** (July 1980).

Clark, Duncan, and Brian McMahon: *Preventive Medicine,* Little, Brown, Boston, 1967.

Dachelet, C., and T. Sullivan,: "Autonomy in Practice," *Nurse Practitioner J,* Mar.: 1979.

Davis, M., et al.: *The Relaxation and Stress Reduction Workbook,* New Harbinger, Richmond, Cal., 1980.

De Castro, Fernando, et al.: *The Pediatric Nurse Practitioner,* Mosby, St. Louis, 1976.

Dubos, R.: *Man Adapting,* Yale University Press, New Haven, 1965.

————: *Mirage of Health: Utopias, Progress, and Biological Change,* Harper and Row, New York, 1959.

————: *So Human an Animal,* Scribner, New York, 1968.

Dunn, H. L.: "High Level Wellness for Man and Society," *Amer J Pub Health* **49**:786-692 (1959).

DuVall, Evelyn M.: *Marriage and Family Development,* 5th ed., Lippincott, Philadelphia, 1977.

Ehrenreich, B., and D. English: "For Her Own Good," *Mother Jones,* August 1978.

Engel, G.: *Psychological Development in Health and Disease,* Saunders, Philadelphia, 1962.

Fredricks, Carlton: *Eating Right for You,* Grosset and Dunlap, New York, 1972.

Freeman, Ruth B., and Janet Heinrich: *Community Health Nursing Practice,* 2d ed., Saunders, Philadelphia, 1981.

French, Ruth: *Dynamics of Health Care,* 3d ed., McGraw-Hill, New York, 1979.

Fry, P. W.: "The Scientific Method and Its Impact on Holistic Health," *Advances in Nurs Sci* **2**:1-7 (1980).

Gerrard, D. M.: "Is There Any Value in Western Medical History?" *Wellness Workbook,* Part 4: *Health Professions,* Wellness Resource Center, Mill Valley, Cal., 1977.

Haggerty, R.: "Changing Life Styles to Improve Health," *Preventive Med* **6**:276-89 (1979).

Harms, Valerie: "What Is Holistic Medicine, Anyway?" *Ms.,* March 1978.

Harris, D. M., and S. Guten: "Health-Protective Behavior: An Explanatory Study," *Health and Soc Behavior* **20**:17-29 (1979).

Hastings, A.: *Health for the Whole Person,* Westview Press, 1980.

Hayes-Bautista, D.: "Holistic Health Care," *Social Policy,* March/April 1977.

Hettler, B.: "Wellness Promotion on a University Campus," *Advances in Nurs Sci* **2**:84-91 (1980).

Holleran, P.: "A Holistic Model of Individual and Family Health Based upon a Continuum of Choice," *Advances in Nurs Sci* **3**:27 (1981).

Holmes, T. H., and R. H. Rahe: "The Social Readjustment Rating Scale," *J Psychosomatic Res* **11**:213 (1967).

Hurlock, E. B.: *Child Development,* McGraw-Hill, New York, 1972.

Johnson, D.: "A Philosophy of Nursing," *Nurs Outlook* **7**:198-200 (1959).

Kaslof, Leslie: *Holistic Dimensions in Healing,* Doubleday, New York, 1978.

Keller, M.: "Toward a Definition of Health," *Advances in Nurs Sci* **4**:43-64 (1981).

Kim, M. J., and D. A. Moritz: *Classification of Nursing Diagnoses: Proceedings of the Third and Fourth National Conferences,* McGraw-Hill, New York, 1982.

Krieger, D.: *The Use of Therapeutic Touch,* Prentice-Hall, Englewood Cliffs, N. J., 1959.

————: *Foundations for Holistic Nursing Practices: The Renaissance Nurse,* Lippincott, Philadelphia, 1981.

LaPatra, Jack: *Healing—The Coming Revolution in Holistic Medicine,* McGraw-Hill, New York, 1978.

Leahy, K. M., M. M. Cobb, and M. C. Jones: *Community Health Nursing,* 4th ed., McGraw-Hill, New York, 1982.

Lenihan, J., and W. Fletcher: *Health and Environment,* Blackie, Glasgow, 1972.

Leonard, G.: "Holistic Health Revolution," *New West,* May 10, 1976.

Levine, M.: "Holistic Nursing," *Nursing Clinics of North America* **6**:253-263 (June 1971).

Lovejoy, N.: "Biofeedback: A Growing Role in Holistic Health," *Advances in Nurs Sci* **2**:83-94 (1980).

Luce, G. G.: *Body Time,* Random House, New York, 1971.

Mastal, M. F., and H. Hammond: "Analysis and Expansion of the Roy Adaptation Model: A Contribution to Holistic Nursing," *Advances in Nurs Sci* **2**:71-81 (1980).

Mauksch, I.: *Primary Care: A Contemporary Nursing Perspective,* Grune and Stratton, New York, 1981.

McCusker, J., and G. Marrow: "The Relationship of Health. Locus of Control to Preventive Health Behavior and Health Beliefs," *Patient Counseling and Health Education,* 1980, pp. 146-150.

Miller, J.: "Cultural Factors in Health," *South African Nurs J,* Oct. 1977.

Milsum, J. H.: "Health Risk Factor Reduction and Life Style Change," *Advances in Nurs Sci* 3:1-13 (1980).

Moyer, N. C.: "Health Promotion and Assessment of Health Habits in the Elderly," *Advances in Nurs Sci* 3:51-58 (1981).

Narayan, S., and D. Joslin: "Crisis Theory and Intervention: A Critique of the Medical Model and a Holistic Nursing Model," *Advances in Nurs Sci* 2:27-39 (1980).

Natalini, J. J.: "The Human Body as a Biological Clock," *Amer J Nurs,* July 1977.

Neugarten, B. L.: "Continuities and Discontinuities of Psychological Issues into Adult Life," *Human Development* 12:121-130 (1969).

Nightingale, Florence: *Notes on Nursing,* Harrison and Sons, London, 1860.

Orem, Dorothea: *Nursing: Concepts of Practice,* 2d ed., McGraw-Hill, New York, 1971.

Orlando, Ida: *The Dynamic Nurse-Patient Relationship,* Putnam, New York, 1981.

Oyle, Irving: *The Healing Mind,* Celestial Arts, Millbrae, Cal., 1975.

Parkerson, G. R., S. H. Gehlbach, et al.: "The Duke–U.C. Health Profile: An Adult Health Status Instrument for Primary Care," *Med Care* 19(1981).

Pelletier, K.: *Mind as Healer, Mind as Slayer,* Delta, New York, 1977.

Price, Sylvia, and Lorraine Wilson: *Pathophysiology: Clinical Concepts of Disease Process,* 2d ed., McGraw-Hill, New York, 1982.

Rice, B., et al.: "Beyond IQ," *Psychology Today,* September 1979.

Richardson, Henry B.: *Patients Have Families,* Commonwealth Fund, New York, 1948.

Rogers, Martha: *Theoretical Basis of Nursing,* Lippincott, New York, 1971.

Roy, Callista: "Adaptation: A Conceptual Framework for Nursing," *Nurs Outlook,* 18:42-45 (1970).

Selye, H.: *The Stress of Life,* McGraw-Hill, New York, 1956.

———: *Stress without Distress,* Signet Books and Lippincott, New York, 1974.

Singer, R. B., and L. Levinson: *Medical Risks,* Lexington Books, Lexington, Mass., 1976.

Strasser, J. A.: "Urban Transient Women," *Amer J Nurs* 12:2076-2079 (1978).

Terris, M.: "Approaches to an Epidemiology of Health," *J Public Health* 65:1037-1045 (1975).

Tom, C. K., and D. M. Lanuza: "Nursing Assessment of Biological Rhythms," *Nurs Clinics of North America,* December 1976.

Travis, J.: *Wellness Workbook,* Wellness Resource Center, Mill Valley, Cal., 1977.

U. S. Bureau of the Census: *1970 Census of Population,* U. S. Government Printing Office, Washington, D.C., 1973.

U. S. Department of Health, Education, and Welfare: *Healthy People: Surgeon General's Report on Health Promotion and Disease Prevention,* U. S. Government Printing Office, Washington, D.C., 1974.

U. S. Department of Health and Human Services, Health Resources Administration: *GMENAC Report,* Vols. I-VII, U. S. Government Printing Office, Washington, D.C., 1980.

Vandenberg, S. G.: "The Hereditary Ability Study: Hereditary Components in a Psychological Test Battery," *Amer J Hum Genet* 14:220-37 (1962).

Ward, B., and R. Dubos: *Only One Earth,* Norton, New York, 1972.

Watson, Jean: *Nursing—The Philosophy and Science of Caring,* Little, Brown, Boston, 1979.

Weinstein, M., and H. Fienberg: *Clinical Decision Analysis,* Saunders, Philadelphia, 1980.

Wiedenbach, Ernestine: *Clinical Nursing: Helping Art,* Springer, New York, 1964.

Wilson, R., M. Wingender, et al.: "Effects of Health Hazard Appraisal Inventory on Practices of College Students," *Health Educ,* Jan-Feb 1980.

BEHAVORIAL DEVELOPMENT

CHAPTER TWO

Joan McParland
Karen A. Szymanski
Mary Kolassa Lepley

The process of growth and development from childhood to adulthood is characterized by physical as well as behavioral changes. The nurse providing holistic care must have a broad understanding of normal patterns within both of these areas in order to complete a thorough assessment of the client. This chapter addresses behavioral development that can be assessed by observing and analyzing behavior patterns.

Aspects of behavioral development include psychological, social, and emotional development.

DEFINITION OF BEHAVIOR

Various definitions have been given to the term *behavior,* and one which seems most simple, yet complete, is Wiedenbach's:

> Behavior is the individual's response, both verbal and nonverbal, to a stimulus.[1]

The response is based on genetic endowment as well as the sum of all the client's past environmental experiences with parents and other significant people in one's life. Behavior is learned during the process of growth and development throughout the life span. Other environmental variables which can affect behavior include culture, health state, nutritional status, child-rearing practices, social class, and school and work experiences.

Many behaviors are learned through interaction with the environment.

PRINCIPLES OF BEHAVIORAL DEVELOPMENT

Just as physical development follows a normal sequence from conception, behavioral development also occurs in *identifiable stages.* For example, the female preschooler spends many hours imitating behaviors of her mother when "playing house." Thus, the child learns through observation, imitation, and play certain mothering behaviors. These learned behaviors will, most likely, be repeated in later years when the child becomes a mother figure. If the child never has a female role model (mother or other significant caretaker), this can influence her behavioral responses to mothering later in life. Behaviors may have to be learned through other role models such as nursery nurses or friends with children or through trial and error. If in addition nurturing behaviors are not experienced during childhood, the girl may find it difficult to nurture future offspring, thus potentially jeopardizing the maternal-infant bonding process.[2]

Another characteristic of behavioral and physical development is that of *readiness.* A certain maturational state must be reached before certain behaviors can be performed. For example, eye-hand coordination, fine motor skill, and dexterity must be present before a child can learn to write. Early manipulation of utensils and efforts at scribbling

Behavioral development normally occurs in identifiable stages across the life span.

Behaviors can be learned from role modeling.

A certain maturational readiness must be attained in order to perform certain behaviors.

provide initial opportunities for learning. Thus, more complex and more refined behaviors build upon simple and more general learned behaviors.

Behavioral development can also be assessed from a *motivational perspective.* Certain theorists believe that behaviors develop or change as a result of a person's motivation to achieve a goal. For example, an adolescent may demonstrate very disciplined study habits related to school because he or she knows that high academic achievement will probably gain him or her admission to college. Therefore, the motivation to achieve high grades has a specific purpose, and behaviors are regulated accordingly. Certainly environmental factors, such as cultural influences, may also have an impact on a person's inherent motivation. Thus, interacting variables must be recognized as influencing behavior patterns.

Chess and coworkers[3] provided documentation for two essential and basic concepts about behavior through extensive longitudinal studies of children's individual behavior:

1 Each child has his or her own specific, individual behavioral and *temperamental style,* which is identifiable in the first week of life and may persist throughout life.

2 Behavior becomes understandable through clarification of the *interaction between a particular child and a particular set of parents or caretakers.*

Thus, certain behavioral characteristics are present so early in a child's life that one might speculate that they are innate and that they may even determine reactions to imposed parental and environmental influences. In other words, a person has a continual effect on his or her world, as well as the world having a continual effect on the person.

TEMPERAMENT

Further understanding of behavior can be gained by identifying temperamental qualities which represent the basic style which characterizes a person's behavior. Thomas, Chess, and Birch[4] made a major contribution when they were able to accurately classify infants' behavior under nine headings:

1 *Activity level:* From early infancy some babies are more active than others.

2 *Biological regularity:* Babies are found to differ significantly in the regularity of their biological functioning (crying, feeding, sleeping, and elimination).

3 *Approach or withdrawal as a characteristic response to a new situation:* When introduced to a new stimulus pattern (for example, people, food, toys, or procedure), some babies readily adapt, while others withdraw or pull away.

4 *Adaptability to change in routine:* Some babies easily and quickly alter behavior to fit the mother's desired new routine, while others accommodate more slowly to change.

5 *Level of sensory threshold:* Babies with a high "sensory threshold" do not startle at loud noises or bright lights or react to being wet or soiled. Babies with a low sensory threshold startle quickly and cry almost immediately with soiling.

Highlights

Behaviors can be influenced by one's motivations.

Interacting factors, such as culture, child-rearing practices, and motivation, can influence behavior patterns.

One's temperamental style can be identified at birth.

Parent-child interactions should be analyzed when assessing behavior.

Infant temperament can be classified according to the following:

1 Activity level

2 Biological regularity

3 Approach or withdrawal response

4 Adaptability

5 Response to sensory stimuli

6 *Positive or negative mood:* Some babies are mostly happy and smiling and coo when awakened, while others are generally fussy and cry when they are held or put down.

7 *Intensity of response (in terms of the amount of physical energy displayed):* Some babies demonstrate tremendous energy in response to pleasurable and painful activities, while other babies show less energy.

8 *Distractability:* Some babies are better able to concentrate on feedings and visual stimuli no matter what else is happening around them.

9 *Persistence and attention span:* There is great variation in infants' abilities to persist in an activity or to resume an activity after interruption.

These nine categories represent a characteristic way of classifying infants' temperaments as "easy," "slow to warm up," or "difficult." One temperamental style is not necessarily better than or more normal than another, but it certainly will have an effect on behavior manifested in any given situation. As the infant matures through childhood and into adulthood, patterns of functioning may remain fairly consistent as a consequence of temperament. However, the child's temperament is susceptible to change, and in the course of development environmental circumstances, such as parenting practices, may heighten, diminish, or modify reactions and behavior. An awareness of the child's temperament by parents, family, and health care providers may help one understand and work more effectively with the child. This becomes apparent in the following case study.

As a baby, Cathy was not easily consoled by cuddling, she fussed often despite attempts by her parents to meet basic needs such as feeding and diaper changing, and she displayed a low sensory threshold. She was easily awakened by even the slightest noises, and changes in daily routines by her mother left her irritable. By age 3, Cathy's mother reported that she would not go to bed unless persistently coaxed and that she did not want to sleep by herself or in her own bed. The parents remained continuously supportive of Cathy through infancy and toddlerhood and usually gave in to her wants and desires with some restrictions. They would read Cathy bedtime stories and would allow her to fall asleep in whatever room they were sitting in so that she would not be frightened, and later they would move her into her own room. Cathy's strong need to remain close to her parents and their ability to provide love and an environment conducive to the development of trust and autonomy within limits fostered Cathy's normal growth and development. By age 4, Cathy was a more secure child emotionally and was able to sleep alone and go to bed without a fuss. She responded well to disciplining by her parents and had formed social relationships with other children her age.

On the basis of temperament, a child may be considered "easy," "slow to warm up," or "difficult."

Even though some might consider Cathy to be a "difficult child," Cathy's parents seemed to understand her temperament and managed to use parenting techniques which worked effectively with her. In retrospect, the parents considered Cathy to be a lovable and enjoyable child. They were able to accept her behavioral individuality and adapt situations to meet her needs.

PSYCHOSOCIAL DEVELOPMENT

Besides temperament, the psychosocial development of the child and adult causes one to behave in a unique way in various life situations.

Psychosocial development directs behavioral responses.

This development involves sequential stages through which a child's personality passes in the process of becoming an adult. Just as physical or motor skills are acquired at each stage of development (i.e., sitting up at 6 months, walking by 15 months, and running well by 24 months), the psychosocial aspects develop in a relatively predictable pattern. Each succeeding stage draws on the accomplishments of the previous stage, so that as one developmental stage is completed, more positive growth occurs. It is the constancy of the process that allows the nurse to evaluate the client to determine if normal progress is taking place.

In order to more clearly understand psychosocial growth and development, the nurse must first understand theoretical approaches describing this sequential process. The most frequently cited theoretical systems which cover the life span include (1) psychoanalytical theories as represented by Freud and Erikson, (2) developmental theories of Gesell, Lewin, Piaget, Kohlberg, Cumming and Henry, Havighurst, and Neugarten, and (3) behavioristic (social learning) theories described by Sears, Bijou and Baer, and Heider.

Psychoanalytical Theories

Sigmund Freud

The theories of Freud[5] build upon a framework which is dynamic, systematic, and comprehensive in the way it defines psychosocial development and behavior. The aim of therapy is to help the person being treated work through present conflicts or the incompleted developmental level so that he or she might move effectively into the natural stage of mature development.

The dynamic force is called the *libido* or *life force*. Initially, Freud viewed this force as primarily sexual in nature. However, by broadening the scope, the libido can be seen as a motivating force behind behavior. A person strives for self-preservation and pleasure in general, as well as for survival of the species. A mature person can further channel gratification in creative endeavors.

Freud's systematic framework incorporates four major stages of development: (1) the oral stage, (2) the anal stage, (3) the phallic stage, further subdivided into Oedipal or Electra and latency, and (4) the genital stage. This theory of psychosexual development aims to explain personality organization.

The *oral stage* encompasses the first year of life. Energy which may be considered sexual in nature is concentrated around the mouth, lips, and tongue, thereby providing oral gratification.

If the infant's major need of feeding is met by a loving mother who also provides protection and comfort, then healthy development will occur. The infant becomes secure and is able to form stable relationships with caretakers, which will allow him or her to proceed to greater independence and move on to the second stage of development.

During the *anal stage,* the child begins to manifest a primary egotistical nature. Gratification is obtained through exploration of the body, leading to autoerotic pleasures. Energy is concentrated around the rectum and anus through the expulsion and retention of feces and the exercising of associated muscle groups. Pleasure is also derived from the emotional satisfaction of being in control of one's bodily functions, as well as the sensuality associated with the anal erogenous area. Since toilet training is the primary task at this time, the child may experience conflict or ambivalence when "holding on" (conforming to the toileting demands of the parents) or "letting go" (satisfying instinctual drives). If

Behavioral development can be examined using various theoretical approaches.

Freud's theories provide a foundation for the psychoanalytical approach to analyzing behavior.

The *libido* is a motivating force behind behavior.

In Freud's framework, a person passes through four stages: (1) oral, (2) anal, (3) phallic, and (4) genital.

Egotism is noted during the anal stage.

Toilet training is the primary developmental task to be mastered during the anal stage.

the experience of toilet training is favorable, the child's personality matures appropriately.

The *phallic stage* begins at about age 3 and continues until puberty. With resolution of the anal stage, autoerotic pleasures are now gained through self-stimulation of the genitalia. This behavior leads to primitive feelings of sexuality which the child directs mainly at the opposite-sex parent. A rivalry between the child and the same-sex parent ensues in an effort to win the attentions and love of the other parent.

The *Oedipal complex* is the sexual feelings that a boy experiences for his mother and the rivalry that he feels toward his father. The male child wants mother for himself and attempts to intrude between his parents. The *Electra complex* is basically the same situation in reverse for the girl, but is complicated by a feeling of ambivalence toward the mother. For the girl, the mother represents not only a rival but also a caregiver. The normal resolution of these complexes is the child's identification with the parent of the same sex. Final resolution occurs in adolescence when the child relinquishes the parent of the opposite sex as a love object and is ready to turn to an outside love object of the opposite sex.

Since the child has learned that he or she cannot freely indulge sexual feelings and desires but must control them to a certain degree, the formation of a conscience takes place. At this point the child moves into a period of psychosexual *latency,* during which time sexual impulses are repressed. The child, who is now 6 or 7 years old, seeks pleasure from the external world through peer relationships, school achievements, and relations with the adult world. Energy and interest are concentrated on intellectual and physical pursuits.

As the child approaches puberty, physiological sexual changes bring on a renewal of sexual issues and interest. Now in the *genital stage* of Freud's framework, the adolescent struggles for independence from parents and seeks love relationships that eventually lead to mature sexual encounters with a love object or person. Thus, puberty is thought to create the pleasure-seeking aim of reproduction through sexual encounter. Upon reaching the genital stage, the child has passed successfully through each of the earlier stages.

Freud has identified three primary structures of personality that evolve in a developmental sequence in the process of acquiring emotional organization and control: the id, ego, and superego.

The *id* is the agency of the mind which houses the instinctual forces associated with the earliest developmental stage. It remains primarily unconscious but makes itself felt through thoughts, desires, and sensations. It operates on the "pleasure principle," seeking immediate gratification for all its desires. The gratification of these desires is controlled by the ego and superego.

The *ego* operates on the "reality principle." It assesses such factors as safety, time, and possibility when deciding which demands and the extent to which these demands of the id and superego will be satisfied. The ego develops autonomy or the capacity for self-regulation from the interaction of the id with the environment. The ability of the ego to deal with the demands of the id and of the superego to maintain contact with reality is referred to as *ego strength.* The ego may also be labeled the *conscious* or *will.*

The *superego* is the agency of the mind frequently referred to as the *conscience.* Like the ego, it develops through the influence of the environment, especially the parenting figures. The child attempts to please the parents to gain love and views punishment as a loss of love, thereby using the parents' values as limits. If the child has resolved the Oedipal or Electra complex, he or she is on the way to developing a superego. Thus, an ethical-moral dimension of personality develops.

As can readily be seen, the ego is a pivotal point in a healthy person. It is through the internal conflicts of these structures and the resulting balance that behavior is produced. The ego's strength in controlling the id's and superego's demands determines the so-called normality of the resulting behavior and satisfactory progression through psychosocial development.

Erik Erikson

Erikson's theory of development[6] is more psychosocial in nature than is Freud's. He considers the influence society and its representatives exert on the developing person. Erikson stresses the ego and its growth. The ego is the central process which guards the organism against shock by enabling it to anticipate internal and external dangers and to deal with change while maintaining a sense of continuity. He has divided a person's development into eight stages with a crisis to be resolved in each stage. Resolution of each crisis can be toward a negative or positive pole. The closer the resolution falls toward the positive pole, the better the chance the succeeding stage will be positively resolved, culminating in a healthy personality.

Erikson strongly believes in the interaction of physical and psychological development.

In Erikson's first stage, the *oral stage,* the infant is completely dependent on others to satisfy necessary wants. The task to be resolved is trust versus mistrust. Trust is attained by the parenting figures' response to the child's needs. The more consistently the needs are met, the more secure the child feels, and therefore the more likely the child will be to trust others. This trust is necessary before the child can enter the next stage.

Erikson's eight stages of personality development are the following:

I Trust versus mistrust

In the second stage, *early childhood,* the child's physical maturation allows a greater freedom to explore the environment, to become independent, and to make a choice, and thus the child is able to develop autonomy. During this time the parenting figures must establish limits to prevent the child from engaging in meaningless experiments which may overwhelm him or her, but at the same time they must not prevent exploration, thereby hindering development. In this stage the child also begins to experience and explore others' reaction to him or her and to delay gratification in order to experience positive feedback.

II Autonomy versus shame and doubt.

In the *play age,* the third stage, the child's initiative is developed by undertaking and planning a task independently. With initiative the child is more likely to forget failures and to approach new tasks with more directness. If the child receives disapproval for independent action, guilt rather than initiative will be attained. At this age, the child learns to interact with others in play (cooperative play) and not just to play alongside others (parallel play) as was the norm in the previous stage.

III Initiative versus guilt

The fourth stage, *school age,* is a time when either industry or inferiority is gained. Industry refers to a feeling of accomplishment that one has the mental and/or physical prowess needed to win the approval of family, teachers, and peers. If this feeling of accomplishment is not present, the child may develop a sense of inferiority and withdraw from family, peers, and competition with others.

IV Industry versus inferiority

In *adolescence,* the fifth stage, the task is to find a sense of identity, and if this is not achieved, role diffusion results. Adolescence is a transitional stage when the values, drives, skills, and ambitions of childhood must be reviewed and redefined in the framework of concrete opportunities and approaching adulthood. Adolescents must establish their own identity. To do so they must modify parental values with which they are not comfortable, choose a lifestyle of their own, and determine where they

V Identity and repudiation versus identity diffusion

are headed. Basically, they must feel personal satisfaction in who they are. Adolescents usually stay in a peer group as a way of assisting themselves in shaping this identity.

Unlike Freud, Erikson continued his stages beyond adolescence. His sixth stage, *young adulthood,* is a time when a person is able to reach out to form friendships and to develop an intimate relationship with another. The other polarity is isolation. This occurs when a person cannot form friendships, is dissatisfied with oneself, and is unable to commit oneself to a partnership because of an inability to develop and live by compromises without loss of ego.

In *adulthood,* the seventh stage, the task is generativity versus stagnation. The adult is concerned with guidance of the next generation. If one's life is satisfying, interests can turn outward to community activities, friends, and hobbies.

The last stage, *mature age,* brings either integrity or despair. A person who feels comfortable with the past can face old age and death with the feeling that life has been worthwhile. Despair occurs when the ego has no satisfying feelings to draw on.

Developmental Theories

Arnold Gesell*

Arnold Gesell,[7] as a maturational theorist, emphasizes the family as the pivotal center at which the interaction of inner and cultural forces comes to the most significant expression. The household is a cultural workshop for transmitting the social inheritance: a democratic household fosters a way of life which respects the individuality of the growing child. The child as an organism and the environment as a culture are inseparable. Each reacts to the other. The reactions of the child are primary: he must do his own growing. The culture helps him to achieve his developmental potentialities, helps him to learn, but the process of acculturation is limited by the child's natural growth process.

The child's personality is a product of slow and gradual growth. His nervous system matures by stages and natural sequences. All of his abilities, including his moral thoughts, are subject to laws of growth.

Gesell espoused a developmental philosophy of child care that is

. . . sensitive to the relativities of growth and maturity. It takes its point of departure from the child's nature and needs. It acknowledges the profound forces of racial and familial inheritance which determine the growth sequences and the distinctive growth pattern of each individual child. It envisages the problem of acculturation in terms of growth; but this increases rather than relaxes the responsibility of cultural guidance. Developmental guidance at a conscious level demands an active use of intelligence to understand the laws and mechanisms of the growth process.[8]

Gesell discusses the dynamics of the growth complex as an overview of total unitary action with the system in dynamic flow. The outstanding features are the following:

Day cycle: Growth is a self-renewing, self-perpetuating, and self-expanding process which occurs every day.

Self-regulatory fluctuations: The living growth complex during the period of infancy and childhood is in a state of formative instability

*From Mary Jane Amundson, in Mary Tudor (ed.), *Child Development,* McGraw-Hill, New York, 1981, pp. 124–128. Used by permission.

VI Intimacy and solidarity versus isolation

VII Generativity versus self-absorption or stagnation

VIII Integrity versus despair

Family, child, and culture are interacting forces in facilitating the child's development.

Outstanding features of the growth complex as defined by Gesell are its day cycle, self-regulatory fluctuations, and constitutional individuality.

combined with a progressive movement toward stability. The growing organism oscillates along a spiral course toward maturity.

Constitutional individuality: Each child has a distinct mode of growth which is unique and which is also highly characteristic.[9]

Gesell emphasized a passionate regard for the individual, which he maintained was crucial to a truly democratic orientation to life. A corollary of this stress on the importance of the individual is the concept of individual differences. Yet, paradoxically, it is here that Gesell seems to have been most generally misinterpreted. This stems from the organization of most of his books in terms of the continued stress on ages and stages of behavioral development throughout childhood and adolescence.[10]

Kurt Lewin*

Kurt Lewin's point of view is called *topological field theory* and is based on his concept of *life space,* which consists of those selected aspects of the environment which stand out for the individual as psychologically meaningful.[11] He viewed the life space as a region marked with *routes* and *barriers.* Routes lead to goal objects with positive and negative *valences,* which indicate attractiveness or repulsion. The person in the field is moved or immobilized by the action of these valences along the pathways that are open to him, representing courses of action. Lewin was less interested in how a life space comes to be constituted as it is than in its structure at the moment of action. He saw the life space becoming progressively more differentiated in the course of development and conceived of regression as a dedifferentiation of the life space. It does not seem incompatible with his views to assume that the life space also undergoes qualitative reorganization and reintegration as development proceeds.[12]

Lewin's field theory is postulated as a restatement and refinement of naïve theory. A basic concept is life space—which includes the sum of all the facts that determine the person's behavior at a given time. These contemporary facts are directly relevant to the behavior and are divided into two large classes: those that describe the environment and those that describe the person.

The psychological environment is defined in terms of its effect on behavior. All parts of the psychological environment influence the person's behavior, and therefore the environment is a description of the external situation as it affects behavior, which is not physical activity but merely a change in the psychological environment. Behavior is a means for attaining some goal; it is viewed as locomotion in the direction of the goal within some defined space (region). The environment is described in geometrical terms. It is composed of regions which may correspond to varied psychological events, activities of the individual, group memberships, or physical areas. The arrangement of the regions in the psychological environment is called the *cognitive structure.* Lewin postulated the existence of psychological forces in the environment. The movement of the person from one region to another was explained in terms of a force on the person in the first region in the direction of the second region. Any force must have a point of application, a strength, and a direction. A valence represents a force field that is manifested in a particular force on a particular person and may be positive or negative. If there are many

Highlights

A basic concept in Lewin's theory is "life space"—the sum of all the facts that determine the person's behavior at a given time.

The psychological environment is defined in terms of its effect on behavior.

Behavior is a means for attaining some goal.

*Ibid.

different regions with valences, there may be various forces upon the person, some which may be in the same direction and reinforce one another and some which may be in different directions and conflict with one another.

Needs of the person are correlated to forces in the psychological environment. The effect of a need system in a state of tension is that some region in the environment acquires a positive valence. Consequently, there is a force on the person in the direction of that region. Directed action to satisfy this need is one possible consequence, or the need may remain latent until the appropriate goal becomes available.

The basic assumption is that development involves an increase in the number of regions and an increase in the strength of the boundaries of these regions. The aspects of development include the following:

As the child grows older, he exhibits a greater variety of behavior.

Behavior becomes increasingly guided by a governing purpose, a main theme.

The psychological environment of the child expands both in area covered and in time span.

Growth of the child involves change in the dependence of his activities on one another.

An increase occurs in realism, which is identified by its psychological properties, not by external reality.[13]

As the individual grows older, a greater variety of behaviors is exhibited.

Jean Piaget*

According to Jean Piaget's theory,[14] the major forces which facilitate the developmental process are: maturational forces; results of experience and environment; results of explicit and implicit teaching of the child by others in the environment; and the process of equilibration (cognitive development and particularly the development of organized belief systems).[15]

Unorganized belief systems contain inherent self-contradictions and conflict; force is set up to harmonize the child's ideas one with another and is the process of equilibration.

Piaget, a French biologist, begins from the point of view that as all organisms adapt to their environment, they must possess some form of structure or organization which makes the adaptation possible at all. Thus he views organization and adaptation as the basic invariants of functioning. Adaptation is further subdivided into two closely interwoven components, *assimilation* and *accommodation*.

A person possesses some form of structure or organization which makes adaptation to the environment possible.

Assimilation involves changing the elements in the situation (e.g., experience or food) so that they can be incorporated into the structure of the organism (e.g., intellectual or digestive systems) in order that the individual may adapt to the situation. Accommodation implies modifying the structures of the organism so that the organism can adapt to the situation. Assimilation and accommodation are also regarded as functional invariants. For Piaget, every intellectual act necessitates some intellectual structure, while intellectual functioning is characterized by assimilation and accommodation.

Two important components of adaptation are assimilation and accommodation.

As the baby interacts with his environment, he builds up sequences of actions, or patterns of behavior, called *schemata* which have definite structure. In the postinfancy period, the term schema refers to mental actions and intellectual structures. In assimilation, the child has to absorb new experiences into his existing schemata, whereas in accommoda-

*Ibid.

tion there is the modification of existing schemata or the buildup of new ones. But once new experience is assimilated, the child's schemata become more complex, and because of this, accommodations of even greater complexity are possible. Changes in the schemata brought about by attempts at accommodation and reorganization brought about independently of external stimulation together ensure schemata of greater complexity and hence intellectual growth.

Piaget has provided much evidence to suggest that there is a fixed sequence of stages in the growth of thought and that thinking at one stage is qualitatively different from that of another.[16] The age at which children reach the stages varies because of the educational and cultural backgrounds, the degree of intellectual stimulation they receive, and heredity.

These stages, described in Lovell,[17] include the sensorimotor period, the preoperational stage, concrete operational thought, and formal operational thought.

Sensorimotor period In the first 21 months or so of life, the schemata built up need the direct support of information obtained through the senses and through motor action. Each element in the schema comes into being at the exact moment when other aspects of the environment provide the necessary support for it. During the development of sensorimotor intelligence, there is a growth of the more specialized intellectual achievements, e.g., the sensorimotor construction of causality, imitation, objects, play, space, and time. It is during this period that the basic schemata are elaborated for dealing with the environment, as in the case of space when the child adjusts his actions to reach near and distant objects and the case of time when he adjusts his actions to catch a swinging rattle.

Preoperational stage The child moves from the stage of sensorimotor intelligence into what Piaget calls the preoperational stage of thought, when he can differentiate a *signifier* (an image or a word) from a significate (what it is the signifier stands for) and call forth the one to represent the other. The capacity to make this differentiation and to be able to make an act of reference is termed the symbolic function. With the onset of language, the nature of the child's intelligence greatly changes. *Representational thought* can grasp a number of events as a coherent whole, whereas, at the level of sensorimotor intelligence, successive actions and perceptual states are linked one by one. Representational thought provides the child with a less transient and far more flexible model of the outside world and extends the range of thought well outside the present environment, for he is no longer dependent on action and immediate perception for thought.

Between 2 and 4 years of age intellectual development seems to consist largely in the building up of this representational activity and in differentiating image and language, on the one hand, from action and reality, on the other. Between ages 4 and $5\frac{1}{2}$ years, the child is more able to examine and set about a specific task, adapt his intelligence to it, and commence to reason about more difficult everyday problems. Even so, one of the marked characteristics of thought at this stage is its tendency to center on some striking feature of the object about which he is reasoning to the exclusion of other relevant aspects, with the result that the reasoning is distorted. The child is also incapable of seeing a situation from other than a personal point of view. However, around $5\frac{1}{2}$ years of age, the rigid and irreversible intellectual structures begin to become more flexible, and there is a transition to the next stage of thought.

Highlights

Piaget's theory of cognitive development includes 4 stages: (1) sensorimotor, (2) preoperational, (3) concrete operational thought, and (4) formal operational thought.

In the sensorimotor stage information obtained through the senses and motor action support development.

In the preoperational stage the child can differentiate an image or a word from what it stands for (for example, an object) and can name an object not in sight.

The child uses "representational thought."

Situations are viewed egotistically.

Piaget calls the overall 4- to 7-year-old period one of *intuitive thought*. The term intuition indicates the rather isolated and sporadic actions in the mind which occasionally give a foretaste of later systematized thinking but which do not yet coalesce into an integrated system of thought, as they do when operational thought sets in.

Concrete operational thought   At this stage the child's logical thought extends only to objects and events of firsthand reality. The child is able to take into account two contrasting features, e.g., height and width, which could balance and compensate for any distortion brought about by concentrating on one aspect of the situation. At 7 to 8, the schemata which have developed are different in kind from those present at 4 to 5 years of age. The capacity to reason and understand demands a higher-order schema which permits a simultaneous grasp of successive sequences in the mind. The child can now look at his own thinking and monitor it. Also, for any action in his mind, he can now understand that there are other actions that will give the same result. There is now learning with understanding. In Piaget's system, when mental actions have a definite and strong structure, they are termed operations. Thus any action which is an integral part of an organized network of related action is an operation. In Piaget's view, concrete operational thought must possess certain properties, which are *closure, reversibility, associativity,* and *identity*.

Formal operational thought   As the child becomes better at organizing and structuring data with the methods of concrete operational thought, he becomes aware that such methods do not lead to a logically exhaustive solution to his problems. The adolescent, due to the maturation of the central nervous system and the continued interaction with the cultural milieu together with the resulting feedback, can now produce more complex operations when faced with certain kinds of data or situations. The adolescent can set up a number of *hypotheses* and establish which are compatible with the evidence in front of him.

Piaget argues that the age of onset of formal thought is relative to the culture pattern, for in some undeveloped societies, adolescents do not appear to attain this level of thought.[18] So beyond some minimum ages, perhaps set by neurophysiological factors, the level of an individual's thinking may be a product of the progressive acceleration of individual development under the influence of education and culture.

For Piaget, there are four major influences affecting intellectual growth; these are briefly listed below.[19]

1 Biological factors, which probably determine the unfolding of the stages of intellectual growth in a fixed sequence.

2 *Equilibration* (the process of bringing assimilation and accommodation into balanced coordination) or autoregulation factors, which probably lie at the origin of mental operations themselves.

3 General factors resulting from socialization, which arise through exchanges, discussions, agreements, and oppositions in social intercourse between children or between children and adults. Such influences operate to a greater or lesser extent in all cultures, and they are closely linked to the equilibration factor since the general coordination of actions concern the interindividual as well as the intraindividual.

4 Factors related to education and cultural transmission, which differ greatly from one society to another.

Highlights

In the stage of concrete operational thought, the child's thought is more logical and there is learning with understanding.

Operations are mental actions which have a definite and strong structure.

When the child reaches the stage of formal operational thought, maturation and sociocultural interaction increase and the child can generate hypotheses and use reasoning in formal thought.

Piaget established that intellectual development follows a predictable pattern.[20]

All development proceeds in a unitary direction.

Developmental progressions are in order and can readily be described by criteria marking distinct developmental phases.

There are distinct organizational differences between childhood and adult behavior in all areas of human functioning.

All mature aspects of behavior have their beginnings in infant behavior and evolve through all subsequent patterns of development.

All developmental trends are interrelated and interdependent; developmental maturity means the final and total integration of all the developmental trends.

Lawrence Kohlberg*

Kohlberg's major contribution to the study of human development has been his insight into the development of *moral behavior*.[21] Morality indicates a set of rules for determining one's social actions which have been internalized by the individual. The rules tend to be related to the culture and are internalized because of some inner motivation.

Kohlberg has identified three levels which include a total of six definite and universal stages of development in moral thought.[22] These stages are the products of interactional experience between the child and the world, experience which leads to a restructuring of the child's own organization rather than to the direct imposition of the culture's pattern upon the child. Throughout life the organism receives enormous inputs of information from which he reconstructs his image of the world. In early infancy, the messages he receives are largely undifferentiated sounds, lights, and feelings, but with growth comes consciousness and ability to distinguish people and objects. Growth and the experiences of life bring to the child an expansion in his image of the world of things and human relationships. A child is not born with values but forms them in his relationships with his family and his culture. The value systems of a culture are transmitted in the processes of that culture by the information inputs which the culture generates.

Level I—preconventional—ages 4 to 10 in American middle-class culture Moral value resides in external, quasiphysical happenings, in bad acts, or in quasiphysical needs rather than in persons and standards. The two stages emphasize punishment and obedience orientation and a nonquestioning deference to superior power. Right action consists of that which instrumentally satisfies one's own needs of others.

Level II—conventional—preadolescence Moral value resides in performing good or right rules in maintaining the conventional order and expectancies of others. The two stages focus on orientation to interpersonal relations of mutuality and to approval, affection, and helpfulness. Correct behavior consists of doing one's duty, showing respect for authority, conforming to the fixed rules, and maintaining the given social order for its own sake.

Level III—postconventional—adolescence Moral values reside in conformity by the self to shared or shareable standards, rights, or duties. Within these two stages, orientation is to internal decisions of conscience but without clear rational or universal principles. The growth within

*Ibid.

Piaget established that intellectual development follows a predictable pattern.

One's culture and inner motivations influence moral development.

Relationships with family and culture assist one in formulating values.

Cognitive understanding of moral concepts influences the internalization of moral rules.

this level is toward ethical principles appealing to logic, comprehensiveness, universality, and consistency. Kohlberg concludes that something like the internalization of moral rules depends closely upon the cognitive growth of moral concepts and that conscience develops late. He also states that social class and the extent of participation in peer group activities is related to moral development quite independently of IQ.

Elaine Cumming and William Henry*

Psychological and social changes during the aging process are closely united, and they have a significant impact on each other. It is difficult to explain mental processes, behavior, and feelings without the perspective of social roles, positions, and norms. A theory of aging that is purely social or psychological would be most unusual, and it is more appropriate to approach these aging factors as *psychosocial* theories. Probably the most controversial and widely discussed is the *disengagement theory*, developed by Elaine Cumming and William Henry.[23, 24] This theory views aging as a process whereby society and the individual gradually withdraw, or disengage, from each other, to the mutual satisfaction and benefit of both. The benefit to individuals is that they can reflect and be centered on themselves, having been freed from societal roles. The value of disengagement for society is that some orderly means is established for the transfer of power from the old to the young, making it possible for society to continue functioning after its individual members have died.

The theory does not indicate whether it is society or the individual who is responsible for initiating the disengagement process, but one may readily detect several difficulties with the premise. Many older persons are highly satisfied to remain engaged and do not want their primary satisfaction to be derived from reflection on younger years. Senators, supreme court judges, and college professors are among those who commonly derive satisfaction and provide a valuable service for society by not disengaging. Since the health of the individual, cultural practices, societal norms, and other factors influence the degree to which a person will participate in society during the later years, some critics of this theory claim that disengagement would not be necessary if society improved the health care and financial means of the aged and increased the acceptance, opportunities, and respect afforded them.

A careful examination of the population studied in the development of the disengagement theory indicates certain of its limitations. The disengagement pattern which Cumming and Henry described was based on a study of 172 middle-class persons between the ages of 48 and 68. This group was wealthier, better educated, and of higher occupational and residential prestige than the general aged population. No blacks or chronically ill persons were involved in the study. Caution is advisable in generalizing for the entire aged population from findings based on less than 200 persons who are not representative of the average aged person. While nurses should appreciate that some older individuals may wish to disengage from the mainstream of society, this is not necessarily a process to be expected from all aged persons.

Robert Havighurst†

At the opposite pole from the disengagement theory, Havighurst proposes the *activity theory* [which] proclaims that an older person should continue a middle-aged life-style, denying the existence of old age as long as possible, and that society should apply the same norms to old age as it does to middle age and not advocate diminishing activity, inter-

*From Charlotte Eliopoulos, *Gerontological Nursing,* Harper & Row, New York, 1979, pp. 30–32. Used by permission.
†Ibid.

The disengagement theory postulates that the individual gradually withdraws from society as aging occurs, as reflected in certain behaviors.

The activity theory suggests that the individual remain active and involved in society as aging occurs.

est, and involvement as its members grow old.[25] This theory suggests ways of maintaining activity in the presence of multiple losses associated with the aging process—including substituting intellectual activities for physical activities when physical capacity is reduced, replacing the work role with other roles when retirement occurs, and establishing new friendships when old ones are lost. Declining health, loss of roles, reduced income, a shrinking circle of friends, and other obstacles to maintaining an active life are to be resisted and overcome instead of being accepted.

This theory is not without merit. Activity is generally assumed to be more desirable than inactivity as it facilitates physical, mental, and social well-being. Like a self-fulfilling prophecy, the expectation of a continued active state during old age may be realized. Because of society's currently negative view of inactivity and "acting old," it is probably best to encourage an active life-style among the aged, consistent with society's values. Also supportive of the activity theory is the reluctance of many older persons to accept themselves as old, although one of its problems is the assumption that most older people desire and are able to maintain a middle-aged life-style. Some want their world to shrink to accommodate their decreasing capacities or their preference for less active roles. Many lack the physical, emotional, social, or economic resources to continue active roles in society. Aged people who are expected to maintain an active middle-aged life-style on a retirement income of less than half that of middle-aged people may wonder if society isn't giving them conflicting messages. The results and consequences of multiple expectations to remain active that cannot be fulfilled by the aging individual still need to be researched.

Bernice Neugarten*

The *developmental theory* of aging, also referred to as the *continuity theory,* relates the factors of personality and predisposition toward certain actions in old age to similar factors during other phases of the life cycle.[26] Personality and basic patterns of behavior are said to be unchanged as the individual ages. The activist at age 20 will most likely be an activist at age 70. On the other hand, the young recluse will probably not be active in the mainstream of society when he or she ages. Concepts and patterns developed over a lifetime will determine whether an individual remains engaged and active or becomes disengaged and inactive. The recognition that the unique features of each individual allow for multiple adaptations to aging and that the potential exists for a variety of reactions gives this theory reality and support. Aging is a complex process, and the developmental theory considers these complexities to a greater extent than most other theories. While the implications and impact of this promising theory are uncertain, since it is in an early stage of research, it should be closely followed.

Several other theories, although less developed, need mentioning. One theory (Rose, 1965) views the aged as a subculture whose members are typically forced to interact primarily with each other, due to their negative treatment by society. One problem with this theory is that it is not valid for all social classes of aged people. A similar theory (Streib, 1965) views the aged as a minority group which, like the handicapped and certain racial groups, has visible characteristics that are discriminated against—the signs of being old. Aged persons who do not display such characteristics and are able to maintain a youthful appearance are less discriminated against. This is not valid in all circumstances, however, since older individuals possessing great wealth, status, or fame are often the subjects of admiration rather than discrimination.

*Ibid.

The developmental or continuity theory of aging suggests that the individual will remain engaged or become disengaged in society based on lifetime patterns (behavior) and concepts.

To an extent, the biological, psychological, and social processes of aging are interrelated and interdependent. Frequently, loss of a social role alters an individual's drives and speeds physical decline, and poor health forces retirement from work, promoting social isolation and the development of a weakened self-concept. While certain changes occur independently, as separate events, most are closely associated with other age-related factors. It is impractical, therefore, to subscribe solely to one theory of aging. Wise nurses will be eclectic in choosing the aging theories they will utilize in the care of older adults; they will also be cognizant of the limitations of these theories.

Behavioristic (Social Learning) Theories*

Robert Sears

Sears founded a theory of social learning and socialization[27] of the child on the basis of psychoanalytic hypotheses and placed the causal explanations and theoretical justifications of these hypotheses within the stimulus-response framework.[28] Sears focuses upon those aspects of behavior which are overt and can be measured; for Sears, personality development can best be measured through *action* and *social interaction*. He is primarily concerned with evaluating active behavior from this perspective: an emphasis on the learning experience of an individual that results from an action sequence—i.e., the learning effects of the stimulus-response sequence—in which each effect of an action can become the learned cause of future behavior. Action is instigated by a drive that is strong enough to impel the individual to respond to a cue, or stimulus. Initially, all stimuli are associated with primary, or innate, drives such as hunger. The satisfaction or frustration that results from the behavior prompted by these primary drives leads the individual to adopt additional behaviors. During this interactive process, the individual learns new modes of behavior, the satisfactory results of which serve to reinforce the achieving behavior. Constant reinforcement of specific actions, in turn, give rise to new, or learned, drives and to primary-drive equivalents; these are the secondary drives. These secondary drives arise from the social influences on development. Development may be considered a continuous, orderly sequence of conditions which create actions, new motives for actions, and eventual patterns of behavior.

As long as everyday social life proceeds as if developmental phases were a reality, all social learning tends to proceed in comparable patterns. All human functioning must be seen as the result of the interactive effects of all the influences, both constitutional and experiential, that have impinged on the individual. Social behavior depends almost exclusively upon the impact of others, rather than upon any internal developmental processes.[29] Early training of the infant distinctly implies an expectancy of different levels of readiness. Therefore, social conditions dictate the existence of developmental phases, regardless of whether they are based upon dependent fact.

Sears relates each of the following to the three developmental phases which he outlines.[30]

Meaning of the particular phase

Place of primary needs

*From Mary Jane Amundson, in Mary Tudor (ed.), *Child Development,* McGraw-Hill, New York, 1981, pp. 121–124. Used by permission.

According to Sears, personality development is best measured through action and social interaction.

Development creates actions, new motives for actions, and eventual patterns of behavior.

Place of secondary motivational systems

Five major motivational systems in development (dependence, feeding, toileting, sex, and aggression)

Important processes in development (identification, play, motility, reasoning, and conscience)

Social factors (parent's own status, sex, ordinal position, class, education, and cultural heritage)

Phase I—rudimentary behavior: Native needs and early-infancy learning The first phase connects the biological endowment of the newborn child with the endowment of the social environment. This phase introduces the infant to the environment and provides the foundation for ever-increasing interactions with the environment.

During the early months of a child's life, his environmental experience has not yet directed his learning. An infant's behavior in the first 10 to 16 months of his life involves his attempts to reduce inner tension originating from his inner drives. The way in which these innate needs are met introduces environmental learning experiences. When the infant's behavior tends toward specific goal-directed behavior, each completed action which brings about a reduction in tension is the one which is most likely to be repeated again whenever the tension arises. Successful development is characterized by a decrease in autism and innate need-centered actions and by an increase in dyadic, socially centered behavior. Early child development investigates three essential areas:

Sears describes three developmental phases: (1) native needs and early-infancy learning, (2) family-centered learning, and (3) extrafamilial learning.

The first phase deals with rudimentary behavior and the early interaction between child and environment.

1 The conditions for a child's motivational system to be learned

2 The circumstances in which parents and other environmental factors reinforce a child's learning

3 The products or behavioral patterns of a child's learning

Sears' learning theory classifies dependency as a central component of learning. Rewarding reinforcement in all dyadic situations depends upon the child's having consistent contacts with one or more persons. Both child and mother have their repertoire of significant actions which serve to stimulate responses from the other which will be compatible with their own expectancies.

Aggression, on the basis of Sears' early research on the frustration-aggression hypothesis, is a consequence of frustration. Aggression readily becomes an early and vital aspect of learned behavior because frustration occurs from the very moment the infant experiences discomfort or pain and delay in finding relief from the unpleasant experience. Aggression, usually manifested through anger, is primarily a response to this frustration.

Phase II—secondary motivational systems: Family-centered learning Socialization begins to take place during this second phase, when primary needs continue to motivate the child. Aspects of the undisciplined life of the infant become subject to the rigors of parental training. Primary needs are gradually incorporated into repeatedly reinforced social learning or secondary drives. From now on these secondary drives will be the child's main motives to action, unless social environment fails to provide the necessary reinforcement. Social learning depends upon replacing previous learning with newer experiences that are based upon more appropriate satisfaction rather than upon avoiding unpleasant experiences or upon a fear of consequence.

The second phase deals with secondary motivational systems in which learning is family-centered. The most significant influence comes from the mother or father and gradually there is a transition to more independent, self-initiated behavior.

Early-childhood development is essentially anchored in the satisfaction gained from the learned dependency upon the mothering person. As the child grows older, a sensitive mother looks upon excessive emotional dependency as behavior which should be altered. Slowly, the child learns to gratify his dependency drive by performing actions that he previously anticipated and demanded from his mother (imitation). The child discovers a new source of gratification in the very process of self-initiated imitation, which eventually leads from imitation of behavioral sequences to acting like another person. He may behave as if he possesses the psychological properties and skills of another. A nonmotivational system, identification, emerges and becomes a goal response.

Phase III—secondary motivational system: Extrafamilial learning By the time the young child is chronologically and developmentally ready for school, he is ready to absorb from a world which lies beyond that of his family. His new and wider environment helps him to achieve social, religious, and eventually political and economic values. All acquisitions of later value judgments are based on his earlier incorporations of his parents' behavior and what he has learned from his parents' teaching.

Highlights

The third phase deals with secondary motivational systems in which socialization is greatest outside the family environment.

Sidney Bijou and Donald Baer

In Bijou and Baer's analysis, development is defined as the progressive changes in the way an organism's behavior interacts with the environment and is limited to the observable, recordable instances of the responses of the developing child and to the specific events which operate on him and thus make up his environment.[31]

Changes in behavior are dependent on interactions with the environment according to Bijou and Baer.

The child is conceptualized as an interrelated cluster of responses and stimuli. The environment is conceived as events acting on the child: some specific stimuli and some setting events. The child and his environment interact continuously from fertilization until death. The psychological development of a child, therefore, is made up of progressive changes in the different ways of interacting with the environment. Progressive development is dependent upon opportunities and circumstances in the present and in the past. The circumstances are physical, chemical, organismic, and social. The influences may be analyzed in their physical and functional dimensions.

The theory proceeds by the following chain:

The developing child is adequately conceptualized as a source of responses, which fall into two functional classes: *respondents,* which are controlled primarily by preceding eliciting stimulation and which are largely insensitive to consequent stimulation, and *operants,* which are controlled primarily by consequent stimulation. The attachment of operant responses to preceding (discriminative) stimuli is dependent upon the stimulus consequence of behavior previously made in the presence of these *discriminative stimuli.* Some responses may share attributes of both respondents and operants.

Initial understanding of the child's development next requires analysis of the child's environment, which is conceptualized as a source both of *eliciting stimuli,* controlling his respondents, and of *reinforcing stimuli,* which can control his operants.

Subsequent analysis of the child's development proceeds by listing the ways in which respondents are attached to new eliciting stimuli and detached from old ones, through respondent conditioning and extinction. Similarly, a listing is made of the ways in which operants are strengthened or weakened through various reinforcement contingencies and discriminated to various stimuli which reliably mark occasions on which these contingencies hold. Some respondents are called emotional, and the conditioned eliciting stimuli for them may be provided by people and hence are social. Some of the operants strengthened are manipulatory, and some of their discriminative stimuli consist of the size, distance, weight, and motion of objects; hence, this development is perceptual-motor. Some of the operants are vocal, as are some of the respondents. The discriminative stimuli, reinforcing stimuli, and conditioned eliciting stimuli typically are both objects and the behavior of people. Hence, this development is both cultural and linguistic.

Highlights

Emotional, perceptual-motor, and cultural and linguistic development are based on varying stimuli (people and objects) in the environment. There are discriminative, eliciting, and reinforcing stimuli.

The processes of the discrimination and generalization of stimuli are applied throughout these sequences of development. Thus, the child's operants and respondents may be attached to classes of eliciting and discriminative stimuli. These classes may have varying breadths, depending upon the variety of conditioning and extinction procedures applied to them. Consequently, the child's manipulatory and verbal behaviors seem to deal in classes; this phenomenon, coupled with the complexity of discriminative stimuli possible in discriminating operants, typically gives the label "intellectual" to such behaviors.

The equation of discriminative stimuli to secondary reinforcers suggests that many discriminative stimuli will play an important role in strengthening and weakening operant behaviors in the child's future development. Some of these discriminative stimuli consist of the behavior of people (typically parents) and thus give rise to social reinforcers: attention, affection, approval, achievement, pride, status, etc. Again the preceding principles are applied but now to the case of social reinforcement, offered for what are therefore social behaviors under social discriminative stimuli.

Behaviors are called respondents and operants, which are strengthened or weakened by stimuli.

In all these steps, the scheduling of eliciting, discriminative, and reinforcing stimuli, to one another and to responses, is applied. This gives an explanation for characteristic modes of response which distinguish children: typical rates, the use of steady responding or bursts of activity, resistance to extinction, and the likelihood of pausing after reinforcement.

The cultural environment, or, more exactly, the members of the community, starts out with a human infant formed and endowed along species lines, but capable of behavioral training in many directions. From this raw material, the culture proceeds to make, in so far as it can, a product acceptable to itself. It does this by training: by reinforcing the behavior it desires and extinguishing others, by making some natural and social stimuli into discriminative stimuli and ignoring others, by differentiating out this or that specific response or chain of responses, such as manners and attitudes, and by conditioning emotional and anxiety reactions to some stimuli and not others. It teaches the individual what he may and may not do, giving him norms and ranges of social behavior that are permissive or prescriptive or prohibitive. It teaches him the language he is to speak; it gives him his standards of beauty and art, of good and bad conduct; it sets before him a picture of the ideal personality that he is to imitate and strive to be. In all this, the fundamental laws of behavior are to be found.[32]

The cultural environment teaches the individual how to act by reinforcing desirable behavior and extinguishing undesirable behavior.

Fritz Heider

The *naïve theory* of development is concerned with the various concepts that are thought to underlie voluntary action. Several sources of interaction included are personal wants, ulterior reasons, the promptings of sentimental attachment, the inclination to accede to requests, obedience to commands, and moral obligations. Intentional behavior is viewed as stemming from the person himself, as being active rather than passive in its nature. However, naïve psychology also conceptualized the events that impinge on the person and arouse feelings and reactions.[33]

The theory contains a complex set of assumptions and laws that govern much of our understanding of other people. Briefly, these are as follows:

According to naïve theory human behavior is cognitively directed and depends on inherent motivations and interaction with the environment.

Nearly all human behavior is cognitively directed, that is, directed toward the attainment of goals which must be cognized before they can become operative. This cognition is seen as a natural process depending merely upon the exposure of the person to the external world.

Differences in the behavior of different people depend upon differences in motivation, which in turn depend upon differences in dispositional characteristics.

As well as being motivated by appropriate goal objects, people also respond to external pressure or imposition, which may arouse hostility, gratitude, fear, and other reactions. These feelings and their accompanying behavioral consequences are reasonably predictable. Two other classes of psychological mechanisms, according to commonsense theory, are sentiments and feelings of moral obligation.[34]

Related to development and change, Heider's primary concern is with the naïve theory of social behavior as based on a mixture of these two assumptions:

1 In certain fundamental aspects, *human behavior is innate* and appears without training. These include self-evident actions, e.g., perception, instrumental actions, and emotional reactions.

2 In other important respects, children are not like adults because they are uninformed and untaught. Areas that give meaning to experience, such as information, meanings, and values, are seen as acquired.[35]

Naïve psychology is not a stated theory but a body of beliefs about human behavior. Commonsense beliefs are the ground from which theories of human behavior may grow but are equally the ground in which literary criticism, the historian's understanding of social processes, and the theologian's ideas of the relation of God to people are rooted.

Summary

Each of the theories of psychosocial development just discussed provides a differing approach to examining and assessing a person's development. Terminology and phase-stage descriptions vary in each. However, there is a unifying core that runs throughout the theories. All of the theorists stress an orderly, sequential process in development, with complexity increasing as the person matures and masters the lower-level tasks. In order to continue normal development, tasks or phases must build upon one another. Problems occur if there is failure to complete a particular task or phase. Each theory is dynamic in that it postulates a need for growth on the part of the person. Thus, development is seen as a multidimensional process that proceeds in an orderly way and depends on major interaction between heredity and environment.

There are many common threads among theories of psychosocial development.

Psychoanalytical, developmental and behavioristic theories all provide a framework for assessing normal behavior patterns across the life span.

OTHER INFLUENCES ON BEHAVIORAL DEVELOPMENT

In addition to the effects of temperament and psychosocial development on behavior, there are numerous other variables which exert influence on a person's behavioral development. These include the formation of an identity, values, role identification, and sexuality.

Self-Identity

The formation of a self-identity, which incorporates self-image and body image, is an ongoing process from infancy, with the major focus in adolescence. Adolescence, a transitional period between childhood dreams and values and adulthood's opportunities and values, is a time in which one attempts to find a sense of continuity between past and future and between what one feels oneself to be and what one thinks others expect one to be. In this search the resulting behaviors and ideas often precipitate a conflict between the parents and the adolescent. In many respects this stage parallels Erikson's second stage of development, early childhood. In both, the urge toward independence with a concurrent desire to remain dependent creates ambivalence which results in the adolescent insisting on being treated as an adult one day and a child another day. In both stages, the person's exposure to outside influence increases, eventually leading the person to experiment with different identities prior to making any final decisions.

Self-identity develops across the life span with major strides occurring in adolescence.

George Mead views the development of self occurring as the capacity to interact with others evolves.[36] This process, like most aspects of development, is gradual and proceeds from the simple to the complex. Identity is found in two ways, through the life experiences of the person and through feedback of others with whom the person interacts. The quality of the resolution of each stage of development provides a clue to the self-identity being formed. The closer the resolutions are to the positive pole the more normal the self-identity and the better the self-image.

Social and environmental experience influences the development of self-identity.

"Feedback" deals with the reactions of significant others to the person's behavior. Mead describes this as "social interaction which allows the individual to see himself as others see him."[37] Thus the reflected appraisals of parents or significant other people shape the types of behaviors engaged in, the values incorporated into the personality structure, and the sense of morality developed. Not until adolescence (defined according to tasks to be accomplished, not age boundaries) does the process tend to become disruptive.

What emerges in adolescence are behaviors, values, and sexual actions which seemingly are an open defiance of parental teachings and guidance. This negative view of the adolescent turmoil can be altered by thinking of these actions as a sign that the person is entering a transition period and is heading toward maturity. At this time the peer group provides an important support for the adolescent. It is here that values, ideas, and behaviors can be tested and discarded without fear of belittling, and while maintaining a sense of identification.

Conflicts normally occur during one's struggle to establish an identity.

Adolescence can be said to have ended when a person has become self-supporting in a chosen occupation and has formed a value system and lifestyle with which he or she feels comfortable. Again, the emphasis is on completion of tasks rather than age boundaries. In today's society the above tasks are often not completed until the mid twenties. This does not signal abnormality; rather when examined by today's standards this delay in completing these tasks is to be expected. One consequence of more formal education being required for many occupations is that society has also extended the period of financial dependency and, to some degree, emotional dependency on the parents. The point to remember is that a person's behavior and completion or noncompletion of the tasks required must be examined within the framework of society as a whole and within the person's immediate cultural values and expectations.

The formation of an identity continues after adolescence; however, the basis or sense of identity which is needed to accomplish the tasks of later life must be established in adolescence. Erikson uses the term *beyond identity* to signify the continuation of identity formation after adolescence and also to signify that some forms of identity crises can occur in later stages.[38] In his book *Dimensions of a New Identity*, Erikson summarizes how identity is employed from the period of adolescence onward.

Identity formation continues after adolescence.

> In youth you find out what you care to do and who you care to be . . . In young adulthood you learn whom you care to be with . . . In adulthood you learn to know what and whom you can take care of . . .[39]

In summary, the formation of a self-identity is an ongoing process which receives the most attention in that period defined as adolescence. Identity forms by tapping past experiences and using the reactions of significant other persons as a guideline. The formation of a self-identity is:

> . . . a process of simultaneous reflection and observation, a process taking place on all levels of mental function by which the individual judges himself in the light of what he perceives to be the way in which others judge him in comparison to themselves . . . while he judges their way of judging him in the light of how he perceives himself . . .[40]

Values

An infant is not born with a set of values, a sense of morality, or an understanding of the roles to be assumed in life. These are learned by one as development occurs. The culture into which one is acclimated does not always impose its values on the child, rather the child adjusts and reorganizes his or her framework to society's influences. This adjustment occurs through the parenting figures' approval or disapproval and is transmitted via the folklores, myths, and fairy tales of the society. Developmentally it has been shown that the child seeks the approval of parents or significant other people. According to the feedback received, the child adjusts overt behaviors. Positive feedback reinforces the behavior, while negative feedback prompts the child to extinguish the behavior.

Behaviors reflect the values of the person.

The culture into which one is socialized is dynamic. It is a process by which a person adapts to the environment, and the culture also ensures its continuity by passing on the whole to succeeding generations.[41] Values, though abstract, are strongly influenced by culture. It is also important for the nurse to remember that clients' value systems also extend to their perceptions of health. Goldstein incorporates values into his definition of health:

A direct relationship can be seen between behavior and culture.

> . . . a condition related to a mental attitude by which the individual has to value what is essential for his life. "Health" thus appears as a value; its value consists in the individual's capacity to actualize his nature to the degree that, for him at least, it is essential.[42]

Role Identification

A role is defined as patterns of acts leading toward specific goals. The different roles which a person assumes can be said to consist of four stages: the anticipatory stage, the honeymoon stage, the plateau stage, and the disengagement-termination stage.[43]

Highlights

The anticipatory stage is the time during which the child receives the developmental training which socializes the child into those roles approved by the culture. Role expectations are transmitted through others and are clarified for the child from feedback received. This stage is also experienced before the assumption of any new role by the adult, for example, the engagement period marking the transition from a single state to a marital role or the months of pregnancy before parenthood begins. Though the anticipatory period is a defined period of time, preparation for the roles being assumed is part of the socialization of the child.[44]

There are four stages in role identification: (1) anticipatory, (2) honeymoon, (3) plateau, and (4) disengagement-termination.

The honeymoon stage is that undefined time immediately after the full responsibilities of any role are assumed. The end of this stage is difficult to define, since it blends with the next stage. However, it can be said that this is the adjustment period to a new role. The plateau stage is reached when the role responsibilities are being fully exercised, and adaptation to these responsibilities has occurred.[45]

The last stage, disengagement-termination, signals the need for change and further adaptation. This is the period preceding the end of a given role and includes its actual termination.[46] The period before a divorce and during the divorce itself is an example. This stage also overlaps the anticipatory stage. The engagement period before marriage anticipates a new role but also signals the end of a familiar one. This dual process means the person must draw on existing defenses to cope with the stresses.

Since a person assumes many roles simultaneously, especially in adulthood, many changes can occur in roles the client is experiencing. These potential stresses, when combined with other anxiety-producing events, can exhaust the person's ability to adapt unless intervention and support are given.

Changes in roles can cause stress in the client.

Sexuality

Human sexuality begins at birth. During adolescence it is brought into focus for two major reasons. The first deals with the tasks of adolescence, which are a review and critique of all components of oneself; the second is a consequence of the physiological maturation of the emerging young adult. What could only be performed in fantasy can now be performed in reality. A person lives one's sexual life in society, and a balance between one's needs, other's needs, and society's expectations must be struck.[47]

See Chaps. 5 to 14 for discussion of sexuality across the life span.

Defining what is normal is difficult, since as sexual norms change to fit society's needs, there is usually a gap between the initiation of change and its acceptance by society. Early Israelite tribes were polygamous until some males were left without female partners. The Greeks regarded sex as a natural pleasure to be enjoyed until Alexander the Great's conquest of India, Egypt, and Mesopotamia. These cultures' glorification of celibacy and self-denial placed sex and pleasure under a shadow of guilt and condemnation[48] which has been promulgated by Christianity. Freud startled the Victorian era by his theory of sexuality in the child, but he was also a victim of his cultural mores because he could not extend these feelings of sexuality to the adult woman.[49]

Technological value and interpersonal changes (family and support systems) in today's society bring additional pressure on adolescents and young adults in defining their sexual values. The child has absorbed the family's values on sexual behavior, gender identification, and associated gender behavior. Anna Freud maintains that the first year of life is the

The child's unique relationships with parents, siblings, and peers contribute to the child's sexuality.

crucial step in sexual development. She feels this is when instincts develop and the capacity for being able to love or not being able to love is determined.[50]

Developmentally, the infant gains sexual clues from the manner in which he or she is handled by the parenting figures. In early childhood, gender identity is established (differences in sex gender are noted by the child), and the family reinforces gender-related behavior which is considered acceptable. This occurs by the response of the parents to the child, the type of play the child is encouraged and permitted to engage in, and the response of significant other people to the child. School experiences further define gender-appropriate behaviors. Teachers respond to students according to their own gender-appropriate behavior orientation. Girls may be told that certain subjects, such as math, are unfeminine. This message may be carried over into adolescence by equating interest and ability in technical areas with a loss of femininity and/or loss of popularity.

Children also form an idea of sex from the sex information or lack of information given to them, the manner in which it is taught, and the parents' reactions to sex play and sex curiosity. Activities which are normal for the child, such as masturbation, exhibitionism (displaying one's nude body), and voyeurism (looking at another's nude body for pleasure) still have myths surrounding them. For example, despite reports from sex researchers that masturbatory activity is a common way of seeking pleasure, some believe it to be a sign of mental disorder, to cause fatigue and physical debilitation, or to be an activity that only the immature engage in.[51]

Another influence on the child's developing sexual awareness and value system are the clues from the mass media. Television shows, commercials, and printed materials all convey a message. Stories may have the female needing to be rescued by the male; advertisements may subtly convey the message that a certain product makes one more attractive and thus more popular.

By adolescence a person must review sexual values, ideas, and behaviors which have been developed by social, emotional, and physical conditioning as well as by sexual experiences. However, strong physiological changes and peer group pressure may push the person into physical experimentation with sex before one has had an opportunity to place into perspective feelings of intimacy and physical pleasures. If this occurs, the person's resulting feelings have an impact on his or her developing sexual values, future sexual behaviors and self-identity. If negative feelings result, support and intervention are indicated to help the person to examine present behaviors, future implications, and ways to change current actions.

Defenses which a person can employ and which enable one to step back from internal and external pressures are asceticism and intellectualization. Asceticism occurs when antagonism toward the resurging sexual instincts brings about a repression more severe than normally seen. However, this repudiation of sexual instincts spreads to all pleasures.[52] Gradually as the ego activates or develops other defense mechanisms to cope with the sexual instinct the person relinquishes this defense.

Intellectualization is not an attempt to solve the problems raised by sexual instincts; rather it is an indication that an alertness exists to translate the instinctual demands into an abstract process as they are perceived.[53] The result is that sexuality is regarded as a process with no emotional components or personal meaning for the person. Though this defense may also be relinquished as the person's ego finds other coping mechanisms, it may be carried over into adulthood by some people and used to separate out the emotional component of most situations.

Gender identity is established in early childhood.

Exploratory sexual behaviors normally occur during development.

The mass media can influence one's ideas about sexuality.

During adolescence the individual reviews his or her sexual values, ideas, and behavior.

The adolescent or young adult must try to integrate boy or girl sexual identification with man or woman sexual identification. Normal resolution of this conflict results in a sexual code which includes a sexual identity, sexual feelings, and sexual behaviors and practices with which one is comfortable despite potential or actual conflict with family, peers, and society.

THE FAMILY AND ITS INFLUENCE ON BEHAVIOR

Overview of Family Networks

The twentieth century nuclear family usually consists of a man and woman joined in a socially sanctioned union and their children. In most cases, the children are the biological offspring of the spouses, but, as in the case of adopted children in our society, they need not be biologically related. The family is also a "social system . . . in that it is an organization or assemblage of objects united in some form of regular interaction or interdependence . . . . The family as a social system is not a closed system, existing in isolation. Rather, it is an open system which sustains relationships with other systems in the total transactional field."[54]

The family relates to other systems in society, specifically to the economic subsystems, the political systems, the local community, and the respective value systems associated with them. "It is in the interchange between the family and the community that individuals attain their identity, while the family gains approval for their conformity to the social value system."[55]

The family relates to other systems in society, and interchange occurs.

The internal functions of the family are generally considered to be the socialization of children, "basic personality formation, status-conferral and tension-management functions for an individual member."[56] In order to relate to the external social systems as well as satisfy the family's internal needs, other tasks are necessary and are sometimes considered functional problems. These problems are termed "task performance, family leadership, integration and solidarity, and pattern-maintenance."[57] They are considered problems in terms of current and continuing changes in cultural values. All of these functions are broad and there is overlapping between the family and society's influence. Not only does society influence the nuclear family, but the products (children) of the nuclear family affect society by their behavior.

The family is responsible for socialization of children.

A less mechanical approach to the function of the nuclear family is proposed by Ackerman. He views the family as "the basic unit of growth and experience, fulfillment or failure. It is also the basic unit of illness and health."[58] Ackerman looks at some of the problems that can disrupt the function of the family unit. From within, the family must adjust to a wide range of vicissitudes that affect the relations of each family member to each other. Under favorable conditions the emotions of love and loyalty prevail and family harmony is maintained. Under conditions of excessive tension and conflict, mutual antagonism and hatred are aroused and the integrity of the family is threatened.

The family is the basic unit of growth, experience, and fulfillment.

In order to function successfully, the family must "solve its problems, maintain unity and balanced role relations, execute its necessary functions and learn and grow in a creative direction."[59] These processes are similar to issues facing a person as he or she progresses through the stages of growth and development.

Ackerman, like Bell and Vogel, ascribes to the notion that the family must function as an open system with society. He goes on to state that some families, for a variety of reasons, become "closed corporations,"

The family network should be an open system.

shutting their members within and reducing to a minimum any significant interchange with the outside world. This design affects the member's image of people in the wider world as being the same or different or friendly or menacing. It molds the pattern of emotional receptivity toward outside persons or strangers; it may foster attitudes of warm, trusting welcome or of suspicion, fear, rejection, and hostility.[60] It is apparent that the closed corporation family is not adequately fulfilling its functional tasks and that the successful family network is an open system.

Hess and Handel view the major function of the family as providing ways for persons to be separate. As well as focusing on individuality, they are also concerned with family interactions.

> In their mutual interaction the family members develop more or less adequate understanding of one another, collaborating in their effort to establish consensus and to negotiate uncertainty. The family's life together is an endless process of movement in and around consensual understanding, from attachment to conflict to withdrawal—and over again. Separations and connectedness are the underlying conditions of a family's life, and its common task is to give form to both.[61]

The family fails functionally if it is unable to deal with the ways that members become separate and connected. Functional failures are the bases for family dysfunction, while successful family functioning is the basis of mental health. All of the cited tasks of the family are influenced by society as well as the individual identity of each member. The family's role in personality development and socialization of its youth has a profound impact on the adult's ability to cope with stress. As Handel and Hess point out, communication patterns within the family can enhance one's ability to cope with issues related to separation. If a family has not succeeded in teaching its members to successfully cope with intimacy and separation, its members will not be able to cope with the rapid changes in our society or the various role changes inherent in young adulthood.

Effective communication patterns are extremely important to family functioning.

The Family and Its Role in Mental Health

Ackerman views the adult as the reflection of his or her own personal identity, which is inseparable from group experiences—particularly the family. The family socializes its youth to assume the responsibilities of adulthood, and the success of this process is dependent upon numerous factors. The family is viewed as the major influence in mental health, as it provides the medium for managing conflict and anxiety as well as serves as an intermediary between its members and society. The identity of the family and its youth is an evolutionary process which eventually provides the unit with methods for coping with stress. Effective adaptation requires, therefore, a favorable balance between the need to protect sameness and continuity and the need to accommodate to change.[62] This balance enhances one's ability to develop a personality that is flexible, yet stable in its ability to cope with conflict. It also creates a unit in which its members are free to grow and become individualized. This process of adaptation consists of "specific patterns for role relations that provide satisfactions, avenues of solution of conflict, support for a needed self-image and a buttressing of crucial forms of defenses against anxiety."[63]

Other important factors in the socialization process are the family's role in providing not only the basic needs of its members but also affectional bonds, psychic integrity, patterns for sexual roles, opportunities to evolve a personal identity, training for integration into social roles and

The family has a major influence on the development of good mental health in its members.

their related responsibilities, and support for individual learning, creativity, and initiative.[64] The psychic integrity of a person involves the development of a repertoire of healthy defense mechanisms. Ackerman equates defense mechanisms with some disappointments in acquiring satisfaction, as these enhance one's ability to tolerate frustration, and "the acceptance of less than complete fulfillment are essential to emotional growth. Without these there would be an insufficient spur to new experience and new achievement."[65] His thesis supports the contention that anxiety is growth-producing. The behavior of the adult is goal-directed and is based on one's personal identity and value orientation which is learned in the family's socialization process. If a person is able to tolerate frustration, he or she will certainly seek pleasure and avoid pain, but the goal of pleasure should be related to learning through one's exploration and mastery of various role changes in adulthood.

We cannot overlook the impact of society on the family in its function of socialization. Ackerman, like Toffler, contends that there are negative forces in our culture which are a hindrance to the success of most of our current families' tasks.

> The relations of person and society in our time are characterized by a confusion of norms, a lack of clarity as to what society expects of the individual in the fulfillment of social roles. With this is associated a widespread tendency toward loneliness. One of the outstanding characteristics in our society is the individual's emotional isolation and lack of security in group living. The need for group belongingness is profound, but the thwarting of this need is extensive.[66]

If in fact our highly mobile and technological society is not providing clarity regarding norms for one's social role and related behavior, one must question how any family, as an open system, can succeed in socializing its youth. Mental health is associated with a personality that is flexible and able to select aspects of the dominant values of their family and society which provide one's coping repertoire with some stability. If our values change too rapidly, then there is very little security available to reinforce one's personal identity. It is evident that alienation is a by-product of our society and that in the future different family networks may be seen. Additional resources may also be needed to assist families in their functions.

The Impact of Rapid Change on the Family

In order for members of our society to avoid adaptive collapse in the face of rapid technological changes and the related value shifts in our society, they must be socialized in such a manner that they have a wider repertoire of coping methods. Some feel that early in childhood, issues related to attachment and separation should be scrutinized; it is even suggested that our youth need to learn early in life how to cope with transience. This notion has a profound impact on the family's role in personality development. One logical conclusion of this suggestion is that less emphasis should be placed on maternal-infant bonding and greater emphasis on learning to disrelate and separate.

Another effect of rapid change in our society is the conclusion that the twentieth century nuclear family is ineffective in its socialization process. Many think we will eventually see the disintegration of the family as we now know it. On the other hand, others feel that the turbulence in our society will drive people deeper into their families, and marriage will be viewed as at least one stable structure in their lives. "Ac-

Highlights

See Defense Mechanisms for further discussion of the various methods people use to direct stress and anxiety into constructive channels.

Society impacts on family functioning.

Family members must learn to cope with rapid change.

Controversy exists as to whether the family will continue to endure as it is currently.

cording to this view, the family serves as one's portable roots, anchoring one against the storm of change. In short, the more transient and novel the environment, the more important the family will become."[67]

Another difference in families that can be anticipated is a loss of their ability to transmit society's values to their youth. Unless the nuclear family experiments with different structures, it may become an isolated, closed system. Toffler cites some of the varieties of structures which can enhance the family's ability to transmit values. Communal groupings, which are becoming more popular, seem to reduce a person's and the family's sense of alienation. Therefore,

> . . . childless marriages, professional parenthood, post-retirement childbearing, corporate families, communes, geriatric group marriages, homosexual family units, polygamy—are a few of the forms and practices with which innovative minorities will experiment in the decades ahead.[68]

In conclusion, it appears that, as health providers, it is difficult at best to assess the norms of family structure and function. The nuclear family has been the prototype of our society since the industrial revolution, but it is hard to predict the forms our families of the future will assume. We can assume that various practices in the family will evolve, and our role is to assess, nonjudgmentally, how successful these groups are in the task of socializing their youth to function successfully in our superindustrial society.

BEHAVIORAL REACTIONS TO CHANGE, LOSS, AND STRESS

The twentieth century nuclear family has less control over the transmission of values, beliefs, and traditions to their children. Our specialized and fragmented socialization processes have changed the roles of family members and have subjected them to other multiple changes. This situation has many implications in terms of developmental tasks at all ages but is particularly relevant for the child, adolescent, and young adult. In order to assist clients in dealing with rapid and multiple changes, nurses must familiarize themselves with reactions to change, loss, grief, and anxiety and must incorporate this knowledge into their assessment of behavioral development.

Change as a Loss

The person who is dealing with any change often experiences stress, loss, and anxiety, which require coping and adaptation. *Loss* is defined as a real or threatened separation from a loved one, work, a body part, skills, or possessions. Changes in physiological functioning, role, status, and body image and even successes also constitute a loss. *Grief* is the emotional reaction to a loss, while *mourning* is the painful process of giving up the lost object and reinvesting one's energies in another role or person.

Losses occur at all stages of growth and development. Some theorists think that our initial experience with loss occurs when we are separated from the security of the womb at birth and that each developmental task represents a loss as well as success in the accomplishment of new skills. Successful resolution of a loss can promote growth in terms of adaptation as the person acquires a wider variety of healthy coping mechanisms. The mourning process is one of the most distressing emotional tasks that a person must endure. Persons face this process daily in our highly mobile, changing society. Therefore, it is important to recognize normal grief reactions, as they occur daily.

Family structure may change to meet the needs of a changing society.

Rapid and multiple changes require one to be able to make adjustments in an effective way.

Change may cause one to experience stress, loss, and anxiety, which are reflected in behavior.

Loss occurs at all stages of growth and development.

The overview of theories on loss and grief has a historic perspective, and it should be noted that some early theorists focus only on the actual death of a parent or significant other person. Currently, it is assumed that these theories are applicable not only to separation by death but to all real or threatened changes and separations.

Normal Grief Reactions

Grief is a universal phenomenon. Switzer states that "grief has as its core experience an acute attack of anxiety, precipitated by the external event of the death of a person with whom one is emotionally involved, and that other behavioral responses are dynamically related to the anxiety."[69] This theory is acceptable, but the notion of "death" as the precursor of anxiety can be modified to incorporate any loss. The grief process does not differ in relation to the respective loss, as change and separation can precipitate the same emotional experiences.

Freud differentiates between melancholia and mourning as a matter of kind rather than degree, with a premorbid personality composition at the root of a melancholic reaction to a loss. He feels that both states are associated with profound pain and that similar symptoms are seen in both the normal and pathological state, but that a lowering of one's self-image is absent in mourning and is the critical diagnostic factor between the two. One might refute this distinction, which he calls "a lowering of the self-image regarding feelings to a degree that finds utterances in self-reproaches and self-revilings."[70] The mere fact that all people have ambivalent feelings toward the loss would lead one to conclude that guilt and self-reproach, to a limited degree, are part of the normal grief process. On the other hand, Freud links ambivalence with separation from a loved one rather than a loss through death of a loved one, which leads one to believe that the nature or type of loss is also a differentiating factor in mourning or melancholia. It is probable that there is no difference between the feelings evoked by separation, change, or death; only a difference in the degree of anxiety.

Siggins describes the process involved in normal grief work as a working through of an affect which if released in its full strength, would overwhelm the ego. Fenichel maintains that "grief is plainly a postponed and apportioned mitigation, the taming of that wild and self-destructive kind of affect which can still be observed in a child's panic upon the disappearance of its mother. . . ."[71] Once again a relationship is seen between change, separation, anxiety, and the feelings evoked by death.

Lindemann, on the other hand, describes the symptoms which are common to the normal grief process. These include "sensations of somatic distress occurring in waves lasting from twenty minutes to an hour at a time, a feeling of tightness in the throat, choking with shortness of breath, a need for sighing, an empty feeling in the abdomen with lack of muscular power, and an intense subjective distress described as tension or mental pain."[72] He also cites the presence of some psychic phenomena, emotional distance from others, preoccupation with the lost object, feelings of guilt, self-reproach, some anger and irritability with others, and aimless activity.

All of the authors who write about grief concur that certain steps must be accomplished to successfully complete the grief process. The goal of grief as stated by Engel is to "extricate oneself from the bondage to the deceased and [work] at finding new patterns of rewarding interactions."[73] "Deceased" is equated here with change and separation. Engel also speaks to the stages of grief that are common to all grief work. The first stage is *shock and disbelief,* wherein the person is stunned and feels numb. This is felt to be a defense against all feelings, particularly anxiety, which might evoke the reality of the loss. The second stage is *developing awareness,* in which the reality of the loss is allowed into conscious awareness. In this stage somatic symptoms occur along with anger which is usually displaced. Crying is typical, along with some emotional regression. The third stage is called *restitution* and is considered the period in which the work of mourning occurs. In this stage the rituals for the dead must be attended to; viewing the body and leaving of remains at a cemetery force the awareness of the loss into consciousness. The last stage is *resolving the loss.* The major work in this stage is intrapsychic for the mourner. Many months are required for this stage as the mourner attempts to deal with the "painful void" created by the loss. Initially, the lost object becomes idealized and all negative feelings are repressed. From idealization, the mourner moves to identification with the positive qualities of the dead person, until eventually the mourner becomes progressively less preoccupied with the dead person.

Engel feels that the successful work of mourning takes a year or more. The clearest evidence of successful healing is the ability to remember comfortably and realistically both the pleasures and disappointments of the lost relationship. All theorists agree that any extreme in the *degree* of the normal grief process is pathognomonic, e.g., appearances of traits of the deceased in the behavior of the bereaved, particularly symptoms present during the terminal illness.

Successful resolution of loss results in one being able to remember both pleasures and disappointments regarding the lost object.

The process of mourning will differ in intensity and duration in relation to the degree of importance the lost object had for the client; i.e., if marriage was the basis for the person's sense of identity, then divorce will be a major loss. If the work of grief is not accomplished, all subsequent *threats* of loss or change will reactivate the unresolved loss. In such cases, people tend to form pathological, binding relationships and are unable to tolerate any form of separation. This in turn can interfere with growth and development, family structure, and personal achievements. It is also important to keep in mind that there are many obstacles to successful grief work: the age of the mourner, the age of the lost object, the number of significant other people, and most important, multiple and rapid losses. Another obstacle to grieving is the ability to tolerate the anxiety aroused by a loss.

Normal Anxiety Reactions

Human beings are adaptive organisms, and as such, employ various resources to facilitate adaptation. One resource is anxiety, which can be defined as an energy which forces us to behave in some manner. It is a vague subjective feeling that something is wrong although no specific event can be identified which causes this uneasiness. Anxiety arises when there is a threat to the physical or psychological well-being of the organism. Anxiety cannot be seen, but behavioral manifestations indicate the level of anxiety one is experiencing as well as the person's ability to adapt to this experience. Anxiety can be used constructively or destructively and is considered healthy when it provides us the opportunity to develop new defense mechanisms which in turn facilitate growth. Conversely, it is destructive when our repertoire of defenses proves inadequate for adaptation. In this case, we are unable to use new methods of coping and regression occurs. Every person in a new situation must either master anxiety or become a slave to it.

Anxiety as a motivating force can be traced through all stages of development. In infancy threats to the child's biological well-being

Anxiety can be a reaction used to facilitate adaptation.

Anxiety is manifested in behavioral reactions such as restlessness and fidgeting and in physiological responses such as increased heart rate and sweating.

create anxiety and lead to the behavioral manifestations of crying and restlessness. The child's anxiety is relieved by maternal or paternal interventions. By the age of approximately 6 months the child may develop "stranger anxiety." This feeling of discomfort evoked by unfamiliar faces is relieved by seeking the familiar, which is usually the maternal or paternal figure. By the time the child is a toddler, he or she has sufficiently mastered stranger anxiety to become curious about the environment and himself or herself in relation to that environment. As the child attempts to become more autonomous, the gap between wishes and reality creates "basic anxiety."[74] This anxiety is aroused by the conflict between dependency on and hostility toward the parent who is setting limits on his or her independence. It is felt that the hostility toward the parent evokes fears of helplessness and isolation as the child learns that he or she is not yet capable of being completely independent.

Separation anxiety may also appear in toddlerhood as the child fears abandonment by the mother or father. This anxiety seems to be related to the conflict between the dependency and hostility described above, as well as the child's reaction to the conflict. The behavior related to this anxiety may be seen in the child's attempts to symbolically shut out mother or father, i.e., "closing the door on her or him." These attempts are temporary, as the child's anxiety prompts him or her to seek maternal or paternal comfort and alleviate this feeling. Another manifestation of separation anxiety is the transient fears about drains or vacuum cleaners, which are viewed as objects used by the parent to discard undesirable objects. Some think that these fears arise from the child's concern that mother or father will retaliate against the child's hostile impulses. These conflicts are usually resolved by the child's wish to please and receive maternal or paternal love, which counterbalances the hostility. At this stage of development, it is felt that all anxiety is generated by external forces. In other words, a significant maternal or paternal figure disapproved or did not give the child comfort. Also, most symptoms of anxiety are transient and center around issues related to feeding, sleeping, and elimination.

As the child enters the phallic stage (as described by Freud) of development, anxiety is now aroused by both external and internal events. The fear of parental disapproval and the desire to be loved have brought about the acquisition of an ego and superego. Disapproval now generates superego anxiety as the child evaluates self against the standards of the parents. Castration anxiety also appears in boys at this time. According to Freud, the male feels that anyone who does not have a penis lost it as a result of parental retaliation against sexual impulses. This anxiety is reinforced by the prohibition against masturbation and exhibitionism, which are both common and normal behaviors at this age. These activities provide not only pleasure but reassurance in the intactness of the genitals.

In the latency period the child shows increasing sophistication in defenses, and external manifestations of anxiety diminish. There is an increase in socially acceptable behavior, in conformity to social mores, and in the child's self-esteem, which are related to physical and intellectual accomplishments. All of these events reinforce the acquired defenses against anxiety. The anxiety in adolescence is multifaceted and related to the transition between childhood and adulthood. The adult's overt manifestation of anxiety is similar to that of the child in the latency stage. The adult's repertoire of defenses is usually complex and stable, though certainly not static.[75]

This overview of the development of normal anxiety demonstrates that each person reacts to danger in ways specific to one's own personal

Anxiety can be seen across the life span.

Examples of anxieties seen in childhood include separation anxiety, stranger anxiety, and castration anxiety.

history. Each person employs specific defenses to protect the self from danger, to master anxiety, and to find solutions to emotional conflicts. The ability to do this depends on innate tendencies, experiences in early years, and current events. Therefore, each person can tolerate different amounts of stress, loss, and anxiety. In assessing a client's ability to manage anxiety, all of these issues must be kept in mind. Some ego characteristics in the adult which can be assessed and which are thought to be important indexes of a sound ability to tolerate anxiety are (1) a high tolerance for frustration, (2) a good potential for sublimation, and (3) a strong urge to complete developmental tasks. If one is unable to manage change, loss, grief, and anxiety, deviations in psychological or physiological functioning may occur.

Highlights

There are individual differences in reactions to anxiety and in the ability to tolerate varying degrees of anxiety.

Defense Mechanisms

During the process of development a person learns various methods to direct the stress and anxiety felt into constructive channels. These methods, called *defense mechanisms,* are used to reach what Piaget calls the *state of equilibrium* and to complete Erikson's and Freud's stages of development.

Defense mechanisms assist one in dealing with anxiety and stress.

Defense mechanisms are defined as the methods employed by the ego to deal with the tensions resulting from ungratified basic drives or super-ego disapproval. Sigmund Freud first used the term defense mechanism in the late 1800s to define the ego's means of defending itself. Though he later ascribed this function to the defense known as *regression,* he reverted back to his original definition in the 1920s.[76] Anna Freud has consolidated and amplified her father's analysis of defense mechanisms in her writing *The Ego and the Mechanisms of Defense.*[77]

Anna Freud has listed three motives which activate the ego's defenses: superego anxiety, objective anxiety, and instinctual anxiety. *Superego anxiety* is created when the superego seeks to block the gratification of an instinctual desire. The conflict is between the id and the superego, with the ego as moderator. *Objective anxiety* is motivated by dread of the outside world; specifically, the child fears to gratify an instinctual desire because he or she has been forbidden by a significant other person (someone important to the child). The last motive is *instinctual anxiety.* Here the ego, having assessed the gratification of an instinctual desire as inappropriate, begins protecting the individual. The conflict is between the id and the ego.[78]

Superego anxiety, objective anxiety, and instinctual anxiety activate ego defenses.

Developmentally, objective anxiety governs the child from the period of complete dependency on others, through the time when the ego is being formed, until latency. During latency the ego becomes motivated by superego anxiety rather than objective anxiety. This shift occurs as the superego grows and the child becomes less dependent on the parenting figures. Now the child does not fear losing parental love as much as conflicting with the growing but rigid superego. Finally in puberty when the focus shifts to physiological sexual changes that are accompanied by a concurrent increase in sexual impulses, instinctual anxiety triggers the ego's defenses.[79]

In addition to the usual repertoire of defenses available to the adolescent, Anna Freud has established two additional ones used by the adolescent in an attempt to control and master the instinctual desires. The first, asceticism, is the attempt to control instinctual desires by repudiation and the second, intellectualization, is the attempt to control the instincts by thought.[80]

See Sexuality for a discussion of asceticism and intellectualization.

Defense mechanisms do not just appear. They are learned as the need arises. A person will continue to employ the usual repertoire as long as they work. Only when the defenses are not successful does a person seek new defenses to deal with stress and anxiety. Newly acquired defenses do not necessarily displace old defenses, since they are rarely used in isolation. For example, if a person denies the occurrence of a given event, that event is maintained in the unconscious by repression. It is only through the acquisition of new, more complex defenses that a person is able to progress through and adapt to the new stresses facing him or her in each developmental stage.

Common defense mechanisms are listed in Table 2-1. The table is divided into three categories: those mechanisms always compatible with mental health, those which may lead to pathogenesis if overused, and those always pathogenic. As can readily be seen the majority of defenses fall into the second category. These become pathogenic when "(1) they . . . seriously restrict the functions of the ego and the freedom of the child, (2) they . . . impede further development, (3) they . . . alienate the child from other people and (4) they . . . distort his view of reality."[81] Only one defense mechanism is normal regardless of how often it is used; likewise there are two defenses whose use always is considered pathological. These pathological defenses involve handling conflicts by exhibiting physical symptoms involving the functions of the body.

Table 2-1 lists several defense mechanisms used by persons in situations of stress and anxiety.

Managing Anxiety and Coping with Stress

Anxiety as a motivating force in human development may be considered a healthy stressor which generates various physiological and psychological responses. The responses to stressors are defined as *the state of stress*, the "sum of all the nonspecific effects" as well as the "consequence of any

Anxiety can be a healthy stressor throughout human development.

Table 2-1
Defense Mechanisms

Always normal:	
Sublimation	Channeling frustrated sexual and/or hostile desires into constructive outlets.
May lead to pathogenesis:	
Compensation	Covering up a weakness or making up for frustration in one area by overgratification in another.
Denial	Refusing to perceive or face reality or to allow it into the conscious.
Displacement	Discharging pent-up feelings, usually of a hostile nature, onto an object other than the original one which aroused the emotion.
Identification or introjection	Increasing feelings of worth by identifying with and incorporating into self values and traits of an admired person.
Isolation or dissociation	Separating the affective component from the factual component of a situation and keeping them in separate compartments.
Projection	Placing blame for difficulties or attributing to others one's own negative, hostile, unacceptable feelings.
Rationalization	Attempting to prove that one's behavior is justifiable and thus worthy of self.
Reaction formation	Preventing unacceptable desires from being expressed by exaggerating opposite attitudes and types of behavior and using them as barriers.
Regression	Retreating to earlier developmental levels under stressful situations.
Repression	Preventing dangerous or painful thoughts from entering consciousness.
Always pathological:	
Conversion	Exhibiting physical symptoms involving portions of the body innervated by the sensory and/or motor nerves.
Somatization	Exhibiting physical symptoms involving portions of the body innervated by the sympathetic and/or parasympathetic system(s).

demand made upon the body."[82] Stressors are various factors which have an impact on the organism; they may be activity, drugs, bacteria, or pleasurable events. The essence of stress is its nonspecific character. There is no absolute process of selectivity in either emotional or physical reactions within the organism. On the other hand, stress is a reality which occurs daily in our lives and, like anxiety, demands that one react. This reaction is behavior, which may be constructive or destructive.

Coping with stress involves a defensive stance, and the resolution is determined by various internal and external factors which impinge on the organism. This may account for Hans Selye's contention that each person will not react in the same manner to a similar stressor. Although there is no specific cause and effect relationship between stressors and stress, his theory does allow one to make some general predictions about the effect of stress on clients' physical and emotional status. The general adaptation syndrome described by Selye is an interdependent, three-step process equated with the state of stress. It consists of the alarm reaction, the stage of resistance, and the stage of exhaustion. "In a nutshell, the response to stress has a tripartite mechanism consisting of: (1) the direct effect of the stress upon the body; (2) internal responses which stimulate tissue-defense; and (3) internal responses which stimulate tissue-surrender by inhibiting defense. Resistance and adaptation depend on a proper balance of these three factors."[83]

Selye, like the theorists on loss and grief, thinks that the intensity of the stressor modifies the response. Just as the importance of the loss determines the intensity of the grief reaction, the intensity of the stressor determines the intensity of the reaction. ". . . it is not necessary for all three stages to develop before we can speak of General Adaptation Syndrome. Only the most severe stress leads eventually to the stage of exhaustion and death."[84] There are numerous stressors in everyday life which produce only the first two reactions; in other words, most people learn to cope as part of their socialization process and their acquired genetic composition and, consequently, are able to cope effectively with stressors throughout each day without becoming emotionally or physically exhausted. "In the course of a normal human life, everybody goes through these first two stages many, many times. Otherwise we could never become adapted to perform all the activities and resist all the injuries which are man's lot."[85] Selye appears to be referring not only to the stresses inherent in the process of normal growth and development but also to the stress associated with change, loss, grief, and anxiety.

Selye concludes that the ultimate cause of physical or emotional exhaustion is frustration or "unsuccessful struggles which leave irreversible chemical scars" on the organism.[86] In other words, the inability to find new and healthy coping mechanisms in the face of change, loss, and stress can cause irreversible physical or emotional damage. Alvin Toffler reinforces the thesis that change and its related anxiety are a basic component of successful growth and development when he says "to eliminate [stress] and adaptive reactions would be to eliminate all change, including growth, self development, maturation. It presupposes complete stasis; change is not merely necessary to life, it is life; by the same token, life is adaptation."[87] Anxiety and stress are motivating forces in human development. Although there exists the possibility of risking complete adaptive exhaustion in persons and groups by the current rapid technological changes occurring daily, change and anxiety are necessary for a more complex and sophisticated society.

An important role of the nurse is to counsel clients to look carefully at the rate and meaning of changes which are occurring in their life.

Highlights

Stress affects a person physically and emotionally.

Selye's general adaptation syndrome consists of the following stages: alarm reaction, resistance, and exhaustion.

Individuals learn to cope with stress as part of their socialization process.

Anxiety and stress are motivating forces in human development.

Selye advises us to carefully examine our optimum stress level and plan our changes accordingly. Clients must be assisted in learning more about their ability to cope with changes and stress. Selye's general adaptation syndrome is only one way of viewing the management of anxiety. His model can be a useful tool for assessing the client's ability to adapt to the stress associated with rapid change, loss, grief, and anxiety.

In conclusion, Table 2-2 can be used when assessing clients' behaviors to grief, stress, or change and their impact on health. Selye's theory is also applicable in assessing the broader scope of human development. He relates the general adaptation syndrome to human growth and development as follows:

> Whatever demand is made upon us, we proceed through (1) the initial alarm reaction of surprise and anxiety because of our inexperience in dealing with

Highlights

See Table 2-2 when assessing clients' behaviors related to grief, stress, or change.

Table 2-2

Application of the Assessment Process to Grief and Stress Reactions

Stages in a grief reaction†	General adaptation syndrome*	Behavioral manifestations	Nursing assessment
Shock and disbelief	Alarm reaction signals anxiety	Increased heart rate Tightness in throat Shortness of breath Sighing Dry mouth Denial Changes in level of concentration Stunned or numb appearance Lack of a verbal response Response in monosyllables	Assess previous experiences with loss Assess significance of loss, age of bereaved, etc.
	Resistance	More defense mechanisms called into play	Assess repertoire of coping mechanisms and support systems
Developing awareness (reality of loss allowed into conscious awareness)		Denial lifting Restlessness Weeping Increased anxiety Increase in somatic symptoms Changes in sleeping, eating, and activities of daily living Anger (usually displaced) Mild regression Guilt Withdrawal	
Restitution		Behavior similar to above but more preoccupied with lost object Usually rituals for loss performed Anxiety mild or moderate in intensity Client vulnerable and open to learn	Assess need for learning new coping behaviors, i.e., sublimation
Resolving the loss		Repression of negative feelings for lost object Idealizing lost object Identification with positive qualities of lost object Eventually less preoccupied with loss	Reassess resolution and coping at varying intervals
	Exhaustion	Somatic symptoms similar to those of lost object prior to loss or separation Abrupt early substitution of loss with similar object Client unable to adapt to loss and anxiety Defenses not working Psychoneurotic disorders Psychophysiological disorders Psychosis	Assess for extremes in degree of behavioral reactions

*Hans Selye's theory about an organism's three-stage response to stress.
†The four stages of grief cited by George Engel that a person goes through during grief work.

a new situation; (2) the stage of resistance when we have learned to cope with the task efficiently and without undue commotion; (3) the stage of exhaustion, a depletion of energy reserves which leads to fatigue . . . ; these three stages, which repeat themselves throughout life whenever we are faced with a demand, are surprisingly similar to the lability of inexperienced childhood, the stable resistance of adulthood, and the final exhaustion of senility and death.[88]

SUMMARY

Human beings are adaptive organisms. A healthy child or adult has the capacity to change and maintain health both physically and psychologically. A mentally healthy person as defined by Marie Jahoda is one who

. . . actively masters his environment, shows a certain unity of personality, and is able to perceive the world and himself correctly.[89]

This chapter has discussed many of the components and behaviors which lead toward a mentally healthy adult. The child's growth has been traced developmentally with emphasis placed on the importance of the physical and sociocultural environment and those in it. The view that loss is growth-producing has also been presented. Growth (change) cannot occur without a sense of loss and the resolution of the resulting grief associated with loss.

Saying one is mentally healthy does not imply that one is always happy. Rather, the healthy person is able to meet life's stresses, using the defenses available or developing new ones if necessary. The healthy person thinks well of and is able to accept himself or herself, sees his or her strengths and weaknesses, and does not rely on only one attribute for his or her self-esteem. He or she realizes that self-esteem is multifaceted.

The healthy person has developed a social network; he or she can relate to others and can live in society. But a healthy person can also make his or her own decisions, can weigh the implications of these in the context of his or her needs, the needs of others, and the needs of society, and can maintain an awareness of the reaction of others to these decisions.

Response to stress means growth in the mentally healthy person. Adaptation is not easy in today's world with its many changes which challenge established values. The impact of rapid change should be carefully monitored. One method for enhancing our ability to adapt is to anticipate changes, scrutinize their importance, and attempt to gradualize them.

REFERENCES

1. Wiedenbach, Ernestine: *Clinical Nursing: A Helping Art,* Springer, New York, 1964.

2. Bowlby, John: "The Making and Breaking of Affectional Bonds." *Br J Psychiatry,* **130:**201–210 (1977).

3. Chess, Stella, Alexander Thomas and Herbert C. Birch: *Behavioral Individuality in Early Childhood,* New York University Press, New York, 1963.

4. Thomas, Alexander, Stella Chess, and Herbert C. Birch: *Temperament and the Behavior Disorders of Children,* New York University Press, New York, 1968.

5. Freud, Sigmund: *Basic Writings of S. Freud,* A. A. Brill (ed.), Random House, New York, 1938.

6. Erikson, Erik: *Childhood and Society,* Norton, New York, 1950.

7. Gesell, Arnold, and F. Ilg: *Infant and Child in the Culture of Today,* Harper, New York, 1943.

8. Ibid., p. 289.

9. Ibid., p. 291.

10. Rebelsky, F., and L. Dorman (eds.): *Child Development and Behavior,* Knopf, New York, 1970, p. 7.

11. Lewin, Kurt: "Behavior and Development as a Function of the Total Situation," in L. Carmichael (ed.), *Manual of Child Psychology,* Wiley, New York, 1954.

12. Stone, L. J., and J. Church: *Childhood and Adolescence,* Random House, New York, 1973, pp. 404–405.

13. Baldwin, A.: *Theories of Child Development,* Wiley, New York, 1968, pp. 117–119.

14. Piaget, Jean: *The Origins of Intelligence in Children,* International Universities Press, New York, 1952.

15. Baldwin, *Theories of Child Development,* p. 296.

16. Lovell, K.: *An Introduction to Human Development,* Macmillan, New York, 1969, p. 23.

17. Ibid., pp. 24–33.

18. Ibid., p. 35.

19. Ibid., p. 38.

20. Maier, H. W.: *Three Theories of Child Development,* Harper & Row, New York, 1969, pp. 141–142.

21. Kohlberg, Lawrence, and C. Gilligan: "The Adolescent as a Philosopher: The Discovery of Self in a Postconventional World," *Daedalus,* vol. 100, no. 4, p. 1051 (Fall 1971).

22. Sutterly, D. C., and G. F. Donnelly: *Perspectives in Human Development,* Lippincott, Philadelphia, 1973, p. 226.

23. Cumming, Elaine, and William E. Henry: *Growing Old: The Process of Disengagement,* Basic Books, New York, 1961.

24. Cumming, Elaine: "New Thoughts on the Theory of Disengagement," in Robert Kastenbaum (ed.), *New Thoughts on Old Age,* Springer, New York, 1964.

25. Havighurst, Robert J.: "Successful Aging," in Richard H. Williams, Clark Tibbitts, and Wilma Donahue (eds.), *Processes of Aging,* vol. I, Atherton, New York, 1963.

26. Neugarten, Bernice L.: *Personality in Middle and Later Life,* Atherton, New York, 1964.

27. Sears, R. R., E. E. Maccoby, and H. Lenin: *Patterns of Child Rearing,* Harper & Row, New York, 1957.

28. Maier, *Three Theories of Child Development,* p. 437.

29. Ibid., p. 146.

30. Ibid., pp. 155–175.

31. Bijou, S., and D. Baer: *Child Development—A Systematic and Empirical Theory,* Appleton-Century-Crofts, New York, 1961, pp. 83–85.

32. Keller, F. S., and W. N. Schoenfeld: *Principles of Psychology,* Appleton-Century-Crofts, New York, 1950, pp. 364–366.

33. Baldwin, *Theories of Child Development,* p. 26.

34. Ibid., pp. 35–36.

35. Ibid., p. 36.

36. George Herbert Mead: *Mind, Self and Society,* University of Chicago Press, Chicago, 1934, p. 136.

37. Ibid. p. 136.

38. Erik H. Erikson: *Identity: Youth and Crisis,* Norton, New York, 1968, p. 135.

39. Erik H. Erikson: *Dimensions of a New Identity,* Norton, New York, 1973, p. 124.

40. Erikson, *Identity: Youth and Crisis,* p. 22.

41. Mead, Margaret: *Continuities in Cultural Evaluation,* Yale University Press, New Haven, 1964, p. 36.

42. Goldstein, K.: "Health As Value," in A. Maslow (ed.), *New Knowledge in Human Values,* Regnery, Chicago, 1959, pp. 178–188.

43. Rossi, Alice S.: "Transition to Parenthood" in William C. Sze (ed.), *Human Life Cycle,* Jason Aronson, New York, 1975, pp. 509–510.

44. Ibid., p. 509.

45. Ibid., p. 510.

46. Ibid.

47. Resnick, H. L. P., and Marvin E. Wolfgang (eds.): *Sexual Behaviors,* Little, Brown, Boston, 1972, p. 41.

48. McCary, James Leslie: *Human Sexuality,* Van Nostrand, New York, 1978, p. 10.

49. Gagnon, John H., and William Simon: *Sexual Conduct,* Aldine, Chicago, 1973, p. 29.

50. Freud, Anna: *The Ego and the Mechanisms of Defense,* International Universities Press, New York, 1946, p. 139.

51. McCary, *Human Sexuality,* p. 152.

52. Freud, *The Ego and the Mechanisms of Defense,* p. 154.

53. Ibid., p. 162.

54. Bell, Norman W., and Ezra F. Vogel (eds.): *A Modern Introduction to the Family,* Free Press, Glencoe, Ill., 1968, pp. 2–6.

55. Ibid., p. 10.

56. Ibid., p. 12.

57. Ibid., p. 19.

58. Ackerman, Nathan: *The Psychodynamics of Family Life,* Basic Books, New York, 1958.

59. Ibid., p. 100.

60. Ibid., p. 342.

61. Hess, Robert, and George Handel: "The Family as a Psychosocial Organization," in Gerald Handel (ed.), *The Psychosocial Interior of the Family,* Aldine, Chicago, 1967, pp. 10–24.

62. Ackerman, *Psychodynamics,* p. 85.

63. Ibid., p. 86.

64. Ibid., p. 19.

65. Ibid., p. 20.

66. Ibid., p. 65.

67. Toffler, Alvin: *Future Shock,* Random House, New York, 1970, p. 239.

68. Ibid., p. 249.

69. Switzer, David: *The Dynamics of Grief,* Abingdon, Nashville, 1970, p. 143.

70. Freud, Sigmund: "Mourning and Melancholia," in James Stachey (ed.), *The Complete Psychological Works of Sigmund Freud,* vol. XIV: *1914–1916,* Hogarth, London, 1957, pp. 237–259.

71. Siggins, Lorraine D.: "Mourning: A Critical Survey of the Literature," *Int J Psychiatry,* 3: 418–430 (1967).

72. Lindemann, Erich: "Symptomatology and Management of Acute Grief," in Howard Parad (ed.), *Crisis Intervention: Selected Readings,* Family Service Association of America, New York, 1965, pp. 2–19.

73. Engel, George: "Grief and Grieving," *Am J Nurs,* **64**(9):93–98(1964).

74. Horney, Karen: *The Neurotic Personality of Our Time,* Norton, New York, 1937, pp. 94–95.

75. Wiedman, George (ed.): *Personality Development and Deviation,* International Universities Press, New York, 1975, pp. 40–123.

76. Freud, *The Ego and The Mechanisms of Defense,* p. 42.

77. Ibid., p. 42.

78. Ibid., pp. 54–60.

79. Ibid., pp. 143–148.

80. Ibid., pp. 154, 163.

81. Kessler, Jane W.: *Psychopathology of Childhood,* Prentice-Hall, Englewood Cliffs, New Jersey, 1966, p. 66.

82. Selye, Hans: *The Stress of Life,* McGraw-Hill, New York, 1956, p. 42.

83. Ibid., p. 47.

84. Ibid., p. 64.

85. Ibid.

86. Selye, Hans: *Stress Without Distress,* Signet Books, New York, 1974, p. 94.

87. Toffler, *Future Shock,* p. 342.

88. Selye, *Stress Without Distress,* p. 78.

89. Erikson, *Identity: Youth and Crisis,* p. 92.

BIBLIOGRAPHY

Books

Ackerman, Nathan: *The Psychodynamics of Family Life,* Basic Books, New York, 1958.

Bell, Norman, and Ezra Vogel: *A Modern Introduction to the Family,* revised ed., The Free Press, New York, 1968.

Erikson, Erik H.: *Childhood and Society,* Norton, New York, 1963.

———: *Dimensions of a New Identity,* Norton, New York, 1973.

———: *Identity: Youth and Crisis,* Norton, New York, 1965.

————: *Insight and Responsibility,* Norton, New York, 1964.

Freud, Anna: *The Ego and the Mechanisms of Defense,* International Universities Press, New York, 1966.

Freud, Sigmund: *General Psychological Theory,* Crowell-Collier, New York, 1963.

Gagnon, John H., and William Simon: *Sexual Conduct,* Aldine, Chicago, 1975.

Hess, Robert, and George Handel (eds.): *The Psychosocial Interior of the Family,* Aldine, Chicago, 1967.

Horney, Karen: *The Neurotic Personality of Our Time,* Norton, New York, 1937.

Jones, Dorothy, Claire Dunbar, and Mary Jirovec: *Medical-Surgical Nursing,* 2d ed., McGraw-Hill, New York, 1982.

Kessler, Jane W.: *Psychopathology of Childhood,* Prentice-Hall, Englewood Cliffs, N.J., 1966.

Kimmel, Douglas C.: *Adulthood and Aging,* John Wiley, New York, 1974.

Lennart, Levi (ed.): *Emotions: Their Parameters and Measures,* Raven Press, New York, 1975.

Lidz, Theodore: *The Family and Human Adaptation,* International Universities Press, New York, 1963.

Mead, Margaret: *Continuities in Cultural Evolution,* Yale University Press, New Haven, 1964.

McCary, James Leslie: *Human Sexuality,* Van Nostrand, New York, 1978.

Parad, Howard (ed.): *Crisis Intervention,* Family Service Association of America, New York, 1965.

Piaget, Jean: *The Origins of Intelligence in Childhood,* International Universities Press, New York, 1952.

———— and Barbel Inhelder: *The Psychology of the Child,* Basic Books, New York, 1969.

Resnick, H. L. P., and Marvin E. Wolfgang: *Sexual Behaviors,* Little, Brown, Boston, 1972.

Rogers, Carl: *On Encounter Groups,* Harper & Row, New York, 1970.

Selye, Hans: *The Stress of Life,* McGraw-Hill, New York, 1956.

————: *Stress without Distress,* New American Library, New York, 1974.

Simmel, George: *Conflict and the Web of Group Affiliations,* Free Press, New York, 1955.

Strachey, James (ed.): *The Complete Psychological Works of Sigmund Freud,* vol. XIV, *1914–1916,* Hogarth Press, London, 1957.

————: *The Complete Psychological Works of Sigmund Freud,* vol. XIX, *1923,* Hogarth Press, London, 1963.

————: *The Complete Psychological Works of Sigmund Freud,* vol. XXII, *1932–1936,* Hogarth Press, London, 1966.

Sutterly, Doris Cook, and Gloria Ferraro Donnelly: *Perspectives in Human Development,* Lippincott, Philadelphia, 1973.

Switzer, David: *The Dynamics of Grief,* Abingdon Press, New York, 1970.

Toffler, Alvin: *Future Shock,* Bantam Books, New York, 1971.

Wiedman, George (ed.): *Personality Development and Deviation,* International Universities Press, New York, 1975.

Yalom, Irvin D.: *The Theory and Practice of Group Psychotherapy,* Basic Books, New York, 1975.

Articles

Donne, John: "Devotions upon Emergent Occasions: Meditation XVII," in M. H. Abrams et al. (eds.), *Norton Anthology of English Literature,* Norton, New York, 1968, pp. 916–917.

Engel, George: "Grief and Grieving," *Amer J Nurs* 64:9 (September 1964), pp. 150–158.

Gillies, Dee Ann, and Irene Alyn: "Psychosocial Assessment and Intervention," Chap. 5, *Patient Assessment and Management by the Nurse Practitioner,* Saunders, Philadelphia, 1976, pp. 150–158.

Keniston, Kenneth: "Youth as a Stage of Life," in William C. Sze (ed.), *Human Life Cycle,* Jason Aronson, New York, 1975, pp. 331–350.

Lindemann, Eric: "Symptomatology and Management of Acute Grief," in Howard Parad (ed.), *Crisis Intervention,* Family Service Association of America, New York, 1965, pp. 2–19.

Rossi, Alice S.: "Transition to Childhood," in William C. Sze (ed.), *Human Life Cycle,* Jason Aronson, New York, 1975, pp. 505–530.

Siggins, Lorraine: "Mourning: A Critical Survey of the Literature," *Int J Psychiatry* 3: 418–430 (May 1967).

ESTABLISHING A DATA BASE: THE HEALTH HISTORY

CHAPTER THREE

Mary Kolassa Lepley

In recent years the nurse has relied on the history-taking format of medicine when compiling the data base for nursing practice. Although this format has allowed the nurse to collect much data, it has proved inadequate because it focuses on illness and does not always consider the whole person. Further, nursing's contribution to the health care delivery system is not reflected in the medical tool.

Chapter 1 discusses in depth a philosophical approach to the client as a whole unit. This chapter proposes a mechanism for data collection that the professional nurse can use in providing quality health care to clients in a variety of settings. The tool to be discussed in this chapter reflects both a nursing and a holistic philosophy and permits a thorough, systematic, and continuous assessment of the whole person—body, mind, and spirit.

THE HEALTH HISTORY: SETTING THE STAGE

The health history provides a compilation of subjective data acquired during the client-nurse interview. The nurse collects a health-oriented data base by observing and questioning the client about the interrelated categories that make up the health history. This enables the nurse to assess or judge the client's total health state. The health history further provides the baseline data for nursing diagnoses, management of health care, and evaluation of nursing care. Through concise and systematic recording of all data by the nurse, the health history serves as the basis for an ongoing record of the client's progressive state of well-being. Data collected on subsequent visits can be added to the health history as the client moves through the health care system.

Assessment is the first step in the nursing process.

See Table 3-2 for the format of the health history.

THE CLIENT ROLE

The term *client* is used to refer to the consumer of health care because it implies decision-making powers. Traditionally, the label of *patient* has been used by health care professionals in settings of both wellness and illness. *Patient* implies a person who is ill and who is more likely to be a dependent receiver of health care. Since a consumer has the right to be involved in planning and deciding health care which may affect him or her physically, socially, or psychologically, *client* is a more appropriate label. It implies autonomy and responsible participation in formulating goals for health promotion, health maintenance, and disease prevention. To further ensure a holistic approach to care, the nurse must determine how the client views his or her role. If the client believes it to be subservient to the role of health care providers, it is the nurse's responsibility to help the person adjust to the role of client and take on a more active role in his or her health care.

The term *client* will be used throughout this book to refer to the consumer of health care.

ENTRY INTO THE HEALTH CARE DELIVERY SYSTEM

Highlights

Refer to page 88 for a more detailed discussion of entry into the health care system.
From forty-five minutes to 1 hour should be an adequate time to collect required data.

The reason for entry into a health care system varies among clients, and this must be considered by the nurse. The nurse should determine if the client is seeking health maintenance, health promotion, or disease prevention.

For example, if a client seeks a routine health visit, the nurse will need to schedule adequate time for the interview with the client and/or caretaker so that a thorough health history may be collected. If the informant is made to feel rushed or treated as "just another case," the result may be an inaccurate or partial data base. On the other hand, clients entering the system on an unscheduled visit may not always be able to participate in extensive data collection. If a thorough data base is needed, a future visit may be necessary in order to complete the entire health history.

FACTORS INFLUENCING THE NURSE-CLIENT ENCOUNTER

Before discussing components of the health history, the nurse must consider factors which are critical to the data collection process. These factors include:

1 Appraising the informant
2 Establishing trust
3 Assuring confidentiality
4 Planning the setting
5 Determining time boundaries
6 Identifying mental set

Appraising the Informant

The nurse must judge if the client or other informant is giving accurate data during the health history taking process. The client is considered to be the primary data source, while other informants providing data about the client are secondary data sources.

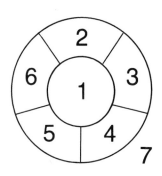

1, Primary source (client); 2, relatives; 3, friends; 4, health care professionals; 5, records; 6, other; 7, secondary sources.

Primary Data Source

Since the client's own account of health history data is fundamental to health assessment, he or she is considered to be the *primary data source*. In many instances, only the client can relate in detail personal information that may affect the health state. However, a client's reliability and accuracy as a primary informer may not always be accurate, so the nurse must evaluate the client's general competency. Factors such as age, intellectual ability, and congenital or related health limitations may all contribute to the collection of a limited data base.

In order to enhance the data collection process, the nurse should try to simplify language. This is especially important when seeking information from children. Parents or caretakers present during data gathering can be asked to explain terms commonly used by the child when discussing body parts, body processes, and health conditions or problems. The nurse may also use pictures and drawings to help clarify questions and information for the child.

Adults with varying intellectual ability may also require careful questioning in order to elicit accurate information. For example, a 25-

Validate rephrasing to assure understanding.

year-old man who has only an elementary education may have difficulty understanding specific health care terminology. As with the child, questions and terms may need to be simplified or even rephrased to ensure adequate understanding. In addition, a continuous clarification process developed between the nurse and client will help assure mutual understanding of a question's meaning and the significance of the client's response.

Secondary Data Sources

Secondary data sources may be used to substantiate a client's history or to provide additional data. These additional sources of information may include parents, relatives, friends, previous clinic or hospital records, and other health care providers.

The adolescent client may provide a partial data base, with additional data being provided by the caretaker.

If the client is an infant or a very small child, the informant will usually be the mother, father, or other caretaker. When such a situation occurs, the nurse will direct questions to the caretaker after establishing that the secondary source is reliable. If the nurse is seeing the infant or child for the first time, previous health care records such as immunization schedules must be submitted by the caretaker. The nurse may also obtain previous hospital records on the child's birth and neonatal period before the initial interview. These records will provide background data, reduce redundant questioning of the caretaker, and give the nurse additional data which can be validated during the interview. If other health care providers have been involved with the child in the past, the nurse may solicit information from them as well. All possible sources of information should be identified and used so that the nurse will have a more holistic picture of the child's overall health state.

When interviewing senior citizens or adults with physical or behavioral limitations, the nurse may find that the client is only partially reliable. Because of the aging process, the older adult may be confused or forgetful at times, especially about relating dates, remote events, or occurrences accurately. Consequently, the nurse must identify and use all other possible secondary data sources, such as relatives, friends, and previous health records, to obtain a more complete data base.

Establishing Trust

Most relationships are built on trust, and the client-nurse relationship is no exception. *Trust* is the basis of open and effective communication, which allows a person to freely express inner feelings and thoughts.

Convey a feeling of trust to the client.

Frequently the client may trust the nurse because of the role he or she occupies as a health care provider. However, effective use of the communication process to enhance open communication will result in the development of a trusting relationship, more positive sharing of information, and more productive planning for the client's health promotion.

In the past, clients had little control over selection of providers and were often placed into a situation of relinquishing data in order to reap the benefits of the health care provider. Today clients are taking a more active role in their health care, rejecting relationships that are superficial, and selecting health care providers with whom they can establish a more trusting relationship. The client will seek out the nurse who conveys warmth, empathy, and congruence and genuineness in a caring relationship.

The client usually takes a *risk* in trusting the nurse with health history data.

Warmth

Warmth implies that the relationship is unconditional. The nurse imparts a caring attitude through both verbal and nonverbal expressions.

An unconditional relationship is without limitations or requirements.

Such a phrase as, "I really want you to be satisfied with your care; it is important to me," communicates a sense of genuine caring and infers warmth. A soft tone of voice and direct eye contact are nonverbal expressions which provide additional feelings of caring and enhance trust.

Empathy

Empathy refers to the nurse's ability to develop sensitivity to the client's feelings, emotions, and experiences and to communicate this understanding to another person. Most people have known emotions such as anger, frustration, joy, sadness, satisfaction, success, and the like. Knowledge of these reactions can be used by the nurse as a foundation for developing and relating to the client empathetically. In addition, this knowledge can create an environment that will allow the client to share personal feelings more readily.

The nurse draws on personal experiences in learning to be empathetic.

Congruence and Genuineness

Congruence and genuineness are conveyed to the client when the nurse is open, honest, and truthful about the client's health state and health care matters. The following response is an example: "I know you are making an effort to follow good health habits; I would like to commend you for your efforts."

Carl Rogers developed the concept of congruence.

Refer to pages 77 to 84 for additional techniques which enhance development of trust.

Assuring Confidentiality

Confidentiality is a characteristic of the trusting relationship. It requires that the nurse not disclose information communicated by the client to any other person unless it benefits the client's health state.

The client comes to the nurse prepared to reveal both personal and private information. How the nurse receives and uses this information is of prime concern. The nurse needs to assure the client that all information will be used with utmost discretion within the health care system and only to benefit the client's health state. Clients who have had little contact with health care providers or have experienced negative encounters will be especially skeptical. The nurse can ease these feelings of distrust by reassuring the client that confidentiality will be maintained. As contact with the nurse continues, the client will be able to gain confidence in the nurse as a primary provider of health care.

The nurse may ask the client to indicate specifically those persons who are to be given client data.

If confidentiality must be violated for any reason, the client has the right to be informed.

Planning the Setting

The health history may be collected in a variety of physical settings, e.g., hospital, clinic, office, home, day care center, and school. Therefore, it is important that the setting be conducive to the free exchange of information between client and nurse.

A quiet and comfortable area, not congested with other clients and health providers, offers a setting conducive to data collection. Minimizing the number of distractions or interruptions which might occur during the encounter will enhance the interaction between nurse and client.

Although it may not be possible to conduct the interview in a private room, it is crucial that the nurse speak softly and directly with the client. Comfortable seating arrangements, good lighting, and optimum room temperature without drafts will also make the environment more adaptable to conversation.

Arranging the chairs in a face-to-face position decreases the chance that others will overhear the encounter and is an ideal way to convey to the client a feeling of caring and genuine interest in what he or she has to

The nurse prepares the area before the client's arrival.

say. Too often nurses stand over a client who is in a bed or on an examining table. Such a position makes it difficult to maintain eye-to-eye contact and also puts the client in what appears to be a subordinate position. This should be avoided whenever possible.

When talking with small children it is important to "come down to their level." To toddlers or preschoolers, standing adults appear to tower far above them. To avoid this, the nurse should create an environment where both sit at an equal level. Developing sensitivity to how children view the world will facilitate the nurse's ability to communicate with most children.

The *atmosphere* refers to the psychological setting established by the nurse. It is an integral component of the setting. The elements of trust, confidentiality, and genuine caring should be a part of the atmosphere conveyed to the client. Maintaining a calm, unhurried environment will further enhance the atmosphere and facilitate the data-gathering process.

Determining Time Boundaries

Deciding when to collect data is as important as the elements that surround the information-gathering process. Timing the interview so as not to exhaust or unnecessarily detain the client is especially important. A lengthy interview may jeopardize the accuracy and relevancy of the data obtained. A nurse noting behavior in the client that suggests restlessness should inquire whether the client would like to postpone further questioning until another time. Allowing the client to set the pace of the interview is often appropriate, and the nurse should impose limits only when absolutely necessary.

Restless behaviors can include lack of eye contact, fidgeting with hands, and frequent body repositioning.

If the client begins to ramble, the nurse should redirect conversation back to the original topic.

Children often have a short attention span and will find it quite difficult to concentrate during an interview. Frequent breaks that include diversionary activities such as games may make it easier for the nurse to complete the interviewing process with the child and/or the caretaker. Aging adults may also need to have their interviews scheduled into two or more time sequences to avoid exhaustion and undue stress. The nurse should try to determine a client's behavior and collect data within time boundaries that are comfortable for the nurse and the client.

The nurse who is abrupt, interrupts the client, frequently looks at a watch, or attempts to do a variety of technical tasks while trying to elicit pertinent data may be conveying a hurried approach, lack of interest in the situation, or lack of concern for the client. Such cues quickly alert the client that the nurse is not really interested in hearing what the client is saying. Consequently, the nurse may collect an incomplete data base, which may lead to inaccuracies in the nursing diagnosis. On the other hand, an accurate and complete data base will be enhanced by alertness, attentiveness to detail, a calm voice, and an unhurried manner.

Collection of accurate data is enhanced by the nurse's attentive and thoughtful behavior.

Identifying Mental Set

The mental set of both the client and the nurse may affect the outcome of the interview. *Mental set* is how one thinks and what one believes about a situation. The nurse must determine the client's mental set on health beliefs and health care. The nurse's mental set may also be an important factor in determining care provided to a client.

The nurse comes to the interview with a broad theoretical knowledge base learned through formal and informal education, a philosophy of nursing care, a system of values and beliefs, and very specific expectations about the outcome of the interview. All these factors will influence the professional nurse's role. Likewise, the client brings to the situation past experiences with the health care delivery system, the potential threat of unconfirmed disease, a philosophy of life which may include specific beliefs about health, a value system, and expectations about the encounter with the nurse. All these factors will influence the client and become part of each member's mental set. By using principles of the holistic philosophy to guide the interviewing, the nurse is able to maintain a nonjudgmental attitude regarding client responses, to acknowledge those components that come together to form the whole person, and to collect, interpret, and process data as the client intended. By maintaining an interaction free from imposition of values on the client, listening carefully, and validating information, the nurse should be able to obtain helpful data from which a plan of care can evolve. By continuously monitoring one's mental set and the client's, the outcome of the nurse-client interview will be significantly enhanced.

See Chap. 1.

THE COMMUNICATION PROCESS

Communication is a necessary part of living and is learned through experience. The way people learn to communicate as children and young adults is an integral part of the maturation process.

> Human communication is . . . the process whereby we generate and transmit meaning . . . the process of eliciting responses to stimuli . . . the means by which we present ourselves to the world . . . the matrix for all life's activities and the essential ingredient of all nursing functions . . . both an art and a science.[1]

> To question the importance of communication in our personal, professional and political lives would be as foolhardy as to question our need for air and water. Man is a social animal, and his very existence depends upon his ability to communicate with himself, with others, and with his environment.[2]

Effective communication skills are critical to the data-collection process.

The nurse learns through experience which communication techniques will elicit the most data and aid in enhancing the client's health state. The most effective climate in which to learn how to communicate with a client and to conduct a health history interview is in settings where the nurse encounters actual clients. As the nurse develops effective communication skills, communication patterns can be expanded to a variety of professional encounters. The nurse should become familiar with verbal and nonverbal language, the communication contract, and factors that affect the communication process.

Verbal and Nonverbal Language

The communication process is characterized by verbal and nonverbal language. From birth, human beings begin to communicate verbally—first through crying, then through babbling and imitating sounds, then to words and phrases, and finally to sentences and the written word. Along with this progressive development of verbal language comes nonverbal language development. This includes the progression from nonspecific gross motor movements to fine adaptive motor skills, the progression from direct, focused eye-to-eye contact to socially defined eye movements, and the learning of facial expressions and body gestures that are culturally and socially determined.

See Body Language.

The meanings of verbal and nonverbal communication are in the sender as well as in the receiver of the message. The volume, tone of

See Fig. 3-1 depicting communication.

voice, and rate of speaking affect the message's meaning. Words and sentences provoke visual images and auditory, olfactory, and tactile sensations. With such an array of communicative messages, it is amazing that information is interpreted so quickly and accurately. As a person matures, cultural development along with expanding cognitive and emotional abilities aid in the interpretation of messages. Infants, children, and adults are all capable of interpretation—applying meaning to verbal and nonverbal messages.[3]

Verbal language is the single most important tool used by the nurse to interview the client and to compile data. Effective verbal communication is an active process that involves a reciprocal interchange through speaking and listening. Ideas and feelings expressed by the nurse and the client during the interview provide significant information and enhance the effectiveness of the data-collecting process. (See Fig. 3-1.)

If the nurse uses the appropriate communication techniques at the right moment during the interview, the client will perceive questions and other verbal cues through all sensory levels as they were intended and respond with the desired information. When the nurse is keenly attentive to the client, the messages will be seen and heard accurately and interpreted correctly. This attentiveness will likewise communicate to the client the nurse's sensitivity and sincerity and facilitate the development of a trusting relationship. Imparting to the client that he or she is important and that *all* data are vital to promoting a health state is essential to the holistic approach.

The Communication Contract

Before initiating the actual interview, the nurse and the client should have a basic understanding of the goals of the interviewing process and mutually agree to the content or focus of the discussion. This may be in the form of an implied or an explicit communication contract.

Implied Contract

An implied communication contract is based on general assumptions and expectations held by each party participating in the binding agreement. Rules are unwritten and may be derived from cultural upbringing, social influence, educational background, and one's own system of values and beliefs.[4] Most nurse-client relationships operate under such a contract because of the role positions that the nurse and the client occupy.

For example, the nurse's role might be one of a health care provider to the client, with all the rights and privileges that go with such a role. The nurse may thus expect the client to share all pertinent information that will contribute to a nursing diagnosis on the client's health state.

However, the client may have other suppositions. Assumption of the sick role, as it is called by Parsons and Lederer, suggests that responsibility for one's physical condition is relinquished and that the client submits to a dependent position and is dominated by the nurse.[5,6] In this instance the client expects the nurse to make all the decisions for and about health care. Under such conditions, there is great potential for role strain because of possible incongruence of role expectations between the nurse and the client and for misunderstandings over conditions of the unwritten contract. Because of its obvious limitations, the implied contract is a less than desirable format to use for data collection.

Explicit Contract

The explicit communication contract is usually written, somewhat formal, and agreed to by each party. This binding agreement presents a clear idea of the purpose for which the contract was devised. Both par-

Implicit in the communication process is an intact central nervous system (CNS).

Listening is a critical element of the communication process.

An implied contract may be improved on by verbalizing that which is implied so that nurse and client may reach agreement.

Figure 3-1 Communication. The sender relays a verbal or nonverbal message to the receiver, who in turn responds to the sender through a feedback message.

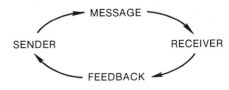

ties share in the responsibility to fulfill the commitments of the contract. There is no hidden agenda, and the potential for developing role strain is minimized, since each person knows what to expect from the other. The explicit communication contract has the further advantages of allaying client anxiety and of removing misconceptions or fantasies the client may have about the health interview.[7] Therefore, it is highly recommended that an explicit communication contract be devised between the nurse and client to clarify the purpose of the encounter (Table 3-1).

The explicit contract in Table 3-1 may be adapted to meet individual client needs.

Factors That Affect the Communication Process

The nurse who is learning to communicate as a professional must be aware of and able to recognize variables that may positively or negatively affect communicating with a client. The list of variables that influence communication is innumerable; therefore, only the most common will be addressed.

See texts specifically written on communication for additional discussion; see Bibliography.

Culture

As a health care provider, the nurse frequently comes into contact with clients of varying ethnic, racial, and cultural backgrounds. Because U.S. society is mobile, homogenous groups no longer reside in specific geographical areas. The nurse must be able to adapt to encounters with persons of differing cultural or ethnic backgrounds. Ethnicity, race, or culture may dictate certain norms, roles, customs, values, traditions, and unique symbolic behaviors which may affect the way the client interacts with the nurse. For example, Native Americans (American Indians) customarily conceal emotions and refrain from verbalizing physical discomfort. In such a situation the nurse may embarrass or offend the client with direct, probing questions about the health state. Thus, communication style must be adapted to that of the client so that a productive interaction results.

See Chap. 1 for definitions of ethnicity and culture.

Specific language barriers may also relate to differences in race or ethnic background. The client may speak a different language or have different meanings for similar phrases or words. The nurse may need to enlist the assistance of an interpreter or secondary data source so that communication is not stifled and pertinent information can be elicited.

Language

Semantic expressions, as in slang or jargon, are heavily used in Western society, yet such linguistic patterns may be easily misunderstood and misinterpreted or even offend the listener.

Nurses frequently use technical language or jargon that clients may not understand. For example, a client may not understand when the nurse says, "What are your dietary patterns?" The question, "What do you usually eat for breakfast, lunch, and dinner?" is more clear and precise. Since the intent of communication is to generate understanding, the nurse must be keenly aware when selecting vocabulary to avoid using semantic expressions.

The nurse must validate the perceived meaning of messages communicated by the client.

Table 3-1
Components of the Explicit Communication Contract

Names of the participating parties
Date, time, and location of the interview and subsequent examinations
Plans for scheduling future meetings
Expected behaviors of the nurse and the client identified
Conditions for referrals or consultations with other health care providers
Acknowledgements of decision-making powers of parties concerned
Rules on documentation of assessments and findings

Hearing, Vision, and Speech Variations

With hearing, vision, and speech losses, as in the case of a vision- or hearing-impaired client or a deaf-mute, the nurse should explore comfortable ways to facilitate the communication process. It may be adequate to verbalize or to use pencil and paper, but if sign language and/or lipreading is the preferred method of communication, the nurse should enlist the assistance of a person trained in sign language and lipreading for accuracy. Often the nurse can save time and decrease stress in clients if such resources are found early in professional practice so that they can be easily contacted when needed.

THE INTERVIEW

The goals of a successful interview are (1) to establish a trusting relationship with the client, (2) to elicit pertinent information about the client's health state, and (3) to assess verbal and nonverbal behavior that will indicate needed nursing intervention.

The nurse often finds that initial interviews are difficult to conduct and require much more thought and planning than expected. Initial interviews should be supervised by a skilled professional so that the beginner can receive constructive feedback immediately after each interview. With conscientious practice and experimentation with various communication techniques, the nurse will become both comfortable and proficient with client interviews.

Introduction

The nurse opens the interview with a cordial greeting, stating the client's name and title. The client should then be allowed the same opportunity of introduction. The nurse then proceeds to describe briefly his or her role in relation to the client and indicates that a health history will be taken. The nurse should discuss with the client both the purpose of the health history and how information to be collected will be used. The client can then be given an opportunity to ask questions freely.

Observations

Age, sex, race, and physical appearance are often the first cues that the nurse notes about the client. These nonverbal cues will evoke a general overall impression of the client's state of health and denote outstanding characteristics that may help direct the interview. The nurse should use keen observational skills, as well as other sensory modalities, in order to process all pertinent data elicited during this initial encounter.

When focusing specifically on the client's physical appearance, the nurse simultaneously begins to establish a rapport, which may be enhanced by introductory conversation. Making the client as comfortable as possible will facilitate the subsequent interview and physical examination. The nurse should note the client's general manner of dress, posture, gait, body movements, breath odor, state of nutrition, stature, and skin condition and coloring at this time.

Body Language

Body language is an important form of nonverbal communication that provides significant data to the attentive nurse. It can include "any nonreflexive or reflexive movement of a part, or all of the body, used by a person to communicate an emotional message to the outside world."[8]

If the nurse is unable to communicate with the client because of hearing, vision, or speech variations, assistance should be gained through a resource person.

Clarifying roles helps to make the client's expectations of the health provider more realistic.

See Chap. 4.

The nurse must watch the client and listen closely when making observations.

See Chap. 4.

See Verbal and Nonverbal Communication.

Expressions of body language, e.g., gestures, facial expressions, eye movements, and posturing, are signals that alert the nurse to explore their meaning. The client may not be comfortable verbalizing emotions, attitudes, or feelings but may provide the nurse with a wealth of data through nonverbal cues (see the following example).

An adolescent girl sits observing the interaction between the nurse and her mother. The girl appears poised; she sits quietly with her hands in her lap and her legs crossed and watches pleasantly. As soon as her mother leaves the room she begins to slouch in the chair, and her facial expression changes to one of disgust.

What does this situation reveal about the relationship between the girl and her mother? The nurse should pursue the use of body language in an attempt to interpret these nonverbal cues.

In many instances, messages are sent and received through body language. The client may actually contradict direct verbal communication through a gesture or a facial expression. The observant nurse will recognize cues and will include them as part of the data-collection process.

Territoriality

Territoriality is another concept related to body language that has been clinically studied, and results are applicable to nursing. Reportedly, every person strives to maintain a personal space or territory, no matter how close the setting. An important part of how people relate to one another is reflected in how one's space is defended and how a person approaches another person's area.

Dr. Edward T. Hall studied humans' personal space and coined the word "proxemics" to describe his theories and observations about "zones of territory" and how they are used. Within this conceptual framework he identified four distinct zones: intimate distance, personal distance, social distance, and public distance. Each has both a "close phase" and a "far phase," which reflect human interaction that, in most instances, is culturally defined.[9]

Intimate Distance

Intimate distance is labeled "close" if actual physical contact occurs and "far" if a distance of 6 to 18 inches (15 to 45 cm) is maintained. During the nurse-client interview or physical examination, intimate distance occurs frequently. The nurse may be positioned next to the client at a far intimate distance while completing the health history and may engage in close intimate contact during the physical examination. Generally, these distances are acceptable in health care situations, especially if nurse and client are comfortable with their respective roles.

It is important for the beginning practitioner to explore personal feelings about such distances, since ambiguous feelings about touching a client may result in an awkward approach to the total assessment. Likewise, the client may communicate nonverbally a sense of shyness exhibited by difficulty in exposing certain body parts. When this occurs, the nurse may need to explain procedures ahead of time and actually ask permission to examine or to make physical contact.

When working with toddlers, preschoolers, and school-age children, the nurse must be keenly aware of body language cues from children that indicate resistance to encroachment on their territory. Younger children are just beginning to explore their bodies, and many feelings are bound

One interpretation of this behavior could be that the girl respects her mother and does not wish to displease her.

The four zones of territory can be applied in the nurse-client encounter: (1) intimate distance, (2) personal distance, (3) social distance, and (4) public distance.

A client of the opposite sex may be embarrassed by physical contact.

It may be important to prepare the client for invasion of personal space.

up in their need to define their own sexuality. Reassurance and assistance from a parent or caretaker may be necessary for the child in order for the nurse to complete data collection.

School-age children are usually quite cooperative, especially if equipment and procedures are made familiar to them before an interview and examination. However, the nurse must continue to be alert for verbal or nonverbal cues that indicate uncomfortable reactions and to respond accordingly.

Sensory stimuli are sharpened at an intimate distance and may provide additional data and clues for nursing diagnosis. Normal body odors, visual alertness and clarity, projection of voice, and responses to tactile sensations are relevant assessments. The nurse should be conscious of his or her own sensory stimuli and how they might be interpreted by the client. Strong perfumes, hair sprays, or deodorants may be offensive and even induce nausea in the client. Volume and tone of voice should be low so that the nurse does not compromise the client's auditory perception. A pleasant-smelling mouthwash may be used to counteract breath odors, and gum-chewing is not recommended.

Personal Distance
Personal distance is labeled "close" at $1\frac{1}{2}$ to $2\frac{1}{2}$ feet (45 to 75 cm) and "far" if a distance of $2\frac{1}{2}$ to 4 feet (75 to 130 cm) is maintained. The nurse may use the close personal distance for the client interview, especially if it is noted from nonverbal cues that the client is uncomfortable with intimate distance. Parts of the physical examination that require focusing on a larger area, such as symmetry of extremities, may best be done at the far personal distance. Entering the client's personal space may also be threatening, making adequate preparation vital.

Social Distance
Social distance is labeled "close" at 4 to 7 feet (130 to 210 cm) and "far" at 7 to 12 feet (210 to 360 cm). Close social distance is more impersonal, whereas far social distance is more formal. A nurse who is standing at close social distance may cause the seated client to feel dominated. Sensory stimuli become more weak at the close range and are usually lost at the far range, with the exception of visual and auditory stimuli. Visual contact becomes important at far social distance, and direct eye contact should be maintained during conversation. Social distance is most often observed in a clinic or hospital waiting room, where clients are usually not required to communicate with health care providers.

Public Distance
Public distance is labeled "close" at 12 to 25 feet (360 to 750 cm) and "far" at 25 feet (750 cm) or more. Public distance does not allow for ease of communication and substantially limits the nurse's view of certain physical and nonverbal client cues. The nurse can use close public distance effectively when assessing the client's gait and gross motor movement. The use of the Snellen chart for an eye examination is another example of close public distance, since screening requires a distance of 20 feet (600 cm) for accuracy. Working with a variety of clients, the nurse may discover other verbal or nonverbal communications that are best elicited or observed using public distance.

Interviewing Techniques

The experienced nurse-interviewer draws on a broad knowledge base of the communication process to successfully conduct an interview and com-

Tensing of muscles and defensive arm and leg movements are frequent nonverbal reactions in children.

Continue to assess sensory stimuli, since they remain sharp at a personal distance.

See Chap. 4.

Various other nonverbal characteristics will be discussed in Client Profile/Biographical Data and in General Appearance, Chap. 4.

plete the health history. Communicating with a variety of clients of varying ages will greatly increase the development of interviewing skills. Using techniques that have been clinically studied and applied in many previous situations will also help both the novice and the experienced interviewer conduct the interview.

Several authors have described various techniques such as questioning, silence, and reflecting which have been used to aid the client in moving toward long- and/or short-term health goals. Each of these techniques can be applied to the interviewing process. Each will be discussed briefly in the following pages.[10–17]

Highlights

Twenty-two interviewing techniques are discussed on the following pages.

Questioning

The quality and structuring of questions unequivocally influence the quality of the client's response.

This statement suggests that the nurse must take into account his or her own personality as a controlling factor that influences the interview. A nurse who is highly structured and formal may show these characteristics in the interview. One nurse, for example, may develop a systematic questionnaire which includes a separate category for each area of data that is essential to nursing assessment, while the nurse who is less formal may develop a more flexible, open-ended, and informal approach to data collection. The latter method is often preferred, since it allows the client some control in choosing the order of the questions. With the more structured method the client may not have such control. Nevertheless, there are advantages and disadvantages to both methods of questioning. The effective interviewer will quickly learn to adapt personality and personal style to each client situation.

The nurse's personality may influence the success of the interview.

The sequence and phrasing of the questions also affect the flow of the interview.[18]

Regardless of the method of questioning, the nurse should move logically from one component of the history to the next. This gives the client time to concentrate on one subject and complete one idea before moving on to another subject.

Accuracy in obtaining all the facts will be enhanced by an organized method of questioning.

Using the format of this chapter, it is recommended that the nurse begin the interview by first focusing on the client profile, which includes biographic data, and then moving progressively to more personal areas. Questions which move from the general to the more specific and intimate will allow for mutual discussion and help facilitate data collection. This strategy provides for a more personal approach initially and allows the client needed time to develop a trusting relationship so that intimate questions are less embarrassing.

The nurse should use simple vocabulary, avoid stereotyping, not be judgmental or opinionated, and complete the interview with an attitude of support, thus enhancing the interviewing process.

Using Silence

Silence encourages the client to verbalize. It allows time for both the nurse and the client to ponder questions and answers and thus slows the pace of the communication. It provides an opportunity to organize thoughts and allows time for the nurse to observe nonverbal communication.

If silence is prolonged the client may become uncomfortable.

Accepting

The nurse indicates recognition of the client's thoughts and feelings through verbal and nonverbal cues. Even though the nurse may agree or disagree with the client, he or she should attempt to remain nonjudgmental. A simple yes or "I follow what you said," as well as nonverbal

The nurse should remain nonjudgmental in interacting with clients.

gestures such as nodding and raising the eyebrows, communicate a sense of understanding to the client.

Giving Recognition

The nurse recognizes the client as a person throughout the interaction and attempts to make the client feel comfortable at the onset of the interview. Statements such as "Good morning, Mr. Jones," or "You look well-rested and cheerful," give recognition to the whole person.

As the interview progresses, the nurse may recognize specific statements or behaviors exhibited by the client. Statements such as, "You sound as if . . . ," "It appears to me that . . . ," and "You seem quite uncomfortable when . . ." acknowledge the client's efforts to communicate.

The client's self-esteem may be enhanced through recognition.

Offering Self

The client must feel that the nurse can be trusted with all the information conveyed during the interview. By "offering self," the nurse indicates an interest in the client's situation and a willingness to help the client attain satisfaction. The nurse may offer self through physical presence, by being genuine and warm, or by indicating a willingness to assist the client with a health-related task.

See Establishing Trust.

Giving Broad Openings

Offering the client an opportunity to speak freely can be facilitated by the use of broad openings. For example, the nurse may say, "Why don't you begin by telling me the purpose of your visit today," "Are there other things bothering you?" or "What else would you like to share with me?" Such statements indicate that the client should take the initiative to speak.

Freedom of response is encouraged through use of broad openings.

Offering General Leads

The nurse can also facilitate communication by allowing the client to continue to direct the discussion and cover areas that are of personal significance. The nurse is less verbal at this time in an attempt to give the client time to respond more completely. Responses such as, "Continue, please," "And then what happened?" and "Tell me about your concerns" keep the nurse's verbal interaction at a minimum and the client's at a maximum.

Placing Event in Time or Sequence

The nurse may need to clarify the exact time of an event, predisposing factors that led to an event, or relationships associated with a certain event in order to (1) determine the problem, (2) make the correct nursing diagnosis, (3) determine cause and effect, and (4) solve the problem more accurately. Questions to facilitate this process include "What factors seemed to have led up to . . . ?" "Did this reaction ever happen before or after . . . ?" "Do you recall a previous pattern of events when you responded this way?" "Can you associate this problem with any other significant event occurring in your life?" Such questions allow the client to respond with specific data about the timing or sequence of an event.

The nurse will often have to construct questions around events and circumstances in order to obtain more precise data.

Making Observations

The nurse may state personal observations in order to encourage mutual understanding or to facilitate the client's awareness of a situation. The client may be sending nonverbal cues unconsciously, and the nurse may deem it appropriate to bring these to the client's attention. Such responses as "I sense that you are in pain sometimes," "Did you know that you are continuously bringing up your job?" or "Am I correct in saying

The nursing observations verbalized must not threaten the client's self-awareness.

that what you are experiencing now is different from before?" may be used. These phrases may help to clarify issues, allow the client to know how others are reacting to what is being said, and help validate verbal and nonverbal cues.

Encouraging Description of Perceptions

In order to clarify what the client perceives during the data collection process, the nurse may ask, "How do you feel about that?" "What do you think I mean when I said . . . ?" This type of questioning helps to broaden the nurse's understanding of why the client may be confused, concerned, in doubt, or apprehensive about a subject area and provides an opportunity to clarify data and avoid misperceptions.

Encouraging Comparisons

The nurse may wish to have the client compare ideas, experiences, or relationships by noting similarities and differences in other events affecting the health state. Questions such as "Do you see any differences between your present health and that of three months ago; can you tell me about them?" "Does this present problem resemble a previous medical condition?" and "In what way is it similar or dissimilar?" help to clarify issues and make the client become more aware of associations between various factors that may cause a particular problem.

Comparisons may enhance the data base collected.

Restating

By restating or repeating the context of an area of discussion, the nurse can convey whether the client has effectively communicated an idea. Restating also ensures clarity of understanding.

For example:

Client: "My medication was prescribed to be taken 4 times per day."

Nurse: "Do you mean that you take your medication every 6 hours each day?"

Client: "No. I take the medication at 7 A.M., 11 A.M., 4 P.M., and 9 P.M."

In this situation the nurse could have made an inaccurate assumption. By clarifying the situation with the client, the nurse ensures that data will be recorded correctly. Restating may also encourage the client to continue the discussion of the current topic.

The nurse may restate the client's words verbatim to promote clarity.

Reflecting

The technique of reflection can be used by the nurse to direct questions, concerns, feelings, and ideas back to the client so that thoughts can be reevaluated. Reflecting also indicates to the client that the nurse accepts statements already made as valuable information. The following interaction demonstrates reflection.

Client: "Have I provided you with enough information about my family history?"

Nurse: "Do you feel that you have been thorough in sharing this information?"

Note that while the nurse maintains a nonjudgmental attitude, the client is being allowed time to reflect on what has been said and to control the conclusion of the discussion. Should the client think of additional data, it can be added at this time.

Reflection acknowledges that the client has a right to opinions and decisions.

Focusing

The nurse usually concentrates on a single point in the discussion to emphasize its importance to the client and to encourage the significance of certain health components. For example, the nurse might say, "The influence of your occupation on your health is worth exploring more closely. Do you realize that working with asbestos creates certain problems that over time may affect your breathing?" The nurse here implies to the client that occupation can influence the health state and that more data are needed for assessment. The client can then be directed to provide additional information through specific questioning.

Giving Information

The technique of giving information provides a teaching opportunity for the nurse. By sharing information and facts with the client, active involvement in determining health care needs can be facilitated. In addition, teaching helps to build a trusting relationship and enables the client to become more involved in decision making on health care. As data collection progresses, the nurse may also want to share information about the remainder of the health history interview and physical examination. This helps to prepare the client for subsequent discussions.

Information is given in terms of what and how much the client can handle.

Seeking Clarification

As has been stated, it is important to the client's health maintenance and health promotion that the nurse understand verbal and nonverbal communications. Statements by the nurse such as "I'm not sure what you mean" or "Why would you say that is significant?" can help clarify vague areas and enhance interpretations by encouraging the client to explain further. If statements still do not appear clear, the nurse should not dwell on the subject any further, since that may cause the client to withdraw. Instead, the nurse should consider other ways to gain the data, such as through secondary sources.

Early in the interview the client should also be encouraged to seek clarification.

Presenting Reality

Occasionally the client will make statements that suggest an unrealistic perception about health or health care. The nurse should encourage the client to evaluate and reconsider these ideas and offer an alternative, more realistic response. Responses by the nurse such as "That's an unusual idea," "I'm not sure I can believe that," or "Do you really think that is possible?" may help the client to reflect on what has been said. With some assistance, thoughts can be clarified so that a more realistic response can be presented.

Seeking Consensual Validation

Consensual validation is a technique that provides for mutual understanding between the nurse and the client during the communication process. Since many variables can influence perceptions and affect data collection, the nurse must determine if the client's words, ideas, and concepts are sending the intended message. Statements such as, "Tell me if I'm interpreting what you say correctly," "Do you mean that you are unsatisfied with your present eating habits?" or "Are you using this word to infer criticism of your health care?" may be used to help clarify perceptions. Through consensual validation, the nurse indicates to the client that clarity is essential for accurate assessment and the client in turn provides the needed data to validate the nurse's perceptions.

The nurse should be aware that a statement may have a different meaning for the client.

Verbalizing the Implied

It is necessary for the nurse to be able to base assessments and plans for health care on factual data. Therefore, to avoid having to make inferences rather than accurate interpretations, the nurse should direct the client to verbalize that which is implied. For example,

Expanding on a client's thoughts and perceptions will help to clarify and validate data.

Client: "Well, my financial status may be influencing my health, but I doubt it."

Nurse: "Do you think your finances allow you to purchase enough food for an adequate diet?" "Do you think your inadequate income causes you stress?"

This type of response helps the client to clarify data and shows that the nurse is attentive to information offered by the client. In addition, it may give the nurse and client new insights on the cause of a particular problem.

Encouraging Evaluation

In order for the client to be an active participant in making decisions about personal health care, the client must evaluate contributing data and plans for health care along with the nurse. Personal feelings and values as they relate to significant persons and health care providers must also be addressed. Statements such as, "Do you think this will be effective for you?" or "How will this influence your present routine?" suggest an opportunity for client evaluation. Clients who have had difficulty adhering to a particular therapeutic plan in the past should be asked to define realistic plans for achieving a goal. For example, the nurse may feel that an overweight client could lose 5 lb (2.25 kg) in 2 weeks, while for the client, a more realistic goal is 2 lb (0.90 kg).

Attempting to Translate Nonverbal Cues

In certain situations it becomes important for the nurse to translate the nonverbal cues received from the client. This may be necessary when the client's verbal communication is incongruent with the nonverbal gestures or when the client's statements are meaningless to the nurse. For example, if a male client states, "I have a good relationship with my children" but his eyes seem distant and sad when he says this, the nurse might respond, "You seem to feel lonely; do you see your children often?" Through this response the nurse is attempting to give the client a chance to talk about his children in an effort to clarify the apparent incongruence between verbal responses and nonverbal cues.

Suggesting Collaboration

As with evaluation, the client should be allowed to collaborate with the nurse on as many health care issues as possible. The client who is encouraged to take responsibility for personal well-being will certainly benefit in the future. Through collaboration, the nurse can anticipate that the client will be more likely to adhere to recommended health regimens, practice health maintenance behaviors, and seek preventive care because of personal involvement in discussions on health care.

Summarizing

Summarizing should occur at the end of each part of the health assessment. With the completion of the health history, and the validation of the physical examination, important points of the encounter can be emphasized for greater understanding. A sense of closure is a positive feeling for both the client and the nurse. Emotions, impressions, and perceptions have been shared, and factual data have been gathered. By summarizing all that has happened during the encounter, the nurse promotes comprehension of the significant interchange that has occurred.

The foregoing discussion of interviewing techniques has been presented in order to aid the nurse in developing communication skills. Some techniques will be successful with certain clients, while other techniques will not. The conscientious nurse will try various approaches and determine those which work best.

Factors that Block Communication

Now that the nurse knows what techniques facilitate communication, it is also important to be able to recognize verbal errors that block communication. These blocks include changing the subject, giving advice and/or false reassurance, jumping to conclusions or making decisions for the client, being repetitious, and using facts inappropriately. When any one of these factors occurs during communication between the nurse and client, it may limit the success of the verbal interaction.

Changing the Subject

Changing the subject occurs when there is an abrupt shift in the focus of the conversation; another subject is introduced before ending the one being discussed, preventing the client from completing a thought. The following is an example of changing the subject:

Nurse: "How do you relax after a stressful day at work?"

Client: "I usually go home and have a glass of wine and read the paper."

Nurse: "Don't you think physical exercise would be better than drinking wine?"

The nurse has changed the subject from stress to alcohol consumption and exercise without inquiring further about the effects of stress on the client. A better response by the nurse would be, "Do you think the wine relaxes you enough so that stress does not adversely affect you physically or emotionally?"

By finishing one subject before going on to the next, communication is enhanced and potentially significant data are not omitted.

Giving Advice

Giving advice or false reassurance may also hinder the data-collection process. It occurs when the nurse responds to a part of a conversation with the client by providing input inappropriately. The client may resent such techniques and thus withdraw from the communication process. The nurse may also jeopardize the trusting relationship that leads to openness and sharing.

An example of inappropriately giving advice follows:

Client: "I don't know whether I should continue with my job, considering the risks to my health."

Nurse: "If I were you, I would change jobs immediately. It's not worth it to take the risk."

A better response by the nurse would be:

Nurse: "What do you see as your alternatives to the situation?"

Instead of giving advice, the nurse is encouraging the client to solve the situation.

Occasionally the client will ask for advice from the nurse, but before responding, the nurse should try to determine if the client has already come to a conclusion. Supporting the client's decision once it has been determined is usually the best approach.

Jumping to Conclusions

Jumping to conclusions or making decisions prematurely may result in an inaccurate judgment or an error in recording the data. For example:

Client: "I have smoked two packs of cigarettes a day for 15 years."

Nurse: "I'm sure you want to quit smoking. Why don't you stop now?"

By jumping to such a conclusion, the nurse has not allowed the client to verbalize feelings completely and has also made a value judgment. The nurse should provide the client with adequate time to share feelings and answer questions. If this does not occur, the nurse may make a decision on the client's health care based on an inadequate data base.

Repetitiveness

Repetitiveness is usually annoying. It bombards the client with too many cues for one idea. Some redundancy may be necessary in certain instances, but the nurse must use good judgment when using this technique. For example:

Nurse: "Has your physician limited your intake of high-cholesterol foods?"

Client: "Yes. My physician has prescribed a strict diet, which I follow faithfully. It includes only poultry, fish and veal, fruits, vegetables, and special bread."

Nurse: "You know, high-cholesterol foods are not good for your heart and lead to obesity. I think you should watch your weight."

Such repetition by the nurse may be interpreted as "preaching" and result in the client's "tuning out." A more appropriate response by the nurse would be one that supports the client's efforts to watch the diet and limit cholesterol intake.

Inappropriate Use of Facts

Inappropriate use of nursing or health-related facts can be deceiving to the client. This often occurs when the nurse is attempting to change the client's attitude or behavior, especially when either conflicts with the nurse's own values. The major problem is that it compromises the trusting relationship, which may further jeopardize the client's faith in health care providers. The client may also be swayed to change attitude and behavior in order to please the nurse. Note the following example:

Nursing and health-related facts must be clearly understood by the client in order to promote health.

Client: "The only exercise I get during the day is walking about my office. Sometimes I'll walk 1 or 2 miles on a weekend."

Nurse: "Mr. Jones, you really need more exercise to improve your health. At your age of 45, activity is important for your cardiovascular system and to prevent overweight. I exercise by running every day."

In this situation the nurse has criticized Mr. Jones for his lack of exercise and has implied that he might take up running to benefit his heart and weight. A better approach would be to discuss in detail how the heart is affected by exercise and weight and then to discern Mr. Jones's feelings about the subject and his readiness to change habits.

Summary

The application of the communication process is essential to data collection and to the completion of the nursing assessment. The nurse must remain cognizant of the various interviewing techniques that can be applied to facilitate communication in diverse health care settings when working with clients and families.

Use of appropriate communication techniques will enhance data collection and accurate nursing assessment.

THE HEALTH HISTORY: FORMAT

The format for the health history is contained in Table 3-2. Using the general approach to the client and the appropriate setting and applying the elements of the interviewing process, the nurse is ready to begin the

The format for the health history is contained in Table 3-2.

Table 3-2
Health History Format

Client profile/biographical data
    Client's name
    Address
    Sex
    Age and birthdate
    Place of birth
    Race and nationality
    Marital status
    Religion
    Occupation
    Social Security number
Health Perception/Health Management
    Current health status/health habits
    Past health status
        Birth history
        Growth and development
        Common childhood illnesses
        Immunizations
        Previous hospitalizations
        Accidents or injuries
        Allergies or allergic reactions
    Family history
    Value and belief patterns
Life patterns/lifestyles
    Age
    Race
    Heredity
    Culture
    Growth and development
        Physical capabilities
        Cognitive capabilities
        Social capabilities
        Emotional capabilities
    Behavioral development
    Biological rhythms/including Sleep/Rest Patterns and Elimination Patterns
    Environmental factors
    Economics
    Community resources
Roles and relationship patterns
    Family life
    Occupation
    Societal relationships
Self-perception/self-concept patterns

Cognitive/perceptual patterns
    Sensory perception (hearing, vision)
    Education
    Intelligence
    Pain perception
Sexuality/reproductive patterns

Nutritional/metabolic patterns
    24-hr recall
    Basic four food groups
    Recommended daily dietary allowances
    Food intake record
Exercise/activity patterns

Coping patterns/stress tolerance patterns

---

data-collection process. Each component of the health history found in Table 3-2 will be discussed in the pages to follow.

    It is important to note that the nursing assessment is an essential element in the formulation of a nursing diagnosis and in all subsequent health care planning with the client. Therefore, the nurse must be able to elicit effectively a sound data base from the client, since all future client encounters will be based on this foundation.

Review the steps of the nursing process presented in Chap. 1: (1) assessment, (2) diagnosis, (3) goals, and (4) evaluation of outcomes.

Phases of Establishing A Data Base

The health history can be completed in two phases: the data-collection phase and the recording of the data on the client's permanent record.

Data-collection Phase

Collection of data results from the nurse-client interview. Using the information that has been presented up to this point in the chapter, the nurse should organize thoughts and approaches in order to compile data on each component of the history. Since various pattern areas can influence the client's health state collectively, each area must be addressed during the interviewing process.

See Data Collection in Chap. 1.

See Chap. 1 for a discussion of the functional assessment model.

Recording Phase

Recording will occur when all data have been collected and after the nurse and client have departed company. It is recommended that the nurse refrain from recording data while it is actually being collected, since this may induce stress in the client and possibly cause the nurse to overlook important observations and cues. If the interview is especially lengthy, the nurse may take brief notes during the process if this is explained to the client.

See Recording the Health History Data.

Notes may be necessary when completing data on the past health status, family history, and review of body components.

Entry into the Health Care System

Before completing the client profile, the nurse should identify the client's reason for entry into the health care delivery system. The nurse should have the client describe his or her own perception of health and why he or she is seeking health care. By using a holistic approach to questioning, the nurse may discover that the client's reason for entry is related to health promotion, health maintenance, or disease prevention rather than to restoration of health because of a specific problem.

Generally there are four main reasons a client enters the health care system: (1) referral, (2) annual physical, (3) follow-up appointment, or (4) school or occupational requirements.

Referral

Often clients are referred by another health care provider or person in the community. Other nurses or various physicians, psychologists, and other specialists may refer a child or an adult for health assessment and physical examination. Likewise, teachers or colleagues may refer a person for health assessment.

A client who follows through on a referral probably values the opinions of others regarding health.

Annual Physical

Many clients routinely schedule an annual physical examination with their health care provider. Others are reminded to have an annual physical as part of their insurance plan. Whatever the motivation, the nurse should encourage this behavior.

Follow-up Appointment

A client may need to see a health care provider for follow-up examinations after an initial visit. The nature of the visit should also be noted.

School or Occupational Requirements

Often a child must have a physical examination with developmental screening before entering school. This is done to (1) ensure that immunizations are up to date, (2) guarantee that the child will not be exposing others to an illness, (3) verify that the child is physically and developmentally ready for school, and (4) verify that hearing, vision, language, and motor and social skills are not delayed.

An employer may require health screening and a physical examination before hiring a person. This protects the employer, since certain occupations may be mentally or physically stressful to certain persons. Further, it decreases the risk to the employer of having to pay worker's compensation for an illness, disability, or specific health need identified shortly after the new employee has been hired.

Components of the Health History

Many components interact to make up the health history. Therefore, it is necessary to collect data about each component so that the nurse will have a complete picture of the client's health state.

Client Profile/Biographical Data

The client profile includes the following biographical data:

1 Name
2 Address
3 Sex
4 Age and birthdate
5 Place of birth
6 Race and nationality
7 Marital status
8 Religion
9 Occupation
10 Social Security number

The client may record this information on the permanent record before the initial appointment with the nurse. In some settings a secretary or clerk may gather this data, or it may be sent to the client's home to be completed and returned.

Client's Name The client's full name is recorded, using first, middle, and last names. A woman's maiden name must also be recorded. For a married couple whose last names differ, the nurse should record both spouses' last names. When interviewing a child whose last name differs from the legal parent or guardian, both names should be recorded. Such precise client identification ensures accuracy and also facilitates filing and retrieval of records for future reference. In one facility there may be numerous clients with the same last name; therefore, it is essential to keep names accurately recorded.

Address The client's current mailing address is recorded. If the person is planning to move in the near future, a forwarding address should also be obtained so that future contacts may be possible.

If the client has home and work telephone numbers, both should be recorded. If possible, the nurse should also record the address and/or telephone number of a relative or close friend who could contact the client in an emergency. The client's home address may also provide the nurse with additional data about economic status and environmental setting. Often certain neighborhoods within a geographical area are commonly known to be low, middle, or upper class. The nurse can use this knowl-

The nurse will record verbatim the client's stated reason for seeking health care.

Refer to Table 3-2 for the health history format.

If the client is a child, the parent may record or report information.

Addresses change frequently in today's mobile society.

edge of the community to help direct future questions. Other factors, including location of housing, should be determined, since environmental issues may affect the client's health state.

Sex The client's sex is simply noted as male or female.

Age and Birth Date Stated age and birth date should be noted and checked against one another for any discrepancy. Occasionally a client may err when giving a birth date. Therefore, the nurse should figure the birth date based on age to ensure accuracy in recording data.

Place of Birth The place of birth, including city, county, and state, should be carefully noted. Frequently, a birthplace can provide clues to cultural background, localized exposure to certain noxious environmental forces, or common illnesses known to be prevalent in specific areas and regions of the country.

Race and Nationality The client's race and nationality are important data, since they may be of diagnostic significance in certain health problems. For example, variations in skin color or in musculoskeletal structure may be observed during assessment; however, knowledge of race or nationality can make potentially abnormal findings well within normal limits. In addition, cultural background, an inherent component of race and nationality, will reflect important data and may influence future teaching strategies used by the nurse.

See Race.

Marital Status Marital status is generally recorded as single, married, widowed, or divorced. Each category may provide information on the client's lifestyle and help identify potential or actual support systems. If a client is single, widowed, or divorced, further data should be sought on any significant relationships. Research suggests that relationships are essential for everyone; therefore, absence of relationships may result in loneliness and could cause stress, thus affecting the client's health state. It is often assumed that a married status implies that a meaningful relationship with another person exists. This may not always be the case; therefore, careful evaluation of all relationships, including a marital situation, must be tactfully but accurately evaluated. Determination of the number of children or other dependents who pose economic responsibility should also be identified.

Note the length of years spent in each state, especially widowed or divorced, since time and perception of loss can affect health.

Religious Affiliation The client's religious affiliation may be an additional influencing factor on health state. A person's health beliefs, values, and attitudes can be closely linked to and influenced by religion. For example, some people believe that when they become ill, they are being punished by God for some wrongdoing earlier in life. This can create a problem for the client and may lead to delayed healing or the seeking out of nonprofessional health care through "religious healing." Although the latter may prove helpful for some, it may not influence the client's health perception.

See Health Status Perception.

Religion may also directly affect both treatment of health problems and compliance with health care regimes. Most members of the Jehovah's Witness Congregation, for example, directly refuse the administration of blood components to any family member even in the face of impending death, because of religious beliefs. Therefore, health care is affected.

In addition, religion can dictate health patterns for its followers, as in the case of circumcision. Followers of the Jewish faith often enlist a rabbi to perform circumcision of all male offspring as part of a special religious ceremony. Most other circumcisions of male infants are performed by an obstetrician.

As these examples show, the potential influence of religion on the client often relates to life experiences and should be viewed as integral to the health history.

The nurse must thoroughly assess religion as an integral component of the biographical data.

Occupation Current occupation will differ among clients. Today, job opportunities, improved pay scales, flexibility of hours, mobility, and lifestyle all influence job selection. These factors may result in a client who works in an area in which he or she was not previously trained or educated. In other instances, a person may follow the same career throughout a lifetime. Whatever the situation, data on current place of employment, as well as on previous work experiences, should be identified. In addition, a description of the work setting and potential occupational hazards should be noted and adequately assessed and evaluated later in the interview.

Note the client's current occupation and usual occupation if they differ.

Social Security Number The Social Security number is used as a means of identification and also makes easy the retrieval of client records. It should be clearly noted on a specific place on the client's record for quick access.

Accuracy in recording the Social Security number is essential.

Health Perception / Health Management
How a person perceives and maintains health reveals much about that person's biological and psychological properties and sociological and cultural values, beliefs, and attitudes. It is essential to recall that a definition of health is based on self-knowledge about health and illness and interpretation of that knowledge. Depending on that definition, a client may demonstrate a wide and variable range of health behaviors. The nurse must learn to recognize the client behavior appropriate to states of wellness.

See the discussion on concepts of health and the philosophy of holistic health in Chap. 1.

Frequently clients seek health care only when they perceive that deviations or changes have occurred in their health state.

See Chap. 1 for a definition of wellness.

Steele and McBroom state that health behaviors are "preventive behaviors, consisting of the utilization of health services for the assumed purpose of maintaining or improving one's health and avoiding the effects of illness."[19] This definition might be broadened to incorporate the idea that health behaviors could include the client who has a known health problem and is seeking resolution to that problem. The nurse must keep in mind that the client's health status perception is an important reflection of the perceived value of health behaviors.

Questions to elicit data

1 How would you define health?

2 What do you do routinely to maintain your health?

3 Do you believe that health is a priority in your life? What is more important? What is less important?

4 What makes you feel less healthy? When? Is there a pattern to these feelings?

5 Do you wait for certain signs or symptoms to appear before seeking health care?

6 Do you have home remedies for treatment of certain signs or symptoms?

7 What alternatives to health care do you use?

8 What made you decide to seek health care today?

The nurse may wish to record notes when eliciting these data to avoid any omissions.

Signs are objective responses; *symptoms* are subjective responses generated by the client. Signs are validated by physical examination.

9 Do you feel that it is important to be included in decision making regarding your health care?

10 Do you trust health care professionals when it comes to managing your care?

11 How do you decide if you are not healthy?

12 Do you believe health care is your right? Do you feel comfortable seeking health care?

13 What is it like to be a client of the health care system?

14 Do you believe that you have any responsibilities as a client (e.g., to self, to health care providers, in following health care recommendations, or in decision making)?

15 Do you understand what is expected of you as a client?

16 Can you identify your expectations of the nurse, doctor, health care delivery system?

17 Has your family been included in your health care? How?

Highlights

Present questions so that the client is encouraged to answer thoroughly.

If the client is a child, direct questions to the parent or caretaker, since his or her perceptions and values influence the child.

Understanding the client's own perception of role facilitates articulation of the nurse's role with the client's role. As a result, the potential for an optimal outcome of health care will be enhanced.

It is also essential that the nurse make his or her role clear to the client; see Holism and the Nursing Process in Chap. 1.

Current Health Status and Health Habits Further delineation of health status perception includes collecting data on the client's current health status and health habits. Determination of these variables provides clarification of the individual's perception of his or her present state of health. Specific interviewing questions can be used to focus the client's attention on various aspects of the topic.

Questions to elicit data

1 How would you describe your present health condition?

2 Do you feel that your health is compromised in any way? If so, how?

3 What aspects of your health state do you feel good about?

The nurse should adapt questions on health status to individual situations.

When questioning the client about health habits, the nurse should use discretion so as not to offend the client or place value judgments on client behavior. When questioning a child, it is important to verify answers with the parent or caretaker unless data are revealed to the nurse "in confidence."

See Health Habits in Chap. 1.

See Nutritional Patterns.

See sleep patterns in Biological Rhythms.

Questions to elicit data

1 Do you smoke tobacco (cigarettes, cigars, pipe)? How many packs a day or how much a day? How long have you been smoking regularly? Have you tried to quit?

2 How does smoking or smoke in the air affect you?

3 Do you use street drugs (e.g., marijuana, heroin, cocaine, speed, angel dust)? How much a day? How often? For how long? Have you ever noticed any side-effects? Would you like to quit using the drug(s) at any time?

4 Do you use any drugs or medications prescribed by a physician? Do you use nonprescription (over-the-counter) drugs? How often? For what purpose?

Children or adolescents may be unwilling to share personal information unless certain that the nurse will keep it confidential, or use it to facilitate health care.

5 How do you maintain personal hygiene (such as skin, dental, eye, and foot care)?

Highlights

Depending on the client's answers, the nurse may make a preliminary judgment on whether the client requires health maintenance, health promotion, or restoration of health. Further data collection will confirm the nurse's assessment.

Past Health Status To obtain a more accurate historical profile, an assessment of the client's previous health status is essential. The following data should be included, appropriate to the client's age:

1 Birth history
2 Growth and development
3 Common childhood illnesses
4 Immunizations
5 Previous hospitalizations
6 Accidents or injuries
7 Allergies or allergic reactions

The present health state of an adult or child usually depends on past health conditions.

The nurse should take notes so that data are not forgotten.

Birth History The birth history is divided into prenatal, natal, and postnatal periods. The prenatal period spans conception to birth and includes significant data on the mother's health during pregnancy. The natal period is the time surrounding the actual birth, and labor and delivery information is noted. The postnatal period refers to the period from birth through 2 weeks of age. The birth history may influence one's life and how one ages. Those physical, behavioral, and psychological parameters that occur at birth should be recorded carefully.

See Chap. 5 for a discussion of prenatal and postnatal periods.

See Chap. 11 for a discussion of the natal period.

Growth and Development Collecting data on growth and development is essential whether the client is a child, an adolescent, or an adult. Growth measurements include weight and height. Head and chest circumferences are also taken in children. Growth is expected to occur progressively with age. Development is usually evaluated with standardized screening tools. Past strengths and weaknesses should be noted.

See Chaps. 5 through 14, which discuss growth and development specific to each age.

Common Childhood Illnesses Mention of common childhood illnesses will alert the nurse to potential factors that put the client at risk for present or future health problems. The client or informant should be questioned about illnesses such as measles, mumps, rubella, diphtheria, pertussis, tetanus, smallpox, streptococcal infections and rheumatic fever, and poliomyelitis. If a positive response is elicited, the nurse should then request specific details about the event and/or age of onset, treatment, and health care follow-up.

Immunizations Recently national emphasis has been placed on immunizing infants and children against many of the common childhood illnesses. Polio and diphtheria, once prevalent in the United States and elsewhere, are now almost nonexistent because of successful immunization programs. Because these and other diseases are now extremely rare, there appears to be a somewhat relaxed attitude among Americans about immunization of children. Hence, the nurse must stress the need for immunization.

See Chaps. 5 through 14 for immunization schedules.

In questioning the client or informant, the nurse should seek data about when and where immunizations were received and what, if any, adverse reactions or side-effects occurred. If the client has never been immunized, the nurse should consider developing an immunization schedule as soon as possible.

Previous Hospitalizations The nurse should gather the following information concerning previous hospitalization:

1 Reason for admission

2 Place of admission

3 Length of stay

4 Surgical procedures undergone

5 Other

For each category, the nurse should ask questions that will further determine needed data. Questions about the success of the treatment, development of complications, present effects of hospitalizations, and follow-up care will elicit specific information. When necessary, past hospital records may be used to obtain a more complete background on a specific hospitalization.

Accidents or Injuries All accidents and injuries should be fully listed and described, including the time, place, and events surrounding the incident. In addition, the overall impact of the accident or injury on the client's health state should be determined and evaluated accordingly.

Allergies or Allergic Reactions Many people are allergic to a variety of substances within the environment. Therefore, it is important for the nurse to determine these materials and their overall impact on the client's health state.

Specific allergic reactions to foods, drugs or medications, inhalants such as pollens, insects or animals, and other environmental agents or contactants should be carefully noted. The nurse should ask the client to

Table 3-3
Family History

Relative	Age, yr	General Health; Disease	Cause of Death, Age
Maternal			
Grandmother		Good	Heart failure, 86
Grandfather	90	Fair; arthritis	
Aunt	65	Good; obese	
Uncle		Poor; hypertension, heart disease	Heart attack, 57
Paternal			
Grandmother		Poor; diabetes	Complications of diabetes, 50
Grandfather	77	Heavy smoker; lung cancer	

Familial or Inherited Disorders	Client	Relative
Heart disease		
Hypertension		
Arteriosclerosis		
Coronary artery disease		
Blood disorders		
Renal disease		
Cancer		
Diabetes mellitus		
Obesity		
Arthritis		
Gout		
Mental illness		
Epilepsy		
Migraine		
Allergies		
Anemia		

describe the timing of occurrence, the reaction to the causative factor, and the treatment which is used to obtain relief. If the client has undergone specific testing to isolate allergens, determining when and how this was done and the results obtained will be of great importance.

If the client is unaware of allergies to any of the above categories, the nurse should rephrase questions to elicit data about common allergic-type symptoms that occur with allergic reactions. Examples of questions that may provide data about potential allergic reactions denied earlier by the client are "Do you ever develop watery, itchy eyes after exposure to . . . ?" "Have you ever had a skin rash develop after eating certain foods?" "Do you experience nasal congestion or difficult breathing after contact with certain animals?"

In addition to allergic responses to elements within the environment, it is important to ask specifically if the client was ever treated with an antibiotic (e.g., penicillin) or received a blood transfusion. Since allergic reactions to both are not uncommon, it is as important to know the reaction as it is to know that the person has taken the drug and has not had a reaction.

Allergic responses can include sneezing, itching, nasal congestion, watery eyes, difficulty in breathing, fever, chills, skin rash, and irritability.

Family History Questions about the client's family should include information about maternal and paternal grandparents and continue inquiries in descending chronological order. Parents, aunts, uncles, cousins, and siblings are included. Table 3-3 contains a sample chart that the nurse might use to record data on family history.

When familial tendencies or inherited disorders are present, detailed data are collected. Since there are innumerable inherited disorders, a checklist of the main ones is incorporated into the chart in Table 3-3.

Genetically transmitted disorders (such as sickle cell anemia or hemophilia) should be identified, since risk of recurrence in offspring is possible. Recording of data in a family tree (Fig. 3-2) is another method

Discussion of family is expanded in Chap. 2.

See Chap. 1 for a discussion on family history.

The client may be referred for genetic counseling.

Figure 3-2 Family tree.

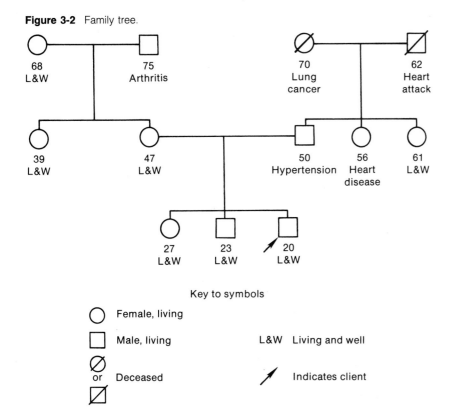

Key to symbols

○ Female, living

□ Male, living   L&W Living and well

⊘ or ⊠ Deceased   ↗ Indicates client

of completing the family history. Visual representation may assist the client in recognizing the influence of the family history on his or her health status. Whatever method is used to collect family history, it is important that it be thoroughly completed, since the data elicited can help to identify populations at risk and determine preventive health teaching.

Life Patterns and Lifestyle

Discussion of lifestyle refers to those patterns that make up a person's way of socially, psychologically, physically, and culturally interacting with the environment. This component of the health history includes personal characteristics (e.g., age, race, heredity), patterns of growth and development (including behavioral development), and other factors that are part of a person's daily existence. Data collection should be thorough, since factors can affect the client's health status.

Age The nurse should assess variables related to age that may affect health care.

Questions to elicit data

1 Are you satisfied with your present age? Do you wish you were older or younger? Why?
2 What do you fear most about aging?
3 What age did you enjoy the most? Why?
4 Do you feel that your health is currently good? Explain.
5 How do you plan to stay healthy as you get older? Do you look forward to retirement? What are your plans for retirement?

Race The nurse will have noted racial characteristics when collecting biographical data. As a lifestyle factor, race can be further assessed.

Questions to elicit data

1 What effects does your race have on your lifestyle?
2 Do you think your race affects your health? How?
3 Do you know of any health problems you have that can be related to your race? Any problems in family members?
4 Are there any preventive health measures you (need to) follow because of your race? Describe.

Heredity The data collected in the family history will provide the nurse with the basis for further inquiry into heredity.

Questions to elicit data

1 Do you know of any familial tendencies toward disease?
2 Do you have a family history of any genetic disorder?
3 Are you at all concerned about having children with physical or mental defects? Why?
4 Do you have any relatives (maternal and paternal) with a physical or mental defect?

Accurate determination of familial health problems will help identify risk population and direct preventive health education.

See Age in Chap. 1.

See data collected on Exercise-activity Patterns and health habits.

See Culture, Family Life, and Nutrition.

See Family History.

Concerns about the effects of genetic defects apply to clients of childbearing age.

Data obtained using the above questions is integrated with family history data to complete this part of the assessment. Both should be used to determine factors that will enhance health and reveal potential risk factors.

Culture   It is important that the nurse know certain values, attitudes, acts, and patterns of perceiving the world that have special cultural meaning for a client, since these may affect the client's health state. The guidelines below should be helpful.

1 Determine the meaning of communication patterns. Language and the thought patterns that result from language are influenced by culture. Vocabulary, body language, and voice qualities vary within a culture and convey specific meanings. A preschooler may say, for example, "I don't eat medicines unless Mommy gives them to me, because she said they will make me sick." This child has learned that medicines are not toys and that the amount taken must be controlled by the mother. This is health teaching that is valued by the mother and conveyed to her child through language.

2 Determine how the client obtains and uses resources in the environment to maintain physical welfare. For example, one person may consider food and housing as a priority and spend a paycheck purchasing such items, while another may consider clothing as a priority and spend money on this because of the desire to convey to others that he or she can afford nice clothes. Such diversity in value systems reflects cultural influence.

3 Determine how family roles and relationships influence the client's attitudes toward health and the ability to follow health practices. A single, teenage girl, for example, may be sexually active but does not practice birth control because she fears that her parents may find out. She is taking a risk of becoming pregnant. The girl is influenced by the cultural norms of her peers to have sex and, at the same time, is aware of her parents' attitude toward teenage sexual behavior. The situation results in conflict for the girl, thus potentially jeopardizing her health state.

In many situations the nurse will find that culture has a great influence on the client's health attitudes and health behaviors.

Growth and Development   When assessing client growth, development, and maturation, the nurse will want to focus on four major areas: physical, cognitive, social, and emotional capabilities. Throughout the remaining chapters of the text, unique characteristics of each stage of development will be elaborated on.

   Physical Capabilities   Physical capabilities include gross and fine motor skills that depend on intact skeletomuscular and neurological systems. Since these two systems are highly interactive, they can be assessed continuously throughout the physical examination. Data collected later on activity will add to the assessment. Developmental screening tests and age-specific general assessment tools provide further information. Questions related to physical strength, stamina, fatigue, and pain are important components to include in the data collection.

   Cognitive Capabilities   Thought, perception, understanding, and reasoning are the cognitive capabilities assessed. Throughout the interview the nurse should be evaluating the client's capabilities in respond-

See Culture, Chap. 1, when assessing the client's culture.

Children are affected by culture through child-rearing practices.

The client learns to meet basic needs through cultural experiences.

Family roles and relationships can affect the health beliefs a person adopts.

See Chaps. 1 and 5 through 14 for more specific and complete data across the life span.

See Chap. 4 and the sections on growth and development in Chaps. 5 through 14.

See Cognitive/Perceptual Patterns for further detail.

ing to questions and conveying information. Assessment of neurological status throughout the physical examination will provide more definite information.

Social Capabilities Social capabilities include establishing harmonious relationships or affiliations with one's family, friends, and others. The beginnings of these social interactions take place at birth through mother-father-child attachment processes. Development depends on continued reinforcement of positive social encounters throughout the life span. Data collected earlier on family life can be incorporated into this assessment of relationships.

Some developmental assessment tools, such as the Denver Developmental Screening Test (DDST), provide methods for more detailed evaluation. The nurse should use whatever tools are available for collecting data.

Emotional Capabilities Emotional capabilities comprise one's awareness and application of affect and feelings to other people and situations encountered during daily life. The person learns to be responsive to inner feelings as well as to others' feelings, develops coping abilities to deal with accomplishments and stresses, and assumes responsibility for his or her behavior.

The nurse assesses these capabilities throughout the interviewing process. Also, data collected on sexuality patterns will provide insight into the client's emotional stability.

Questions to elicit data

1 Do you feel that you are emotionally stable? How do you usually cope with stress?

2 How do you identify stressors?

3 Do you have any difficulty coping with daily stresses?

4 Do you see (or have you ever seen) a psychiatrist or psychologist for counseling or treatment?

5 Do you feel good about yourself as a person? How do you act when you are happy? When you are sad?

Answers to the above questions will increase the nurse's perception of the client's emotional sense of well-being. It is important for the nurse to observe and assess behavior patterns because data will provide insight into the client's self-concept, motivations, and means of adapting or coping in daily life. Since norms for behavioral development have been established based on various theorists (e.g., Freud, Erikson, Piaget), the nurse can use these norms as a frame of reference when compiling data. Chaps. 5 through 14 also give specific information about the unique patterns of behavior identified in each age group across the life span, and these chapters should be referred to in order to further verify norms of behavioral development.

Biological Rhythms Biological rhythms which can be assessed by the nurse include patterns of sleep and waking, elimination, food intake (nutrition), vital signs, the menstrual cycle, mood, and activity. These regularly recurring processes may indicate the client's state of well-being (e.g., vital signs) or may have an influence on the client's health state (e.g., alteration in the sleep-wakefulness cycle). Thus, it is important that the nurse attempt to identify circadian, ultradian, and infradian rhythms and to assess their impact on the client.

See Chaps. 5 through 14 for age-specific assessment on social abilities.

Most developmental assessment tools pertain only to children. See Chaps. 5 through 14.

See Chaps. 5 through 14 for age-specific assessments related to emotions and coping responses.

See Coping Patterns and Stress Tolerance Patterns.

Self-perception/conception patterns influence emotions.

See Chap. 2 for a complete discussion of behavioral development.

Tom has validated interview questions related to biological rhythms which can be incorporated into the health history by the nurse.[20] These questions are divided into subjective data (client-related) and objective data (observed by the nurse) and are contained in Table 3-4. Once data are interpreted, validated, and evaluated, the nurse may be able to assist the client with appropriate interventions.

It is important to remember during assessment that infants' and children's rhythms differ from those of adults, and rhythms of various functions develop circadian periodicity at different times after birth.[21]

Also, it may be difficult for the nurse to collect the objective data as identified by Tom. This data requires direct assessment over 24 to 72 hours minimum. However, the nurse could request that the client keep a detailed record for a specified time at home and submit the data at a subsequent health visit.

Data on the menstrual cycle are also useful.

Questions to elicit data

1 Do you ever experience physical or emotional changes before your menstrual period? Describe. Do these affect your ability to function as usual?

2 Do you experience behavioral swings during your menstrual cycle? Describe.

3 Do you ever experience severe cramps, nausea, or diarrhea (all symptoms of dysmenorrhea) during your menstrual period? Do you use medication to treat these symptoms?

4 How do these premenstrual and menstrual changes affect family and work relationships?

Highlights

See Biological Rhythms in Chap. 1 and Chaps. 5 to 14 for age-specific information.

Body rhythms can be altered by changes in time zones, stress, and shift work.

Both the premenstrual syndrome and dysmenorrhea are considered to be physiological disorders caused by hormonal imbalances.

Table 3-4
Tool for Assessing Circadian Rhythms

Subjective data
  Would you consider yourself a "day" person or a "night" person?
  If you had your choice, would you go to bed after midnight or much earlier?
  What time do you usually go to bed and get up in the morning?
  How does it make you feel when you are forced to change these habits, e.g., because of your job, long-distance travel, or hospitalization?
  Do you feel sociable and cheerful or antisocial and grumpy when you first get up? If you are grumpy and irritable, how long does this last?
  Do you have a "best" or a "worst" time of day? What makes you classify it as best or worst?
  Do you have any physical complaints that you notice? Do these correlate with when you feel best or worst?
  How many meals do you eat a day? What times do you usually eat them? When do you eat your largest meal?
  How often do you usually urinate during a day? Do you get up at night to void? How often do you move your bowels? Is this a regular pattern for you? What do you do to keep elimination patterns regular?
  Do you perspire? When? How much?
  How many hours of sleep do you require to feel good? Do you awaken during your sleep cycle? Why? Can you fall back to sleep? Do you take naps? What helps you to fall asleep?
  Do you ever have recurring dreams during sleep? Do the dreams frighten or awaken you?
Objective data
  Daily peaks and troughs on temperature, pulse, and respiration and blood pressure graphic records
  Urinary excretory patterns (quantity and frequency in relation to time of day)
  Consistent behavior patterns (cheerful, alert, energetic, and verbose or irritable, quiet, less alert, and lethargic) in relation to time of day
  Environment, e.g., lighting schedule activity—rest schedule, meal times, presence of clocks or other time cues
  Medication patterns (name of drug, quantity, and frequency in relation to time of day)

Source: Adapted from Cheryl K. Tom, "Nursing Assessment of Biological Rhythms," *Nurs Clin North Am* **11:**621–630 (1976).

Environmental Factors Information about the type of environment the client lives in is important to the nurse in planning health care.

Highlights

See the discussion on Environmental Factors in Chap. 1.

Questions to elicit data

1 How are you affected by the weather and climate in your home environment?

2 Do seasonal changes affect your health in any way? Describe.

3 Do you have running water in your home? Is it city water? Is it fluoridated? Approximately how many cups of water do you drink in a day? Do you know of any factory waste products that are contaminating your water supply? Do you drink bottled or spring water?

4 Do you live in a densely populated area? Is there much pollution (industrial, air, wastes, automobile)? How are you affected by air pollution?

5 Do you smoke? How are you affected by smoke? Do members of your family smoke?

See questions posed about smoking in Health Habits.

6 Are you exposed to any air pollutants in your home or work environments (such as aerosols and fumes)? Describe.

7 Describe your home and work environments with regard to noise levels, lighting, air quality, and number of persons who share those environments.

Assessment of potential noxious factors in the client's environment is also necessary to promote wellness and, possibly, to prevent disease.

See Environmental Factors, Occupation, and Nutritional Patterns for questions that pertain to this assessment.

Questions to elicit data

1 What do you feel are the most significant pollutants or noxious factors you are exposed to daily?

2 Do you think that air, water, soil, and noise pollution affect your health? How?

3 What do you do to help prevent these different kinds of pollution?

4 Are you politically involved in fighting pollution? Do you make your feelings known to legislators?

5 How close is your home to a nuclear power plant? Does this concern you?

6 Did your mother ever take diethylstilbestrol (DES) to prevent threatened abortion in pregnancy?

7 How do you protect yourself from sun exposure? Do you use a sunscreen?

8 How do you prevent pollution or hazards in your home? At work? In school? In your neighborhood?

9 How do you protect against food-pollution hazards?

10 How do you protect against noise pollution from a stereo, television, appliances, or heavy equipment?

11 What do you teach your children about pollution?

12 What preventive health measures do you follow to counteract the potential adverse effects of pollution?

Economics The nurse should then collect economic data.

Highlights

See Economics in Chap. 1.

Questions included in the occupational history may apply.

Questions to elicit data

1 What is your major source of income?
2 Is your income adequate for purchasing necessities such as food, clothing, and household items?
3 Can you identify any financial worries, such as large bills?
4 Is your spouse employed? If you are living with someone, do you share expenses?
5 Do you have money saved in case of an emergency?
6 Do you have a health insurance policy? Does it cover your family? Do you understand your policy?
7 Do you have any outstanding medical bills?
8 How will you pay for your health care today?
9 Do you have supplemental forms of income?
10 Do you collect welfare money?
11 Do you worry about not having enough money to buy things?
12 How would you describe your current financial status?

Community Resources When assessing the client's knowledge or use of community resources, the nurse must ask specific questions based on personal knowledge of what is available.

See Community Resources in Chap. 1.

Questions to elicit data

1 Do you use or have you ever used an association, organization, a foundation or society that is health related (e.g., March of Dimes, Red Cross, American Heart Association)?
2 Do you use neighborhood health clinics? For what purpose?
3 Have you ever been visited at home by a public health nurse? Why?
4 Have you sought or received financial assistance from any health-related group in your community?
5 Do you feel that you could benefit from any particular community resource? Which one? Why?
6 Would you like a referral to any community resource?

If the client is totally unaware of community resources available, the nurse should note this during assessment.

Roles and Relationship Patterns

Inherent in the assessment of roles and relationship patterns is exploration of a client's role (e.g., provider, father, mother) and the responsibilities of that particular role within the context of the person's current lifestyle. This includes gathering data about the client's occupational history. Family support systems, family dynamics, and societal relationships that may influence this pattern area should also be assessed.

Questions to elicit data

1 What do you consider your role(s) to be within your family and society?

2 Have there been any major changes in your roles and/or responsibilities recently? Explain.

3 Do you foresee changes in the coming years? Have you begun to prepare for any of these changes?

4 Describe your relationship with your children. Do you plan to expand your family? Are your parenting patterns different from those of your parents? Explain.

Family Life The status one holds in the family and the roles one performs may affect health and the ability to adapt to challenging and changing situations. Determining these roles, as well as family relationships that may be supportive or restrictive, may contribute to overall compliance to a plan of care.

When exploring family relationships, the nurse must keep in mind that this is very personal information. Questions must not be probing; they should be straightforward.

Questions to elicit data

1 What is your family composition? Who is the most significant person in your life?

2 Elicit data on roles of members. Who works? Who does household chores? Who pays the bills? Who is head of the household?

3 Do you depend on relatives (significant others) for any type of help or support?

4 Who makes the major decisions that affect family members?

5 Is family income adequate for buying goods and services?

6 How do you resolve conflicts?

7 How do you and your family cope with stress (e.g., emotional, financial, compromising health)?

8 What preventive health care do you and/or your family participate in?

9 How do you and your family react to illness of members?

10 How do you deal with health care emergencies?

11 Do you have a primary health care provider?

12 Do you and your family do activities (leisure, religious) together? How often? Describe.

13 How do family customs and beliefs affect your lifestyle?

See Chap. 2 for more indepth discussion of family.

When assessing families, the ideal would be to actually observe family functioning in the home.

Occupation In collecting occupational history data from both adults and children, the goals are (1) to identify all information that may help in recognizing past and present occupational hazards, (2) to evaluate client satisfaction and productivity in a job, (3) to identify stressors that may adversely affect physical, psychological, social, and emotional health, and (4) to assist the client with ways to cope with hazards, problems, or stressors.

See Occupation in Chap. 1.

Questions to elicit data

1 Are you happy with your occupation and your position?

2 Do you gain personal satisfaction from your work situation?

3 Do you think your work environment is safe?

4 Are there health hazards? Describe any preventive measures used by your employer to help reduce these hazards.

5 Does your employer provide health insurance, health screening facilities, and health services for employees?

6 Can you take time off from work when ill or for routine health visits? How many sick days did you take this past year?

7 Are you aware of the effects on health of such occupational contaminants as chemicals, plastics, detergents, pesticides, aerosols, solvents, exhaust, explosives, radiation, anesthetics, and the like?

8 Do you believe that certain contaminants can be carried home and thus be hazardous to family members (e.g., asbestos)?

9 Do you believe certain occupational contacts can affect your reproduction or children you may conceive? How?

10 Does your work cause stress? How does this affect you?

11 Is your income adequate?

12 How do you travel to and from work? What is the distance? Does traveling bother you?

13 If the client is a housewife the nurse should ask, What does your typical day involve? Does your role cause any stress? Describe.

For children, adolescents, and young adults, school is a major occupation. Therefore, when interviewing these clients the nurse may pose questions on school attendance. Questions should be phrased appropriately and clearly for the age of the client.

Questions to elicit data

1 Do you enjoy school? What are your favorite subjects?

2 Are you involved in sports or other activities? Do you find this enjoyable?

3 Do you have favorite games or activities?

4 Do you think your school and play environments are safe? Why?

5 Does your school have a health service and a school nurse? What does the nurse do?

6 What things in your school and play environments may be harmful to your health?

7 Do you think that you can become ill because of school, school-related activities, or play activities? How?

Societal Relationships Depending on the client's age and reason for seeking health care, the nurse may need to alter the style of questioning about societal relationships.

See Societal Relationships in Chap. 1.

Questions to elicit data

1 What do you perceive your social status to be?

2 What is your status or position at work?

3 Do you supervise other employees? How do you feel about this?

4 Are you a member of any work-related committees, clubs, unions, or organizations?

5 Do you hold a leadership position? Describe.

6 What other organizations are you a member of (e.g., church, school)? What is your position?

7 Are you excused from work (or committees, clubs, church) and other responsibilities when you feel ill?

8 Do you participate in mass screening or optional health treatment programs? How often?

9 How do you think government influences your health care?

Self-Perception and Self-Concept Patterns

When assessing client self-perception and self-concept patterns, the nurse examines the client's self-knowledge and attitudes and includes a description of the client's self-image in relation to personal appearance and competence (cognitive, affective, and psychomotor). Data collected should reflect a person's values and personal sense of worth as well as personal goals and opportunities for achievement.

Some of the data collected about life patterns may reinforce data collected here.

Questions to elicit data

1 Do you feel good about yourself? Do you feel comfortable with the way you look and feel?

2 How would you describe yourself to another person? Your physical appearance? Your personality?

3 What would you describe as your strengths and weaknesses?

4 Are there things you would like to change about yourself? Describe.

5 Are you pleased with your accomplishments so far? Describe.

6 Do you have future goals you would like to achieve? Would you like to accomplish these in 5 years? In 10 years?

Cognitive and Perceptual Patterns

Exploration of a client's sensory perceptions (including vision, hearing, taste, smell, and touch) and cognitive abilities, based on education and intelligence, are components of this pattern area. Use of prosthetics (e.g., eyeglasses, hearing aids) should be noted, and the regularity of their use described. Also, the client should be asked to describe pain perception and pain tolerance and comfort measures used to promote relaxation.

Sensory Perception

Questions to elicit data

1 Vision

How would you describe your vision? Do you wear glasses? Do you see as well as you did 5 years ago? Have you ever experienced eye pain, itching, headache, or any problems with your eyes? Does anyone in your family have eye problems? When was your last eye examination?

2 Hearing

How well do you hear? Describe. Have you experienced any changes in your hearing in the past 5 years? Does anyone in your family have hearing problems? Do you use any type of hearing aid or device? When was your last hearing examination?

Questions exploring sensory perception also provide data about the client's neurological status.

3 Taste
Describe your sense of taste. Have you noticed changes in your sense of taste in the past 5 years? Describe.

4 Smell
Can you smell all odors in your environment, such as food and flowers? Have you noted any changes in your ability to detect odors? Describe.

5 Touch
Describe your sense of touch. Do you lack feeling in any area or part of your body? Have you experienced any changes in your ability to feel when touching or being touched? Describe. Do you think you are very sensitive to pain? When you experience pain, how do you handle it?

Education Education is reflected in intellectual ability relative to age. During the interviewing process, the nurse should continually assess the client's reasoning powers, capacity of understanding, and competency in engaging in abstract thought.

When interviewing children about their educational process, the nurse must be aware of the child's intellectual and developmental levels. Questions should provide for evaluation of interests in school, achievement records, motivation to learn, and future interests in continued education.

See Education in Chap. 1.

Education may affect the client's understanding of the health process and ability to follow a health care regimen.

Questions to elicit data

1 What grade have you completed or what is your highest earned degree?

2 Do (did) you enjoy school?

3 What are (were) your favorite subjects?

4 Do (did) you receive good grades?

5 Did you ever receive any achievement awards?

6 How would you describe your memory? How long can you pay attention to something before becoming distracted?

7 Will your education prepare you for an occupation?

8 Do you have any areas of difficulty in your studies? Is there a particular way you learn more easily than another?

9 Do you think an education is important?

Intelligence As discussed in Chap. 1, intelligence can be measured by various achievement tests. This information, however, is not always completely reliable or readily available. Therefore, during the interviewing process the nurse should assess indications of mature learning and thinking capacity. This is reflected in the client's ability to communicate requested data to the nurse.

More specifically, the nurse should appraise the client's following abilities:

See Occupation and Education; also see Chaps. 5 through 14 for patterns of intellectual development across the life span.

1 To perform motor tasks during physical examination (e.g., writing, picking up an object, walking)

2 To follow directions when given a task or asked a question

3 To communicate verbally and nonverbally appropriate to the situation

4 To relate to the nurse with acceptable social behavior and mannerisms

See Chap. 4 for assessment of intellectual abilities during the physical examination.

Sexuality and Reproductive Patterns

Discussions related to sexuality and reproduction are important but can be threatening to the client. Therefore, it is essential that the nurse approach assessment sensitively. Significant considerations include the client's perceived satisfaction with his or her sexuality, female reproductive patterns, male and female premenopausal or postmenopausal state, and menstrual patterns. The client should be asked to note perceived problems within this pattern area and to determine how long the problems have persisted. Dating patterns and a person's approach to social interaction can be explored as appropriate.

The nurse should pose questions to the client that will elicit data about sexual identification, self-concept, self-esteem, and related patterns of behavior.

See Chap. 2 for an indepth discussion of sexuality.

Questions to elicit data

1 How do you feel about yourself?

2 Are you satisfied with your physical appearance or would you like to change it?

3 What makes you feel as though you are male (female)?

4 Are you sexually active? For how long?

5 Do you have an enjoyable sexual relationship? Do you have the same partner?

6 Are you satisfied with your knowledge of sex? Would you like more information?

7 Do you use birth control methods? What? When? How often?

8 Did you have a good relationship with your mother and father? Did they provide you with sex education?

9 Do you have children? What do you teach them about sex?

10 Do you ever feel discriminated against because of your sex? Describe.

11 How do you think your sex/sexuality affects your health?

12 Have you ever had venereal disease? If so, what treatment did you receive?

Females

13 Describe your menstrual cycle (onset of menses, duration, last menstrual period, any problems).

14 Have you ever been pregnant (abortions, miscarriages, number of living children)? Did you enjoy being pregnant? Were your pregnancy and delivery uncomplicated?

15 Do you examine your breasts regularly? How often?

16 What was the date of your last Pap smear?

17 Have you experienced menopause? Describe. What are your expectations if it has not occurred?

Males

18 Do you ever experience problems with intercourse?

19 Do you have any feelings about male menopause?

20 Do you examine your testes?

Nutritional Patterns

The depth of nutritional information gathered will depend on the purpose of the client's health care visit. The client's age and sex and body size,

See Nutrition in Chap. 1.

Highlights

The nurse must approach the discussion of sexuality very sensitively.

It should be noted whether the client is heterosexual, bisexual, or homosexual.

See Chap. 11 for discussion of menstrual history and pregnancy.

composition, and surface area should be considered. Note that additional nutritional requirements must be met during infancy, adolescence, and pregnancy, since these are periods of increased growth and development.

Data may be collected using one or all of the following as guidelines: (1) the 24-hour recall, (2) the basic four food groups, (3) the recommended daily dietary allowances (RDA), (4) a food intake record, and (5) other miscellaneous information.

Twenty-four-hour Recall If the client's general condition is good and weight is appropriate for age and height (Table 3-5), the nurse may ask for only a 24-hour recall of the client's dietary intake. This method is simple and practical and does not require extensive recall.

Questions to elicit data

1 What did you consume at each regular meal and between meals, including beverages, during the past 24 hours?

2 What was the quantity of each item? Estimate using familiar household weights and measures.

3 Does this represent a typical day's intake?

Highlights

This part of data collection may take 30 minutes or more.

See Recommended Daily Dietary Allowances.

The 24-hour recall of food intake may not provide a totally accurate picture because of lack of memory, day-to-day variations in meal patterns, and feelings about the importance of food to health.

Table 3-5
Adult Height and Weight [Desirable weights in pounds according to height and frame (in indoor clothing)]

Height (with 1-inch heels)		Frame		
ft	in	Small	Medium	Large
		Men aged 25 and over		
5	2	112–120	118–129	126–141
5	3	115–123	121–133	129–144
5	4	118–126	124–136	132–148
5	5	121–129	127–139	135–152
5	6	124–133	130–143	138–156
5	7	128–137	134–147	142–161
5	8	132–141	138–152	147–166
5	9	136–145	142–156	151–170
5	10	140–150	146–160	155–174
5	11	144–154	150–165	159–179
6	0	148–158	154–170	164–184
6	1	152–162	158–175	168–189
6	2	156–167	162–180	173–194
6	3	160–171	167–185	178–199
6	4	164–175	172–190	182–204
		Women aged 25 and over*		
4	10	92–98	96–107	104–119
4	11	94–101	98–110	106–122
5	0	96–104	101–113	109–125
5	1	99–107	104–116	112–128
5	2	102–110	107–119	115–131
5	3	105–113	110–122	118–134
5	4	108–116	113–126	121–138
5	5	111–119	116–130	125–142
5	6	114–123	120–135	129–146
5	7	118–127	124–139	133–150
5	8	122–131	128–143	137–154
5	9	126–135	132–147	141–158
5	10	130–140	136–151	145–163
5	11	134–144	140–155	149–168
6	0	138–148	144–159	153–173

*For girls between 18 and 25, subtract 1 lb for each year under 25.
Source: Metropolitan Life Insurance Company, New York.

The nurse should then compare the client's diet to the basic four food groups and the RDA for adequacy and note any discrepancy.

Basic Four Food Groups Table A-15 describes the basic four food groups, indicating the nutrient pattern to be followed and the recommended quantity or serving size. Using the data obtained from the client's 24-hour recall, the nurse can compare the intake of essential food. "Empty-calorie" foods are not found among the four food groups, since they do not contribute to good health.

Recommended Daily Dietary Allowances The 24-hour recall is compared to the RDA (see Table A-12). The client's diet is then determined to be adequate or inadequate, depending on the way the allowances are met.

Food Intake Record A food intake record of 3 to 7 days will provide more detailed and accurate information about the client's nutritional history. Since eating patterns vary daily, it is important to include both weekdays and a weekend day.

For the recording the client is asked to list each food and beverage (including alcohol) as it is consumed throughout each day. Estimation of actual food amounts using weights and household measures is required. Again, the nurse can use the RDA and the basic four food groups to analyze nutrient and food content.

The nurse may find any or all of the following factors useful to the assessment of nutritional patterns:

1 The client's eating schedule, e.g., time of day, place, and speed of eating, food likes and dislikes, appetite
2 The effect of emotions and mood swings on appetite
3 The accessibility and availability of foods to the client
4 The client's shopping practices, e.g., use of a shopping list
5 Available cooking equipment and cooking methods; who cooks
6 The use of preservatives, additives, snack foods, dietary supplements, and fortified foods
7 Whether the client eats alone or with others
8 Whether the client's weight is appropriate for age and height (see Table 3-5)
9 Dietary and cultural patterns affecting nutritional patterns
10 Conditions that may affect the client's ability to eat or digest foods, e.g., ability to swallow, condition of teeth, use of dentures
11 The effect of alcohol consumption on appetite and/or dietary patterns

In summary, the nutritional assessment is significant, since it reflects the client's general health condition.

Exercise and Activity Patterns

The regularity with which a person moves about in carrying out activities of daily living in part determines his or her ability to expend energy

See Tables A-15 and A-12.

A food composition table is needed to approximate nutrient content.

Foods high in fat, oil, or sugar offer little nutrient value and are "empty-calorie" foods.

See the recommended daily dietary allowances in the Appendix.

In the food intake record the client is asked to record each item immediately after consumption to ensure greater accuracy.

The nurse should question the client about miscellaneous information only if it enhances the dietary assessment, since this is time consuming.

through activity. In addition, the type, quality, and frequency (regularity) of a planned exercise regimen and the types of activities that promote rest and relaxation further help to describe exercise-activity patterns. Use of leisure time should also be included as part of the client's activity pattern.

Questions to elicit data

1 What is your usual pattern of activity during the day?

2 Do you have a special exercise program? What is it? How long have you been doing it?

3 What do you feel are the benefits of physical exercise?

4 What physical activities do you enjoy most?

5 How do you determine how much activity you can tolerate? How do you feel after exercising?

6 Do you know what your heart rate is at rest and during strenuous activity?

7 Does your rate, rhythm, and depth of breathing increase with exercise?

8 Do you know what good body mechanics are?

9 What do you do on your days off from work or school?

10 Have you ever had restrictions placed on your activities because of health problems?

11 What information would you like to have about exercise?

12 Describe your leisure time activities. Do you prefer to spend time alone?

See Exercise Activity in Chap. 1.

For an exercise to be considered a pattern, it must be done at least three to four times a week.

Coping Patterns and Stress Tolerance Patterns

Exploration of the client's coping and stress tolerance patterns should reflect personality ability to handle daily stresses and life crises. Analysis of a person's capacity to resist those factors that can disrupt personal lifestyles and self-integrity should also be determined. In addition, assessment of this pattern area should include the client's (as well as the nurse's) perception of actual or potential stressors within the client's environment and reflect the client's behavior responses to stress(ors) and the processes used to cope with stress.

When assessing stress, the nurse is most interested in collecting data for use in the prevention of potential health problems.

Data collected on other patterns may be useful during this part of the assessment.

Questions to elicit data

1 How would you define stress in yourself? Identify situations that have caused you stress.

2 How do you respond physically and mentally to stressful situations?

3 Do you feel that you can handle stress? How? Do you handle stress well?

4 Does stress ever interfere with your family relationships or your work? How?

5 What stresses have you experienced during the past year? How did you deal with these? Did these stresses cause significant changes for you?

6 Do you think stress can be healthy or unhealthy?

7 How do you think stress affects your health? What do you do to relax?

8 Do you have someone special who helps you deal with stress in your daily life?

9 What makes you happy? What makes you sad?

10 Is it easy for you to express your emotions?

11 Has there been a significant loss in your life? How did you handle this loss? Do you feel that you have resolved this loss?

12 Have you experienced many recent changes in your life? Do you expect any? Would you like to make some life changes?

13 Do you feel you are coping well with your life at this point? Describe.

Review of Body Components

The review of body components enables the nurse to systematically and quickly question the client about each of the body's major anatomical and physiological parts. This will provide a means of cross-referencing data already collected during the health history and may alert the nurse to important subjective data that was previously omitted or missed or validate that data already collected.

The components covered in the review are the same that will be physically examined. See Chap. 4.

The review is usually covered from a head-to-toe (cephalad-to-caudad) approach, and the client should be given enough time to provide a thoughtful response. Since the list of information to be collected is fairly long and often difficult to remember, it may be helpful for the nurse to keep this review of body components on a card so that referral can be made, thus assuring completeness. Also, the nurse will want to take notes as each component is discussed, so that significant data will not be omitted when it comes time to record the client's entire health history.

The review of body components is subjective data; the physical examination is objective data.

Chaps. 5 through 14 address age-specific normal findings present during the review of body components.

The narrative format should emphasize the health functioning and maintenance of each body part as well as perceived problems identified by the client. If any problems are noted, further data should be elicited on any interventions that were carried out to resolve the problem(s).

The following example of the review of body components should assist the nurse in collecting data.

Avoid repetitious questioning if data were already assessed thoroughly during the health history interview.

General appearance: weight 125 lb, height 5'6 inches, well hydrated, normal pigmentation, no rashes, some skin dryness due to climate

Head: headaches occur during stress (relieved by meditation)

Hair: good distribution of shiny, silky strands of brown hair

Face: happy affect, symmetrical features, clear complexion

Eyes: clear vision, eyes sensitive to air pollution, which causes watering and itching, no corrective lenses, last examination 3 years ago

Ears: good hearing, no history of infections

Nose and sinuses: good sense of smell, sensitive to pollen, which causes sinus blockage (relieved by oral [PO] decongestants)

Mouth: sense of taste good, few dental caries, speech pattern clear and precise, oral hygiene 2 times per day, last dental check 6 months ago

Throat: occasional sore throat during winter months, infections infrequent

Neck: good range of motion

Lungs: does not smoke, tolerates vigorous physical exercise with mild shortness of breath, no chest pain

Heart: does aerobic exercises 3 times per week, not aware of any current problems, heart murmur as a child resolved at age 4

Breasts: does routine breast examination once a month, no masses

Abdomen: good appetite, no pain

Kidneys and bladder: regular urinary excretion without burning or frequency

Bowels, rectum, and anus: regular pattern of elimination every 2 to 3 days, occasional constipation relieved by increased roughage in diet

Genitalia: well developed, no discharge, no history of venereal disease

Extremities: good range of motion, physically active, occasional pain in the right knee due to an old ski injury 4 years ago, no numbness

Summary

Upon completing the health history interview, the nurse will have accumulated large amounts of data. Based on these subjective data, the nurse will have formulated impressions about the client's health status and will probably recognize which data are the most significant. The nurse may want to make additional notes on areas of the client's history that need further assessment.

Performing the physical examination will provide the nurse with objective data to complete the assessment process. Once the nurse has a total picture of the client's health status, nursing diagnoses may be formulated to describe the client's condition or problems, if any exist. From that point, the diagnosis provides a focus for developing goals for the client related to health maintenance, health promotion, or disease prevention. As the nurse continues to solve problems with the client (an active participant in decision making), together they can identify a desired outcome for health care.

The outcome indicates progress toward promoting health and resolving potential or actual problems. Once the desired outcome is known, plans of care (goals or interventions) can be identified and implemented. At a later time the nurse should evaluate the client's health state to validate resolution or to indicate that the desired outcome(s) was achieved. Thus, the nurse will have applied the nursing process to health assessment.

Recording the Health History Data

Now that the nurse has finished the client interview, all data collected are entered in the client's record as soon as possible. This record becomes a permanent, legal document that is accessible to all members of the health care team; thus, it should be complete and reflect the nurse's collaborative role with team members.

Highlights

Questions related to client skin and neurological status should be integrated into the review of body components.

Accuracy, succinctness, and thoroughness are of utmost importance when recording data.

The nurse should follow certain principles in recording the health history:

1 Review the data collected and organize it in the format of the health history. Only the most important and relevant items are recorded. Be objective, concise, and specific.

2 For clarity, write clearly and use accurate sentence structure. When computers are available, information should be concise.

3 Record data in enough detail to include all information that is relevant to each category.

4 Use the health history format and label specific entries so that they can be easily located by the reader.

5 Use only common abbreviations and symbols that will be understood by various health care professionals.

6 Date and sign the client's record, since it becomes a legal document. This will also facilitate future identification of the nurse.

When recording data, avoid repetitious content.

Record data in the client's own words.

Record all assessments. Avoid introductory phrases.

An example of a common abbreviation is qid; it means *four times a day*.

One tool for client care management that is widely used in a variety of health care settings is Weed's problem-oriented record (POR) system.[22] With this format, client information can be recorded in an organized and systematic way by any member of the health care team. The system consists of four essential components:

1 Establishing a data base: subjective information obtained during the health history, e.g., the client profile, health status perceptions, and functional pattern areas, and objective information obtained from physical examination and laboratory data.

2 Formulating a problem list: impressions and diagnoses emerge and provide the key to all information in the record. This category correlates with nursing diagnoses.

3 Delineating specific plans or goals: for each problem listed, goals should be directed toward health promotion, health maintenance, and disease prevention or resolution.

4 Follow-up of each problem: the problem is evaluated at a later time to determine progress toward achievement of goals or resolution.

To use the POR system, the nurse must (1) establish a data base, (2) formulate nursing diagnoses, (3) delineate goals, and (4) evaluate interventions.

As the client's health status changes, the problem list is updated. If more information is obtained through nursing assessments, problem titles may change as diagnoses evolve. New problems or conditions thus may be identified and added. Problems terminate when goals are achieved, i.e., problems are resolved.

Since the client's permanent record is updated by various health professionals (nurses, physicians, social workers, nutritionists), problems identified are numbered and titles remain consistent. In this way, the system is standardized, and clinical judgments, rationale, and results are all readily discernible.

The narrative notes for each problem are written on the POR and follow the SOAP format below:

S = subjective data

O = objective data

A = assessment, i.e., analysis of data resulting in a diagnosis

P = plan, i.e., goal-directed outcomes

See Table 3-6 for application of the SOAP format to an identified nursing diagnosis.

Table 3-6
Application of the SOAP Format

Nutritional Deficit
- S: "I skip breakfast, eat a salad and fruit for lunch, and have a large dinner of meat and vegetables. But I really would like to learn about good nutrition."
- O: 25-year-old female, height 5′ 8″, weight 118 lb; average daily caloric intake 1400 calories; based on requirements of basic four food groups, deficient in milk, meat, and bread and cereal groups; RDA requirements not met for protein, vitamins A, D, and B_6, thiamin, riboflavin, calcium, and iron; income adequate to purchase foods.
- A: Inadequate nutritional intake
- P: Counsel on the components of a well-balanced diet
  Balance food intake by scheduling three meals a day plus an afternoon and evening snack
  Develop a meal plan based on the four food groups and RDA
  Instruct client on how to keep a daily diary of food intake for 2 wk
  Schedule a follow-up appointment to reassess nutritional status

Since the physician's subjective and objective data focus more on disease, assessments and plans will be directed toward prevention, cure, and alleviation of disease; the nurse, however, will perform nursing assessments, interpret data (using nursing diagnoses), develop nursing care plans, and evaluate outcomes by focusing on the client's functional abilities. An example of how the nurse can record an identified functional problem using the SOAP format is contained in Table 3-6. From this example it can be seen that one category from the health history is diagnosed as not optimal. The nurse uses the POR as a tool for recording the deficiency in the SOAP format. Thus, a functional problem has been identified, and plans have been made to resolve the problem, which will be reevaluated later.

Such use of the POR will not only assist the nurse in documenting client information but will also lead to improved health care and the ability to audit client records and verify results.

REFERENCES

1. Margaret L. Pluckhan, *Human Communication: The Matrix of Nursing,* McGraw-Hill, New York, 1978, pp. ix, x.

2. Ibid., p. 14.

3. Ibid., p. 19.

4. Ibid., p. 104.

5. Talcott Parsons, *The Social System,* The Free Press, New York, 1951.

6. Henry Lederer, "How the Sick View Their World," *J Soc Issues,* 4–15 (August 1952).

7. Pluckhan, op. cit., pp. 104–105.

8. Julius Faust, *Body Language,* M. Evans, New York, 1970, p. 2.

9. Edward T. Hall, "Proxemics. A Study of Man's Spatial Relationship," in *Man's Image in Medicine and Anthropology,* International University Press, New York, 1963.

10. Arthur W. Combs, Donald L. Avila, and William W. Purkey, *Helping Relationships: Basic Concepts for the Helping Professions,* 2d ed., Allyn and Bacon, Boston, 1978.

11. P. Goldin and B. Russell, "Therapeutic Communications," *Am J Nurs* **69:**1928–1930 (September 1969).

12. J. Hays and K. Larsen, *Interacting with Patients,* Macmillan, New York, 1963.

13. Loretta Bermosk, "Interviewing: A Key to Therapeutic Communication in Nursing Practice," *Nurs Clin North Am* **1:**205–214 (1966).

14. Hildegarde Peplau, *Basic Principles of Patient Counseling,* Smith, Kline and French Laboratories, Philadelphia, 1969.

15. Annette Garrett, *Interviewing: Its Principles and Methods,* Family Service Association of America, New York, 1972.

16. William D. Brooks and Philip Emmert, *Interpersonal Communication,* William C. Brown, Dubuque, 1976.

17. Kim Giffin and Bobby R. Patton, *Fundamentals of Interpersonal Communication,* Harper & Row, New York, 1971.

18. Pluckhan, op. cit., p. 143.

19. J. L. Steele and W. H. McBroom, "Conceptual and Empirical Dimensions of Health Behavior," *J Health Soc Behav,* **13:**382–392 (December 1972).

20. Cheryl K. Tom, "Nursing Assessment of Biological Rhythms," *Nurs Clin North Am* **11:**621–630, (December 1976).

21. Theodor Hellbrügge, "The Development of Circadian Rhythms in Infants," *Cold Spring Harbor Symposia on Quantitative Biology,* **25:**311–323, 1960.

22. L. Weed, "Medical Records that Guide and Teach," *N Engl J Med* 278:593, 1969.

BIBLIOGRAPHY

Aamodt, Agnes M.: "Culture," in Ann L. Clark (ed.), *Culture, Childbearing, Health Professionals,* Davis, Philadelphia, 1978.

Anthony, E. J., and Theresa Benedek: *Parenthood: Its Psychology and Psychopathology,* Little, Brown, Boston, 1970.

Ardrey, Robert: *The Territorial Imperative,* Atheneum, New York, 1966.

Aschoff, J.: "Exogenous and Endogenous Components in Circadian Rhythms," *Cold Spring Harbor Symposia on Quantitative Biology,* **25:**11–28, 1960.

Bassler, Sandra Furman: "Origins of Biological Rhythms," *Nurs Clin North Am* **11:**575–582 (December 1976).

Battistella, R. M.: "The Right to Adequate Health Care, *Nurs Dig,* (January-February 1976).

Bentz, J. M.: "Missed Meaning in Nurse/Patient Communication," *Am J Matern Child Nurs* **5:**55–7 (January-February 1980).

Biddle, B. J., and E. J. Thomas: *Role Theory: Concepts and Research,* Wiley, New York, 1966.

Birdwhistell, Ray L.: *Kinesics and Context: Essays on Body Motion Communication,* University of Pennsylvania Press, Philadelphia, 1970.

Brown, F. A., Jr. et al.: *The Biological Clock: Two Views,* Academic Press, New York, 1970.

Burns, E. M.: "Critical Issues in Social Health Policies: Today and Tomorrow," *Man and Medicine,* **1:**205 (Spring 1976).

Byrne, Marjorie, and Lida Thompson: *Key Concepts for the Study and Practice of Nursing,* Mosby, St. Louis, 1972.

Carpenter, C. R.: "Territoriality: A Review of Concepts and Problems," in *Behavior and Evolution,* Yale University Press, New Haven, 1958.

Chinn, Peggy: *Child Health Maintenance,* 2d ed., Mosby, St. Louis, 1979.

Conroy, R. T., and J. H. Mills: *Human Circadian Rhythms,* Churchill, London, 1970.

Craig, Grace: *Human Development,* Prentice-Hall, Englewood Cliffs, N.J., 1976.

Crawford, Charles O. (ed.): *Health and the Family: A Medical-Sociological Analysis,* Macmillan, New York, 1971.

Duvall, Evelyn Millis: *Marriage and Family Development,* 5th ed., Lippincott, Philadelphia, 1977.

Felton, Geraldine: "Body Rhythm Effects on Rotating Work Shifts," *Nursing Digest,* **4:**29–32 (1976).

Gilmore, G. D.: "Planning for Family Wellness," *Health Education* **10:**12–16 (September-October 1979).

Gordon, James S.: *Final Report to the President's Commission on Mental Health of the Special Study on Alternative Mental Health Services,* U.S. Government Printing Office, Washington, D.C., 1978.

Gordon, Marjory: "Assessing Activity Tolerance," *Am J Nurs* **76:**72–75 (January 1976).

Hall, Edward T.: *The Silent Language,* Doubleday, New York, 1959.

Hall, Edward T.: *The Hidden Dimension,* Doubleday, New York, 1966.

Havighurst, R. J.: *Developmental Tasks and Education,* 3d ed., David McKay, New York, 1972.

Hewitt, F. S.: "The Nurse and Patient: Communication Skills," *Nursing Times* **77** (suppl.): 17–20 (May 1981).

Hewitt, Helan E., and Betty L. Pesznecker: "Blocks to Communication with Patients," *Am J Nurs* **64**:102–103 (July 1964).

Hill, M. M.: "When the Patient Is the Family," *Am J Nurs* **81**:536–538 (March 1981).

Hill, Reuben: *Family Development over Three Generations,* Harvard University Press, Cambridge, 1971.

Howard, Rosanne Beatrice, and Nancie Harvey Herbold: *Nutrition in Clinical Care,* McGraw-Hill, New York, 1978.

Hudson, R. Lofton: "How and How Not to Communicate," *The Denver Post,* September 24, 1978, pp. 51, 53, 55.

Kaslof, Leslie J.: *Wholistic Dimensions in Healing, A Resource Guide,* Doubleday, New York, 1978.

Katchadourian, Herant A., and Donald T. Lunde: *Fundamentals of Human Sexuality,* Holt, New York, 1972.

Kiesing, R. M.: "Theories of Culture," in B. J. Siegel, A. R. Beals and S. A. Taylor (eds.), *Annual Review of Anthropology,* Annual Reviews, Palo Alto, 1974, pp. 73–97.

Kubler-Ross, Elisabeth: "What Is It Like to Be Dying?" *Am J Nurs* **71**:54 (January 1971).

Luce, Gay Gaer: "Biological Rhythms in Psychiatry and Medicine," National Institutes of Mental Health, Public Health Services Publication no. 2088, Washington, D.C., 1970.

Mays, R. M.: "Primary Health Care and the Black Family," *Nurs Prac,* **4**:13–15, 20–21 (November-December 1979).

Meyer, Evelyn E., and Peter Sainsbury (eds.): *Promoting Health in the Human Environment,* World Health Organization, 1975.

Mills, John (ed.): *Biological Aspects of Circadian Rhythms,* Plenum Press, New York, 1973.

Murray, Ruth Beckmann, and Judith Proctor Zentner: *Nursing Assessment and Health Promotion Through the Life Span,* 2d ed., Prentice-Hall, Englewood Cliffs, N.J., 1979.

Myco, F.: "Circadian Rhythms: Clocking in," *Nurs Mirror,* **152**:32–34 (April 1981).

Nash, J.: *Developmental Psychology: A Psychobiological Approach,* Prentice-Hall, Englewood Cliffs, N.J., 1970.

Newman, B. M., and P. R. Newman: *Development through Life,* Dorsey Press, Homewood, Ill., 1975.

Pender, Nola: "The Influence of Personal Attitudes and the Expectations of Others on the Occurrence of Health-Promoting Behaviors in Adults," American Nurses' Association Publication D-67:3, 1979.

Pender, Nola: "A Conceptual Model for Preventive Health Behavior," *Nurs Outlook* **23**:385–390 (1975).

Peters, Ruanne, H. Benson, and D. Porter: "Daily Relaxation Breaks in a Working Population: Effects on Self Reported Measures of Health Performance and Well-Being," *Am J Public Health* **67**:946–953 (1977).

Rackovsky, I.: "Nurses, Nursing and Culture," *Supervisor Nurse,* **11**:20–22 (July 1980).

Rogers, C. R.: "Communication: Its Blocking and Its Facilitation," in S. I. Hayakawa (ed.), *Language, Meaning and Maturity,* Harper and Brothers, New York, 1954.

Ross, M.: "Nursing the Well Elderly," *Can Nurse,* **77**:50–55 (May 1981).

Rothberg, J. S.: "Why Nursing Diagnosis?" *Am J Nurs* **67**:1040–1042 (1967).

Ruffin, J. E.: "Changing Perspectives on Ethnicity and Health," American Nurses' Association Publication M-27:1–45, 1979.

Sarbin, T. R., and V. L. Allen: "Role Theory," in G. Lindzey and E. Aronson (eds.), *The Handbook of Social Psychology,* vol. 1, Addison-Wesley, Reading, Pa., 1968.

Sedgwick, R., et al.: "Focus on Health: Family Health Assessment," *Nurse Practitioner,* **6**:37–45, 54 (March-April 1981).

Selby, Philip: *Health in 1980–1990: A Predictive Study Based on International Inquiry,* Karger, Basel, 1974.

Serafini, Patricia: "Nursing Assessment in Industry," *Am J Public Health* **66**:755–760 (1976).

Shaw, M. E., and P. R. Costanze: *Theories of Social Psychology,* McGraw-Hill, New York, 1970.

Sterman, M. B., and Toke Hoppenbrouwers: "The Development of Sleep-Waking and Rest-Activity Patterns from Fetus to Adult," in M. B. Sterman, et al. (eds.), *Brain Development and Behavior,* Academic Press, New York, 1971.

Sussman, Marvin B.: "Family Systems in the 1970's: Analysis, Policies and Programs," *Anns Am Acad,* **396**:(July 1971).

Tudor, Mary: *Child Development,* McGraw-Hill, New York, 1981.

Volpe, P.: *Man, Nature and Society, An Introduction to Biology,* William C. Brown, Dubuque, 1975.

Wahl, P. R.: "Therapeutic Relationships with the Elderly," *Journal of Gerontological Nursing,* **6:**260–266 (May 1980).

Wilson, Robert: *The Sociology of Health, An Introduction,* Random House, New York, 1970.

Wu, Ruth: *Behavior and Illness,* Prentice-Hall, Englewood Cliffs, N.J., 1973.

Wu, Ruth: *Job Safety and Health,* vol. 3, U.S. Department of Labor, Occupational Safety and Health Administration, 1975, p. 7.

Dorothy A. Jones

Chap. 4 contains a complete discussion of the physical examination, using a head-to-toe approach.

The techniques of inspection, palpation, percussion, and auscultation are used to organize the examination of each body part.

The narrative discussion presented in the left column ties in with the photography and visual information in the middle column.

The Highlight column is used to emphasize critical information. It can also serve as a place to make notes.

This column can be used for note taking.

Diagnostic Tests are presented in each chapter following the physical examination sections and in the appendix as well.

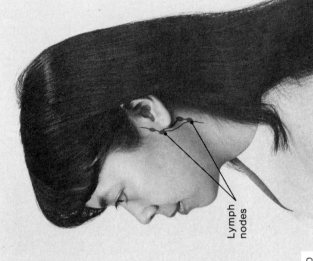

b

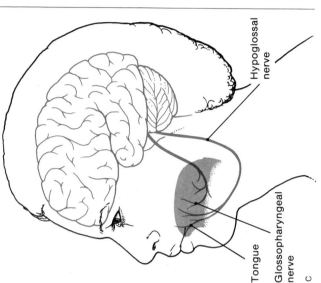

Lymph nodes

Hypoglossal nerve

Tongue

Glossopharyngeal nerve

c

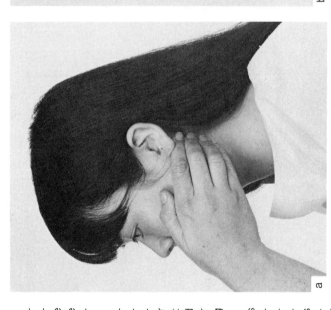

a

INTRODUCTION

This chapter presents a complete discussion of the normal physical examination. Young adults appear in many of the photographs, since it is during this age period that physical growth and development peaks.

A head-to-toe approach is used throughout this and subsequent chapters in discussing the physical examination. Information about the examination is further organized under four major headings: inspection, palpation, percussion, and auscultation. These four heads appear as appropriate to the body part being assessed.

Information about the examination is presented in three columns. The left-hand column contains the narrative discussion. In the wide middle column, photographs, drawings, charts, and tables illustrate the discussion. Where possible, the actual examination is pictured on the left side of this column (a) and specific anatomy is pictured on the right (b). In the righthand column appear highlights which direct the reader's attention to important information in the discussion and illustrations. New information may appear in the Highlights column to emphasize a critical point; this column is also used for cross references to other parts of the chapter or book. It may also be used for taking notes.

Throughout the chapter, the second color emphasizes specific anatomical structures or other important information (c).

The chapter is organized in the following sequence:

Equipment
Techniques of the Physical Examination
The Physical Examination (head to toe) including preparation of the client
Diagnostic Tests

TECHNIQUES OF THE PHYSICAL EXAMINATION

There are five techniques that may be used by the examiner to obtain clinical data during the examination of a client. These techniques are inspection or observation, palpation, percussion, auscultation and use of the senses.

Senses

Use of the senses can provide the examiner with additional information about the client. Sight, touch, smell, hearing, and taste can be used whenever appropriate to collect additional data (a).

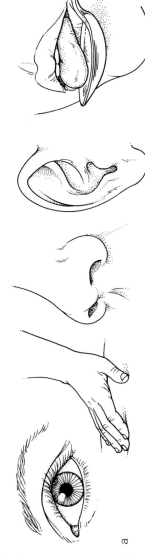

a

Inspection

Inspection involves critically viewing a client during all phases of the physical examination. The process begins when the examiner first meets the client and ends following the completion of the examination. While the technique of inspection is heavily used during the initial phase of the interaction between the examiner and the client, it will also be used to collect additional data throughout the physical examination (b).

The client should be made as comfortable as possible during inspection. The examination room should be warm and well lit to help obtain the most accurate data.

Inspection provides the examiner with a wealth of information about a client and is one of the most valuable examining techniques.

Both the client and the examiner will be asked to use the senses during the examination.

The examiner should be continually alert for visual cues that may suggest the need for additional examination and exploration.

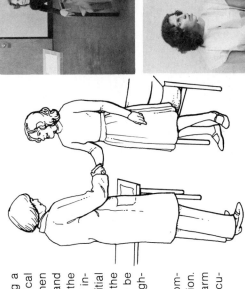
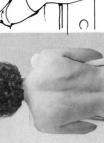
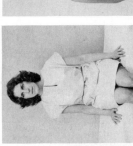
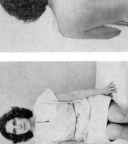

b

To obtain the most accurate data, the examiner should be sure that the area to be palpated is fully exposed.

Palpation

Palpation is a technique used to examine accessible body parts through effective use of the sense of touch. The size, symmetry, and location of an organ can be learned and an evaluation of that organ's function made through use of the examiner's hands.

The *palm* of the hand is used most effectively to determine sound vibrations (especially in the area of metacarpal joints) (a).

The *back* (dorsum) of the hand is sensitive to changes in body temperature (b).

When an area is being palpated, the client should be relaxed and comfortable (c). The examiner should be certain that the room temperature is comfortable. The examiner's hands should be warm to prevent client discomfort and/or alteration in skin texture.

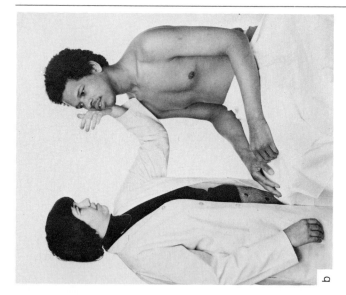

a

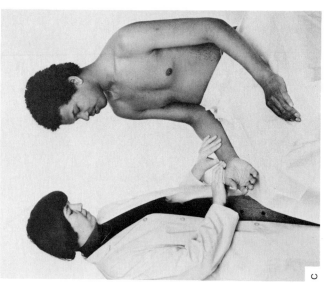

b

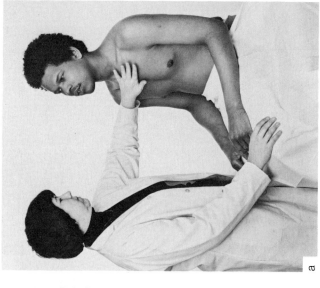

c

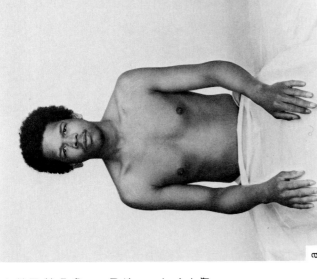
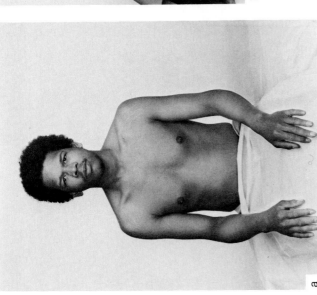
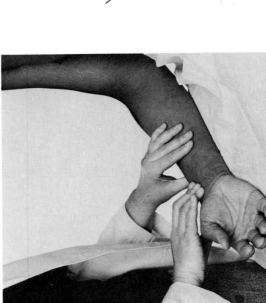

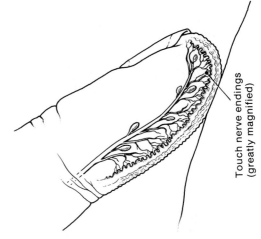

Touch nerve endings (greatly magnified)

The position of the client during palpation will depend upon the body part being examined. When the thyroid gland is being palpated, the client would most likely be sitting (a). When the abdomen is being examined, the client would be lying down.

When palpating the abdomen, having the client bend the knees may relax abdominal muscles (b).

Palpation techniques will differ according to the body part being examined. Usually the palpation is slow and deliberate, progressing from the exertion of light to deep pressure.

Light palpation requires use of the finger tips to obtain information (c). The finger tips contain many nerve endings concentrated within a limited space, making this area particularly sensitive to light touch (d).

Light palpation is most effectively used when examining organs near the skin surface (e.g., lymph nodes), or when checking skin turgor or pulsations (e.g., radial or temporal pulses.)

If the client is tense during abdominal palpation, taking deep breaths will help to increase relaxation.

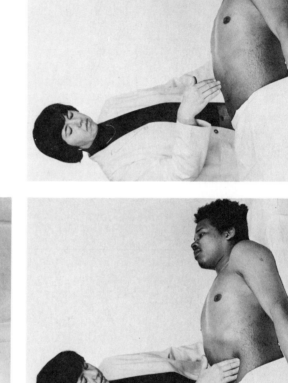

Deep palpation requires the use of both hands to examine deep lying structures (organs such as the liver or kidneys).

To perform deep palpation, the examiner places one hand directly over the area to be examined and relaxes it completely.

The upper hand is then placed completely over the relaxed lower hand. Pressure is applied from the upper hand in order to guide the lower hand as it examines the structure below it (a).

When palpating any body structure, the examiner should look for variation in organ size, density, contour and texture.

When palpating organs such as the kidneys or lungs, bilateral evaluation is important, since the additional data help the examiner to detect changes and validate findings.

An additional technique, called rebound palpation, may be used to examine a specific body area.

In this technique, the client is asked to recline. The examiner exerts pressure with the tips of the fingers on the abdomen (b) and releases quickly by removing hand (c). Normally, pain should not be felt.

Percussion

Percussion is the voluntary striking, thumping, or tapping of a body surface, primarily the chest and abdomen, which results in the production of a sound or touch vibration (a). The vibrations produced in one area are compared with sounds produced in the surrounding tissue. Solids, liquids, air, and gases all transmit differing sounds.

Percussion is used to determine:

1 *Density* of an area, structure, or organ (b)

2 *Location* of an organ

3 *Boundaries* of an organ in relation to surrounding structures

4 *Size and shape* (contour of the underlying structure)

It is important to note that when percussing an area, movement should progress in a logical sequence, e.g., top to bottom (c and d) or from areas of greater resonance to those of less resonance.

Highlights

The examining area should be quiet during percussion.

The position of the client during percussion will be determined by the body part being examined.

It is easier to perceive differences in sounds when moving from areas of greater resonance to those of less resonance.

PHYSICAL EXAMINATION

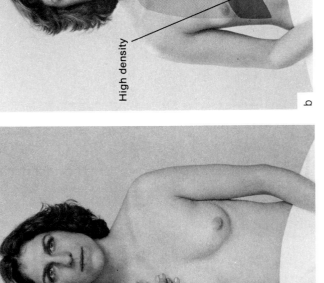

a

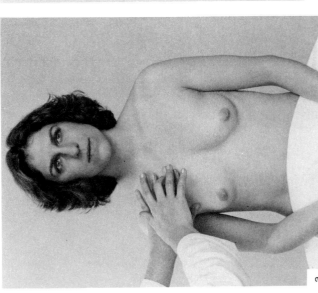

c

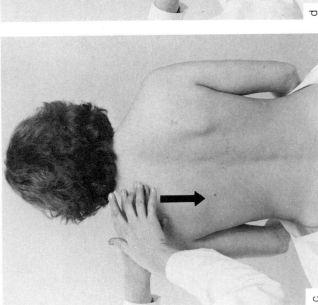

b

Low density

High density

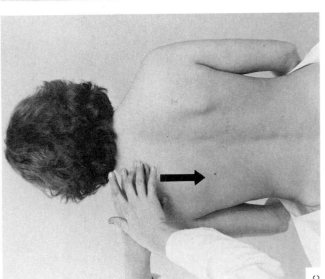

d

Highlights

The pleximeter receives vibrations only from the tissue it is in close contact with.

The fingernail of the plexor finger must be trimmed to prevent injury to the pleximeter during percussion.

Excess fat tissue can lessen the striking percussion blow and decrease or distort the overall sounds produced. Increasing the force exerted against the body surface (by using the thumb) may generate more accurate data.

Fist percussion is used where there is increased tissue dullness and rather than producing a sound, tissue vibration is felt.

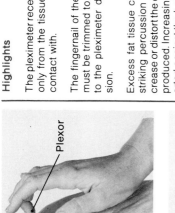

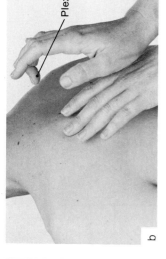

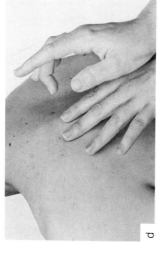

a

b

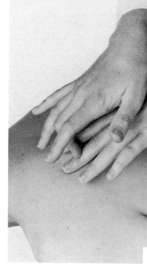

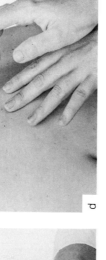

c

d

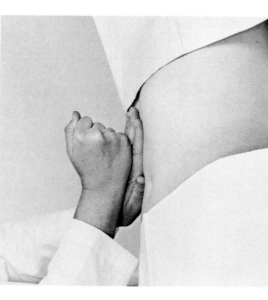

e

The **pleximeter** (middle finger of left hand) is placed directly on the body surface, while the remaining fingers and the palm of the hands are relaxed and kept off the skin (a).

While the pleximeter is pressed firmly against, the skin, the **plexor** (the middle finger of the other hand) is bent slightly before being used to strike a sharp, quick blow to the distal phalanx of the pleximeter (the area between the cuticle and first joint) (b).

It is important to note that the speed and force of the striking movement is produced by the flexed wrist action of the striking hand.

The hand is flexed back on the fore arm and then moved forward, sharply to deliver the striking blow (c).

This finger must be removed quickly after each strike to avoid diminishing the quality of the sound being transmitted (d).

Fist percussing

In this technique a blow is given directly to a body surface by a fisted hand. This type of blow will produce a response or sensation within the client that results from tissue vibration. The technique is frequently used when examining the liver or kidneys. The striking blow is delivered either directly to the body surface being examined or indirectly to the dorsum surface of the other hand (e).

Highlights

The greater the amplitude of a sound wave the louder the sound.

Low pitch sounds occur with slower vibration, while high pitch sounds occur with faster vibration.

The more air found within tissue the deeper and louder the sound, and the longer the duration of the sound.

The less variation in sound, the flatter the sound.

The duller the sound, the shorter its duration.

Hyperresonance refers to an intense booming sound, with a lower pitch than normal resonance. This sound is usually not heard in the healthy adult.

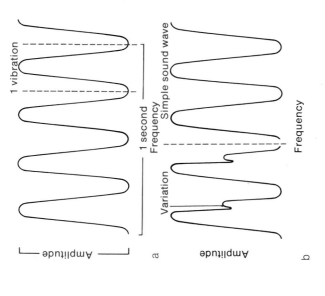

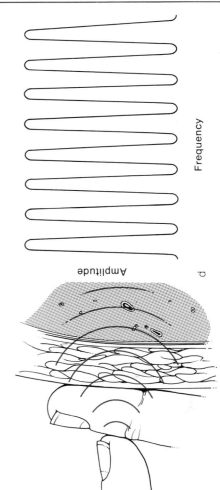

Character of sound Sound varies according to intensity or loudness, frequency or pitch, quality, and duration.

Intensity or *loudness*: the amplitude or volume of a sound.

Frequency: the number of vibrations that occur per second. *Pitch* is determined by the frequency of sound (a).

Quality or *timbre*: variations in the loudness and pitch within a sound wave which help to distinguish one tone from another (b).

Duration: the length of time a sound is sustained.

Types of sounds The variation in sounds produced during percussion is determined by the degree of density present in the body part being examined.

Resonance: the sound produced over those body parts containing both air and mass such as the lung (c). The sound is easily audible and has a low to moderate pitch (d).

Highlights

Tympany is often likened to the sound produced by a kettledrum.

When tissue is more solid, the sounds produced will be fainter, higher-pitched, and of shorter duration.

Tympany: a more musical sound heard over body parts containing air (e.g., bowels [a]). It is a high-pitched, hollow sound of long duration (b).

Flat: a short sound that does not resonate. The pitch is higher than that heard in dullness (d). It is heard generally over those body parts that normally contain a solid mass (e.g., muscle in arm or leg [c]).

Dull: a medium-pitched thudlike sound with diminished loudness (f). It is usually heard in areas of increased density (e.g. liver [e]).

Auscultation

Auscultation is the technique of listening to a sound produced by a particular body organ, for example the heart, lungs, or abdominal viscera.

Immediate auscultation is achieved by the examiner placing an ear against the particular body surface being examined (a). Frequently the sounds heard lack clarity because of interference from environmental noise.

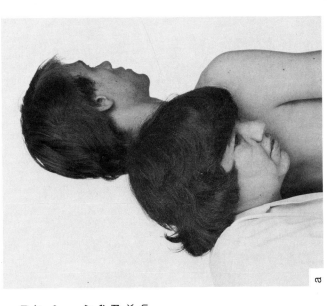

a

Mediated auscultation is achieved by placing a stethoscope against the body organ being examined (b).

The *bell* ((c) of the stethoscope is used to pick up low-pitched sounds (e.g., those from abdominal viscera).

The bell should be placed lightly against the body surface. If pressure is exerted, the skin may swell and act as a diaphragm and disrupt the transmission of the low-pitched sound.

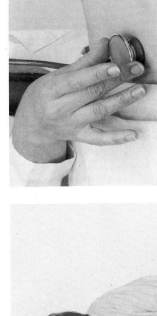

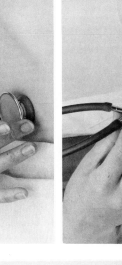

b

c

Highlights

Comfort in using data obtained by auscultation requires practice.

Since the parameters of normal sounds vary from person to person, time, practice, and experience are required to perfect use of the technique.

Refer to p. 130, Fig. b, for discussion on the use of the stethoscope.

Sounds auscultated are often of low intensity.

The *diaphragm* of the stethoscope is used to detect high-pitched sounds (e.g., from heart or lungs). It should be placed in full contact with a body surface (b).

To avoid extraneous noise, movement of the stethoscope against the body surface should be prevented.

The sounds that can be auscultated and the characteristics of each of these sounds are similar to those discussed under percussion.

Highlights

For the most accurate results, auscultation should be performed on an exposed body surface.

The position of the client during auscultation is determined by the body part being examined.

The stethoscope should be warmed to body temperature to avoid client discomfort.

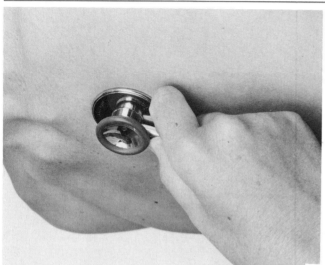

Refer to p. 125, for a discussion of type and characteristics of sounds produced.

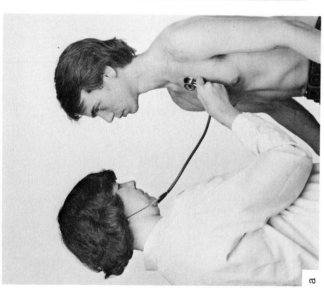

a

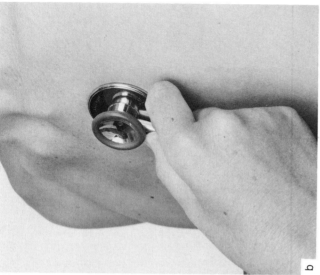

b

EQUIPMENT

There are a variety of resources used to assist the nurse in determining the client's health and bodily function.

The following discussion will focus on those pieces of equipment most frequently used by the nurse to collect data.

The Examining Room

Basic equipment found in an examining room (a) includes the examining table, a stool, an examining lamp, and a stand or table with the following general supplies: tape measure, thermometer, tongue blades, flashlight, gloves, watch with a second hand, cotton balls, pins, alcohol, basins, etc. The room should also be furnished with a sphygmomanometer for measuring blood pressure, either portable or fixed to the examining room wall.

Culture tubes, paper and pencil, culture plates, and hemastick, urine test tablets or dipsticks, along with slides may be available for more extensive laboratory tests (b).

Light touch sensation can be determined by use of cotton wisp.

Soft brushes can be used to assess client's perception of light touch.

The sharp edge of a pin can be used to assess pain perception.

The examining room should be fully equipped and ready for use with each client.

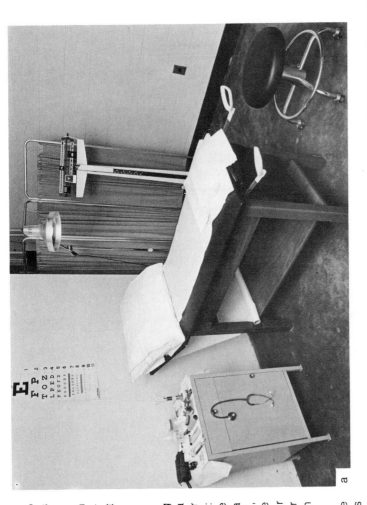

a

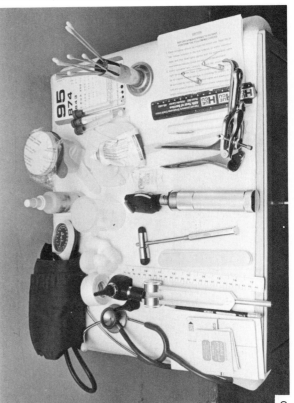

b

Highlights

The bell portion of the stethoscope is used to hear low-pitched sounds.

The diaphragm portion of the stethoscope is used to hear high pitched sound.

Refer to the techniques section of Chap. 4 for further information on stethoscopes.

There are two types of sphygmomanometers: mercury and aneroid.

Refer to the techniques section of Chap. 4 for further information on blood pressure.

Cuffs come in several widths and should cover at least one-third and not more than two-thirds of the upper arm.

When the cuff of a mercury gravity sphygmomanometer is inflated, the column of mercury rises.

The sphygmomanometer is used in conjunction with a stethoscope to evaluate the client's blood pressure.

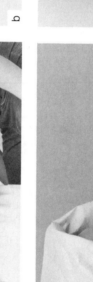

b

Diaphragm

Bell

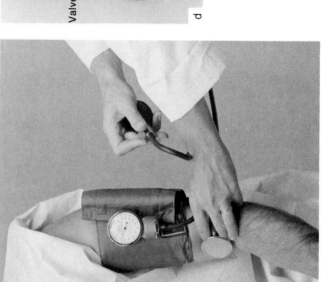

Manometer

Cuff

Bulb

Valve

d

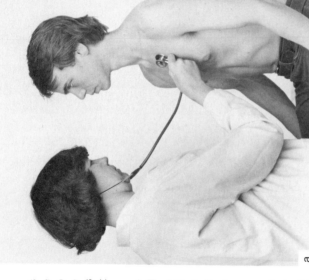

a

c

The Equipment

Stethoscope

A stethoscope is used to pick up sounds not ordinarily heard by the ear (a). The examiner fits the earpieces snuggly into the ears. The tubing of the stethoscope - 25 to 30 cm (10 to 12 inches) long - is flexible and thick enough to filter out noise from the outside.

The chestpiece contains two components (b). The *bell* portion picks up all sounds, especially low-pitched sound. The *diaphragm* portion picks up all sounds, but more specifically high-pitched sounds. The stethoscope is used when auscultating the heart, lungs, and abdomen.

Sphygmomanometer

A sphygmomanometer is used to measure diastolic and systolic blood pressures (c). This instrument consists of an inflatable cuff and two tubes, one of which leads to a bulb used to inflate the cuff, the other of which leads to a manometer. The manometer registers pressure in the cuff and may be either a mercury gravity type or the aneroid type shown here (d).

The examiner obtains a blood pressure reading by placing the cuff around the client's upper arm.

As the cuff is inflated the pressure indicated on the aneroid dial rises. The cuff should be inflated to approximately 20 to 30 mmHg beyond the point where the client's pulse is obliterated. The bell of the stethoscope is placed over the artery and air is then released, using the valve on the bulb.

The first sound heard is recorded as the diastolic pressure (e.g., 110/). The point at which the sound becomes soft and muffled before disappearing is recorded as the systolic pressure (e.g., /70).

Highlights

The otoscope is used to inspect the external auditory canal and the tympanic membrane.

In children, the posterior inferior auricle is grasped and pulled downward away from the body.

The base of the otoscope can be held in an upright or inverted position.

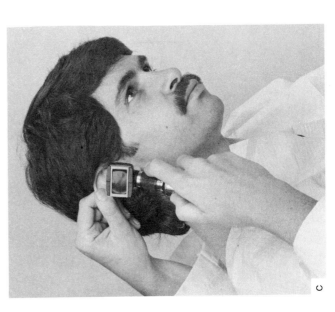

b

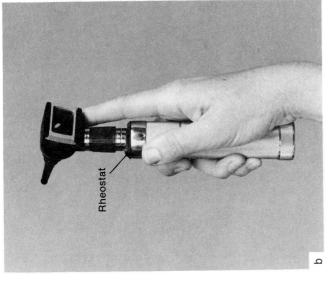

a

c

Otoscope

The otoscope is used to illuminate the external auditory canal and tympanic membrane. The otoscope head inserts into a battery operated instrument which forms the base of the otoscope (a). This base also serves as a handle to be used by the examiner during the assessment. The otoscope can be turned on by pressing down on the rheostat clockwise (b). The examiner can control the amount of light used to look at the ear simply by turning this mechanism.

The otoscope is usually held in the dominant hand. The examiner grasps the superior portion of the client's auricle and pulls it slightly away from the body, upward and outward (c). This helps to straighten the canal prior to insertion of the speculum into the external canal.

A variety of speculum sizes are available to accommodate the client's ear size. The correct size is determined by client comfort and adequate visibility. Care should be taken to ensure smooth, gentle insertion and removal of the speculum to avoid injury.

The ears should be examined bilaterally and the speculum cleansed in an antiseptic solution after each use.

Ophthalmoscope

The ophthalmoscope is used to illuminate the structures of the internal eye for viewing and examination (a). An ophthalmoscope head replaces the otoscope head used previously and attaches to the male adapter of the battery-operated base (b).

To secure its position, the ophthalmoscope head is inserted downward into the handle and turned clockwise until it fits tightly in the socket. To turn the light on, a button found at the neck of the handle (the rheostat) is depressed and turned clockwise until the desired light intensity is achieved.

The head of the ophthalmoscope contains five structures: the viewing aperture; the lens selector dial; the lens indicator (illuminated); a front surface mirror window; and an aperture-setting lever or dial (c).

After turning on the light, the examiner can select the aperture to be used to admit the light by adjusting the aperture lever to the desired position.

To bring the image being viewed into focus, the examiner rotates the lens selector dial until the object is clear.

The illuminated lens indicator is used to assist in further clarifying an object.

The lens indicator is marked with numbers called **diopters**. The black numbers have a positive value (0 to +40) and the red numbers have a negative value (0 to -20).

The lens indicator helps to compensate for myopia (near-sightedness) and hyperopia (far-sightedness), but not astigmatism. The examiner holding the ophthalmoscope in one hand, and 5 cm in front of the client, can rotate the lens indicator until the focus is clear (d).

Highlights

The ophthalmoscope is used to view internal eye structures.

The head of the ophthalmoscope contains:

- a viewing aperture
- a lens selector dial
- an illuminated lens indicator
- a front mirror surface window
- an aperture setting lever
- a bifocal setting (not all have this)

It should be noted that the placement of the various components of the ophthalmoscope may vary with the brand model used.

To bring an image into view, the examiner adjusts the aperture and rotates the lens selector dial until the object is clear.

The lens indicator is marked in diopters. Black numbers have a positive value, red numbers a negative value.

The hyperopic eye will require greater focusing in the plus sphere for clarity, the myopic eye in the negative sphere.

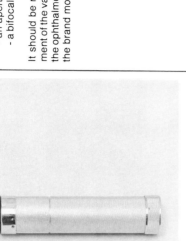

a

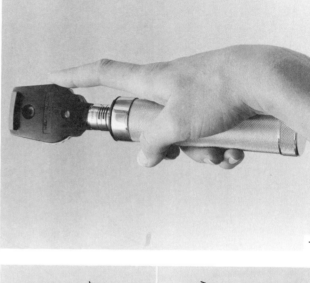

b

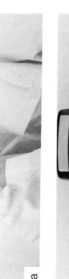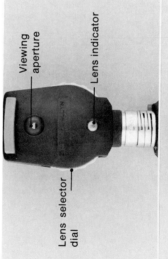

Viewing aperture

Lens indicator

Lens selector dial

Mirror window

Aperture selection dial

c

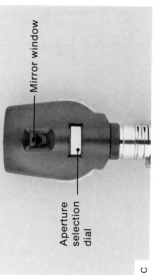

d

Highlights

The viewing aperture contains five apertures:

- a large aperture
- a small aperture
- a red free filter
- the grid
- the streak or split

The red free light excludes red rays from the viewing field, permitting better assessment of the eye vessels and surrounding tissue.

The fixation pattern is a pattern containing an open center with thin lines which permits improved viewing of the macula.

For a complete discussion of the examination using the ophthalmascope refer to the discussion of the eye.

Refer to examination of the nose for further discussion of the use of the nasal speculum.

The viewing aperture contains five different apertures (a): the large aperture (used for dilated pupils), the small aperture (used for undilated pupils), the red free filter or green beam (used to examine the optic disk; if hemorrhage were present it would appear black, while melanin deposits would appear gray), the grid (used to determine the fixating pattern and relating the characteristics of that pattern when estimating changes in the fundus), and the slit or streak aperture (used to examine the anterior segment of the eye for levels of lesions, e.g., tumors).

It is essential that the batteries in the handle of the instrument be recharged daily to allow for maximal light intensity.

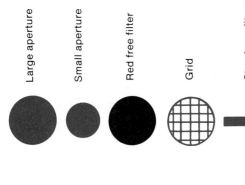

Large aperture

Small aperture

Red free filter

Grid

Streak or slit aperture

a

Nasal Speculum

A nasal speculum is used to inspect the internal nasal structures (b). With the client's head tilted backward, the examiner holds the speculum in the dominant hand and in the closed position. The speculum is inserted into the nasal orifice and gently opened when in place (c). Following the viewing of the nasal canal, the speculum should be closed prior to removal.

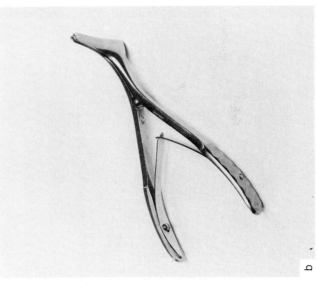

b

c

An audiometer may be used to test hearing, but is a more specialized test and may not be performed during a routine examination.

Refer to discussion of the ear for a description of the Rinne test.

Refer to measurement section in chapter for further discussion of skin fold measures.

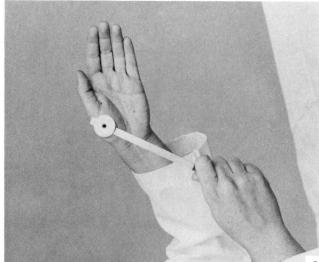

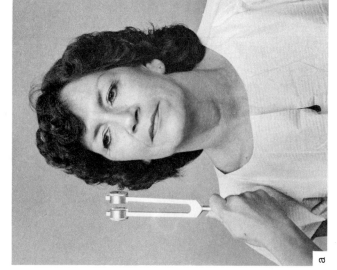

a

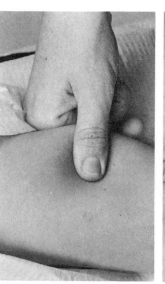

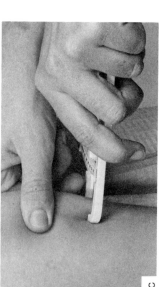

b

c

Tuning Fork

A tuning fork is used to evaluate auditory bone and air conduction. The fork frequencies are between 500 to 1,000 cps. The examiner holds the fork below the two upper prongs and above the terminal point at the base of the tuning fork (a). The two prongs are activated by quickly tapping them on the knuckle or heel of the hand (b). This causes vibrations of the fork and the test of hearing can be performed (Rinne test).

Bone conduction and the sensivity of bony prominences in the body can also be assessed using the tuning fork.

Fat Calipers

Fat calipers are used to determine excessive accumulation of adipose tissue. The examiner holds specially calibrated calipers and compresses them, opening the upper portion of the calipers. The examiner pinches the client's skin in a fatty area (e.g., over the posterior portion of the upper arm), places the calipers around the pinched tissue, and takes a reading to measure the actual amount of fatty tissue (c).

Reflex or Percussion Hammer

The percussion hammer is used to assess reflexes of the upper and lower extremities (a). There are a variety of hammers, but all will have a solid chrome single stem base and a rubber tip (b).

The examiner holds the hammer in the dominant hand between the thumb and index finger, and uses a striking motion for assessment. The examiner can either place the thumb of the free hand over the area to be assessed and strike the thumb, or strike the client's skin directly.

Vaginal Speculum

The vaginal speculum is used to assist in the inspection of the vaginal canal. There are two types of metal speculums used, the Graves and the Pederson.

The Graves speculum is most commonly used (c). It comes in a variety of sizes: 3½ to 5 inches long and ¾ to 1½ inches wide.

The examiner places the index and middle fingers of the nondominant hand into the vagina and spreads the fingers. Pressure is then exerted toward the posterior vaginal wall.

The speculum is held closed in the examiner's dominant hand with the blades held between the middle and index fingers (d). The client is asked to bear down to increase the opening of the vaginal canal and relax the surrounding musculature.

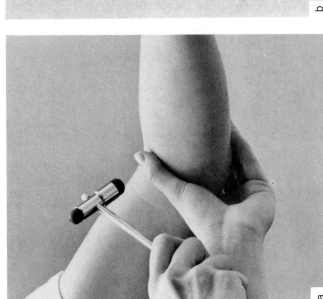

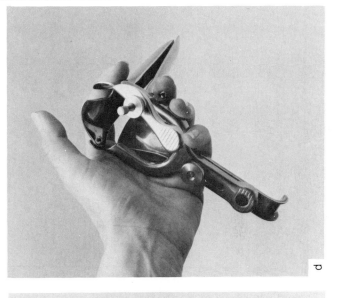

a

b

c

d

Highlights

Refer to discussion of the extremities for more information on palpation of reflexes.

The Graves and Pederson vaginal speculums are used to examine the internal vaginal canal.

Disposable vaginal speculums are available, but may be uncomfortable to the client.

To warm the speculum it should be run under warm water.

Vaginal speculums are sized to accommodate the unique physical anatomical structures of each client.

The client is asked to bear down prior to insertion of the speculum into the vaginal canal to increase the vaginal opening and relax the musculature.

The vaginal speculum is first inserted in an oblique position and then rotated to a transverse position.

During insertion and withdrawal of the vaginal speculum the blades of the instrument should remain closed to prevent trauma to the vaginal wall.

The speculum may need to be reinserted at different angles in order to view the cervix.

The gum stimulator is used to evaluate the gum tissue surrounding each tooth structure.

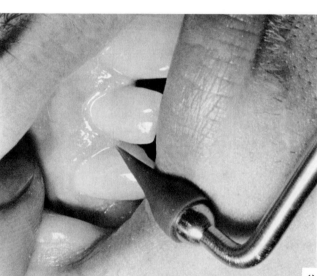

c

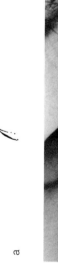

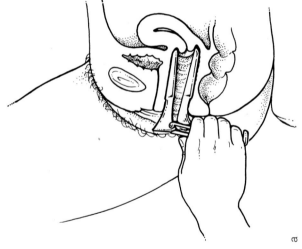

b

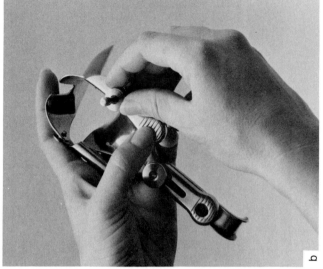

a

The speculum blade is then inserted obliquely into the canal until the end of the speculum reaches the end of the examiner's fingers still in the vagina. The examiner gently rotates the closed speculum to a transverse position (at a 45° angle with the examination table), and removes the fingers. The speculum is then advanced completely into the vaginal canal (a).

The lever located on the base of the speculum is depressed, thereby opening the speculum blades (b). This action should be performed gently. Expansion of the blades allows for viewing of the vaginal canal and cervix.

If the cervix is not immediately in view, the blades should be closed, the speculum withdrawn halfway, and then reinserted in a different angle.

When the cervix is visible the depressed lever can be locked in the open position for further examination.

Before withdrawing the speculum, it is unlocked and the blades are closed.

Gum Stimulator

A gum stimulator is a rubber-tipped instrument used to assess the gums and surrounding tooth structure. Holding the stimulator in the dominant hand the examiner places the tip of the stimulator between and at the base of each tooth and in a gentle rotating motion stimulates the gum area (c).

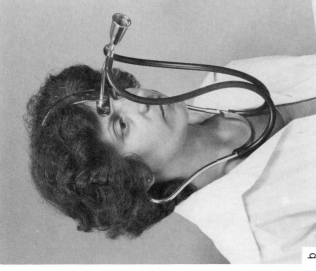

a

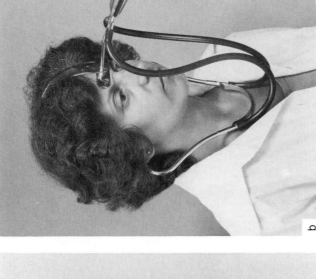

b

Miscellaneous Equipment

The following pieces of equipment may be used during the physical examination depending upon the particular examiner, the setting, and client:

1 Anoscope - used to view the internal anal canal

2 Tonometer - used to measure intraocular pressure (a)

3 Fetascope - used to auscultate fetal heart beat (b)

4 Pelvimeter - used to measure pelvic width

5 Goniometer - used to measure joint movement

Summary

The various pieces of equipment assist the nurse in obtaining additional data about the client's physical health. Personal skill in utilizing the equipment will determine the reliability of results obtained. While equipment helps validate the nurse's subjective and objective assessment, it in no way replaces the importance of other means of data collection.

When observing the client the examiner should note the total picture ("gestalt," or whole) presented by the client, as this will provide cues which will help direct the examination.

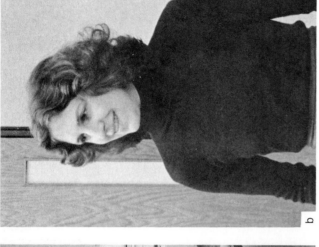

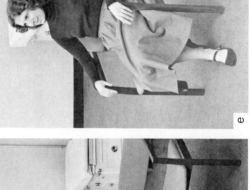

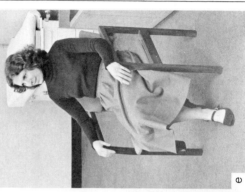

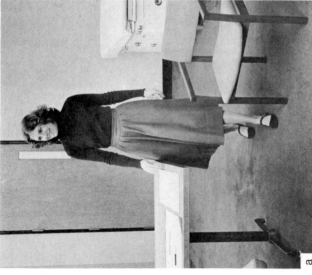

Changes in facial expression may indicate discomfort and should be explored as the interaction progresses.

Complete assessment of gums and teeth are found under mouth examination.

GENERAL APPEARANCE

Initial observations begin when the client first enters the examining room (a). There are four major areas that can be observed and inspected at this time. These are general appearance, stature, movement and demeanor. The client's height, weight, and vital signs should also be measured at this time.

Appearance

1 *Skin color:* Refers to the general tone of the skin, and the pigmentation and health of the tissue. Cultural uniqueness should also be noted. The skin should be intact, with color and tone appropriate to the client.

2 *Appearance:* Includes the appropriateness of the client's dress, general grooming, hair growth patterns, and personal hygiene.

3 *Facial expression:* Assess the general expression of the face noting the eye contact established between the client and examiner.

4 *Nutrition:* Refers to the state of nourishment and fluid intake. Fat distribution (as observed) should be even throughout the body. In addition, the gums should be pink and the relative absence of cavities noted.

The general appearance of the teeth, the speech pattern, and the movement of the mouth can also be observed at this time.

Stature

1 *Symmetry:* The overall size of body parts (e.g., arms, legs, head). Each part should be in relative proportion to one another (c).

2 *Posture:* The client should hold the body in an erect and comfortable position when in a standing or sitting position (d), (e).

Highlights

Refer to the section on Measurement for evalution of height and weight.

The client's body movements should be smooth and coordinated when walking and seated.

When observing movement and coordination, the examiner can assess the intactness of the neurological system. Refer to the section on examination of the extremities.

The client should be fairly relaxed and composed during the interaction.

Dramatic alteration in tone of voice may be significant and should be further investigated.

Fidgety movements, anxiety, and minimal eye contact may be noted if client is tense.

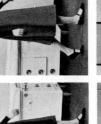
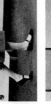
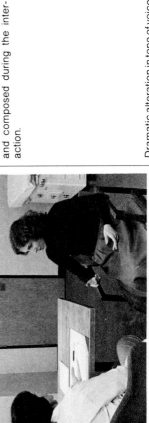
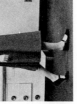
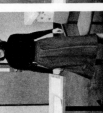
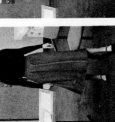
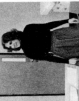
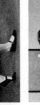
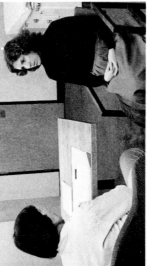
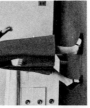
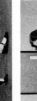
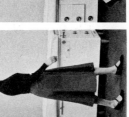
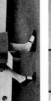
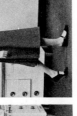
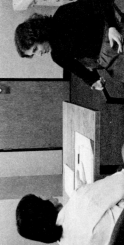
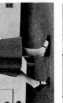
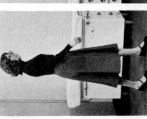
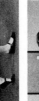
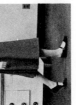
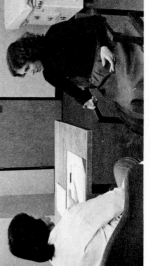
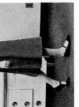
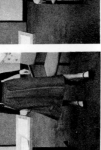
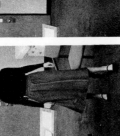
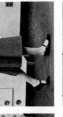
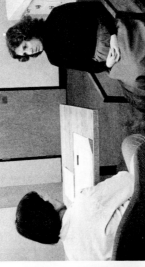
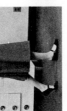
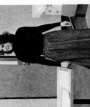
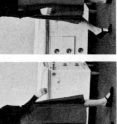
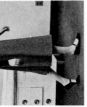
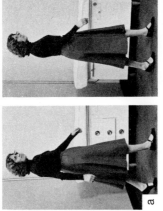

3 *Body build*: The overall distribution of body fat and bone structure should be evaluated. Measurements of height and body weight should be incorporated into the evaluation of an individual's build.

Movement

1 *Gait*: When walking, the client's movements should be coordinated and posture well balanced (a).

2 *Range of motion*: Note the smooth, coordinated movements of body parts from the time the client enters the room until seated. Mobility of each body part should allow for uninhibited movements in a variety of directions (b).

Demeanor

1 *Composure*: The client should appear comfortable during the interaction with the examiner. Facial expression can also be observed at this time (c).

2 *Mental status*: The client should be attentive to the examiner and aware of the surroundings. Responses to questions should be appropriate and given immediately. The level of the client's comprehension should be evaluated during the interaction.

3 *Speech*: The client should speak at a well-paced rate; the pronounciation of words and expression of thoughts and ideas should be clear and understandable. Potential language problems can be identified at this time and measures taken (eg. interpreter) to insure accurate reporting.

4 *Disposition*: The client's mood and general responses should be observed. Normally, the client should be willing to respond in a pleasant manner to questions asked by the examiner.

Highlights

Various scales have been developed for interpreting body weight in relation to height and body frame. The examiner should use the same scale consistently.

Conversion 1 lb. = .4545 kg

A measuring tape may be used to determine height if a scale is unavailable.

b DESIRABLE WEIGHTS
For Women 25-59 Years of Age

Height* Feet Inches		Small Frame	Medium Frame	Large Frame
4	10	102-111	109-121	118-131
4	11	103-113	111-123	120-134
5	0	104-115	113-126	122-137
5	1	106-118	115-129	125-140
5	2	108-121	118-132	128-143
5	3	111-124	121-135	131-147
5	4	114-127	124-138	134-151
5	5	117-130	127-141	137-155
5	6	120-133	130-144	140-159
5	7	123-136	133-147	143-163
5	8	126-139	136-150	146-167
5	9	129-142	139-153	149-170
5	10	132-145	142-156	152-173
5	11	135-148	145-159	155-176
6	0	138-151	148-162	158-179

*with shoes on, 1-inch heels

For Men 25-59 years of Age

Height* Feet Inches		Small Frame	Medium Frame	Large Frame
5	2	128-134	131-141	138-150
5	3	130-136	133-143	140-153
5	4	132-138	135-145	142-156
5	5	134-140	137-148	144-160
5	6	136-142	139-151	146-164
5	7	138-145	142-154	149-168
5	8	140-148	145-157	152-172
5	9	142-151	148-160	155-176
5	10	144-154	151-163	158-180
5	11	146-157	154-166	161-184
6	0	149-160	157-170	164-188
6	1	152-164	160-174	168-192
6	2	155-168	164-178	172-197
6	3	158-172	167-182	176-202
6	4	162-176	171-187	181-207

*with shoes on, 1-inch heels

SOURCE:
Metropolitan Life Insurance Co. 1983

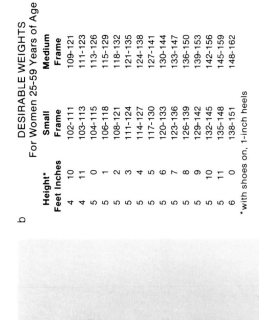

a

c

Measurements

Measurements include the further delineation of physical parameters that affect the general health of an individual. Body weight, height, and evaluation of vital signs are included in this assessment.

Body weight Each client's weight differs because of such influences as nutrition, heredity, height, fat distribution, and bone structure. Parameters for average weight measurements of various age groups are included in Chaps. 5 to 14. Table b describes the weight parameters for men and women 25 years and older as established by the Metropolitan Life Insurance Company.

An individual should be weighed on a standardized balanced scale. Ideally, the client should remove all clothes before being weighed. If this is not possible, the person should remove shoes and have weight recorded (a). the client should be weighed with the same clothing if repeated measures are needed.

Weight is recorded in pounds or kilograms.

Height An individual's height is the measure of the standing length of the body structure. It is influenced by many factors including culture and heredity. Height is measured on a standard scale, with the client standing erect (c). Usually the shoes are removed. A head piece which extends from the measuring pole is used to increase the accuracy of the measurement.

Height is usually recorded in feet and inches.

Highlights

Palpation of the carotid arteries is discussed under the Examination of the Neck.

Palpation of the radial, brachial, and dorsalis pedis pulses are discussed under the Examination of the Extremities.

Trained athletes may have a pulse rate as low as 50 beats per minute.

Women tend to have a pulse rate that is normally 5 to 10 beats faster than men.

The elderly generally have a slower pulse rate.

Variations in pulse rate will be noted as appropriate throughout the text.

Body temperature is regulated by the hypothalmus.

The body (hypothalmus) responds to changes in body temperature and regulates it by conserving heat (e.g., increasing temperature) or lowering heat (e.g., by perspiration).

Conversion Farenheit to Celsius
$F - 32 \times 5/9 = C$ or
$C = F - 32/1.8$

Conversion Celsius to Farenheit
$9/5C + 32 = F$ or $F = (C \times 1.8) + 32$

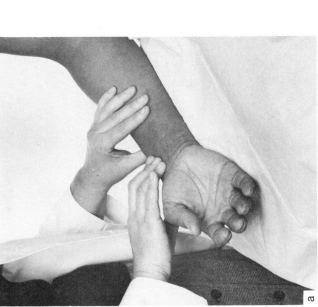

b

Pulse rate   This is the measurement of an arterial pulsation (or wave) conducted by the left ventricle through the aorta to the periphery. It also provides an evaluation of cardiac functioning and efficiency. Pulses can be measured (palpated) over various peripheral sites (b).

Peripheral pulses can be obtained by a monitoring device or, more commonly, through direct palpation. Using a palmar surface of the fingertips the examiner places the hand over the artery to be assessed (a) and counts the pulsations for 1 minute. Normally, the pulse has a regular rhythm and a rate of 60 to 100 beats per minute. Pulse rate is recorded as the actual number of beats per minute.

a

Temperature   The body needs heat for metabolic functioning to occur at the cellular level. Body temperature is measured by glass thermometry or an electric probe (c). It can be assessed through oral, rectal, or axillary measurements and is recorded in degrees Farenheit (F) or degrees Centigrade (C). Normal body temperature ranges from 97 to 99.6°F with an average of 98.6°F (37°C).

Normally, biological rhythms, exercise, medications, the environment, age, and hormonal changes can affect body temperatures.

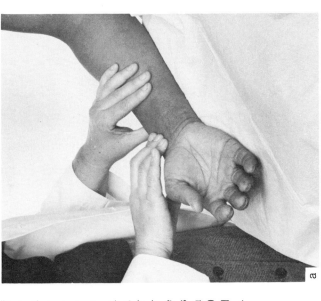

c

Refer to the discussion under examination of the Lungs for a more complete assessment of respirations.

Pulse pressure is the difference between systolic and diastolic blood pressure.

Aneroid needle and mercury manometers are used to measure blood pressure.

Mercury manometers are more accurate but all need to be calibrated routinely.

Respiration   The rate at which air is exchanged (inspired and expired) should be measured. This is usually accomplished by counting the actual number of respirations taken by an individual during a period of 1 minute. In the adult at rest, the respiratory rate is approximately 16 to 20 respirations per minute (a).

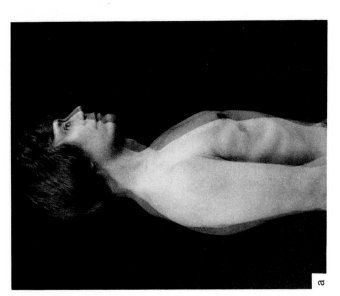

a

Blood pressure   This is the force exerted by the blood against the wall of an artery as the heart contracts (systole) and relaxes (diastole). The pressure is generated by the pumping action of the heart modified by the peripheral resistance of the arteries (b). This pressure is assessed indirectly by applying measured pressure to the overlying tissue, which is sufficient to occlude the artery.

It can be measured by a manometer which is assumed equal to the intraarterial pressure.

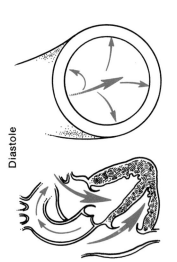

Diastole

Systole

b

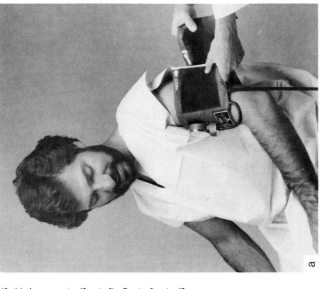

a

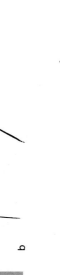

b

Turbulence

c

To measure blood pressure a cuff is placed over at least one-third and not more than two-thirds of the upper arm or leg (a).

The bladder of the cuff should fit completely around the arm or leg. The cuff is then inflated until pulse is obliterated. This is usually 30 mmHg, beyond the point at which the actual pulse is no longer audible. The bell of the stethoscope is then placed over the artery being assessed to pick up low-frequency Korotkoff sounds as the cuff is deflated (b).

The phenomena of noise associated with turbulent blood flow through the vessels permits the examiner to indirectly measure the pressure of the blood inside the artery. The turbulence created results in the production of *Korotkoff sounds* (c).

There are five phases to this sound:
Phase I - First heard; clear tapping sounds increasing in intensity (systolic pressure reading);
Phase II - During further deflation of the cuff a softer sound appears (replaces Phase I);
Phase III - Sharper sounds, less marked than Phase II;
Phase IV - Sudden change in sound from Phase III to a soft muffled sound with flowing quality;
Phase V - All sounds disappear.

Normal variations in blood pressure will be noted when various age groups are discussed throughout the text.

In normal and healthy individuals up to 25% of the total mass of the body can consist of fat cells in quantities large enough to form adipose tissue. Some of this fat is located internally, surrounding organs such as the kidney. However, more than half of the fat is found subcutaneously where it "blankets" the individual.

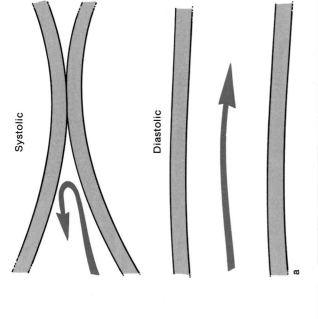

Systolic

Diastolic

a

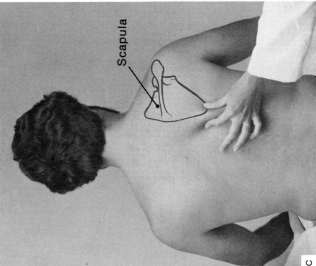

Scapula

c

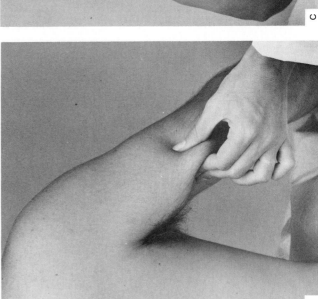

b

Systolic pressure is equal to that pressure which occludes blood flow (a). It is measured at the point exactly before which sounds of turbulent flow are heard.

Diastolic pressure is equal to that pressure at which no sounds of turbulence are heard (a).

The normal systolic blood pressure ranges between 95 and 140 mm Hg with an average reading of 120 mm Hg. The normal diastolic blood pressure ranges between 60 and 90 mm Hg with a mean reading of 80 mm Hg.

Measurement of Skinfold Thickness

The measurement of fat density can be obtained through several measures (eg. soft tissue roentgenograms). However the most practical, and relatively inexpensive measure is the assessment of skinfold thickness using fat calipers.

There are two body sites used routinely to measure skinfold thickness, the *triceps site* and the *subscapular site*. These sites are easily accessible in the general physical examination and have a layer of fat of relatively uniform thickness that may provide accurate measurement of general body subcutaneous fat.

The triceps site is over the triceps muscle halfway between the elbow and the acromial process of the scapula. The skinfold measurement should be parallel to the longitudinal axis of the upper arm (b).

The subscapular site is located 1 cm below the inferior angle of the scapula in line with the natural cleavage lines of the skin (c).

There are several areas of the body where the adipose tissue may be lifted or pulled out with the fingers to form a skinfold.

The technique used in making skinfold measurements is not difficult. There are several types of calipers manufactured for skinfold measurement. Each type varies in cost and includes directions for accurate calibration of the instrument.

When taking a skinfold measurement, the skin should be lifted by grasping firmly between the thumb and forefinger. A well defined "fold" should be formed without causing the client discomfort (a).

The calipers should be placed on the skin at a point where the two fold surfaces are approximately parallel. It is recommended that the skinfold be lifted about 1 cm from the site where the calipers are placed and the skinfold measured (b).

Skinfold thickness measurements should be compared against the most recent graphic distribution scales provided by the U.S. Dept. of HEW. Assessment of relative subcutaneous fat which indicates the growth pattern of individual clients may be made in percentiles. Table c demonstrates the range of skinfold thickness measures for the triceps site.

Highlights

Other sites that may also be used to measure skinfold thickness are the following:

midaxillary site - in the midaxillary line midway between the nipple and the umbilicus, with the fold perpendicular to the midaxillary line.

suprailiac site - above the iliac crest in the midaxillary line, with the fold perpendicular to the midaxillary line.

medial calf site - on the medial aspect of the leg near its greatest circumference, with the fold parallel to the long axis of the leg.

If the calipers are unavailable for use in measuring skinfold thickness, an approximation may be made. When the skin is lifted for measurement at the routine sites, the skinfold should not be wider than one-half inch. If more than one-half inch separates the examiner's fingers, it is likely that the client is obese.

References:

U.S. Dept. HEW. Vital and Health Statistics: *Skinfold Thickness of Youths 12-17 Years*, Series II, No. 132, January 1974.

Brozek, J.: the Measurement of Body Composition, M.F.A. Montagu, ed., *An Introduction to Physical Anthropology*, Charles C. Thomas Publishers, Springfield, Illinois, 1960, pp. 637-686.

Table c from Frisancho, A.: Triceps skinfold and upper arm muscle size norms for assessment of nutritional status, Am. J. Clin. Nutr. **27**:1052, 1974.

This table is based on results of the Ten-State Nutrition Survey of white males and females, 1968-1970.

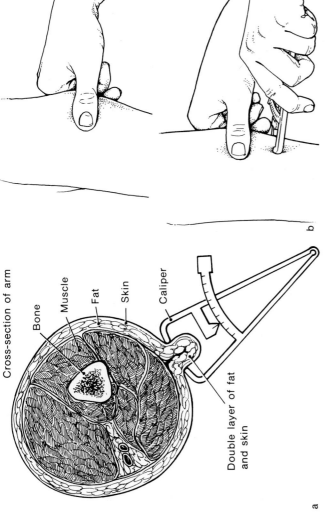

Cross-section of arm

Bone

Muscle

Fat

Skin

Caliper

Double layer of fat and skin

a

b

Table c—Percentile for Skinfold Measurement

Triceps skinfold percentile, mm

Age group	Age midpoint, years	5th	15th	50th	85th	95th
Females						
0.0-0.4	0.3	4	5	8	12	13
0.5-1.4	1	6	7	9	12	15
1.5-2.4	2	6	7	10	13	15
2.5-3.4	3	6	7	10	12	14
3.5-4.4	4	5	7	10	12	14
4.5-5.4	5	6	7	10	13	16
5.5-6.4	6	6	7	10	12	15
6.5-7.4	7	6	7	10	13	17
7.5-8.4	8	6	7	10	15	17
8.5-9.4	9	6	7	11	17	24
9.5-10.4	10	6	8	12	19	24
10.5-11.4	11	7	8	12	20	29
11.5-12.4	12	6	9	13	20	25
12.5-13.4	13	7	9	14	23	30
13.5-14.4	14	8	10	15	22	28
14.4-15.4	15	8	11	16	24	30
15.5-16.4	16	8	10	15	23	27
16.5-17.4	17	9	12	16	26	31
17.5-24.4	21	9	12	17	25	31
24.5-34.4	30	9	12	19	29	36
34.5-44.4	40	10	14	22	32	39
Males						
0.0-0.4	0.3	4	5	8	12	15
0.5-1.4	1	5	7	9	13	15
1.5-2.4	2	5	7	10	13	14
2.5-3.4	3	6	7	9	12	14
3.5-4.4	4	5	6	9	12	14
4.5-5.4	5	5	6	8	12	16
5.5-6.4	6	5	6	8	11	15
6.5-7.4	7	4	6	8	11	14
7.5-8.4	8	5	6	8	12	17
8.5-9.4	9	5	6	9	14	19
9.5-10.4	10	5	6	10	16	22
10.5-11.4	11	6	7	10	17	25
11.5-12.4	12	5	7	11	19	26
12.5-13.4	13	5	6	10	18	25
13.5-14.4	14	5	6	10	17	22
14.4-15.4	15	4	6	9	19	26
15.5-16.4	16	4	5	9	20	27
16.5-17.4	17	4	5	10	14	20
17.5-24.4	21	4	5	10	18	25
24.5-34.4	30	4	6	11	21	28
34.5-44.4	40	4	6	12	22	28

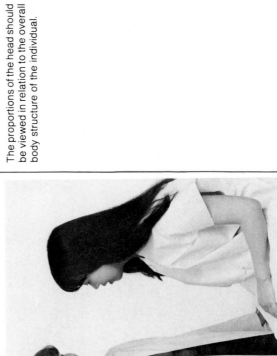

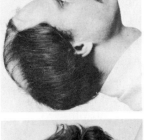
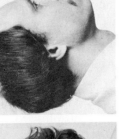

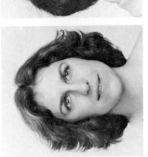
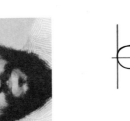
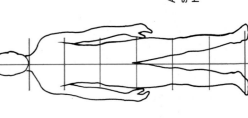

Approximately seven head heights tall

HEAD

Examination of the head focuses upon the bony structure of the skull and the tissues and organs related to it.

The assessment begins with overall observation of the head and its structural framework, the skull, and includes separate examinations of the scalp, face, nose, mouth, eyes, and ears (a).

Inspection and palpation are the main techniques used in examining the head. Percussion and auscultation are used only in special areas discussed later.

Inspection

To examine the head and its related structures, place the client in an upright position facing the examiner.

The examiner first observes the overall appearance, proportion, and symmetry of the head in relation to body structure (b).

Normally, the head is symmetrical, with the skull and face in balance (c).

The size and shape of the head will vary from client to client.

Skull

The skull is a bony framework which protects underlying structures and gives shape and form to the head (a).

Inspection

The skull has several bony prominences which form the boundaries of the skull wall.

These boundaries include the frontal bone, the parietal bone, the occipital bone, the mastoid process, and the facial bones: the maxilla, mandible, and zygomatic bone (cheekbone) (b).

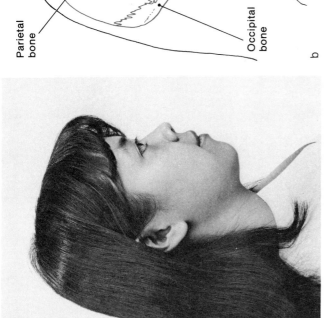

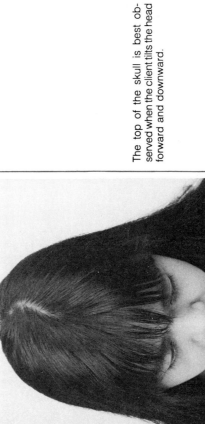

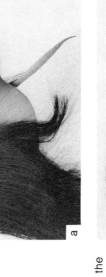

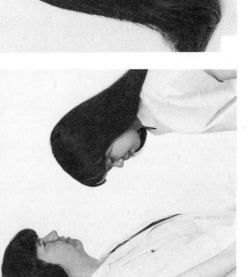

To observe the top of the skull, ask the client to tilt the head forward and downward (c). The examiner then notes the shape and roundness of the skull (d).

Scalp

The superior and lateral portions of the skull are referred to as the scalp. The examination of the scalp includes assessment of the hair, skin, and related bony prominences of the skull.

Inspection

Examination of the scalp occurs with the client in a seated position. The room should be well lit, and the examiner should stand behind the client to obtain a clear view.

The distribution of a client's hair may affect the identification of scalp landmarks.

If a hairpiece is being worn, the examiner should ask that it be removed so that the scalp can be clearly viewed.

The boundaries of the scalp extend from the frontal bony prominence posteriorly to the occipital bone and laterally to the mastoid processes.

The examiner separates the hair to observe the scalp (a). Normally the scalp is clean and smooth and is often lighter in color than the skin. There should be no interruption in skin integrity.

The hair should be separated in different sections in order to inspect the entire surface of the scalp.

Palpation

When palpating the scalp and hair, have the client remain in a seated position.

To palpate the scalp, the examiner again separates the hair, thereby making the scalp visible.

Then, in a gentle, light, rotary motion, the fingertips of the examiner are used to feel the scalp and bony structures beneath it.

Palpation should begin at the frontal bone moving posteriorly to the occipital bone (b), and then, from the top of the skull, laterally along the coronal suture to the mastoid process (c).

Refer to Fig. b on p. 147 for anatomy of skull.

During palpation the scalp should move freely. The surface should be smooth and consistent, with no significant depressions or elevations present.

Complaints of tenderness or discomfort during palpation should be explored.

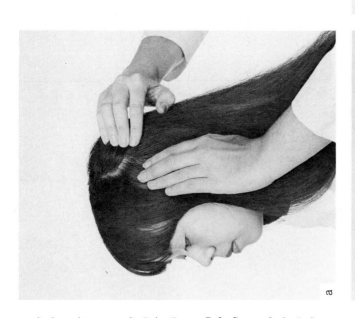

a

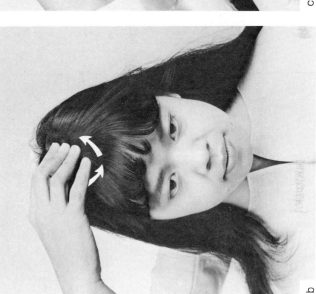

b

c

Highlights

General hair distribution over the entire body surface will be discussed as appropriate.

The use of hair color should be noted.

Hair distribution is often greater in males than in females.

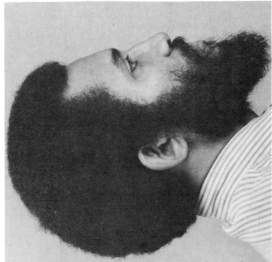

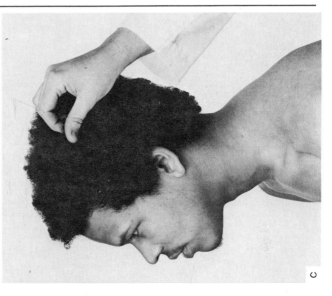

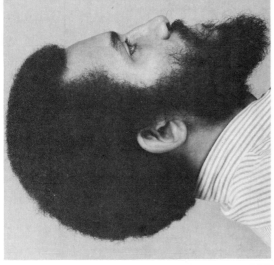

a

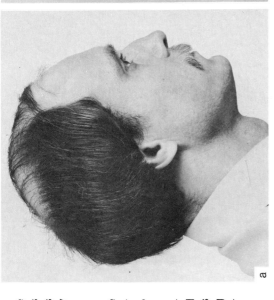

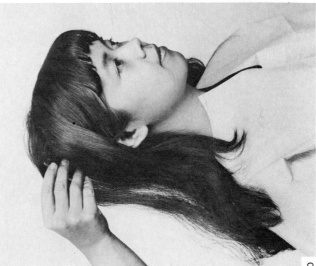

c

b

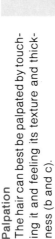

Hair

The hair provides a covering for the scalp. There is a wide variation in what is considered normal hair distribution. This factor should be assessed individually for each client (a).

Inspection

With the client in a seated position, the examiner should inspect the hair in relation to its overall distribution. Normally, the hair will cover the entire scalp.

The general flow, texture, thickness, luster, and appearance of the hair should be observed carefully. These qualities will vary from client to client depending upon genetic characteristics and personal hygiene.

Palpation

The hair can best be palpated by touching it and feeling its texture and thickness (b and c).

Clean hair will feel silky and smooth to touch. The amount and the texture of hair will help determine thickness.

The examiner should be alert to changes in facial expression throughout the entire physical examination, as these changes may provide cues that will require further exploration.

Facial symmetry will vary from client to client.

FACE

Examination of the face includes the assessment of the facial bones and of the related tissues and organs. The examiner will quickly observe that facial structure varies widely from client to client. The face is often the mirror of a person's emotions and feelings. Facial expression can change from moment to moment and will often reflect moods and personal feelings.

Inspection

The client remains seated and is gowned. The room should be well lit so that the skin and facial expressions can be clearly observed.

The examiner standing a foot or two in front of the client can best observe the bilateral symmetry of the face and the position of the facial structures (a).

The examiner may observe the client and then engage in conversation, noting the coordination of facial movement as the client responds (b).

The face is generally symmetrical and in proportion to the skull (c).

The shape and size of the face are determined by the bone structures that lie beneath the surface of the skin.

These structures include the frontal bone, the eye orbit, the nasal bone, the zygomatic bone, the maxilla, and the mandible. They form the boundaries of the face and will be referred to throughout the examination (d).

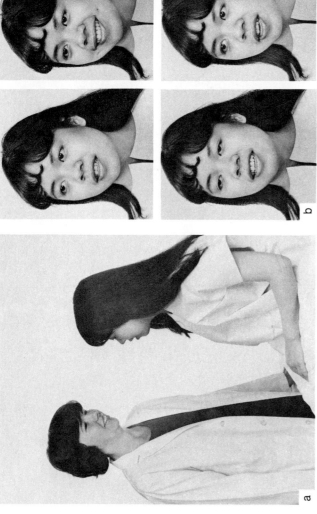

a

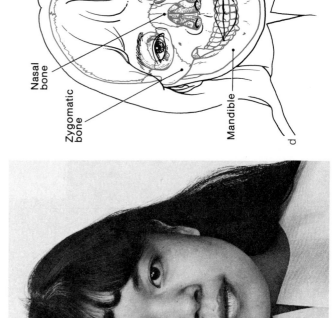

b

c

d

Frontal bone

Eye orbit

Maxilla

Nasal bone

Zygomatic bone

Mandible

In addition to the bony structures of the face there are additional facial components which help to give shape and form to the face. These include the forehead, eyebrows, eyes, nose, mouth, and ears.

The *forehead* is inspected in terms of its general organization (a). Frowning may cause changes in the forehead surface and wrinkles there can reflect behavioral disposition. Wrinkling of the forehead tissue may also accompany aging.

The *eyebrows* are normally in an equidistant position over each eye. Hair distribution over each eye. Hair distribution should be within normal limits for males and females (b).

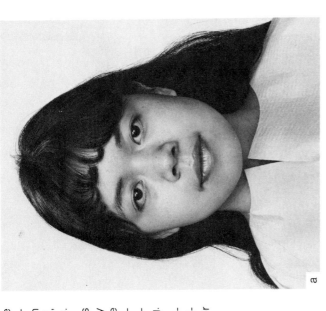

a

b

The *eyes* should lie at the same level on either side of the nose (c). The size and shape of the eyes and all facial components are racially and genetically determined.

The *palpebral* fissures (the openings between the eyelids) can be observed by looking directly into the eyes of the client. Normally they are equal in length (d).

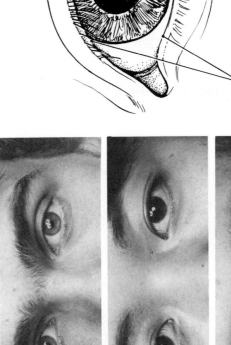

Palpebral fissure

c

A more complete discussion of the eyes is found on p. 160.

When the eyes are opened, the upper lids should be kept in position and drooping should not be present.

A more complete discussion of the nose is found on p. 189.

The shape and symmetry of mouths will vary between sexes and among cultural groups.

These folds may be more obvious in the elderly individual.

Mild acne may be a normal facial marking during various stages of growth and development.

Hemangeomas are reddish-brown discolorations commonly called birthmarks. They may appear on the face or other body parts.

Facial scarring or the elevation of facial skin in specific areas due to acne should be noted by the examiner.

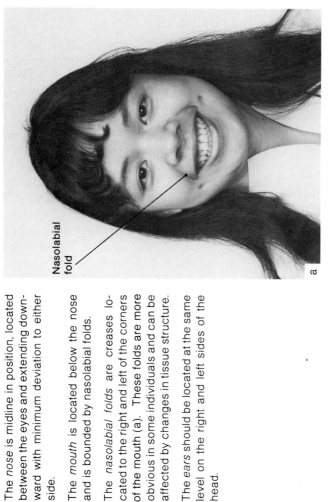

Nasolabial fold

a

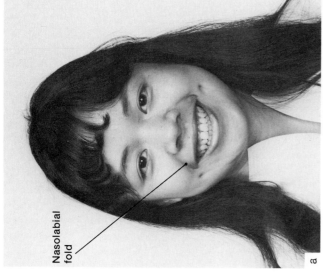

b

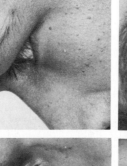
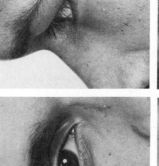

c

The *nose* is midline in position, located between the eyes and extending downward with minimum deviation to either side.

The *mouth* is located below the nose and is bounded by nasolabial folds.

The *nasolabial folds* are creases located to the right and left of the corners of the mouth (a). These folds are more obvious in some individuals and can be affected by changes in tissue structure.

The *ears* should be located at the same level on the right and left sides of the head.

To observe facial changes as well as special markings, it may be necessary to have the client tilt the head to increase the amount of light to various facial angles (b).

General markings on the skin, including moles, freckles, and birthmarks, should be noted. The examiner should cite the location of these markings in relation to other facial structures (c).

Skin color is both culturally and genetically determined. The examiner should observe the general tone and texture of the skin.

Highlights

Hormonal influences may also affect the presence of facial hair in the female.

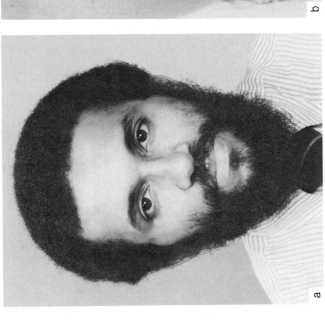

a

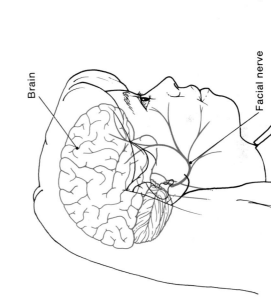

b

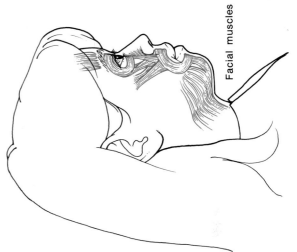

c

Brain

Facial nerve

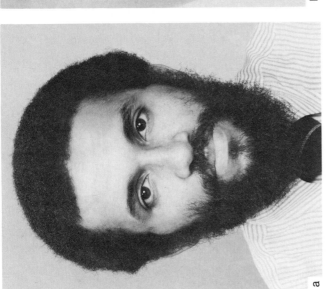

d

Facial muscles

Hair distribution over the face will vary between males and females. A beard, sideburns, or a moustache are often seen in the male (a).

Facial hair distribution in the female is generally not as obvious as in the male (b). However, there are some ethnic groups where facial hair is considered to be normal for the female.

The VIIth cranial nerve is called the facial nerve (c) and provides sensory and motor innervation to the facial muscles (d).

To test the strength and function of this nerve, the examiner asks the client to complete specific tasks and then observes the individual's facial responses.

The client remains seated and is asked to:

1 *Raise and lower the eyebrows:* Normally both brows should move in an upward and then downward movement at the same time (a).

2 *Frown:* Changes in facial expression and wrinkling of the forehead are noted during this activity (b).

3 *Close eyes tightly:* The client is asked to squint and tighten the facial muscles and keep both eyes tightly closed (c).

4 *Puff the cheeks:* The examiner notes the bilateral expansion of the client's cheeks as the mouth fills with air (d).

5 *Show the teeth:* The client is asked to exaggerate mouth opening while making teeth visible to the examiner (e).

6 *Smile:* The bilateral movement of the mouth and cheeks is observed as the client smiles (f).

Normally, there is no spastic movement of the face during the examination of the facial nerve.

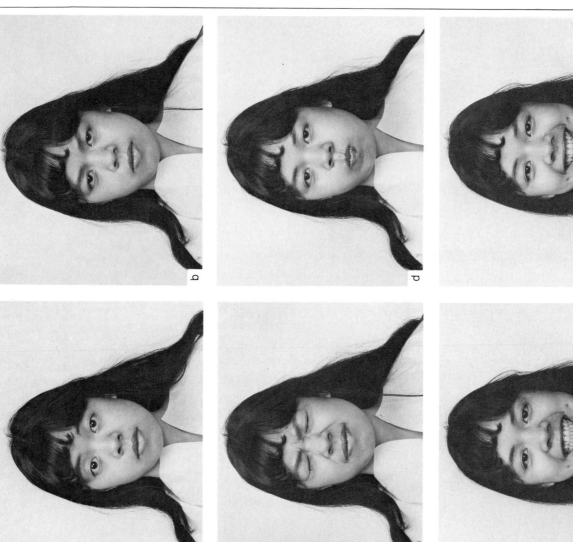

Facial scarring or elevation of
facial skin (e.g., due to acne) may
require further assessment.

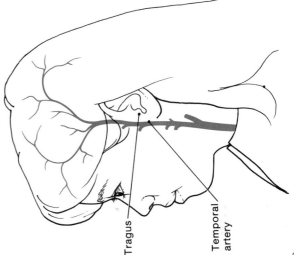

Tragus

Temporal
artery

c

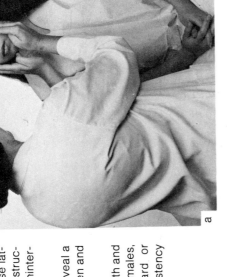

a

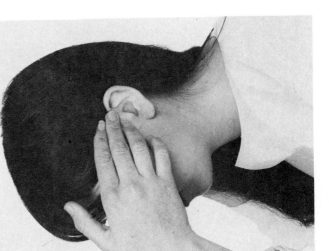

b

Palpation

To palpate the bony structures of the
face the examiner remains in the same
position, a foot or two in front of the
seated client. Using the fingertips, the
examiner begins the bilateral examination of the face, moving from the forehead to the chin and from the nose laterally (a). Generally, the facial structures are firm and intact and uninterrupted in continuity.

Palpation of the facial skin will reveal a
texture that can vary between men and
women.

Generally, the facial skin is smooth and
soft, and has good elasticity. In males,
the presence of a heavy beard or
moustache will alter this consistency
over the specific areas.

The *temporal artery* is one source of
blood supply to the face and can be
easily palpated. This artery is anterior to
the *tragus* of the ear (b and c).

The examiner, using the fingertips lightly, palpates the artery. Normally, pulsations are rhythmic and can range between 60 to 100 beats per minute.

Palpation of the artery should not cause
pain or reveal tenderness or hardness.

A complete discussion of nodes (i.e., sub occipital, pre/post auricular, tonsilar, mandibular, and sub mental) appears on pages 222 and 223.

Bilateral examination of the Vth cranial is essential in order to insure the accuracy of the results.

The masseter muscle is referred to as the muscle of mastication.

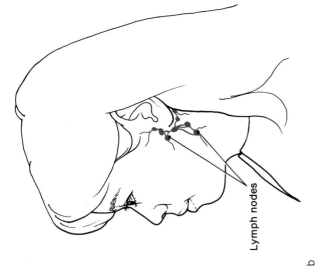

a

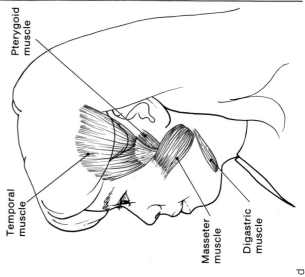

Lymph nodes

b

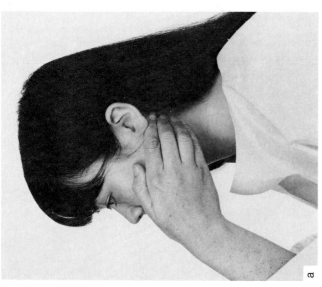

Brain

Origin of trigeminal nerve

c

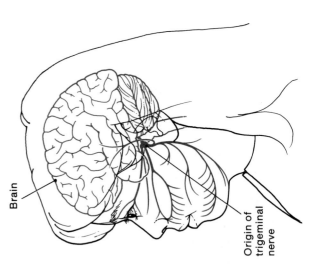

Pterygoid muscle

Temporal muscle

Masseter muscle

Digastric muscle

d

Several lymph nodes are present in the facial area. Normally, these nodes are not palpable (a). Fig. b points out the location of some nodes for reference.

When the examiner palpates over the nodal areas no discomfort should be felt by the client.

During palpation, the trigeminal nerve can be tested to assess its intactness. The *trigeminal nerve*, or *Vth cranial nerve*, originates at the base of the brain. It divides into three major nerves and has both sensory and motor fibers (c).

The motor fibers provide innervation of the masseter, temporal, pterygoid, and digastric muscles (d).

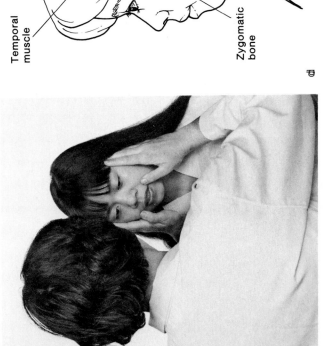

Masseter muscle

b

Temporal muscle

Zygomatic bone

d

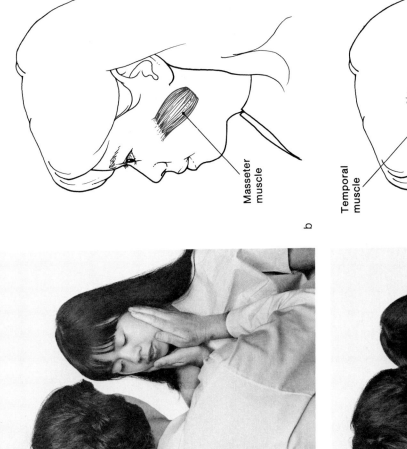

a

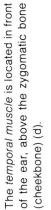

c

To test these muscles, the client is asked to bite down as hard as possible. The examiner palpates the *masseter muscle* (b) by placing a hand on each side of the face above the angle of the jaw while the client is biting down (a). Note the general muscle size, strength (bilateral), and symmetry of the musculature.

The *temporal muscle* is located in front of the ear, above the zygomatic bone (cheekbone) (d).

To palpate the temporal muscle, the examiner places one hand on each side of the head in the temporal area and asks the client to bite down (c). Again, the size, shape, and symmetry of the muscle is noted.

When examining facial muscles, the size, shape and symmetry should be noted bilaterally.

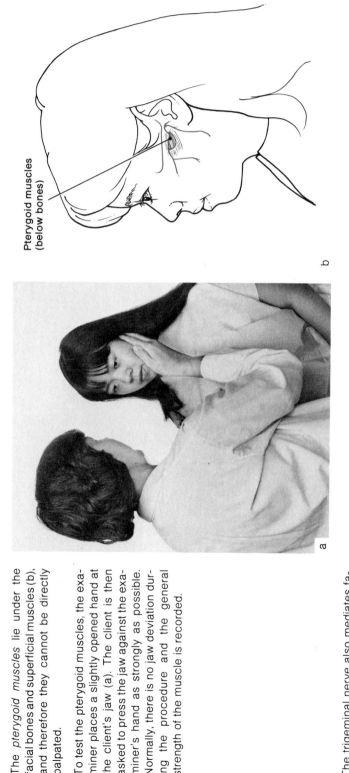

a

Pterygoid muscles (below bones)

b

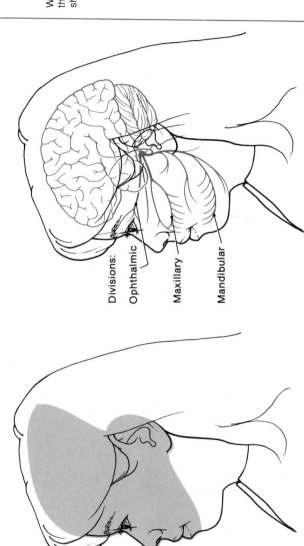

c

Divisions:
Ophthalmic
Maxillary
Mandibular

d

The *pterygoid muscles* lie under the facial bones and superficial muscles (b), and therefore they cannot be directly palpated.

To test the pterygoid muscles, the examiner places a slightly opened hand at the client's jaw (a). The client is then asked to press the jaw against the examiner's hand as strongly as possible. Normally, there is no jaw deviation during the procedure and the general strength of the muscle is recorded.

The trigeminal nerve also mediates facial sensation in response to touch, pain, temperature change, and vibration.

Sensory innervation is provided by this nerve to the skin of the face and the anterior half of the scalp, the eye, the external ear, and internal structures of the mouth and nose (c).

The nerve branches into three main divisions in order to provide sensory stimulation to the areas noted above. These are the ophthalmic, maxillary, and mandibular divisions (d).

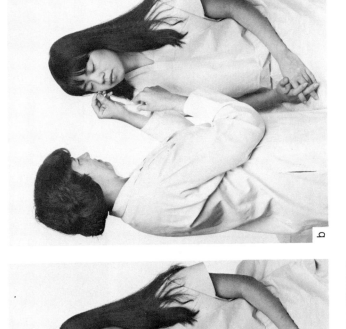

a

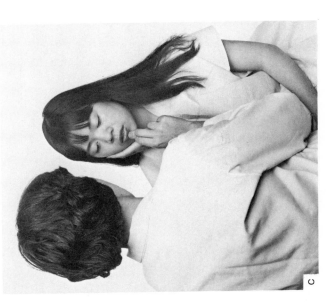

b

c

To test sensory innervation by the trigeminal nerve, the examiner will stimulate each area with hot and cold instruments and with soft touches and pinpricks. The client remains in a sitting position and is asked to close the eyes during the procedure to eliminate visual input.

To test temperature perception, hot and cold test tubes are alternately placed on the face (a).

Normally, the client will be able to distinguish changes in temperature.

To test for sensitivity to a soft touch, cotton wisps are used and alternated with pinpricks to determine presence or absence of pain sensation (b).

Normally, the client will be able to distinguish pain from soft touch with complete accuracy.

The trigeminal nerve also contains afferent fibers of the corneal reflex. This will be tested during the examination of the eye.

Afferent and efferent fibers also affect the jaw closure reflex. To test this reflex (called the maxillary reflex or "jaw jerk"), the examiner places one hand directly on the midline portion of the chin, below the lip with the client's mouth open slightly (c). Using the fingers of the other hand, the examiner taps the thumb. Normally, if the reflex is intact, the mandible will raise, thereby closing the mouth. The response, however, is hard to elicit.

The examination of the eye is complex and often reflects the physical as well as the emotional/spiritual health of the individual.

Eyes should be aligned with one another and positioned to the right and left of the nose.

The shape of the eyes are genetically influenced and vary with each client.

EYE

The examination of the eye is complex and includes the testing of visual acuity, assessment of the ocular structures, evaluation of visual fields, extraocular movements, testing of ocular reflexes and the ophthalmoscopic examination. The client's general state of physical and emotional health will often be reflected in the eyes. Inspection, palpation, and ophthalmoscopic examination are the techniques used to elicit data.

Inspection

In general, the client remains seated comfortably at the end or the side of the examining table (a). The examiner will change positions throughout the examination.

Extraocular Structures

To inspect the general appearance and the position of the ocular structures, the examiner stands directly in front of the client. Normally, the eyes are symmetrical, parallel, full, bright, and set to the right and left of the nasal bone. The shape of the eyes is influenced by racial or genetic characteristics and therefore will vary from client to client (b).

The eyes are located in orbits formed by the bones of the face (c). The *orbital roof* is formed by the sphenoid and frontal bones; the *medial wall* by the maxilla, lacrimal and sphenoid bones, and the *lateral wall* by the zygomatic and sphenoid bones.

The *lacrimal groove* is located in front of the medial wall and contains the lacrimal sac.

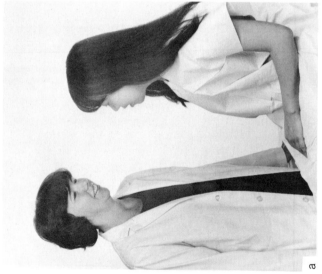

a

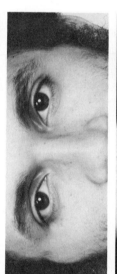
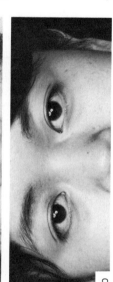
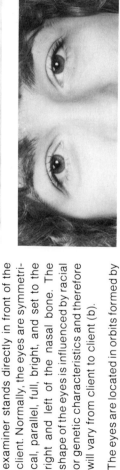

b

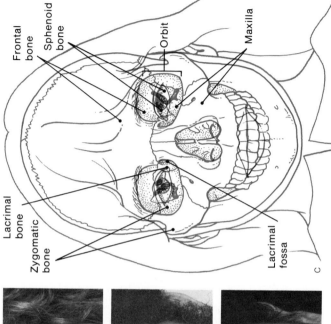

Frontal bone

Sphenoid bone

Orbit

Maxilla

Lacrimal bone

Zygomatic bone

Lacrimal fossa

c

The upper and lower eyelids are separated by a palpebral fissure.

Normally, the upper eyelid will open and close freely and completely.

The punctum is the only tear structure seen on initial inspection.

The color and fullness of the eyelashes varies with each client. Normally, the fullness of the eyelashes diminishes with age.

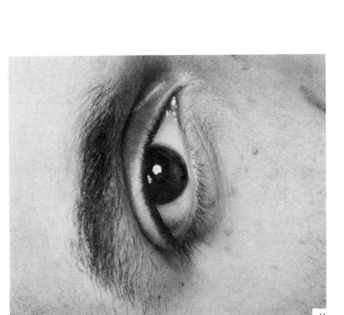

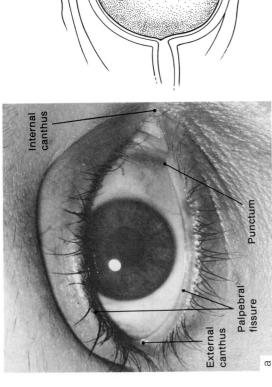

The upper and lower *eyelids* are separated by the *palpebral fissure*. The two angles of the fissure are called the *external* (temporal) and *internal* (nasal) *canthi*. The inner canthus contains the *punctum* which is responsible for lacrimal duct drainage (a).

The *upper eyelids* extend upward from the fissure to the bony orbit and join with forehead skin. The shape of the lid is maintained by muscles, ligaments, and the fibrous tarsal plates (b). Normally, the upper eyelids open and close completely and do not droop or lag.

The *lower eyelids* extend downward, are shorter, and do not fold. They join the facial skin below the lower orbital area.

The skin surrounding both eye lids generally is smooth, continuous, and of similar color to facial skin. Facial markings (eg. pigmentation), may be noted, and should be investigated if skin integrity is interrupted.

The margins of the eyelids contain the hair follicles of the *eyelashes*, and *sebaceous glands*. The color and fullness of eyelashes varies with each client. Normally eyelashes are evenly distributed and have an outward curve. Eyelashes decrease in fullness as the client ages.

Eyebrows are located above each eye. The quantity, distribution and color of eyebrows are individually and genetically determined. Normally, eyebrow color is similar to that of the client's genetic hair coloring. Fullness of the eyebrow will vary with each individual, with males frequently having thicker brows (c). Eyebrows can become coarse and thin with aging.

Ocular Structures

In viewing the eye structures, the client remains seated in a well lit room. The examiner may utilize a penlight to aid in the inspection of these structures.

The *cornea* is smooth, moist, transparent tissue, that covers the pupil and iris. The structure connects with the conjunctiva at the point of the *limbus* (a). The cornea is extremely sensitive to touch, and is innervated by the ophthalmic branch of the fifth cranial nerve. The cornea can be visualized by using a penlight directly into and to the side of the anterior eye. Normally, the structure should appear shiny, bright, transparent and smooth. The anterior chamber can be inspected along with corneal illumination. The chamber should appear transparent. Usually, the anterior chamber is best assessed by lateral or side view illumination. The *anterior chamber* is bounded laterally by the sclera and the ciliary body; anteriorly by the cornea; and posteriorly by the iris and that part of the lens within the pupil opening (b). It is filled with fluid produced by the ciliary body.

Fluid moves out of the anterior chamber through the *canal of Schlemm*, located at the angle of that chamber.

A *tonometer* is used to evaluate intraocular pressure (c). Tonometry readings are often performed routinely on individuals over 40 years of age. A complete discussion is found in Chap. 13.

Highlights

The cornea is extremely sensitive to touch due to innervation by the ophthalmic branch of the 5th cranial nerve (see palpation).

Upon inspection, the cornea should appear shiny, bright, transparent and smooth.

The anterior chamber can best be assessed from a lateral position. Normally, it is transparent.

The anterior chamber contains a fluid produced by the ciliary body.

Intraocular pressure is determined by the rate of aqueous production and resistance to aqueous outflow throughout the angle of the anterior chamber (canal of Schlemm). (Refer to discussion of the Eye in middle adulthood chapter.)

Figure b adapted from Dorothy A. Jones et al, Medical-Surgical Nursing, A Conceptual Approach, 2nd ed., McGraw-Hill, 1982, p. 1187, Fig. 32-1. Used with permission of McGraw-Hill Book Company.

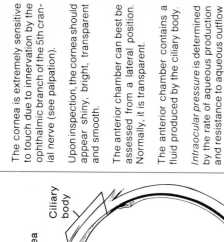

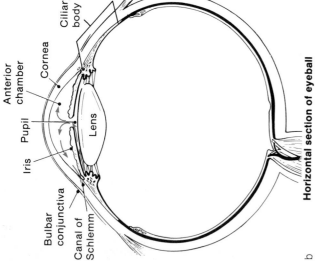

Horizontal section of eyeball

b

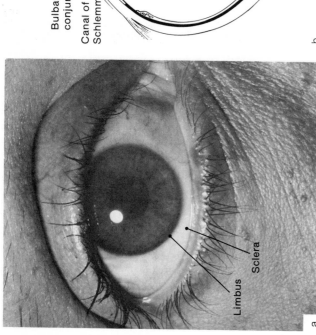

Sclera

Limbus

a

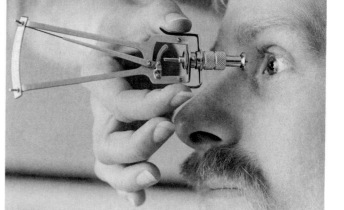

c

Highlights

Upon inspection the iris should appear flat.

In black individuals dark pigmentation (small dots) may be observed in the sclera.

The conjunctiva covers the anterior eye and sclera and lines the eyelids.

The caruncle is a small fleshy elevation located in the nasal corner of the conjunctiva.

Closing the eyelids contracts the orbicularis muscle and prevents eyelid eversion.

To inspect the conjunctiva lining, the upper lid must be inverted.

Fat deposits may be observed beneath the sclera and show through the membrane as a yellowish color at the periphery.

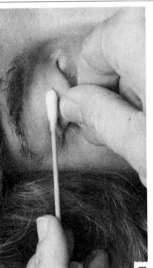

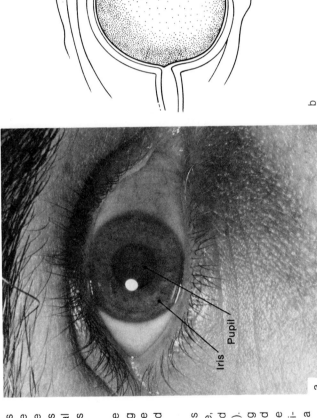

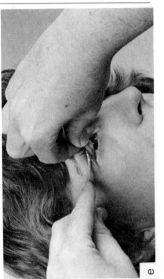

The *iris* surrounds the pupil and is inspected for color and shape (a). These factors vary with each individual and are usually genetically influenced. The iris can also be inspected during corneal illumination. From a lateral view, the iris should appear flat.

The *sclera* is the white portion of the anterior eye. The *conjunctiva* is a lining that covers the anterior portion of the eyes, the lids (palpebral portions), and the sclera (bulbous portion) (b).

To assess the conjunctiva the client is asked to look up, down and to the side, as the examiner holds the lower lid downward against the bony orbit (c). The white sclera is usually visible along with the clear conjunctiva. Small blood vessels may also be observed in the conjunctiva. The color of the conjunctival tissue varies, but will usually have a pink to reddish coloration.

To inspect the upper conjunctival lining, it is necessary to invert the upper eyelid. To accomplish this, the client is asked to look down while keeping the lids slightly open. The examiner then grasps the upper eyelashes and gently pulls downward. A cotton tipped applicator is then placed directly on the eyelid (1 cm) (d).

While holding the eyelashes, the examiner exerts a gentle downward pressure on the applicator. This action inverts the lid.

During inspection, the lashes are held in place against the bony orbit, directly below the eyebrow (e). Normally, the upper lid conjunctival lining will appear shiny, pink to reddish color, and smooth.

Tears lubricate as well as cleanse the anterior eye surface.

Tears are drained from the eyes through the puncta, lacrimal ducts and lacrimal sac into the nasolacrimal duct.

The plural of punctum is **puncta.**

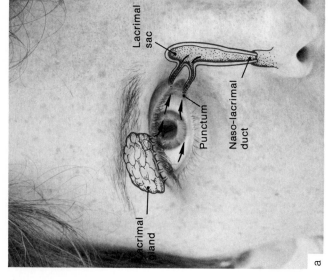

a

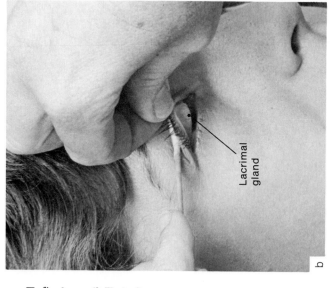

b

While the upper conjunctiva is being examined, part of the lacrimal mechanism can also be inspected. The eyelids aid in lubricating the anterior eyeball and protect it from injury. Blinking serves to distribute tears, and lubricate as well as cleanse the anterior eye surface. The lacrimal or tear glands, along with the puncta (a), the naso-lacrimal duct and the lacrimal sac, are responsible for tear production and removal.

Lacrimal glands are located within the bony orbit, and provide secretions as needed to moisten the conjunctiva.

Tears drain from the eyes through the *puncta* into the *lacrimal ducts* and *lacrimal sac* (also located within the bony orbit) into the *naso-lacrimal duct* to the nose.

To examine the lacrimal gland, the examiner should elevate the temporal aspect of the upper lid and ask the client to look down and to the opposite side.

Normally, a small portion of the lacrimal gland can be seen (b). Usually the tissue observed is smooth and continuous, without bulging.

After the area is inspected the eyelid is returned to its downward position and the applicator is removed. The procedure is then repeated on the opposite eye.

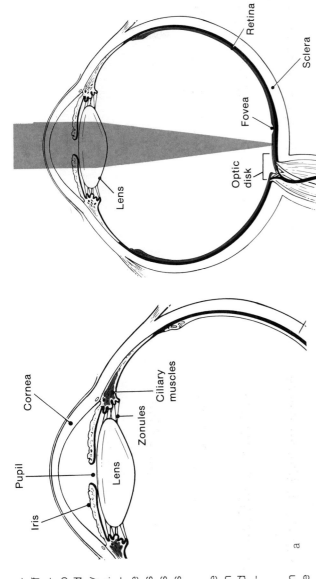

a

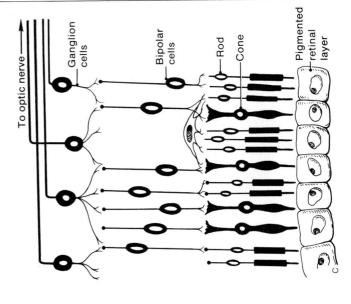

b

Right eye

c

To optic nerve →

Ganglion cells

Bipolar cells

Rod
Cone

Pigmented retinal layer

Highlights

The lens is the center of the eyes' refractory system and is normally transparent.

The lens contains epithelial cells covered by an elastic membrane called a lens capsule.

Figures a and b adapted from Dorothy A. Jones, et. al., Medical-Surgical Nursing, A Conceptual Approach, McGraw-Hill, 1982, p. 1187, fig. 32-1. Used with permission of McGraw-Hill Book Company.

Objects seen by the retina are formed upsidedown and reversed, right to left.

Rods and cones are sometimes referred to as neurosensory receptors.

Rods are responsible for vision in the dark.

The cones contain pigment sensitive to colors (blue, red and green light waves).

The *lens* is located at the pupillary opening, behind the iris (a). It is the center of the eyes' refractory system and is normally transparent. The lens contains no nerves or blood vessels. It is composed of epithelial cells, which are covered by an elastic membrane (*lens capsule*). The lens is attached around its periphery to muscles which control its size (thickness). Fibers that connect the lens to the muscles are called *zonules*. This enables the lens to adjust to and focus on objects close up and at a distance.

The lens can be assessed during the ophthalmoscopic examination. It can also be evaluated through direct and lateral illumination. Normally, the structure should be transparent.

The remaining ocular structures are in the interior eye, visible in part during the ophthalmoscopic examination. These structures will be discussed since tests of visual acuity (which follow) measure their function.

The *retina* is the light sensitive portion of the eye. It lines the interior surface of the eyeball (b).

The amount of light that reaches the retina is determined by the coordinated function of the muscles of the iris and ciliary body.

Rods and cones are found in the retina (c). They are sometimes called the *neurosensory receptors.*

The *rods* are responsible for vision in the dark. This is due to the presence of a pigment called *rhodopsin* which bleaches when light is present.

The *cones* contain pigment sensitive to blue, red and green light waves.

Along with neurosensory receptors, the retina contains three specialized sites which contribute to vision. They are the fovea centralis, the macula, and the blind spot (a).

The *fovea centralis* is a slight depression on the retina. The area contains a heavy concentration of cones, making it the point of central vision and acute color vision.

The *macula* is a yellow area surrounding the fovea, and is composed mostly of cones. It appears slightly darker than the normal surrounding retinal area and it is the area of most acute vision.

The *optic disk* is sometimes called the *blind spot*. It is that site at which the optic nerve leaves the eye and goes to the brain. This area is located in the upper nasal quadrant of the visual field and does not register a visual image.

Vision

Seeing or vision occurs in a most dynamic way. When light is presented to the retina, the neurosensory receptors are stimulated and impulses are conducted to the optic nerve (CN II). Fibers from each eye move to a point called the *optic chiasm* (b). Here, medial fibers from the nasal (inner) half of the retina cross to the opposite side in the chiasm. Lateral (outer) fibers from the retina remain on the same side of the chiasm.

Vision is produced as a result of the nerve tracts entering the visual cortex of the occipital lobe.

Assessment of the internal eye structures and vision itself is discussed under Visual Acuity.

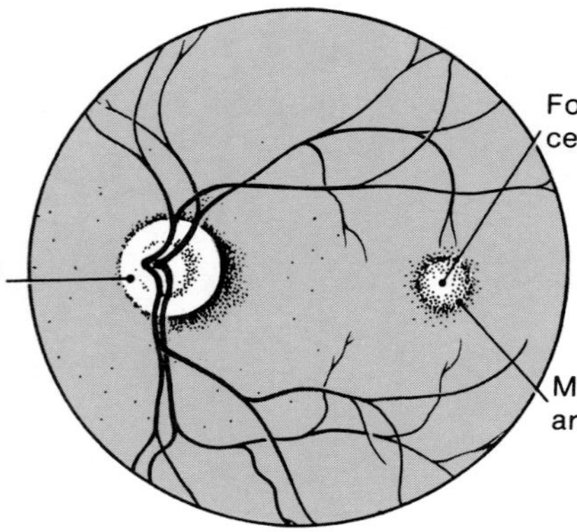

Highlights

The retina contains three sites which contribute to its function:

1 the fovea centralis
2 the macula
3 the blind spot

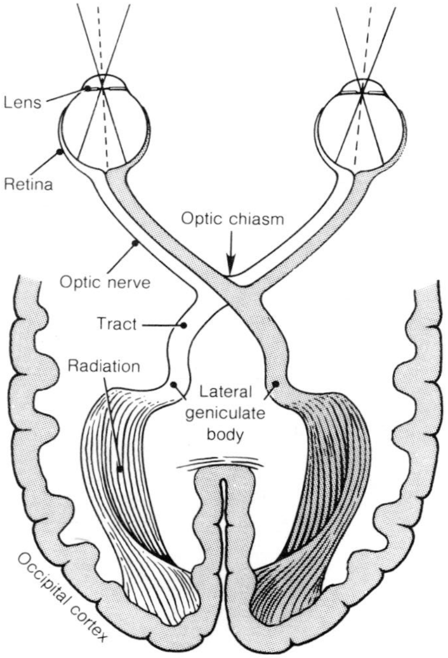

The fovea centralis is the point of central and acute color vision.

The macula is the area of most acute vision.

The blind spot is sometimes called the optic disk.

The blind spot does not register a visual image.

The optic chiasm is the point at which ocular nerve fibers move toward medial fibers and cross to opposite sides.

Vision is produced when nerve fibers enter the visual cortex of the brain's occipital lobe.

Figure b adapted from Dorothy A. Jones, et. al., Medical-Surgical Nursing, A Conceptual Approach, McGraw-Hill, 1978, p. 1182, fig. 34-3. Used with permission of McGraw-Hill Book Company.

Fovea centralis
Macular area
Optic disc

a

Lens
Retina
Optic nerve
Optic chiasm
Tract
Radiation
Lateral geniculate body
Occipital cortex

b

Visual Acuity Vision can be evaluated in terms of three components (a):

1 The ability of the eye to focus and accommodate

2 The intactness of the optic nerve (CN II) to receive and transmit an image

3 The ability of the cerebral cortex to receive and interpret an image.

The clarity and transparency of a client's ocular structures (e.g. cornea, anterior chamber, and the lens), as well as the adequacy of an individual's central vision (e.g. retina) are essential for visual acuity and accuracy.

Visual acuity can be tested in several ways. The most common test used is the standardized Snellen eye chart. The chart contains rows of letters in various sizes which the client reads aloud.

To complete the test the client is asked to stand or sit at a distance of 20 feet from the chart (b). The chart is usually placed on a flat surface (e.g. the wall) to facilitate readibility. When possible the chart should be covered prior to its use, to avoid memorization of letters.

The client is initially asked to cover one eye with a cardboard or other opaque cover. Fingers should never be used as they can cause blurring. With the room well lit the client is asked to read those lines indicated by the examiner.

The examiner may ask the client to read a specific line or to read from the top line and move downward from right to left as each line is scanned.

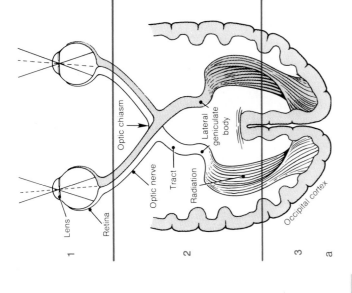

Vision is evaluated in terms of

1 the ability of the eye to focus and accommodate

2 nerve intactness (CN II)

3 the competence of the cerebral cortex to receive and interpret an image

Visual acuity is often assessed through the use of the Snellen eye chart.

The Snellen chart should be placed on a flat surface for easy reading and covered, when not is use, to avoid memorization.

Fingers should never be used to cover the eyes as they may cause blurring and falsely affect acuity.

Figure a adapted from Dorothy A. Jones, et. al., Medical-Surgical Nursing, A Conceptual Approach, McGraw-Hill, 1978, p. 1182, fig. 34-3. Used with permission of McGraw-Hill Book Company.

A numerator and denominator are used to record the client's measure of visual acuity (a). The *numerator* is 20 and equals the distance between the Snellen chart and the client's location (standing or sitting) at the standard distance (20 feet). The *denominator* equals the distance at which the normal eye is able to read the letters on the chart. The number on the chart opposite the last line the client can read is recorded as the *denominator*.

In the normal eye, measure of visual acuity is recorded at 20/20.

Persons who use corrective lenses should be assessed with and without lenses to determine visual acuity and evaluate the lenses being used.

The examination is repeated on the opposite eye and recorded as described above.

A gross assessment of near or close-up vision can be determined by having the client read a newspaper clipping or a smaller (hand-held) version of the Snellen chart (b). This measure will help to determine the ability of the lens to focus at a distance and close-up. Normally, the client should be able to read the close-up material with complete accuracy and uninterrupted flow.

The client can also be asked to further test visual acuity by correctly identifying the number of fingers being held up by the examiner (c). Distinguishing light from dark is another measure of visual competence.

While the results of performance on the Snellen chart is recorded as numerator and denominator, it is not a fraction in it's truest sense.

The number opposite the last line the client has read is recorded as the denominator.

A 20/50 reading means that the client sees at 20 feet what the normal person sees at 50 feet.

The larger the denominator the poorer the vision.

When the opposite eye is tested the client may be asked to read the Snellen chart from left to right.

Gross assessment of visual acuity can be achieved by having the client read a newspaper clipping.

$$\frac{20}{25}$$

F E L O

$$\frac{20}{20}$$ Numerator
Denominator

D L F P C

$$\frac{20}{15}$$

L E F O I

$$\frac{20}{13}$$

F D P L T

a

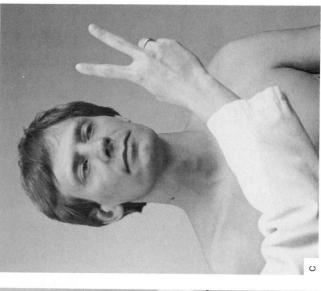

b

c

Highlights

Visual pathways can be evaluated by testing peripheral vision.

When testing peripheral vision the object should be slightly vibrated, since the eye picks up moving objects more quickly.

The client's temporal visual field may be more extensive than the examiner's during assessment of peripheral vision.

Testing peripheral vision provides a crude estimate of an individual's visual field.

Visual pathways can be evaluated (in part) by testing *peripheral vision*. To test peripheral vision, the client and examiner face each other, with their eyes at the same level. Using a cardboard cover or the hand, both cover one eye so that the eye opposite each other is open. The examiner stands (or sits) two feet from the client. The client is asked to look ahead, then at equal distance from both the examiner and client, the examiner brings an object (e.g. pencil) in from the periphery to the central vision area (a). The client is asked to note when the moving object is first seen.

The procedure is repeated in a clockwise or circular fashion at 45° angles so that total peripheral vision is tested (b). The client's peripheral vision is compared with the examiner's. It should be noted that the client's temporal visual field may be more extensive than the examiner's during assessment of peripheral vision.

As shown in this chart (c), temporal peripheral vision is more extensive than nasal peripheral vision. When the measurement is taken with the straight line of gaze at 0°, normal superior vertical peripheral vision is at about a 45° angle and temporal vision is at an 85° angle.

The procedure is repeated on the opposite eye and the tested eye of the examiner and client is covered.

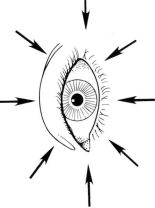

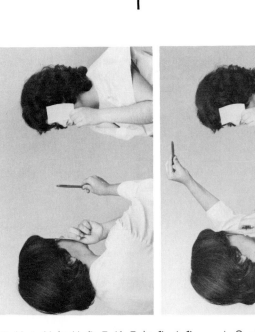

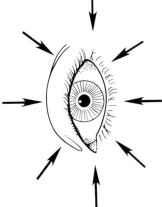

Extraocular Movements

Further determination of eye function and symmetry (parallelism) can be evaluated by inspecting ocular movements. Located posterior and between the roof and lateral wall of the eye is the *superior orbital fissure* (a). This area contains the arterial and venous blood supply as well as those cranial nerves i.e., oculomotor, (CN III), the trochlear (CN IV), and the abducens (CN VI) nerve, which facilitate eye movement.

Six muscles are responsible for eye movement (b). They include the four rectus muscles, the superior, inferior, and the lateral and medial attached to the vertical and the horizontal meridians of the orbital axis respectively. The superior and inferior oblique muscles also facilitate eye movement and the return of ocular motion to a central position.

The *superior oblique* and *lateral rectus muscles* are supplied by the 4th and 6th cranial nerve. The *superior, inferior,* and *medial recti muscles* along with the *inferior oblique* muscles are served by the 3rd cranial nerve.

When the medial rectus muscle contracts and the lateral rectus muscle relaxes, adduction results (c).

Contraction of the superior rectus muscle assisted by the inferior oblique muscles, results in a pulling action leading to elevation and inversion of the eye. The pulling of the inferior rectus muscle assisted by the superior oblique muscles, results in depression or extorsion of the eye.

To test extraocular muscle function the examiner uses three tests. These include the six cardinal positions of gaze, the Hirschberg test, and the cover-uncover test.

Cranial Nerves - 3, 4 and 6 interact to affect eye movement.

The optic foramen is the opening through which the optic nerve and ophthalmic artery travel into the orbit.

The muscles affecting eye movement include the superior, inferior, lateral and medial recti muscles, and the superior and inferior oblique muscles.

To test extraocular muscle function the examiner uses three tests:

1 the six cardinal positions of gaze
2 the Hirschberg test
3 the cover-uncover test

Right orbit

a

b

c

Positions of gaze The range of extra-ocular eye movements can best be examined through assessment of the six cardinal positions of gaze.

To test these movements, the examiner stands in front of the seated client. An object (e.g., a pencil or the examiner's finger) is held 12 to 18 inches away and the client is asked to follow the motions created with a gaze (a).

The distance of the object held in front of the client should be adjusted so that it is clearly visible to the client. The examiner may request that the client fix the gaze briefly at the extreme point of each movement presented. The gaze should remain steady at these extreme points.

The object should be moved to the left, upward to the left of midline, downward to the left of midline, to the right, upward to the right of midline and downward to the right of midline (b). Normally, extra-ocular movements should be smooth, continuous, parallel, and uninterrupted. The procedure is then repeated on the opposite eye.

The Hirschberg test This test is used to assess ocular muscle strength and alignment (parallelism) of the eye. With the examining room darkened, the client is asked to look straight ahead while the examiner shines a penlight from a distance of 30 cm (about 12 inches) to 60 cm (about 2 feet), into both corneas. Normally, a dot of light will be noted on the cornea's shiny surface at a similar position in both eyes. (e.g., 9 o'clock position [c]). A response to this test within normal limits indicates muscle balance, alignment and symmetry.

Highlights

The *six cardinal positions of gaze* are tested by movement of an object in a clockwise direction.

Extraocular movement should be smooth, parallel, continuous and uninterrupted.

The *Hirschberg test* is used to evaluate the muscle strength and eye symmetry.

PHYSICAL EXAMINATION

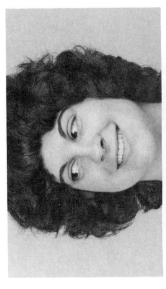
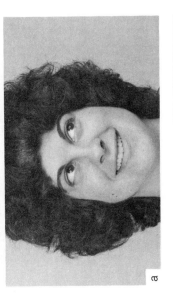

a

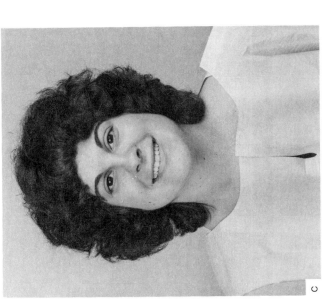

c

b

Highlights

The *cover-uncover test* is used to assess muscle strength and binocular vision.

During the cover-uncover test the eye that was covered should not move when cover is removed.

Pupil testing involves the assessment of cranial nerves III, IV and VI.

Pupil size is affected by the amount of light entering the eye.

Cover-uncover test This test is used to assess muscle strength and binocular vision. The seated client is asked to fix the vision on a specific object within 30 cm (one foot) in front of the eyes (e.g., the examiner's hair or nose).

The examiner covers one of the client's eyes with a blank piece of cardboard (or other eye cover), and examines the eye that is uncovered, observing the eye's ability to fix on the specific object (a). Following this observation, the cover is removed from the opposite eye. The examiner notes the movement of that eye (b). Normally, if the muscles are intact, the eye should be focused and therefore eye movement will not be observed.

The procedure is then repeated with the opposite eye.

Pupil Testing Testing of the pupils involves the assessment of three cranial nerves (CN II, IV, VI).

Normally, pupils are round and equal in size (c). Pupils dilate when sympathetic fibers are stimulated and constrict when parasympathetic fibers are stimulated.

Pupil size is usually affected by the amount of light that enters the pupil opening. Increasing amounts of light cause the pupil to constrict; decreasing amounts of light cause dilation of the pupil.

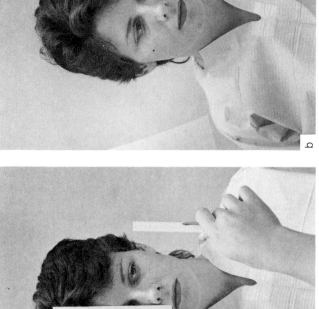

a

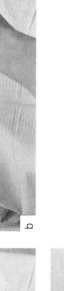

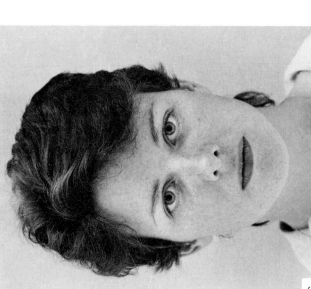

b

c

An individual's pupillary reaction is assessed through direct and consensual light response.

Normal pupil functioning can be recorded as **PERRLA** (**P**upils **E**qual **R**ound **R**eactive to **L**ight and **A**ccommodation).

The rapidity with which a pupil responds to light varies with each client.

To test *convergence constriction,* the client focuses on an object (e.g. pencil) placed directly in front of the eyes and follows it as it moves toward the bridge of the client's nose.

Depcoria - congenital abnormality in the shape of the pupils.

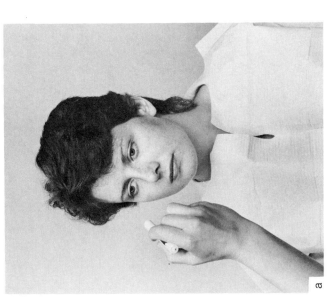

a

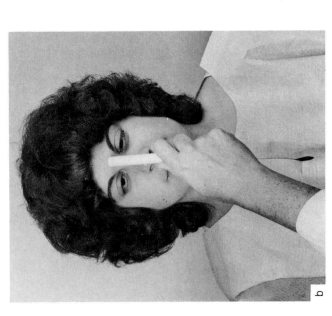

b

Assessing the client's response to light can be accomplished in two ways: first through *direct light,* then by *consensual light.*

To assess the client's response to *direct light* the room is darkened. A penlight is beamed toward the side of the eye by the examiner and then gradually moved directly into the anterior portion of the external eye (a).

The lighted eye is assessed for direct pupillary constriction. Simultaneously, the opposite eye is observed to determine if *consensual constriction* has occurred. The procedure is then repeated in the opposite eye.

Normally, both direct and consensual responses should be present. The rate of pupillary constriction may vary with each client.

The examiner may wish to test *convergence constriction* (or accommodation) of the eye muscles also at this time. To accomplish this the examiner asks the client to once again follow the finger or pencil movement held 30 cm (or 12 inches) to 60 cm (or 18 inches) in front of the client. The examiner brings the object toward the bridge of the individual's nose (b). Normally, both eyes will converge simultaneously on the object. The constriction of the pupils and synchronous convergence of the eyes should persist until the object is approximately 3 to 6 inches from the nose.

Refer to equipment section of Chap. 4 for a discussion of the ophthalmoscope.

Visualizing objects at a distance normally results in pupillary dilatation.

The client may remove contact lenses during the eye examination but it is not essential.

Ophthalmic dilators (e.g., 1% cyclogel or 10% phenylephrine hydrochloride) may be used to facilitate pupillary dilitation.

Eye drops should not be used to dilate the pupil in the presence of glaucoma.

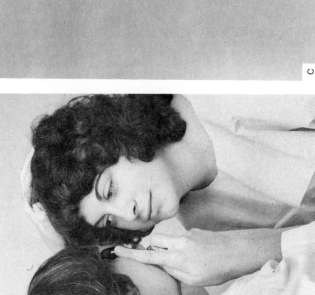

c

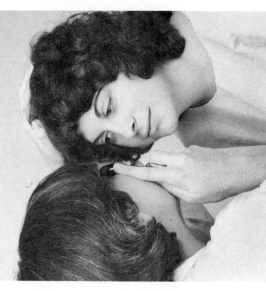

b

Superotemporal vein and arteriole

Fovea centralis

Macular area

Inferotemporal vein and arteriole

Superonasal arteriole and vein

Optic disc

Inferonasal arteriole and vein

a

Ophthalmoscopic Examination

The ophthalmoscopic examination involves the use of an ophthalmoscope (refer to equipment section) to visualize the color, clarity and size of the internal eye particularly, the retina, macula, and the optic disk (a). In addition, the color and size of the arteries and veins are also observed.

With the client seated and the room darkened, the examiner instructs the client to stare at a fixed object at a distant point. This action causes the pupil to dilate and prevents excessive eye movements.

Facing the client, the examiner places the ophthalmoscope in the right hand and holds it against the right eye for visualization of the client's right eye (b). When examining the client's left eye the procedure is reversed.

The examiner can place the opposite hand (in this case the left hand) above the client's eyebrow for stability.

Bracing the ophthalmoscope against the examiner's face the examiner turns the scope light on. The examiner's index finger is then placed on the lens disc to facilitate easy rotation as needed (c). The lens should be at 0, initially.

The examiner then looks through the viewing hole to begin the examination. Standing approximately about 15° lateral to the client's line of vision, the ophthalmoscope light is shone into the eye (a). This allows for the visualization of the "red reflex" or orange-red coloration that appears on the pupil when light is directed toward it.

The examiner then moves as a unit with the ophthalmoscope toward the light reflex (and the client). The retina and other structures can then be inspected.

The lens dial can be rotated to +15 to +20 to view the patency of the anterior chamber. By slowly moving the lens dial back to 0 the vitreous body can be observed for its transparency.

The color of the retina is normally of a reddish-orange. The area has a rich blood supply and contains slight pigmentation on the posterior layers.

There are four sets of retinal vessels (artery and vein) which emerge from the optic disk (b). These sets of vessels supply distinct retinal regions (namely the superonasal, inferotemporal, the inferonasal and superotemporal).

Blood vessels are often the first structures seen on inspection of the internal eye. The vessels tend to be narrower near the periphery and increase in diameter as they reach the optic disk. Normally, the walls of the vessels are transparent. The arteries are bright red and smaller than the veins. Arteries also have a narrow light reflex, veins do not (c).

Since the optic disk is not immediately seen, blood vessels are identified peripherally and followed centrally until they converge with other vessels. The optic disk is usually observed.

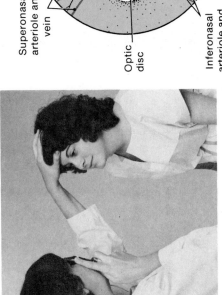

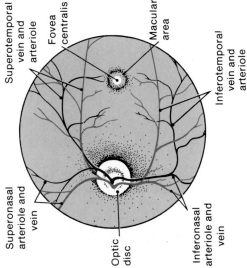

Superotemporal vein and arteriole

Fovea centralis

Macular area

Inferotemporal vein and arteriole

Superonasal arteriole and vein

Optic disc

Inferonasal arteriole and vein

b

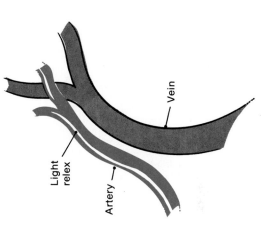

Light reflex

Artery

Vein

c

The client may blink during the eye examination. If excessive, the examiner may choose to stabilize the upper lid against the orbital rim.

If the "red-reflex" is lost, back away from the client and re-direct the light until the reflex is observed.

The eyeball is filled with a thick gelatinous substance called the **vitreous body**.

There are four sets of blood vessels (arteries and veins) which supply the retinal regions. They are:

1 superonasal
2 inferotemporal
3 inferonasal
4 superotemporal

Blood vessels are often seen on initial inspection of the eye.

The average ratio of arteries to vein is 2:3 or 4:5.

Blood vessels tend to be narrower in the periphery, increasing in size as they near the optic disk.

The *optic disk* is found on the nasal half of the retina and has sharp lines which isolate it from the retina. It is about 1.5 mm in diameter and is round (to oval) shaped. Its color ranges from a pink shade to creamy yellow. The examiner can usually distinguish the disk from the retina because it is lighter in color (a).

The optic disk can range from round to oval shape.

In dark skinned persons, pigmentation may be seen around the margins of the disk. In addition, a grayish tissue coloration may be seen in some individuals on the temporal side, near the disk.

The optic disk and retinal background vary from client to client, being lighter in light haired people and darker in dark haired people.

The *physiologic cup* (or depression) can be seen slightly temporal to the central portion of the disk. It appears slightly lighter in color than the disk and does not extend to the disk borders.

The physiologic cup is a depression on the disk that is a whittish-yellow coloration.

The retinal area surrounding the fovea centralis (point of central vision) is called the *macula*. This area is slightly darker in appearance than the retinal tissue and contains no observable blood vessel. It is nourished by vessels from the choroid area.

The macular area contains no observable blood vessels and is nourished by vessels from the choroid area.

To visualize the macula, the client is asked to look directly into the light from the ophthalmoscope.

Examination of the retina usually proceeds in an organized manner (e.g., clockwise). Changes regarding the structure are recorded in terms of their location from the disk (b).

The distance from the disk and the size of other findings are estimated in terms of disk diameters (DD); or as distance from the disk in relation to a clock position.

The procedure is repeated on the opposite eye and findings recorded.

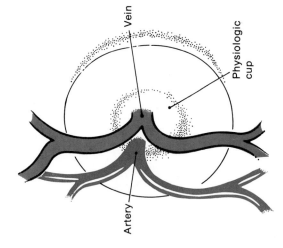

a

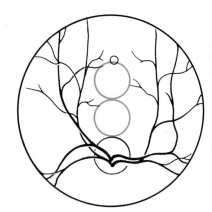

Fovea – two optic disks diameters (2 DD) at 3:00 on temporal side

b

Palpation

The *lacrimal sac and nasolacrimal duct* can be palpated by pressing directly over the medial aspect of the lower lid inside the orbital rim (a). Normally, the area should be pain free to touch, with no excessive tearing noted.

The ophthalmic division of the fifth cranial nerve (CN V) innervates the cornea. Intactness of this nerve is assessed by testing the *corneal reflex.*

The client is asked to look to the right or left. The examiner then takes the wisp of cotton and lightly brushes the lateral side of the cornea of the eye opposite to the direction in which the client is looking (b). Normally the client should blink when this procedure is performed.

Following an extensive eye examination, the client should be given an opportunity to relax before directly proceeding to the next part of the assessment.

Highlights

To palpate the lacrimal sac and ducts the examiner presses directly over the nares.

Normally, there should be no discomfort or excessive tearing during palpation of the tear ducts.

The ophthalmic division of the fifth cranial nerve is responsible for the corneal reflex.

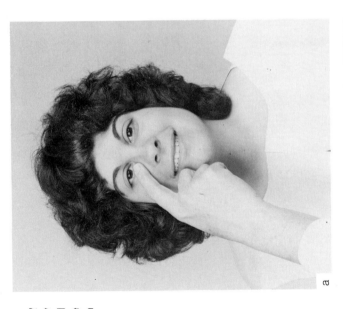

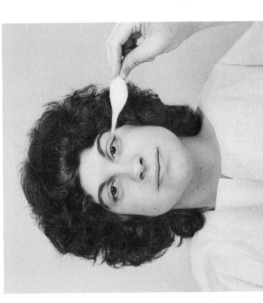

EAR

The ear is the sensory organ of hearing and balance. Examination of the ear includes assessment of the external, middle, and inner ear (a). Inspection and palpation are the main techniques used in this examination. The otoscope, tuning fork, and watch are used to assess all of the components of the ear. The examination of the external, middle and inner ear is a continuous process that has been separated out for emphasis only.

The External Ear

The external ear contains two components, the auricle, or pinna, and the external auditory canal. While the mastoid process is not a part of the external ear structure, it is usually examined at this time.

Inspection and palpation are used to examine the external ear.

Inspection

When the external ear is being examined, the client should be seated with the examiner directly facing the client's side (b).

The *auricle* or *pinna* of the ear is the structure first inspected. The auricle is composed of cartilage to which the perichondrium and skin adhere closely. This structure is bounded at the bottom by the *lobule* (soft tissue), anteriorly by the *tragus* and the *crus of the helix*, and posteriorly by the *helix*, *antihelix*, and the *triangular fossa* (c).

The auricle is normally a clearly defined structure. While the size and shape of the auricle will vary with each individual, it should be in proportion to body size, and be symmetrical. It is usually similar in color to the client's facial skin.

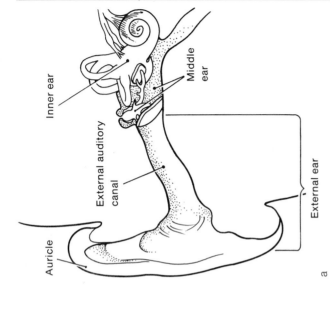

a

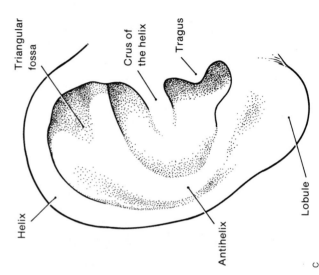

Triangular fossa

Crus of the helix

Tragus

Helix

Antihelix

Lobule

c

Inner ear

Middle ear

External auditory canal

External ear

Auricle

b

Highlights

Refer to equipment section for a discussion of instruments.

The auricle contains many curved structures which help trap sound waves.

Inspection of both auricles is required to determine position, symmetry, and size.

The skin of the external ear should be examined thoroughly, including the posterior and lateral surfaces, to assess its intactness.

It is important to observe the position of the external ear in children (refer to Chap. 5).

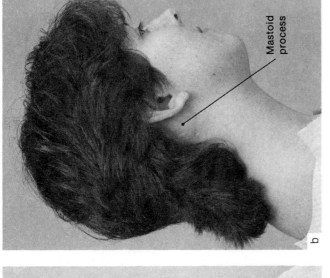

a

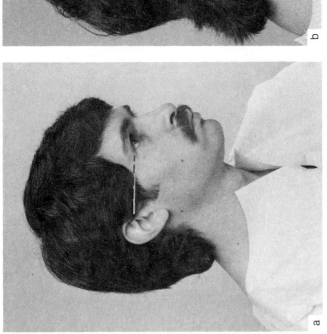

c

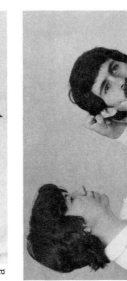

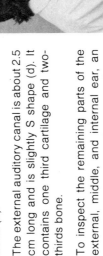

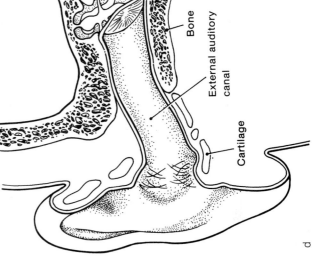

Bone

External auditory canal

Cartilage

d

b

Mastoid process

The lobule may be connected to the facial skin or hang unattached to the skin surface.

To determine the position of the ear, the examiner should find the point where the superior portion of the helix attaches to the scalp, then run an imaginary line from the helix to the lateral angle of the eye (a). Vertical variation in the line should run horizontally with little or no downward deviation.

The mastoid process is a bony prominence located behind the lower part of the auricle (b). While it is not directly connected to the auricle, it can be inspected at this time. Normally, the skin surface, although slightly protruding, is smooth and similar in color to the surrounding facial skin.

The opening of the *external auditory canal* should be clear, dry, open, and should follow the normal contour of the canal (c).

The external auditory canal is about 2.5 cm long and is slightly S shape (d). It contains one third cartilage and two-thirds bone.

To inspect the remaining parts of the external, middle, and internal ear, an otoscope will be used. Before moving to the use of the otoscope the examiner should palpate the auricle and mastoid process.

Palpation

Initially, the auricle can be examined by holding it between the examiner's thumb and four fingers and pulling gently on the structure. This action should not be painful. Normally, the structure is firm and mobile, and contains smooth ridges (a).

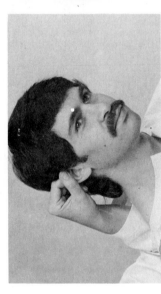

The examiner should then fold the ear forward to palpate behind the ear easily (b). After this action the examiner should release the auricle. Normally, the structure will return to its usual position without assistance.

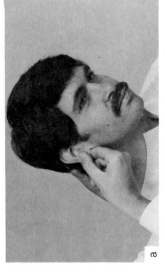

The external auditory canal entrance can be palpated for structure and softness of skin surface (c).

The mastoid process is then carefully palpated (d) using the deep palpation over the entire area. Normally, the area is firm and intact, with a slight protuberance and clearly defined ridges. The skin covering the structure is smooth and continuous and is similar in color to the facial skin.

Highlights

Good room lighting is needed when inspecting and palpating the auricle.

It is very important to include palpation of the mastoid process in the examination of the external ear.

Palpation of the mastoid should not be painful. If it is, further examination is needed.

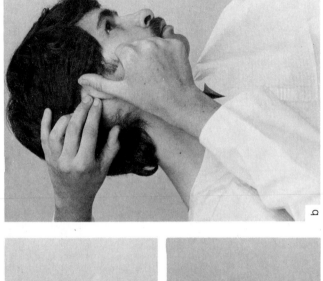

a

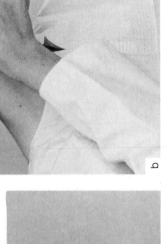

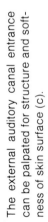

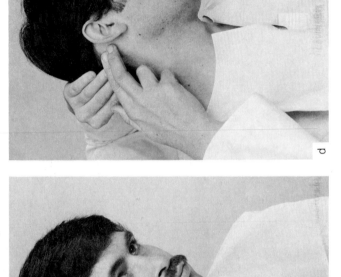

b

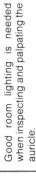

c

d

Inspection (assisted)

Before inserting the otoscope into the external auditory canal, ask the client to tip the head toward the opposite shoulder (away from the examiner) (a).

This action is taken to improve the visibility of the auditory canal by creating a more horizontal plane.

Depending upon the size of the canal, attach the largest speculum to the otoscope that the client can accommodate.

Should the client experience pain during insertion of the otoscope it must be removed and a smaller speculum used.

Refer to p. 131 under Equipment Section for a more complete discussion of the otoscope.

When inserting the otoscope in children the auricle should be pulled downward.

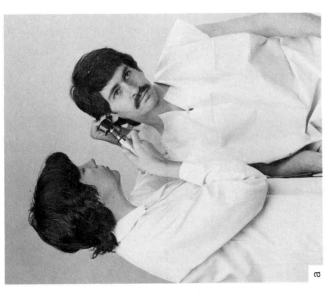

The examiner holds the otoscope in the palm of the hand and uses the opposite hand to pull the auricle upward and backward (b). This action helps to straighten the canal and increase visibility. The light at the end of the speculum will help to view the canal.

The membranous covering of the inner two-thirds of the external auditory canal will normally appear smooth and a slightly deeper pink than the skin surrounding the auricle. The membrane is thin, and small intact blood vessels may be visible.

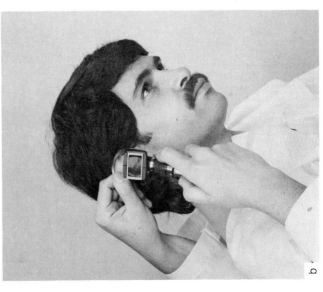

Middle Ear

As the examination of the auditory canal continues, the examiner, using the otoscope, will see a translucent covering at the end of the canal called the **tympanic membrane** (or eardrum). This membrane separates the external ear from the middle ear (a). The area of the middle ear is small, and filled with air. It is located within the temporal bone. The auditory ossicles are sometimes referred to as the **malleus, incus,** and **stapes** (b).

There are several openings into the middle ear. These include:

The opening from the external auditory meatus covered by the tympanic membrane

The opening connecting the middle ear with the Eustachian tube

The openings into the inner ear through the oval window and the round window

Inspection

Examination of the middle ear is achieved through the use of the otoscope with the client remaining in a seated position (c).

The components of the middle ear are not accessible to examination. However, inspection of the tympanic membrane can provide significant information about the status of the middle ear.

The middle ear has several functions. It transmits sounds across to the inner ear, it protects fragile auditory structures from intense vibrations, and it prevents rupture of the tympanic membrane by equalizing air pressure.

The Eustachian tube extends from the pharynx to the middle ear and opens during swallowing and yawning and helps equalize pressure.

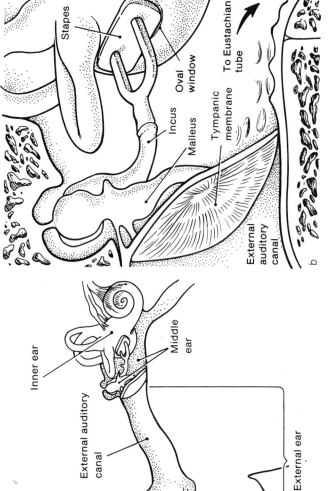

a

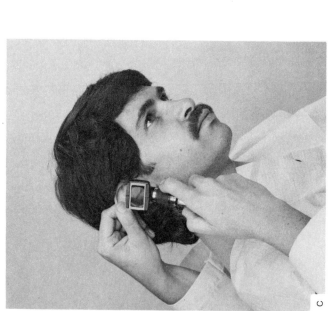

b

c

Three ossicles found in the middle ear are the malleus, the incus and the stapes.

The membrane is made up of fibrous tissue, mucous membrane, and layers of skin. It is normally shiny, and translucent, and is pearl gray in color. The eardrum appears to be pulled inward toward its center due to the action of the malleus, one of three ossicles functioning in the middle ear (a).

The short process of the malleus originates in the superior part of the drum, protrudes into the eardrum above the handle of the malleus, and continues downward to the *umbo*. The umbo is located at the point where the membrane is most concave. Upon examination, the umbo is seen as a dense, whitish streak through the transparent membrane.

The light reflex will vary from a bright to a dim light.

Most of the membrane (drum) appears taut and evenly distributed. This is referred to as the **pars tensa**. The tautness of the pars tensa creates a cone of light referred to as **light reflex.** The point of the light reflex is directed downward below the umbo (a point of maximal concavity of the drum) and toward the periphery of the drum. The **pars flaccida** is located at the upper portion of the pars tensa and appears less taut.

The white light reflex, the umbo, the long and short processes of the malleus, and the malleolar folds are sometimes referred to as "landmarks" present during examination of the eardrum.

A ring of dense fibrous tissue called the **tympanic ring** or **annulus** surrounds the periphery of the tympanic membrane. The annulus will appear well defined, whitish gray and denser than the rest of the eardrum. It should surround the eardrum without interruption. The anterior and posterior **malleolar folds** are two additional folds located at the superior portion of the membrane. The examiner may also note a varying number of blood vessels present. When observed, these vessels are usually regular, smooth, and intact (b).

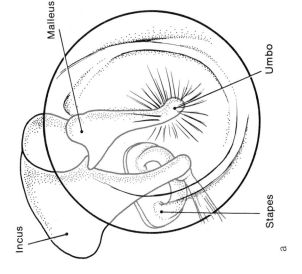

Malleus

Incus

Umbo

Stapes

a

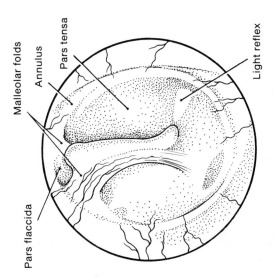

Malleolar folds

Pars flaccida

Annulus

Pars tensa

Light reflex

b

184

The vestibule and semicircular canals are the organs of equilibrium and balance.

The cochlea houses the essential organs of hearing.

The organ of Corti is found within the coiled structure of the cochlea.

Inner Ear

The inner ear is not accessible to inspection (a). The area is composed of a bony labyrinth and within this structure, a membranous labyrinth. The bony labyrinth is composed of three parts, the *vestibule*, the *semicircular canals*, and the *cochlea* (a). The two major functions of the inner ear structures include hearing (vestibule and semicircular canals) and balance (cochlea).

Hearing

Normally, hearing occurs when sound waves enter through the auricle into the external auditory canal. These sound waves then cause the tympanic membrane to vibrate. The sound vibration then enters the middle ear, travels across the malleus, incus, and stapes, to the oval window and to the inner ear. The sound then travels through the fluid of the coiled structure called the cochlea, to the *round window*, where the vibration dissipates. The sensitive hair cells within the *organ of Corti and membrane of Corti* are set into action by the vibrations present (b). As the organ of Corti is activated, it stimulates impulses in the sensory endings of the cochlea branch of the auditory nerves (CNVIII), hearing then occurs (c).

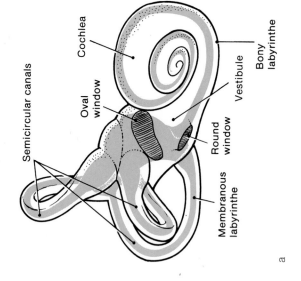

a

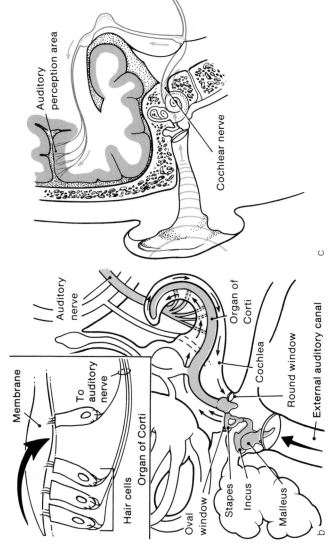

b

c

Inspection

While the inner ear cannot be directly seen, there are several tests that can be done to determine the intactness of the auditory nerve. These include:

1 Voice test
2 Watch-tick test
3 Tuning fork test
4 Rinne's test

Voice test The client remains seated and is asked to close both eyes. The examiner stands to one side, approximately 2 feet from the client, who covers the opposite ear (a). The examiner then whispers a word such as a number, color, or name into the client's ear. The examiner can regulate the whisper into a soft, medium, or loud whisper.

Whispered sounds are high-pitched. The examiner repeats the same word with the regular spoken voice and notes the responses. The procedure is then repeated in the opposite ear. Normally, the whispered sound should be heard equally well in both ears.

Watch-Tick Test The watch-tick test also assesses the client's ability to hear high-pitched sounds. The client is again seated and is asked to cover the opposite ear. The watch is held at the same distance, audible to the examiner (b). The client is asked to respond "yes" if sound is heard and "no" if it is not. The procedure is repeated with the opposite ear. Normally, the ticking watch is accurately heard in both ears.

The watch can also be held close to the client and gradually moved away until no longer audible to the client. The same procedure is repeated on the opposite ear and the distance compared.

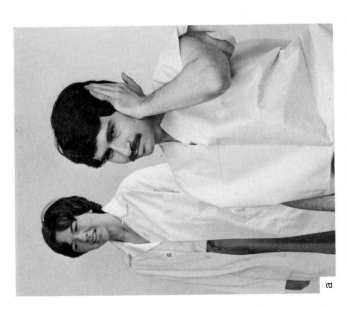

a

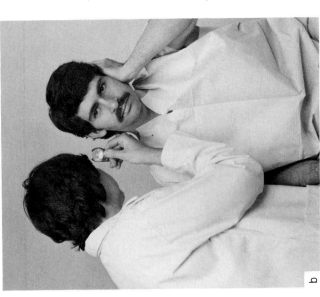

b

Highlights

The intactness of the auditory nerve can be assessed through tests such as the voice test, watch-tick test, and the Rinne test.

The clients are asked to close their eyes during the voice test to prevent lip reading.

Whispered sounds usually are higher-pitched sounds (refer to sound pitch, p. 125).

Poor response to the voice test will require a more extensive hearing evaluation.

The watch-tick test can only determine high frequency sounds.

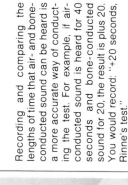

To set the tuning fork into vibration, pinch the ends of the fork and release suddenly or tap the tuning fork against the hand (knuckle portion).

In conductive hearing loss sound is louder in the affected ear.

Bone conduction refers to sound to the cochlea (CNVIII) that is transmitted through the bones of the skull.

Air conduction refers to sound transmitted through the ear canal through the processes of the middle and inner ear to the cochlea and auditory nerve.

Recording and comparing the lengths of time that air- and bone-conducted sound can be heard is a more accurate way of conducting the test. For example, if air-conducted sound is heard for 40 seconds and bone-conducted sound for 20, the result is plus 20. You would record: "+20 seconds, Rinne's test."

In *mild* hearing loss air-conducted sound will be heard longer, but not twice as long as bone-conducted sound.

Tuning Fork

The tuning fork is used to determine conductive or sensorineural hearing loss. There are sensory hearing tests which utilize a tuning fork to determine sound perception. These are, Weber's test, Rinne's test, and Schwaback's test.

Weber's Test The Weber Test is commonly used to test for lateralization of hearing. The client remains seated while the examiner places the stem of a vibrating tuning fork against the midline portion of the client's skull (a). The client is then asked to indicate if the vibrating sound is heard and if the sound is louder either in the right or left ear.

Normally, the sound is equally loud in both ears.

The Rinne's Test With the client in a seated position, the examiner places the handle of a vibrating tuning fork against the mastoid process behind one ear (b). The client is asked to indicate verbally or through a hand signal when a sound is no longer heard.

The examiner then removes the still-vibrating tuning fork and places it near the anterior ear surface (c). The client is asked to indicate if the sound is heard and to signal accordingly when the sound ceases. When this occurs, the examiner may wish to hold the tuning fork against his or her own ear to see if there is any residual sound present. This procedure is then repeated on the opposite ear.

Normally, the client will hear the tuning fork twice as long when sound is conducted by air as opposed to bone. When the client hears air-conducted sound (tuning fork held by the ear) longer than bone-conducted sound (tuning fork over the mastoid process), the Rinne's test is positive.

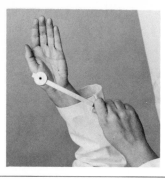

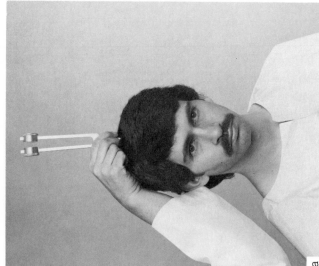

a

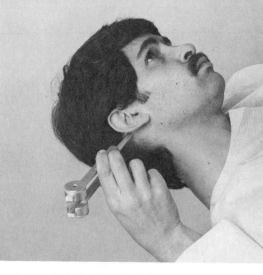

b

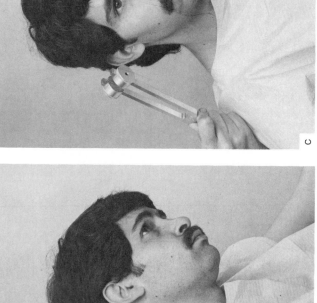

c

If there are differences in the lengths of time that the client and examiner hear the sounds, then Schwaback's test may indicate nerve damage or bone loss.

The Schwaback test is used to compare the client's hearing against the examiner's.

Schwaback's Test In Schwaback's test the examiner sets the tuning fork into vibration and alternately places the fork first over the client's mastoid process (a) and then over the examiner's. This process continues until both cease hearing the sound. If there is no hearing loss present in either individual, it is expected that both will cease hearing the sounds at the same time.

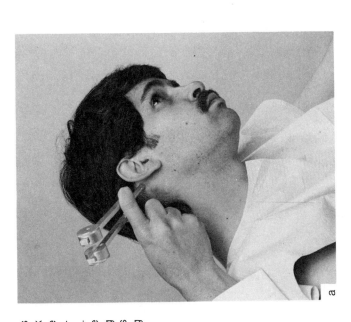

a

Balance

There are neurons contained within the vestibular portion of the auditory nerve which send fibers to the neuro-epithelium of the semicircular canals. The nerve fibers synapse with motion receptors in specialized areas of the canals (b). Movement of the head causes fluid in the canals to flow past the receptors, which then send messages to the medulla, cerebellum and spinal cord (vestibular spinal tract). These messages inform the brain, eyes and postural muscles (c) of the change in position of the head, enabling the body to maintain balance.

There are several tests for vestibular function that can be used by the examiner to determine a client's sense of balance. The first is the labyrinthine falling test and the second is a positioning determination.

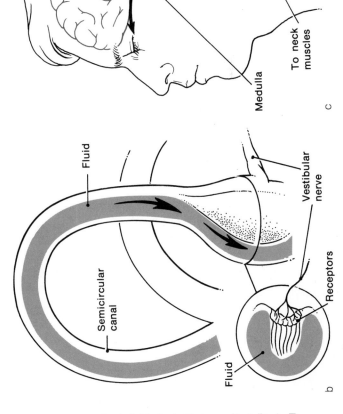

b

c

When the examiner places his or her arms around the client, it provides a sense of reassurance to the individual and prevents injury should the client start to fall.

The Romberg Test is also a test of the client's proprioceptive system.

Test for specific vestibular function, however, Caloric (Ba'ra'ny's Test) Rotational (Nylen-Ba'ra'ny's Test) and Electric (electronstagmography) stimuli are used if alterations in balance are present.

Labyrinthine Falling Tests The client is asked to stand with the toes and heels placed together. The examiner then stands alongside the client with his or her arms surrounding but not touching the client. (This test is sometimes referred to as the Romberg Test.)

The client is then asked to close both eyes (a). Although some individuals may waver slightly, they should maintain their erect position and not fall for at least 5 seconds.

Position Determination The client is asked to sit comfortably, face the examiner and close both eyes (b). Again the client should maintain an erect position with no or slight swaying. The client should be aware of the surrounding environment and his or her position in relation to it.

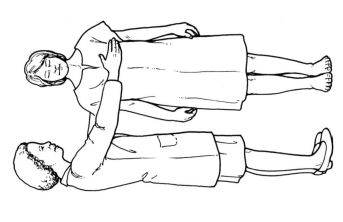

a

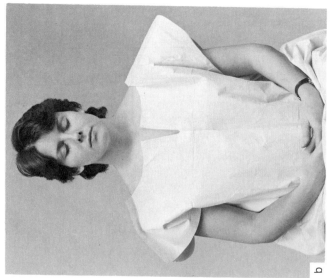

b

NOSE

The nose is readily accessible to examination. It can be assessed as part of the facial examination or evaluated as a separate entity. For purposes of examination, the nose is divided into the *external* and *internal* nose.

Inspection

To inspect the *external nose*, the client is seated in an upright position and facing the examiner.

The external nose is triangular in shape, although the size, shape (contour), and profile of the nose will vary from client to client (a).

The external nose is usually in a midline position bounded by the forehead at the *glabella*, its uppermost angle, and laterally by the facial structures. The *dorsum nasi* is formed by the midline joining together of the lateral sides of the external nose. These structures should be intact and clearly defined (b).

The lateral surface extends down and around the lower portion of the nasal tip to form the fatty fibrous tissue of the *ala nasi*. The *tip* of the nose is formed by cartilage and fibrous tissue at the free angle at the lower portion of the structure.

When inspecting the base of the nose, two openings called **nares** are observed to the right and left of the midline structure known as the **columella**.

The nasal framework is composed of both bone and cartilage. The upper third of the structure is *bone*, while the remaining two-thirds contain *cartilage* (c).

When examining the nose, it is important to have the room well lit for adequate viewing.

Variations in the size and shape of the nose are influenced by race, sex, and genetics.

The upper portion of the *dorsum nasi* is also called the *bridge* of the nose.

The columella extends into the internal nose to form the **nasal septum**.

Surgery on the nasal structures may alter facial appearance.

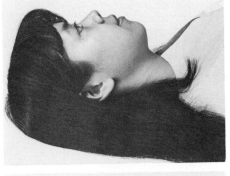

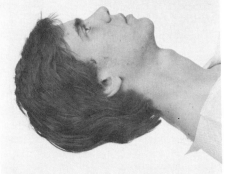

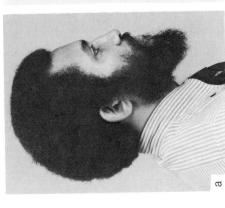

a

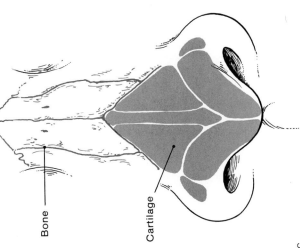

Glabella
Bridge
Dorsum nasi
Nares
Ala nasi
Columella

b

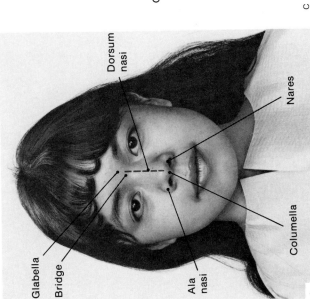

Bone
Cartilage

c

To inspect the general nasal framework, the examiner may ask the client to change the position of the head to increase visibility of a particular structure.

The external nose should appear proportionate to other facial structures.

Nasal symmetry is assessed by having the examiner identify the nasal septum and then observe its relationship with the other nasal structures. To accomplish this, the client tilts the head backward and looks at the ceiling (a).

The examiner observes the movement of the *ala nasi* during respiration to determine nasal flaring. Normally, there should be free bilateral expansion of the nasi on inspiration (b).

To inspect the *internal nose*, the client should remain sitting erect. The examiner should stand or sit facing the client, changing the position when necessary for a better view of the nasal structures.

Inspection of the internal nasal structures begins at the nares. Each nares continues posteriorly into the nasal chamber forming the right and left nasal passages (c).

Alteration in the continuity of the nasal framework may be influenced by past traumatic injury or congenital deformity and should be investigated.

It is important to note that the septum is rarely perfectly straight. However, the septum should not be significantly deviated.

The nasal passages are equally divided by the nasal septum.

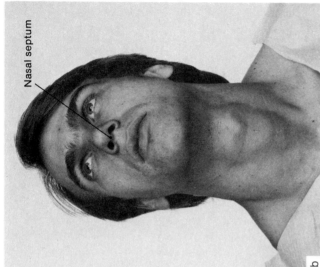

Ala nasi

a

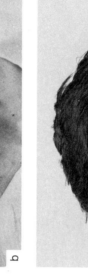

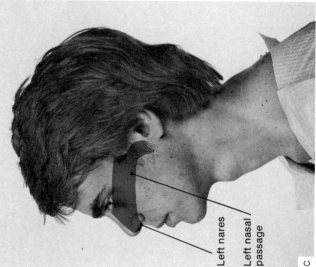

Nasal septum

b

Left nares

Left nasal passage

c

At any time, one nasal passage may be more patent than the other.

A mirror can be held in front of each nares during expiration. If the chamber is patent, clouding of the mirror will occur as the warm air reaches the mirror surface.

The client should be supported during position change to avoid losing balance.

Use of the nasal speculum is discussed on p. 133.

An otoscope with a short, wide attachment piece may also be used to inspect the internal nose.

The examiner's right hand is placed on the client's head to allow for the free movement and to improve inspection of the nasal orifice.

The nasal mucosa is often redder in color than oral mucosa.

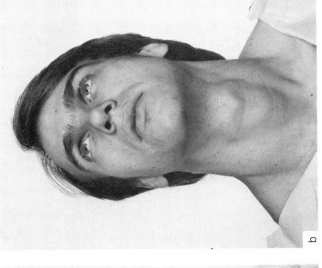

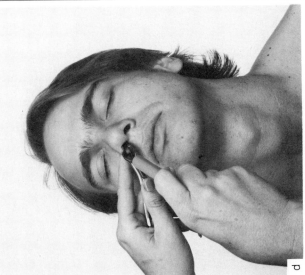

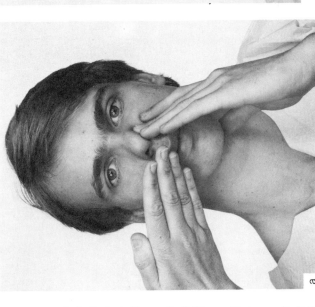

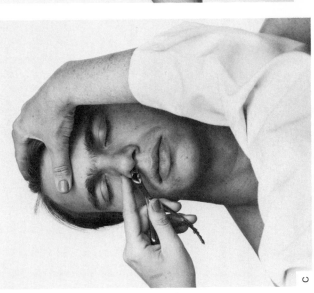

Normally, each passage is patent and free of drainage. To assess nasal patency the client is asked to close the mouth and apply pressure against one nostril, using the fingers. The client is then instructed to exhale forcefully. The procedure is repeated by occluding the opposite passage. Normally, the examiner is able to hear and feel the unobstructed movement of air from each nasal chamber (a).

The client should tilt the head slightly backward to allow the examiner to see into the anterior vestibule of the internal nose (b).

To look into the internal nose and related structures, a nasal speculum and penlight will be used.

A head mirror may also be used to view internal nasal structures, but is usually not required during an uncomplicated examination.

The client should be relaxed and comfortably seated. The examiner places the right hand on the client's head (thumb on forehead) as demonstrated in the photograph (c).

The examiner then inserts the nasal speculum into the nares holding the instrument in the left hand. The speculum can be opened as widely (anterior-posterior) as the client will tolerate. The examiner should avoid hitting the septum with the tip of the speculum, as it could cause pain. Note that the forefinger of the left hand is used to guide the speculum along the lateral wall.

The walls of the internal nose are only lined with a mucous membrane. Normally, the mucosa is pink, moist, and smooth. A penlight may be used to increase visibility of internal structures (d).

Kiesselbach's plexus is the site where nose bleeds most frequently occur.

The nasal septum is a cartilaginous structure which becomes the medial wall of the right and left nasal passages.

It is common to observe slight nasal deviation in adults.

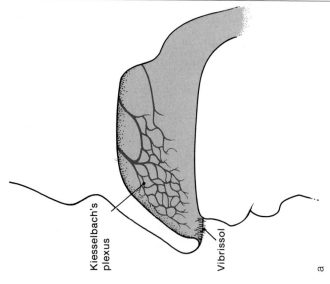

Kiesselbach's plexus

Vibrissol

a

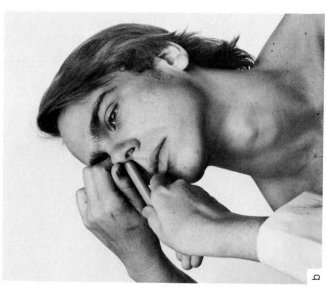

b

Inside the nares and continuing along the anterior passage is a hair lining (cilia or vibrissol) which helps filter inspired air as it enters the upper respiratory tract. The amount of hair visible at the entrance to the passage varies from client to client.

The anterior portion of the septum contains a highly vascular area called **Kiesselbach's plexus** (a).

To inspect the internal septum, tilt the client's head backward slightly. Place a thumb softly against the tip of the client's nose and push it upward.

A penlight is then inserted into the nasal chamber with the light directed upward and toward the septum. This allows for illumination of the septum which can be clearly seen by the examiner looking into the opposite chamber (b). Normally the septum is clear and transparent.

Highlights

To view the choana, the examiner inserts a postnasal mirror into the client's mouth and extends it posteriorly toward the pharyngeal wall. With the use of illumination the examiner can adjust the mirror to see various aspects of the choana.

This procedure is usually completed by an ear, nose and throat specialist.

Normally, the turbinates are a deep pink color.

The inferior turbinate is the largest and is located in the lower lateral wall of the internal nose and varies in size.

The middle turbinate can normally be seen by inspecting the anterior nose.

The nasolacrimal duct, which drains tears from the eye, empties into the inferior meatus.

The 1st cranial nerve is the olfactory nerve.

When selecting an aroma for a client to identify, be sure it is a familiar substance.

The client should be able to correctly identify the substance being used.

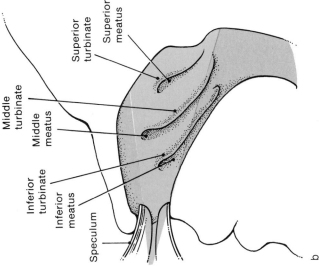

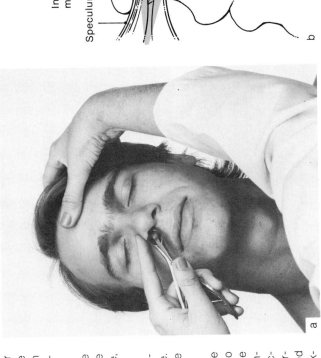

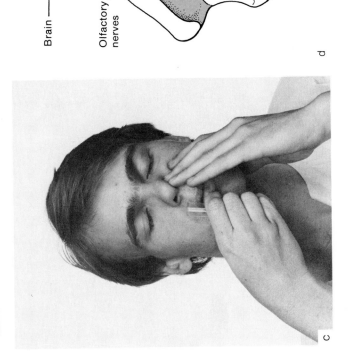

The **choana** is located in the posterior portion of each nasal chamber. It is the opening through which air is drawn from the nasal chamber into the upper respiratory tract.

The internal nose also contains three curved bony structures. These are the superior, middle, and inferior conchae, or *turbinates*.

The turbinates are parallel to one another on the lateral wall of the nose. They humidify, clean, and regulate the temperature of inspired air.

Beneath each turbinate is a groove called a *meatus*. The sinuses drain into these grooves. The three meatuses are called superior, middle, and inferior. Inspection of the turbinates can be accomplished during viewing of the internal nose. With the speculum fully opened and the head of the client tilted backward, the turbinates can be seen (a).

The turbinates and meatuses are clearly visible and move freely (b). They are normally deep pink in color.

The *olfactory nerve* receptors (1st cranial nerve) are found above the superior turbinate in the roof of the nasal cavity (d).

These receptor cells transmit impulses for smell to the temporal lobe of the brain.

To test the functioning of the olfactory nerves, the client is asked to close his eyes and occlude one nares by pressing one finger against one nostril (c).

A strong-smelling substance such as coffee, alcohol, or ammonia is placed in a test tube and held directly in front of the client's unobstructed nostril. The client is then asked to correctly identify the material.

Palpation

During palpation the client remains in a seated position.

The examiner, standing to the client's side places one hand on the client's head to increase balance and to ensure accuracy of findings.

The external nasal structure is palpated initially (a). The nasal bone and cartilage are palpated and continuity and absence of tenderness are noted.

The soft tissue primarily located at the ridges and nares is also palpated to evaluate tissue structure (b). Normally, this area is soft to the touch.

The Paranasal Sinuses

The **paranasal sinuses** are hollow, air-filled cavities lined with mucous membrane. Each sinus contains a drainage tract which allows for the exit of fluids should they accumulate. Normally, there is little or no drainage present in the nasal sinus. Inspection and palpation are techniques used to assess the sinuses.

Inspection

The paranasal sinuses are found within the bones of the skull and communicate with the nasal cavity. The frontal, maxillary, ethmoid, and sphenoid sinuses are components of the paranasal sinuses (c). The frontal and maxillary sinuses are most accessible to examination (d).

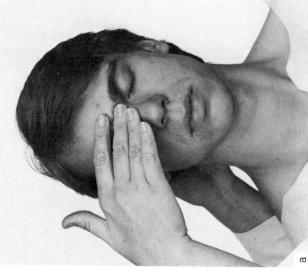

a

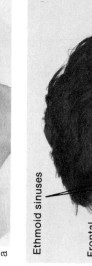

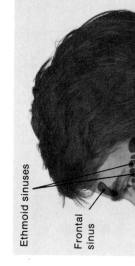

b

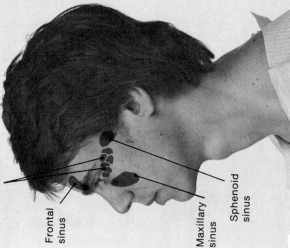

Ethmoid sinuses

Frontal sinus

Maxillary sinus

Sphenoid sinus

c

Frontal sinuses

Maxillary sinuses

d

The paranasal sinuses affect voice resonance and warm, moisten, and contribute to filtering air.

The paranasal sinuses all drain into the nasal cavity.

The frontal, maxillary, and anterior and middle ethmoid sinuses drain into the middle meatus.

Care should be taken to use a clean penlight each time the maxillary sinuses are inspected.

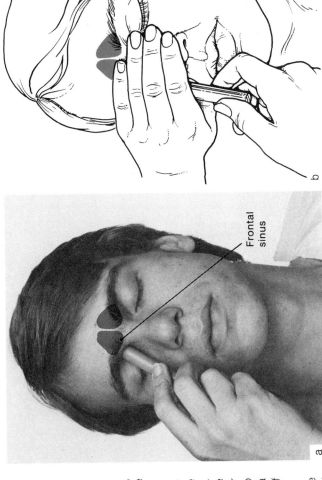

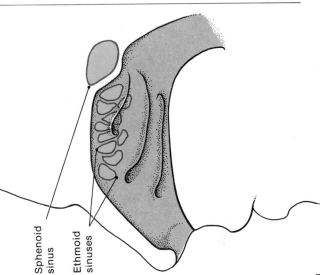

Frontal sinus

a

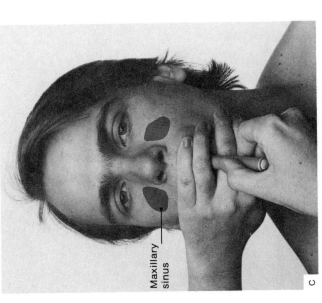

Maxillary sinus

c

b

Sphenoid sinus

Ethmoid sinuses

d

The *frontal and maxillary sinuses* are inspected by illumination.

During this part of the examination the client remains seated, facing the examiner. The examining room is darkened and a penlight is used to illuminate the sinus area.

The *frontal sinuses* are paired sinuses, located on either side of the bridge of the nose, deep to the eyebrows.

To inspect the frontal sinus the examiner places the penlight on either side of the nasal bridge below the eyebrows. The penlight is directed upward (a). The examiner then places the free hand over the nasal bone and end of penlight to block out excess light. Normally, a reddish-pink glow appears in the area of the frontal sinuses (b).

The *maxillary sinuses* are located above the right and left upper molar area and below the zygomatic bone.

To inspect the maxillary sinus a penlight is inserted directly into the oral cavity and directed toward the roof of the mouth. The client is asked to close the lips around the penlight and the examiner covers the mouth with the free hand (c), and observes the light response. Normally, there should be a pinkish-red glow in the area of the maxillary sinus.

The sphenoid and ethmoid sinuses are not accessible to examination, but, as they may be involved in sinus problems their location is noted here for reference.

The *ethmoid sinuses* are found in the lateral walls of the nasal passages above the middle turbinates (d).

The *sphenoid sinuses* are posterior to the ethmoid sinuses and above and behind the superior turbinate (d).

PHYSICAL EXAMINATION

Highlights

Bilateral examination of both the frontal and maxillary sinuses is performed to compare responses over each area. Normally, no difference is recorded.

Palpation of the frontal bone directly above the eyebrow may be used to assess the frontal sinuses.

Palpation

During palpation of the sinuses, the client remains seated. When examining the frontal sinuses, the examiner places one hand on the forehead to stabilize the head and puts the first two fingers of the free hand into the superior part of each orbital socket beneath the eyebrows (a). Pressure is then exerted upward against the bone surface. Normally, no discomfort is caused by this procedure.

Palpation of the maxillary sinuses is accomplished by placing the tips of the right and left fingers directly beneath the right and left cheekbone (b). Using gentle pressure over the maxillary sinus area, both cheeks are stimulated simultaneously. Normally, this procedure does not cause pain or discomfort.

Palpation of the maxillary sinuses may also be performed with the first two fingers of one hand (c).

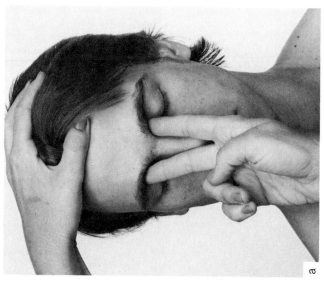

a

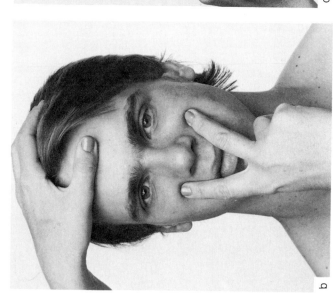

c

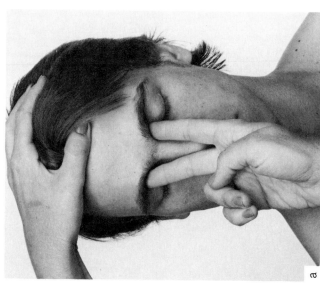

b

MOUTH

Examination of the mouth begins with the assessment of the external structures of the mandible, cheeks, and lips and moves into the oral cavity for inspection of the buccal mucosa, the teeth and gums, the tongue, and the oropharynx. The client and the examiner should be seated and facing one another. It is important that the examiner and client be at the same level (a).

A tongue blade, gum stimulator, oral mirror, penlight, gauze pad, and gloves will be utilized during the examination. Inspection and palpation will be the main techniques used to collect data.

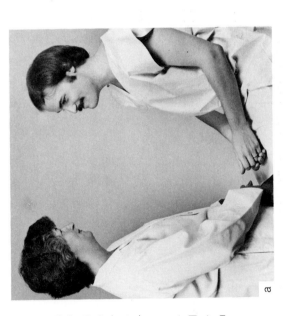

a

Cheeks

The cheeks provide skin covering for the bony structures of the face. The color and texture of the skin will vary according to race, age, and sex.

Inspection

When observing the cheeks, the examiner should note skin texture, color, and symmetry (b). Normally, the cheeks are smooth in females and may be somewhat rougher in males depending upon hair distribution. The buccinator muscle is an important component of the cheeks (c). It aids in chewing by holding food close to the teeth.

Palpation

Palpation of the right and left cheek by the examiner helps to determine the skin texture as well as general health of tissue. Normally, the tissue will return to normal position after light squeezing.

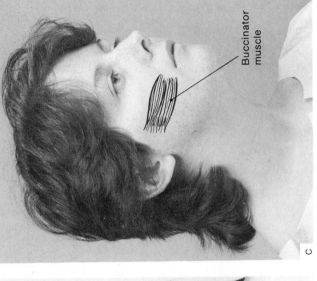

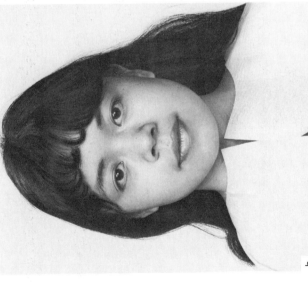

Buccinator muscle

c

b

The examiner should observe the general external symmetry of the lower half of the face when the client's mouth is closed.

The cheeks expand to allow for initial storage of food during digestion.

Information about nutrition and body hydration can be gathered during the inspection of facial skin.

Alterations in facial skin integrity (eg. moles) or birthmarks may be noted during the facial inspection and should be explored with the client, as appropriate.

Refer to Fig. c, p. 178, for location of the tragus of the ear.

During the opening and closing of the jaw the sound of the temporomandibular should not be audible.

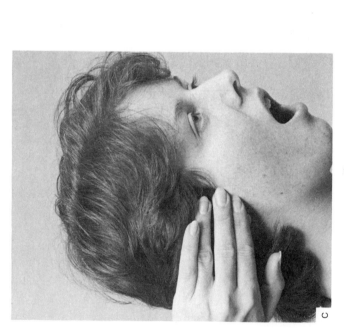

b

Mandible

Temporomandibular joint

Tragus

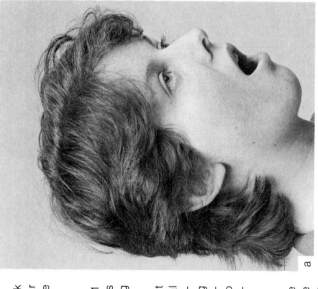

a

c

Mandible

The mandible forms the bony framework of the mouth. Assessment of mandibular movements (a) should precede the examination of the lips.

Inspection

The temporomandibular joint, located 1 cm anterior to the tragus of the ear, is responsible for the opening and closing of the mouth (b).

To inspect jaw movement ask the client to open and close the mouth several times. This process should be completed with ease and comfort. During this movement note the even approximation of the upper and lower jaw to each other. There should be no protrusion of the jaw observed.

Palpation

The temporomandibular joint can be palpated by applying direct pressure over the joint area. The examiner places the second, third, and fourth fingers of each hand on the right and left side of the face, in front of the ear, and exerts light pressure (c). The client is asked to open and close the mouth in uninterrupted movements. Normally, there should be free, comfortable, smooth, and continuous movement at the joint site with good approximation of the lips upon complete closure.

Lips

The lips are the fleshy rim of the mouth. They provide entry to the oral cavity, aid in the digestive process by removing food from utensils, and contribute to word formation in speaking.

Inspection

When inspecting the lips, the examiner will observe a wide variation in the size and shape of the lips (a). In all individuals, the point where the upper and lower lip meet should be noted. This is commonly called the *commissure*. The right and left commissures should appear level with each other (b).

In most clients the lips form a natural arch, with the upper and lower lips symmetrical and proportionate to one another. The color and shape of the lips will vary among clients. Normally, the lip surface is pink, smooth, and moist.

The **orbicularis oris**, a band of muscle fibers, surrounds the mouth and is innervated by the VIIth cranial nerve (d). Stimulation of this nerve results in the closure and protrusion of the lips.

To test the intactness of the VIIth cranial nerve, ask the client to whistle (c). Normally, you will note the equal closure and protrusion of both lips.

It is important to observe the client speaking. The examiner should focus attention upon the movement of the lips at this time. Normally, the lips will move freely.

The color of the lips will vary in shade, depending upon race.

Female clients should remove makeup when their lips are being examined to improve visibity and increase the accuracy of the assessment.

The orbicularis oris is a band of muscle fibers surrounding the mouth and innervated by the VII cranial nerve.

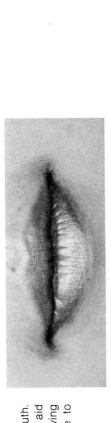

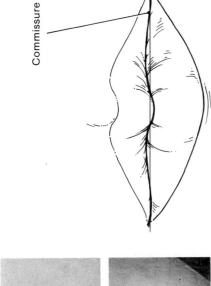

a

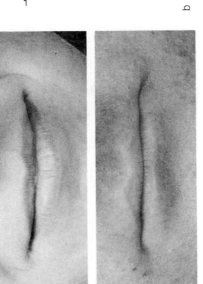

Commissure

b

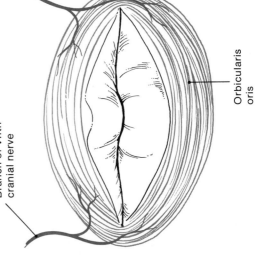

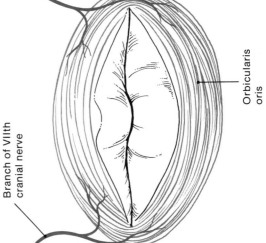

Branch of VIIth cranial nerve

Orbicularis oris

c

d

The *vestibule* is the space bounded externally by the lips and cheeks and separated from the oral cavity by the teeth.

Gloves may be used by the examiner instead of a gauze pad when inspecting the inner structures of the mouth.

The lips are lined with a smooth, pink mucous membrane on both internal surfaces of the lips. The labial glands, small whitish-yellow patches, can be observed on the inner surface of the lips. These glands provide secretion that keeps this area moist. The presence of blood vessels may also be observed at this time.

The **labial frenulum** is a thin fold of mucous membrane which secures the lower lip to the gum. To inspect this area the examiner places a gauze pad on the client's lower lip and pulls it gently downward (a). The inner surface of the lips can then be observed.

The **maxillary mucobuccal fold** is the band that secures the upper lip to the gum (b). To inspect this area a procedure similar to that outlined above is followed with the exception of pulling the lip upward.

Palpation

For palpation of the lips the client faces the examiner and keeps the lips relaxed and slightly open. The examiner palpates the lips by placing the lip surface between the gloved thumb and index finger while gently exerting pressure over the areas along the upper and lower lip surfaces (c). Normally, these areas are soft and smooth, and the skin surface is continuous and uninterrupted.

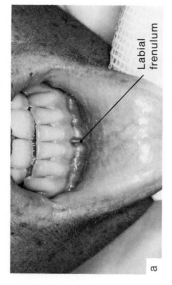

a

Labial frenulum

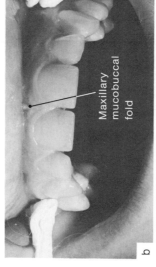

b

Maxillary mucobuccal fold

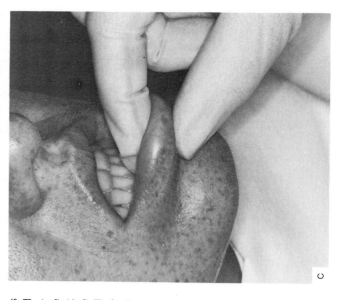

c

Teeth and Gums

The author acknowledges the assistance of Maureen E. Burns, Dental Technician with the preparation of this section of Chapter 4.

The teeth separate the internal surface of the cheeks and lips from the oral cavity. They aid in digestion by preparing food for swallowing and contribute to taste perception by stimulating the release of chemical substances during chewing.

To examine the teeth and gums keep the client in a seated position facing the examiner (a). A pair of gloves, an oral mirror, and a rubber-tipped gum stimulator are needed to complete the examination.

Inspection

To inspect the teeth, ask the client to close the mouth in a normal position and expose the teeth. The bite is observed, and the position of the upper and lower teeth during forced occlusion is noted (b). In a normal bite, the upper teeth protrude slightly in front of the lower teeth (c). Note arrangement, number, and condition of the observable teeth at this time.

Highlights

The examiner may wish to place a gloved hand in client's mouth to examine the approximation of molars while in occlusion.

In an uncorrected occlusion the examiner may note protrusion of upper or lower teeth, or note teeth out of alignment.

Tea, cigarettes, and certain medications (e.g. antibiotics) may stain teeth. Cleaning can remove the staining in most cases.

The use of fluoride may result in a brownish discoloration of the teeth.

Chronic exposure to lead may cause the development of a black line along the gum margin.

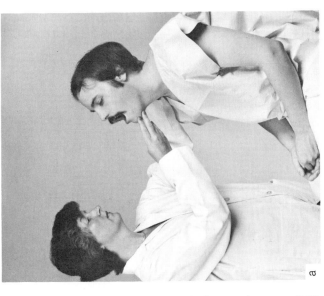

a

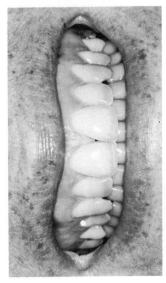

b

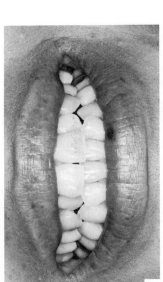

c

Highlights

The term *dental caries* refers to the presence of decay within a tooth.

If third year molars have not yet erupted, a space may be noted in the area.

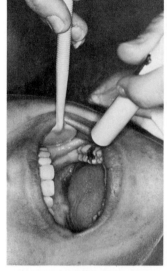

b

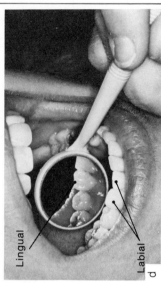

Lingual

Labial

d

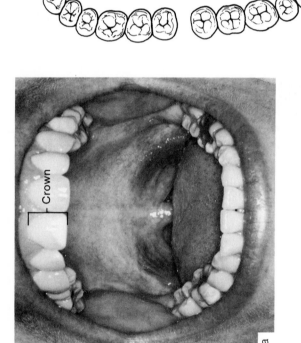

a

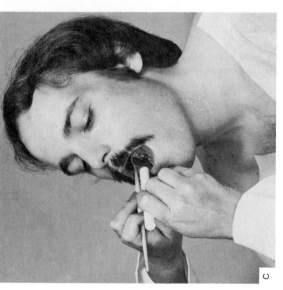

c

The color of each tooth is then noted. The exposed portion of the tooth is called the crown. The normal crown is white in color, although the degree of whiteness may vary with each client.

The shape of teeth will vary with each client and the type of tooth being inspected (a). Age, wear of teeth, and general dental health will also contribute to the teeth's shape and structure.

Each individual has a maximum of 32 teeth (b). Missing teeth and malpositioned teeth should be noted and their locations recorded.

Malposition of the third year molars may be seen frequently. Often this is due to limited growth space.

Using a penlight and oral mirror the examiner can inspect the lingual and labial aspect as well as the biting surface of each tooth (c and d).

The examiner may also note dental restorations, such as crowns, jackets, inlays, and fillings. The number of restorations will vary with each client according to general dental health.

With the client's mouth still in an open position, the buccal mucosa of the oral vestibule can be examined (a). Using a penlight the inner cheek walls can be assessed. Normally, this surface is smooth, pink, and continuous. The saliva normally present will lubricate the surface.

Stensen's duct is the duct that carries the secretions of the parotid gland (b). The opening of Stensen's duct is located in a small protrusion on the cheek approximately opposite the upper second molar. This duct opening normally is small and whitish-yellow or light pink in color. It is soft and patent and is accessible to palpation.

The **gingiva** (gums) is the fibrous and mucosal covering of the periodontal ligaments and bone structure of the tooth and assessing it is a critical part of the oral examination (c).

The gingiva is subdivided into two components called the free and attached gingiva (d). The *free gingiva* forms a collar around the neck of the tooth, and the *attached gingiva* adheres firmly to the underlying bone and tooth and extends to the *mucogingival junction*. The gap between the free gingiva and the tooth is called the *gingival sulcus*. The sulcus and tooth surface near the free gingiva should be free of plaque. Normally, the gingiva is clearly defined around the margin of each tooth and is pale pink, firm, and slightly stippled.

The client should be asked to remove dentures or other removable prostheses from the mouth to allow for a thorough gum assessment.

In blacks, the gums may appear bluish in color and may contain brown pigmentation.

The mucogingival junction is the point at which pale pink, firm gingiva meets darker, loosely attached mucosa.

Stippled means dotted or irregular in surface like orange peel.

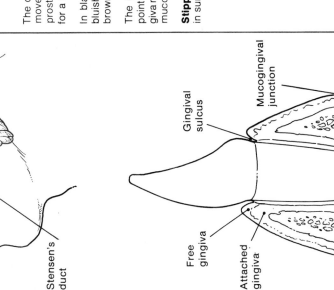

Parotid gland

Stensen's duct

b

Gingival sulcus

Mucogingival junction

Free gingiva

Attached gingiva

d

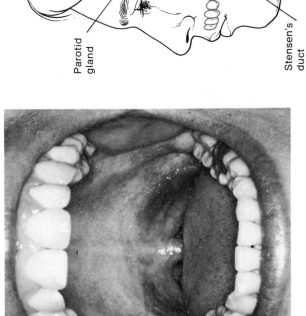

a

c

The use of drugs, or the presence of tooth decay or stress, may result in gum bleeding. During pregnancy, some women develop "pregnancy gingivitis" or bleeding gums.

Palpation

Palpation of teeth and gums involves the application of the examiner's fingertips to the oral tissue to determine the mobility of teeth and the health of gums. Gloves should be used during this part of the examination. Each tooth is checked for movement by holding the index finger to the front surface and the thumb to the back surface of the tooth and moving it gently. The teeth should not be movable (a).

The examiner should then move the fingers along the anterior and posterior gum surface (b). Normally, this surface is stippled and firm. Bleeding should *not* be noted during this procedure.

A gum stimulator can also be used to evaluate the state of tissue. To complete this procedure, insert the tip of the stimulator between each tooth (c) directly below the neck of the tooth. Then stimulate the tissue with a gentle rotary motion (d). Normally, bleeding or discomfort is not present.

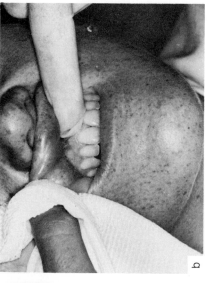

b

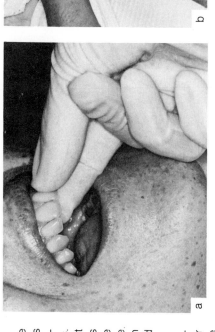

a

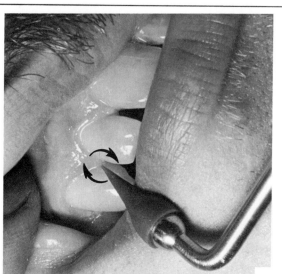

d

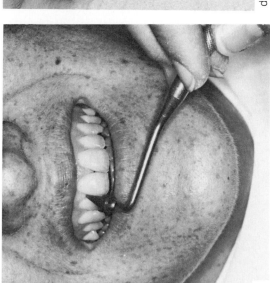

c

The size of the tongue will vary from client to client. However, its size should be proportional to other structures within the oral cavity.

Normally, an individual's general state of hydration can be determined by evaluating the moistness of the tongue's surface.

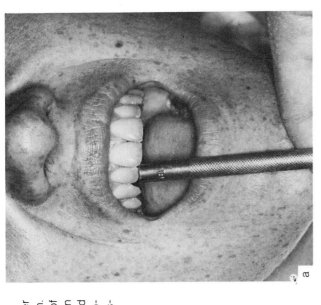

a

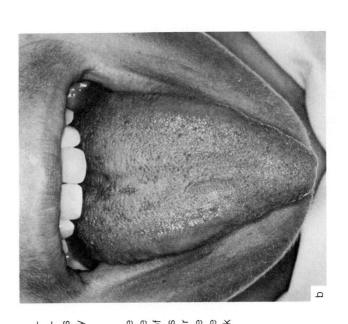

b

Percussion

To percuss the teeth, the examiner should ask the client to open the mouth. Then tap each tooth with the blunt end of the gum stimulator with a gentle motion (a). The tooth normally has a dull sound when tapped with a metal rod. This tapping motion should not cause any discomfort to the client.

Tongue

The tongue is a curved, flexible muscular structure located within the mandible. It is composed of striated muscles and contains both glands and fatty tissue.

Inspection

To inspect the anterior portion of the tongue, ask the client to extend the tongue forward (b). The tip (or apex) of the tongue is thin and narrow and rests against the surface of the lower incisor teeth. The dorsal surface of the tongue extends from the tip of the tongue to the epiglottis. Normally, the tongue is pink and moistened by saliva.

Highlights

The **fungiform papillae** contain cells that serve to remove bacteria and food that normally form on the tongue's surface.

Slight tremors may be observed in the elderly during forward extension of the tongue.

The anterior two-thirds of the dorsal surface of the tongue has many small protrusions called **papillae**, which contribute to the rough appearance of the tongue's surface (a).

The posterior one-third of the tongue surface is slightly uneven and covered with a slightly thinner mucosa than is the anterior portion.

The anterior and posterior tongue surfaces are separated by a V-shaped landmark called the **sulcus terminalis**.

The papillae contained in this area are called **vallate** or **circumvallate papillae**. These papillae are round, discrete eminences and are the largest of the tongue's papillae.

The tongue receives motor innervation by the hypoglossal and glossopharyngeal nerves (c).

To inspect the hypoglossal nerve ask the client to extend and retract the tongue in continuous movements (b). If the nerve is intact, there will be strong, symmetrical, coordinated, and unlimited movement during this activity. When extended forward, the tongue should be located in a midline position with no deviations or tremors observed.

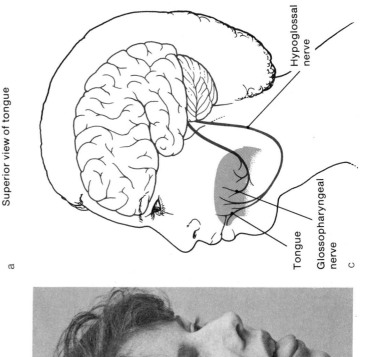

Sulcus terminalis

Vallate papillae

Papillae

Superior view of tongue

a

Hypoglossal nerve

Tongue

Glossopharyngeal nerve

c

b

The hypoglossal nerve also influences additional tongue movements. The client should be able to touch the hard palate (located in the roof of the mouth) with the tongue. During this movement the examiner can observe the ventral (floor) surface of the tongue (a). Normally, this area is smooth, with large veins apparent because of a thinner membraneous covering.

With the tongue still in that position, additional structures within the oral cavity can be examined. These include the *lingual frenulum*, the *submandibular ducts*, and the *sublingual fold* (b).

The **lingual frenulum** is a fold of mucous membrane that joins the tongue to the floor of the mouth. The **submandibular ducts** (Wharton's ducts) open at the side of the frenulum on the floor of the mouth.

The sublingual salivary gland is the smallest of the three main salivary glands and is located on the floor of the mouth. This gland combines with mucous membrane to form the **sublingual fold**. This fold contains many small openings which help moisten the oral cavity.

The glossopharyngeal nerve (IXth cranial nerve) and facial nerve (VIIth cranial nerve) are the sensory receptors responsible for taste (d).

To test the intactness of these nerves, a substance, such as salt or sugar, can be placed on the anterior and posterior surfaces of the tongue (c). The client is then asked to determine the source of taste being experienced.

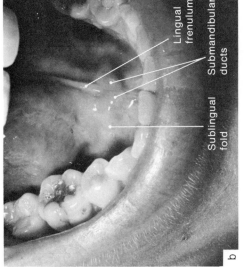

a

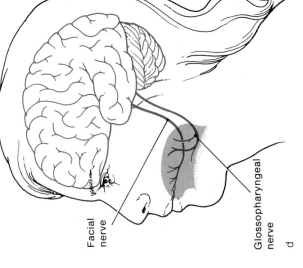

Lingual frenulum

Submandibular ducts

Sublingual fold

b

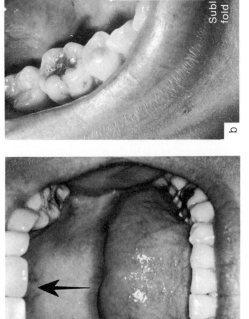

c

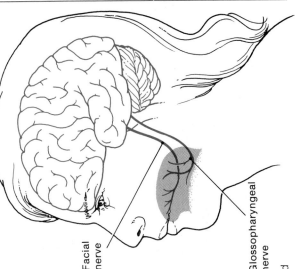

Facial nerve

Glossopharyngeal nerve

d

The lingual frenulum, the submandibular ducts, and the sublingual fold can be inspected during the examination of the ventral surface of the tongue.

Different parts of the tongue surface are able to distinguish certain tastes more effectively than others.

Bitter

Sour

Salt

Sweet

Taste buds are present over the entire surface of the tongue, and occasionally on the posterior surfaces of the epiglottis and the soft palate.

Highlights

When palpating the tongue, ask the client to keep the tongue inside the mouth to reduce muscle tension.

During palpation of the tongue, the salivary glands and submaxillary ducts can be palpated.

The nasopharynx terminates at the base of the oropharynx.

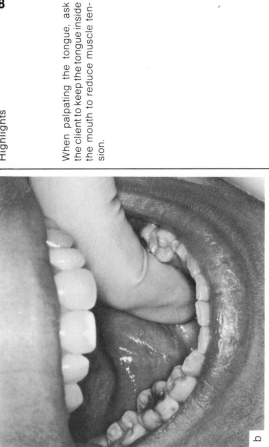

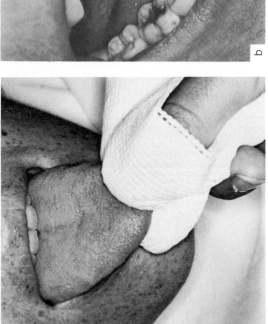

a

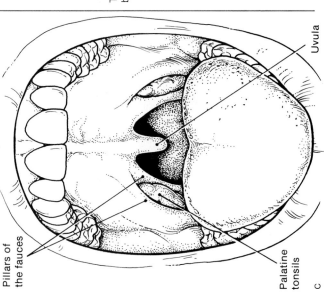

Uvula

Pillars of the fauces

Palatine tonsils

c

Palpation

To palpate the posterior and lateral tongue surface, ask the client to extend the tongue forward and place a 4 by 4 inch gauze around the tip of the tongue. Hold the tongue in hand (a). Move the tongue freely from the right to left, examining the borders of the tongue surface, the posterior surface containing papillae. It is smooth, with no interruptions in the surface present. The margins of the tongue should be smooth and intact.

Using gloves, the examiner can gently but firmly palpate the tongue on both the dorsal and ventral surfaces.

The floor of the mouth is formed by the mandibular bone, which can be easily palpated (b). The membrane on this surface is loose and easily movable and is moistened by saliva. The region of the sublingual salivary glands and submaxillary ducts should be palpated for smoothness and patency. Manual examination of the remaining oral mucosa and, cheeks can also be completed at this time.

Oropharynx

The **oropharynx** is that part of the pharynx that communicates directly with the oral cavity. Structures in the oropharynx include the *uvula*, the *pillars of the fauces*, and the *palatine tonsils* (c). Examination of the roof of the mouth (hard and soft palates) is a natural prelude to examination of the oropharynx; therefore both will be discussed here.

Inspection

To inspect the oropharynx, a tongue blade should be used (a). The tip of the blade is placed in the middle of the tongue, with the end of the blade held between the examiner's thumb on the lower surface and the index and third finger on the top of the blade. This position will allow the examiner to push down and pull forward on the blade, increasing the visibility of the oropharynx. At this time the hard and soft palates can be examined (b).

When assessing the hard and soft palate, tilt the client's head backward.

The **hard palate** is seen as a bony structure, covered by a mucous membrane. The surface is rough, irregular in appearance and pale pink in color (c).

After examining the hard palate, move on to the soft palate which is located just posterior to it. The soft palate is a deeper pink in color and is covered by a thinner mucosa. Because of this, blood vessels may be observed.

The tongue blade should be placed near the V-shaped sulcus terminalis to inspect the oropharynx.

The presence of rugae, wrinkles or folds in the mucosa, contributes to the uneven appearance of the hard palate.

A bony protuberance called the *torus* may be observed during the examination of the hard palate.

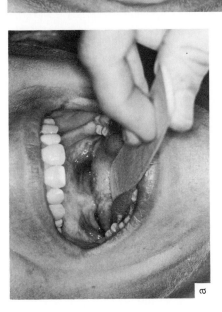

a

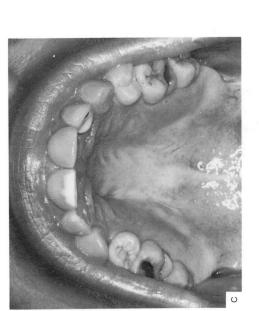

c

b

Hard palate

Soft palate

Tonsils may contain crypts which can collect oral debris and become infected.

Some clients will be very sensitive to the stimulation of the gag reflex. Use caution to avoid causing vomiting.

Eliciting the gag reflex insures the intactness of the IXth and Xth cranial nerves.

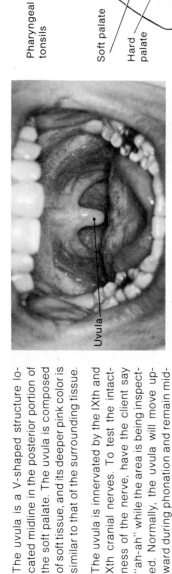

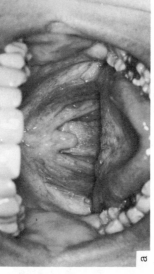

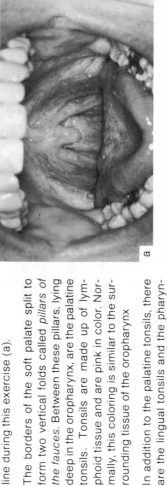

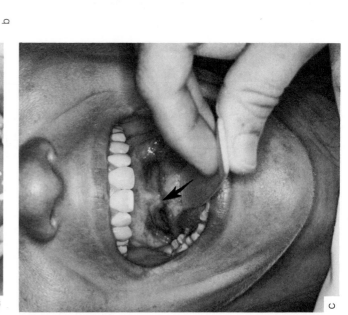

Pharyngeal tonsils

Soft palate

Hard palate

Palatine tonsils

Lingual tonsils

b

Uvula

a

c

The uvula is a V-shaped structure located midline in the posterior portion of the soft palate. The uvula is composed of soft tissue, and its deeper pink color is similar to that of the surrounding tissue.

The uvula is innervated by the IXth and Xth cranial nerves. To test the intactness of the nerve, have the client say "ah-ah" while the area is being inspected. Normally, the uvula will move upward during phonation and remain midline during this exercise (a).

The borders of the soft palate split to form two vertical folds called *pillars of the fauces*. Between these pillars, lying deep in the oropharynx, are the palatine tonsils. Tonsils are made up of lymphoid tissue and are pink in color. Normally, this coloring is similar to the surrounding tissue of the oropharynx (b).

In addition to the palatine tonsils, there are the lingual tonsils and the pharyngeal tonsils, or adenoids (b).

Before removing the tongue blade, the *gag reflex* should be elicited. The examiner gently moves the tongue blade back toward the posterior oropharynx to stimulate the gagging response (c). Eliciting this response ensures the intactness of the IXth and Xth cranial nerves.

NECK

The examination of the neck includes assessment of the neck muscles, carotid arteries and jugular veins, the thyroid gland and trachea (b).

When the neck area is being examined, the client should be seated at the side edge of the table, facing the examiner (a). As the examination progresses both the client and the examiner will change positions as indicated in the discussion to follow.

Assessment data obtained through examination of the neck and surrounding areas can best be obtained through inspection, palpation, and auscultation.

Inspection

The neck area is initially inspected for some general features. These include skin color, tone, and intactness, and the symmetry, size, and shape of the neck.

The color of the skin is similar to the skin shade of the face. Skin surrounding the neck is intact, conforming to the underlying structures of the neck (e.g., the cervical spine and neck muscles).

The size and shape of the neck will vary with each individual (c). The age, sex, and general growth and development patterns of each person, along with the inherited predispositions (e.g., varieties of bone structure and tissue distribution), will directly affect the size and shape of the neck.

In the elderly there may be a sagging of skin tissue around the neck area due to a decrease in muscle tone. If the client is overweight there may be an excess amount of skin folds around the neck area, due to increased adipose tissue.

Highlights

During the examination of the neck, the techniques of inspection, palpation and auscultation are used to obtain data.

The color of the skin around the neck is similar to that of the surrounding tissue and conforms in shape to the underlying structures.

The size and shape of the neck can vary with each client.

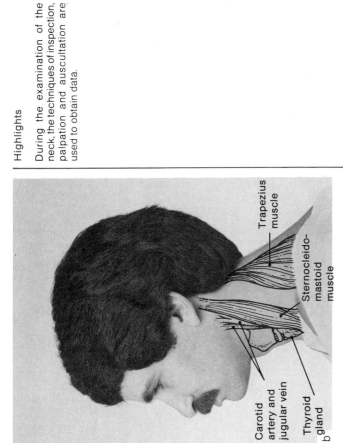

a

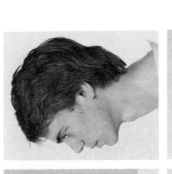
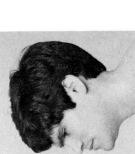

Trapezius muscle

Sternocleido-mastoid muscle

Carotid artery and jugular vein

Thyroid gland

b

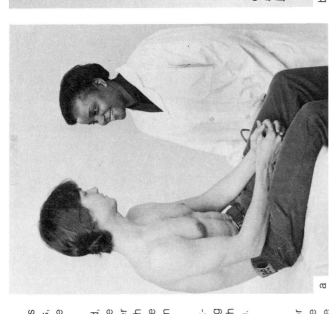

c

In healthy adults the neck may appear asymmetrical due to fat deposits.

The sternocleidomastoid and trapezius muscles are used as landmarks to assess neck symmetry.

The anterior and posterior triangles are two divisions of the sternocleidomastoid muscles found on each side of the neck.

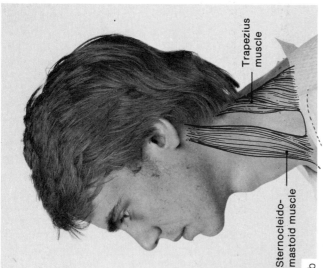

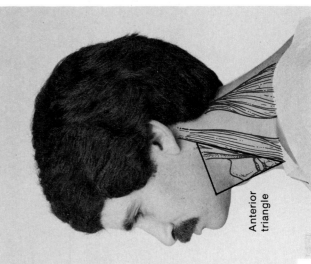

b

Trapezius muscle

Sternocleido-mastoid muscle

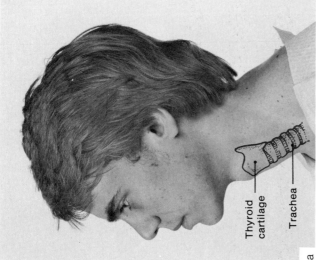

a

Thyroid cartilage

Trachea

c

Anterior triangle

Usually, the neck is round and smooth covered with uninterrupted skin. There is an overall symmetry to the neck with a slight bulging over the trachea and related cartilage (a).

When inspecting the neck, it should be observed for symmetry, while held in its normal position. Usually the neck is symmetrical and centered in relation to the head and surrounding structures.

The neck muscles are inspected for development and symmetry. These neck muscles are the sternocleidomastoid and trapezius muscles (b).

The sternocleidomastoid muscle extends from the mastoid process (behind the external ear), to the upper sternum and the proximal portion of the clavicle. This muscle is frequently used as a landmark of the neck.

The sternocleidomastoid muscles divide each side of the neck into an anterior and a posterior triangle.

The *anterior triangle* is formed by the mandible (superiorly), the sternocleidomastoid muscle (laterally) and the midline of the trachea (medially) (c). The thyroid gland, the trachea, and anterior cervical nodes are found within the anterior angle. Running parallel with the sternocleidomastoid muscle is the carotid artery.

Highlights

The trapezius muscles (two) are flat, large, and of trapezoid shape.

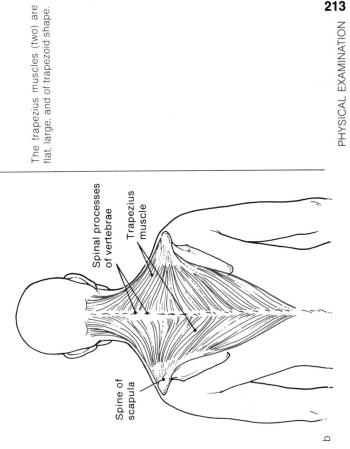

The *posterior triangle* is formed by the clavicle (at the base), the trapezius muscle (medially), and the sternocleidomastoid muscle (laterally) (a). Posterior cervical lymph nodes are also found in this triangle.

The trapezius muscles (two) are flat, large and triangular in shape. This muscle begins at the occipital bone of the skull, the cervical vertebrae and the thoracic vertebrae and inserts on the clavicle and the spine of the scapula (b).

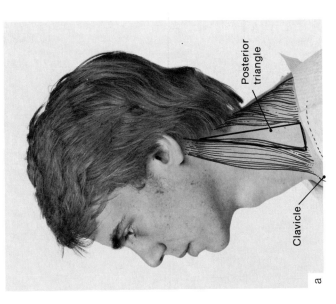

Both the sternocleidomastoid muscles and the trapezius muscles are innervated by CN XI.

The trapezius and sternocleiodomastoid muscles are tested for motion and strength.

The sternocleidomastoid muscles and trapezius muscles are innervated by cranial nerve XI (b). To test the intactness of CN XI and neck movement the client is asked to move the head in several directions.

First the client (with the mouth closed) is asked to flex the head downward until the chin rests upon the chest (a). Normally, this should occur in smooth movement with no resistance or discomfort present.

Next the client is asked to turn the head to the right side (laterally) about 90° and flex the head until the chin reaches the right shoulder (c). The procedure is then repeated on the left side. Again, the normal response should be smooth and uninterrupted movements, with no discomfort. The head can also be extended backwards to rest upon the shoulders in an effort to observe full range of motion of the neck musculature.

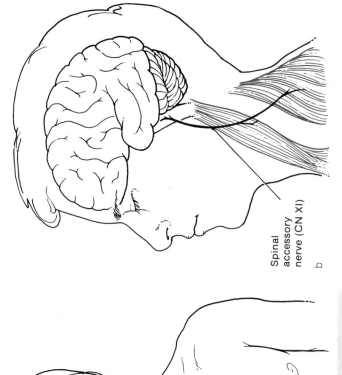

a

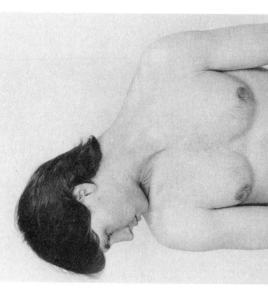

c

Spinal
accessory
nerve (CN XI)

b

The thyroid cartilage is the largest of the cartilagenous structures of the neck.

The thyroid gland contains two lobes, joined together by an isthmus.

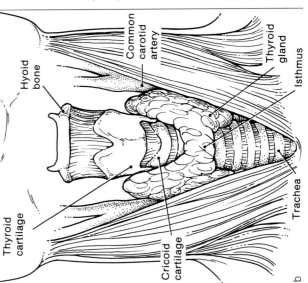

b

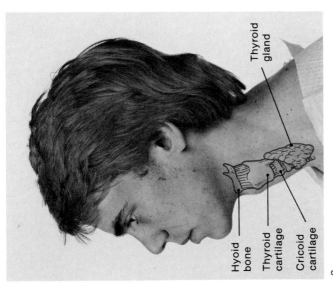

a

Additional structures in the neck inspected for symmetry, intactness, and movement, include the hyoid bone, the thyroid cartilage, the cricoid cartilage and the thyroid gland (a).

The *hyoid bone* is located below the mandible at an angle with the floor of the mouth. Below, the shield shaped *thyroid cartilage* is found. This structure is notched at its superior edge, and is at the level of the bifurcation of the common carotid artery into the internal and external carotid arteries (b).

The *cricoid cartilage* is located below the thyroid cartilage and is the uppermost of the *tracheal rings* which follow

The *thyroid gland* is located in the middle of the anterior aspect of the neck and contains two irregular, cone shaped lobes. These lobes, situated laterally, are joined on the lower portion of the lobes and medially by an isthmus. This connection spans across the trachea and cricoid cartilage.

The *trachea* is located directly below the thyroid gland, protected by the tracheal rings.

When inspecting these structures, the examiner should stand directly in front of the client observing the lower neck area in particular. It is essential that good lighting shine on the area so that subtle neck movements can be accurately observed.

The client is given a glass of water and asked to swallow normally: first with the head in a normal position, then with the head slightly extended (a).

The movement of the cartilage during swallowing should be smooth and continuous. The trachea, thyroid and larynx will rise with swallowing (b). The trachea should be in a midline position and with no unusual bulging of tissue observed.

Examination of *blood vessels* in the neck includes the assessment of veins and arteries. Usually, the jugular veins and the carotid arteries are the focus of this assessment.

The jugular veins are made up of two components: internal and external jugular veins (c). The *internal jugular veins* are large and are located deep within the sternocleidomastoid muscles and close to carotid arteries. The *external jugular veins* are superficial and can be observed above the clavicle and the juncture of the sternocleidomastoid muscles. Blood from the jugular veins empties into the superior vena cava.

Bilateral evaluation of the internal and external jugular veins can be performed in an indirect way, to determine venous return and filling volume. These important parameters help to evaluate the quality of cardiac performance.

Inspection of the cartilagenous structures of the neck can best be observed by asking the client to swallow sips of water and observing neck movement.

The trachea should be in a midline position.

The internal and external jugular veins are inspected bilaterally for quality of pulsation and pressure.

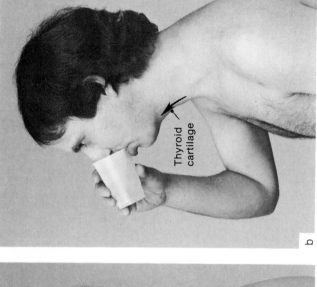

a

b

Thyroid cartilage

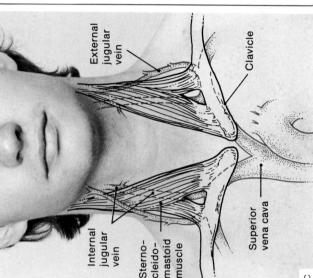

External jugular vein

Clavicle

Internal jugular vein

Sterno-cleido-mastoid muscle

Superior vena cava

c

Venous pulsations are usually not observed while the client is seated.

When the client is in a sitting position, there are no obvious pulsations present. Therefore, to assess for *venous pulsations* in the area of the jugular vein the client assumes a supine position (a).

The client should remove all clothing from around the neck and thorax to permit increased visibility. A blanket can be used but should not create excessive changes in the neck's contour.

When the client is in a supine position the trunk is elevated at a 45° angle and the body is in alignment, a venous pulse can be seen.

Venous pulsations may become more visible if the client's head is turned away from the side being examined. The examiner places a penlight directly above the clavicle and over the sternocleidomastoid muscle (b).

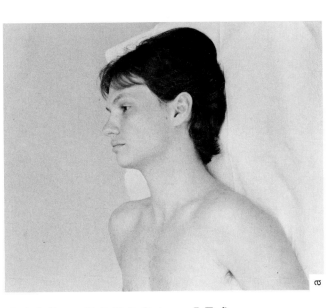

a

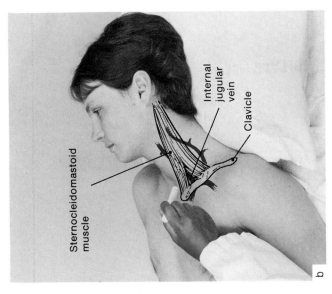

b

Sternocleidomastoid muscle

Internal jugular vein

Clavicle

When the right atrium contracts and forces blood into the right ventricle, there is a brief backflow of blood into the vena cava. This action normally results in a *venous pulse wave* (a).

The pulse wave consists of three positive components (a, c, v) and two negative components (x and y).

The **a wave** is the most peaked of the three positive waves and is the result of atrial contractions. This wave is most sensitive to alterations in blood flow from the right atrium to the right ventricle.

The **c wave** is the result of carotid artery pulsation and retrograde transmission of the pulse wave occurring concurrently.

The **v wave** reflects increased volume (filling) in the vena cava and right atrium. During this time the tricuspid valve is closed. This increase in pressure is reflected in the jugular veins as the v wave.

The **x descent wave** is a negative wave produced during ventricular systole and by atrial diastole. It is a result of a downward displacement of the ventricle.

The **y descent wave** occurs as the tricuspid valve opens and the blood from the right atrium goes into the right ventricles.

Pulse waves are usually observed as a slow, "wavelike" continuous movement. These waves can be observed when the heart rate is usually below 90.

Normal venous pulse wave consists of three positive waves a, c and v and two negative waves x and y.

The v wave is also referred to as the passive filling wave.

The x descent wave is present during ventricular systole and atrial diastole.

The y wave occurs as the tricuspid valve opens and blood goes from the right atrium to the right ventricle.

The venous pulsations are "wavelike" and continuous movements.

Venous wave formation may be affected by inspiration.

Refer to heart section of Chap. 4 for further discussion on blood flow through heart.

Systole	Diastole

a c x v   a c x y v

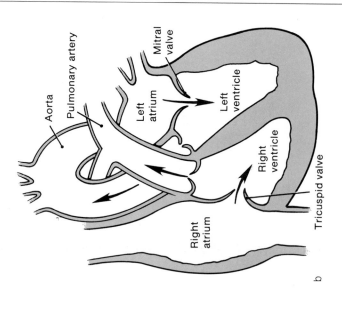

Aorta
Pulmonary artery
Mitral valve
Left atrium
Left ventricle
Right atrium
Right ventricle
Tricuspid valve

b

Highlights

The height of pressure within the veins is determined by measuring venous pressure.

The sternal angle (or angle of Louis) is used as a point of reference.

The distance between the sternal angle and the highest level of jugular pulsation is measured in centimeters.

The normal height of the jugular veins is normally 1 to 2 cm above the clavicle.

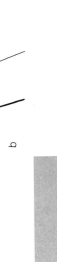

Sternal angle

Atria

b

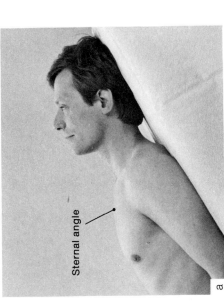

Sternal angle

a

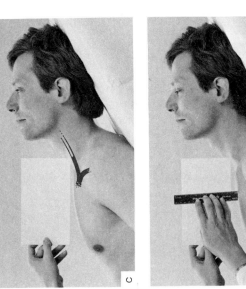

c

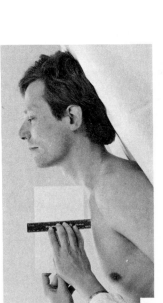

d

The *venous pressure* may be established by both direct and indirect measurements. The indirect measurement will be discussed since it is most frequently used during a routine physical examination.

To measure venous pressure indirectly, the examiner should first establish a reliable landmark for the level of the atrium. The sternal angle (angle of Louis) is frequently used to determine this reference point (a and b).

The client remains lying down with the head slightly elevated 30° to 45° from the horizontal surface. The distance in height between the sternal angle and the highest point of internal jugular vein pulsation is measured in centimeters in the following way.

Using a piece of paper, the examiner establishes the horizontal level of the client's point of highest venous pulsation (c). If internal venous pulsation is not visible, the point at which the external jugular vein appears collapsed can be used as a reference point.

A centimeter ruler is then placed at the sternal angle perpendicular to the horizontal plane to establish the vertical measure (d).

The height of the jugular venous pulsation is normally 1 to 2 cm above the clavicle.

When the height of the pulsation is more then 3 to 4 cm above the sternal angle, it is considered abnormal.

The *carotid pulses* are parallel to the internal jugular veins (a) and are often used to determine the rate and general force of the arterial pulses.

To inspect the carotid pulses the client is seated facing the examiner (b). The neck is then inspected for carotid pulsations. Normally, there may be a smooth, slight rhythmic impulse noted; usually it is synchronous with the S₁ heart sound.

The examiner may choose to assess the neck vessels later in the examination to avoid having the client continually change positions.

Carotid pulses are not affected by inspiration or change in position.

The carotid pulsations are normally smooth, with a synchronous rhythmic impulse.

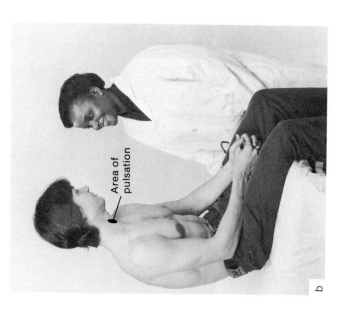

Trapezius muscle

Sternocleido-mastoid muscle

Carotid artery and jugular vein

Thyroid gland

a

Area of pulsation

b

Palpation

The neck muscles can be palpated to assess their strength and intactness.

The strength of the sternocleidomastoid muscles can be tested with the client in a seated position. The examiner places a hand against the side of the client's face. The client is then asked to turn the head toward and against the resistance (a). Normally, the examiner can feel the strength being exerted. The procedure can be repeated on the opposite side of the face and the strength noted. Usually the strength is bilaterally equal.

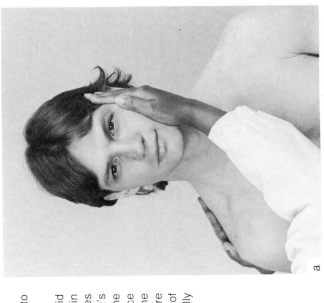

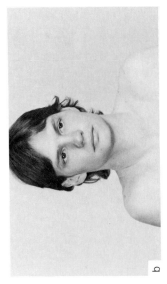

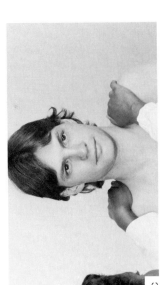

Trapezius muscle strength is measured by asking the client to sit in a relaxed position and shrug the shoulders (b). Normally, this should occur without interruption and cause no discomfort. To test the strength of these muscles the examiner places the hands on the client's shoulders. The client then continues to shrug the shoulders against the resistance exerted by the examiner's hands (c). Normally, there should be equal and strong resistance offered.

Highlights

Numerous lymph nodes are found in chains throughout the neck region.

The thyrolinguofacial chain drains such areas as the parotid gland, palatine tonsils, nose, submaxillary glands, and thyroid gland.

The nodes in the neck are located in the anterior and posterior neck triangles.

In addition to nodes found in triangles of the neck, the *preauricular node* (in front of the ear) and *post auricular* located behind the ear, may be included in the examination.

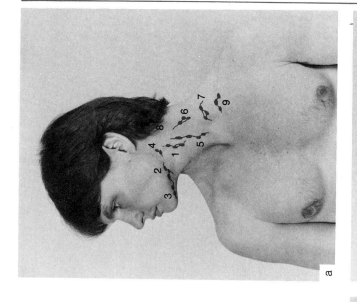

a

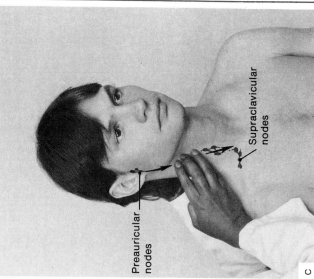

Preauricular nodes

Supraclavicular nodes

c

There are numerous *lymph nodes* found in the neck. These nodes are generally grouped and referred to as chains (a). These chains include the following:

1 The *superficial cervical chain* is found above and anterior to the sternocleidomastoid muscle.

2 The *submandibular chain* is located below the mandible.

3 The *submental chain* is located below the mandible, near the chin.

4 The *thyrolinguofacial chain* is located deep behind the angle of the mandible.

5 The *deep cervical chains* are located behind the sternocleidomastoid muscles and associated with deep structures including the thyroid gland, larynx, and internal jugular vein.

6 The *spinal accessory nerve chain* is associated with the IXth cranial nerve.

7 The *transverse cervical artery chain* follows the transverse cervical artery and vein.

8 The *occipital chain* is located at the posterior base of the skull.

9 The *supraclavicular chain* is located above and deep to the clavicle.

The chains included in the examination can be located by finding the anterior and posterior triangles (b).

Nodes are best palpated in a sequence starting above the neck with the preauricular nodes and progressing downward to the supraclavicular nodes (c).

Posterior triangle

Anterior triangle

b

Highlights

The posterior triangle includes the occipital, superficial cervical, deep cervical, spinal and supraclavicular node chains.

Normally, nodes are not palpable regardless of the chain being examined.

Within the anterior triangle, the *superficial cervical*, the *submental*, the *submandibular*, and the *thyrolinguofacial* nodes or node chains are found (a).

The posterior triangle (b) includes the *occipital* nodes (located posteriorly at the skull base); the *transverse cervical chain*; the *deep cervical chain* (located deep to the sternocleidomastoid near the internal jugular vein and difficult to reach by examination); the *spinal accessory nerve chain*; and the *supraclavicular* (found deep to the clavicle and sternocleidomastoid area).

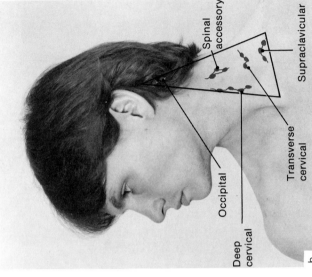

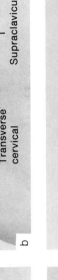

a

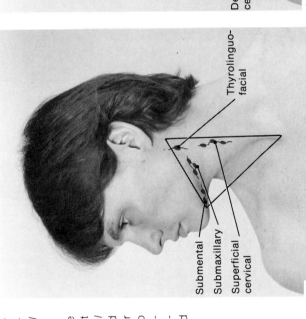

b

Submental
Submaxillary
Superficial cervical

Thyrolinguofacial

Spinal accessory
Supraclavicular
Transverse cervical
Occipital
Deep cervical

When palpating the neck for the presence of nodes, the examiner should place the pads of the index and middle fingers on the client's skin, moving the underlying tissue gently. Generally the neck is examined one side at a time (c). Normally, nodes are not palpable.

Additional techniques may also be used to examine the nodes in the anterior triangle, the submental, submandibular, and sublingual nodes. The client remaining seated, is asked to flex the head forward or move it to the side in order to ease tension and facilitate the examination. The examiner than places one hand on back of the client's head for balance and the fingertips of the other hand under the mandible. The skin and underlying subcutaneous tissue is then moved laterally over the mandible (ramus) to identify nodes if present (d).

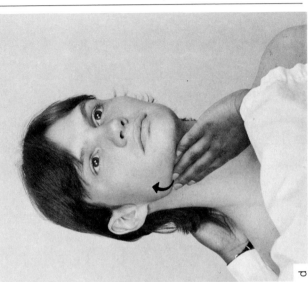

c

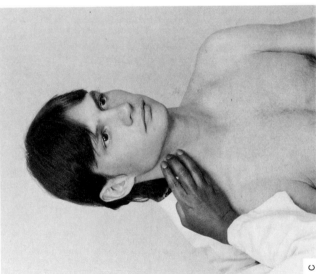

d

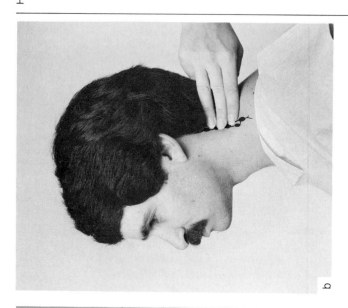

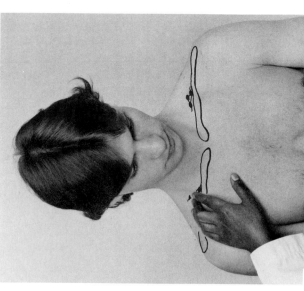

When examining the submandibular nodes the examiner, who may be gloved, can place the index finger on the inside floor of the client's mouth and the thumb over the ramus of the mandible. The tissue lying between the examiner's fingers is then rotated gently to determine the presence of nodes (a).

Nodes in the posterior triangle (e.g. the occipital node) are examined in a fashion similar to that of the anterior nodes. However, the examining fingers move posteriorly into the triangle to assess the area (b).

When examining nodes in the supraclavicular or scalene region, the client remains seated facing the examiner, usually with the head flexed slightly forward.

When examining the left side of these chains, the examiner uses the right index finger and places it in a hooked or somewhat rounded manner over the clavicle and lateral to the sternocleidomastoid muscle (c). Using a gentle rotating movement, first light and then deep, the area can be explored fully. The procedure is reversed to examine the client's right side.

Normally, even when the examination for nodes is more specific, the results are negative. At times small, mobile, and clearly defined nontender nodes may be detected in healthy individuals.

If the examiner is uncertain of the findings, the size, shape, number, and tenderness of nodes should be referred for further assessment.

Small, mobile, and clearly defined nodes may be found in healthy clients. If the examiner is uncertain of the findings, referral and follow-up are essential.

A posterior and anterior approach can be used to palpate the thyroid gland and related structures.

Normally, the thyroid gland is not palpated.

When using a posterior approach the examiner stands behind the client.

The thyroid and attached trachea will rise upon swallowing.

During displacement of the thyroid cartilage, the lobes should not be enlarged, tender or asymmetrical.

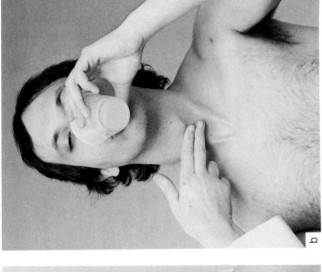

a

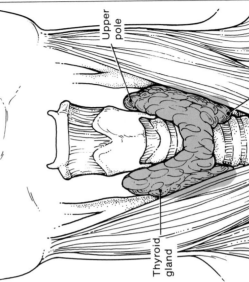

b

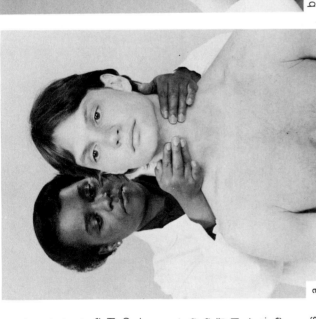

c

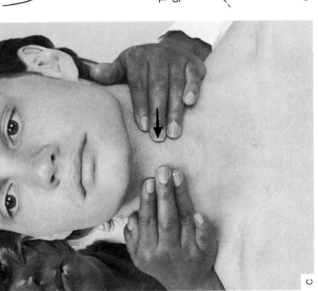

d

Upper pole

Lower pole

Thyroid gland

The thyroid and related structures can be palpated using two approaches: a posterior or an anterior approach. Normally, the thyroid gland cannot be palpated. However, in extremely thin individuals, it may on occasion be palpable.

When using the posterior approach, the examiner stands behind the seated client (a). The individual is asked to lower the head slightly to facilitate relaxation of the neck muscles.

The examiner places the tips of the fingers directly on the lower portion of the neck, in the area of the trachea. The client is then asked to swallow sips of water. Normally, the examiner will feel the normal rise of the thyroid and attached trachea during this maneuver (b). However, the thyroid gland will not be palpated.

Next, each lobe of the thyroid gland is palpated along with surrounding neck structures. The client is asked to turn the head slightly in the direction being examined. When the right lobe is to be examined, the client's head is turned slightly to the right. To facilitate the examination, the client will also be asked to swallow sips of water during palpation.

The examiner places the fingertips of the left hand on the neck, slightly displacing the thyroid cartilage to the right. The examiner's right fingers are used to palpate the lateral cartilage area for any enlargements or changes in structure (c).

The thyroid isthmus is then palpated, followed by the lower poles of the lateral lobes, then the upper poles (d). Normally, there should be no enlargements, tenderness, asymmetry or discomfort noted during this procedure.

The thyroid lobes should be palpated bilaterally.

When using the anterior approach, the examiner assesses the thyroid gland while standing in front of the client.

The thyroid gland can also be palpated by having the examiner place the thumb deep into and behind the sternocleidomastoid muscles, while the index and middle fingers are placed into the front portion of the muscle (a). Normally, there should be no muscle enlargement noted as the area is palpated.

Both maneuvers are repeated to examine the left lobe. Again, there should be no discomfort upon cartilage displacement and no lobe enlargement palpated.

When using the *anterior approach* to palpate the thyroid gland, the client remains seated and the examiner stands in front of the individual. Again, the client's head remains slightly flexed downward and in the direction of the lobe being palpated.

The examiner places the palm or surfaces of the index and middle fingers over the cricoid cartilage (b). The client is asked to swallow sips of water and the smooth upward movement of the thyroid is assessed.

The lobes are palpated anteriorly by displacing the thyroid cartilage to the left with the left hand and examining the lateral lower and upper lobes with the right hand (c). The procedure is repeated to assess the right lobe. Normally, there should be no discomfort or asymmetry or tenderness experienced during the procedure or enlargements palpated.

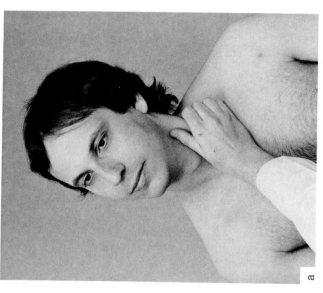

a

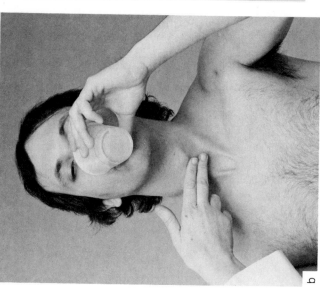

b

c

The trachea can be palpated at this time by having the examiner place a finger on the trachea in the area of the sternal notch (a). The examiner then slips the finger off the trachea to the right and then to the left side. Normally, there should be no deviation to either side present.

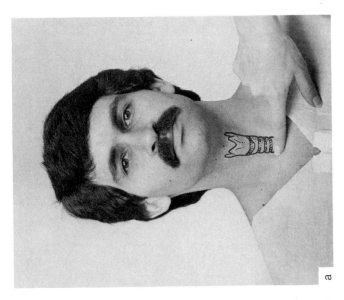

The carotid pulses are palpated one side at a time to avoid pressure or occlusion of the carotid sinus. Using the tips of the forefingers the examiner (standing to the side of the client) places the hand below and to the center of the angle of the jaw and the edge of the sternocleidomastoid muscle (b).

The neck muscles should be relaxed during the process. To accomplish this ask the client to turn the head slightly toward the side being examined. The carotid pulse should be assessed for amplitude, contour, duration, and rate. Normally, the pulse has a smooth rapid upstroke followed by a less palpable downstroke (dicrotic notch) downstroke.

The rate is normally 60 to 100 beats per minute occurring at regular intervals with a force or amplitude determined by the overall quality of the impulse. Arterial pulse pressure is usually elevated to between 30 and 40 mmHg.

Arterial pulses should be assessed on the opposite side of the body and the findings compared.

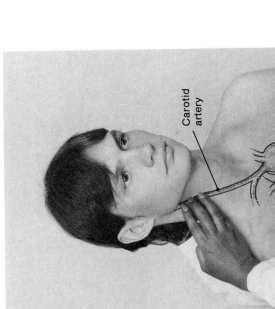

Carotid artery

To avoid confusing venous and arterial pulsation, the examiner can lightly palpate carotid pulses on one side of the neck while observing the venous wave on the opposite side. This action is best observed with the client in a reclining position and therefore may be assessed later in the examination (a).

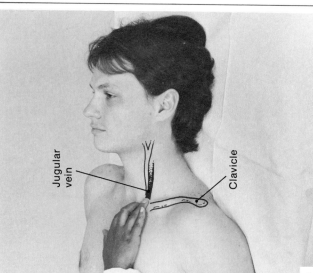

a

Jugular vein pulsations can be eliminated by applying gentle pressure over the vein at the base of the neck, above the clavicle (b). This action normally blocks the retrograde transmission of the venous pulse wave.

Refer to discussion on palpation of venous pressure. (p. 219)

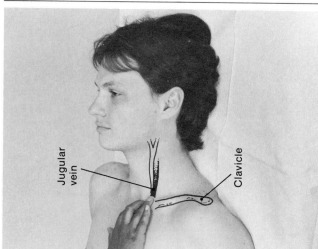

Jugular vein

Clavicle

b

With the client lying down, the examiner gently places the palm of the hand in the upper right quadrant of the abdomen (in the vicinity of the liver) and exerts manual pressure for about 30 seconds to 1 minute (c). This procedure stimulates the *hepatojugular reflux* and in the normal client results in very little (if any) elevation in jugular venous pressure.

Stimulation of the hepatojugular reflex normally results in very little elevation in venous pressure.

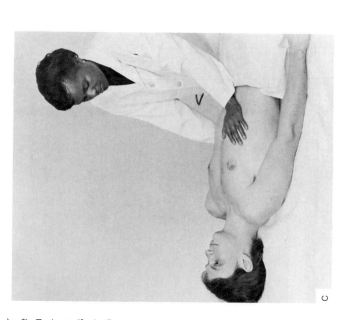

c

Auscultation

In order to determine the flow of blood through the arteries, auscultation is employed. With the client seated or lying down the examiner places the bell of the stethoscope at the base of the neck over the carotid artery (a). The client is asked to hold his or her breath and the examiner listens carefully. Normally, the sound is smooth, regular, and uninterrupted.

Normally, there should not be vibrations (bruits) heard over the thyroid area.

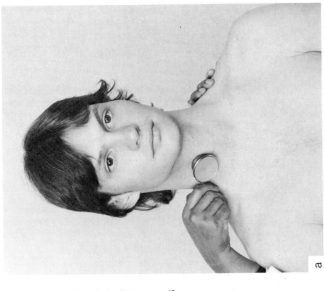

a

Highlights

The bell of the stethoscope is used to auscultate the carotid arteries in order to pick up abnormal low-pitched sounds (e.g., bruits).

Highlights

Examination of the thorax is followed by assessments of the lungs, heart, and breasts.

Examination of the thorax includes inspection of the anterior, posterior, and lateral chest wall.

When examining females, the posterior thorax may be examined before the anterior surface.

THORAX

The examination of the thorax includes inspection of the thoracic landmarks as well as the assessment of the lungs and the heart. Since the anterior chest wall is included in this assessment, examination of the breasts will also be discussed.

Inspection

To facilitate the examination of the underlying structures of the thorax (i.e., heart and lungs), inspection of the anatomical structure and landmarks is critical.

During inspection of the thorax, the client should usually be sitting at the side of the examining table, facing the examiner (a).

The client should remove all clothing (including jewelry) from the waist to the neck. In female clients a drape may be used to ensure personal privacy.

There are four areas of the chest that should always be examined during each phase of the thoracic examination: the anterior, posterior, right lateral, and left lateral chest wall (b). The sequence used is decided by the examiner. When examining females, the posterior thorax may be assessed before the anterior surface (c).

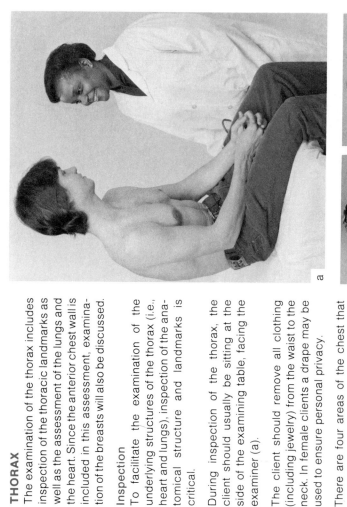

a

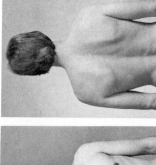

b

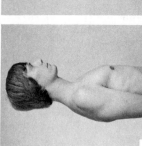

c

The client's posture and body alignment also influence chest movement.

As the examination begins, the size, shape, and symmetry of the chest are observed (a). The surface of the chest wall along with the identification of hair distribution, skin contour, and texture are also evaluated. Nutritional status and skin color can also be evaluated through chest inspection. Slope of the ribs should also be noted.

Normally, the surface of the chest (anterior, posterior, and lateral) is smooth and continuous. It is similar in color to the surrounding skin. The hair distribution over the chest varies; hair is most obvious in males. Axillary hair is present in both males and females.

The size and shape of the chest wall should be in proportion to the rest of the body.

To evaluate thoracic symmetry, the examiner should note the position of the shoulders and the bilateral movement of the chest wall during normal respiration. In the normal adult, the shoulders should be located at the same position to the right and left of the body.

In some adults one shoulder is slightly higher than the other. The clavicle should not be overly prominent (b).

When observing the client's chest wall at close range, the examiner may note a greater development of either the right or left side of the chest wall. This is normal and is often associated with right-and/or left-sided dominance.

Evaluation of the anterior-posterior diameter of the chest wall is made by inspecting the right and left lateral views of the chest (c).

In the normal adult there is usually a greater (about 2 times) lateral than anterior-posterior diameter (d).

Often the individual's body weight influences the prominence of the clavicle. In a thin person the clavicle may be more prominent. In an obese person it is much less obvious.

Greater development of either the right or left side of the chest wall is not uncommon and may be associated with right or left sided dominance.

The anterior-posterior diameter of the chest increases during aging.

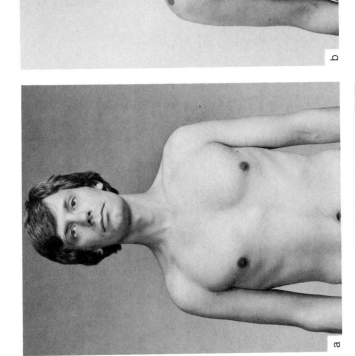

a

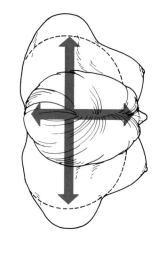

Clavicle

b

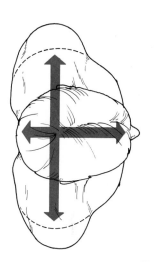

c

d

Highlights

The anterior chest wall contains three important landmarks: the midsternal line, and the right and left midclavicular lines.

Additional anterior surface landmarks include the right and left sternal borders, the suprasternal notch the supraclavicular fossa, and the angle of Louis.

The normal spine should be straight upon a lateral view, slightly convex superiorly, and concave inferiorly.

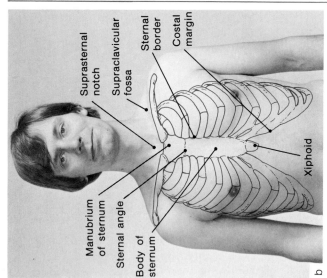

a

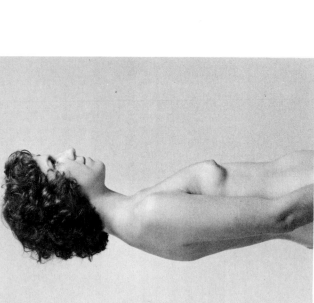

Suprasternal notch
Supraclavicular fossa
Sternal border
Costal margin
Manubrium of sternum
Sternal angle
Body of sternum
Xiphoid

b

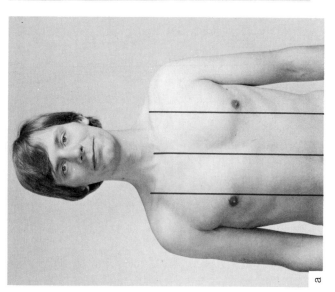

c

Additional landmarks can be identified to help the examiner relate physical findings more accurately. The use of imaginary vertical lines drawn on the chest wall can help the examiner locate various physical structures more easily.

The *anterior surface* contains three vertical lines (a). The midsternal line is located in the middle of the sternum and extends downward to the xiphoid process. The midclavicular line begins at the middle of each clavicle and extends downward toward the base of the thoracic cage.

Anterior thoracic landmarks include the right and left sternal borders, the suprasternal notch, the supraclavicular fossa, the costal margin, and the sternal angle, sometimes referred to as the angle of Louis (b).

The *angle of Louis* is located at the junction of the manubrium and the costal cartilage of the second rib.

The *supraclavicular fossa* is a depressed area located directly above the clavicle.

The *suprasternal notch* is the depression found above the manubrium.

The *posterior thorax* can be inspected by observing the spine and expansion of the posterior chest wall. The spine should be straight upon a lateral view, slightly convex superiorly and concave inferiorly (c).

Highlights

The spinous processes are best observed when the client moves forward.

The vertebra prominens is an accessible landmark when examining the posterior ribs. It is the spinous process of the 7th cervical vertebra.

The identification of the spinous processes may help to facilitate the examination of the posterior ribs and/or the vertebrae.

The *spinous processes* are best determined if the client bends forward slightly flexing the spine (a). Care must be taken to protect the client from falling forward and losing balance.

The *vertebra prominens* (7th cervical vertebrae) serves as an accessible landmark to aid the examiner in inspecting the posterior ribs and vertebra.

In order to find the vertebra prominens the client should be asked to flex the neck slightly forward. The spinous process of the 7th cervical vertebra is the most prominent spinous process observed at the base of the neck. It projects downward from the body of C7 and overlies the first rib (b).

The examiner should be aware of the fact that spinous process T1 overlies rib T2, T2 overlies T3, etc. This will be important when the examiner is attempting to count the number of ribs present in the well adult.

The ribs can also be numbered in relation to the scapulae. The 7th rib is found approximately at the inferior angle of the scapula (c).

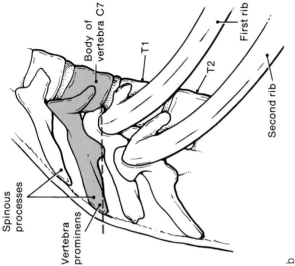

a

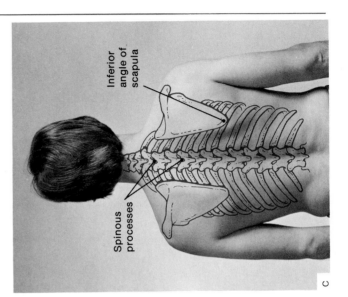

b

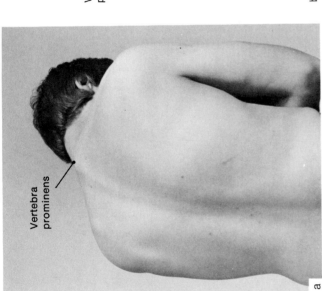

c

Highlights

Imaginary lines identified on the chest wall facilitate examination of the chest wall.

The lines on the posterior chest wall include the midspinal and scapular lines.

The anterior, posterior, and midaxillary lines are three significant lines used on the lateral chest wall to identify specific landmarks.

The landmarks identified on the posterior chest wall can be identified in relation to the three imaginary lines, the midspinal line and the scapular lines (a). The midspinal line travels downward along the spinous processes of the vertebrae. The right and left scapular lines run parallel to the spine (vertebrae) through the inferior angle of the scapula.

In order to obtain an accurate inspection of these posterior lines the examiner must be sure the client is sitting erect with the hands at the side.

The lateral chest wall also contains three imaginary lines: the anterior axillary line, the posterior axillary line, and the midaxillary line. The anterior line extends downward from the axillary folds found along the anterior lateral chest wall. The posterior axillary line extends downward from the posterior lateral folds. The midaxillary line is located at the midaxilla point, and extends from the apex of the axilla downward (b).

When locating the midaxillary line, the client's arm should be placed in an abducted position, away from the lateral chest wall at an angle no greater than 90 degrees.

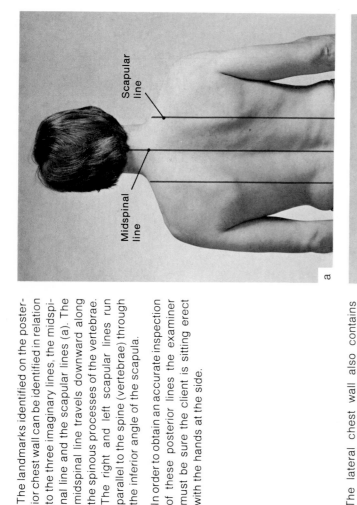

Scapular line

Midspinal line

a

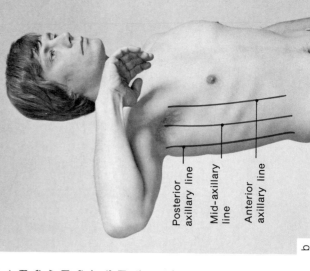

Posterior axillary line

Mid-axillary line

Anterior axillary line

b

Palpation

Palpation is used for further assessment of the integrity of the thoracic cage, the surrounding musculature and for initial evaluation of bronchial patency. To complete this assessment the client continues to remain seated at the side of the examining table. This will allow the examiner continued access to the anterior and posterior thoracic surfaces. As always with palpation, skin temperature, texture, and turgor should be assessed. Normally, the skin should be cool to touch, smooth and continuous.

Assessing skin turgor over the upper anterior thoracic cage can be one of the best indicators of normal hydration status of a client. This can be accomplished by slightly squeezing the skin on the chest wall between the thumb and index finger, then releasing it (a). In the well hydrated individual the skin should return to its normal position.

Palpation should occur in an orderly fashion beginning at the apices, and moving to the posterior, anterior, and lateral chest. The trachea should be midline in the suprasternal notch, equidistant from the sternocleidomastoid muscle and clavicles (b).

The various muscles and soft tissue areas can be palpated at this time including the trapezius, sternocleidomastoid, latissimus dorsi, pectoralis, rectus abdominus and finally the intercostal muscles (c). These structures should be smooth and firm and have appropriate tone.

Refer to the measurement section in Chap. 4 for discussion of ranges for body temeprature.

Skin turgor can best be assessed over the anterior chest wall.

Refer to the section on examination of trachea for additional data.

Evaluation of muscle groups (eg., the trapezius and intercostal muscles) can be accomplished during palpation of the thorax.

Highlights

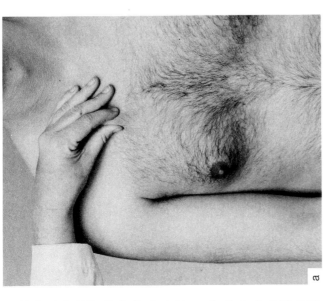

a

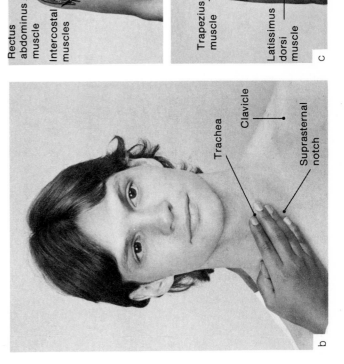

Pectoralis
muscle

Rectus
abdominus
muscle

Intercostal
muscles

Trapezius
muscle

Latissimus
dorsi
muscle

c

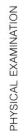

Trachea

Clavicle

Suprasternal
notch

b

PHYSICAL EXAMINATION

Palpation of the intercostal spaces begins at the angle of Louis.

Palpation of the *intercostal spaces* can follow this initial assessment. The examiner begins by initially identifying the angle of Louis (or sternal angle). The bony structure felt directly to the side is the second rib.

In order to identify additional ribs and intercostal spaces on the anterior chest wall, the examiner places the index finger on the space above the second rib and the middle finger, below the second rib and begins to count (a). The space above the second rib is the first intercostal space; the space below is the second intercostal space. The examiner continues to count downward in an oblique line, lateral to the edge of the sternum (b).

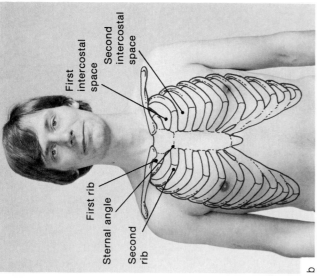

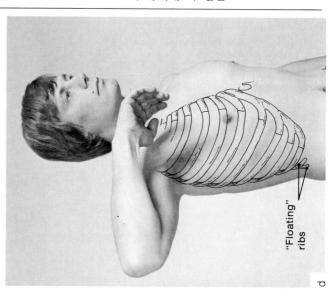

First intercostal space

Second rib

Second intercostal space

First intercostal space

Second intercostal space

First rib

Sternal angle

Second rib

b

The bony structures — clavicles, sternum, ribs, scapula, and spinous processes — are painfree when palpated.

Intercostal spaces may be difficult to palpate in obese clients.

The intercostal spaces contain intercostal muscles and appear flat, and slightly depressed in relation to the ribs and related structures (c).

When palpating the intercostal spaces, they should be smooth and pain-free to the touch. In obese clients, these spaces will be difficult to determine because of excess adipose tissue. In thin clients, these spaces are easily found.

During palpation of the interspaces, the related ribs of the thoracic cage are also assessed.

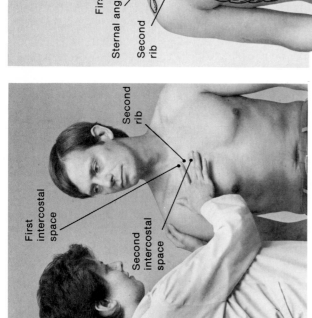

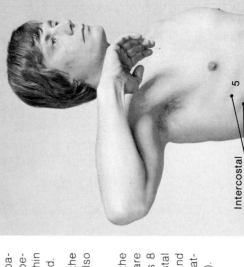

5

6

7

Intercostal spaces

c

"Floating" ribs

d

The first seven ribs articulate with costal cartilage; ribs 8 to 10 are attached to the costal cartilage above the 7th rib.

The 11th and 12th ribs are "free floating" and can be palpated laterally.

The first seven ribs articulate with the costal cartilage. The remaining ribs are positioned in the following way: ribs 8 through 10 are attached to the costal cartilage above the 7th rib; the 11th and 12th ribs are referred to as "free floating" and can be palpated laterally (d).

Highlights

The manubriosternal junction is located at the level of the 5th thoracic vertebra.

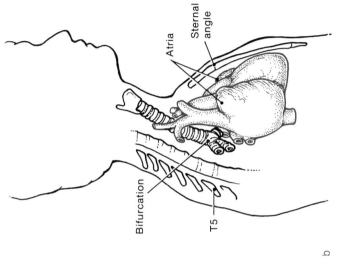

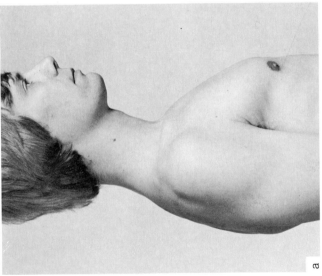

a

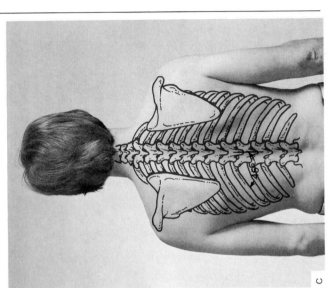

Sternal angle

Atria

Bifurcation

T5

b

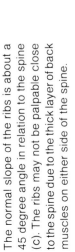

c

It is also important to remember that the manubriosternal junction (sternal angle) is located at the same level as the 5th thoracic vertebra, the bifurcation of the trachea, and the upper level of the atria of the heart (a and b).

The normal slope of the ribs is about a 45 degree angle in relation to the spine (c). The ribs may not be palpable close to the spine due to the thick layer of back muscles on either side of the spine.

The scapulae should be on the same level.

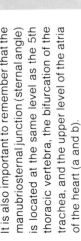

Careful explanation of the components of the lung examination will
be needed in order to have the full
cooperation of the client and to
ensure the accuracy of the data
collected.

Examination of the lungs is best
accomplished with the client
seated.

Note the posture of the client as he
or she sits, and the ease of
breathing.

Symmetry of chest movement can
best be observed with the client in
a recumbent position.

The rise and fall of the chest wall
should be regular, symmetrical,
and equal.

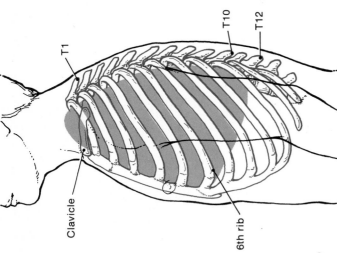

T1

T10

T12

Clavicle

6th rib

b

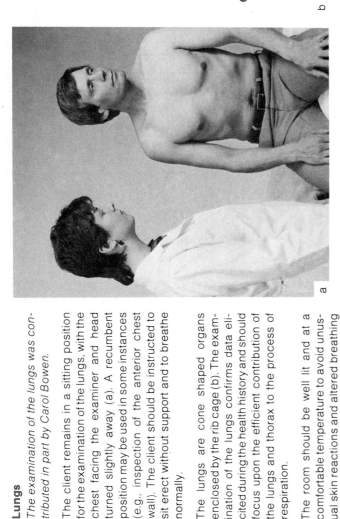

a

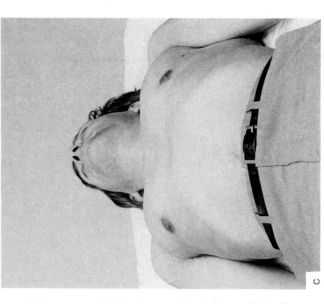

c

Lungs

*The examination of the lungs was con-
tributed in part by Carol Bowen.*

The client remains in a sitting position
for the examination of the lungs, with the
chest facing the examiner and head
turned slightly away (a). A recumbent
position may be used in some instances
(e.g., inspection of the anterior chest
wall). The client should be instructed to
sit erect without support and to breathe
normally.

The lungs are cone shaped organs
enclosed by the rib cage (b). The examination of the lungs confirms data elicited during the health history and should
focus upon the efficient contribution of
the lungs and thorax to the process of
respiration.

The room should be well lit and at a
comfortable temperature to avoid unusual skin reactions and altered breathing
responses.

The examination will proceed from
inspection to palpation, percussion, and
then auscultation.

Inspection

During inspection of the anterior chest,
the client may be asked to lie down.
Alterations in the symmetry of chest wall
movement can best be observed with
the client in a recumbent position (c).

The examiner observes the rate, rhythm
(regularity), and amplitude of respiratory
excursion. The total configuration of the
chest movement during respiration is
noted at this time.

The normal rise and fall of the chest wall
should be equal and symmetrical. Expansion of the thoracic cavity should be
even.

Normally, respirations are between 16 to 20 breaths per minute. As the examiner observes the client, the rate, rhythm, and depth of each respiration should be carefully observed.

The client should be asked to inspire, and the examiner observes the movement of the rib cage, the degree of chest expansion, and the intercostal movement (a). There should be no obvious bulging or retraction of the rib cage noted.

During inspiration, the diaphragm will move downward. The contraction of the intercostal muscles results in the upward and outward movement of the thoracic cavity, thereby causing an increase in intrathoracic volume and a decrease in intrathoracic pressure. As a result, air is then drawn into the lungs (b).

Women usually breathe costally or by using thoracic movement. Men (and children) usually breathe diaphragmatically (c).

During inspection of respirations, the width of the subcostal angle is usually less than 90 degrees (d). The angle normally widens on inspiration; however, in the healthy adult, this movement is minimal.

The ribs normally move slightly forward beyond the sternum during inspiration.

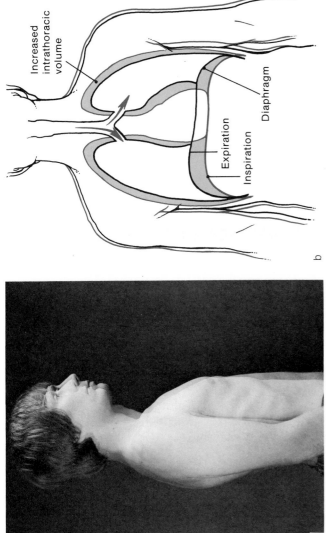

a

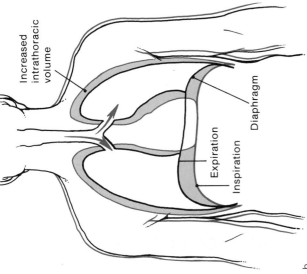

Increased intrathoracic volume

Expiration
Inspiration

Diaphragm

b

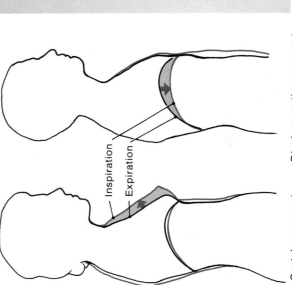

Sternocleido-mastoid muscle

Trapezius

External intercostal muscles

Costal angle

Anterior scalene muscle

Diaphragm

d

Costal movement

Inspiration
Expiration

Diaphragmatic movement

c

Highlights

Respirations occur normally between 16 to 20 breaths per minute.

Inspiration occurs with the downward movement of the diaphragm, and contraction of the intercostal muscles, which increases the intrathoracic volume, and decreases the intrathoracic pressure thereby drawing air into the lungs.

Women breathe costally; males diaphragmatically.

Highlights

During expiration there is relaxation of the diaphragmatic and intercostal muscles and return of the ribs and diaphragm to normal position compressing the lungs and forcing air outward.

It is important to note the length of the expiratory phase.

Observation of the client's respiratory movements permit careful inspection of the muscle and bone structures that are affected by the process.

Gas exchange in the lungs occurs between the alveoli and arterial blood supply.

Figure d adapted from Dorothy A. Jones, et al., Medical-Surgical Nursing, A Conceptual Approach, McGraw-Hill, 1982, p. 761.

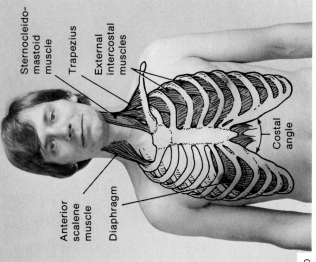

Sternocleidomastoid muscle

Trapezius

External intercostal muscles

Anterior scalene muscle

Diaphragm

Costal angle

b

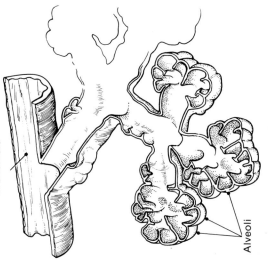

Bronchiole

Alveoli

d

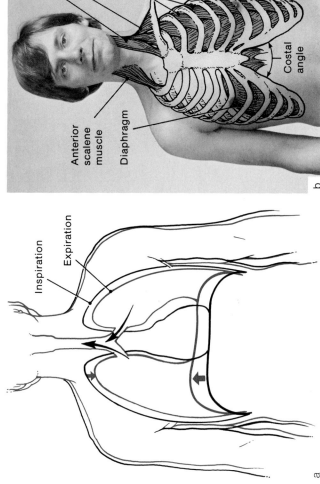

Inspiration

Expiration

a

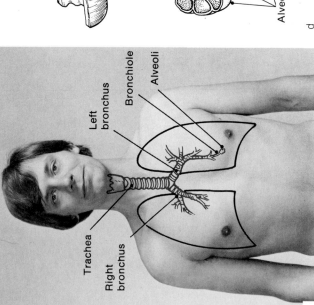

Trachea

Right bronchus

Left bronchus

Bronchiole

Alveoli

c

During expiration the reverse process occurs. There is a relaxation of the diaphragmatic and intercostal muscles The diaphragm and the ribs return to their original placement. With this action the lungs are compressed, forcing the air contained in the lungs to the outside (a).

Expiration is normally longer than inspiration.

The examiner should caution the client to avoid exaggerated rising and lowering of the chest wall during deep inspiration. This can distort the chest movement and lead to misinterpretation of cues. The examiner can instruct the client to breathe normally to help diminish this potential distortion.

During the entire respiratory process, the use of the *accessory muscles — trapezius, anterior scalene,* and *sternocleidomastoid* (b) — should be observed. Normally, there are no accessory muscles used during the respirations of a healthy adult.

The relationship of the respiratory process to the various structures of the thoracic cage should also be observed.

Normally, the trachea is midline, carrying the air into the main bronchus which bifurcates into right and left bronchi (c). This bifurcation takes place at the level of the sternal angle anteriorly and at the 4th thoracic spine posteriorly. The bronchi become smaller tubes, the *bronchioles,* and finally the air is carried into the periphery of the lungs into the alveoli where the actual gas exchange occurs (d).

Highlights

Palpation of the chest wall should proceed without discomfort for the client.

The posterior chest wall is usually used to measure expansion.

Chest wall expansion can also be performed on the anterior chest at the costal margin but is of less value.
During chest expansion there should be an upward and outward movement observed (3 to 5 cm).

Fremitus is sound produced as air passes through a patent airway causing the lungs and chest wall to vibrate.

Palpation

During palpation, thoracic expansion and lung density (fremitis) are assessed.

Thoracic expansion Palpation is particularly useful in assessing respiratory expansion. The flexibility and movement of the lungs and thoracic cage during inhalation is noticed first in inspection.

During palpation, the examiner can examine expansion from the anterior and/or posterior position. The posterior assessment is more frequently used.

As the posterior wall examination progresses, the examiner places the thumbs to the right and left of the spine at the level of the 10th rib. The palms of the hands are spread laterally over the lower posterior chest surface (a). The client is then asked to breathe deeply. As the person inhales, the examiner's fingers move as the thoracic cage expands. The distance between the thumbs increases on respiration, and can then be measured. The thumbs should move an equal distance slightly upward and outward. Normally this distance is 3 to 5 cm.

Fremitus Fremitus is produced by air that passes through a patent respiratory system resulting in vibrations of the lungs and chest wall (b). The vibrations can be assessed during palpation, usually through the posterior chest wall. Fremitus can also be assessed during percussion and auscultation (see discussion below).

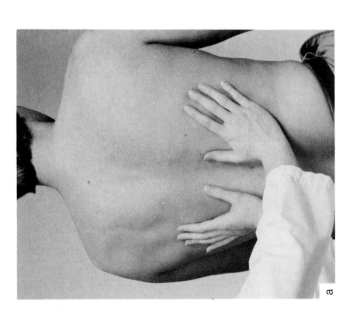

a

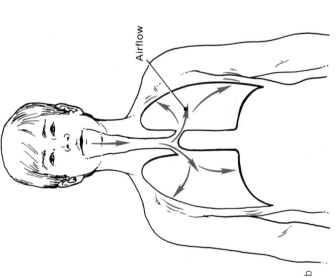

Airflow

b

The right lung contains 3 lobes; the left lung contains 2 lobes.

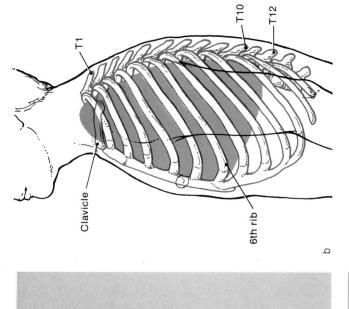

b

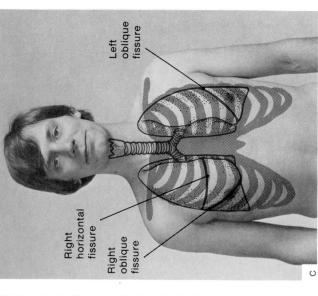

a

c

This is the beginning of evaluation of air movement in the lungs. Therefore, it is important to be mindful of the anatomy of the lungs in relation to the bony structures discussed earlier (a). Further identification of landmarks (related to lung borders) will aid in the description of findings.

The apices, or tops of the lungs, extend approximately 1½ inches above the clavicles anteriorly and T_1 posteriorly (b). The anterior inferior border lies at the 6th rib on the midclavicular line.

Laterally, the lung extends from the axilla to the 8th rib at the midaxillary line. On the posterior thorax, T_{10} and T_{12} mark the lower border depending on degree of expiration and inspiration respectively.

The right lung is composed of 3 lobes while the left contains 2 (c). To visualize this concept, a three-dimensional lung model is helpful. Both lungs have oblique or diagonal lung fissures which extend from the third thoracic vertebrae laterally and down toward to the 5th rib at the midaxillary line. They continue anteriorly and medially to the 6th rib at the right and left midclavicular line.

The right lung is further divided by a horizontal fissure that extends from the 5th rib at the right midaxillary line horizontally to the 4th rib at the right sternal border, creating a middle lobe. The air passage in this lobe must be evaluated anteriorly as it is practically impossible to do from the posterior chest.

Highlights

The lung lobes are enclosed by a visceral pleura.

The parietal pleura is in contact with the diaphragm and the inferior lung borders.

Between the parietal and visceral pleura there is a small amount of lubricating fluid to permit easy respiratory movement.

The spoken voice is transmitted through the trachea, bronchi, bronchioles, and alveoli.

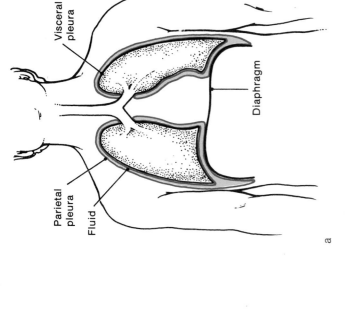

Visceral pleura

Parietal pleura

Fluid

Diaphragm

a

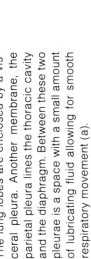

b

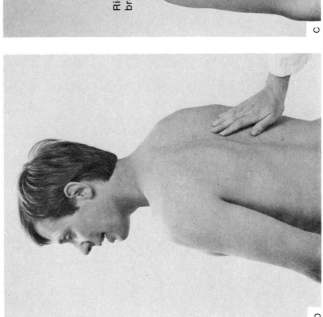

Left bronchus

Bronchiole

Alveoli

Trachea

Right bronchus

c

The lung lobes are enclosed by a visceral pleura. Another membrane, the parietal pleura lines the thoracic cavity and the diaphragm. Between these two pleurae is a space with a small amount of lubricating fluid allowing for smooth respiratory movement (a).

The spoken voice is transmitted through the trachea, bronchi, bronchioles, and alveoli (c). The sound waves set the thoracic cage in motion acting as a large resonator. This produces vibrations in the chest wall which can be felt by the hands of the examiner (b). This is called vocal or *tactile* fremitus.

To determine fremitus, the examiner places the hand over the lung lobes and the intercostal spaces to assess the quality of the sound being transmitted. There are three possible hand positions:

1 Use of the palmar base of the fingers against the chest wall (a)

2 Use of the ulnar aspect of the hand or closed fist against the chest wall (b)

3 Use of one or two hands directly against the chest wall (c)

In any of these positions, the examiner palpates symmetrically, applying adequate and equal pressure. The hands are placed as parallel to the ribs as possible.

With the examiner's hands in place, the client is asked to repeat numbers ("1, 2, 3, 99") or phrases ("ee, ee").

Fremitus is most prominent over areas where bronchi are closest to the chest wall. This will vary greatly in individuals depending on the intensity and pitch of the voice, increasing as intensity of the voices increases and pitch drops.

Fremitus is usually symmetrical except for slightly greater intensity over the right upper lobe. It is forceful in the second intercostal space at the sternal border near the area of bronchial bifurcation (d).

The examination should move methodically from the upper to the lower border of the lungs, comparing right with the left side.

Fremitus can be felt on the anterior chest, but the posterior wall is most frequently used. A more complete assessment of lung density and determination of lung borders can best be evaluated using the posterior position.

Assessment of fremitus can be determined as the examiner places the hand over the posterior chest wall while the client repeats phrases such as "1, 2, 99" or "ee, ee."

Fremitus is most prominent over areas where the bronchi are closest to the chest wall.

Fremitus is usually symmetrical, slightly greater in intensity over the right lung.

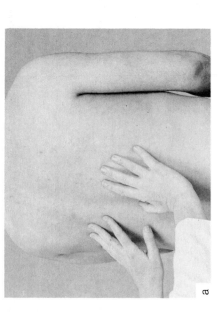

a

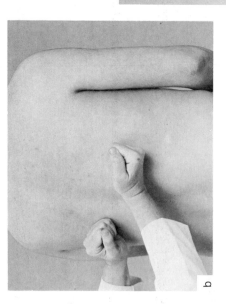

b

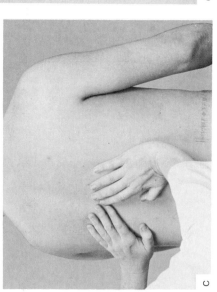

d

Bronchial bifurcation

c

Highlights

Percussion of the lungs is used to determine density.

Percussion of the posterior chest wall usually occurs before percussion of the anterior wall.

There are two methods for percussion:

1 immediate — the examiner strikes the object to percuss directly with the palmar aspect of the 2d, 3d, and 4th fingers together or with the palmar aspect of the tip of the middle finger.

2 mediate — the striking of an object held against the area to be percussed.

The client is asked to bend forward during percussion to increase lung exposure.

When percussing the chest wall, it is essential to compare both the right and left sides.

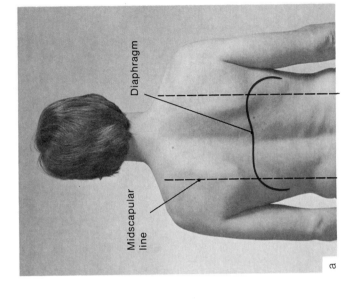

a

Diaphragm

Midscapular line

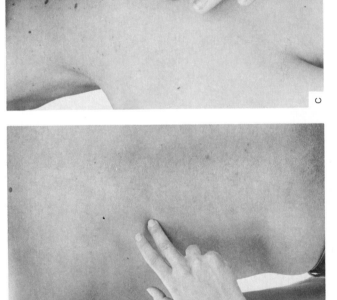

c

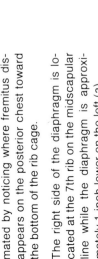

b

The level of the diaphragm can be estimated by noticing where fremitus disappears on the posterior chest toward the bottom of the rib cage.

The right side of the diaphragm is located at the 7th rib on the midscapular line while the diaphragm is approximately 1 inch lower on the left (a).

Percussion

Percussion is the light tapping of the body to determine position, size, and density of an underlying structure or cavity. In the case of the respiratory system, it is primarily used to determine the relative amounts of air, liquid, or solid in the lungs, and also to determine position and boundaries of organs. The depth of penetration of sound is approximately 5 to 7 cm.

Percussion of the chest wall can be accomplished with the client remaining seated. Usually the posterior chest is percussed before the anterior surface.

Two methods are used to percuss the chest wall: *immediate* (or direct) percussion (b) and *mediated* (or indirect) percussion (c). Mediated percussion is most often used.

Highlights

During percussion it is important to be aware of the underlying anatomical structures that will alter resonance (eg. the heart produces a dull note).

Percussion should occur in a logical, upper to lower order.

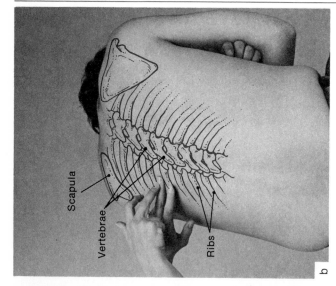

a

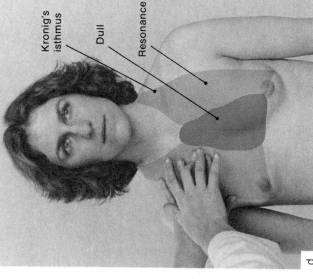

b

Scapula

Vertebrae

Ribs

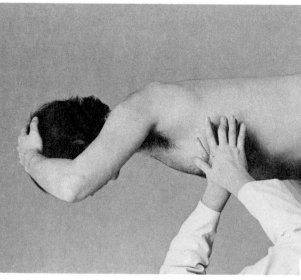

c

Kronig's isthmus

Dull

Resonance

d

The normal percussion note is usually resonance.

To begin percussion, the client should bend forward with arms folded in front (a). In this position, the scapulae move laterally thereby exposing more of the lung. Then percuss symmetrically at 5 cm intervals upper to lower, left to right, and right to left.

When percussing, the examiner should avoid the bony areas (b) and be certain to percuss the interspaces, comparing one side to the other. The examiner should also listen for the intensity, pitch, quality, and duration of the note percussed.

After percussing the posterior chest, the client raises the arms and the lateral chest is percussed (c). Next, percuss the anterior chest beginning with the apices and moving down.

In percussing the anterior chest, it may be necessary to gently displace female breasts. Note that the bony areas will sound flat and that the heart will produce a dull percussion note (d). Normal heart tissue produces areas of dullness to the left of the sternum from the third to fifth interspace.

It is important to percuss anteriorly to properly evaluate the middle right lobe of the lung.

When percussing the apices, there is usually a 5 cm area of resonance located between the neck and the shoulder muscles (Kronig's isthmus) (d).

Unless otherwise noted, the normal percussion note is resonant throughout. It is essential when percussing for resonance, that intensity, pitch, quality, and duration of sound be measured bilaterally on all surfaces of the chest wall.

Finally, it is important to measure diaphragmatic excursion during percussion. A centimeter ruler and pen will be needed for this.

After instructing the client to inhale deeply and hold the breath in, the examiner percusses down along the midscapular line until the lower lung edge is identified (a) and marks it using a washable pen marker. The change in percussion note will help identify the border.

The client next takes a few normal respirations. After this, the examiner asks the client to exhale completely and hold, and percusses up from the earlier marker point to this point, measuring the distance between the two points (b). This represents the excursion of the lungs; normally, this distance is 3 to 5 cm. Like the measurement of expansion, measurement of excursion is usually done on the posterior chest. Both right and left sides of the chest must be measured.

Auscultation

Auscultation of the lungs is accomplished through the use of a stethoscope or via the ear directly. When using the stethoscope, place the diaphragm against the surface to be examined (c). The examination should be approached in an organized fashion to include apices, posterior, lateral, and anterior chest wall.

Diaphragmatic excursion should be measured during percussion (normally, it is 3 to 5 cm).

Auscultation should proceed from the apices to the posterior, lateral, and anterior chest wall.

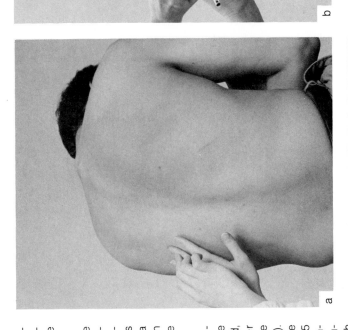

a

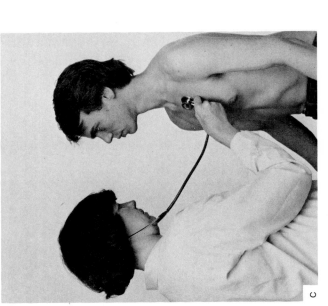

b

c

When using the stethoscope, place it tightly held against the chest as movement of the instrument will interfere with proper assessment of the sounds (movement of muscle or hair may distort the sound the examiner hears).

The client should be seated and instructed to breathe through the mouth more deeply and slowly than is the normal pattern. As the examiner moves the stethoscope from upper to lower, left to right sides of the chest (a), air movement will be picked up as the air passes through various areas of the tracheobronchial tree. The breath sounds differ in various areas of the lung due to the change in the anatomy, proximity of the underlying structures to the chest wall, and the thickness of the chest wall.

Normally, inspiration is heard longer than expiration (5:2). Inspiration is not truly longer but additional expiration is simply not heard. Sometimes expiration may be completely inaudible.

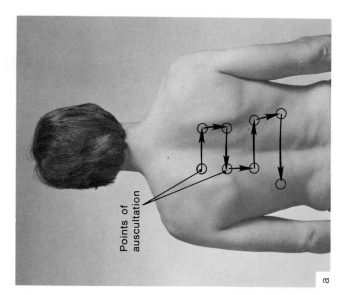

Points of auscultation

a

Vesicular sounds are normally heard over most of the lungs.

Exaggerated vesicular breath sounds can exist in thin people and children and during exercise. The expiratory phase may be more prominent as well.

Bronchovesicular sounds are normally heard anteriorly at the sternal borders, and between the scapulae, at the right medial apex.

Characteristics of Breath Sounds

Type	Location	Duration		Pitch	Intensity
		Inspiration	Expiration		
Vesicular	Peripheral lung	5 : 2		Low	Soft
Bronchovesicular	First and second intercostal space at sternal borders and over major bronchi	1 : 1		Moderate	Moderate
Bronchial	Over trachea	5 : 6		High	Loud

Vesicular breath sounds (b), normally heard over most of the lung, are the result of air moving through the entire lung space. These sounds have been described as gently rushing, breezy, or swishy, soft, and low pitched.

Bronchovesicular sounds (c) are a second type of breath sound resulting from air movement particularly through the bronchial tree. Normally they are heard over the bronchi at the sternal borders at the second interspace anteriorly, between the scapulae posteriorly and at the right medial apex. Here inspiration will be equal to expiration, the sounds are of moderate pitch and intensity.

The third type of sound — bronchial or tracheal (d) — is heard over the trachea. These sounds are high pitched and loud with expiration, and equal to or longer than inspiration.

b

c

d

Bronchial or tracheal sounds are heard over the trachea.

The stethoscope can also be used to evaluate fremitus.

Direct mediation of breath sounds can occur when the examiner places the ear over the client's chest wall to assess sound and air transmission.

The final sound which a stethoscope can help to evaluate is similar to that of tactile fremitus. Again, the client is asked to say "1, 2, 3 or 99" or "ee, ee." The sound will be loudest medially and softest in the periphery, changing with the thickness of the chest (a). Voice sounds are heard best over the trachea and bronchi. Speech is a distinct noise. *Bronchophony*, or exaggerated voice sound is normal over the trachea and right upper lobe posteriorly.

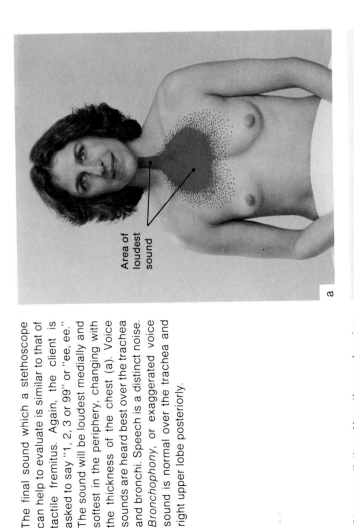

Area of loudest sound

a

Direct mediation of breath sounds using the ear can be accomplished by placing the ear directly over the chest wall (b). The client repeats the breathing response as noted above and the examiner notes the results. This technique is rarely used in adults because it is limited in its accuracy.

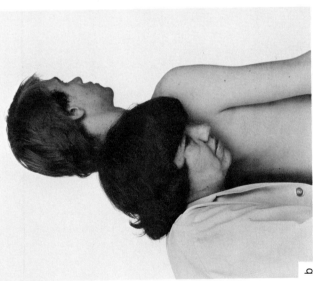

b

Evaluation of cardiac function can also be determined by assessing pulses, venous pressure, skin and nail color is discussed in the extremities and neck section.

Percussion is no longer used to outline the size of the heart.

The position of the heart is oblique, one-third to the right and two-thirds to the left of the midclavicular line.

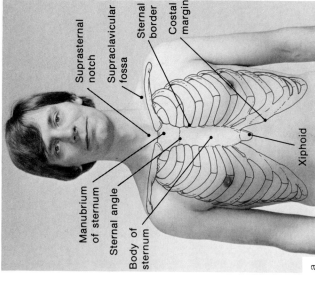

a

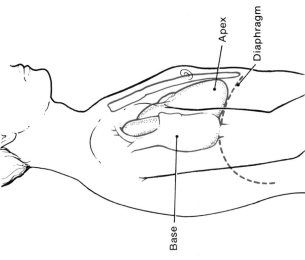

c

Heart

Contributed by Margaret Allen Murphy.
R.N., C.

The examination of the heart includes assessment of the anterior and left lateral surfaces of the chest wall.

Heart sounds associated with adequate blood flow and the pumping action of the heart are evaluated to determine the level of function of the individual's cardiovascular system.

The landmarks identified during inspection of the thorax (a) are used as reference points for inspection of the heart. (See Thorax).

The examination sequence is inspection, followed by palpation and auscultation.

Inspection

The initial inspection focuses on topical movements related to the pumping action of the chambers of the heart.

The heart is located in the middle and left areas of the chest wall. The upper, posterior portion extends slightly to the right and left of the sternum and is referred to as the **base** (b). The heart is tilted forward resting upon the diaphragm (c). The **apex** or lower anterior portion of the heart comes in contact with the chest wall at the fifth left intercostal space, just medial to the midclavicular line.

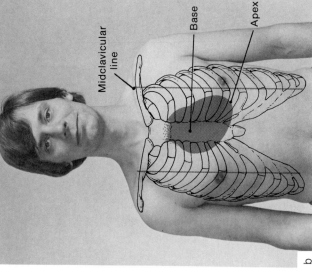

b

Adequate exposure of the anterior chest and good lighting is required to evaluate movements of the chest wall.

During inspection of the anterior chest wall, the client is asked to lie in a supine position, stripped to the waist and with all jewelry removed (a). Adequate tangential lighting enables the examiner to see pulsations of the anterior chest wall. A regular pulsation showing a uniform thrust is associated with regular heart rhythm. This is the only pulsation normally seen on the chest wall and is noted inside or at the midclavicular line at the fifth left intercostal space. The pulsation is reflective of apical pulsation and is referred to as the **Point of Maximum Impulse** (PMI).

Adequacy of heart action is reflected in the coloring of the skin of the trunk and limbs. The skin should have a pink cast to it.

Palpation

Information about the apical impulse obtained by inspection is validated by palpation. It is best felt with the client lying on the left side and the examiner facing the client (b).

The examiner places the fleshy pad of one finger over the point on the left anterior chest where the impulse was seen on inspection. The apical impulse (PMI) feels like a rhythmical light tap against the examiner's finger and should be timed (number of beats per minute). The normal range is 60 to 100 beats per minute.

The healthy client at rest will have a quiet chest; the only movement seen or felt will be the apical impulse as described. The skin of the trunk and limbs is pink, warm and firm to the touch. Pinched gently between the fingers, it feels pliable and returns to a smooth surface immediately when released (c).

Palpation of the apex beat is accomplished by holding the fleshy pad of one finger against the chest wall where the impulse was seen on inspection. It is between 60 to 80 beats per minute. The pulsation may not be present in 50 percent of normal adults since breast tissue or obesity may obscure the apex beat otherwise known as the point of maximum intensity (PMI).

The apical impulse lasts less than one-half of the ventricular systole.

Tissue hydration and hydrostatic pressure is maintained by normal blood volume and rate of transport, which is controled by the pumping action of the heart.

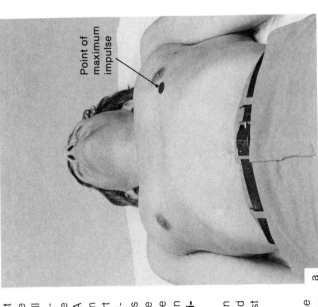

Point of maximum impulse

a

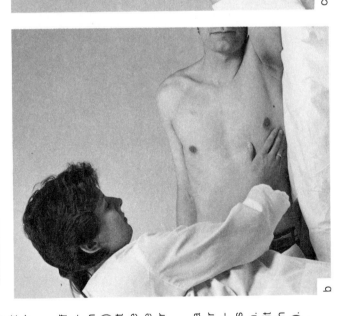

c

b

PHYSICAL EXAMINATION

Highlights

The wall of the left ventricle is thicker than the right ventricle.

The atria are often shown as being on top of the ventricles for schematic purposes (b) but are actually located behind the anteriorly placed ventricles (a).

Heart sounds are represented here as "lubb-dubb."

The first heart sound (lubb) is caused by two actions - closing of the mitral valve and closing of the tricuspid valve.

The second heart sound (dubb) is caused by two actions - closing of the pulmonic valve and closing of the aortic valve.

Figure d adapted from Dorothy A. Jones, et al., Medical-Surgical Nursing, A Conceptual Approach, McGraw-Hill, 1982, p. 852, fig. 23-16. Used with permission of McGraw-Hill Book Company.

Auscultation

The heart consists of four chambers: the two posterior atria and two anterior ventricles. The left and right ventricles are divided by the interventricular *septum*. The right heart receives unoxygenated blood returning from the general circulation by way of the superior and inferior vena cava. Blood is then pumped through the tricuspid valve into the right ventricle. From the ventricle, blood enters the pulmonary artery and is transported to the lungs to be oxygenated (b). This cycle generates the sound associated with the tricuspid component of the first heart sound (lubb), and the pulmonic component of the second heart sound (dubb).

The left atrium receives oxygenated blood from the lungs through the pulmonary veins and pumps it through the mitral valve into the left ventricle. From the ventricle it is pumped into the general circulation through the aorta (b). This cycle generates the sounds associated with the mitral component of the first heart sound (lubb) and the aortic component of the second heart sound (dubb).

The pumping action of the heart chambers is rhythmical, with one-way valves keeping the blood moving through the chambers of the heart in only one direction (c). Muscle bundles called the *trabeculae carnae* line the anterior and inferior ventricle walls and work with other muscles (e.g., *papillary*) and valves to help control and direct blood flow (d).

The *atrioventricular* valves (mitral and tricuspid) prevent reverse flow between the atria and ventricles. The *semilunar valves*, (pulmonic and aortic) prevent reverse flow between the ventricles and the pulmonary artery and aorta.

a

Left atrium
Left ventricle
Right ventricle
Right atrium

b

Lung
Left atrium
Left ventricle
Right ventricle
Superior vena cava
Right atrium
Inferior vena cava

c

Pulmonic valve
Increased pressure in ventricle closes valve
Right atrium
Tricuspid valve
Right ventricle

d

Posterolateral mitral leaflet
Anteromedial mitral leaflet
Chordae tendineae
Trabeculae carneae
Papillary muscle

The aortic area (A) is located at the right intercostal space along the right sternal border.

The pulmonic area (P) is located at second left intercostal space along the left sternal border.

The tricuspid area (T) is located at the fourth and fifth intercostal space along the left sternal border.

The mitral area (M) is located at the site of maximum impulse.

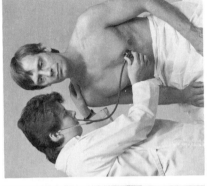

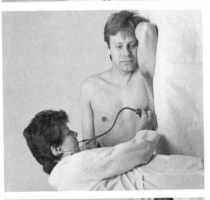

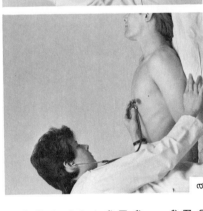

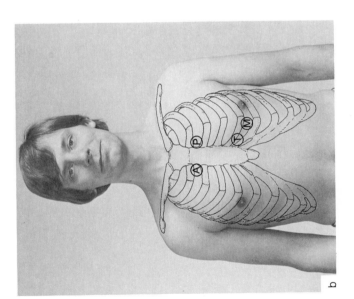

a

b

The sounds generated by the pumping of the heart are transmitted through the chest wall and can be amplified with the aid of a stethoscope. Sequentially positioning the client in supine, left-lateral, and sitting, (leaning slight forward) positions (a) allows the examiner to compare the heart sounds at rest, with the left side of the heart thrust forward, and with the right ventricle in contact with the chest wall.

The areas of the anterior chest where heart sounds can be selectively heard with the greatest intensity have been classically described. The names of these "listening posts" indicate the valvular sound predominantly transmitted to that position or area (b).

The sound of the aortic valve closing after the oxygenated blood leaves the left ventricle is transmitted best to the aortic area (A) - the second intercostal space along the right sternal border. The sound of the pulmonic valve closing after the blood leaves the right ventricle is transmitted to the pulmonic area (P) - the second intercostal space along the left sternal border.

The sound of the tricuspid valve closing as ventricular pressure builds with ventricular filling is transmitted to the tricuspid area (T) - the fourth and fifth intercostal spaces along left sternal border.

The sound of the mitral valve closing as ventricular pressure builds with ventricular filling is transmitted to mitral area (M) - the cardiac apex.

Highlights

Normally, only the (S₁) first and (S₂) second heart sounds (lubb-dubb) are heard upon auscultation.

Auscultation begins with the client in the supine position (a). The flow of blood through the heart chambers and vessels is usually smooth and quiet. Normally, the closing of the mitral and tricuspid valves before systole (first heart sound, S₁) and the closing of the aortic and pulmonic at the end of systole (second heart sound, S₂) are audible. These are characteristic heart (lubb-dubb) sounds.

Systole - contraction of heart; ejection of blood; occurs between first and second heart sounds.

Systole occurs as the pressure within the ventricles rises and blood flows into them from the atria. The ventricles begin to contract causing the atrioventricular valves to shut (lubb). As the ventricles contract, intraventricular pressure exceeds the pressure in the aorta and pulmonary artery causing the aortic and pulmonic valves to open silently and blood to fill those vessels (b). At the end of *systole* the pressure in the ventricles has decreased due to the outflow of blood, and the pressure in the arteries has increased. The pulmonic and aortic valves close at this point (c).

Diastole - relaxation of the cardiac cycle allows for filling of atrium; cardiac dilatation.

When the ventricles relax, the atrioventricular valves open, and ventricular filling once again takes place (d). This is commonly called *diastole*.

a

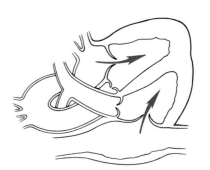

Diastole

b

Systole

c

d

The heart sounds heard in the T and M area (apex) will accentuate the first heart sound.

The heart sounds heard in the P and A area will accentuate the second heart sound.

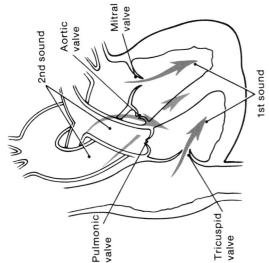

2nd sound

Aortic valve

Mitral valve

Pulmonic valve

Tricuspid valve

1st sound

b

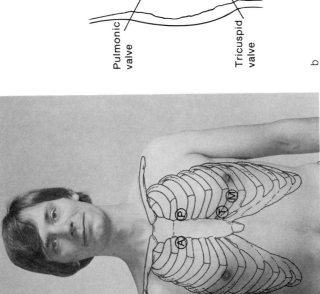

a

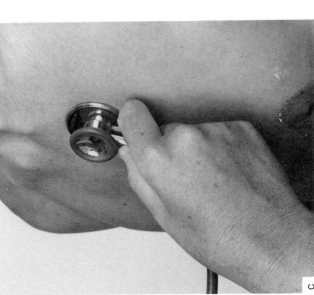

c

The first heart sound occurs with the closing of the mitral (M) and tricuspid (T) valves at the end of the ventricular filling.

The second heart sound occurs with the closing of the aortic (A) and pulmonic (P) valve at the end of systole (a).

Heart sounds radiate in the same direction as blood flow (b) therefore the first heart sound is heard (T and M) louder and longer and with a lower pitch at the apex. The second heart sound (A and P) is heard with greater intensity at the base.

With the stethoscope placed firmly against chest wall using the diaphragm (c), the examiner listens through several cycles of inspiration and expiration moving the stethoscope to each area (A, P, T, M). At each site, the examiner listens with the diaphragm followed by listening with the bell. The bell should be held lightly against the chest wall for the best sound.

Respiration affects events on the right side of the heart much more than those on the left.

Changes produced by respiration are only for two or three beats at the begining of inspiration and should be listened for during continuous respirations, not with held breath.

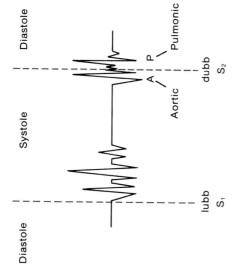

Diastole   Systole   Diastole

lubb   dubb
S_1 S_2

Aortic   A   P   Pulmonic

a

Since events of the left side of the heart take place slightly before those on the right, the mitral and aortic valves close slightly before the tricuspid and pulmonary valves. Usually the difference is not detectible by ear, but can be demonstrated in a picture of the wave form generated by the sounds (a).

During inspiration, however, negative pressure within the chest causes a greater amount of right ventricular filling then during expiration. This delays the closing of the pulmonic valve sufficiently so that the split sound can be detected by the ear with aid of the stethoscope.

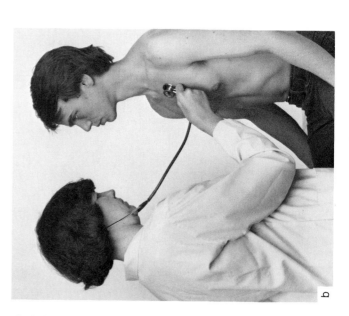

b

This physiologic (normal) splitting of S_2 with inspiration is heard best using the diaphragm of the stethoscope with the client in the sitting position (b).

Another sound which may be heard in the chest of a thin young adult is called a third heart sound or S_3 (a). It disappears after age 30. The sound of S_3 is a low-pitched thud heard best with the bell of the stethoscope on expiration. It is associated with early ventricular filling and is thought to occur when the mitral and tricuspid valves open and a large volume of blood falls into the relaxed ventricle during diastole.

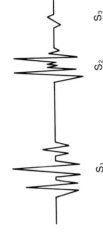

S_1 S_2 S_3

This sound is best heard with the client in the supine position (b). The examiner listens at T and M. The client is then asked to turn on the left side (c). The examiner holds the bell of the stethoscope in position over the site where the extra sound has been heard and listens again. The client is then asked to sit up and lean forward while the examiner holds the stethoscope in the position (d). The client is asked finally to return to the supine position and the examiner listens again. Return to the supine position increases ventricular filling sounds.

An S_3 is common in hyperkinetic states, i.e., exercise, pregnancy and mild to moderate anxiety.

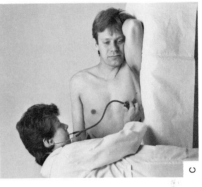

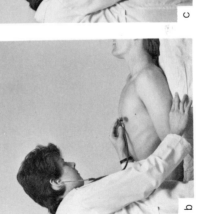

a

b

c

d

Highlights

A third heart sound may be heard in thin young adults under age 30.

The two normal heart sounds plus an S_3 sounds like "lubb-dubb-uh." It is heard best at the mitral area.

Normal hyperkinetic states include exercise, pregnancy, and mild to moderate anxiety. Each can produce an S_3 sound.

An audible S_3 frequently develops in pregnancy by the 30th week due to increased blood volume (hyperkinetic state).

The two normal heart sounds plus an S₄ sound like "Tuh-lubb-dubb".

Sudden recumbency will accentuate ventricular filling of sounds S₃ and S₄.

Functional murmurs may be heard in young adults because the heart and valves are small and blood velocity is great.

Murmurs are of longer duration than other heart sounds. Functional heart murmurs are heard in the middle of systole and are always associated with other entirely normal findings.

Functional heart murmurs are heard best in the pulmonic area and along the left sternal border.

Functional murmurs decrease when the client is in the sitting position.

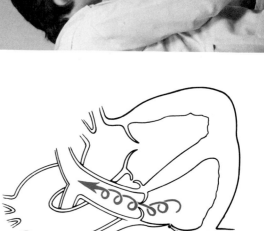

S₄ S₁ S₂ S₃

a

Atrioventricular valve closed

b

c

A sound which can sometimes be heard in the normal adult over age 50 is called a fourth sound or S₄ (a). The sound of S₄ is also low-pitched, but quiet and soft. It is heard best with the bell of the stethoscope on inspiration. It is thought to occur when most of the blood is in the relaxed ventricle and the atrium contracts, forcing the last bit of blood into a ventricle which has lost some of its elasticity–due to aging. The examiner listens for S₄ in the same manner described for S₃.

Another sound which can sometimes be heard in the normal chest is a functional or innocent murmur. It is heard in children and young adults because the heart is small and its valves are small and the blood flow velocity is great.

These murmurs are called **functional heart murmurs**. They have a blowing quality, increase with held expiration, and decrease when the patient sits up. They are benign and tend to disappear with age.

The sound of turbulence may be heard particularly when the blood rushes into the pulmonary artery and/or the aorta during systole (b).

Standing to the right of the supine client the examiner listens with the bell and the diaphragm of the stethoscope at the left sternal border from the pulmonic area to the end of the sternum, as well as at the neck and apex to detect any radiation (c). This procedure is repeated with the client in the left lateral position and with the client sitting, leaning forward facing the examiner.

Breast

Contributed by Meredith Censullo, R.N., M.S.N.

Examination of the breast provides for assessment data acquired by inspection and palpation. During the examination the examiner should emphasize the technique, position, and rationale for each stage of the process, including normal expectations and variations. The examiner should encourage the client to perform a self breast examination (SBE) on a routine monthly basis, a day or two after the end of the menstrual period (a). At this time the breasts are the smallest, non-tender and the glandular tissue is least congested.

Inspection

To inspect the breast the client is seated, facing the examiner, nude to the waist in a well lighted room. The examiner should stand directly in front of the client with full view of upper torso (b). The general appearance of the breast should then be observed noting specifically the size, symmetry, contour, texture of the skin, color, vascular patterning present and the appearance of the nipple and areola (c).

Self Breast Examination

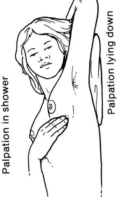
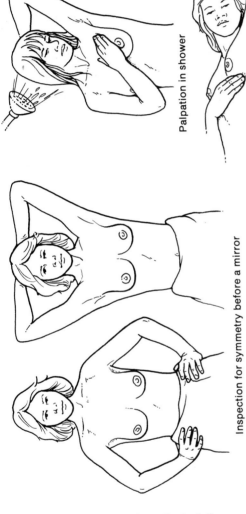

Inspection for symmetry before a mirror

Palpation in shower

Palpation lying down

a

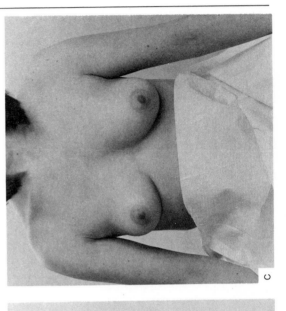

b

c

Highlights

SBE = Self Breast Examination

The examiner should determine if the client knows how to perform a SBE.

The client's ability to perform a SBE can be determined through return demonstration.

Breast examination can be performed during bathing as water and soap can ease movement through maneuvers.

Highlights

The *tail of Spence* is frequently the site of breast tumors.

The breasts are located between the second and sixth ribs, bounded by the sternum and midaxillary line. In the upper lateral quadrant of the breast is a projection of breast tissue into the axilla called the *tail of Spence* (a).

The breast is composed of glandular tissue and is supported by fibrous tissue. *Cooper's ligaments* are bands of fibrous tissue which are found within breast tissue (b). Eventually these ligaments attach to the muscle of the chest wall. The bulk of the breast is fatty tissue located in *superficial* and *retromammary* areas. The proportion of glandular, fibrous and fatty tissue varies with age, state of nutrition, past and family history, menstrual and pregnancy history, and lactation and hormonal experiences.

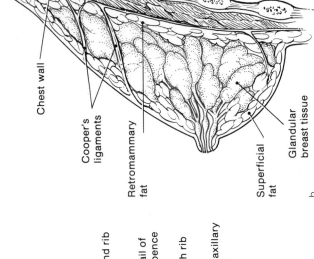

a

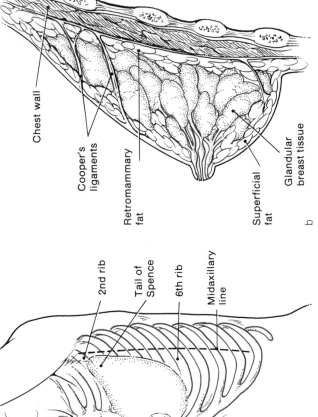

b

There are approximately 15-25 lobes contained within each breast. These lobes contain the *acini cells* which are responsible for milk production. The lobes divide into a network of smaller lobules (20-40) containing collecting ducts which terminate in the nipple (c).

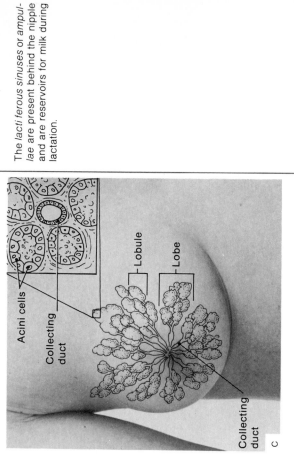

c

The breast should be inspected with the client sitting with (a) arms at sides; (b) arms elevated; (c) hands presented against hips, and (d) sitting or standing, bending over with arms outstretched.

The size of breast varies with each individual. In addition one breast is often larger than the other.

Change in size: (eg. shrunken breasts). *Asymmetry:* irregular contour, indicated by indentation or puckering; *Fixation:* breasts do not move equally (look for bilateral symmetry of nipples when client changes position of her arms); *change in surface:* thickened texture, puckered (orange-peel appearance, indicates edema); *Ulcerations, inflammation or elevated skin temperature in nonpostpartum women; or change in pattern,* dilated subcutaneous veins in nonpregnant women are all variations which require further investigation.

Supernumerary nipples (accompanied by areola and/or glandular tissue) found along embryological milk-line are not considered abnormal.

Nipples (in absence of pregnancy, postpartum, breast feeding or sexual manipulation) that are red, ulcerated, thickened, with discharge, or having a shape other than round, are abnormal variations and require further investigation.

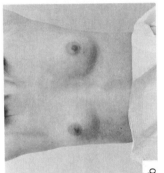
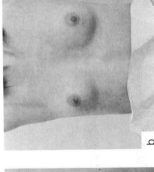
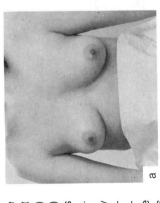

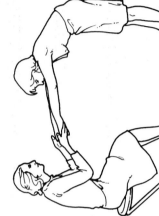
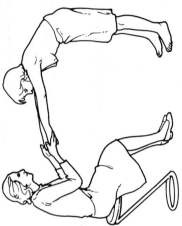

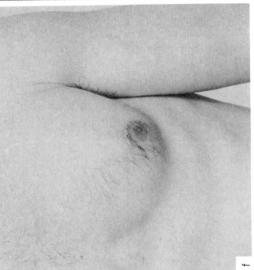

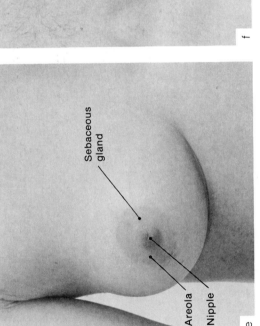

Sebaceous gland

Areola
Nipple

Inspect the breast with the woman in the following positions: (a) sitting, arms at her sides; (b) sitting, arms elevated; (c) sitting, hands pressed against hips; (d) sitting or standing, bending over, arms outstretched, supported by the examiner.

Normal breasts are mobile and fall freely from the chest wall. They appear bilaterally symmetrical. Breast sizes varies, with one breast often larger than the other. Small, large and pendulous breasts fall within normal limits.

Normally, the tissue covering breast is smooth, similar in appearance to the skin of the abdomen or back. Bilateral linear blue coloring of the skin indicates underlying vascular structures. In addition a pale to whitish striae can be observed following stretching.

Areolae are pigmented areas surrounding the nipples. Normal color ranges from pink to brown, with minimally demarcated margins. The areola surface contains sebaceous glands (which appear as papillae in an asymmetric pattern), and hair follicles around the periphery (e).

Nipples are circular, located in the center of the areola. They consist of pigmented, erectile tissue. The nipples may protrude, be flush with surrounding tissue or inverted. Their surface is fine and smooth and contains milk duct openings.

The male breast consists of a nipple and areola (f). Beneath the surface is a thin disc of breast tissue that usually is not distinguishable from the surrounding tissue.

Palpation

The breast contains many lymph nodes that head into a lymphatic drainage system. Palpation of the axillary nodes and breast tissue is accomplished with the client initially in a sitting position and then lying down.

While the client remains seated, the examiner then palpates the subclavicular, supraclavicular (a), and axillary lymph nodes.

Normally, lymph drains to the supraclavicular (located above the clavicle towards midline) and subclavicular nodes (located below the clavicle [b]). To palpate these areas, the client places her arms at her side and the examiner assesses the nodes on both sides of the body.

There are three areas of axillary nodes (c). *Pectoral nodes* are inside the anterior axillary fold, along the lower border of the pectoralis major. The *subscapular nodes* are deep within the posterior axillary fold along the lateral border of the scapula. The *lateral axillary nodes* are felt along the upper humerus.

To palpate for axillary lymph nodes, the examiner supports the client's arm, thereby relaxing the pectoral muscles. With the other hand, thoroughly and gently palpate the entire area reaching deep into the axilla (d). The examiner can better feel the nodes, by compressing the tissue against the muscle wall. The client's arm should be moved through the full range of motion while palpating. This will improve the accuracy of the examination by increasing the surface area being examined. Normally, lymph nodes are not palpated.

Highlights

The *cutaneous, areolar* and *deep lymphatic drainage systems* are three examples of lymphatic drainage from the breast. They drain areas such as breast skin, areolae and nipples and mammary tissue respectively.

With the client sitting and arms at the side the pectoral, subscapular and lateral axillary nodes are examined bilaterally.

When examining the nodes be certain the muscles are relaxed so as to avoid missing changes. Some examiners use soapy water on the breast to facilitate the ease with which the fingers move to palpate breast tissue.

Palpable nodes should be investigated further.

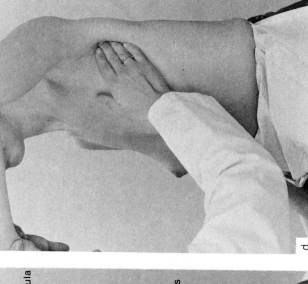

b

Clavicle

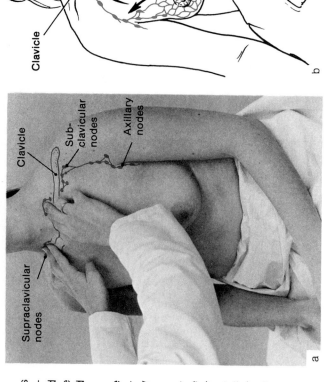

Clavicle

Subclavicular nodes

Axillary nodes

Supraclavicular nodes

a

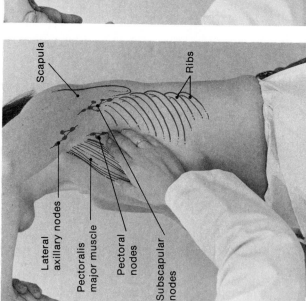

Scapula

Ribs

Lateral axillary nodes

Pectoralis major muscle

Pectoral nodes

Subscapular nodes

c

d

All four quadrants of the breast should be examined in a logical approach to insure a thorough palpation of each area.

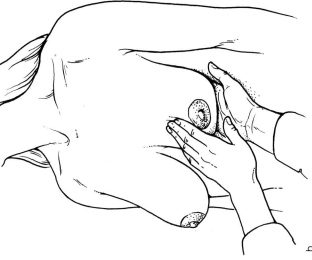

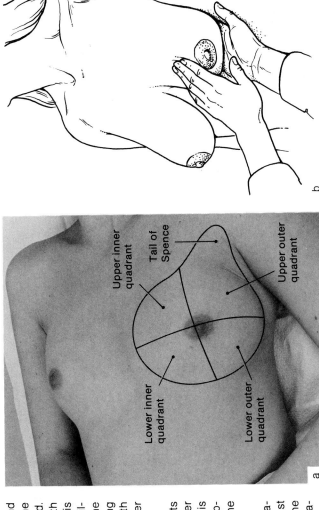

a

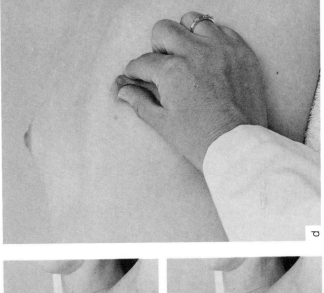

b

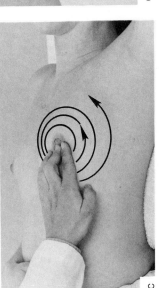

d

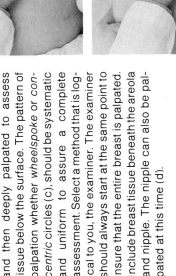

c

Upper inner quadrant

Tail of Spence

Upper outer quadrant

Lower inner quadrant

Lower outer quadrant

Next, direct the client to lie down and raise the arm above the head on the same side as the breast to be palpated. A small pillow can be placed beneath the shoulder on the same side. This spreads the breast tissue medially, facilitating access to the outer layer of the breast. Again, palpate gently, covering every square inch of breast tissue with particular attention to the upper, outer quadrant and tail of Spence.

Each breast is divided into 4 quadrants (the upper outer; upper inner; lower inner; lower outer [a]). Each quadrant is palpated starting in a systematic approach from the lateral areas to the center.

If the breasts are pendulous, the examiner may have to support the breast with one hand while examining the quadrants of the other (bimanual palpation [b]).

To palpate breast tissue, the examiner uses the flat portion of the fingers in a rotary motion, which compresses the breast tissue against the chest wall. The breast tissue is palpated gently at first and then deeply palpated to assess tissue below the surface. The pattern of palpation whether *wheelspoke* or *concentric circles* (c), should be systematic and uniform to assure a complete assessment. Select a method that is logical to you, the examiner. The examiner should always start at the same point to insure that the entire breast is palpated. Include breast tissue beneath the areola and nipple. The nipple can also be palpated at this time (d).

Highlights

Tenderness of breast tissue may be present during menses.

Should masses or changes be noted in the breast tissue, the examiner should diagram location of mass, define the breast in quadrant, describe location, size in centimeters, shape, consistency, moveability, degree of deliniation, erythema, dimpling of edge of the mass in duration of nipple, discharge and tenderness.

Significant findings in examining the male breast require further investigation.

The presence of smooth, firm, mobile, discs of breast tissue surrounding the areola (temporarily present in normal puberty) is called *gynecomastia*.

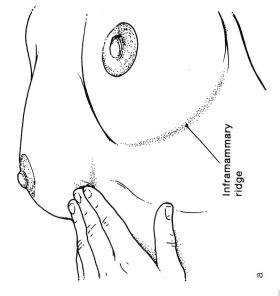

Inframammary ridge

a

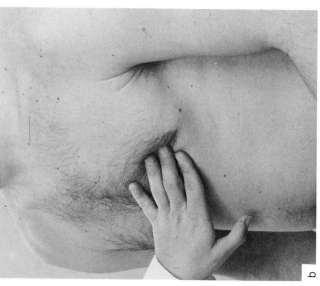

b

Normally, the female breast feels soft to touch. Breast tissue in the young woman is firm and elastic and non-tender. In normal glandular tissue, one feels a fine nodularity throughout. Generalized coarse nodularity is common when progesterone is present. A transverse ridge (inframammary ridge) along the lower border of the breast is normally found in large breasts (a). Breast tissue in the elderly that feels stringy or granular is also normal.

When palpating the male nipple and areola, tissue should feel soft, nonnodular (b). Obese client may have enlarged breasts. It is important to distinguish between fatty tissue and firm discs of glandular enlargement.

ABDOMEN

Contributions to this section made by Mary Ellen Maguire R.N., C., M.S.W.

The examination of the abdomen includes the assessment of the bowels, liver, spleen, stomach, gallbladder, pancreas, kidney and abdominal blood vessels (a). When the abdomen is being examined, the standard order of examination differs, with inspection followed by auscultation, palpation and percussion. If auscultation followed the movement and stimulation of percussion and palpation during the abdominal examination, it might result in false interpretation of bowel sounds.

The equipment necessary for abdominal examination is a marking pencil, a tape measure or ruler, and a stethoscope.

Specific anatomical landmarks are used by the examiner during the examination. Two common methods to describe abdominal findings result from dividing the abdomen into sections. The first, and most often used approach, divides the abdomen into four sections: right upper quadrant (RUQ), right lower quadrant (RLQ), left upper quadrant (LUQ), and left lower quadrant (LLQ) (b).

The second method divides the abdomen into nine sections. These nine sections and related regions (epigastric, umbilical and hypogastric or suprapubic) are shown in Fig. c.

Highlights

The techniques of the abdominal examination follows the sequence of inspection, auscultation, percussion and palpation.

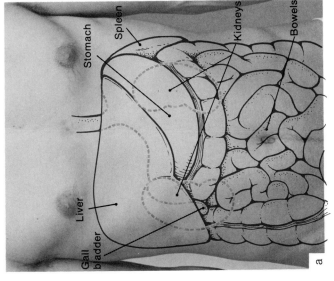

a

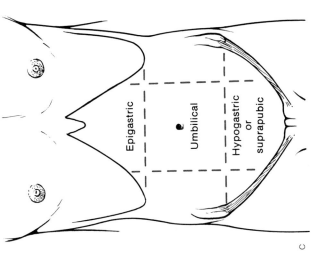

c

b

Inspection

To examine the abdomen place the client in a supine position with hands at the sides. To facilitate the examination, the client must have an empty bladder and should be instructed to breathe slowly through the mouth. Drape the client to ensure warmth and comfort, and prevent tensing of the abdominal muscles. With the abdomen fully exposed unobstructed observation can be made.

When inspecting the abdomen, the client should be relaxed (bladder emptied); warm and comfortable, with the abdomen fully exposed.

Room temperature should also be warm to prevent shivering and tensing of the abdominal muscles.

Shivering or tensing of abdominal muscles can cause misinterpretation of data.

A small pillow under the head and another under the flexed knees will enhance muscle relaxation (a). A relaxed client is essential for an accurate abdominal examination. The client can be further relaxed by the examiner's support and explanations.

The examiner should stand and then sit at the right side of the client, looking across the fully exposed abdomen (b). This enables the examiner to observe the abdomen for symmetry, hair distribution, distention, skin condition, contour, and unusual protuberances. The client is instructed to take deep breaths to allow the examiner to look for changes in symmetry or contour. Organ enlargement may become evident during deep inspiration. Normally, these changes are not present.

The examiner stands and then sits at the right side of the client to inspect the fully exposed abdomen

The abdomen is inspected for size, shape, contour and symmetry.

Contour of the abdomen and the absence of symmetry (including distention, masses, peristalsis, respiratory movements, and pulsations) are also observed.

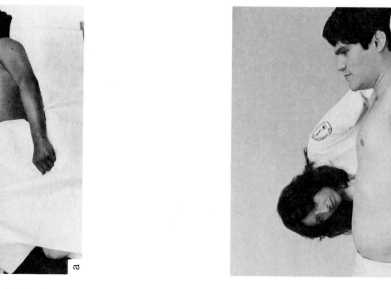

a

b

Contour will differ from client to client. Evaluation of contour is determined by inspecting the area from the rib margin to the pubic bone. With the client in a recumbent position, contour is observed (a). Normal abdominal contour can be described as *flat*, often seen in youths, athletic clients, or elderly, thin clients; *rounded*, more often found in the female than the male and due to excess subcutaneous fat and poor muscle tone; *protuberant*, often a descriptor for an obese abdomen; and *scaphoid*, or concave, found in underweight clients. Abdominal contour serves as a descriptor of the client's general nutritional status.

Distention, unusual stretching of the abdominal wall, occurring symmetrically or asymmetrically, is not a normal finding and needs further evaluation.

The normal abdomen should remain symmetrical when the client lifts the head and shoulders off the examining table, unsupported (b). This measure will contract the abdominal rectus muscles (c). A ridgelike bulge midline could be an indication of diastasis recti, separation of the rectus muscle layers due to muscle weakness, often associated with obesity. Umbilical or incisional hernias may protrude and should be noted during this maneuver.

Contour of the abdomen differs in each client it may be rounded, protuberant, scaphoid or concave.

Distention of the abdomen requires further evaluation.

When the client contracts the abdominal rectus muscles the abdomen should remain symmetrical.

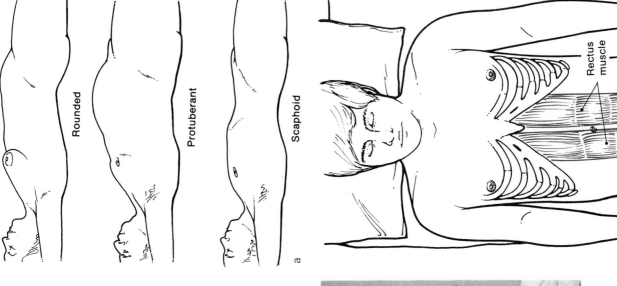

Rounded

Protuberant

Scaphoid

a

Rectus muscle

c

b

Highlights

Skin over the abdominal area should be similar in color to surrounding tissue, smooth and uninterrupted.

Abdominal scars should be described in terms of their size, shape, and location.

Striae - linea albicantes or stretch marks.

Abdominal striae can occur after weight loss or following pregnancy.

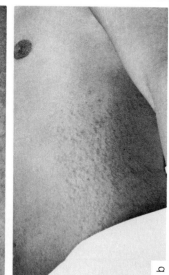

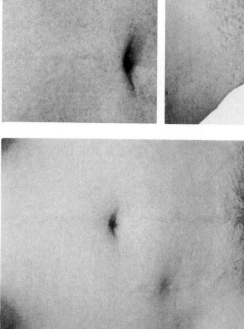

a

b

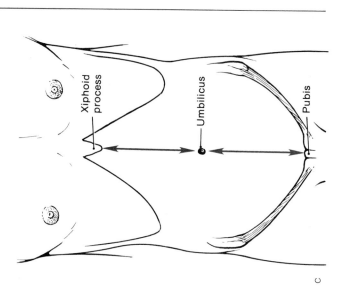

c

Skin The skin is another indicator of general nutritional status. It should be described for general appearance, pigmentation, hydration, elasticity, scars, striae, lesions, venous patterns, and hair distribution. Normally, the color of abdominal skin should be similar to that of surrounding tissue with a soft smooth and uninterrupted surface.

Scars (a) The size and shape of scars should be measured in centimeters and drawn into the appropriate abdominal quadrant.

Striae (linae albicantes) Often referred to as stretch marks, striae are normally pink or blue in color initially, and progress to a silvery white. They appear as lines or streaks on the skin, often in areas of rapid weight gain and loss (b). They occur because of prolonged stretching of elastic fibers of the reticular skin layer. Striae should be described by size, location, and color. Normally, they may be observed after pregnancy or weight loss.

Pigmentation The abdominal surface is often used to compare to other more exposed skin surfaces. It is important to note any unusual pigmentation or discoloration in this area. The length of its presence and changes in color and size should be reported.

Umbilicus The normal umbilicus is positioned midway between the xiphoid process and the pubis (c). The position and shape of the umbilicus may vary (eg., round oval, recessed, protruding) and should be described.

Highlights

Aortic pulsations are sometimes present in clients when inspecting the area of the abdominal area.

It is normal to observe more significant respiratory movements in males particularly at rest.

Abdominal peristaltic movements can be observed with the client in a recumbent and relaxed position.

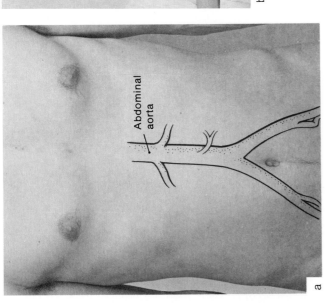

a

b

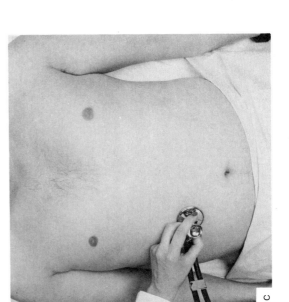

c

Pulsations Aortic pulsations arising over the abdominal aorta are normal though not found in all clients (a).

Respiratory movement The male client normally uses the abdominal muscles for respiration, while the female client normally uses the costal muscles. Therefore it is normal to observe more significant respiratory movement in males, particularly at rest.

Peristalsic movement This movement can be determined by observing the abdomen for several minutes. The client remains in a recumbent, relaxed position and the examiner sits at the client's side (b). Peristaltic (wave like) movements may normally be visible particularly in thin clients. These movements become an abnormal finding when strong contractions are visible through a thick abdominal wall.

Auscultation

When examining the abdomen, auscultation is performed prior to percussion and palpation. This is done because percussion can increase bowel sounds and interfere with the assessment of bowel motility. The diaphragm of the stethoscope is used to auscultate the high-pitched bowel sounds as well as vascular sounds located in the abdominal area (c).

Highlights

Abdominal auscultation precedes palpation and percussion so that increases in bowel sounds created by the above maneuvers will not interfere with the assessment of bowel motility.

Bowel sounds normally occur at a rate of 5 to 20+ per minute.

Bowel sounds are irregular sounds of varying duration.

Decreased or increased bowel sounds reflect changes in bowel motility and should be investigated further.

Bruits are turbulant sounds heard over a dilated or constricted blood vessel. They may be heard in healthy young adults and require further evaluation.

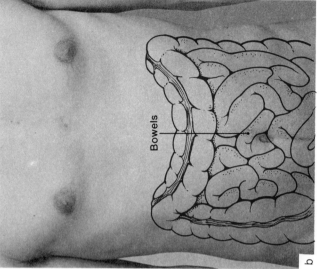

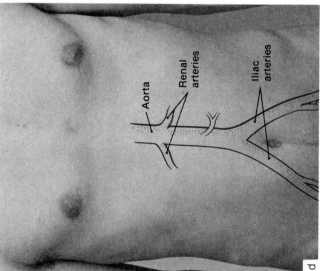

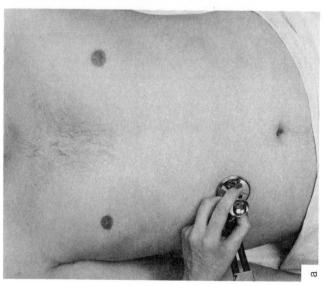

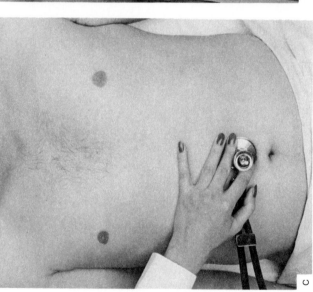

Bowel Sounds Normal bowel sounds occur at rates of 5 to 20+ per minute, and last approximately 0.5 second. These bowel sounds are the sounds of fluid and gas passing through the intestines. They are described as low, dry, rumbling sounds of high-pitched intensity similar to clicks or gurgles. They are often irregular and the duration of the sound may be less than a second to several seconds. The presence of food and the stage of digestion, however, may affect the rate of bowel sounds. It is recommended that the examiner auscultate each quadrant for several minutes before assuming that bowel sounds are absent (a and b).

Abnormal bowel sounds occur in two significant patterns: (1) sounds are absent or extremely soft and widely spaced; (2) sounds occur as waves of loud gurgling, splashing, or tinkling (borborygmi). Such findings require further evaluation.

Vascular Sounds The abdominal aorta and the renal and iliac arteries located beneath the abdominal surface are auscultated for bruits, an abnormal finding (c and d). Rarely, an abnormal venous "hum" may also be auscultated in the periumbilical area. Both findings should be auscultated using both the diaphragm and the bell. If present, the client should be referred for further evaluation.

Percussion

With the client remaining in a comfortable lying position, the abdominal examination continues. The technique of percussion enables the examiner to delineate the border and contours of the solid organs within the abdomen and to outline air in the stomach or bowel. Some examiners prefer to percuss and palpate at the same time when examining and assessing abdominal structures. It is important to develop a systematic pattern of percussion and palpation and use it with all clients, so as to become familiar with the ranges of normal findings (a).

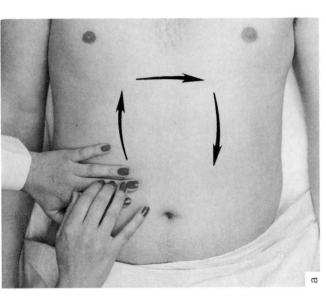

The normal percussion note is tympany, except for dullness over the liver (b) and a small area over the spleen. The tympanic sound is produced due to the fact that air present in the gastrointestinal system will rise to the surface when the client is in a recumbent position (c). Free air in the abdomen also will produce a similar sound. The entire abdomen should be percussed lightly in all four quadrants to assess areas of tympany and dullness.

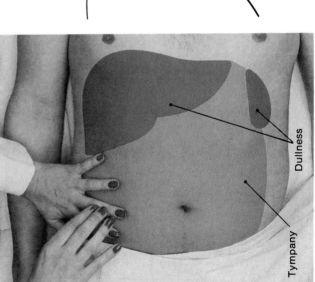

The normal percussion sound of the abdomen is tympany except over the liver and spleen which are dull.

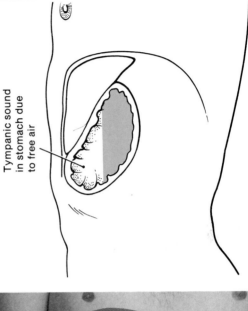

Tympanic sound in stomach due to free air

Liver span measures 6 to 12 cm.

Refer to section on Techniques in this chapter for a discussion of Fist Percussion.

Fist percussion is used to determine tenderness of liver region.

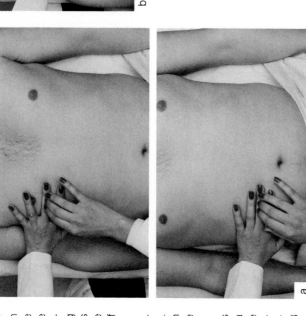

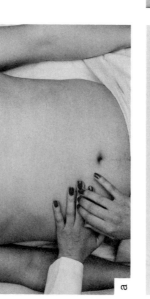

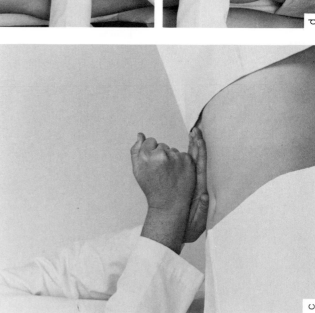

Liver Measurement of liver span begins by percussing for lung resonance in the midclavicular area. To determine this location, the examiner locates the midclavicular line and begins percussing downward (a). The area where lung resonance changes to liver dullness is marked. The fifth to seventh interspace usually is the site of the upper border of liver dullness.

The lower edge of liver dullness is normally located in the right costal margin. The examiner can begin percussion in the right midclavicular line below the umbilicus.

When the percussion note changes from tympany to liver dullness, the area is marked. The distance between the two marks (in centimeters) is then measured (b). The normal liver span measures between 6 and 12 cm, or 4 and 8 cm if percussion is done mid sternally. Liver span is usually greater in the tall or male client than the short or female client.

Fist percussion is a technique that can be used to vibrate tissue rather than percuss it directly. To percuss, the examiner's left hand is placed (palm side) against the right costal margin and striking a blow to the left hand with the ulnar portion of the right fist (c). This should be done on the left and right costal margins for comparison of findings (d). Normally, no tenderness should be present. It is often used to assess the liver. Normally, when the liver is percussed in this manner no tenderness is elicited.

Highlights

Normal splenic dullness is percussed at the level of the 6th or 9th to the 11th rib, just posterior to or at the level of the midaxillary line.

Spleen Normal splenic dullness is percussed at the level of the left 6th or 9th to 11th rib just posterior to the midaxillary line (a and b). Splenic dullness should be described when extending into the normally tympanic area of the gastric air bubble. This would indicate splenic enlargement, an abnormal finding.

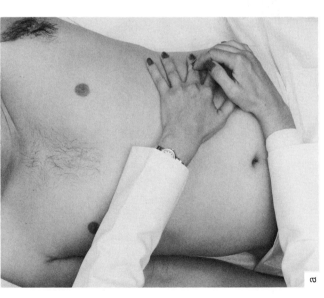
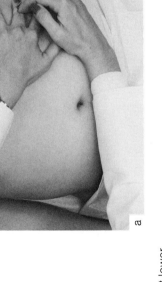

a

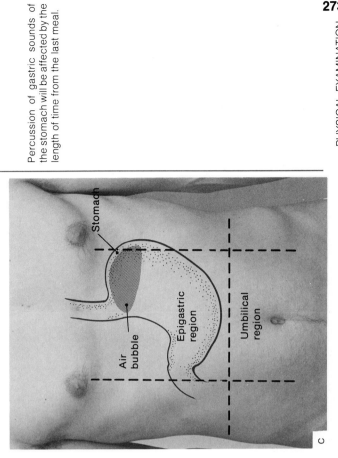

6th rib
10th rib
Spleen
b

Stomach
Air bubble
Epigastric region
Umbilical region
c

Stomach Percussion in the left lower anterior rib cage and the left epigastric region will reveal the deeper lower pitched tympanic note of the gastric air bubble (c). The sounds generated by percussion of the stomach will vary according to when a meal had been eaten.

Palpation

Palpation is used to evaluate the abdominal wall, the abdominal aorta, and the abdominal organs. It may confirm earlier normal findings or provide more information on such abnormal findings as pain, masses, tenderness, or organ enlargement.

To begin palpation, the examiner should stand on the client's right side. The examiner's hands should be warmed before proceeding. The client should be as relaxed as possible to prevent abdominal muscle contraction and resistance (measures to promote relaxation have been described earlier in this discussion [a]).

The abdomen is then examined with first light and then deep palpation in all four quadrants (b). Organs are identified and described as size, shape, position, mobility, consistency, tension, and tenderness. Distance to anatomical landmarks and size should be measured in centimeters, not finger breadths.

Abdominal Reflexes   Before beginning palpation, the examiner should test the abdominal reflexes. Using a sharp object or the metal end of a reflex hammer, lightly but briskly stroke each quadrant of the abdomen toward the umbilicus above and below it (c). The normal reflex will cause the abdominal muscles to contract and the umbilicus to move toward the direction of the stimulus. This reflex can normally be absent in obese clients or in elderly clients who have a flaccid muscle structure.

During palpation it is important that the abdomen be as relaxed as possible.

Refer to section in Chap. 4 under Techniques for a discussion of light and deep palpation.

Normally, abdominal muscles will contract and the umbilicus will move in the direction of the stimulus.

The umbilicus should move freely on palpation returning to normal size and shape.

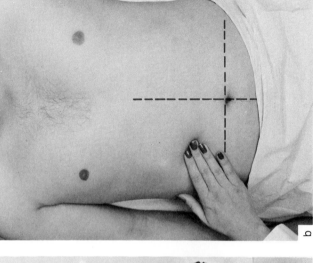

a

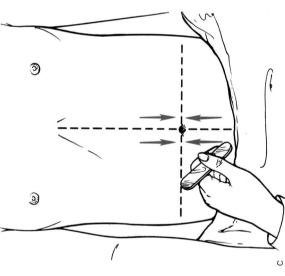

b

c

Light Palpation

For light palpation the examiner uses the fingertip pads and gently explores all four abdominal quadrants by depressing the skin 1 cm with light pressure (a).

In the normal abdomen, organs, masses, or tenderness are not palpable during light palpation. Areas of tenderness should be explored last.

Deep Palpation

Deep palpation may be performed using two methods. The first method is most useful with a relaxed client. The examiner positions the hands as if performing light palpation but deeply palpates all four quadrants to identify the deep abdominal organs. The second method, *bimanual palpation*, is useful when abdominal relaxation is difficult to maintain. The examiner's hands are placed one on top of the other (b). Pressure is exerted with the outside or top hand, while the bottom or underside hand identifies the underlying abdominal structures. The client normally experiences tenderness during deep palpation. Bimanual palpation is also *more* useful with the obese client.

Deep palpation should be performed in an orderly manner to survey the abdominal organs. Normal abdominal structures are occasionally mistaken for masses. Changes caused by a full bladder, bowel segments containing feces, aortic pulsations, the uterus, the common iliac artery, and the sacral promontory may be misinterpreted (c). The normal finding of feces in the ascending or descending colon, or in the cecum, will feel like a boggy, soft, rounded mass. Palpating it may cause cramping.

During light palpation all four quadrants are explored by exerting light pressure (depressing the client's skin 1 cm) over the abdominal surface.

Refer to discussion of deep palpation under *Techniques Used in the Physical Examination.*

The client may normally experience some tenderness during deep palpation.

When palpating the abdomen, normal findings can be changed by such things as a full bladder, or feces in the colon

The examiner should be able to distinguish normal from abnormal findings during the abdominal examination.

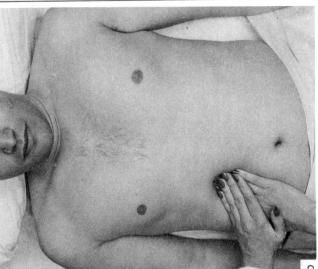

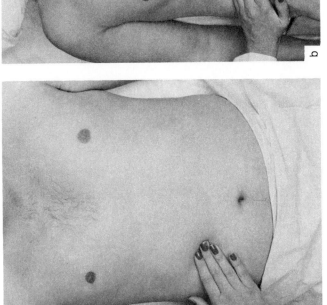

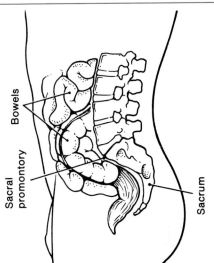

Deep palpation of the liver is used to determine the liver size.

Normally, the liver is usually non-palpable.

Two methods are available to palpate the liver. Normally the liver is not palpable.

If the liver edge is palpable in a healthy person it may be felt in the right costal margin. Usually a palpable liver is found in a thin client.

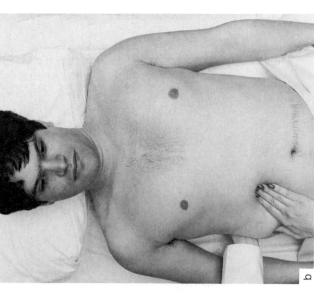

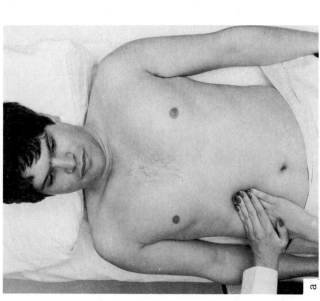

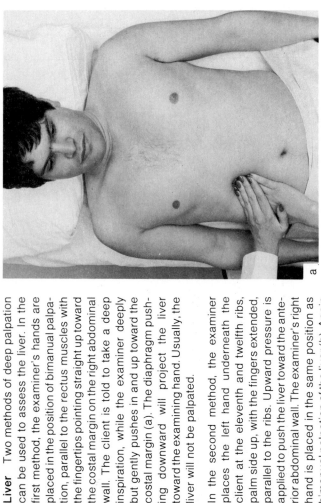

Liver Two methods of deep palpation can be used to assess the liver. In the first method, the examiner's hands are placed in the position of bimanual palpation, parallel to the rectus muscles with the fingertips pointing straight up toward the costal margin on the right abdominal wall. The client is told to take a deep inspiration, while the examiner deeply but gently pushes in and up toward the costal margin (a). The diaphragm pushing downward will project the liver toward the examining hand. Usually, the liver will not be palpated.

In the second method, the examiner places the left hand underneath the client at the eleventh and twelfth ribs, palm side up, with the fingers extended, parallel to the ribs. Upward pressure is applied to push the liver toward the anterior abdominal wall. The examiner's right hand is placed in the same position as bimanual palpation of the liver (b). Again the client is asked to take a deep inspiration, while the examiner presses gently in and up deeply. If the liver is palpable, the examiner will feel it slip under the palpating fingers. The normal palpable liver edge may be felt at the right costal margin and is regular in contour, sharp, and non tender. Frequently, when the normal size liver is palpated, the client is thin.

Normally the liver descends no lower than 1 or 2 cm below the costal margin (c). In most adults the liver is not palpable. A tall client or a client whose diaphragm is lower than is usual may have a normal liver span, although the edge is palpable below the costal margin. Tenderness is tested by fist percussion (refer to earlier discussion).

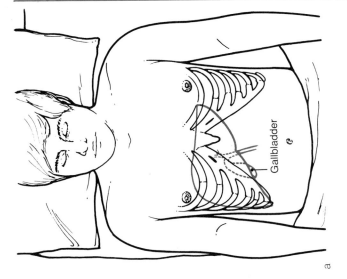

a

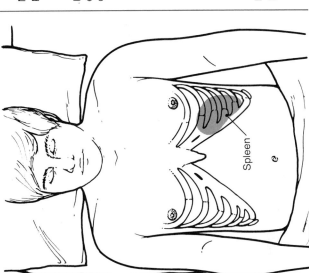

c

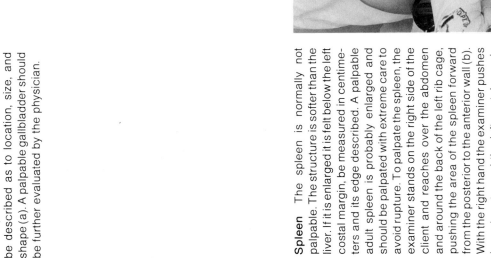

b

Highlights

Normally, the gallbladder is non-palpable.

Normally, the spleen is non-palpable.

If palpable, the spleen is usually enlarged and should be palpated cautiously.

Normally, the pancreas is not palpated.

Gallbladder   Normally the gallbladder is not palpable. If palpated medially or laterally below the liver margin it should be described as to location, size, and shape (a). A palpable gallbladder should be further evaluated by the physician.

Spleen   The spleen is normally not palpable. The structure is softer than the liver. If it is enlarged it is felt below the left costal margin, be measured in centimeters and its edge described. A palpable adult spleen is probably enlarged and should be palpated with extreme care to avoid rupture. To palpate the spleen, the examiner stands on the right side of the client and reaches over the abdomen and around the back of the left rib cage, pushing the area of the spleen forward from the posterior to the anterior wall (b). With the right hand the examiner pushes in and up toward the left costal margin while the client is asked to take a deep inspiration. The spleen, like the liver, will present a sharp edge if palpable (c).

Pancreas   The pancreas is not palpable in the normal client.

Highlights

The abdominal aorta is more easily palpated in the elderly client.

Normally abdominal veins are not seen in the healthy adult.

See section on Techniques for a discussion on rebounding.

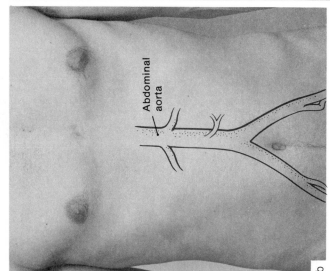

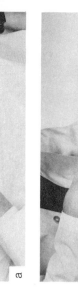

Abdominal aorta

b

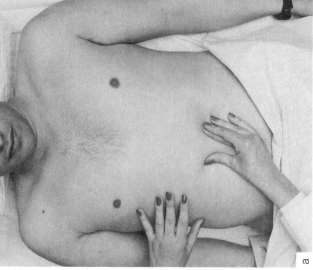

a

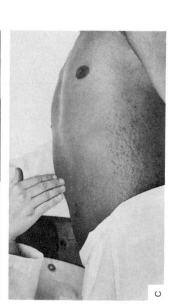

c

Vascular Structures The aorta is normally palpated in the upper abdomen slightly left of the midline (a). The abdominal aorta may be palpated more easily in the elderly or those with a curved spine. It is more difficult to palpate in the young adult. Palpate deeply to delineate the vessels' edges and evaluate the normal pulsations. The normal aorta is less than 4 cm in diameter and is soft and pulsatile from the midepigastric area to the pelvic area (b).

Normally, abdominal veins are not observable on the abdominal surface. In individuals with minimal adipose tissue (thin or malnourished individuals), these veins may be seen.

Rebounding

Rebounding is a technique in which the examiner quickly exerts deep pressure with the fingers over an abdominal area and then quickly releases the fingers from the abdominal surface (c). Normally the client should not experience any discomfort or pain.

Kidney The kidneys normally are not palpable in the adult client, but may be palpable in the aged client or in the client with flaccid abdominal walls. If the kidney is felt, it is described as a solid, firm mass, with a less sharp outline than the liver or spleen. It has no palpable notch as the spleen does. The right kidney lies lower than the left, and is more often palpable (a).

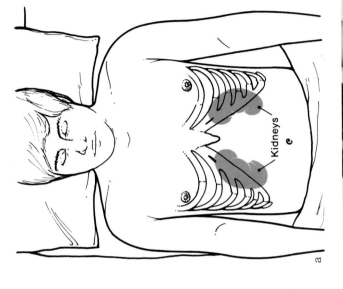

The kidneys may be palpated in the normal elderly client due to loss of muscle tone.

The right kidney is lower than the left kidney, and is more likely to be palpated in the elderly.

To palpate the left and right kidneys the examiner remains on the client's right side. To palpate the right kidney, the examiner places the left hand under the right flank and lifts forward to push the kidney toward the anterior wall. With the right hand the examiner deeply palpates the anterior wall below the right costal margin while the client takes a deep inspiration (b). If the kidney is palpable, the lower pole of the kidney will be felt.

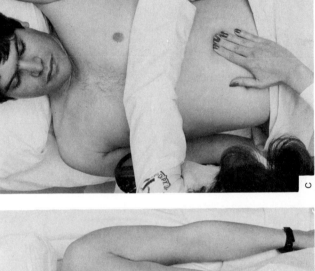

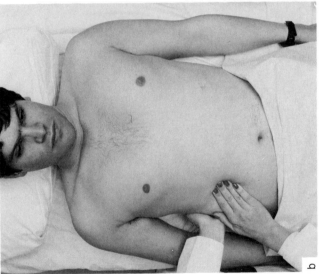

The left kidney is seldom palpable in the normal adult, but should be palpated by the same method used to assess the right kidney (c).

If the kidneys are thought to be palpable, the examiner should percuss the area again to differentiate between liver and spleen findings. The kidneys, because of their deeper location, require a deeper palpation than do the liver and spleen. Abnormal findings should be referred for further assessment.

FEMALE PELVIS

The pelvic examination section prepared by Maureen McRae, R.N.

The examination of the female pelvic anatomy focuses on an assessment of the female reproductive system, pelvic glands and orifices, and related pelvic organs.

It may be performed as part of an annual physical examination, or for diagnosis of pregnancy. It is also performed as part of contraceptive counseling, and when infertility or other gynecological problems are suspected.

Because the focus of pelvic examination includes anatomy which is both physically and psychologically sensitive, the examiner must take care to foster an open and understanding relationship of mutual trust and respect with the client (a).

Related pelvic organs that are included in the pelvic examination are the bladder and the rectum. These structures are included because of their close anatomical position in relation to the reproductive system (b).

The pelvic examination begins with the overall observation of the external genitalia, and moves on to separate and systematic examination of the vestibule, vagina, cervix, uterus, adnexa, and rectum.

Throughout the examination, the client is in the lithotomy position with feet in stirrups (c). The examiner is seated at her feet. The client is gowned and draped to ensure that her privacy and dignity are maintained (d).

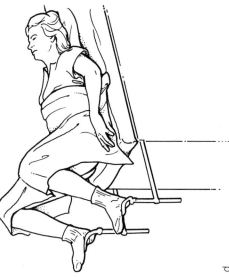

Rectum

Uterus

Adnexa

Vagina

Urethra

Bladder

Symphysis pubis

b

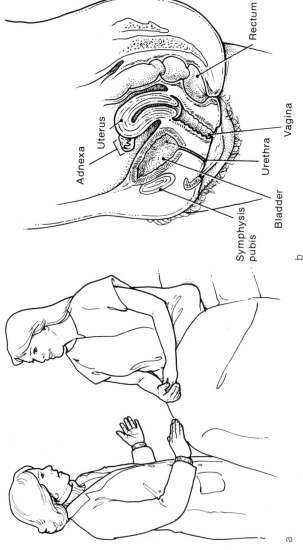

a

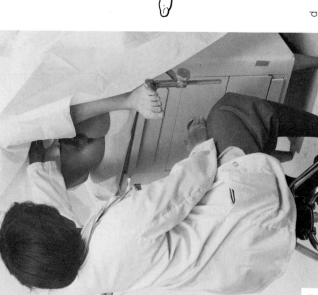

c

d

Inspection and palpation are the main techniques used in the pelvic examination. Inspection is employed for the assessment of external structures, inspection and palpation are used for the assessment of the cervix, and palpation is the technique used for the assessment of the uterus, adnexa, and rectum.

The client may be encouraged to wear shoes and/or stockings during the examination since metal sirrups, if not padded, are cold and uncomfortable (a).

The client should be instructed to empty her bladder before the examination, since a full bladder interferes with the palpation of internal structures and may create unnecessary discomfort.

The bladder is close to the internal reproductive structures, and when distended exerts pressure on these structures.

A pelvic examination adeptly performed, should not cause discomfort.

External Female Reproductive Structures

The female reproductive system is divided into the external structures and the internal structures. *External structures* include those which are visible. They are also referred to as the *vulva*. These structures include the *mons veneris* or *mons pubis, labia majora, labia minora, vestibule, clitoris, vulvovaginal* or *Bartholin's glands, paraurethral* or *Skene's ducts,* and the *perineum* (c).

Inspection

With the client in the lithotomy position, feet in stirrups, legs spread apart as far as comfortably possible, and with the examiner seated at the foot of the examining table approximately one arms length away the examination of the external genitalia can begin (b).

The examination of the pelvis and related structures provides the examiner with an ideal opportunity to teach women about their anatomy. Many women, although they may have had children, are unaware of both the structure and function of their reproductive systems.

The use of a mirror during the pelvic examination allows the client to actively participate.

Slow, deep breathing often helps in relaxation.

Since the examiner is often not visible to the client because of the position of both during the examination, constant communication and explanation of all procedures are crucial.

The vulva is also called the pudendum, from the Latin word meaning "to be ashamed."

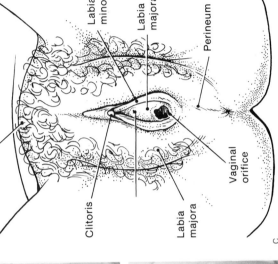

c

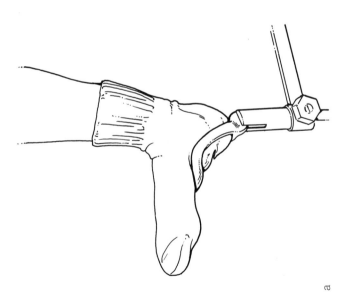

a

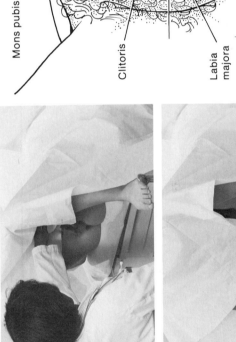

b

Mons pubis

Clitoris

Labia majora

Labia minora

Labia majora

Perineum

Vaginal orifice

The examination of the vulva includes an assessment of the external female genitalia. These structures are visible between the thighs and extend from the area over the symphysis pubis posteriorly to the perineum. Which lies just in front of the rectum. The examiner will observe that the external genitalia are unique to each woman, and vary from woman to woman.

The examiner first observes the overall appearance, symmetry, and general state of hygiene of the vulva, and notes the distribution of pubic hair (a). Normally, the skin is free of lesions and the area is free of vaginal discharge.

In the adult female pubic hair covers the mons pubis and labia majora, and may extend to the abdomen, thighs, and anus. Pubic hair is characteristically coarse and curly.

The **mons pubis (mons veneris)**, which constitutes the upper part of the vulva, is the firm cushion of adipose and connective tissue that lies over the symphysis and the adjoining pelvic bones (b). The overlying skin contains many sebaceous glands and, after puberty, is abundantly covered with hair.

The **labia majora** are the two heavy longitudinal ridges of adipose and connective tissue, heavily pigmented and covered with skin, that form the lateral boundaries of the vulva. They are continuous with and extend downward on each side from the mons veneris and disappear into the perineum posteriorly. The outer surface is covered with hair, while the inner surface of the labium is moist, has numerous sebaceous glands, and is not covered with hair.

Lesions on or around the vulva, interruptions in the skin integrity, or vaginal discharge may require further assessment.

In postmenopausal women, the hair on the labia is thinner and the labia and mons are less full. This occurs as a result of the loss of fatty tissue that coincides with the decrease in estrogen production following menopause.

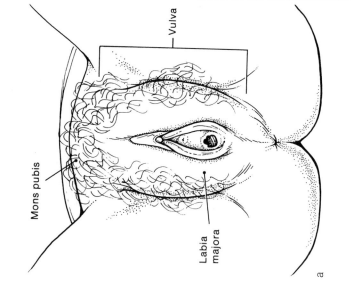

Mons pubis

Labia majora

Vulva

a

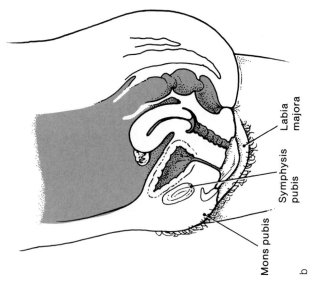

Mons pubis

Symphysis pubis

Labia majora

b

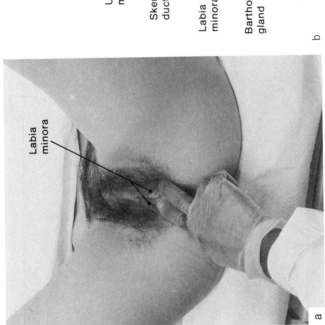

a

To inspect the *labia minora*, the examiner should spread the labia majora apart (a). The labia minora are two thin cutaneous folds lying between and parallel to the labia majora. They normally appear reddish in color, are very vascular, and have a mucous membrane apperance. They are moist and contain sebaceous glands. Anteriorly each labia minus divides into two parts for a short distance and then joins at an angle with the other labium to form a double ridge of tissue around the clitoris.

The labia minora form a hoodlike covering for the clitoris. This covering is termed the **prepuce**, and a band of tissue below it is termed the **frenulum of the clitoris**. The labia minora taper as they extend posteriorly to where they join below the vaginal opening into a thin, flat, transverse fold of tissue called the **fourchet** (b).

The **clitoris** is an elongated, cylindrical body located at the upper aspect of the vulva in the area where the labia minora join anteriorly. It is composed of erectile tissue, contains many blood vessels, and is extremely sensitive. The clitoris varies in size from 2 mm to 1 cm in healthy women. It is usually entirely covered by the labia.

The **vestibule** is the triangular area that becomes visible when the labia minora are spread apart. On inspection the examiner will see the clitoris at the apex of this triangle and the fourchet at its base. Also visible on inspection of the vestibule will be the orifices of the *urethral meatus, Skene's ducts, the vagina,* and *Bartholin's glands*. A depressed space in the tissue between the vaginal opening and the fourchet, the **fossa navicularis,** will be visible at the posterior end of the vestibule.

Prepuce

Clitoris

Frenulum

Vestibule

Urethral meatus

Skene's duct

Labia minora

Bartholin's gland

Fourchet

Fossa navicularis

b

283

PHYSICAL EXAMINATION

Highlights

Skene's ducts are milked during the internal examination by exerting pressure on the anterior vaginal wall as the examining fingers are withdrawn from the vagina. Any discharge from these ducts requires further assessment.

The hymen is a thin membrane which separates the vagina from the vestibule.

Whether or not the hymen is intact will influence the examiner's approach to bimanual examination.

After childbirth the remnants of the hymen look like small tags of mucous membrane around the vaginal orifice; they are called **carunculae myrtiformes** (b).

Bartholin's glands are located at the 5 and 7 o'clock positions in relation to the vaginal orifice.

If these glands are palpable they may be cystic or infected and should be examined further.

Bartholin's glands are also called *vulvovaginal glands*.

The perineal body is the structure that is surgically incised to perform an episiotomy during childbirth. Inspection of this area may reveal an incisional scar.

Hymen

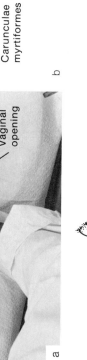

Carunculae myrtiformes

Vaginal opening after childbirth

b

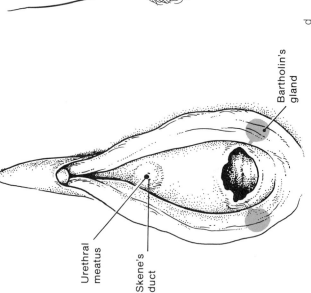

Muscular and fascial pelvic floor

Perineal body

Symphysis pubis

d

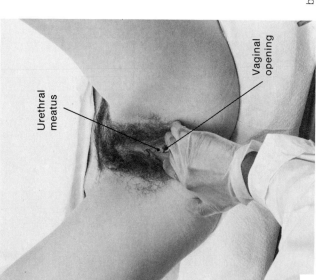

Urethral meatus

Vaginal opening

a

Urethral meatus

Skene's duct

Bartholin's gland

c

Skene's ducts (also called *paraurethral ducts*), are visible during inspection. The examiner will see them on each side of the urethral meatus. They normally have a very small caliber.

The *vaginal orifice* is located in the lower portion of the vestibule (a). It is partly covered by the **hymen**, a membranous tissue which varies in thickness and size in different women (b). The hymen may be quite elastic and stretch considerably, or it may tear easily.

Bartholin's glands are small compound glands situated at the base of the labia majora. Their ducts are visible on each side of the vestibule, posterior and lateral to the margins of the vaginal orifice (c). These glands secrete mucous for lubrication of the vulva. The glands themselves are normally small and are usually not visible or palpable.

The **perineum** is the external surface of the pelvic floor, extending from the arch formed by the pubic bones downward to the anal region. It consists of muscle and fascia which serve as a slinglike support for the pelvic organs (d). The urethra, vagina, and rectum pass between these muscles. The wedge-shaped structure that extends upward from the perineum between the vagina and rectum is called the **perineal body**. The perineal body is stretched and flattened when the vagina is distended during childbirth.

The examiner can inspect the structure and intactness of muscles in the area by asking the client to bear down and strain. Normally, there should be no release of urine or bulging of muscle structures in the perineum.

Internal Female Reproductive Structures

Assessment of the internal female reproductive structures includes inspection of the vagina and cervix, and the related pelvic structure of the rectum. The examiner uses the technique of palpation for the assessment of the uterus and adnexa, and both inspection and palpation for the examination of the rectum.

Inspection

To inspect the vagina, a bivalve speculum is used.

For speculum insertion, the examiner applies a sterile glove to one hand. This is the hand that will insert the speculum and varies with the individual examiner. The examiner inserts the index finger of the gloved hand into the vagina (a). Placing some tension on the posterior fourchet and depressing the perineum slightly, the examiner inserts the speculum downward at a 45 degree angle (b).

Holding the perineum taut helps stabilize the tissues and avoids pulling. Also, this gentle traction helps the examiner to better see the location of the vaginal orifice.

The *vagina* is a potential rather than a real space, a canal-like structure which extends from the lower part of the vulva to the cervix, connecting the external and internal reproductive organs (c). The vagina inclines posteriorly at about a 45 degree angle.

Inspection of the vaginal canal is done while inserting and opening the speculum. The examiner assesses the walls of the vagina for color, tone, and rugae.

Although the vagina and cervix are considered internal structures, both can easily be inspected with the use of a speculum.

Since instrumentation and digital manipulation are required to assess internal structures, the client should be prepared appropriately for digital examination and speculum insertion, as well as for the sensations that accompany these maneuvers.

Speculum insertion requires some skill as well as an appreciation of the anatomy. See Equipment, p. 136. Artificial lubrication of the speculum is rarely necessary, since vaginal secretions normally provide adequate lubrication.

When lubrication of the speculum is required, creams and jellies should be avoided, since they may interfere with vaginal or cervical cytologic examination.

Warm water may be used to warm a metal speculum.

With the client in the lithotomy position, the vagina is not horizontal.

The vagina has both procreative and recreative functions.

Knowledge of the incline of the vagina is important for adequate speculum insertion during examination.

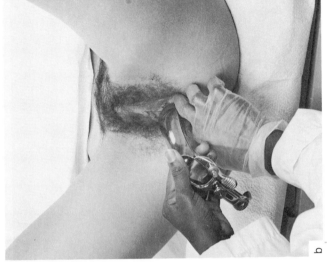

a

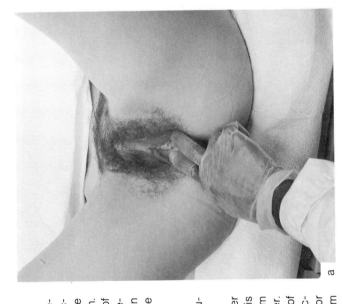

b

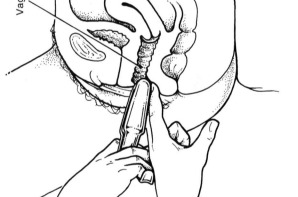

Vagina

c

Highlights

A good light source is essential when examining the vaginal canal.

The vagina is abundantly supplied with blood vessels and lymphatics.

PH of the normal vagina is acid, ranging from 4.0 to 5.0.

Changes in the appearance of the vagina occur normally during pregnancy (Chadwick's sign). See Chap. 12.

The vagina shows changes that occur as a result of changing hormone levels.

The appearance of the vagina mucosa changes with changes in the menstrual cycle and in hormone levels, and in response to sexual excitation.

Ulceration of, or discharge or bleeding from, the cervix requires further assessment.

When the speculum is fixed in the open position, the client may feel the sensation of pulling. The cervix itself is essentially free from sensation.

There are marked changes in the cervix during pregnancy. See Chap. 12.

About one-half of the cervix protrudes into the vagina.

Depending on the time of the examination in relation to the client's menstrual cycle, cervical mucous may appear watery and profuse, connoting normal ovulatory changes.

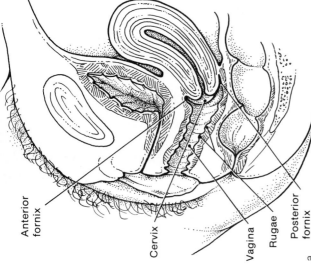

Anterior fornix

Cervix

Vagina

Rugae

Posterior fornix

a

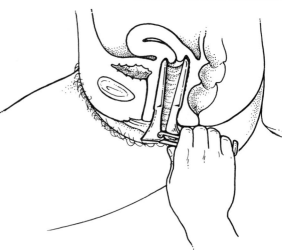

c

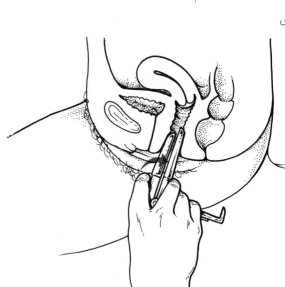

b

The examiner will observe that the vagina is lined with a thick mucous membrane which is pinkish in color and is rugated (a).

The normal vagina is free of lesions and leukorrhea.

In the postmenopausal client, the examiner will find that the normal vagina appears smooth and pale. The rugae are no longer apparent.

Following complete insertion of the speculum, the examiner rotates the speculum to the horizontal plane (b) and gently opens the blades of the speculum by pressing on the lever with the thumb of the gloved hand (c). The examiner then tightens the speculum screw which holds the speculum in an open and fixed position for inspection of the cervix and for the gathering of smears and cultures from both the vagina and cervix when appropriate.

When in the open position, a correctly placed speculum will have blades fitting into the anterior and posterior fornix of the vagina, allowing the examiner to inspect the cervix.

The normal cervix has an internal os which opens into the body of the uterus and an external os which opens into the vagina. It is the external cervical os which is examined by inspection and palpation.

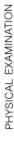

During this phase of the examination, the bladder and rectum are assessed for normalcy. Ask the client to strain. Weakened structures in the bladder (cystocele) and rectum (rectocele) will become apparent if they are present.

Parous: having borne children
Non parous: having borne no children

Palpation is done with the examiner standing at the foot of the table with the elbow of the examining arm supported either on a stool or on the examiner's knee. (Supporting the elbow allows greater sensitivity in the examining fingers.)

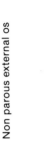

Cervix

External cervical os

Speculum

a

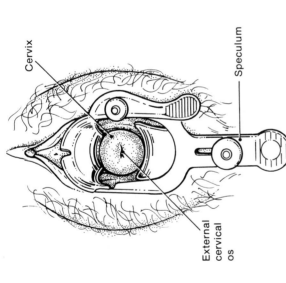

Non parous external os

Parous external os

b

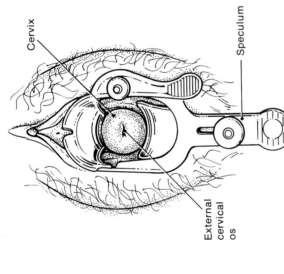

c

The cervix is inspected with the speculum blades fixed in the open position (a). The cervix is examined with the examiner seated at the foot of the examining table, using a good light source. In a woman who has not borne children the normal cervix is round and approximately 2 inches in diameter. The cervix has a small round opening called the external cervical os. In women who have had children, the external cervical os appears as a small transverse opening (b). The examiner inspects the cervix for size, contour, and surface characteristics, and for the configuration of the external os. Pap smears and cultures of the cervix are taken at this time if appropriate. Once inspection is complete, the examiner should withdraw the speculum and once again inspect the vaginal walls.

Palpation

Palpation of the vagina is performed after the cervix is inspected and after the speculum is removed. Using the gloved hand, with the index finger well lubricated, the examiner gently inserts the index finger into the vagina to note whether the hymen is intact. If it is not, then both the index and the middle fingers are used to palpate the vagina (c). The normal vagina will feel free of masses and be free from tenderness. The examiner will palpate a heavy mucous membrane with corrugations (rugae) lining the vaginal canal.

PHYSICAL EXAMINATION

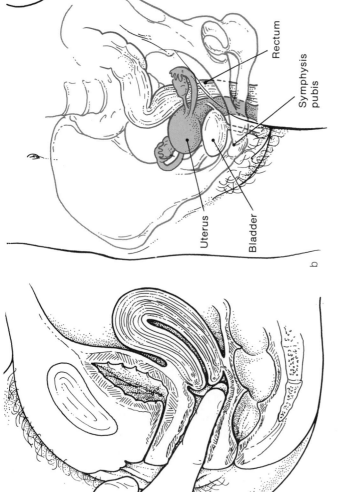

The examiner uses the index and middle finger of the gloved examining hand to enter the vaginal canal and palpate for size, consistency, contour, and dilatation of the cervix (a).

Move the cervix about to determine the degree of freedom of movement and to detect unusual pelvic tenderness. The normal cervix will move freely and such movement should create little discomfort. In some women, a certain amount of cervical dilatation may be normal.

At this time the examiner proceeds to bimanual examination, which requires the use of both hands to palpate the internal reproductive structures.

The *uterus* is the organ in which a fetus develops, and from which it is expelled during childbirth. The uterus is also the organ from which menstruation occurs, and therefore it is under the influence of female hormones. It is a muscular structure situated in the pelvic cavity between the bladder and the rectum (b). It joins with the fallopian tubes on each side near its upper part, which is called the **fundus**. Its lower end, which is called the **cervix**, projects into the vagina (c).

The uterus varies in size with different women, but normally measures approximately 7.5 cm in length, 5 cm in width at the upper part, and 2.5 cm at the antero-posterior diameter. It weighs about 2 ounces.

The uterine cavity is somewhat triangular (pear-shaped) with three openings. Openings at the upper two angles join the fallopian tubes and are called the **cornua**. The lower opening meets the *internal cervical os* (c).

The uterus enlarges tremendously during pregnancy.

Since the uterus is an internal organ, the technique of inspection cannot be used.

Changes in the position of the uterus (e.g., retroverted) should be referred for further examination.

The uterus is palpated bimanually by having the examiner place a gloved hand inside the vagina and the opposite hand placed palm down on the abdomen.

The uterine fundus undergoes marked changes during pregnancy.

Figure b adapted from Dorothy A. Jones, et al., Medical-Surgical Nursing, A Conceptual Approach, McGraw-Hill, 1982, p. 138, fig. 5-15. Used with permission of McGraw-Hill Book Company.

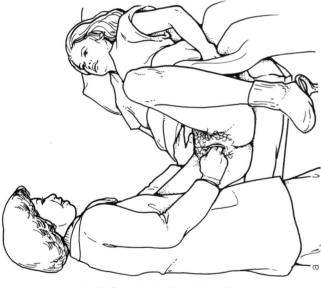

a

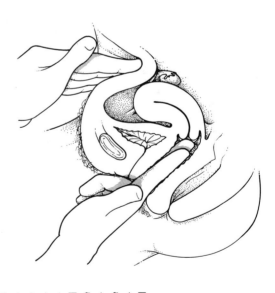

b

The uterus is palpated bimanually. This requires that the examiner use two hands. One is gloved and enters the vagina while the other is ungloved and placed on the client's abdomen (a).

The bare hand is placed palm down on the abdomen with the fingers pointing toward the client's head. The fingers are held together and slightly flexed. The examiner presses firmly against the abdominal wall to displace the lower abdominal and pelvic organs toward the examining fingers that are in the vagina. The hand on the abdomen depresses the fundus of the uterus toward the fingers in the vagina that are resting against the cervix.

Normally, the uterus is free to be brought downward and forward by the hand on the abdomen (b). The examiner palpates both the anterior wall and the fundus of the uterus. The examiner palpates the uterus to determine its position, contour, and mobility, and to reveal any discomfort felt by the client as the uterus is manipulated. The *posterior fornix* is also explored for masses. The normal uterus is free of masses, tenderness, and pain. The fundus is firm and rounded, and relatively smooth.

The adnexa of the uterus includes the two fallopian tubes and the two ovaries. These structures are internal and therefore must be examined by palpation (a).

The *fallopian tubes* are two slender, muscular tubes that extend laterally from the cornua of the uterine cavity to the ovaries. Their length varies from 7 to 14 cm. Each tube has several parts: the interstitial, the isthmus, the ampulla, and the infundibulum (b).

The examiner turns the hand in the vagina so that the palm is upward. The two examining fingers are moved slightly posterior and high into the lateral fornices. The abdominal examining hand then sweeps downward over the fingers in the vagina, attempting to trap the fallopian tube and the ovary between the two examining hands.

The normal fallopian tube is not sensitive, but is so delicate that it usually *cannot* be palpated.

The *ovaries (gonads)* of the female are two small, flattened, oval organs located on each side of the uterus. Each is attached to the lateral wall of the uterus by the ovarian ligament, and to the pelvic wall by a portion of the broad ligament (c). The ovaries perform two main functions; they produce, mature, and extrude ova, and they elaborate hormones. Because of their hormonal functions, they are classified among the endocrine glands of the body.

Figure a adapted from Dorothy A. Jones, et al., Medical-Surgical Nursing, A Conceptual Approach, McGraw-Hill, 1982, p. 138, fig. 5-15b. Used with permission of McGraw-Hill Book Company.

A palpable fallopian tube, especially in the postmenopausal client, requires further assessment.

If unable to palpate the ovary during this maneuver, the examiner may palpate the ovary during rectovaginal examination.

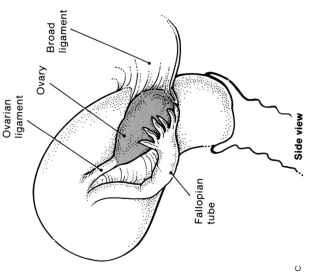

a

b

Infundibulum

Ampulla

Isthmus

Interstitial

Uterus

c

Ovarian ligament

Ovary

Broad ligament

Fallopian tube

Side view

The ovaries are palpated by sliding the abdominal examining hand laterally from the cornua of the uterus (a). The normal ovary will feel small and almond-shaped, and will be mobile. The client will report sensitivity when it is palpated. Size, position, consistency, and contour are noted by the examiner. If unable to palpate the ovary during this maneuver, the examiner may palpate the ovary during rectovaginal examination.

Figure a adapted from Dorothy A. Jones, et al., Medical-Surgical Nursing, A Conceptual Approach, McGraw-Hill, 1982, p. 138, fig. 5-15b. Used with permission of McGraw-Hill Book Company.

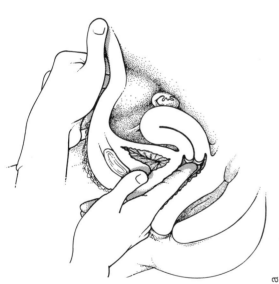

a

The examination of the *rectum* is included in the pelvic examination because of its proximity to pelvic organs. Rectovaginal examination permits palpation of the ovaries, posterior uterine wall, cul-de-sac, and rectum.

The client and the examiner are positioned as for bimanual examination. The lubricated distal finger is inserted into the anus, and the forefinger is placed in the vagina. The perineal body will be in between the two examining fingers (b).

The rectovaginal examination is helpful in clients who cannot tolerate a vaginal examination such as those with small vaginal introitus.

Rectovaginal examination requires much skill and experience. Refer to section on recto/anal examination for further discussion.

Figure b adapted from Dorothy A. Jones, et al., Medical-Surgical Nursing, A Conceptual Approach, McGraw-Hill, 1982, p. 139, fig. 5-16. Used with permission of McGraw-Hill Book Company.

b

The pubic hair (called **escutcheon**) is distributed in a triangular pattern.

The penis is hairless and cylindrical; it is flaccid during the examination.

In the circumsized male, the foreskin is absent and the cone-shaped glans penis is visible.

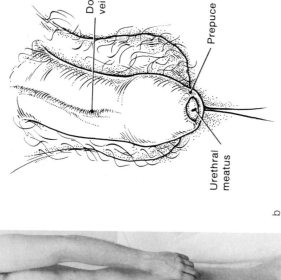

Dorsal vein

Prepuce

Urethral meatus

b

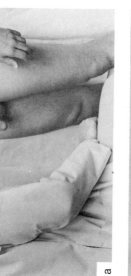

a

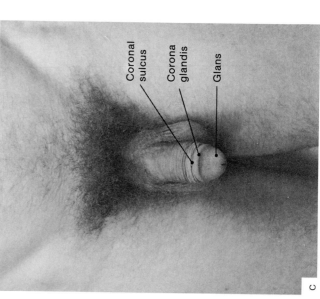

Coronal sulcus

Corona glandis

Glans

c

MALE GENITALIA

Contributions to this section made by Geralyn R. Spollett R.N.C., M.S.

The examination of the male genitalia includes inspection and palpation of the penis, the scrotum (and testicles), and the femoral and inguinal regions.

Inspection

To inspect the male genitalia, the client should be standing with trousers and undershorts removed. The examiner sits directly in front of the client to complete the assessment (a).

The pubic hair (called the **escutcheon**) is coarse and is distributed in a triangular pattern. The amount and texture of pubic hair varies significantly with the race of the client. The usual distribution of hair extends onto the inner sides of the thighs, over the scrotal skin, and frequently in a line toward the umbilicus.

The penis is hairless and cylindrical in shape. It is usually flaccid during the examination. The large and visible dorsal vein is located midline on the dorsum of the penile shaft. Extending from the shaft and surrounding the head of the penis is a free fold of skin known as the **prepuce** or **foreskin** (b). At the tip of the penis, positioned centrally, is the *urethral meatus*. The client can be asked to compress the head of the penis to open the distal end of the urethra for inspection.

In the circumsized client (c), the foreskin is absent, and the cone shaped **glans penis** is visible. The crown formed by the rim of the glans penis is called the **corona glandis**. It is here that the glans joins the penile shaft. Immediately behind the head of the penis is a circular groove called the **coronal sulcus.**

Highlights

The free fold skin surrounding the uncircumcised penis is called the **prepuce** or **foreskin**.

When the foreskin is present, it must be retracted to inspect the exposed surface.

Penile skin during the flaccid state appears wrinkled.

The size and shape of the penis varies from client to client.

The penis in white clients ranges in color from pink to brownish; in blacks, it is light to dark brown.

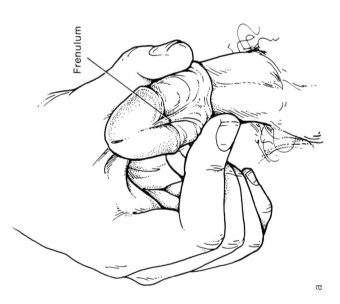

a

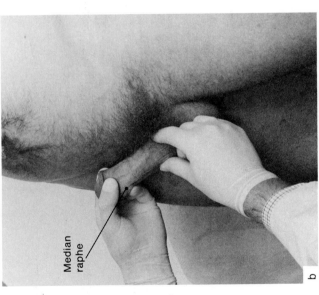

b

A *frenulum* attaches the foreskin to the ventral surface of the glans penis. When the foreskin and frenulum have not been removed by circumcision, it is necessary for the client to retract the foreskin enabling the examiner to inspect the exposed structures (a). After inspection, the foreskin should be reduced to its normal position to avoid possible constriction to the blood and lymphatic vessels in the penis.

In the flaccid state the penile skin is wrinkled. The skin over the glans penis and corona glandis is taut, smooth, and hairless. Usually continuous and uniform over all parts of the penis, the skin of the *median raphe* with its ridge of tissue is the one exception (b).

The size, shape, and coloration of the penis may vary significantly from client to client. It is important for the examiner to establish the norms for the client, and to compare these norms to subsequent changes.

The color of the skin in a white client may range from pink to brownish, and may vary in pigmentation. A black client's penis may appear light to dark brown again with variations in pigmentation.

Highlights

The skin covering the scrotum is rugated and contains small veins.

The size and color of the scrotum varies.

The median raphe acts as a demarcation line which separates the scrotal sac into two sections.

The scrotal sac is separated into two compartments.

The cremasteric or dartos muscle influences the position of the scrotum.

The cremasteric muscle contracts and raises when exposed to cold, and relaxes and lowers when exposed to warmth.

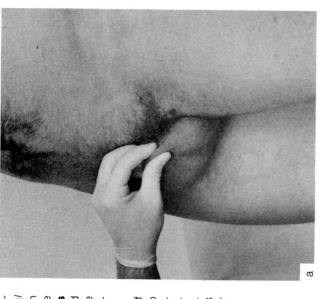

a

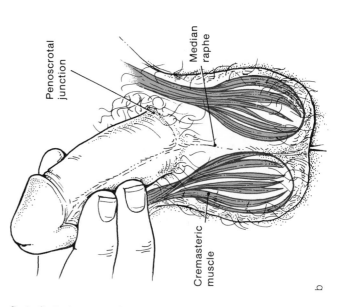

Penoscrotal junction

Median raphe

Cremasteric muscle

b

When the client lifts the penis, the examiner can inspect the *anterior scrotal wall*. The skin covering the scrotum appears rugated. Frequently, minute dilations of veins or **venous ectasias** are visible. The examiner should spread the rugated surface, noting its texture and elasticity (a). The size and coloration of the scrotum will vary.

While it is true that size and coloration of the scrotum varies from individual to individual, the examiner should be cautioned that gross deviations may represent a chronic or congenital disease. Careful description of these findings should be recorded and referred for further diagnosis.

With the client continuing to elevate the penis, the examiner observes the median raphe, a distinct ridge of tissue in the ventral midline of the shaft. At the junction of the shaft and the root of the scrotum is the *penoscrotal junction* (b).

The median raphe acts as a demarcation line, superficially separating the scrotal sac into two sections. Within the scrotal sac, a septum divides the scrotum into two compartments. Due to the greater length of the spermatic cord of the left testis, the left scrotal compartment hangs lower than the right compartment. The muscle tone of the *cremasteric or dartos muscle* influences the position of the scrotum (b). The cremasteric muscle is temperature sensitive, contracting and raising the scrotum when the area is cold, relaxing and lowering the scrotum when the area is warm.

Highlights

The femoral and inguinal canals are potential openings from the abdomen through which abdominal contents can herniate.

The area on the anterior thigh below the inguinal ligament should be inspected for swellings (a). It is in this area that the femoral canal, a potential opening from the abdomen to the anterior thigh, is found (b). The inguinal canal region should also be inspected for swelling. This region lies above the inguinal ligament between the pubic tubercle and the anterior superior iliac spine (b). The inguinal canal is a potential opening from the abdomen through which hernias may protrude. In the normal client no swelling is apparent in either region.

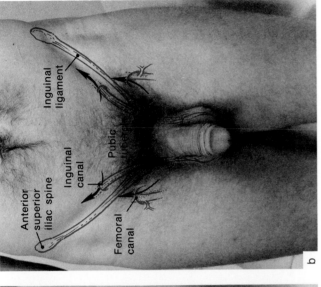

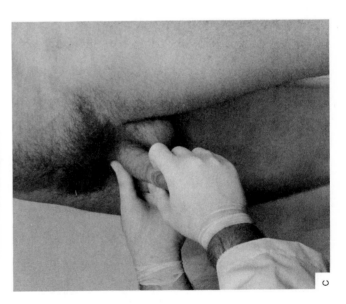

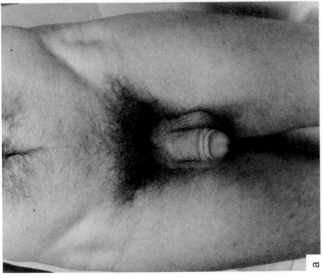

Palpation

Palpation of the penis shaft is performed with the examiner placing the thumb and the first two fingers directly over the penile shaft (c). The shaft feels firm and smooth without areas of induration.

The testis is palpated as a smooth, regular, ovoid mass found in the scrotal sac.

The epididymis is comma shaped and visible as a wedge on the posterior testicular surface.

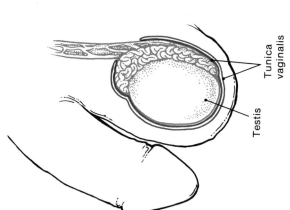

Tunica vaginalis

Testis

b

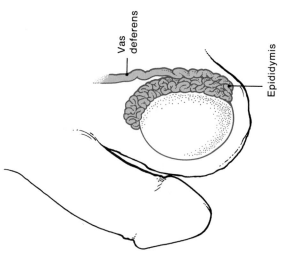

Vas deferens

Epididymis

d

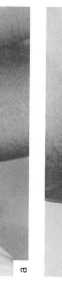

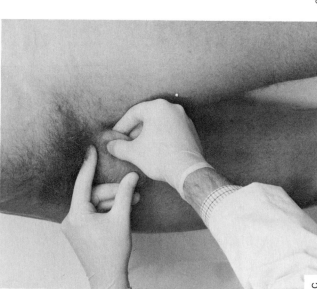

a

c

The examiner usually palpates one scrotal compartment at a time. This is achieved by grasping the scrotum gently between the thumb and the first two fingers (a). The **testis**, an ovoid mass, which is smooth and regular in contour, is the largest, most easily identifiable structure in each of the scrotal compartments (b). Located low in the scrotal compartment, the testis is freely movable and sensitive to pressure. When the testis is squeezed the client will feel a dull aching sensation which radiates to the lower abdomen.

The **tunica vaginalis**, a two-layered membrane surrounding the front and sides of the testis, may fill with fluid, making it difficult to palpate the scrotal contents.

The **epididymis** is a mass of tightly coiled tubules lying vertically upon the posterior surface of the testis (d). Despite its location, it should be readily distinguishable from the testis. It is shaped like a comma, making a visible bulge on the testicular surface. The epididymis is normally not tender to pressure when palpated (c).

Beginning at the tail of the epididymis, the *spermatic cord* can be palpated once again using the thumb and forefinger (a). The spermatic cord contains the **vas deferens** (the duct through which semen travels from the testes), the testicular artery and vein, lymphatics, and nerves (b). The *vasa deferentia* are cordlike, smooth, and movable. The arteries, veins, lymph vessels and nerves are threadlike. In general, the spermatic cord which ascends upward leaving the scrotal sac, has a ropelike quality. Like the epididymis, this tissue is not tender when palpated.

At times the scrotal sac may appear empty. As previously mentioned, the cremasteric muscle can contract raising the scrotal contents. If the contraction is forceful and the external inguinal ring lax, the scrotal contents may actually be pulled into the canal (c).[1] With relaxation of the muscle, the contents will return to their normal position. This rising of the scrotal contents from the scrotal sac is called a **temporary migration**. The examiner confronted with this temporary migration may return to this part of the examination later, checking for a descent of the scrotal contents.

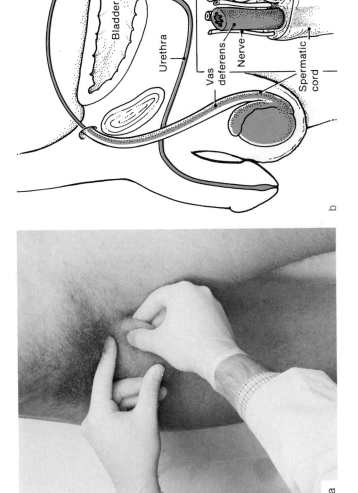

a

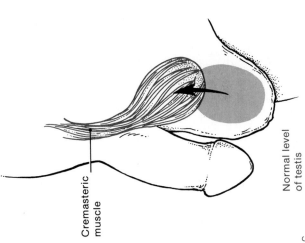

Bladder

Urethra

Vas deferens

Spermatic cord

Nerve

Artery

Veins

b

Cremasteric muscle

Normal level of testis

c

The rising of the scrotal contents from the scrotal sac is called temporary migration.

["Patient Assessment: Examination of the Male Genitalia," **American Journal of Nursing** April 1979, pp. 703.]

Highlights

The femoral canal is usually not palpable. It is located below the inguinal ligament, medial to the femoral artery.

The femoral region should be palpated bilaterally for bulging, tenderness or swelling.

The external inguinal ring is just above and lateral to the pubic tubercle.

The femoral canal is usually not palpable, but is a potential space where hernias may form. To palpate the femoral region the client should be standing facing the examiner who is seated. The examiner should palpate the anterior thigh, first one side, then the other (a). The client can then be asked to bear down. Normally, there should be an absence of swelling, tenderness or bulging noted during the procedure.

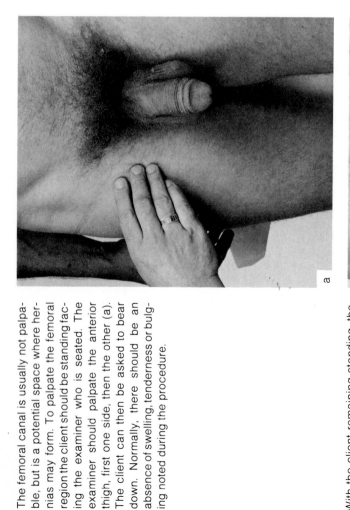

With the client remaining standing, the examiner palpates the inguinal region (b). This area should not exhibit swelling or tenderness upon palpation.

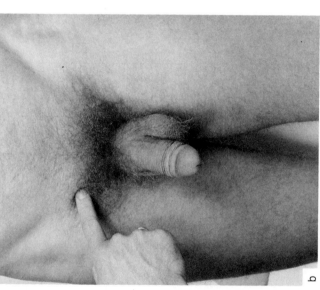

When examining the right inguinal canal, the examiner approaches the client from the right side. The examiner uses the right hand and invaginates loose scrotal skin (a).

With the index finger starting near the bottom of the scrotal sac, the examiner follows the spermatic cord upward to the triangular shaped opening of the external inguinal ring (b). Depending upon the size of this ring, the examiner can follow the inguinal canal. This may not always be possible.

With the examiner's finger at the external inguinal canal or beyond, the client should be asked to bear down as if straining. Normally, there should not be a bulging of tissue felt against the examiner's fingers. This procedure should then be repeated on the opposite side.

Several important lymph nodes are located in the inguinal area and should be palpated at this time (c). They are the superficial inguinal nodes, parallel to the inguinal ligament, and the superficial and deep subinguinal nodes on either side of the femoral canal and femoral artery. The superficial nodes may be palpable but should not be large or tender.

Normally, there should be no protrusion in the inguinal canal during palpation.

The inguinal lymph nodes may be palpated as part of the abdominal examination or as part of the genital examination.

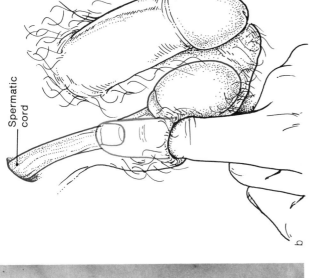

a

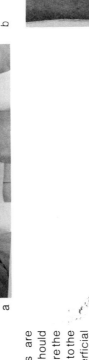

Spermatic cord

b

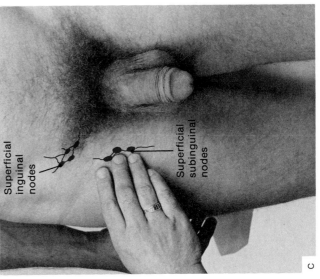

Superficial inguinal nodes

Superficial subinguinal nodes

c

Highlights

There are several positions that may be used during the examination of the recto-anal area. These include the Sim's, knee chest, standing, squatting and lithotomy positions.

The knee-chest position is not used if a speculum is to be used.

The standing position provides for a good examination of the prostate.

The squatting position is often used to reveal rectal prolapse.

ANAL-RECTAL EXAMINATION

The examination of the rectum and anal area includes the assessment of the peri-anal area, the rectum and prostate gland. This examination can be done with the client in a variety of positions. They include the Sim's, knee-chest, standing, squatting and lithotomy positions.

The *Sim's* (or lateral) position is achieved by having the client lie on the left side with the upper (superior) knee flexed and drawn to the chest (a). This position allows adequate examination of the perenium and anal mucosa via inspection and palpation. Palpation of the peritoneal cavity rectally is inadequate in this position as masses tend to fall away from the palpating finger.

The *knee-chest* position occurs with the client on his/her knees and the head and shoulder bent forward resting upon the examination table (b). This position allows for optimal viewing of the rectal anal area particularly if the use of a speculum or other instrument is indicated. If equipment is being used, this position is usually not used.

The *standing position* is accomplished by having the client standing pidgeon-toed with the torso leaning upon a bed or table causing hip flexure (c). The standing position allows effective examination of the prostate gland. It is also an adequate position for speculum examination if needed.

The *squatting position* is achieved by having the client bend the knees and lower the trunk toward the floor (d). The squatting position may be used to determine prolapse. Some lesions of the recto-sigmoid region and pelvis are palpable only from this position.

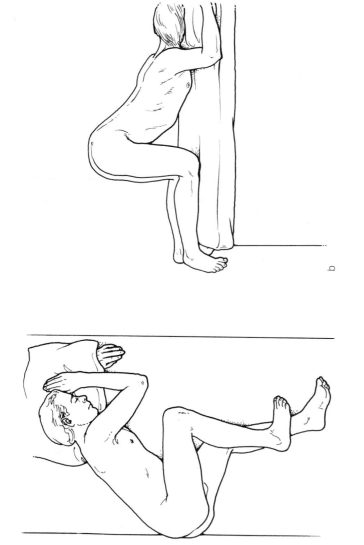

a

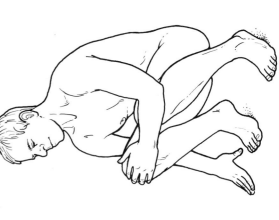

b

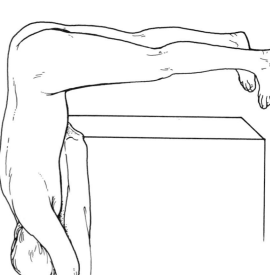

c

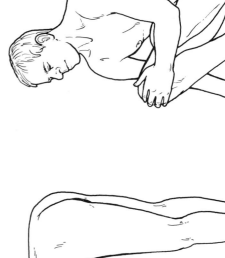

d

The *lithotomy position* is most commonly used in female anal-rectal examination.

The standing position is frequently used with the male anal-rectal examination.

The pigmented area surrounding the anus is redder in children.

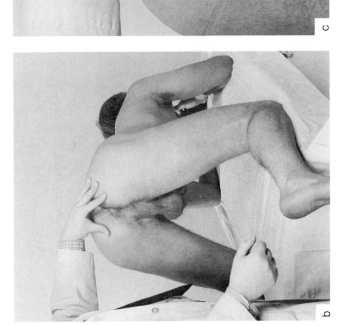

c

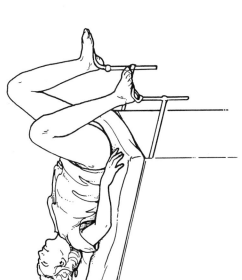

a

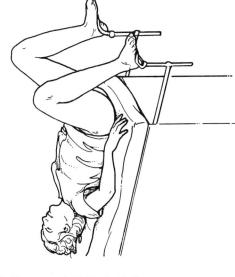

b

The *lithotomy position* occurs when the client is in the supine position with both knees drawn close to the chest (a).

The lithotomy position is convenient to utilize after pelvic examination. The position is good for peritoneal palpation; however, it is not useful if a rectal speculum is to be used.

The lithotomy position is most commonly used with female clients as the rectal examination is an integral part of a total gynecological assessment. The standing position is most commonly used with male clients as it facilitates examination of the prostate gland.

Inspection

To inspect the perianal area, the client assumes one of the positions cited above. The examiner usually stands (but can be seated) in a position that facilitates both direct observation and easy palpation of the rectal-anal area. First the examiner spreads both cheeks of the buttocks apart to observe the anal area (b). Normally, the skin immediately surrounding the anus is more pigmented, a reddish brown, and coarser than the tissue around it. It is usually moist and hairless.

The perianal area should also be inspected for any changes or interruptions in skin integrity caused by fissures or scars. Normally, the skin is continuous and intact (c). Changes in perianal skin integrity can be described in terms of location as positions on the face of a clock with the 12:00 position toward the symphysis pubis and the 6:00 position toward the coccyx.

Highlights

The anal canal is 2.5 to 4 cm long and is the terminal part of the colon.

Retracting the anal skin allows inspection of the mucosa. Normally, the mucosal tissue should be intact, smooth, and free from interruptions of skin integrity or enlarged veins (hemorrhoids).

When the client bears down, the amount of mucosal tissue visible at the anus should not increase.

The pilonidal is the area posterior to the anus. This area is generally not tender to palpation.

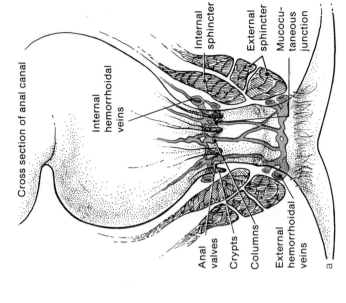

Cross section of anal canal

Internal hemorrhoidal veins

Internal sphincter

External sphincter

Mucocutaneous junction

Anal valves

Crypts

Columns

External hemorrhoidal veins

a

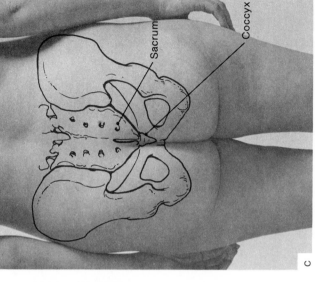

Sacrum

Coccyx

c

b

The anal canal is 2.5 to 4 cm long in the adult and is the terminal part of the colon (a). The internal portion of the canal contains columns of mucosal tissue with spaces between the columns referred to as crypts. Within the columns are the internal hemorrhoidal veins. These veins communicate with each other to form a ring called the *zona hemorrhoidalis*. Between the columns are folds of mucosa known as anal valves.

The anal canal is surrounded by an external sphincter (a voluntary muscle), and an internal sphincter (an involuntary muscle). External hemorrhoidal veins are located in a ring below the external sphincter.

The mucosal lining of the internal anal canal is smooth and moist. It merges with the cutaneous portion of the anal canal at the *mucocutaneous junction*, which can be visualized by exerting tension on each side of the anus.

To inspect the intactness of the anal canal, the client should be asked to bear down as if having a bowel movement (the *valsalva maneuver*). Normally, there should be no prolapse of internal anal canal or rectal tissue during this maneuver (b).

The skin integrity of the sacrococcygeal (pilonidal) area should be inspected next (c). This tissue is smooth and increased hair growth may be observed. Dimples in the skin over the coccyx should be referred.

Palpation

The pilonidal area (the skin over the sacrococcygeal area) must be carefully palpated and should not exhibit edema, induration, or dimples. The area is generally non-tender to palpation.

The external anal sphincter is comprised of a three-loop system of musculature (a), responsible with the internal anal sphincter for securing continence and the ability to defecate.

Palpation of the external anal sphincter involves asking the client to again bear down while the examiner places a gloved lubricated finger directly against the anal verge (b and c). Firm pressure is exerted until the sphincter begins to yield. As this occurs the examiner's finger is slowly inserted further in the direction of the umbilicus as the rectal sphincter relaxes. The pad of the finger should be first inserted and then rotated upon entrance to introduce the fingertip.

The mucosa of the anal canal is smooth and moist. Landmarks to identify include the external and internal anal sphincters, the intersphincteric line and the anal canal. Normally, the examiner can palpate the canal approximately 6 to 10 cm.

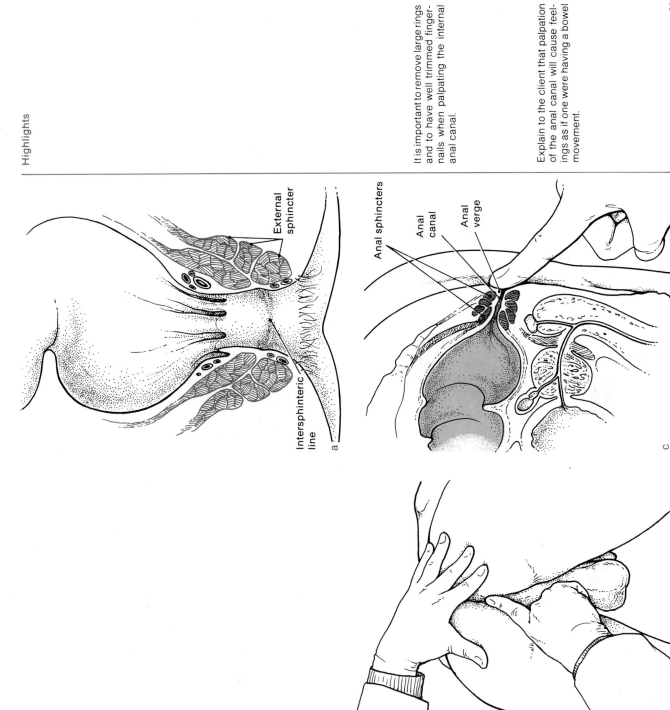

External sphincter

Intersphincteric line

a

Anal sphincters

Anal canal

Anal verge

c

b

It is important to remove large rings and to have well trimmed fingernails when palpating the internal anal canal.

Explain to the client that palpation of the anal canal will cause feelings as if one were having a bowel movement.

Highlights

Hypertonicity of the external sphincter may occur with anxiety, scarring, inflammation or involuntary contractions.

Hypotonic or relaxed external sphincter may occur after rectal surgery, habitual anal intercourse, or neurological deficits.

The bidigital examination of the anal sphincters reveals added data and is helpful in assessing the bulbourethral glands.

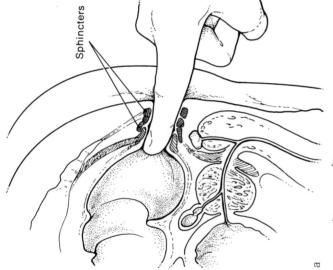

a

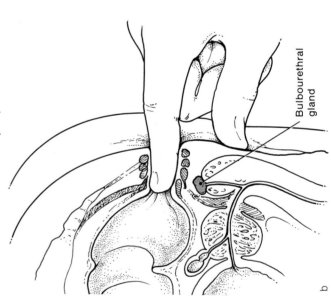

b

Upon insertion of the examining finger through the anal verge, ask the client to tighten the sphincter so that muscle tone and strength can be assessed. The subcutaneous portion of the external sphincter is palpable on the inner aspect of the anal verge (a). The palpating finger should be rotated in order to examine the entire muscular ring. Normally, this is a procedure that is pain free.

The intersphincteric line can be palpated just inside of this muscular ring, marking the junction between the internal and external sphincters. Tone and strength of the internal sphincter should be determined.

Bidigital palpation of the anal sphincters will reveal more data. With the client remaining in the same position, the examiner presses the thumb of the examining hand against the perianal tissue while moving the examining index finger toward it (b). This maneuver is also helpful in assessing the bulbourethral glands.

The rectum is 12 to 14 cm in length and cannot be palpated manually.

The levator ani muscles help control bowel function.

The four semilunar transverse folds or valves hold fecal matter within rectum while flatus passes.

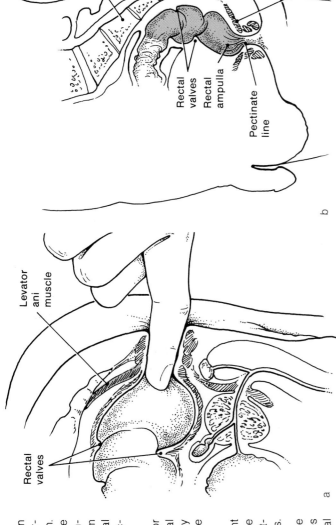

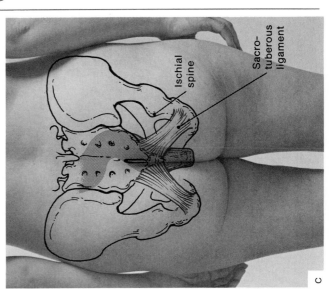

The *rectum* begins at the sigmoid colon at about the level of the third sacral vertebra and ends at the rectoanal junction. Approximately 12 to 14 cm long, the entire rectum cannot be palpated manually. Landmarks to identify the rectum include the rectoanal junction, rectal ampulla, rectal walls, rectal valves, coccyx and sacrum (b).

Palpation of the rectoanal junction, or pectinate line (found above the anal sphincters), can be accomplished by moving the examining finger beyond the sphincters (a).

The *levator ani muscle* (b), an important structure to bowel control, is palpable just inside the rectoanal ring to the lateral posterior aspect of the rectal walls.

Four *semilunar transverse folds* (b), the valves of Houston or the rectal valves can be palpated further along the rectal canal.

Postulated to function as a mechanism for holding fecal matter within the rectum while flatus passes, the rectal valves are often mistaken for intrarectal masses.

The posterior and lateral walls of the rectum may be palpated by rotating the index finger along the rectal canal. The ischial spines and sacrotuberous ligaments may be identified here through palpation (c).

Highlights

Some health care providers advocate self-rectal examination in order to provide improved detection of anal-rectal carcinomas at early stages.

Bimanual palpation is completed on females while in the lithotomy position following the GYN examination.

Bimanual palpation allows the examiner an opportunity to palpate the posterior cervix and uterus; areas not palpable during the routine vaginal examination.

Figure b from Dorothy A. Jones, et al, Medical-Surgical Nursing: A Conceptual Approach, McGraw-Hill Book Company, New York, 1978, p 120.

The posterior wall of the rectum follows the curve of the coccyx and sacrum. The coccyx is palpated to determine mobility and sensation (a). Anal-rectal mucosa must be palpated for smoothness and absence of masses. The posterior rectal walls are the most difficult to evaluate manually due to the distance from the anal verge. While assessing this region, ask the client to bear down so that lesions just beyond the fingertip may be felt if present.

Bimanual palpation

In the female, the rectal examination is usually completed while the client is in the lithotomy position. Bimanual palpation is accomplished by placing the index finger into the vagina and middle finger into the rectum (b). This allows the examiner to palpate the area behind the cervix and posterior uterine surface. These areas are usually not accessible during the routine vaginal examination.

The client is asked to bear down as if straining at stool. Normally, there is no prolapse of cervical or rectal tissue. The surface of the posterior cervix is explored and is smooth and consistant with the surrounding tissue.

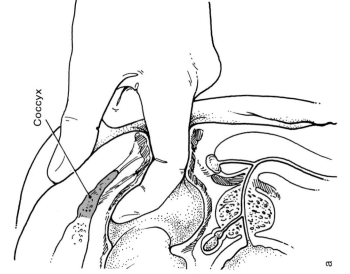

Coccyx

a

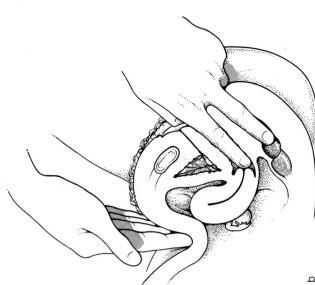

b

Palpation of the Prostate Gland

The prostate gland is a bilobed structure with a normal diameter of approximately 4 cm and length of 2.5 cm. Palpation of the gland can be performed through the anterior wall of the rectal mucosa (a) to assess gland size, shape and consistency. The palpating finger must identify the lateral lobes separated by a central groove, the median sulcus (b). The prostate gland is smooth, firm, without nodules and free from tenderness upon palpation. The urge to urinate is a normal sensation upon palpation of the prostate gland. Again, ask the client to bear down so that a mass not otherwise evident can be palpated. The anterior wall of the rectum should be palpated above the prostate to the area of the seminal vesicles and peritoneal cavity. This region should be free from masses, nodularity and tenderness.

Following the rectal examination, the examiner slowly withdraws the finger. The presence of any feces adhering to the gloved finger should be inspected for color and consistency. The feces should then be tested for occult blood.

The client should then be given tissues for cleansing after the examination has ended for personal hygiene and comfort.

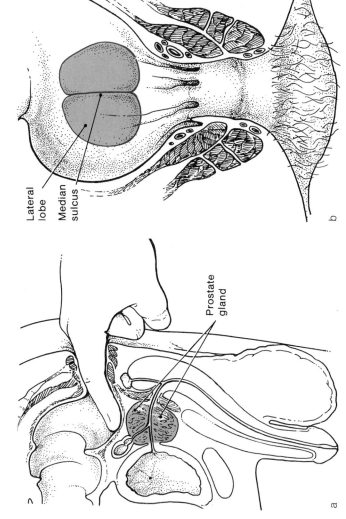

Lateral lobe

Median sulcus

Prostate gland

a

b

Highlights

Palpation of the prostate gland can be accomplished during the rectal examination.

The urge to urinate may normally occur upon palpation of the prostate.

Refer to the descriptions of male genitalia examinations for further discussions.

Guaiac testing is utilized to test feces smear for the detection of occult blood. False positives can be diminshed by requesting client to abstain from red meats three days prior to physical examination.

EXTREMITIES

Contributions to parts of the assessment of the extremities were made by Carol Bowan, R.N., C., M.S.N.

Examination of the extremities is complex. Assessment of the skin and neuromuscular function of the extremities are integrated into the examination of the extremities. Data collection is further complicated by the fact that the extremities are assessed at different times during the course of the examination. Finally, for a portion of the examination, the examiner must rely on the client's subjective interpretation of stimuli (a), rather than on more objective findings such as body temperature.

Inspection and palpation are the two techniques used during this examination.

For purposes of this text, examination of the upper and lower extremities will be discussed together under the two techniques noted above. However, the examiner may find that when using a head to toe approach the upper extremities can be assessed following a general survey of the body and upper body structures (b). The lower extremities can be examined following the abdominal and rectal examinations. Evaluation of the cerebellar function and testing of the sensory system and reflex responses will be included in the examination.

During the course of the examination the client will assume a variety of positions which will be described as they occur. Equipment used includes a reflex hammer, tuning fork, pin, cotton, coin or key, and a tape measure.

The assessment of the extremities is complex, integrating the evaluation of multiple body system functions in the process (e.g., neurological as well as peripheral vascular).

Data received during the examination is frequently the result of a client's subjective responses rather than objective findings.

Upper extremities include shoulder, axilla, arm, elbow, forearm, wrist, hand, fingers (digits).

Lower extremities include buttocks, knee, ankle, foot, toes.

Inspection and palpation are the two techniques most often used during the physical examination.

The client will assume a variety of positions throughout the examination of the extremities.

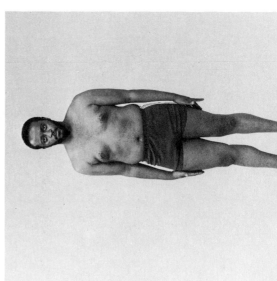

a

b

Inspection

Inspection of the extremities begins at the start of the physical examination with the observance of overall body symmetry, alignment, coordination, and balance. Body posture and stance are examined while the client is standing (a).

The basic support for the body comes from the bones and related skeletal structures. This framework protects the body's organs and tissues from injury, assists in body movement, forms red blood cells, and stores mineral salts.

Bones are classified according to shape: *long* (e.g., humerus, tibia), *short* (e.g., carpal, tarsal), *flat* (e.g., skull), *irregular* (e.g., vertebrae), and *sesamoid* (small, rounded bones, e.g., patella). Almost all types of bones are found in the extremities. Of the 206 bones within the body, 64 are in the upper extremities and 62 are in the lower extremities (including the pelvic girdle) (b).

In general, all bones of the extremities should be in alignment with contour, symmetry, and angulation defined bilaterally.

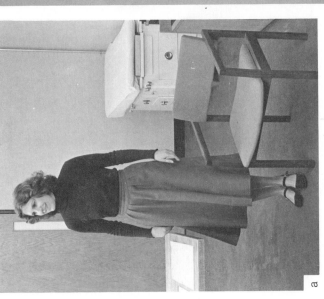

a

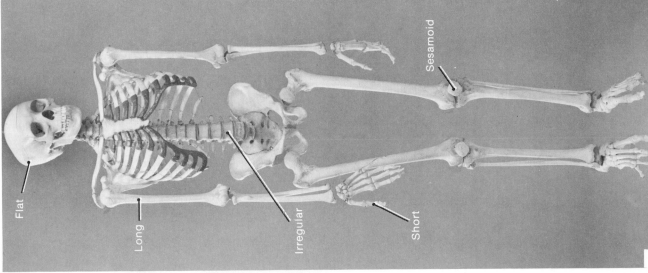

Flat

Long

Irregular

Short

Sesamoid

b

Highlights

Inspection of the extremities occurs at the beginning of the physical examination (refer to General Appearance section).

The bones of the body are classified as long, short, flat, irregular, and sesamoid.

There are approximately 126 bones located in the extremities.

PHYSICAL EXAMINATION

Bone surfaces have certain projections (*processes*) or depressions (*fossae*) which help to join one bone to another, serve as a pathway for vessels and nerves, and act as an attachment for muscles. Other anatomical terms or landmarks used in association with the bones of the extremities include the following (a):

Bone projections (or *processes*) and depressions (*fossae*) help join bones together, serve as a pathway for vessels and nerves and attachments for muscles.

1 *Spine* - sharp, slender projection such as a spinous process

2 *Condyle* - rounded or knucklelike prominence usually found at point of bone articulation

3 *Tubercle* - small rounded process

4 *Tuberosity* - larger rounded process

5 *Trochanter* - large process for attachment to muscle

6 *Head* - terminal enlargement

Anatomical landmarks associated with the bones of the extremities include: processes; spine; condyle; tubercle; tuberosity; trochanter; head.

Inspection of the extremities and overall body framework begins with the client in a standing position. For a more complete view of the upper and lower extremities along with body contour, the client should remove the gown or drape. To prevent discomfort the client can be given a blanket or other covering to use when a specific area is not being assessed.

Inspection of the upper and lower extremities as well as the general bone structure of the body is done to determine symmetry, bilateral equality of length, contour and shape.

The examiner should observe the client from the front and the back to inspect contours. With the client's arms at the side, and standing erect, the length of the extremities should be observed. The arms and legs should be equal in length. The arms can be measured by placing a tape measure from the tip of the acromion process to the tip of the middle finger. The legs are measured from the lower edge of the anterosuperior iliac spine to the tibial malleolus (b).

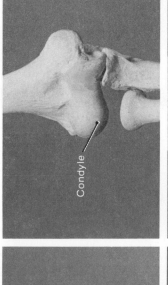

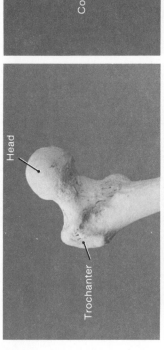

Head

Trochanter

Tubercle

Tuberosity

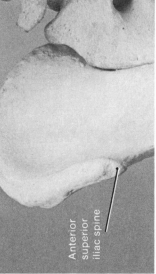

Condyle

Anterior superior iliac spine

a

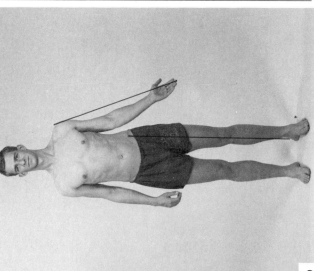

b

Highlights

The relationships of upper and lower extremities to other bone structures (e.g., upper and lower trunk) should be included in the general observation of the client's posture and stance.

The cervical, thoracic, and lumbar curves are composed of 7 cervical, 12 thoracic, and 5 lumbar vertebrae.

The spine should be straight when viewing the client from the back.

The cervical curve is concave, the thoracic curve is convex, and the lumbar curve is concave.

The client moves the body through a range of bending actions to assess flexibility, mobility and balance.

As a client ages there may be diminished flexibility of body movements noted. However, this varies from client to client.

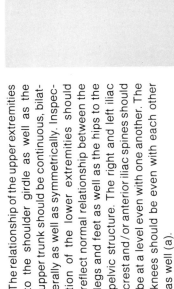

a

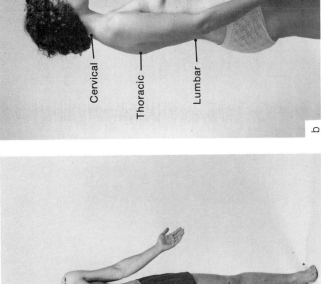

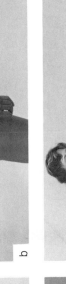

Cervical

Thoracic

Lumbar

b

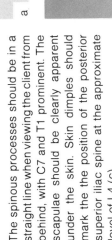

C₇

Scapula

Level of L4

c

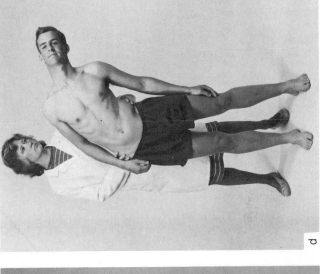

d

The relationship of the upper extremities to the shoulder girdle as well as the upper trunk should be continuous, bilaterally as well as symmetrically. Inspection of the lower extremities should reflect normal relationship between the legs and feet as well as the hips to the pelvic structure. The right and left iliac crest and/or anterior iliac spines should be at a level even with one another. The knees should be even with each other as well (a).

The normal cervical, thoracic, and lumbar curves, which contribute to an individual's posture and body alignment are inspected as the examiner observes the client from all sides. Normally, the cervical curve is concave, the thoracic curve convex, and the lumbar curve, concave (b).

The spinous processes should be in a straight line when viewing the client from behind, with C7 and T1 prominent. The scapulae should be clearly apparent under the skin. Skin dimples should mark the position of the posterior superior iliac spine at the approximate level of L4 (c).

The client is usually able to move the body through the normal range of motion of the spine with ease (d) (see discussion under joints).

The examiner then asks the client to walk across the room or if possible down a corridor and back. The stride is observed as rhythmical, steady, and balanced. The swing of a client's gait is assessed in terms of acceleration, midswing, and deceleration (a). The client's arms usually swing at the sides and in turning, the head and face should lead the body. Steps taken should be a comfortable length, with feet about 2 to 4 inches apart.

To test balance and intactness of motor pathways, the client may be asked to walk a straight line, 10 to 15 feet in length with eyes open and then with eyes closed. The client should be instructed to walk placing one foot directly in front of the other (tandem walking), to walk on the heels, and then walk on the toes. Normally, these actions should be accomplished without losing balance or falling (b).

The *Romberg test* is used to assess proprioception. The client is asked to stand with the feet together and arms at the side. With eyes closed, the client lifts the arms forward with the palms up. The client should be able to hold the arms and body in a steady position with eyes open and eyes closed (c). A healthy client should also be able to hop on either foot in place without losing balance. The examiner should be prepared to protect older individuals or persons having difficulty with these tasks from falling.

Appropriate completion of these maneuvers indicates proper functioning of both the upper motor pathway and the lower motor pathway (d). Further testing of these pathways are done later in the examination.

Highlights

Gait is assessed in terms of stance and swing.

When testing balance, especially in the elderly client, the examiner should be ready to protect the client from falling.

The Romberg test is one proprioception test used to evaluate intactness of the upper and lower motor pathways.

When assessing balance, examination of the inner ear is also of importance. Refer to the examination of the ear.

Upper pathway-motor cortex, corticospinal tract, extrapyramidal tract, cerebellum, cord

Lower pathway-lower motor neuron or anterior horn cell, sensory and motor peripheral nerve, neuromuscular junction in the muscle, competent muscle, functional synapse in the cord

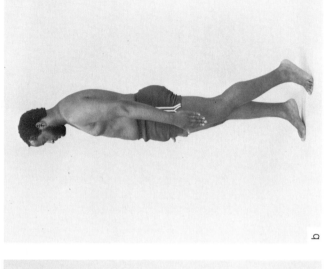

a

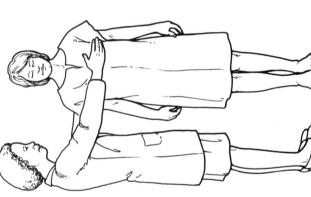

b

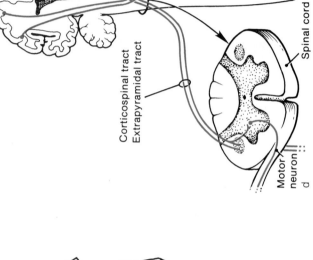

Motor cortex

Corticospinal tract
Extrapyramidal tract

Spinal cord

Motor neuron

d

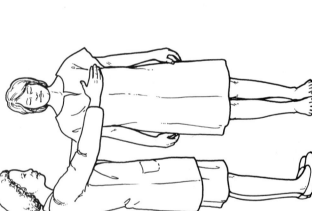

c

Highlights

The client's balance should be maintained erect while sitting.

Throughout the entire examination, the comparison of one extremity to the other, comparison of the distal portion to the proximal portion, and comparison of upper to lower is crucial.

"Aging spots" on the skin (called **lipofucin**) are seen in the elderly.

The angle between the nail and the nail base is normally 160 degrees.

Skin should always be assessed for any abnormal or changing marks and the client referred for further assessment.

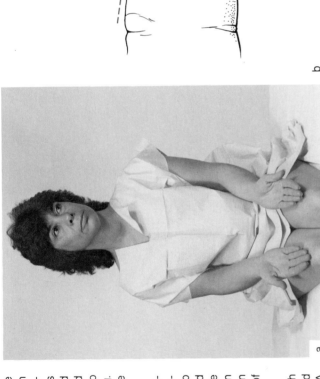

a

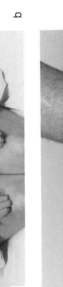

b

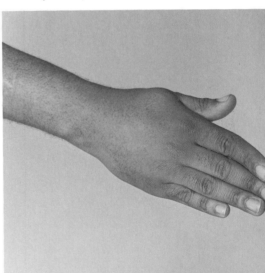

c

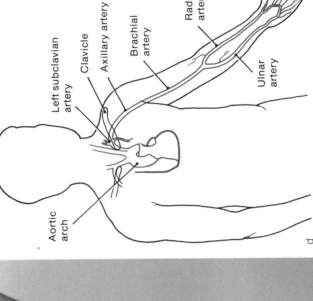

d

After completing these activities, the client should sit on the examination table, facing the examiner and at comfortable distance (approximately arms length). The individual's posture and balance while sitting should be noted. Normally the client should be able to hold the upper body erect without falling. At this time, the extremities should be compared to one another.

Inspection of the *upper extremities* includes evaluation of the skin, blood vessels (veins), joints and muscles. To inspect size and symmetry of hands and arms, the client's hands should be placed palms up. The palmar skin should be smooth and intact and is often lighter than the skin color of the rest of the hand and arm (a).

Nails should appear shiny with smooth edges. The angle between the nail and the nail base is normally 160 degrees. A slight elevation of the skin at the base of the nail is normal (b).

Evaluation of the adequacy of *arterial blood supply* can be observed in the continuity of skin color of the upper extremities with other body parts and assessment of normally pink nail color (c).

The blood supply to the upper extremities originates in a branch from the aortic arch. The name of the artery changes as the artery enters a body part, e.g., when it travels beneath the clavicle, it becomes the *subclavian artery* (d). The subclavian artery becomes the *brachial artery* in the upper arm and divides at the elbow to form the *ulnar* and *radial arteries*.

Veins may be difficult to visualize in the upper extremities of obese clients.

Hair distribution and texture on arms and hands is finer in women than in men.

Inspection of the lower extremities is similar to that described for the upper extremities.

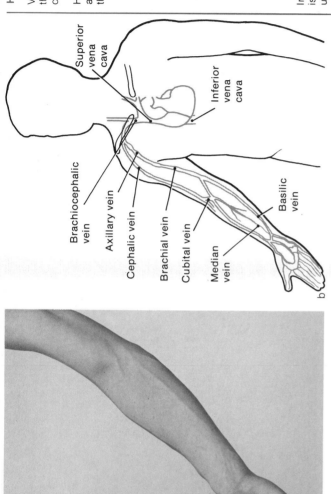

a

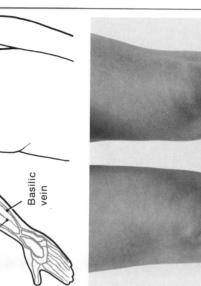

Superior vena cava

Inferior vena cava

Brachiocephalic vein

Axillary vein

Cephalic vein

Brachial vein

Cubital vein

Median vein

Basilic vein

b

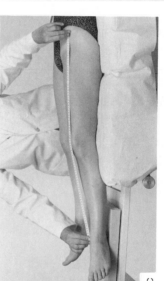

c

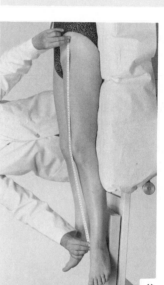

d

The client's *veins* are usually seen in the hands and arms in varying degrees, depending on the individual's age, weight, and the skin thickness (a). In an obese client, veins may not be visible, while in an elderly client, they may be quite prominent due to the loss of the fatty layer of skin.

The major veins of the upper extremities are the *brachiocephalic, cephalic, axillary, brachial, median, cubital, and basilic* (b).

Hair distribution and texture of the hands and arms will vary from client to client. It is important to be aware of recent change in hair distribution (loss or gain). While women will usually have finer body hair than men, older adults may have little or no observable hair.

Inspection of the *lower extremities* is done in much the same fashion as assessment of the upper extremities. Attention should focus on skin, competency of the arteries and veins, muscle mass, joint structure, and range of motion.

With the client lying flat on the examination table, alignment and symmetry of the hips should be noted. Normally, the client should be able to lie comfortably on the table with legs straight. The length of the legs as measured from the anterosuperior iliac spine to the tibial malleolus should be equal bilaterally (c). The skin around the hips and groin area should be smooth and firm. The alignment of the knees should be noted; normally hollows exist on either side of the patella (d).

Highlights

Inspection of skin color in the extremities should be similar bilaterally.

Superficial veins of the leg are visible depending upon age, weight, and skin thickness.

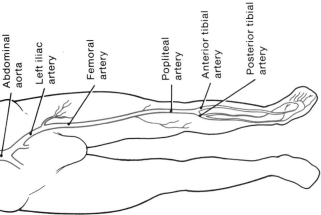

Abdominal aorta

Left iliac artery

Femoral artery

Popliteal artery

Anterior tibial artery

Posterior tibial artery

b

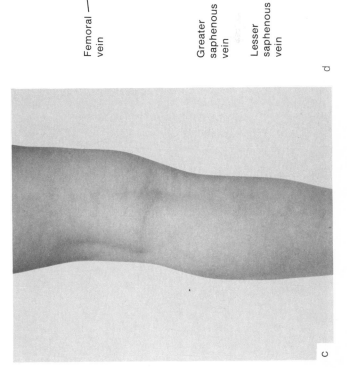

Femoral vein

Greater saphenous vein

Lesser saphenous vein

d

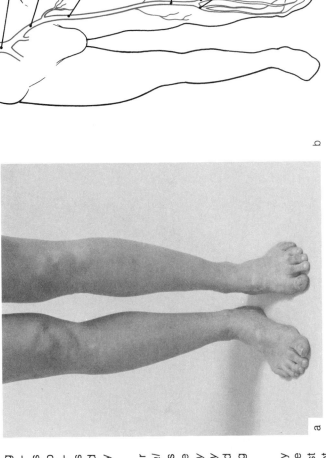

a

c

Examination of the skin on the lower leg is extremely important in regard to functioning of the arteries and veins. Arteries are not visible as they are quite deep within the leg. However, the effectiveness of peripheral arterial circulation is manifested in skin color, which should be similar to that of the rest of the body (a).

The *arterial blood supply* to the lower extremities originates in the *abdominal aorta* and divides below the umbilicus into the *right* and *left iliac arteries*. The iliac artery becomes the *femoral artery* at the upper thigh, the *popliteal artery* behind the knee, and the *anterior* and *posterior tibial arteries* in the lower leg (b).

The prominence of lower extremity veins will vary. Veins tend to be more prominent on the foot, but for the most part, in a normal person veins should not be visible in the upper and lower legs except in the popliteal space (c).

Deep veins responsible for the majority of the blood return from the legs are not visible clinically. The *greater* and *lesser saphenous veins* are the main superficial veins of the leg. They communicate with the deep veins and empty into the femoral vein at the groin (d). The *superficial veins* are visible depending on age, weight of the client, and the thickness of the skin.

Highlights

Hair distribution on the extremities will vary from client to client.

Refer to palpation for measurement of muscle mass.

The joint is the functional unit of the musculoskeletal system.

There are three types of joints:
1. Synarthroses (skull)
2. Amphiarthroses (pubic symphysis)
3. Diarthroses - synovial joints (hip)

Each opposing bone in the joint is covered by cartilage which is attached to a synovial membrane.

The membrane surrounding the synovial cavity contains a lubricating fluid which permits bone movements.

Figure d adapted from Dorothy A. Jones, et al., Medical-Surgical Nursing, A Conceptual Approach, McGraw-Hill, 1982, p. 1209, fig. 32-14. Used with permission of McGraw-Hill Book Company.

Hair is usually present on the lower legs and distributed similarly on either leg. The size, symmetry, and circumference of muscles of the lower extremities including bilateral measurement of the hamstring, abductor, adductor and quadriceps muscles should be determined (a). *Toenails* are whiter than fingernails and perhaps a little thicker. Skin tends to be thicker on the soles of feet but still should be smooth and intact and similar in color to other skin.

The alignment of the toes and ankle bone should be noted. Feet should be slightly externally rotated as the client lies on the table (b).

The **joint** is the primary functional unit of the musculoskeletal system. There are three types of joints in the body (c): *synarthroses* (joints which do not permit movement, e.g., the suture joints of the skull), *amphiarthroses* (joints which are slightly moveable, e.g., pubic symphysis), and the joints which are the focus of the discussion of this chapter, the *diarthroses* or *synovial joints* which are freely moveable.

The basic components of the joints are similar. Each opposing bone in the joint (the bones do not actually touch) is covered by an articular cartilage which is attached to a *synovial membrane* (d). This membrane secretes a lubricating fluid into the joint space which allows for bone movement. Some synovial joints have *articular discs* composed of fibrocartilage which are located between articular cartilage (d). They help minimize impact of shock and allow the joint to respond more quickly to change in pressure.

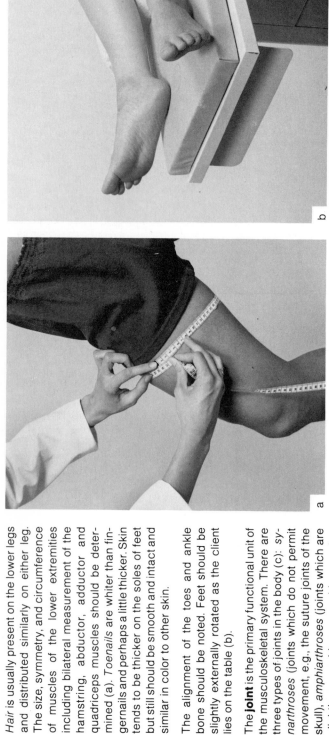

a

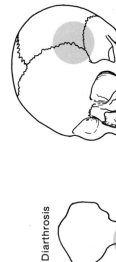

b

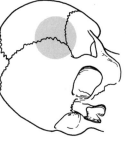

Synarthrosis

Diarthrosis

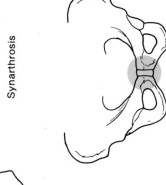

Amphiarthrosis

c

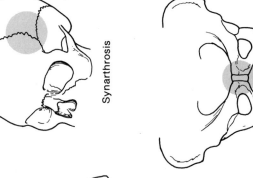

Periosteum

Subchondral bone plate

Articular disc

Articular cartilage

Synovial cavity

Synovium (synovial membrane)

Joint capsule

d

The **bursa**, found within or around the joint is a closed sac of synovial fluid. It is located in the spaces of connective tissue between tendons, ligaments, bones and skin. This sac or bursa facilitates gliding of the skin, muscle, or tendon over a particularly bony surface, e.g., between the skin and patella of the knee (a).

The synovial membrane is supported by a *joint capsule* made of collagen fibers, which in turn is supported by *ligaments*. These ligaments extend directly from bone to bone. The joint is further supported by muscles which are responsible for the degree of a particular joint's movement. It is the support of the muscle groups and ligaments that prevent abnormal joint movement.

There are eight types of movable (synovial) joints (b).

1 *Condyloid joint* - found in the shoulder

2 *Ball and socket joint* - located in the hip joint

3 *Ellipsoid joint* - found in the wrist joint

4 *Hinge joint* - located in joints such as the interphalangeal joint and the elbow joint

5 *Pivot joint* - for example the radioulnar joint (i.e., left-head of the radius, right-the radial notch of the ulna; and the joint in a supinated or pronated position)

6 *Cochlear joint* - a hinge joint which varies slightly from other joints in that the head of the bone is not vertical to the axis of the cylinder, eg., the ankle joint (tibia, fibula, talus)

7 *Saddle joint* - located in the carpometacarpal joint of the thumb

8 *Plane joint* - between tarsal bones of foot.

Highlights

A **ligament** is a structure which supports the joint capsule and extends from bone to bone.

The **bursa**, a joint component, is a sac of synovial fluid found in connective tissue between bones, skin, ligaments and tendons.

Muscle groups and ligaments prevent abnormal joint movement.

There are 8 major movable types of joints. They include:

1 Condyloid joint
2 Ball and socket joint
3 Ellipsoid joint
4 Hinge joint
5 Pivot joint
6 Cochlear joint
7 Saddle Joint
8 Plane joint

PHYSICAL EXAMINATION

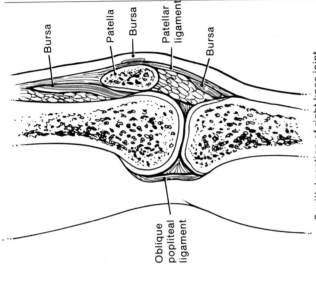

a Sagittal section of right knee joint

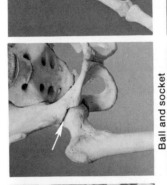
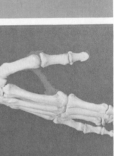
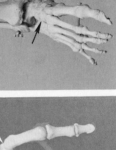
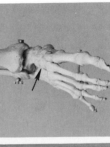
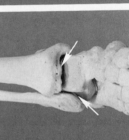
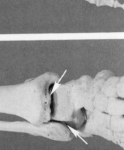
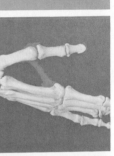
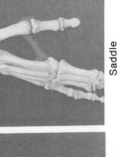

Condyloid
Ball and socket
Pivot
Cochlear
Hinge
Ellipsoid
Plane
Saddle

b

Highlights

Each joint should be inspected for size, contour, symmetry, and mobility.

There are 10 different movements of synovial joints: but not all joints move in all positions.

- flexion
- extension
- abduction
- adduction
- rotation
- circumduction
- supination
- pronation
- eversion
- inversion

There are additional terms that may be used to describe joint movement:

Protraction - moving a part of the body forward on a plane parallel to the ground

Retraction - moving a part of the body backward on a plane parallel to the ground

Elevation - raising a part of the body

Depression - lowering a part of the body

Each joint should be inspected for size, contour, symmetry and mobility. While bony landmarks vary in individual joints, alignment, especially in relation to underlying anatomical features, should be noted.

The synovial joints can move in 10 major directions. Normal joint movements are supported by muscles and ligaments attached to the bones.

Joints should be inspected for the following movements (a):

1 *Flexion* - bending or decreasing the angle between two bones

2 *Extension* - increasing the angle between two bones

3 *Abduction* - moving the bone away from the midline of the body

4 *Adduction* - moving the bone toward the midline

5 *Rotation*- moving the bone around a central axis (the plane of motion is perpendicular to the axis)

6 *Circumduction* - moving the bone so that the end of it describes a circle and the sides a cone

7 *Supination* - moving the bones of the forearm so that the radius and ulna are parallel (if the arm is at the side of the body the palm is moved from a posterior to anterior position)

8 *Pronation* - moving the bones of the forearms so that the radius and ulna are not parallel (if the arm is at the side of the body, the palm is moved from an anterior to a posterior position)

9 *Eversion* - moving the sole of the foot outward at the ankle joint

10 *Inversion* - moving the sole of the foot inward at the ankle joint

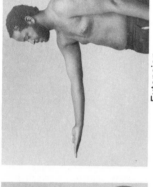

Flexion

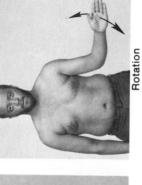
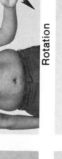

Extension

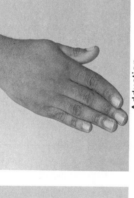

Adduction

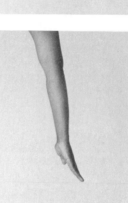

Rotation

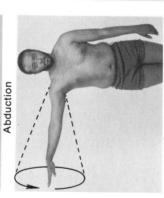

Abduction

Circumduction

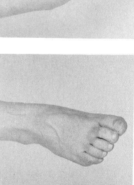

Supination

Pronation

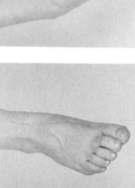
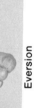

Eversion

Inversion

a

Joint movement should be smooth, uninterrupted and pain free.

Passive joint movement can be facilitated by the examiner.

Range of joint motion will be recorded in degrees.

When the client bends to touch the toes, the lumbar spine changes from concave to convex.

When assessing range of motion of the spine and trunk, care should be taken to prevent the client from falling.

Normally, flexibility decreases with age, although the flexibility of young people may vary greatly as well. Obviously, ease of movement as well as range of movement are considered in evaluating responses.

Lateral bending can occur passively by the examiner placing one hand over the iliac crest, the other on the opposite shoulder thereby forcing lateral movement.

The examiner can facilitate passive rotation by placing one hand on the hip, the other the contralateral shoulder and then pulling both hands in a posterior position.

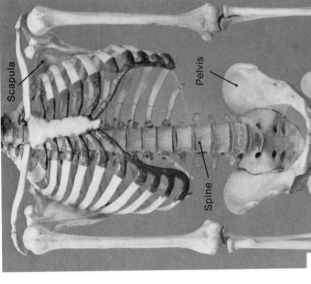

Scapula

Pelvis

Spine

a

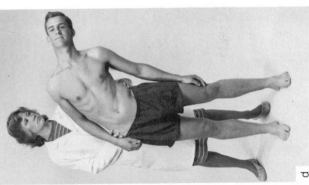

b

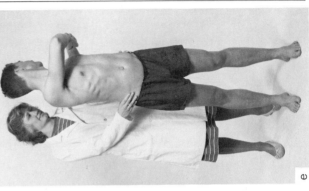

e

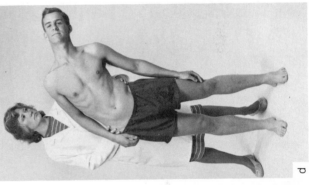

d

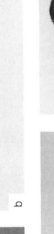

c

Inspection of the joints focuses upon the observation of each joint as it performs a series of range of motion activities. The discussion to follow identifies joints specific to a body part, the structures that articulate in a joint, the joint movement, and the client's activity needed to elicit the movement. Movements should be smooth, uninterrupted, and pain free.

Joint motion will be recorded in degrees. This assumes that prior to execution of the body movement there is a zero (0°) or neutral position. All joint movements should be assessed bilaterally.

Trunk Observation of movement allows for assessment of the spine, the paravertebral muscles, scapulae, and stability of the pelvis (a). Movements include:

1 *flexion* - have the client bend forward in an attempt to touch the toes. Normal range of movement is 75° to 90° (b).

2 *extension* - accomplished by the client assuming an erect, upright position at zero (0°) or natural position.

3 *hyperextension* - achieved by having the client bend the body slightly backward. Normal range is up to 30° (c).

4 *lateral bending* - accomplished by having the client stand erect. The examiner then places hands on the client's hips (iliac crest). The client is asked to bend laterally, first to the right then to the left. Normal range is up to 35° (d).

5 *rotation* - occurs when the client stands straight facing the examiner, then turns to the right and then to the left without moving the position of the pelvis or legs. Normal range is approximately 30°. (e)

Head and Neck Movements of the head and neck are discussed under each respective section in Chap. 4.

Shoulder The *glenohumeral joint* is formed by the humerus and glenoid fossa of the scapula. The articulations between the clavicle and sternum and clavicle and acromion process of the scapula also play a role in shoulder movements (a).

1 *internal rotation* - occurring as the client raises the arm (flexed at the elbow) toward the shoulder. The client's fingers should be pointed toward the floor with palmar surface facing posteriorly. The client then rotates the forearms (forward) anteriorly. Normal range 55° (b).

2 *external rotation* - while the client's arm is at shoulder level, the client rotates the forearm posteriorly (forward and backward). Normal range 40-45° (c).

3 *abduction* - is accomplished by having the client holding the arm and elbow straight; and then upon command, move the arm slightly away from the body extending it upward. Normal range up to 180°.

4 *adduction* - occurs as the client moves the arm (straight at the elbow) from one side of the body across the anterior chest. Normal range 45° (d).

5 *flexion* - the client moves the whole arm forward and up from the neutral position (0°) at the side. Normal range is 180° (e).

6 *extension* - the client moves the arm backward from the neutral position. Normal range is 60°.

Joint movement of the head and neck found under respective headings in Chap. 4.

All of the movements of the shoulder can be put through passive range of motion as the examiner assumes the active role of moving the body part in specific directions.

Movements of the shoulder include:
1. Internal rotation
2. External rotation
3. Abduction
4. Adduction
5. Flexion
6. Extension

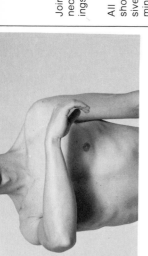

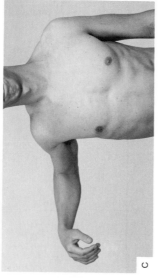

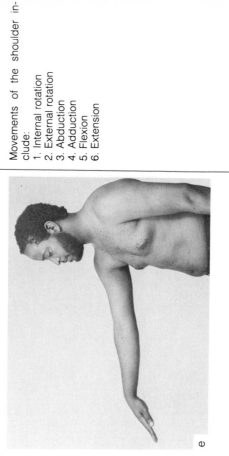

Acromioclavicular joint

Sternoclavicular joint

Glenohumeral joint

a

b

c

e

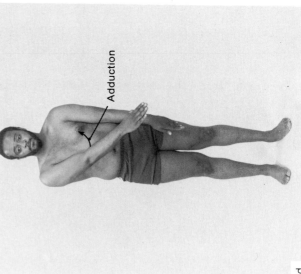

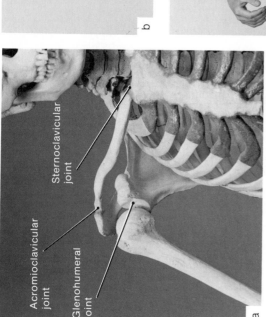

Adduction

d

Elbow Assessment of the elbow involves movement of the articulation
between the humerus, radius and ulna
(a). These movements include:

1 *forward flexion* - occurring as the
client bends the straightened arm
and wrist with the intention of touching the hand to the shoulder. Normal
range is 135° and above (b).

2 *extension* - occurs when the
client straightens the elbow and wrist
from a flexed position to a neutral
point. Normal range 0° (neutral).

3 *supination* - is achieved by having the client rotate the straightened
arm until the palm faces upward.
Normal range is 90° (c).

4 *pronation* - is the reverse of supination. The client with the elbow
flexed at 90° rotates the upward
palmar surface to a downward position. Normal range is 90°.

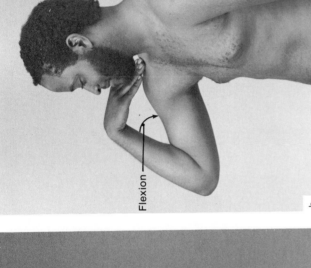

Humerus
Ulna
Radius
a

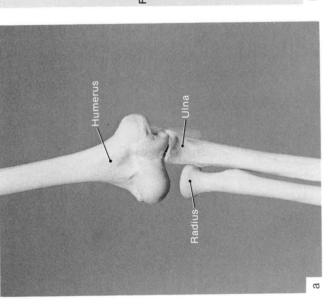

Flexion
b

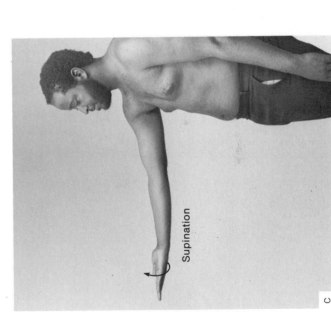

Supination
c

Highlights

Elbow movements are assessed
bilaterally

Movement of the upper extremities
can best be assessed by testing
one side of the body and then the
other.

Movements of the elbow can be
carried out by the examiner (passively) and put through range of
motion activities unassisted by the
client.

Movements of the elbow include:
1. Foward flexion
2. Extension
3. Supination
4. Pronation

Highlights

Wrist assessment involves the evaluation of the radiocarpal joint.

Joint movements of the wrist include flexion, extension, dorsiflexion, ulnar deviation and radial deviation.

Wrist movements are assessed bilaterally.

Movements of the wrist include:
1. Flexion
2. Extension
3. Dorsiflexion
4. Ulnar deviation
5. Radial deviation

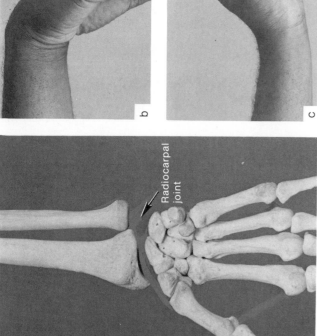

Radiocarpal joint

a

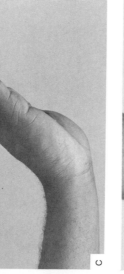

b

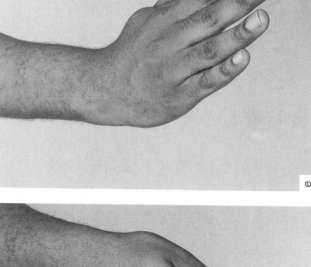

c

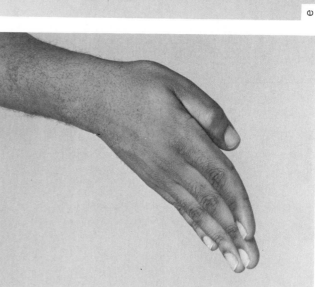

e

d

Wrist Assessment of the wrist involves the evaluation of the radiocarpal joint (a). Inspection of the following movements facilitates evaluation of these joints:

1 *flexion* - occurs as the client bends the wrist from a straight position downward. Normal range is approximately 80-90° (b).

2 *extension* - a neutral position assessed by having the client straighten out hand from a flexed position. The hand should be in alignment with the forearm.

3 *dorsiflexion* - involves the client bending the wrist from a straight position, upward. Normal range is approximately 70° (c).

4 *ulnar deviation*- (abduction) occurs when the client moves the straightened hand from a neutral position outward (toward the ulnar bone). Normal range is approximately 30° (d).

5 *radial deviation* (adduction) - is determined by having the client move the straightened hand from a neutral position inward, toward the radius. Normal range is 20° (e).

Highlights

Evaluation of finger movement includes joint assessment of the metacarpophalangeal, proximal interphalangeal and distal interphalangeal joints.

The examiner can passively evaluate finger flexion by supporting the client's forearm with one hand and closing the client's finger with the other and straightening them to evaluate extension.

Finger movements include:

- flexion
- extension
- hyperextension
- abduction
- adduction

Finger movements are assessed bilaterally.

Fingers Evaluation of finger movement involves the assessment of the metacarpophalangeal, proximal interphalangeal and distal interphalangeal joints (a). This is determined by inspection of the following movements:

1 *flexion* - assessed by having the client make a tight fist. Normal range is 90-100° (b).

2 *extension* - occurs as the client releases the fisted hand and straightens the fingers to a neutral position.

3 *hyperextension* - is achieved by having the client move the fingers from a neutral position, backward (c). Movement should be as a total unit. Normal range is 30° to 45°.

4 *abduction* - occurs when the client moves fingers from a neutral position and then spreads them apart. The range is approximately 20° (d).

5 *adduction* - follows abduction and is the closing of the fingers back to a neutral (0°) position.

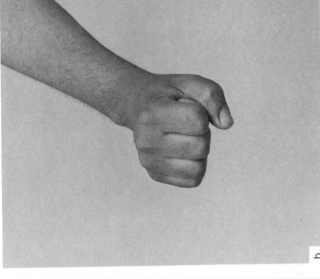

a

Metacarpo-phalangeal joint

Proximal interphalangeal joint

Distal interphalangeal joint

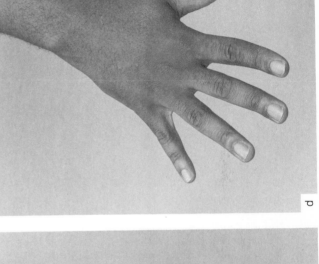

b

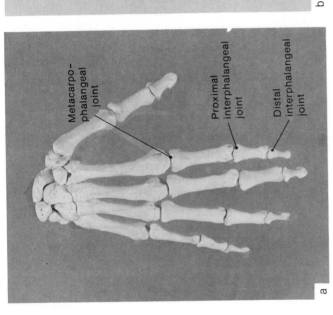

c

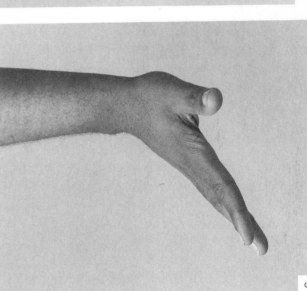

d

Mobility of the thumb is very important in fine manipulation tasks such s grasping writing utensils.

Thumb joint motions include:

- flexion
- extension
- hyperextension
- abduction
- adduction
- oppostion

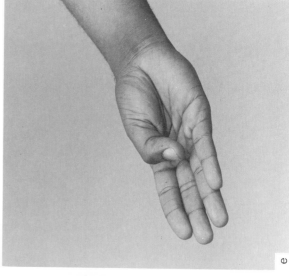

a

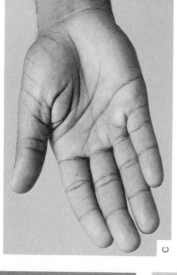

Metacarpo-phalangeal joint

Interphalangeal joint

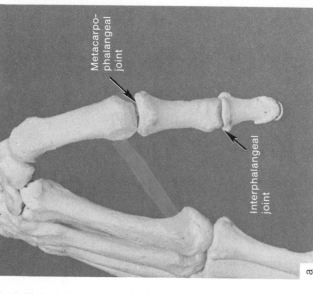

b

c

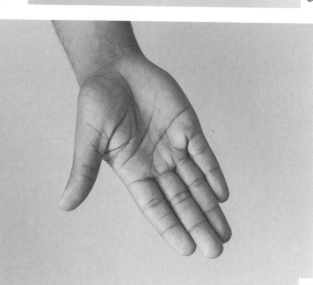

d

e

Thumb Thumb movements are important because they provide the fine manipulation abilities of the hand and support the action of the fingers. Thumb movement is controlled in part by the metacarpophalangeal joint and the interphalangeal joint (a). These joints are involved in the following movements:

1 *flexion* - occurs when the client bends the thumb. Normal range is 50° (metacarpophalangeal joint) to 90° (interphalangeal joint) (b).

2 *extension* - is achieved when the client straightens the thumb and returns it to a neutral (0°) position.

3 *hyperextension* - is achieved when the client extends the thumb backward from a neutral position. Normal range of the interphalangeal joint is 20° (c).

4 *abduction* - occurs as the client moves the thumb upward and away from the palm. Normal range is 70° (d).

5 *adduction* - after the thumb is abducted it is brought back to a neutral position. This is accomplished when the thumb is in alignment with the index finger.

6 *opposition* - can be measured by having the client touch each of the fingers of the same hand with the thumb (e).

Hip The hip joint is the articulation between the acetabulum of the pelvis and the head of the femur (a). To test the range of hip motion the following movements can be enacted:

1 *flexion* - is accomplished with the client standing, the leg held straight and brought toward the chest without bending. Normal range is 45-90° (b).

2 *extension* - occurs with the leg in a flexed position. The client then straighens leg to a neutral position.

3 *abduction* - is examined with the client in a standing or supine position. The leg is moved from a neutral position outward away from the opposite leg. Normal range is 45°.

4 *adduction* - is achieved by having the client bring one leg across the midline as far as possible toward the opposite leg. The procedure is repeated on the opposite leg. The normal range is 20+° (c).

5 *rotation* - occurs with the client standing, turning the foot first inward and then outward. Normal range is 35° (internal) to 45° (external) (d).

Highlights

Flexion and extension of the hip can occur with the client standing or in a supine position with the knee straight or flexed.

Rotation of the hip can occur with the client in a standing and supine position.

Hip movements include:
1. Flexion
2. Extension
3. Abduction
4. Adduction
5. Rotation

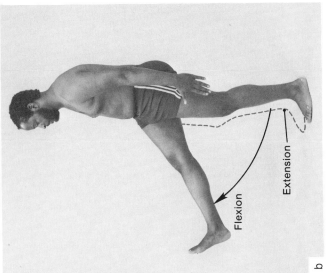

Acetabulum of pelvis

Head of femur

a

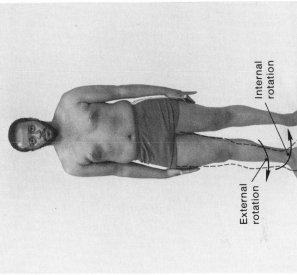

Flexion

Extension

b

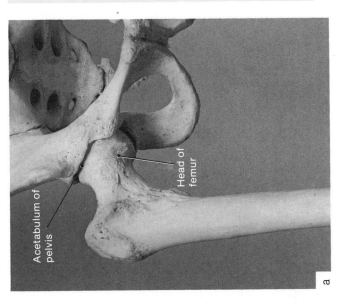

Abduction

Adduction

c

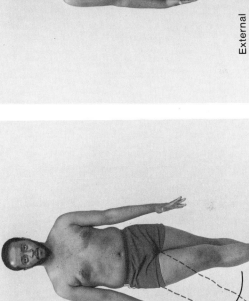

Internal rotation

External rotation

d

Highlights

The anterior and posterior cruciate ligaments give the knee stability.

Knee movements should be assessed bilaterally.

Knee movements include:
1. Flexion
2. Extension

The tibiotalar and talofibular joints are responsible for ankle motion.

When testing ankle movement the client should move one side then the other.

Passive range of ankle movement can occur with the client lying down and the examiner moving the client's foot as described.

Ankle movements include:
1. Dorsi flexion
2. Plantar flexion
3. Inversion
4. Eversion

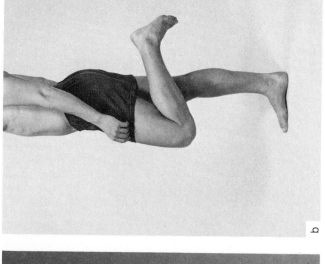

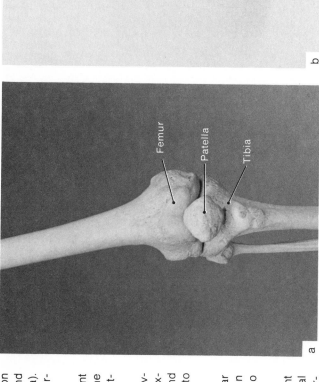

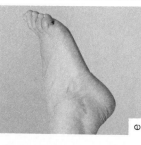

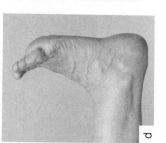

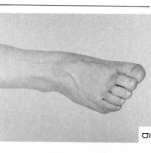

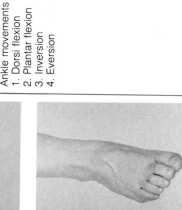

Knee The knee joint is the articulation between the femur and the tibia and includes another bone, the patella (a). Movement of the knee joint is determined by the following motions:

1 *flexion* - occurs with the client standing. The knee is bent with the heel brought upward toward the buttocks. Normal range is 130° (b).

2 *extension* - is achieved by moving the leg from a flexed position. Extension occurs when the knee and leg are straightened and returned to a neutral position.

Ankle The tibiotalar and talofibular joints are responsible for ankle motion (c). The following movements help to evaluate joint function:

1 *dorsiflexion* - occurs as the client brings the foot upward from a neutral position while standing or lying. Normal range is 20° (d).

2 *plantarflexion* - occurs when the client bends the foot downward from a neutral position while standing or lying down. Normal range is 50° (e).

3 *inversion* - involves the client tilting the right and left foot toward one another; the client can be sitting or lying down to complete the procedure. Normal range is 5° (f).

4 *eversion* - occurs while the client is sitting or lying down and both feet are tilted outward. Normal range is approximately 5° (g).

Foot Movement of the forefoot is achieved by tarsometatarsal, intertarsal and intermetatarsal joints (a). These joints are assessed by the following movements:

1 *adduction* - achieved by the examiner placing the hand on the clients heel and the client turning the foot inward. Normal range is 20° (b).

2 *abduction* - occurs again as the examiner stabilizes the heel and the client turns the foot outward from a neutral position. Normal range is 10° (c).

Toes The metatarsophalangeal and interphalangeal joints are located within the toes and allow their movement (d). The following actions help to assess joint function of the toes:

1 *flexion* - occurs when client bends the toes. Normal range is 45° (e).

2 *extension* - is achieved when the flexed toes are straightened and returned to a neutral (0°) position.

3 *abduction* - is accomplished by having the client spread (fan) the toes apart (f).

4 *adduction* - follows abduction and involves returning the toes that were spread apart back together to a neutral position.

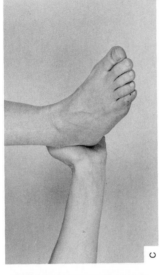

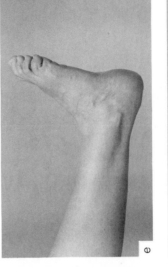

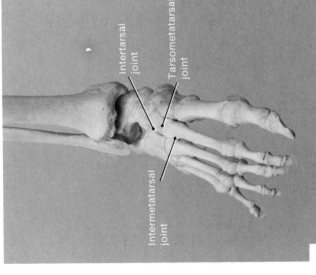

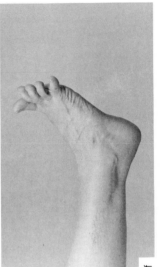

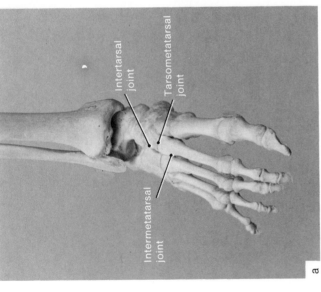

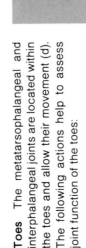

Highlights

The *subtalar* and *transverse tarsal* joints are responsible for inversion and eversion of the foot.

Foot movements include adduction and abduction.

Passive range of ankle, foot and toe movement can be achieved with the examiner placing the hands on the part to be inspected and directing movement as described.

During adduction of the toes they should return to a position where they approximate one another.

Toe movements include:
1. Flexion
2. Extension
3. Abduction
4. Adduction

PHYSICAL EXAMINATION

Highlights

Muscles comprise approximately 40 to 50 percent of body weight.

Muscle fibers of the skeletal system are striated, long and slender.

Muscles are composed of skeletal bundles called *fasciculi*.

Muscles are described in terms of their:

1 action
2 shape
3 origin and insertion
4 number of divisions
5 location
6 direction

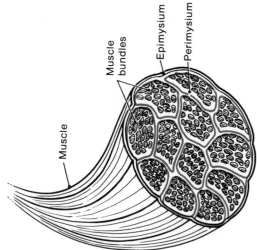

a

b

Muscles give support, move joints, and protect organs. They comprise approximately 40 to 50 percent of the body weight. Muscle fibers of the skeletal system are striated, long and slender.

Each muscle is comprised of a number of bundles called *fasciculi*. The bundles are bound by a sheath called the *perimysium* which is continuous with the *epimysium* or muscle fascia which encloses the entire muscle (a).

Muscles are named according to:

1 action (e.g., supinator)
2 shape (e.g., trapezius)
3 origin and insertion (e.g., sterno-cleidomastoid)
4 number of divisions (e.g., biceps, triceps)
5 location (e.g., tibialis)
6 direction (e.g., longitudinus).

Muscle attachments form the basis for muscle action. The *origin* of a muscle is that end proximal to the axial skeleton. The distal *insertion* is the more moveable attachment (b).

Muscles are inspected for mass and symmetry.

Fasciculations are visible, spontaneous contractions of a muscle group; insufficient to stimulate joint movements.

Muscle mass is determined by bilateral measurement of the circumference of the midpoint of both muscles.

Muscle mass is usually less in women.

Muscle mass can decrease with age.

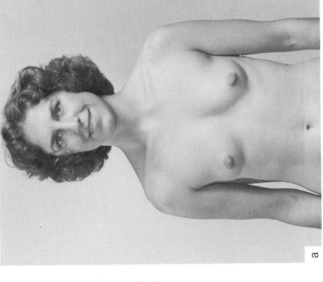

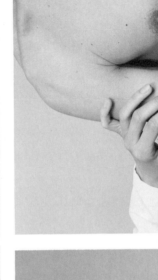

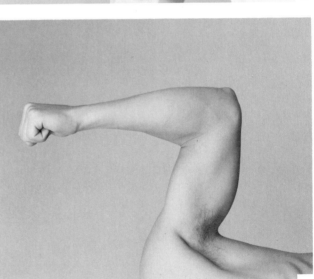

a

b

c

Muscles are inspected for mass and symmetry. Some *fasciculation* of the muscles is normal but is rarely noticed when it occurs.

Determination of normal muscle build is gained only over time by examination of many individuals (a). Variation in determination of bulk is influenced by age, sex, occupation, state of health, and use and disuse. For example, muscle bulk of a professional athlete and a sedentary business executive may differ greatly.

Muscle contour can be assessed by having the client flex the muscle (e.g., biceps) to accent normal roundedness (b).

Muscle mass can be determined by measuring the circumference of the midpoint of the muscle and comparing it with the circumference of the corresponding muscle on the opposite side of the body. (c) A tape measure is placed at midpoint of each muscle group and the reading compared bilaterally. The difference should not be greater than 1 cm.

Muscle mass is usually less in women than in men. Mass may decline in the elderly, but strength does not. Inspection of the joints and muscles is often done at the same time.

Highlights

A discussion of the action of the sternocleidomastoid and trapezius muscles are found under the discussion of the neck.

Only the more commonly discussed muscles have been included here. Additional muscle groups are found in the extremities.

Muscles of the upper extremities are innervated by nerves which branch from the brachial nerve plexus.

The brachial nerve plexus comprises nerves emanating from C_5 through T_1.

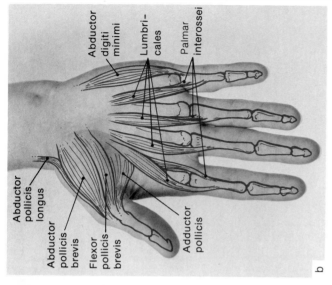

a

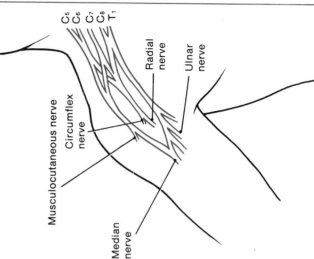

b

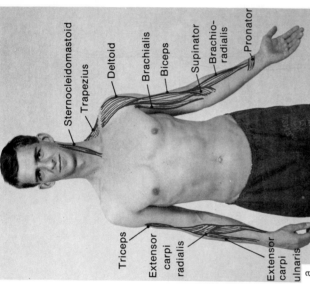

c

The major muscles which move joints of the upper extremities include (a and b):

1 *shoulder* - sternocleidomastoid, deltoid, and trapezius muscles

2 *elbow* - biceps, triceps, brachialis, and brachioradialis muscles

3 *forearm* - pronator and supinator muscles

4 *wrist* - flexor and extensor carpi radialis, and flexor and extensor carpi ulnaris muscles

5 *thumb* - flexor and extensor pollicis brevis and longus, adductor and abductor pollicis, opponens muscles

6 *fingers* - lumbricales, palmar and dorsal interossei, flexor and extensor digitorum, and abductor digiti minimi muscles.

These muscles are innervated by specific nerves which branch from the brachial nerve plexus. This plexus is comprised of nerves emanating from the C_5 through T_1 levels of the spinal cord and influence sensory-motor activity.

The *circumflex* **nerve** innervates the deltoid muscle; the *musculocutaneous nerve* innervates the biceps, brachialis muscles; the *ulnar nerve* innervates some flexors of the forearm and the muscles of the hand; the *median nerve* innervates the flexor muscles; and the *radial nerve* innervates the triceps and extensor muscles of the forearm (c).

Highlights

Muscles of the buttocks vary in size. The size and shape of the right and left gluteal fold should be symmetrical.

The muscles of the lower extremities are innervated by the sacral plexus.

The sciatic nerve originates in the gluteus maximus.

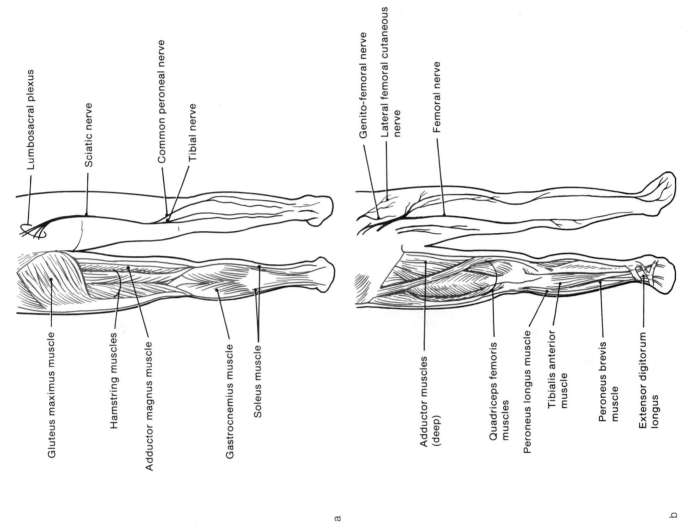

a

Lumbosacral plexus

Sciatic nerve

Common peroneal nerve

Tibial nerve

Gluteus maximus muscle

Hamstring muscles

Adductor magnus muscle

Gastrocnemius muscle

Soleus muscle

b

Genito-femoral nerve

Lateral femoral cutaneous nerve

Femoral nerve

Adductor muscles (deep)

Quadriceps femoris muscles

Peroneus longus muscle

Tibialis anterior muscle

Peroneus brevis muscle

Extensor digitorum longus

The major muscles which move the joints of the lower extremities include (a and b):

1 *hip* - gluteus maximus, medius and minimus, psoas major, iliacus external rotator muscles, quadriceps femoris, hamstrings, and adductor muscles

2 *knee* - quadriceps femoris, and hamstring muscles

3 *ankle* - tibialis anterior, gastrocnemius, and soleus muscles

4 *foot* - tibialis posterior, peroneus longus and brevis muscles

5 *toes* - flexor and extensor hallucis longus and brevis, flexor and extensor digitorum longus and brevis, and the lumbricales muscles.

Muscles of the lower extremities are innervated by the lumbar and sacral plexuses (a and b). The lumbar plexus contains three branches; the femoral nerve, the genito-femoral nerve and the lateral femoral cutaneous nerve.

The genito-femoral nerve supplies the scrotal area and a portion of the thigh. The remaining nerve branches innervate the lateral and anterior skin of the thigh, hips and lower leg and flexor muscles.

The sciatic nerve originates from branches of the lumbar and sacral plexuses beneath the gluteus maximus and descends into the thigh and divides into the tibial and common peroneal nerve.

Highlights

Palpating arterial pulses, skin, muscle tone and strength, and joint movement should be assessed bilaterally.

Peripheral arterial pulses of the upper extremities can be palpated at three points:

    a. the radial artery
    b. the brachial artery
    c. the ulnar artery

Refer to measurements for a discussion of pulses.

Pulse rate is described under measurements [60-100] as beats per minute.

Pulses are graded according to the following scale:

    0 - completely absent
    1 - markedly impaired
    2 - moderately impaired
    3 - slightly impaired
    4 - normal

The popliteal artery is best palpated with the knee flexed.

Palpation

Palpation of the upper extremities includes assessment of the arteries and veins, skin, muscle tone and strength, and joint movement and reflexes.

Arterial pulses can be palpated at three points on the arms. Using the pads of the index and middle fingers, locate the radial artery on the radial side of the wrist, the brachial artery at or above the elbow, and, if possible, the ulnar artery on the ulnar side of the wrist (a).

The *ulnar pulse* is sometimes more difficult to palpate. The pulse on the left side should be compared with the pulse on the right. Pulses should be equal in strength, rate and rhythm and have the same amplitude (height and thrust). Some pulses are obviously stronger than others, but a weak pulse does not necessarily indicate an abnormality. A normal pulse rate is similar bilaterally. The rate is between 60-100 beats.

The *popliteal pulse* can be palpated with the knee in a flexed position. Using both hands and palpating deeply, the examiner should try to feel the pulse with the fingertips. Palpation can be very difficult to feel as the area is less circumscribed and more diffuse. An alternative method is to turn the client on the stomach, flex the knee, and press firmly and deeply into the popliteal space (b). The space should be smooth, with ligaments sometimes palpable (c).

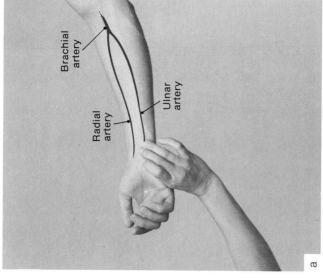

a

Brachial artery

Radial artery

Ulnar artery

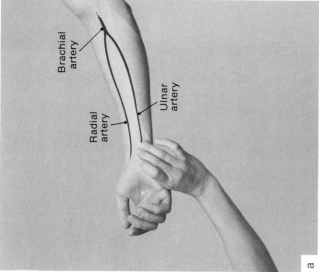

b

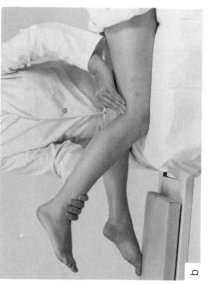

c

The femoral pulses can best be palpated midway between the iliac crest and the symphysis pubis.

The dorsalis pedis and posterior tibialis pulses are difficult to palpate and may be congenitally absent.

Palpation of skin temperature and nail color are two measures used to evaluate circulation to the extremities.

Unexplained changes in skin turgor should be referred for further evaluation.

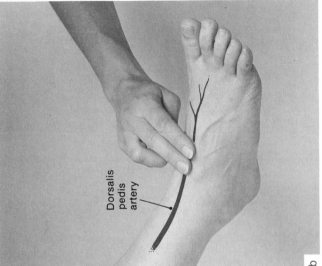

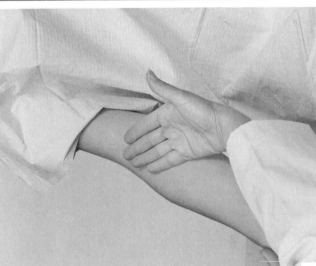

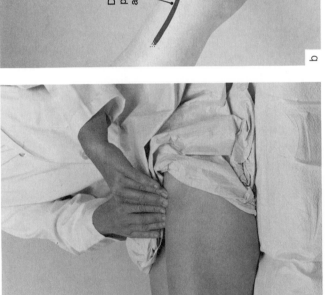

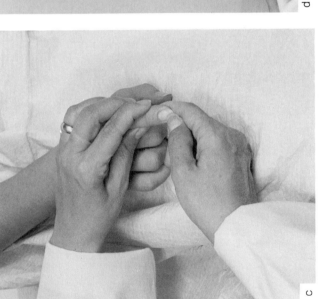

The *femoral pulse* can be palpated midway between the iliac crest and symphysis pubis. Sometimes it is necessary to palpate deeply using both hands (a). Pulses should be equal in strength, amplitude, and shape in both legs.

The *dorsalis pedis pulse* (b), and *posterior tibial pulse* (just behind the medial malleolus of the ankle) are palpated next. Both pulses are sometimes very difficult to feel and may be congenitally absent.

When evaluating circulation in the extremities it is important to look at other aspects of the body such as color of skin and nails. When palpated, nails should blanch but the pink color should return quickly (c). The skin color should be similar to that of the surrounding body tissue and opposing limb.

It is important to palpate skin temperature in the extremities to further evaluate circulation. To accomplish this the back of the examiner's hand is placed directly against the clients skin at various sites (d). The skin should be of equal warmth, bilaterally.

Anxiety, or change in environment may alter skin temperature. This can become . a concern when a difference is found between the two extremities.

The skin can also be palpated to assess hydration. Normally, it should be moist or dry, easy to move. Assessing skin turgor can be determined by pinching the tissue and observing the return to normal position as pressure is released.

Dorsalis
pedis
artery

Palpation of joints and muscle strength should be done systematically comparing the extremities bilaterally.

Refer to palpation of the neck in this chapter for assessment of shoulder and related structures.

The bursa of the elbow lies between the olecranon process and the epicondyles of the humerous.

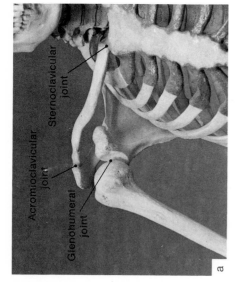

a

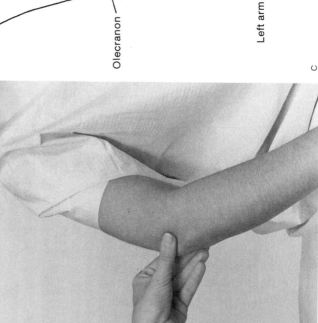

c

b

Palpation of joints should be done systematically, comparing one extremity to the other. This can be accomplished with the client sitting or lying down, depending upon the joint examined.

During palpation, the joints should be free of pain and easily movable. The size of the bones and amount of tissue surrounding the joint also should be noted.

Using the thumb and fingers, the examiner tests the joints of the upper and lower extremities. Assessment of joint and muscles are often performed together. However, for instructional purposes these examinations will be discussed separately.

The *shoulder* joints palpated include the sternoclavicular, the acromioclavicular, and the glenohumeral joints (a). The subacromial and subdeltoid bursae surround and protect this joint. Palpation of the joints and bursae should be completed without any signs of discomfort to the client.

The *elbow* is palpated next. The humerus, ulna, and radius comprise the bony portion of the joint and are enclosed in a synovial membrane. The examiner palpates the medial and lateral epicondyles of the humerus and the olecranon process of the ulna (b).

The elbow is held by the examiner and passively moved in various positions for examination. While a bursa lies between the olecranon process and the skin, the synovial membrane between the olecranon and epicondyles of the humerus, is not palpable. The ulnar nerve can be palpated between the olecranon process and the medial epicondyle (c). The client may experience a tingling sensation when this area is palpated.

Highlights

It is important to assess the extent to which loss of range of motion interferes with activities of daily living. When the ability of the client to carry out these activities is hampered, the loss of movement must be addressed.

The radius articulates with the carpal bones at the wrist.

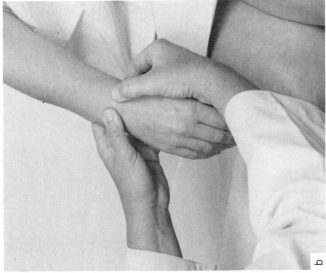

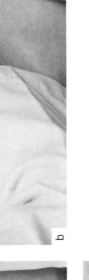

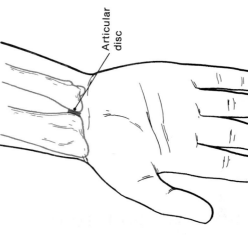

Articular disc

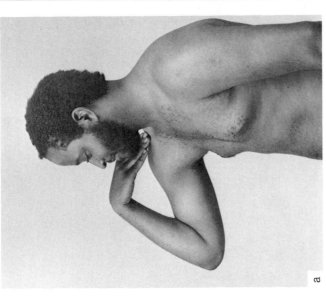

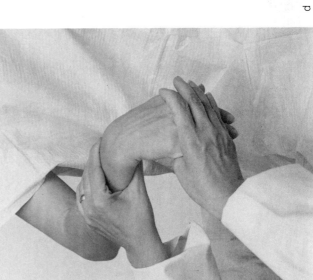

Flexion and extension of the elbow (a) as well as the client's ability to supinate and pronate the elbow should be noted. The examiner can elicit these activities through passive range of motion. (Refer to discussion under inspection of joints.) Movement of the elbow should be free of pain and well coordinated. Palpation of the elbow should be free of discomfort or swelling.

Both the *ulna* and *radius* should be palpated (b), as well as the radial carpal groove on the dorsum of the wrist. The examiner should flex, extend, and deviate the wrist in order to evaluate mobility (c). Normally, the radius articulates with the carpal bones at the wrist. An articular disc separates the radius from the ulna at the wrist joint (d). The bony tips of the ulna and radius can also be palpated at this time. Normally these structures are easily moved and do not elicit pain when examined.

The hip joint is not palpable.

Assessment of the knee is complex.

The suprapatellar pouch should be palpated during the knee assessment.

A synovial membrane encloses the articulating surfaces of the tibia and femur.

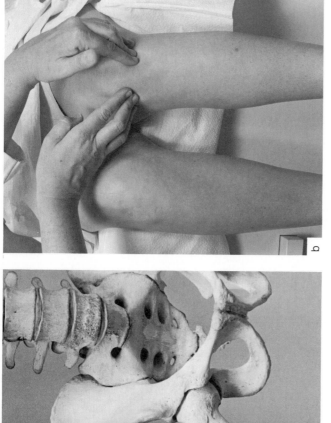

Iliac crest

Greater trochanter

a

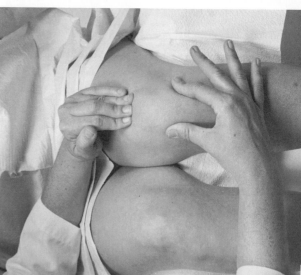

Femur

Patella

Tibia

d

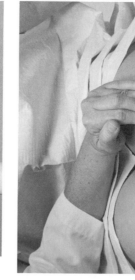

b

c

The *hip joint* is not palpable. However, the greater trochanter of the femur can be felt below the iliac crest (a). Normally, the area should be pain free when palpated.

Examination of the *knee*, a synovial joint, must be done carefully as it is the most complex and delicate of the joints in the body. The knee should be slightly flexed during the examination. The medial lateral epicondyles of the femur, and the patella and the grooves on either side are palpated (b).

The *suprapatellar pouch* is palpated with the examiner placing the thumb over the lateral surface of the joint posterior to the patella. The remaining fingers are placed below the patella forming an arch (c). The contents in between these points is pushed upward and then downward. Normally, this action is free of pain; and fluid should not be present.

A bursa lies between the patella and the skin, but is not palpable normally. Slightly below the patella are the epicondyles of the tibia. Below the lateral tibial epicondyle is the head the fibula. The knee joint is an articulation of the femur, tibia, and patella (d). A synovial membrane encloses the articulating surfaces of the tibia and femur and folds to the patella (*fibular connection*).

The *medial and lateral menisci* are not palpable but aid in the spread of synovial fluid in the knee.

The *medial and lateral collateral* and the *anterior and posterior cruciate* are ligaments that support knee movements.

Palpation of the ankle and the foot is best accomplished with the examiner holding the foot and using the fingertips to assess.

PHYSICAL EXAMINATION

The *medial and lateral menisci* (not palpable), thought to aid in the spread of synovial fluid in the knee, are fibrocartilaginous discs attached to the tibia and the articular capsule (a). Two sets of ligaments are vital to the support and functioning of the knee - the medial and lateral collateral and the anterior and posterior cruciate. Neither is palpable.

Various bursae are located at points in the knee joint. The anterior cruciate limits extension and rotation while the posterior stabilizes the femur against forward dislocation (b). Collateral ligaments prevent lateral dislocation of the knee. Movements of the knee should be painfree, easy, and smooth.

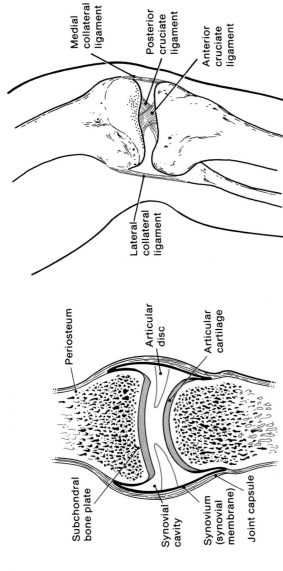

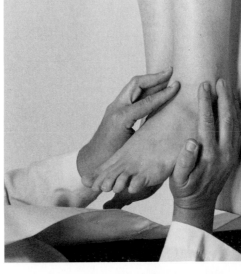

Medial collateral ligament

Posterior cruciate ligament

Anterior cruciate ligament

Lateral collateral ligament

Right knee

b

Periosteum

Articular disc

Articular cartilage

Subchondral bone plate

Synovial cavity

Synovium (synovial membrane)

Joint capsule

a

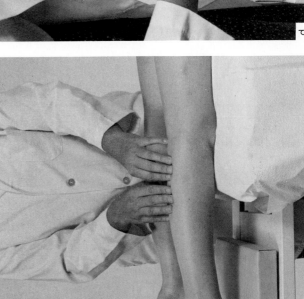

c

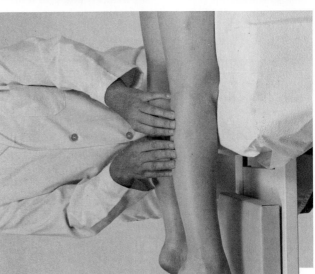

d

The *calf muscle (gastrocnemius)* is palpated by pressing it against the tibia (c). This should be pain free. The examiner should palpate the medial and lateral malleolus of the ankle (d); palpate the *achilles tendon* posteriorly; and flex, extend, evert, and invert the ankle joint. The foot can be stabilized during these procedures by grasping the heel with one hand and palpating with the other.

This should result in smooth non-interrupted movements which are free of pain.

The "longitudinal arch" is an imaginary line which extends from the metatarsal heads to the calcaneous.

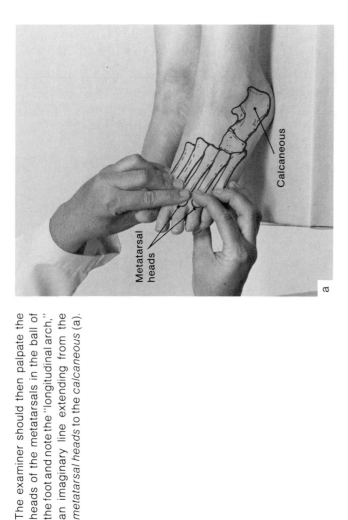

The examiner should then palpate the heads of the metatarsals in the ball of the foot and note the "longitudinal arch," an imaginary line extending from the *metatarsal heads* to the *calcaneous* (a).

Determination of *upper extremity* muscle strength can be evaluated in the assessment of the deltoid, biceps, triceps and wrist and fingers muscles.

Deltoid muscles - the client holds the arms upward and resists attempts by the examiner to push the arms down (b).

Biceps - the client extends the arm(s) and the examiner attempts to flex them (c).

Triceps - the client flexes the arm(s) and the examiner attempts to extend them (d).

Refer to discussion of the neck for palpation of shoulder muscles.

Muscle strength should be assessed bilaterally.

Muscle strength is assessed by determining resistance.

Muscles of the extremities should be assessed bilaterally.

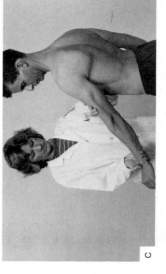

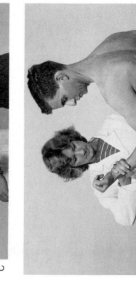

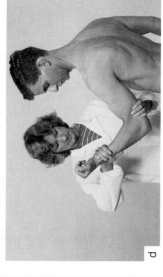

Wrist and finger muscles - the client spreads the fingers out and the examiner attempts to squeeze the fingers closed (a).

In addition, grip can be tested by having the client shake the examiner's hand. The hand and fingers can be held against the examiner's and force exerted.

The finger and wrist joints can be flexed and the examiner can attempt to extend them (b).

Muscle strength of the *lower extremities* can be evaluated by assessing hip strength, hamstrings, adductors, quadriceps, ankle and foot strength.

Hip - the client (in supine position) raises one leg (and then the other) as examiner attempts to hold that leg down (c).

Hamstring muscles - the client flexes the knee while the examiner attempts to straighten out the limb (d).

Quadriceps are muscle groups composed of the vastus lateralis, rectus femoris, vastus medialis and vastus intermedius.

Other muscle groups can be tested, for example, as the client lies on the side and lifts the top leg outward and then brings it closed with opposing resistance applied by the examiner.

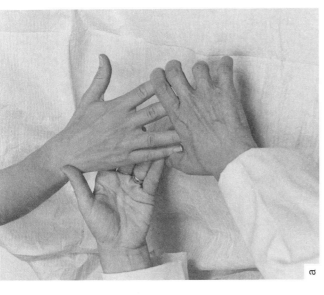

a

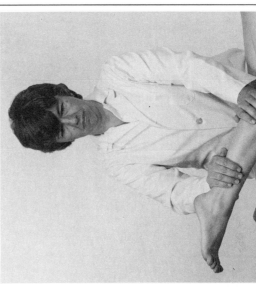

b

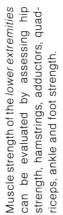

c

d

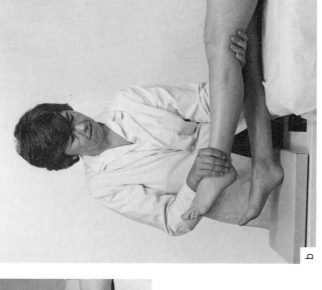

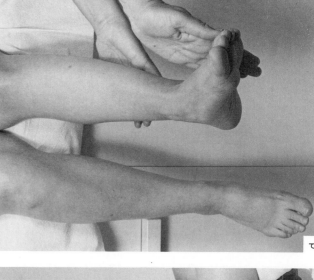

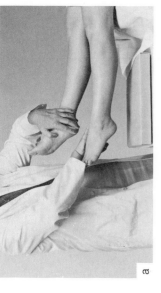

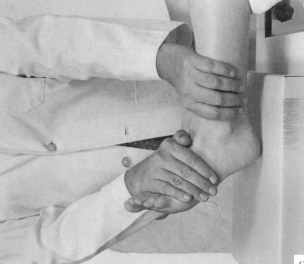

Adductors - can be tested as a group by having the client alternate crossing one leg in front of the other against examiner's resistance (a).

Quadriceps muscles - the client extends the leg and the examiner attempts to flex it (b).

Ankle/foot - the client holds the foot upright exerting forward pressure against the examiner's hand (anteriorly and posteriorly) while the examiner offers resistance (c). The ankle can also be rotated outward with force applied in the opposite direction (d). The toe can be evaluated at this time.

Muscle strength should be evaluated on both sides of the body. Strength is usually greater in the dominant arm and leg. Grading of muscle strength can be recorded as follows:

0 - no contractility (paralysis)

1 - slight contractility

2 - full range of motion with gravity eliminated

3 - full range of motion with gravity

4 - full range of motion against gravity with some resistance

5 - full range of motion with full resistance (optimal normal)

Muscle strength equal to or greater than 3 is considered normal.

Muscle strength is evaluated when resistance is applied to the extremity involved in a range of motion activity.

Muscle strength equal to or greater than 3 is considered normal.

Testing the sensory system can be exhausting and may need to be repeated at a later date if findings are uncertain. In a normal client, however, it is important to test fine motor coordination and proprioception, and sensations including pain, light touch, vibration, and change of position. These are all evaluated by testing the major dermatomes on the arms and legs and the peripheral nerves which innervate the dermatomes (a).

Evaluation of cerebellar function and proprioception should be tested in several ways. The *proprioception system* maintains posture, balance, and acts of coordination. The *posterior columns of the spinal cord* (b) are responsible for transmitting stimuli from the muscles, tendons and joints to the brain.

To assess cerebellar and proprioception function, have the client sit to the side of the examining table. The hands should be placed on the thigh, palms down (pronation). The examiner should then have the client rotate the hand to expose the palmar surface (supination). This action is repeated in a progressive rapid motion (c). Normally, the client can accomplish this task without difficulty.

This test can be used for **dysdiadocho-kinesia** which measures one's ability to terminate movement in one direction and replace it with a movement in an opposite direction.

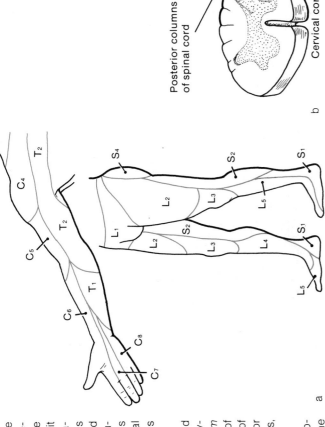

a

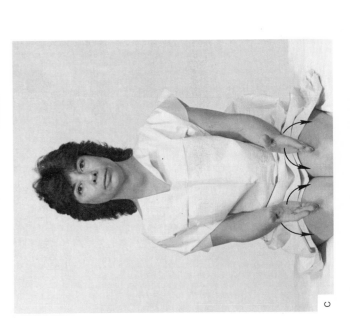

Posterior columns of spinal cord

Cervical cord

b

c

Highlights

When assessing coordination and balance in older adults, movement may be slower and less coordinated.

There are many tests to evaluate the proprioceptive system. All reflect the client's ability to coordinate activities and maintain balance.

Tests used to evaluate proprioception include:

1 the finger-to-finger test
2 knee bending
3 balancing the body while standing on one foot
4 the Romberg test
5 the pronation and supination test

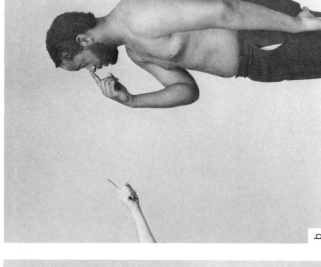

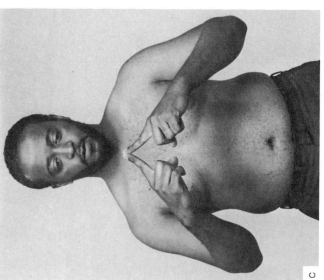

Testing for accuracy and direction of movement can be achieved by asking the client to touch the nose with the index finger using one hand then the other (a). The individual is instructed to close the eyes during the process and repeat the activity with increasing speed. Normally, this is accomplished without discomfort and with accuracy and coordination at all levels of speed.

Another test of proprioception involves asking the client to touch the nose and then touch the finger of the examiner who is standing approximately 18″ away (b). This activity is repeated with increasing speed and should occur with coordinated movements and accuracy.

The finger-to-finger test requires that the client's arms be extended laterally, and the index fingers of both hands brought together (mid-line) (c). This action occurs slowly at first and then rapidly with the eyes open and then closed.

Other activites used to test proprioception include:

a Knee bending without support, normally, balance is maintained as client bends at the knees (a).

b Standing on the one foot for a minimum of 5 seconds with eyes closed, then reversing to the other foot for a minimum of the same time without losing balance (b).

c The *Romberg test* - refer to discussion under inspection of the extremities.

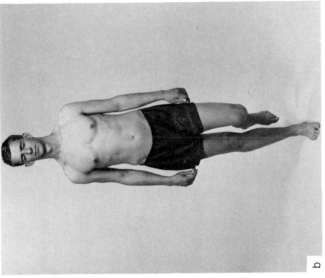

a

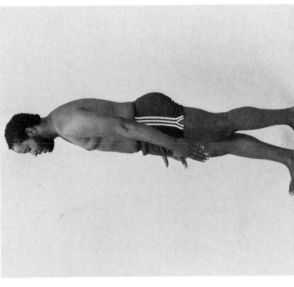

b

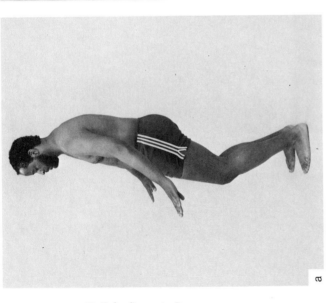

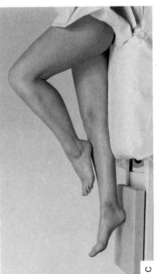

c

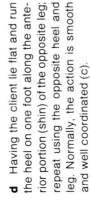
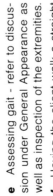

d

d Having the client lie flat and run the heel on one foot along the anterior portion (shin) of the opposite leg; repeat using the opposite heel and leg. Normally, the action is smooth and well coordinated (c).

e Assessing gait - refer to discussion under General Appearance as well as inspection of the extremities.

f Having the client walk a straight line, placing the heel of the leading foot against the toe of the foot that follows (d).

Highlights

Refer to discussion under inspection of the extremities for a discussion of the Romberg test.

Refer to discussion under inspection which describes nerves that innervate the extremities.

PHYSICAL EXAMINATION

To test *sensory function* (e.g., pain, vibration, touch, temperature) the entire skin surface need not be evaluated. However, without forming a specific pattern, the dermatomes and major nerves should be tested.

Light touch: The examiner brushes a piece of cotton or soft brush on the client's skin. The client tells when and where he or she feels the cotton. Light touch is transmitted by both anterior spinothalamic tracts.

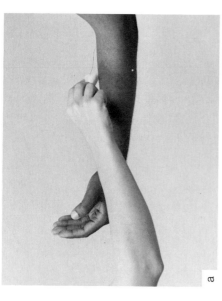

Temperature: Using hot and cold tubes of water, the examiner asks the client to identify the temperature perceived as tubes are placed against the skin. The client is asked to distinguish sensation by telling the examiner that the temperature is "hot" or "cold" (b). Again, various points on the extremities are tested. Normally, the client should be able to distinguish the stimuli at the location where applied.

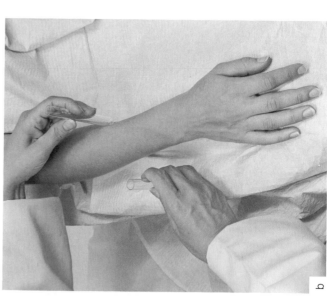

Temperature perception is tested by having the client distinguish between hot and cold.

Testing sensory function is highly dependent upon the client's perception of the stimuli.

Highlights

There are three tests of tactile discrimination:

    a. Stereognosis
    b. Two point discrimination
    c. Extinction

Graphesthesia - the client's ability to perceive a number or letter as outlined in the individual's hand by an examiner.

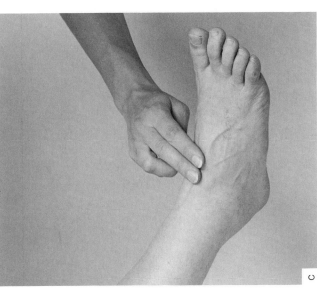

b

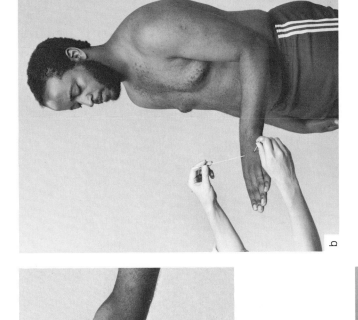

a

c

Tactile discrimination: involves the integration of cortex. Three tests are used to evaluate this integration which involve different action of the sensory system.

a *Stereognosis* - is the ability to recognize an object by touching and handling it. Objects used to test this function should be familiar to the client. (e.g. a coin). The client closes the eyes, and the examiner places the object into the hands (a). The client is instructed to correctly identify the object.

b *Two point discrimination* - involves the individual's ability to discriminate whether one or more areas of the skin are being stimulated at the same time (b). To test this function a pin or other item may be used. The client, with eyes closed, is asked if he or she perceives stimulus at one or more points of the body. Normally, this action will be perceived correctly.

c *Extinction* can be assessed by having the client close both eyes. The examiner touches the client using a light brushing action (e.g., on the back of hands, arm, feet, etc.) and the client reports the side touched (c).

Highlights

The client should be able to differentiate painful stimuli and their location.

Vibrations should be felt in the most distal joints.

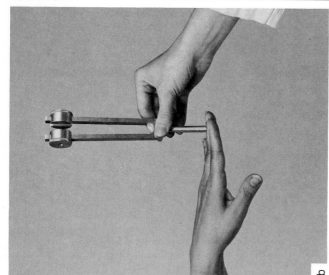

a

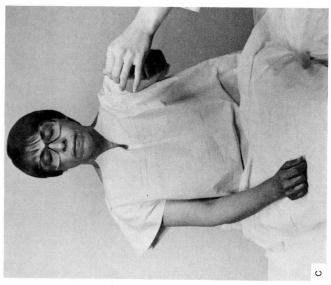

b

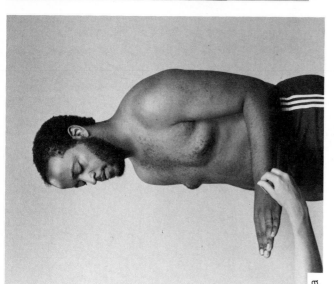

c

Pain – With a pin, the examiner pricks the client lightly on the arms and legs (a). Periodically, the dull end is used to double check accuracy of response. The examiner should determine that the client is able to differentiate sharp from dull before performing the test. The elderly may have decreased sensation in lower legs and feet as a normal aging change.

Vibration – The examiner places a vibrating 200-to-400-cycle tuning fork on the bony prominence of the most distal joints (b). After making sure the client can feel the vibration, the examiner instructs the client to report when he or she no longer feels the sensation on the joints. Often the examiner compares the clients' response to his or her own responses for accuracy. Sometimes, the examiner should stop the vibration of the fork purposefully and ask the client to note when the feeling has stopped. Vibration should be felt in the most distal joints.

Position: With the client's eyes closed, the examiner guides the thumb or great toe in an upward and downward position (c). The client should be able to identify the direction.

The examination of the *reflex system* and the functioning of the reflex arc (a) comes last. The presence of a deep tendon reflex does not indicate proper functioning of the upper motor neurons or higher sensory neurons as the previous testing has done, but rather indicates only an intact lower motor neuron functioning. Components of this process include:

1 the sensory (peripheral) nerve

2 an intact junction (synapse) in the cord

3 motor (peripheral) nerve

4 the neuromuscular junction (synapse in muscle)

5 competent muscle

Deep tendon reflexes - occur when muscles contract as the tendons are stretched. This action reflects the intactness of afferent fibers which arise from the muscle and tendon.

In order to test reflexes, the client should be comfortable and the limb relaxed with the tendon slightly stretched. Holding the reflex hammer (lightly), the examiner briskly and lightly taps the tendon or the bone (b). This tap stimulates a sensory nerve fiber which connects with the motor nerve fiber in the cord and returns to the muscle which then contracts - hence the *reflex arc*. In order to gain a better understanding of a normal reflex, the examiner might test the reflexes of a number of individuals. Reflexes are graded on a scale of 0 to 4+ (0 - ++++).

As with most findings, there is a range of normal results.

In addition to recording reflexes according to the scale, symmetry of reflex can be compared bilaterally.

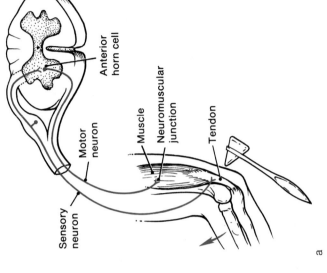

a

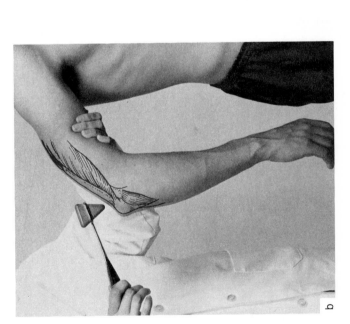

b

Highlights

Examination of the reflexes is performed at the termination of the physical examination.

Deep tendon reflex (DTR) occurs when muscles contract.

Normal reflex action is a jerking movement.

Reflexes are recorded according to a scale which ranges from 0 or no response to 4+ which equals a hyperactive response.

0 - no response

1 - somewhat diminished response; low normal (+)

2 - average, normal (++)

3 - brisker than average; does not indicate pathology (+++)

4 - hyperactive; very brisk (++++)

PHYSICAL EXAMINATION

Pectoralis reflex - can be elicited with the client sitting and holding the arm 6" from the body. The examiner elicits reflex in the shoulder.

Reflexes should be compared bilaterally.

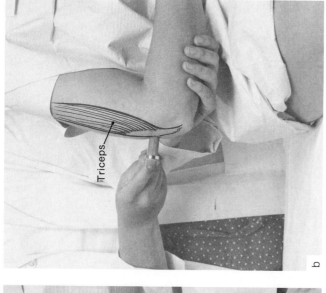

Biceps

a

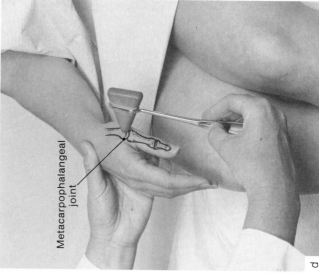

Metacarpophalangeal joint

d

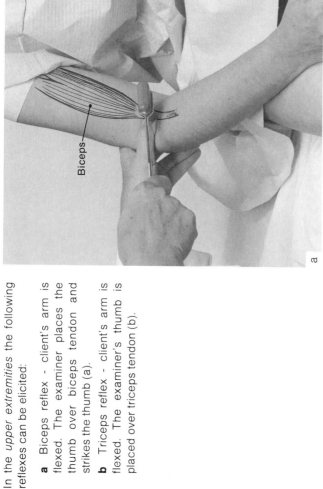

Brachioradialis

c

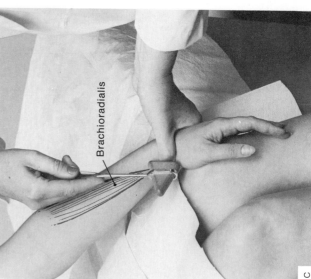

Triceps

b

In the *upper extremities* the following reflexes can be elicited:

a Biceps reflex - client's arm is flexed. The examiner places the thumb over biceps tendon and strikes the thumb (a).

b Triceps reflex - client's arm is flexed. The examiner's thumb is placed over triceps tendon (b).

c Brachioradialis reflex - client's arm is relaxed at the side or on the knee. The examiner's thumb is placed over the radius proximal to the wrist (c).

d Finger and Thumb reflex - client's wrist is relaxed and pronated; the fingertips and metacarpophalangeal joint of the thumb are tapped (d).

In the *lower extremities*:

a Patellar reflex - client is seated with legs hanging over the examining table. The tendon is located directly inferior to the patella (a).

b Plantar reflex - the sole of the client's foot is exposed and a hard object is applied along the lateral surface of the sole from heel to toe (b).

c Ankle reflex - client is seated at the side of the table. The examiner holds the forefoot with one hand, slightly dorsiflexing the foot, and strikes the achilles tendon (c).

The normal response to stimulation of a reflex is a jerking movement. Normally, this action should occur as each reflex is stimulated. In some instances, reflexes may be difficult to elicit. Attention should be paid to the position of the limb and the site at which the reflex is being tapped.

Summary

At the completion of the physical examination, the examiner instructs the client to get dressed. Following this, the examiner shares the findings of the complete health history and physical examination with the client and plans health care accordingly. When necessary, abnormal findings should be followed carefully by the medical physician for evaluation and further assessment.

Recording of all of the data accurately helps the examiner direct care and serves as a basis for further assessment and re-evaluation of the client's health status.

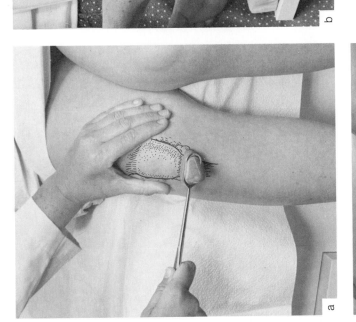

a

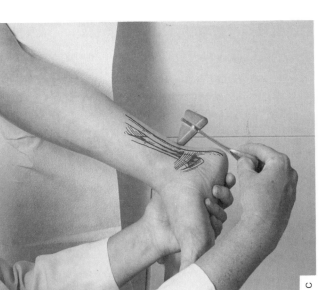

c

b

THE NEONATE CHAPTER FIVE

Phyllis A. Autotte and Mary Kolassa Lepley

The neonatal period (*neo* meaning new [Greek] and *natare* [Latin] meaning to be born) is defined as the first 28 days of life. This period is one of the most critical phases in an individual's life. Neonatal mortality is highest during the first 24 hours of life and accounts for about 40 percent of deaths under 1 year of age.[1] Infant mortality in the United States has steadily declined in the past 25 years because of medical and technological advances; however, the neonatal period continues to be the time of greatest risk (Table 5-1).

Before 1961 a premature infant was defined as a live-born infant weighing 5 lb 8 oz (2500 g) or less at birth. Increased technological advancement has demonstrated the importance of gestational age rather than weight alone as an indicator of risk in the newborn. Therefore, in 1961 the World Health Organization recommended a redefinition of terms: low birth weight was designated to mean infants weighing 5 lb 8 oz or less. Premature infants are born less than 37 weeks after the mother's last menstrual period. These definitions have also been adopted by the American Academy of Pediatrics.

Knowledge of the stages and terms of gestational classification is important in the assessment process of the newborn:

1 *Embryonic period*—the first 12 weeks of life

2 *Fetal stage*—12 weeks to term; *previable*—less than 28 weeks; *viable*—from 28 weeks on

3 *Neonatal period*—the first 28 days of life

4 *Premature*—live-born infant delivered before 37 weeks from the first day of the mother's last menstrual period

5 *Low birth weight*—infant weighing under 5 lb 8 oz

6 *Term*—all infants born with gestational ages from 38 completed weeks up to, but not including, 42 completed weeks

Nurses have a major responsibility in the delivery of health care to neonates.

Gestation refers to the period of pregnancy; the average length of human gestation is 280 days, or 40 weeks.

Table 5-1
Infant Mortality by Age and Color in the United States*

Year	Total			White			All Other		
	<1 yr	<28 days	28 days–11 mo	<1 yr	<28 days	28 days–11 mo	<1 yr	<28 days	28 days–11 mo
1976 (est)	15.1	10.7	4.4	13.4	9.5	3.9	22.1	15.4	6.7
1975	16.1	11.6	4.5	14.2	10.4	3.8	24.2	16.8	7.5
1974	16.7	12.3	4.4	14.8	11.1	3.7	24.9	17.2	7.7
1973	17.7	13.0	4.8	15.8	11.8	3.9	26.2	17.9	8.3
1972†	18.5	13.6	4.8	16.4	12.4	4.0	27.7	19.2	8.5
1971	19.1	14.2	4.9	17.1	13.0	4.0	28.5	19.6	8.9
1970	20.0	15.1	4.9	17.8	13.8	4.0	30.9	21.4	9.5
1960	26.0	18.7	7.3	22.9	17.2	5.7	43.2	26.9	16.4
1950	29.2	20.5	8.7	26.8	19.4	7.4	44.5	27.5	16.9

*For 1976, based on a 10% sample of deaths; for all other years, based on final data. Rates per 1000 live births.
†Based on a 50% sample of deaths.
Source: M. Wegman, "Annual Summary of Vital Statistics—1976," *Pediatrics,* **60:**803 (December 1977). Reprinted with permission.

7 *Preterm*—all infants born before 38 completed weeks

8 *Postterm*—all infants born after 41 completed weeks

THE HEALTH HISTORY

The traditional approach to assessment of the newborn consists of determining health risks and looking for physical problems. The holistic approach does not seek the deficits in the newborn but focuses on each baby's strengths. Health care providers have learned that neonates are able to react to their environment and to elicit distinctive behaviors. They are not all alike. Interactions between baby and parents are important to the neonate's well-being. Parents are encouraged to become active participants in the care of their child and to voice concerns and observations to the nurse. The nurse thus assesses all aspects of health and views the infant as part of a dyad (single parent and infant) or triad (mother, father, and infant) in a unique family situation.

The health history format provides the nurse with a very powerful tool with which to assess the neonate from a multifaceted focus. The individual is seen as a complex of body, mind, and spirit brought into a united whole. The neonate health history provides information for a data base which can be used as a comparison on future visits to a particular health care provider. It emphasizes positive elements which provide for the neonate's well-being, including physical and psychosocial factors and risk factors which could be detrimental to health.

Approach to the Neonate

The interview is the beginning of a trusting relationship between the nurse and the client. In the case of the neonate, most of the verbal interviewing will take place with the parents or caretakers. It is imperative that the nurse use communication skills, develop rapport, and be able to conduct the interview in an unhurried and nonjudgmental manner. Nonverbal communication and its effect on the quality of the interview must be noted. Sensitivity on the part of the nurse will help parents to feel comfortable, which will facilitate discussion of important issues as well as provide the health history information that the nurse is seeking.

See Chap. 3 for a discussion of the Interview.

Setting

The setting for the interview may occur in a hospital, birthing center, well-child clinic, physician's office, or home. Privacy and confidentiality are vital. Having the parents seated provides a comfortable atmosphere.

In the hospital setting, care should be taken to interview at a time when (1) the neonate is not due to feed, (2) the parents are not tired, and (3) visitors are not present. In obstetrical units with unconditional visiting times or provisions for rooming-in, the nurse may arrange with the parent(s) to conduct the interview at a mutually convenient time.

Refer to Chap. 3 for a discussion of the Setting.

The nurse may need to complete the interview in more than one session.

The Interview

It is possible to interview the neonate. Most of the interaction will take place through nonverbal communication on the part of the infant. The nurse must use keen observational skills during the assessment. Verbal communication occurs with the parents or caretakers. The nurse will discuss observations with the parents and encourage their feedback regarding any of their observations while caring for their neonate.

See subsequent discussions of each component of the health history.

Interviewing techniques which will be most useful to the nurse when addressing the parents include questioning, giving broad openings, encouraging description of perceptions, and offering general leads.

See Interviewing Techniques in Chap. 3.

Open-ended questions generally elicit information from the parent's point of view.

Questions to elicit data

1 What can you tell me about your baby?

2 How were your labor and delivery?

3 What kinds of experiences have you had with your baby?

Direct questions resulting in yes or no answers should be used sparingly, since they limit the parent's response. Likewise, the nurse should avoid giving yes or no answers, since they do not usually provide the parents with adequate information.

During interviews a parent will often verbalize concerns about the new baby, e.g., "Is my baby all right?" or "Is my baby acting normally?" The nurse can appropriately give information so that the parent is made aware of the neonate's unique qualities and characteristics.

See Chap. 3 for the technique of giving information.

Client Profile and Biographical Data

Biographical data are recorded by the nurse. The parents' marital status, religion, occupation, and Social Security numbers are recorded, since these data may be important factors in health care of the neonate.

See Biographical Data in Chap. 3.

The parents are further questioned on the reason for bringing the neonate into the health care system. If the nurse is conducting an assessment in the immediate newborn period, the assessment is usually considered routine.

Most newborns cannot be discharged from the hospital without a completed health history.

Health Status Perception

Parents' perceptions of health are recorded next. This is significant data, since the neonate's health care directly depends on parental action. The nurse should phrase questions so that data will reveal how the parents' health beliefs will influence the care they seek for their neonate.

See Perceptions of Health in Chap. 3.

Questions to elicit data

1 Do you have a plan for routine health care for your baby?

2 Do you think you will recognize deviations from healthy behavior in your baby? How?

3 Do you have relatives or friends to turn to when you have questions about your baby's behavior?

Current Health Status and Health Habits

The parents are questioned on what they believe is their baby's current state of health.

Questions to elicit data

1 Do you think your baby is healthy? Why?

2 Describe how you think your baby was affected by labor and delivery.

3 Are you concerned about any areas of your baby's health? Describe.

4 What has your pediatrician told you about your baby?

See Health Habits in Chap. 3.

The neonate's health state can be affected by the health habits of the parents or other persons living with the baby. For example, if the parents follow habits such as personal hygiene, frequent dental checks, nutritious dietary patterns, and no smoking, then the baby will probably benefit. It is important for the nurse to assess what health habits the family follows as they relate to the neonate.

Questions to elicit data

1 Do any family members smoke around the baby? Do you think this can harm the baby? How?

Smoking may be hazardous to the health of the neonate.

2 How often do you change the baby's diapers? How often do you bathe the baby?

3 When do you change the baby's clothes?

4 How often do you wash the baby's feeding items and utensils (such as bottles, nipples, or spoons)?

5 Do you wash items that the baby mouths or sucks on after the items have dropped on the floor?

If the parents or caretakers are unaware of the effects of certain health habits on the neonate, this should be noted during the assessment.

Past Health Status

Data are collected about the prenatal, natal, and postnatal periods. Information will aid in the assessment of the adequacy of the mother's and the neonate's state during pregnancy and the neonate's adaptation to the extrauterine environment.

See Past Health Status in Chap. 3.

Questions to elicit data

Adapt questions to fit the age of the neonate.

Prenatal History

1 What was the pregnancy like? Easy or difficult? Any complications?

2 What is the mother's age and parity, and what were the outcomes of other pregnancies?

3 Was this a planned pregnancy?

4 Did the parents attend prenatal classes in preparation for the birth?

An unplanned pregnancy can be a major stress.

5 Did the mother take any vitamins or drugs during the pregnancy?

6 What did the mother's usual diet consist of and what was her total weight gain during pregnancy?

Weight gain correlates with pregnancy outcome.

Natal History

1 Describe labor and delivery. Were there any complications?

2 Were drugs used during labor or delivery for the mother or baby?

Note length of labor and affect on fetus if known.

3 Was the father present during labor and delivery?

4 What was the condition of the neonate at birth?

5 Did the parents spend time alone with the baby after birth?

Postnatal History

1 Was the baby full term and an appropriate size for gestational age?

2 After birth, did the baby go to the newborn nursery or the intensive care nursery?

3 Did the baby go home with the mother?

4 Did the baby have any problems or complications during the postnatal period?

Neonates who are small or large for gestational age are at risk for problems.

Growth and Development Data are noted from the time of birth to present. The neonate should be gaining weight according to norms. Certain reflexes should also be present during this period. A healthy neonate will establish feeding and sleeping patterns a few days after birth.

See Growth and Development in Chap. 3.

Family History

A complete family history should be compiled. The nurse must keep in mind that neonates may exhibit varying characteristics depending on familial inheritance. For example, some babies may be born with large heads, unusual faces, or unusual behaviors which can be traced to parents or relatives.

See Family History in Chap. 3. Unusual characteristics are frequently within normal limits.

Life Pattern and Lifestyles

Age

All newborns differ in age and other characteristics as well at birth, since the length of gestation varies. A full-term baby usually has much stronger neuromuscular development and more mature reflexes, for example, than a 35-week-gestation baby. Therefore, age gives some insight into the neonate's development.

Note the neonate's chronological as well as gestational age.

Mortality risks also vary with age. The neonate is at the greatest risk for death the first 24 hours of life. Thereafter, the mortality risk declines; however, the greatest number of infant deaths in the United States occurs during the neonatal period. The nurse should assess both chronological and gestational age.

Race

Racial characteristics manifest themselves in a variety of ways, such as the infant's birth weight, rate of growth and development, shape of eyes, and color of skin. Therefore, it is important for the nurse to ask the parents what their race is and how they believe it will affect their baby's health.

See Race in Chap. 3.

Heredity

It is important for the nurse to assess the neonate's heredity, since early detection of problems or confirmation of a normal condition is critical to the neonate's adaptation to life and the family's adjustment to the neonate. Family history data should be recalled by the nurse before questioning about heredity, since these data provide the basis for further inquiry.

See Family History.

The physical examination may confirm the presence of hereditary factors.

1 Do you recognize any family traits in your baby? Describe.

2 Has your baby been diagnosed as having any genetic disorder?

3 Do you think your baby might have any physical or mental defect? Why?

4 What characteristics do you think your baby has inherited from you or any member of your family?

If the nurse detects that the parents are uncomfortable or concerned about responses to questions, this should be noted.

Culture

The birth of a child means different things to people in various cultures. The roles of the father and mother, expectations about the baby, and participation in the care of the baby may be viewed in a variety of acceptable ways. The nurse must determine if there are cultural influences on the parents or caretakers which may affect the health care of the neonate.

Questions to elicit data

1 What does the birth of a child mean to this particular family?

2 Was the father a direct participant during pregnancy and labor and delivery?

The nurse will need to adapt questions to clients of particular cultures.

3 Who will participate in the care and feeding of the child?

4 If the mother is a single parent, what kinds of support systems will be available to her? Who will care for the infant?

5 Who is the disciplinarian in the family? Will this role be shared? What kinds of discipline will be used?

6 How do the parents respond to a crying baby?

Growth and Development

Assessment of growth and development is imperative in the neonatal period to provide baseline data for further serial evaluations as the child grows and develops. Developmental tasks to be accomplished in the first month of life include regulating body temperature in the immediate newborn period, acquiring feeding skills through rooting and sucking reflexes, and acquiring motor skills beginning with head control. The neonate also responds to the environment through visual, auditory, tactile, and taste senses and communicates needs by crying.

See Growth and Development in Chap. 3.

Data collected during physical examination will include areas of growth and development.

The nurse should complete the assessment by involving the parents as much as possible. Since the first month of life is crucial for the neonate and parents to come to know and adjust to one another, the parent's involvement in the assessment process fosters their interest in, and realistic expectations of, their baby.

Physical Capabilities The nurse should assess physical capabilities by questioning the parents and through physical examination. It is important to recall that neonates exhibit a wide range of normal capabilities for a given age. For example, a particular 1-week-old baby may have a strong sucking reflex and breast-feed vigorously, while another may not.

See Physical Examination.

Cognitive Capabilities The nurse should assess cognitive capabilities by noting the neonate's alertness and responses to stimuli in the environment. Since this is a somewhat limited assessment, the nurse must avoid making predictions to parents about future capabilities. Most important, the nurse should assess that the baby (1) regards a human face, (2) is visually alert to bright-colored objects and light, and (3) is auditorily responsive to sounds, e.g., the ringing of a bell.

Highlights

Additional data about cognitive abilities will be noted throughout the physical examination.

Social Capabilities Social capabilities are manifested in the neonate's ability to relate to human interaction. The nurse should note that the baby (1) vocalizes without crying and (2) regards a human face. Some babies will also smile responsively or spontaneously by the end of the first month, and this should be noted.

Emotional Capabilities Emotional capabilities are often difficult to evaluate in the neonate, since the crying state is so predominant during the first month.

See Behavioral Development.

Questions to elicit data

1 Does your baby cuddle when held close?

2 Does your baby stop crying when held, talked to, and cuddled?

3 Does your baby appear satisfied after feedings?

4 Does your baby sleep between feedings? For how long?

5 Do you think your baby is easily frustrated? When?

6 How does your baby seek consolation?

7 Do you give your baby a pacifier? Does your baby like to suck for long periods?

Answers to these questions will increase the nurse's perception of the neonate's ability to cope with the environment and human contact.

Behavioral Development

When assessing behavior in the neonate, the nurse must consider behaviors related to (1) feeding, elimination, and sleep, (2) coping with internal and external stimuli, (3) attachment patterns, and (4) overall adjustment to the extrauterine environment.

Results of studies on neonates and infants have disproved many of the myths once held by parents and health care professionals. Some myths held that a baby was totally dependent on the environment for meeting needs, could not see, hear, or recognize objects for several months, and did not know how to adapt to the environment; another myth held that all babies were alike.[2]

T. Berry Brazelton, a pediatrician and expert in child development, is a pioneer in the assessment of newborn behavior. The result of his work, the Brazelton Neonatal Behavioral Assessment Scale, is an excellent tool for evaluating behavior of a newborn. It can provide important information about the neonate's behavioral patterns, interactions with the environment, and development of attachment behavior with the mother. The scale specifically measures 27 items, including the neonate's neurological capacities, responses to certain stimuli, social behaviors, and self-quieting abilities. It may be used to 1 month of age.[3]

Feeding, elimination, and sleep-wakefulness patterns are also part of behavioral assessment. The nurse can refer to data collected during the assessment of biological rhythms.

Attachment patterns refer to the responses which result from interactions between the neonate and parents or other significant caretakers.

The neonate's sensory capacities and potential for interactive behaviors can be evaluated using Brazelton's scale.

Most studies about attachment have looked at the mother and neonate. Attachment patterns may significantly affect the neonate's physical, psychological, and social growth and development.

According to Klaus, maternal attachment proceeds as follows:[4]

1 Planning the pregnancy
2 Confirming the pregnancy
3 Feeling fetal movement
4 Giving birth
5 Seeing the baby
6 Touching the baby
7 Caretaking

Once the baby is delivered, the most useful way to assess attachment is to observe the reciprocal relationship of the mother and her infant.

Touching has been described by Rubin.[5] Mothers show an orderly progression in the way they explore their infants on first tactile contact. Mothers progress from fingertip touch to palm contact, cradling in the arms, and enfoldment next to the body.

Verbal and visual responses by the mother are also important for stimulating the neonate and facilitating interaction. Studies done by Robson demonstrated that eye-to-eye contact between mother and baby provides the mother with a means for identifying characteristics of her baby and facilitates the attachment.[6]

The nurse will find that the most accurate means of assessing behavior patterns and responses is through actual observation during the data-collection process.

Biological Rhythms

Studies have been done on the neonate's adaptation to biological rhythms, especially the 24-hour circadian rhythm. Hellbrügge has demonstrated that (1) physiological functions develop day and night rhythms independently from each other, (2) day and night rhythms of the different functions become apparent at different times after birth, and (3) the child's maturity at birth is vital for the development of day and night rhythms.[7]

See Table 3-4.

Each baby will develop a unique circadian cycle.

Sleep-Wakefulness Cycle Sleep patterns in the neonate can be a source of parental concern. The evolution of a 24-hour sleep-wakefulness cycle is a developmental task for the neonate and is based on intrinsic rather than extrinsic factors.

Studies on sleep patterns of neonates have shown the existence of wakefulness and basic rest-activity cycles immediately after birth.[8] During the second week of life the day-night periodicity of sleep-wakefulness cycles becomes independent of feeding schedules, and an adult-type sleep pattern appears at about 3 months of age.[9,10]

Battle has demonstrated that sleep contains two cycles: a quiet period with no body or eye movements and an active period of body and rapid eye movements (REM).[11] The REM phase is associated with dreaming. The duration of a sleep cycle is about 90 minutes in the adult and 60 minutes in the normal newborn.

Parmalee and associates have reported that during the first month of life the average neonate spends 15 to 17 hours a day sleeping, with the average sleep period being little more than 4 hours.[12] The longest periods of wakefulness range from 2.39 hours the first week to 3 hours the fourth week.

Parents can be taught to observe the sleep cycles of their baby and use awake times for both feeding and learning.

All authors agree that the establishment of a diurnal cycle of sleep-wakefulness with more sleep at night is related to central nervous system maturity and that a day-night schedule develops later in premature infants than in full-term newborns.

The nurse should assess the neonate's sleep-wakefulness cycle by questioning the parents.

Questions to elicit data

1 How many hours a day does your baby sleep?
2 What is the average length of time of a sleep cycle?
3 What behaviors have you observed as the baby sleeps?
4 What does your baby do while awake?

These data will be incorporated into the total assessment of biological rhythms.

Elimination Patterns Meconium is a thick, greenish black stool composed primarily of cast-off epithelial cells, some secretions from the digestive glands, and swallowed amniotic fluid. Meconium is usually eliminated during the first 24 hours after birth, although passage may be delayed up to 48 hours.[13] Once milk feedings are established, meconium is replaced by transitional greenish brown stools which may contain milk curds. After 3 or 4 days, mild yellow stools are formed. The frequency of stooling in the newborn is closely related to the number of times the baby is fed. Breast-fed babies may have more frequent stools than formula-fed babies. Five to seven stools a day is normal.

Meconium stool is usually eliminated in the first 24 hours after birth.

The newborn usually urinates immediately after birth or shortly thereafter. Kidney function is immature, and the normal neonate's urine contains small amounts of glucose or albumin during the first few days. The first signs of diurnal rhythm in urine excretion occur during the second and third weeks after birth.[14]

To ensure thorough data collection, the nurse should review birth records for elimination patterns in the immediate newborn period. Thereafter, the parents should be questioned about the neonate's usual pattern of urination and stooling.

Questions to elicit data

1 How many wet diapers do you change in a 24-hour period? How many stools does this include?
2 What color is the urine? Does it have an odor? Describe.
3 Does your baby have a strong stream of urine or a dribble?
4 What color are the baby's stools? What is the consistency? Describe the odor.

Assessment of elimination patterns is important to the total evaluation of the neonate's health state.

Temperature At delivery the newborn's body temperature is likely to be the same as the mother's. After delivery there is a transient fall in temperature which is usually resolved in 4 to 8 hours.[15] Because of the initial lability of the neonate's heat-restoring mechanism, special care must be taken to prevent chilling or overheating. Since sweat glands do not begin to function until 1 month of age, the neonate must not be allowed to overheat. Smaller babies have a greater likelihood for labile temperature reactions.

Hellbrügge has shown that up until the fourth week of life, there is little variation in day and night body temperature.[16] After 1 month of age the temperature is higher in the day and lower at night.

Questions to elicit data

1 Do you know how to take your baby's temperature?

2 How do you know if your baby is too warm or too cold other than measuring with a thermometer?

3 How do you judge the amount of clothing to put on your baby?

4 What do you do when your baby is too warm? Too cold?

5 Do you think body temperature influences your baby's health? How?

Metabolic Rhythms Heart rate, respiratory rate, and blood pressure are metabolic rhythms that should be assessed in the neonate during physical examination.

Metabolic rhythms are noted during the physical examination.

During the first 3 weeks after delivery, there is no day-night rhythm to the neonate's heart rate. From the sixth week on the heart rate is lower at night than in the day.[17] The heart rate at birth varies from 100 to 180 beats per minute and stabilizes shortly afterward to 120 to 140 beats per minute. The neonate's respiratory rate varies from 30 to 50 breaths per minute. The blood pressure at birth is about 60 to 90 mmHg systolic and 6 to 20 mmHg diastolic. Both pressures usually rise 2 to 3 mm Hg per year of age.[18]

Parents may notice variations in their baby's breathing patterns, and this should be assessed by the nurse.

Questions to elicit data

1 Do you observe your baby's breathing pattern?

2 Do you ever note changes in your baby's breathing? When? Describe these changes.

3 How do you know if your baby is breathing normally?

The parents' ability to describe to the nurse the neonate's breathing pattern is important to current and future health assessments.

Environmental Factors

The environment of the neonate will affect adjustment to extrauterine life, maturation, and sensorimotor development and thus health care. An infant who is given a safe, comfortable, reasonably clean, and stimulating environment in which to grow and develop will most likely mature quite well. Possible detriments could be a household in which both parents smoke, unsanitary conditions, or the lack of any toys or objects to stimulate vision, hearing, and motor coordination.

If possible, the nurse should make a home visit to assess the neonate's home environment.

Questions to elicit data

1 Where does the family live (home, apartment, motel)?

2 Does the baby sleep in a separate room?

3 Are laundry facilities available?

The nurse may think of additional questions based on answers to these questions.

4 If used, how are bottles cleaned?

5 When traveling, is the baby placed in a car seat?

6 What kinds of objects are used as play things for the baby? Is a mobile hung over the crib? Are rattles and colorful objects used?

Assessment of potential noxious factors in the neonate's environment is necessary to maintain wellness and eliminate threats to health (see Chap. 3).

Questions to elicit data

1 Do you provide a quiet sleeping area for your baby?

2 How do you protect your baby from loud noises and air pollution?

3 How do you protect your baby from sun exposure?

4 Do you use a humidifier in your home or the baby's room?

5 Is the baby exposed to any type of smoking?

Other potential noxious factors discovered during the assessment should be noted.

Economics

The parents' economic status may directly affect their ability to purchase food, clothing, shelter, and health care for their baby. Therefore, the nurse should thoroughly assess the family's economic situation (see Chap. 3).

See Economics in Chap. 3.

Questions to elicit data

1 Is the birth of this baby a financial burden? Describe.

2 How will you manage with the addition of the baby? Do you have a budget?

3 Can you afford health care for your baby? How frequently? Do you have health care insurance?

4 Have you paid your bill for labor and delivery and nursery costs since the baby's birth? How much of this bill was covered by insurance?

The nurse should complete the economic assessment by making a final determination of the family's ability to continue to provide health care for the neonate based on their economic situation.

Community Resources

It is important to the neonate's well-being that the nurse assess the availability and parental use of community resources.

See Community Resources in Chap. 3.

Questions to elicit data

1 Did a public health nurse visit after you came home from the hospital with your new baby? If so, was it helpful?

2 Have you contacted La Leche League to help you with breastfeeding?

3 Do you know of any organizations that provide services to parents of new babies?

4 Do you know of a neighborhood health care clinic close to your home? Would you ever use it for your baby?

Highlights

If the parents or caretakers are unaware of available community resources, the nurse should note this during assessment.

Roles and Relationships

Family Life

A new baby brings joy to most parents and usually requires that they change or adapt their lifestyles and roles to accommodate the addition. The birth of a baby is frequently a crisis for the family as well. Stress and turmoil may exist until each family member learns to adjust to the neonate and to new roles and responsibilities. The nurse will want to assess family life in areas that will affect the health care of the neonate.

See Family Life in Chaps. 2 and 3.

Questions to elicit data

1 Does each family member spend time with the baby? How?

2 Do persons outside the family care for the baby? What directions do you give them?

3 How do you think your life has changed since the baby came home?

4 What new responsibilities do you have for the baby?

5 Do you ever feel frustrated when having to care for the baby?

These questions are in addition to those given in Chap. 3.

The information derived from questioning may provide insight into how the parents relate to the baby, which can have a secondary effect on the neonate's growth, development, and maturation.

Occupation

The parents' occupation and financial status may affect their ability to purchase health care for their neonate. Also, the time spent in an occupation will determine just how much time the parents are able to spend with their baby. This may influence the amount and type of stimulation provided to the baby and possibly some areas of neonatal growth and development. The nurse should determine how the parents' occupations will affect the neonate's health care.

Questions to elicit data

1 If the mother works outside the home, when will she return to work?

2 If the mother is breast-feeding, will she be able to continue?

3 Who will care for the baby if both parents work?

4 What are the health hazards related to the parents' occupations?

5 What kinds of stresses are related to the parents' work?

6 How do parents spend their time with the baby when home from work?

See Chap. 3, for additional questions about occupation.

Societal Relationships

The neonate's health may be indirectly affected by societal characteristics which influence the parents (see Chap. 3).

See Societal Characteristics in Chap. 3.

Sensory Perception

All five of the neonate's senses are functioning at birth. The three which can be readily assessed are vision, hearing, and touch.

Questions to elicit data

1 Have you noticed that your baby focuses on an object or looks for objects?

2 Does your baby respond to loud noises or various sounds by being startled or crying?

3 Does your baby turn toward the direction of sounds?

4 Has your baby had any ear infections?

5 How does your baby respond to touch? Do you stimulate your baby with various textures or skin-to-skin contact?

6 Do you think your baby is sensitive to pain? Why?

Education

The education of the neonate is influenced directly by the parents and indirectly by the environment. For the neonate to learn to vocalize, socialize, and interact with and manipulate the environment, human interaction is necessary.

Parents and caretakers must recognize that the neonate is sensitive to and aware of the world and responsive to it. The newborn learns when to expect food, to distinguish people from objects, and to discriminate the breast nipple from surrounding skin or a bottle. Sensory powers are quite well developed in this first month of life, and the newborn can focus on and follow an object, feel changes in temperature and touch, and distinguish tastes. For the neonate to build on these characteristics, however, parents and caretakers must provide additional stimulation through learning experiences.

Also, the educational level of the neonate's parents will usually influence the care given to the baby and subsequent growth and development. For example, if a mother has learned that talking to her baby will provide visual and auditory stimulation and promote vocalization, the neonate's development will probably be enhanced.

In assessing education the nurse must evaluate the neonate's learning capabilities, what learning experiences are provided for the neonate, and the parents' educational level (see Chap. 3).

See Education in Chap. 3.

It is a myth that the newborn's world is one of confusion. The newborn has the ability to explore and respond to the people and things in the environment.

See Chap. 3 for questions used in eliciting data about education.

Questions to elicit data

1 What types of stimulation are provided to the baby? How does the baby respond?

2 Do you have a mobile hanging over your baby's crib? Does the baby look at it? Does the baby try to touch it?

3 What toys do you use with the baby?

4 How does the baby react to bright colors and noises?

5 Do you cuddle the baby during feedings? Are you breast-feeding?

6 Does the baby focus on your face?

7 What do you think you can teach your baby during this first month of life?

Since there are no tests for evaluating neonatal intellectual ability, the nurse must determine if the baby is responding appropriately to cues given through the environment. An alert, responsive, and happy baby is more than likely receiving adequate educational stimulation. On the other hand, if the baby does not appear alert and responsive, the nurse must determine if the parents or caretakers are providing learning experiences. The nurse must further assess the parents' own educational needs as they relate to care of their baby.

Intelligence

Intelligence is a multifaceted concept of mental capacity. Intelligence includes abstract thinking, visual and auditory memory, causal reasoning, verbal expression, manipulative capacities, and spatial comprehension.[19] In the neonate, intelligence is manifested in motor skills and behavioral reactions in response to sensory experiences.

Piaget's theory of cognitive development places the neonate in phase I of the sensorimotor stage.[20,21] In this phase, operations are at the reflex level, such as rooting, sucking, and swallowing. There is no past or future for the neonate, and awareness of sensations occurs only at the time they are experienced. The neonate has no knowledge of space between self and objects or of causality. Egocentricity predominates, and crying causes needs to be filled.

Environmental factors greatly influence the development of intelligence, which determines the effectiveness of the child's learning. The nurse should stress the importance of early stimulation for the neonate such as touching, holding, cuddling, rocking, and being talked to.

Research indicates that good nutrition prenatally and postnatally is critical to the attainment of intellectual potential.

When assessing the neonate's intelligence, the nurse should evaluate neurological responses, vision, and hearing. This part of the assessment is done during the physical examination. Behavioral responses provide additional data during behavioral assessment.

Questions to elicit data

1 Does your baby watch brightly colored mobiles or objects?
2 How does your baby respond to voices and other sounds?
3 Does your baby have strong sucking and grasp reflexes?
4 Does your baby enjoy the bath?
5 Does your baby vocalize? When? How?
6 Does your baby enjoy skin contact?

After completing questioning, the nurse should explain to parents that data indicate only early intellectual capabilities and that intellectual development will, of course, continue over time.

Sexuality Patterns

The neonate's sex is important for health reasons and also for shaping parental responses. Sexual identity and sexuality are influenced by genetic endowment, culture, and parental attitudes.

See Sex and Sexuality in Chaps. 1 and 2.

Studies indicate differences between male and female neonates. Males have greater muscular strength, lower basal skin conductance, and slower speech development than females. Also, males appear to be more physically active and rigorous and seem to cry more. Such characteristics can influence how the nurse evaluates growth and development. Also, parents must be made aware of potential differences between male and female babies so that health care is not jeopardized.

The neonate's sexuality is greatly influenced by parental expectations of gender-appropriate behavior and attitudes about sexuality in general. Parents relate to their baby within this framework. For example, studies indicate that mothers talk more to female babies than male babies, which may account for females being more verbal than males. Also, parents may show preference for one sex over the other. Pleasure or dissatisfaction shown toward the baby may result from these feelings.

When assessing the sex and sexuality of the neonate, the nurse must keep in mind the above findings.

Questions to elicit data

1 Did you want a boy or girl during pregnancy?

2 Are you now happy about your baby's sex?

3 Whom do you think your baby takes after in looks and behavior?

4 Do you treat this baby differently than your other children? How?

5 Do you think a baby boy or girl is stronger physically? Does this influence how you care for your baby?

6 What expectations do you have of your baby based on sex?

The parents' responses to questions about their baby's sex and sexuality will provide important data about how the parents relate and respond to their child and how they provide for the baby's health care needs.

Nutritional Patterns

A nutritional state which supports normal growth and development is critical to neonatal well-being. An understanding of neonatal nutrition is helpful in approaching the assessment of this factor.

The healthy term neonate should receive $2\frac{1}{2}$ to 3 oz/lb per day (150 to 200 ml/kg per day) of fluids. Caloric requirements usually adequate for growth approximate 110 kcal/kg per day. If the baby is being breast-fed, the diet is considered to be nutritionally sound. In some cases, iron, vitamin D, and fluoride supplements may be recommended for the neonate. In the formula-fed infant, adequate nutrition can be provided with the use of an artificial formula such as Enfamil (Mead Johnson Laboratories), Similac (Ross Laboratories), or SMA (Wyeth Laboratories). Supplemental iron or fluoride may be necessary depending on its content in the formulas and other dietary intake. Early introduction of solid foods (such as cereal) is unnecessary in most cases. This belief is supported by the American Academy of Pediatrics. There is some scientific evidence to substantiate that overfeeding leads to obesity in infants and thus a proneness to obesity in later life. Introducing solid foods too early may cause overfeeding of the neonate.

Advantages to breast feeding are that (1) milk is sterile, (2) milk is rarely allergenic, (3) host-resistant factors including lactoferrin, lysozyme, secretory IgA, lymphocytes, and macrophages are present in significant quantities, and (4) breast-feeding is psychologically beneficial to infant and mother. Many pediatricians now recommend breast-feeding for the first 6 months of life and longer if possible.

Highlights

See Behavioral Development for further discussion of sexuality.

See Family Life, Activity, Education, and Growth and Development when assessing sex and sexuality.

In breast-fed babies, the nutritional value of the breast milk depends on the adequacy of the mother's diet.

In term neonates, a 20 calorie per fluid ounce formula is usually recommended.

Most neonates set their own feeding schedule, which is usually a 3- to 5-hour schedule.

Advantages to bottle-feeding include (1) convenience, (2) the ability to determine the neonate's exact intake, and (3) safety for the neonate if the mother has an infectious disease. Whatever the choice, the nurse should provide support and encouragement.

Nutritional state in the neonate is objectively evaluated by noting weight gain during the first month (see Physical Examination). The nurse may also ask the mother for a 24-hour recall of the number of breast-feedings (or the amounts and type of formula if bottle-feeding). The adequacy of the diet can then be assessed.

In some cases the neonate may be started on solid foods during the first month. Usually the first solid food to be introduced is rice cereal. The nurse must determine the daily amount of cereal taken, as well as milk or formula, in order to assess the neonate's caloric intake and nutritional state.

Other factors to consider in assessing nutrition are the family's nutritional patterns and how these may affect the neonate's state of health. The nurse should collect data about the family's knowledge of the components of good nutrition, the expectations of the parents regarding the neonate's feeding patterns, and if the family uses food as a reward. It is generally believed that parents who eat a well-balanced, nutritious diet will teach their children to do the same.

Exercise and Activity Patterns

During the first month of life the neonate's activity consists of daily patterns of eating, sleeping, and crying. Most motor activity is reflexive. It is important for the family to learn and adjust to the neonate's patterns so that basic needs are met. This usually requires family reorganization. Gradually the baby is incorporated as a family member.

The nurse will want to assess the neonate's patterns of activity and how the family's adjustments may affect the neonate's well-being.

Questions to elicit data

1 How would you describe your baby's daily activity?
2 How have you changed your daily activities since the baby came home?
3 What physical activities do you do with your baby?
4 Do you get adequate rest?
5 Do you spend some recreation time away from your baby?
6 Is the baby included in family activities? Describe.

Coping Patterns and Stress Tolerance

The stresses in the neonate's life are related to physical and psychological needs. The baby cries because of hunger, wetness, or a wish to be put in a different position. Babies normally have fussy periods in the early evening. This may be a time when babies release pent-up energy.

The birth of a baby is a stressful factor in the lives of each set of parents. The relationship of husband and wife will change. When there are young siblings, jealousy may occur. Family routines will be changed, and the first few weeks at home are a time of readjustment. The angelic baby during the day may become a yowling creature in the middle of the night when tired parents want to sleep.

The nurse must assess how the parents perceive the neonate's patterns of stress and responses to stressful situations as well as how the parents feel about and cope with stress in their baby.

Note growth patterns in the neonate by comparing weight and height to percentiles contained in the figures in the Physical Examination.

Using the number of calories per ounce of formula, the nurse can determine caloric intake.

See Table A-15 for a description of the basic four food groups.

Sleep periods usually last 4 to 5 hours. Alert periods will lengthen over time.

See Nutrition and Biological Rhythms.

See Chap. 3 for additional questions about exercise and activity.

The neonate experiences stress related to physical and psychological needs.

The birth of the baby and subsequent care required can be a stress for the parents.

Questions to elicit data

1 Do you think your baby is fussy? If so, why?

2 How often does your baby cry? What do you think are the reasons?

3 Does the baby's crying upset you? How?

4 How do you help your baby deal with frustration or stress?

5 Do you think that you have adjusted well to having this baby? Describe.

6 Do you think caring for your baby will become easier or harder? Why?

If parents and/or caretakers are having difficulty coping with the baby's demands and needs, this should be noted.

Highlights

Additional data on stress may be obtained from previous questions about the neonate's emotional capabilities.

Review of Body Components

A review of the neonate's body components may reveal data that will enhance the actual physical examination. For example, the nurse may ask the parent if the baby becomes startled when hearing a loud noise. Whatever the answer, the nurse would then look for a reconfirming response by examining the neonate. The nurse should question the parents systematically about each body component (see Chap. 3) until all data are collected.

See Review of Body Components in Chap. 3 when collecting data on body components.

SUMMARY

The health assessment provides a multifaceted framework for assessing the neonate by including the total interaction of physical, psychological and sociocultural patterns.

The neonate depends on parents or other caretakers for physical and psychological care as well as for entry into the health care system. Results of studies have demonstrated that the first month of life is when foundations are laid down for the individual's well-being. Each neonate is unique, and individual traits are manifested early in the newborn period. Identifying the steps of the process of maternal-infant attachment as well as neonatal behavioral development are vital parts of the holistic approach.

The importance of including parents in the observation and assessment of their neonate has been emphasized. They should become active participants in the care of their child and share in the decision-making process with the health care provider.

REFERENCES

1. Vaughan Victor and R. James McKay, *Nelson's Textbook of Pediatrics,* 10th ed., Saunders, Philadelphia, 1975, p. 321.

2. Marcene Erickson, *Assessment and Management of Developmental Changes in Children.* Mosby, St. Louis, 1976, p. 49.

3. T. Berry Brazelton, *The Neonatal Behavioral Assessment Scale,* William Heineman, London, 1973.

4. Marshall Klaus and John Kennell, "Mothers Separated from Their Newborn Infants," *Pediatr Clin North Am,* **4:**1020 (November 1970).

5. Reva Rubin, "Maternal Touch," *Nurs Outlook,* **11:**830 (November 1963).

6. Kenneth Robson, "The Role of Eye to Eye Contact in Maternal-Infant Attachment," *Child Psychol Psychiatry,* **8:**25 (January 1967).

7. Theodor Hellbrügge, "The Development of Circadian Rhythms in Infants," *Cold Spring Harbor Symp Quant Biol,* **25:**321–322 (1960).

8. Robert Emde et al., "Human Wakefulness and Biological Rhythms After Birth," *Arch Gen Psychiatry,* **32:**783 (1975).

9. Hellbrügge, "Circadian Rhythms," p. 315.

10. M. B. Sterman et al., *Brain Development and Behavior.* Academic Press, New York, 1971, chap. 11.

11. Constance Battle, "Sleep and Sleep Disturbances in Young Children: Sensible Management Depends Upon Understanding," *Clin Pediatr,* **9:**675–682 (1970).

12. Arthur Parmalee et al., "Sleep Patterns of the Newborn," *Pediatr* **58:**241 (February 1961).

13. Isabel Valadian and Douglas Porter, *Physical Growth and Development from Conception to Maturity,* Little, Brown, Boston, 1977, p. 320.

14. Hellbrügge, "Circadian Rhythms," p. 320.

15. Victor, *Textbook of Pediatrics,* p. 20.

16. Hellbrügge, "Circadian Rhythms," p. 313.

17. Ibid., p. 311.

18. Lewis Barness, *Manual of Pediatric Physical Diagnosis,* Year Book Medical Publishers, Chicago, 1976, p. 17.

19. Victor, *Textbook of Pediatrics,* p. 130.

20. Jean Piaget, *The Origins of Intelligence,* M. Cook (trans.), International University Press, New York, 1952.

21. Herbert Ginsberg and Sylvia Opper, *Piaget's Theory of Intellectual Development,* Prentice-Hall, Englewood Cliffs, N. J., 1969.

22. Heinz Prechtl and David Beintema, *The Neurological Examination of the Full Term Newborn Infant,* The Spastic International Medical Publications (in association with William Heinemann), London, 1965.

23. Virginia Apgar, "A Proposal for a New Method of Evaluation of the Newborn Infant," *Curr Res Anal Anesth,* **32:**260–267 (November–December 1953).

24. Kenneth Holt, *Developmental Paediatrics,* Butterworth's, Reading, Mass., 1977, p. 55.

25. Frederick Battaglia and Lula Lubchenco, "A Practical Classification of Newborn Infants by Weight and Gestational Age," *Pediatr,* **71:**162 (February 1967).

26. Nilly Dubowitz et al., "Clinical Assessment of Gestational Age in the Newborn Infant," *J Pediatr,* **77:**1–10 (January 1970).

BIBLIOGRAPHY

Caplan, Frank: *The First Twelve Months of Life,* Bantam, New York, 1978.

DeChateau, Peter: "The Importance of the Neonatal Period for the Development of Synchrony in the Mother-Infant Dyad—A Review," *Birth and Family Journal,* 4:10–22 (Spring, 1977).

Dubowitz, Nilly: *The Neurological Assessment of the Preterm and Full-Term Newborn Infant,* Lippincott, New York, 1981.

Hunt, J. McVicker: *Intelligence and Experience.* Ronald Press, Chicago, 1961.

Hymovich, Debra: *Child and Family Development: Implications for Primary Health Care,* McGraw-Hill, New York, 1980.

Klaus, Marshall H.: *Parent-Infant Bonding,* 2d ed., St. Louis, Mosby, 1982.

Marx, Gertie F. (ed.): *Clinical Management of Mother and Newborn,* Springer-Verlag, New York, 1979.

Natalini, John: "The Human Body as a Biological Clock," *Am J Nurs,* pp. 1130–1132 (July, 1977).

Oehler, Jerri Maser: *Family Centered Neonatal Nursing Care,* Lippincott, Philadelphia, 1981.

Owen, George: "The Assessment and Recording of Measurements of Growth of Children," *Pediatrics,* 51:461–466 (March, 1973).

Schreiner, Richard L.: *Care of the Newborn,* New York, Ranen Press, 1981.

Smeriglio, Vincent L. (ed.): *Newborns and Parents: Parent-Infant Contact and Newborn Sensory Stimulation,* Lawrence Erlbaum Assoc., Hillsdale, N.J., 1981.

Thomas, Alexander, and Chess, Stella: *Temperament and Development,* Brunner and Mazel, New York, 1977.

Waechter, Eugenia, and Blake, Florence: *Nursing Care of Children,* 9th ed., Lippincott, New York, 1976.

Wieczorek, Rita Reis: *A Conceptual Approach to the Nursing of Children: Health Care From Birth through Adolescence,* Lippincott, Philadelphia, 1981.

Before the nurse examines the neonate, labor and delivery records should be reviewed for significant data which could influence the neonate's health state.

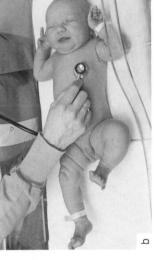

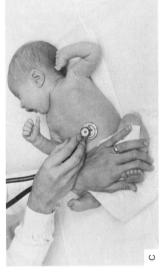

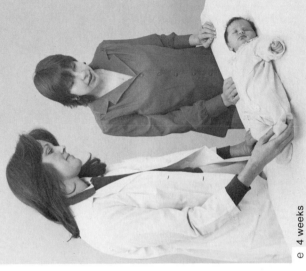

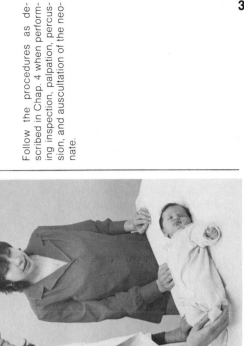

e 4 weeks

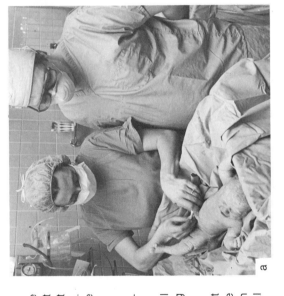

d 12 hours

PHYSICAL EXAMINATION

Within the first month of life the neonate is examined at least three times: (1) at birth (a), (2) approximately 12 hours past birth (b), and (3) at 4 weeks of age (c). During each examination the nurse should assess:

1 Each body component
2 Growth and development parameters
3 Presence of any gross congenital abnormalities (such as missing digits)

Parents should be present for at least one complete examination, since the neonate's future health depends upon the parents' understanding of normal ranges of growth and development.

The physical examination at birth includes certain assessments which are not done on subsequent examinations. These will be discussed in some detail following discussion of the examinations at 12 hours and 4 weeks, in order that the nurse may learn normal findings of a complete examination first.

EXAMINATION AT 12 HOURS AND 4 WEEKS

APPROACH TO THE EXAMINATION

After initial examination at birth, the neonate is given a thorough physical examination by the nurse (d and e). This should be an orderly, systematic process to ensure collection of all significant data related to each body component.

The sequence in which data are collected is usually cephalocaudal (head to toe); however, the actual examination may vary from this sequence due to the state of the baby and the environment.

Follow the procedures as described in Chap. 4 when performing inspection, palpation, percussion, and auscultation of the neonate.

The following guidelines should be used by the examiner preparing to examine a newborn.

1 Provide a warm environment for the neonate using, for example, an overhead radiant heater above the crib (a).

2 Time the examination so that it is performed when the neonate's general condition and vital signs are stable. The examination should be done 1 to 2 hours after feedings.

3 Have a nipple or pacifier (b) on hand to quiet the baby during potentially painful or invasive procedures.

4 Use a soft voice and gentle movements when handling the baby.

5 Approach the exam with clean and warm hands.

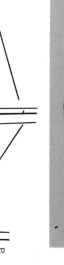

Radiant heater

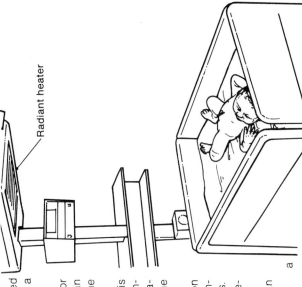

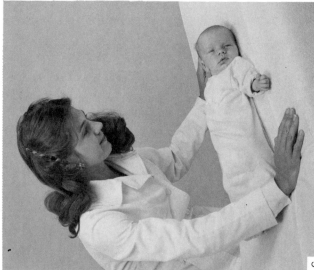

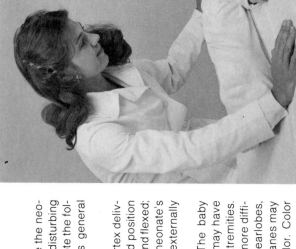

THE EXAMINATION
General Appearance

The examiner should observe the neonate before undressing or disturbing through movement (c), and note the following aspects of the baby's general appearance.

Resting Position After a vertex delivery the neonate lies in a flexed position with arms and legs adducted and flexed; after a breech delivery the neonate's thighs may be abducted and externally rotated.

Generalized Body Color The baby should be generally pink, and may have some acrocyanosis of the extremities. Dark-skinned babies may be more difficult to assess (d), but the lips, earlobes, nailbeds, and mucous membranes may also be checked for pink color. Color may be further assessed during the rest of the examination.

Symmetry of Body Parts The neonate's body parts, such as facial features and extremities, should be symmetrical.

Movements Any spontaneous movements should be noted and described.

State of Consciousness The nurse observes the neonate's state using the Schema of Prechtl and Beintema. The states are:

1 Deep sleep - eyes are closed; breathing regular; no movement (a).

2 Light sleep - eyes are closed; breathing irregular; only small movements (b).

3 Quiet alert - eyes are open but the baby is still and attentive; no large movements (c).

4 Active awake - eyes open; diffuse movement; irregular breathing; vigorous movement (d).

5 Crying - eyes partly or wholly closed; vigorous diffuse movement; crying (e).

When assessing state of consciousness, note that drowsiness is a transition state in which the baby breathes irregularly, and intermittently opens and closes the eyes. This state usually lasts no more than 3 minutes at a time.

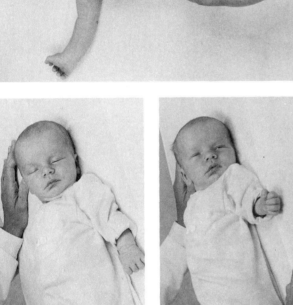

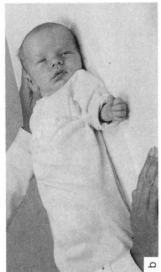

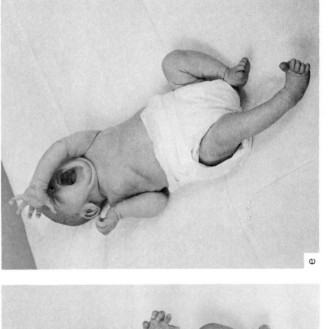

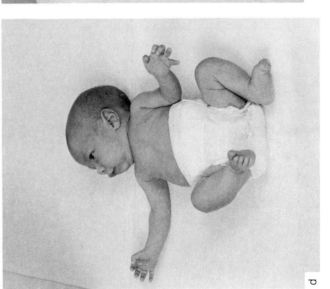

See the discussion of vital signs in the section, Examination at Birth.

After a difficult delivery, a newborn may have bruises or scratches on various parts of the body.

Acrocyanosis is localized cyanosis in peripheral locales, such as hands, feet, or nose.

Acrocyanosis and mottling of skin may normally persist for several weeks after birth.

Mongolian spots eventually disappear during childhood.

Stork bites usually disappear.

Port-wine stains are permanent birthmarks.

Photographs g and h courtesy of Meade Johnson Company.

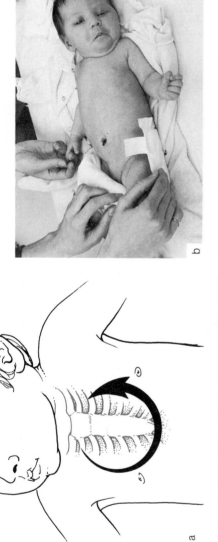

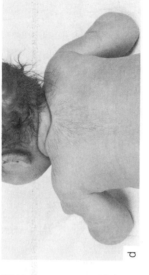

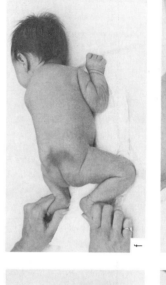

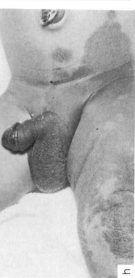

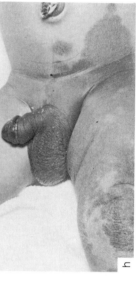

While the baby is still quiet, vital signs should be noted, since disturbing the baby may alter normal heart and respiratory rates and rhythms.

Slip in the stethoscope under the baby's shirt and auscultate the heart beginning at the upper right sternal border and moving counterclockwise (a). Auscultate the lungs, anterior and posterior over all fields.

Next, the examiner should undress the newborn, and inspect the skin in order to further assess color, and check for skin lesions (b).

Normal Variations Many variations, such as those below, are normal.

Vernix caseosa is a white, cheesy substance which protects the skin in utero, and is usually present in varying amounts at birth (c).

Lanugo is fine, downy hair most prevalent on the back and shoulders. The amount varies with gestational age (d).

Mottling of the skin is a lacelike pattern of pale and dark areas, most notably on the extremities (e).

Mongolian spots are large, nondefined, bluish-black areas of pigmentation, usually found over the lumbar region and buttocks, and most common in non-Caucasians (f).

Skin lesions or "spots" that can be seen on the healthy neonate's skin include:

Stork bites are sparse capillary hemangiomas on the upper eyelids, nose, or over the occipital protuberance (g).

Port-wine stains are dense, flat capillary hemangiomas found anywhere on the body (h).

Strawberry nevi may grow for several months, then disappear.

Petechiae are frequently caused by the pressure of labor and delivery on the neonate.

Milia disappear gradually over the first few weeks of life.

Subcutaneous fat necrosis usually disappears.

Photographs a and e courtesy of Meade Johnson Company.

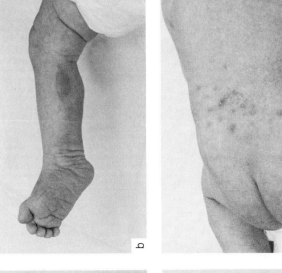

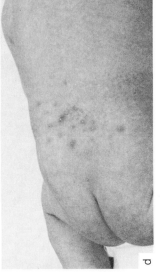

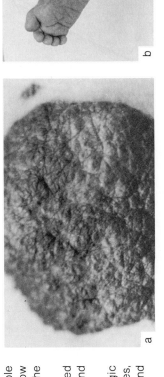

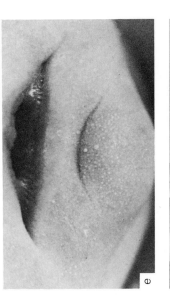

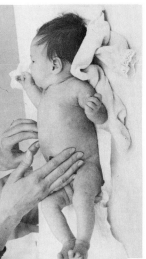

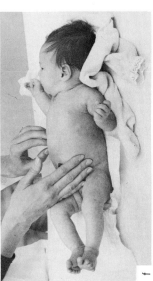

Strawberry nevi are red or purple hemangiomas which frequently grow and become raised anywhere on the body (a).

Cafe-au-lait spots are increased areas of pigmentation usually found on the trunk or extremities (b).

Petechiae are tiny hemorrhagic areas caused by ruptured capillaries, and are usually found on the face and upper trunk (c).

Erythema toxicum (or flea bite rash) is characterized by round, red lesions up to 1 cm in size with central pinpoint, white vesicles or papules. The rash disappears spontaneously (d).

Milia are fine, white spots caused by plugging of the sebaceous glands over the nose, cheeks, and trunk (e).

Subcutaneous fat necrosis is patchy hardening and swelling of subcutaneous tissues found in the scapula region and over the face or buttocks; on palpation the necrosis may feel like small, loose peas under the skin.

Palpation

The examiner should palpate the skin to determine turgor which is present in a well-hydrated neonate.

Texture is usually thin, smooth, and soft to touch, but may be scaly, with varying amounts of desquamation according to gestational age; smooth by 1 to 2 weeks of age (f).

The neonate's head is large relative to body length due to the rapid rate of brain growth during infancy.

Molding refers to the fetal head conforming to the shape of the birth canal.

Normally, two fontanelles are palpable, the anterior and posterior.

Figures a and b courtesy Meade Johnson Company

Head

The examiner should measure head circumference, inspect shape and symmetry, and palpate the sutures and fontanelles of the neonate. Any unusual findings should be noted.

Inspection

The shape and symmetry of the neonate's head (a) varies considerably according to the baby's presentation and position during labor and delivery, and the ability of the bony plates of the skull to shift during the birth process (b). The examiner should note shape through use of descriptive terms such as *elongated* or *round*. The symmetry of the head should also be described.

Palpation

The examiner should palpate sutures and fontanelles to verify their presence and to determine the degree of molding of the head. The following technique is used when palpating the head:

1 Using the index and middle fingers of the right or left hand, the examiner palpates the coronal, sagittal (c), and lambdoidal sutures (d). Overriding of cranial bones may be identified as ridges palpable along the suture lines. Widely spaced sutures may be felt if there is separation of the sutures.

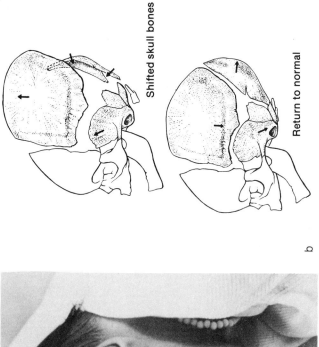

a

Shifted skull bones

Return to normal

b

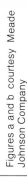

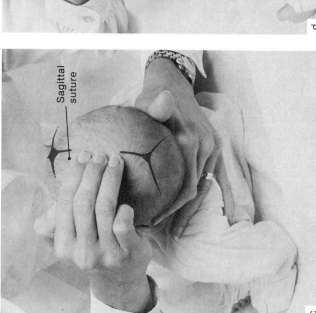

Sagittal suture

c

Lambdoidal suture

d

Fontanelle size varies considerably in the normal neonate.

The anterior fontanelle closes between 12 and 18 months of age.

A pulsating fontanelle is normal.

Crying or coughing may cause increased intracranial pressure which is reflected in a bulging fontanelle.

The posterior fontanelle closes at about 2 months of age.

Caput usually recedes 1 or 2 days after birth.

Cephalohematomas usually require weeks to recede.

Photograph e courtesy of Meade Johnson Company.

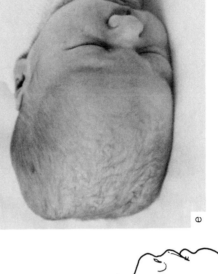

c

Coronal suture

Anterior fontanelle

Sagittal suture

Posterior fontanelle

Lambdoidal suture

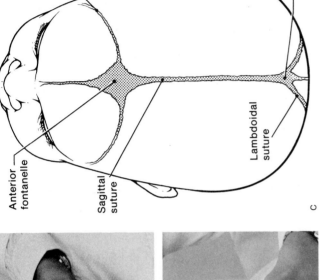

a

b

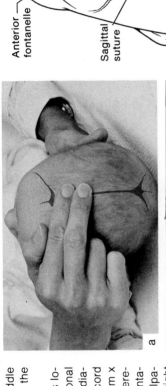

Area of edema

d

e

2 Again using the index and middle fingers, the examiner palpates for the fontanelles.

a The anterior fontanelle (a) is located at the junction of the coronal and sagittal sutures (c), and is diamond-shaped. Measure it and record the size in centimeters (e.g., 2 cm × 1.5 cm). When there is normal cerebrospinal fluid pressure, the fontanelle should feel soft and flat to palpation with the neonate in an upright position and not crying.

b The posterior fontanelle (b), located at the junction of the sagittal and lambdoidal sutures, is usually palpable. Its shape is triangular. Measurement of this fontanelle is unnecessary, unless it is abnormally large.

During inspection or palpation the examiner may identify any of the following normal variations, and these should be noted.

Caput succedaneum: Edema and congestion of subcutaneous tissue, usually over the vertex, which crosses suture lines (d).

Cephalohematoma: A subperiosteal hemorrhage which is noted as an area of swelling limited by suture lines (e).

Lacerations or abrasions: These may be found over the zygomatic arches and preauricular areas and are a result of the use of obstetric forceps during delivery.

Craniotabes: Localized softening of the cranial (usually parietal) bones. Craniotabes are small, shallow, pliable, and springy on palpation.

Face

Inspection

The examiner inspects the face of the neonate for shape and symmetry (a). When awake, the baby should appear alert and responsive. Symmetry of facial features will vary with each baby due to intrauterine position and molding of the head.

One normal variation that may be found during examination is facial (Bell's) palsy or peripheral paralysis of the facial nerve (VIIth cranial nerve). It is manifested by a drooping corner of the neonate's mouth during crying (b), and is caused by use of obstetric forceps.

Bell's palsy is a transient condition.

Hair

Inspection

The examiner inspects the hair and scalp, and notes the presence, quantity, texture, and distribution of the neonate's hair and the condition of the scalp.

The full-term baby usually has fine, silky hair that is evenly distributed over the head (c). The quantity of hair will vary with individual babies (d).

The scalp should be smooth and a normal pink color. Ecchymoses, edema, or lacerations are usually normal variations that are most often due to the delivery process. Any variations should be noted.

The quantity and color of the neonate's hair are partly determined by genetic endowment.

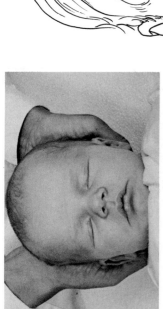

a

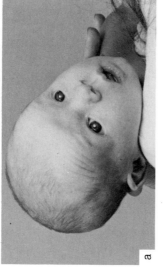

b

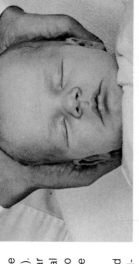

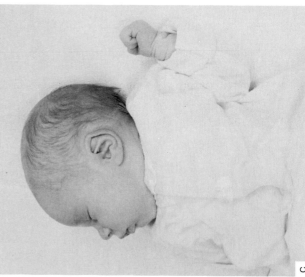

c

d

Eyes

Inspection

The examination of the neonate's eyes includes inspection of position and symmetry. The lids, including eyelashes, should be inspected, as should the tear ducts and glands; the sclera and cornea; the conjunctiva; the pupils, including reaction to light and accommodation (a); the lens; and the fundus. Extraocular movements should be tested.

In the period immediately after birth the eye examination may be delayed due to transient edema of the eyelids caused by trauma during the birth process or by the instillation of prophylactic eye treatments such as silver nitrate (b). Once edema has dissipated, the examiner may proceed.

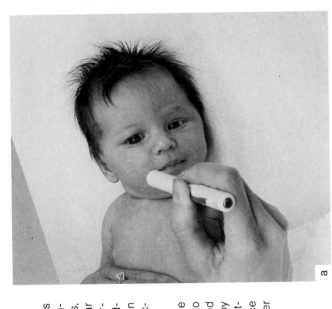

a

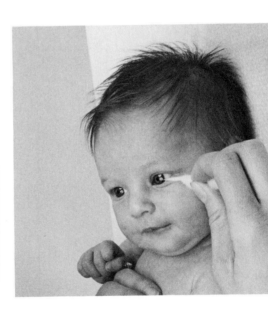

b

The lids should be movable, and lashes should be present on upper and lower lids. The tear ducts and lacrimal glands are not fully functional until 1 to 3 months of age, so tears are frequently not observed in the neonatal period.

The sclera have a bluish tint because they are thin. The cornea should be clear. The corneal reflex can be checked by touching the cornea lightly with a twirled piece of cotton and noting eye closure as a response (c).

The conjunctiva should be pale pink. The size and shape of the pupils are noted, and the pupillary reflex is checked. When a bright light is shined into the baby's eyes, the pupils should constrict.

The iris is usually deep blue in the neonate. Brushfield's spots, which are white specks around the periphery of the iris, may be present in normal neonates.

c

If the examiner has difficulty holding the neonate's eyes open, structure and function of the eyes may be more easily assessed by raising the baby's head or holding the baby upright; this will cause the eyes to open spontaneously.

The eyelids are normally fused up to the 8th month of gestation.

Episcleral and subconjunctival hemorrhages due to birth trauma may be present, and should recede spontaneously.

The final color of the iris usually develops during the first year.

THE NEONATE

The ophthalmoscopic examination of the neonate's eyes should be performed by the examiner (a). The presence of the "red reflex" is assessed. The size and color of the optic disc and macula are noted, as well as the degree of pigmentation of the retina (b). In neonates, the optic disc is frequently pale, the peripheral retinal vessels are not well developed, and the fovelar reflex is absent.

Other reflexes and normal variations to check for during the eye examination include:

Blink reflex: Elicited by shining a bright light into the eyes and observing quick closure of the eyelids.

Doll's-eye test: Performed by moving just the head of the baby in its full range of motion, and noting that the eyes remain stationary, not accommodating to the change in head position (c).

Pseudostrabismus: The neonate's eyes are not held in parallel (d).

Inner epicanthal folds: May be noted in some normal newborns (e).

Setting-sun sign: The irises deviate downward so that part of the white sclera above can be seen under the upper lid margin (f).

Vestibular function test: The examiner holds the baby at arm's length and turns the child slowly in one direction, noting that the eyes look in the direction toward which they are turned; when movement stops, the eyes look in the opposite direction following a few quick, unsustained nystagmoid movements (g).

Highlights

The examiner may need to use mydriatics in order to perform a successful fundiscopic examination of the neonate.

See Chap. 4 for a description of the ophthalmoscopic examination.

The Doll's-eye test reflects immature head-eye coordination.

Pseudostrabismus is transient and may persist to 6 months of age.

The Setting-sun sign is another transient finding in the neonate.

Nystagmoid movements refer to oscillations of the eyeballs.

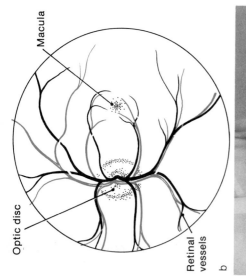

Macula

Optic disc

Retinal vessels

b

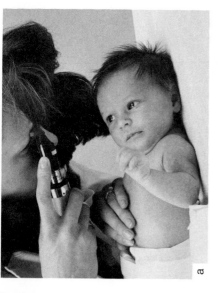

a

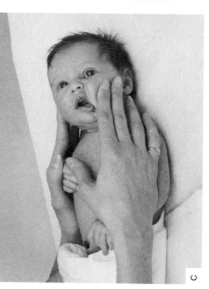

d

c

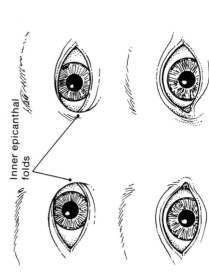

g

Inner epicanthal folds

e

f

Acquisition of normal speech and language development during the first 18 months of life is dependent upon normal hearing.

Perception of sound of various frequencies may be tested in the neonate using items such as a quiet rattle, a bell, and a high-pitched squeeze toy, and noting the neonate's responses.

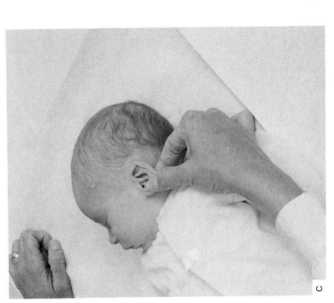

b

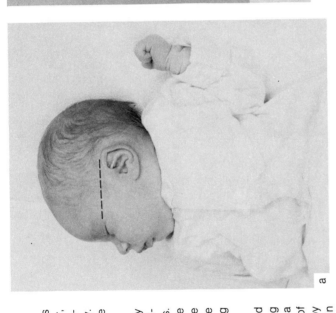

a

c

Ears

Inspection

The examination of the neonate's ears includes inspection of the external ear, external canal, and tympanic membrane, and evaluation of hearing acuity. Position and symmetry should also be assessed.

The external ears of the newborn may be flattened, but there should be well-defined curving of the pinna of both ears. Position and symmetry of the ears are assessed by drawing an imaginary line from the lateral angle of the eye to the upper pinna of the ear and noting placement (a).

Hearing may be tested by making a loud noise, such as a hand clap, and noting the neonate's response, which may be a blink or Moro reflex (b). The mother of the baby should be asked if her baby responds to her voice and to noises in the home. Ask her to describe the responses. More formal testing of hearing acuity requires special equipment and may be done by other health care providers than the nurse.

Palpation

The cartilage of the ears should be firm; recoil should be spontaneous.

The external canal may be plugged with vernix caseosa immediately after birth, but patency must be determined if possible. The examiner should gently pull the pinna away from the head and directly observe the canal (c).

Highlights

The cochlea and vestibule of the ear are anatomically mature at birth.

Otoscopic examination of the neonate is frequently unnecessary, and often postponed until 1 to 3 months of age.

Neonates are obligatory nose breathers.

The newborn can clear partially obstructed nares by sneezing.

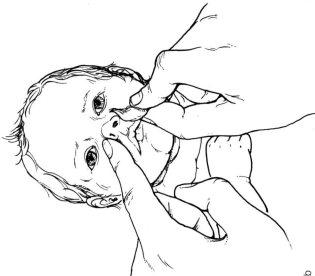

c

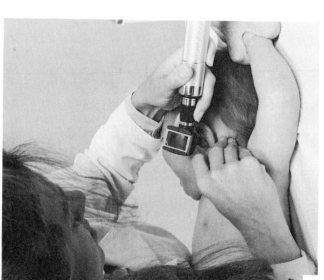

a

b

The tympanic membrane (TM) is difficult to inspect on otoscopic exam for several days past birth due to the small, short canals of the neonate, and the presence of vernix caseosa. Once the vernix has dissipated, the tympanic membrane can be observed and landmarks noted.

To see inside the ear, firmly grip the auricle of the ear and pull down to straighten the upward-curving canal of the baby. Insert the speculum and check the TM for landmarks (a).

Nose

Inspection

The nose of the neonate should be inspected for appearance, shape, patency of nares, color and consistency of mucous membranes, and the presence of any discharge.

The nose may appear flat and the bridge of the nose may be depressed in the newborn period. The examiner tests for patency of each naris by blocking off one and then the other while holding the mouth closed, and holding a piece of cotton in front of the naris (b). If the nares are patent, the cotton will move with each breath. Inhaled blood and amniotic debris may partially obscure observations, so the nose may be gently cleaned with the use of a bulb syringe (c).

Mucous membranes of the nose should be pink and moist. Any discharge coming from the nose should be noted, and the color and consistency described by the examiner.

Sinus

Inspection

The sinuses of the neonate are difficult to assess due to the immaturity of the baby and to the underdevelopment of some of the sinuses at birth. Therefore, the examiner best assesses the sinuses during the examination of the nose, noting unobstructed breathing in the neonate.

The ethmoid and maxillary sinuses are the only paranasal sinuses present at birth (a). The sphenoid and frontal sinuses develop in early childhood. Therefore, routine palpation and percussion are not done in the neonate.

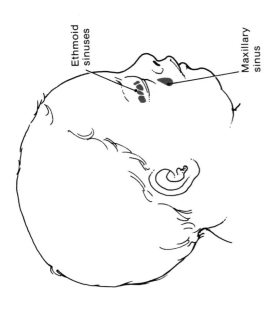

Ethmoid sinuses

Maxillary sinus

Mouth and Throat

Examination of the neonate's mouth includes inspection and palpation of the lips, buccal mucosa, gingiva (gums), hard and soft palates, tongue, posterior pharyngeal wall, and mandible. Symmetry, shape and size of the mouth are also noted.

Inspection

Lips of a normal neonate are pink and moist. A sucking tubercle may be seen in the middle of the upper lip (b). Tubercles usually disappear after weaning from the bottle or breast.

The buccal (cheek) mucosa and gingiva should be pink and moist. Teeth may be present at birth or noted as white areas under the gum line.

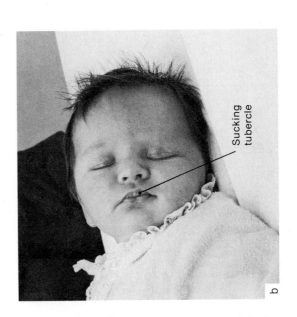

a

Sucking tubercle

b

It is usually easiest to place the neonate in a supine position and examine the mouth with the aid of a light.

The uvular of the soft palate should be midline and should move symmetrically.

The frenulum of the tongue should allow for movement in all directions.

Salivation is scant in the neonate.

The neonate's strong gag reflex can cause regurgitation of stomach contents into the pharynx; therefore, a tongue blade must be used cautiously.

Photographs a and b are courtesy of Meade Johnson Company

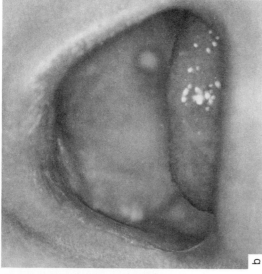

a

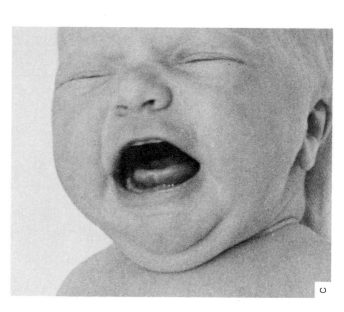

b

c

Normal variations found on examination of the neonate's mouth may include Epstein's pearls which are small, white, epithelial cysts present on the hard palate and alveolar ridge (a), and Bednar's aphthae (b), ulcers or plaques found posteriorly on either side of the midline of the hard palate. They are usually due to sucking.

The tongue of the neonate should be pink, freely movable, and uncoated. An unusually small or large tongue should be noted.

The posterior pharyngeal wall is best examined when the neonate is crying. A tongue blade may be used to depress the tongue and enhance vision. However this procedure may induce a strong gag reflex and should be done cautiously. The pharynx is pale pink and moist in the neonate and tonsillar tissue is not visible.

The size of the mandible is assessed during the examination. If it appears too large or too small in proportion to the rest of the mouth and face, this should be noted.

The healthy neonate's cry should be strong and lusty. This can be evaluated during any opportune time of the physical exam.

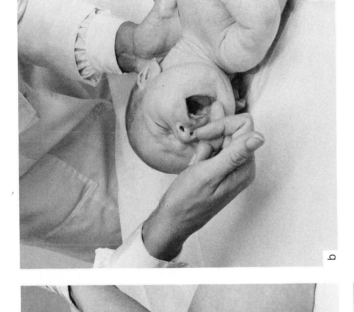

b

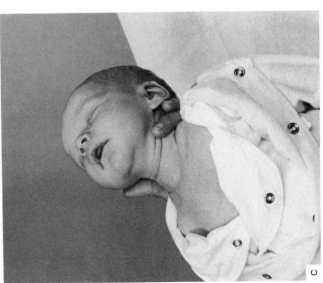

a

c

Palpation

The hard and soft palates should be intact. The examiner may palpate the hard and soft palates by placing a finger in the baby's mouth and feeling the palates as the baby sucks (a).

The rooting and sucking reflexes should be elicited as part of the examination. Their presence, quality, and strength should be evaluated. The rooting reflex is elicited by touching the corners or the middle of the upper and lower lips. The baby responds by opening the mouth and sometimes turning in the direction of the stimulus (b).

The sucking reflex is evaluated by allowing the neonate to suck on the examiner's finger. Movement of the tongue is felt to push the finger up and back. The pattern of the suck is a characteristic burst-pause cycle. Negative pressures of up to 300 mmHg may be generated by the neonate.

Neck

Inspection

Inspect the neck for position, size, symmetry, pulsations, range of motion, and control of movement.

The neck of the neonate is short in relation to the whole body, and may not be visible when the baby is lying down. The examiner may better see the neck by gently lifting the neonate's head and trunk, and allowing the head to fall back (c). The neck should be symmetrical from all angles.

Pulsations may be noted in the carotid region, but these should not be excessive.

Palpation

Palpate the neck to check the location of lymph nodes, the trachea (a), the thyroid gland, and the neck vessels and to test for muscle strength.

The range of motion of the neck including rotation, flexion, and extension, should be checked. Muscle strength can also be evaluated during this maneuver by palpating the various neck muscles. It is also important to palpate the clavicles for intactness since birth trauma may result in fractures.

The cervical lymph nodes may be palpable in the neonate, but are usually less than 5mm in diameter (b). When the trachea is palpated, the examiner should evaluate its midline position. The cartilaginous rings of the trachea may be difficult to distinguish, and so may the thyroid gland. If the examiner is successful in palpating the thyroid, its size, shape, and smoothness should be noted.

Finally, the tonic neck reflex should be checked, since it is important to the neonate's neurologic and motor development. The examiner elicits the reflex by placing the neonate in a supine position, grasping the head with one hand, and turning it to one side. The neonate's arm and leg on the side toward which the head is turned should extend, and the opposite extremities should flex (c). The maneuver should also be done in reverse. This classic fencing position may or may not be present at birth, and is a variable reflex in older neonates and infants. It should be noted if the reflex is present or absent, and if the neonate maintains the tonic neck position constantly. The neonate should demonstrate this reflex only transiently; this means that normal eye-hand coordination will be developed.

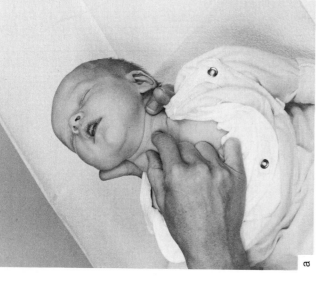

a

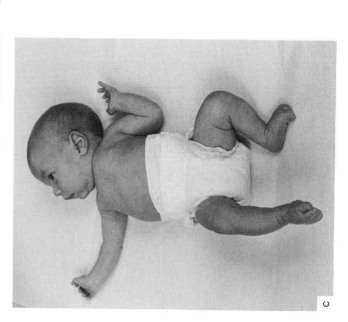

b

Lymph nodes

Thyroid

Trachea

c

Limitation of neck movement in the neonate may be due to birth trauma and hence temporary.

The full-term neonate demonstrates some degree of head control when pulled by the hands up to a sitting position.

The neck of the neonate may be palpated by using the thumb and index finger while supporting the neck and head with the opposite hand.

The tonic neck reflex peaks at 2 to 3 months of age, and should completely disappear by 6 months of age.

A neonate in the fencing position may have difficulty bringing hand to mouth, or to the midline.

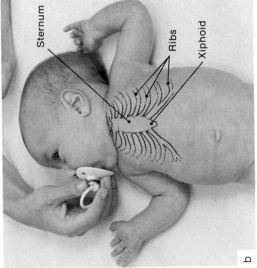

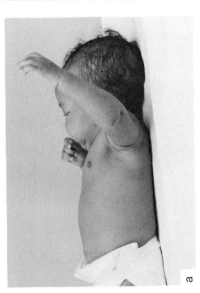

a

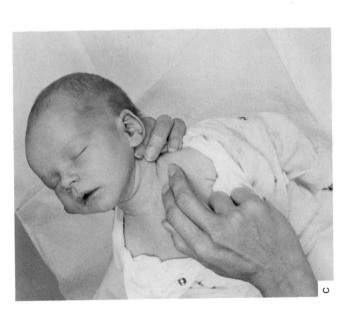

b

Sternum

Ribs

Xiphoid

c

Refer to the Apgar Score for the assessment of initial respiratory effort by the neonate and to the discussion of vital signs for assessing respirations.

Thorax

When examining the thorax of the neonate, the lungs, heart, and breasts will also be inspected, palpated, auscultated, and/or percussed.

Inspection

The chest is inspected for shape, size, and symmetry (a). The neonate's chest is round and the chest wall is relatively thin compared to the adult's. The muscles of the chest are inspected to note their presence, and normal function. The sternum and xiphoid process may be prominent beneath the skin (b). The ribs of the neonate may be noticable on deep inspiration due to the thinness of the chest wall. The movement of the diaphragm should be observed and described.

Palpation

The neonate's clavicles should be palpated for intactness and normal function. Fractures of the clavicles can occur during the birth process due to variations in the fetal position and presentation. Muscles are palpated to determine normal function and strength (c).

Lungs

Inspection

The examiner inspects the chest for lung expansion, symmetry of movements, and the quality, rate, and rhythm of the respirations. Respiratory movements should be symmetrical, abdominal, and are usually irregular in rate, rhythm, and depth during the neonatal period.

Percussion

Percussion of the lung fields is of less value to the assessment due to the small size of the neonate's chest. Localization of vibrations and percussion notes tends to be difficult.

Highlights

The examiner should auscultate with both the bell and diaphragm of the stethoscope.

Refer to the discussion on taking vital signs in the neonate.

During fetal life, circulation of blood and nutrients depends upon four distinct anatomical features: the placenta, a patent ductus venosus, a patent foramen ovale, and a patent ductus arteriosus. The placenta allows for exchange of gases, nutrients, and metabolic wastes. The ductus venosus allows part of the oxygenated blood carried via the umbilical vein to bypass the partially functional liver and proceed on into the inferior vena cava to the right side of the heart. The patent foramen ovale provides a pathway for better oxygenated blood to pass from the right to left atrium into the left ventricle where it is pumped through the aorta to the head and upper extremities. Blood returning to the right atrium and passing into the right ventricle is pumped through the pulmonary artery and then into the descending aorta via the ductus arteriosus. Very little blood flows to the nonfunctioning fetal lungs. From the descending aorta blood returns to the placenta through the umbilical arteries. With the onset of respirations and expansion of the lungs at birth, the foramen ovale, the ductus venosus, and the ductus arteriosus are functionally closed and the circulation changes from the fetal to the adult type. However, permanent anatomical closure of each may not occur until several weeks or months after birth.

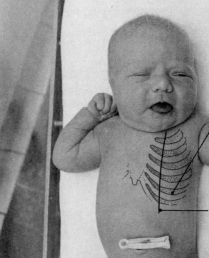

Ductus arteriosus

Foramen ovale

Lung

Inferior vena cava

Descending aorta

O₂ and nutrients

Ductus venosus

Liver

From placenta

Umbilical vein

To placenta

Umbilical arteries

c

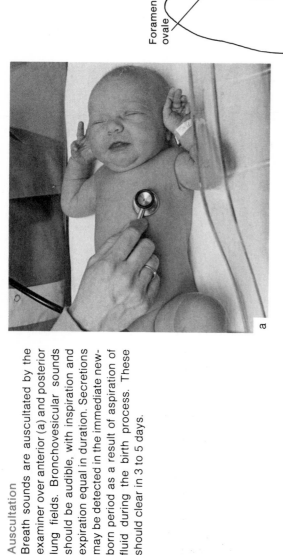

5th interspace

Midclavicular line

a

b

Auscultation

Breath sounds are auscultated by the examiner over anterior (a) and posterior lung fields. Bronchovesicular sounds should be audible, with inspiration and expiration equal in duration. Secretions may be detected in the immediate newborn period as a result of aspiration of fluid during the birth process. These should clear in 3 to 5 days.

Heart

Examination of the heart should include notation of the rate, rhythm, and size, a description of the first and second heart sounds, and palpation of peripheral pulses.

Inspection

Prior to auscultation, palpation, and percussion of the neonate's heart, the examiner inspects the neonate and notes general color, and the location of any pulsations. The baby's color should be pink, indicating adequate circulation. Dark-skinned babies may be more difficult to assess, but the lips, earlobes, nailbeds, and mucous membranes may also be checked for pink color. Pulsations may be visible in the midclavicular line toward the lateral half of the left thorax, near the 5th intercostal space (b).

The examiner must listen carefully when auscultating the heart in order to discern heart sounds from breath sounds.

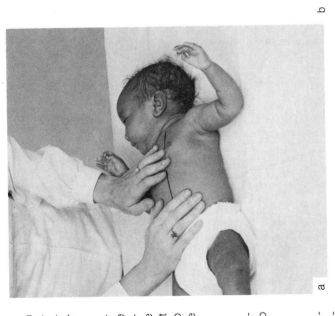

a

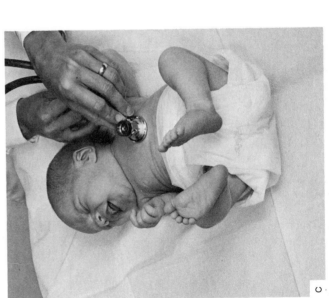

c

b

Palpation

Palpation over the entire precordium should reveal the point of maximal impulse (PMI) in the 3d or 4th left intercostal space just outside the midclavicular line (a).

The femoral, dorsalis pedis, and brachial pulses should be palpated (b). The examiner lightly palpates using one finger, being careful not to obliterate the pulse. It is best to palpate left and right side pulses simultaneously in order to distinguish fullness and equality of the pulsations.

Percussion

Because of the small size of the neonate's chest, percussion of the chest to determine heart size is rarely done.

Auscultation

Auscultation, using the bell and diaphragm of the stethoscope, should reveal a regular rate and rhythm (c). The first (S_1) and second (S_2) heart sounds should be clearly audible, and may be differentiated from breath sounds by palpating a peripheral pulse simultaneously with auscultation. S_1 is usually heard best at the 5th intercostal space, and S_2 at the 2d intercostal space. The second heart sound is often split, reflecting the pulmonic valve closing after the aortic valve. The split frequently widens on inspiration by the neonate.

Transient murmurs (blowing or roaring sounds) may be auscultated in up to 50 percent of neonates during the first 48 hours of life. Some murmurs are due to persistent fetal circulation resulting from late closure of the foramen ovale or the ductus arteriosus. The examiner should note the location of any murmurs heard and describe the sound.

Carotid

Apical

Brachial

Femoral

Dorsalis pedis

Highlights

Refer to the criteria for assessing gestational age when examining the breasts of the neonate.

Secretion from the neonate's breasts is called witch's milk.

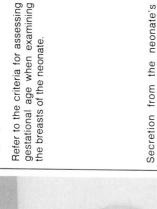

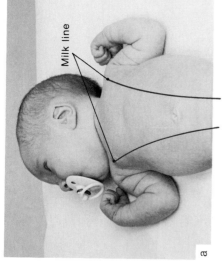

a

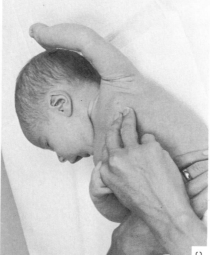

c

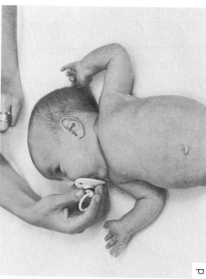

b

d

Breasts

Inspection

The examiner inspects the neonate's breasts, and notes condition, position, and size. Breast enlargement is often seen in either sex in the first few days or weeks of life due to maternal hormones. The examiner may also observe a clear or whitish secretion from the breasts. Either finding should be noted.

Supernumerary (extra) nipples may be found and are considered a normal variation. These nipples occur along the milk line which extends diagonally from the upper outer shoulders to the medial pubic bone. (a)

The color of the neonate's nipples should be pink in white babies and brownish-pink in dark-skinned babies (b).

Palpation

The breast nodule is palpated and the size noted (c). Size reflects gestational age.

Abdomen

Examination of the neonate's abdomen includes assessment of the stomach, liver, spleen, kidneys, bladder, and bowels.

Inspection

When inspecting the abdomen, the examiner should note the size and shape, and any movement (d). The neonate's abdomen is normally rounded and protuberant. Occasionally, peristaltic movements may be visible due to thin abdominal walls. Superficial veins can sometimes be seen.

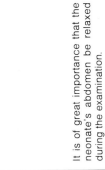

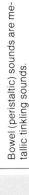

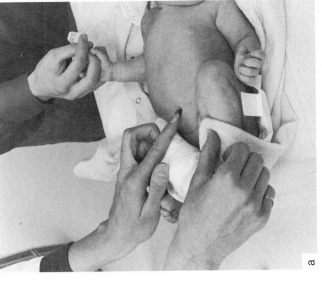

b

The umbilical stump is also inspected (a). In the early neonatal period the examiner should note the number of cord vessels, and the color and condition of the cord. Two small arteries and one larger vein should be present within the Wharton's jelly of the whitish cord (b). By 3 to 4 weeks of age, the central core of the umbilicus is usually covered with skin.

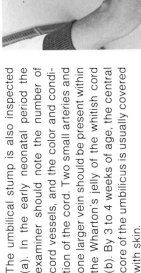

a

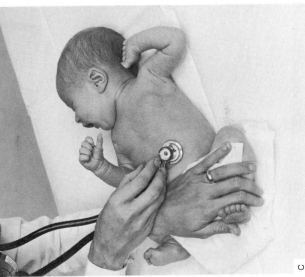

d

Auscultation

Following inspection, the examiner auscultates the abdomen for bowel sounds (c). Normally, peristalsis should be present, while vascular sounds should not exist. Peristaltic sounds may be irregular; therefore it may take 5 minutes or more before sounds are actually heard.

Palpation

Palpation of the abdomen should reveal the location, size, and condition of the neonate's internal organs. The technique used when palpating is the same as that used for the adult. Palpation is made easier if the neonate's abdomen is relaxed. To accomplish this, the examiner flexes the baby's knees (d) or holds the baby's upper back with one hand and flexes the neck while palpating with the other hand.

c

Highlights

The capacity of the neonate's stomach increases with age.

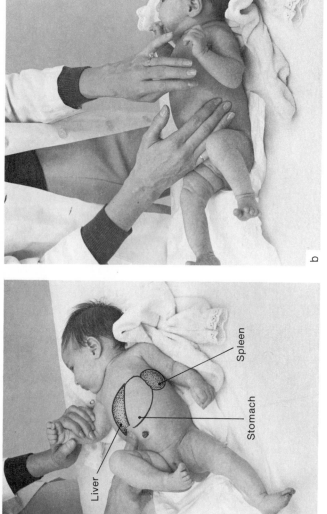

a

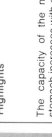

b

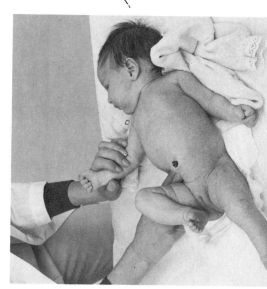

c

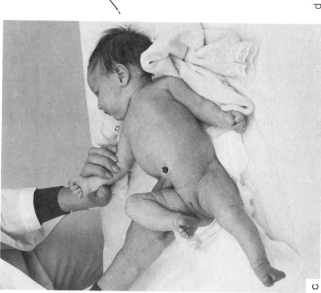

d

Refer to Chap. 4 for discussion of ballottement.

Stomach When palpating the stomach, the neonate is positioned horizontally. The capacity of this organ is approximately 30 to 90 ml at birth. Palpation should reveal the stomach to be located below the diaphragm and between the spleen and the liver, thus occupying a large area of the upper abdomen.

Liver The liver of the neonate fills most of the right upper quadrant of the abdomen. The liver is normally palpated 1 to 2 cm below the right costal margin, although it is also normal for the liver to be located just above this point (a).

Spleen The spleen is palpated at the left costal margin Only the tip of the spleen should normally be felt during this procedure (b).

Kidneys On deep palpation, the kidneys should be felt adjacent to the vertebral column (c). The lower half of the right kidney and the tip of the left kidney normally may be palpated. The technique of ballottement can be used in addition to deep palpation to aid in assessment.

Bladder The urinary bladder will vary in size and position according to the size of the neonate, and the amount of urine contained within (d). Palpation can reveal the presence of the bladder. It will be more easily felt when distended by urine.

Bowels The bowels may be palpated on occasion (a). Two parts of the intestines that may be palpated are the cecum in the right lower quadrant and the sigmoid in the left lower quadrant (b). The examiner further determines normal function of the bowels by noting passage of the first stool, meconium, within 24 hours of birth. The color and consistency of subsequent stools will depend upon the type of feedings the neonate is receiving. Breast-fed babies produce loose, yellow stools, while bottle-fed babies produce more formed yellow stools.

Percussion
The technique of percussion is similar to the examination of the adult in Chap. 4.

Stomach Percussion over the stomach area should result in a tympanic note (c).

Liver When percussing the liver, dullness is usually present over the entire area being examined (c).

Spleen Percussion of the spleen is not usually done in the neonate.

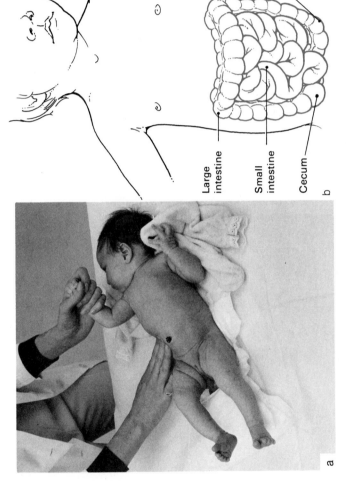

a

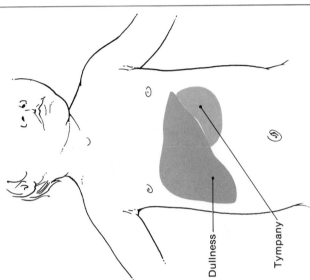

Sigmoid colon

Large intestine

Small intestine

Cecum

b

Dullness

Tympany

c

Refer to Chap. 4 for a description of abdominal sounds.

Kidneys On occasion, the examiner may be able to percuss a kidney in the area of the left midaxillary line (a). The resulting sound is one of dullness.

Bladder Percussion of the bladder can best be accomplished in the area between the symphysis pubis and the umbilicus. When urine is present, a tympanitic note is heard.

Bowels Normally the bowels are difficult to percuss due to the neonate's small pelvis. However, an attempt should be made to carry out this technique when possible.

The final part of the examination of the neonate's abdomen includes assessment of the superficial abdominal reflexes. With the infant in a supine position, the examiner lightly strokes the four quadrants around the umbilicus with a pin or sharp point. The strokes are made diagonally, and form a diamond on the abdomen (b). The expected response is symmetrical movement of the abdominal musculature and umbilicus toward the quadrant which is stroked. It should also be noted if the reflexes are absent.

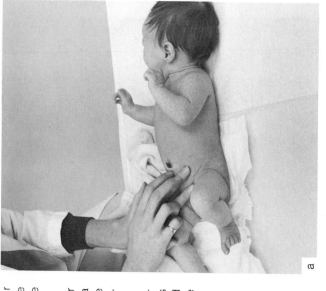

a

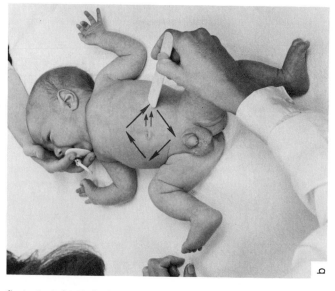

b

Internal structures of the female genitalia include the ovaries, uterus, fallopian tubes, and vagina.

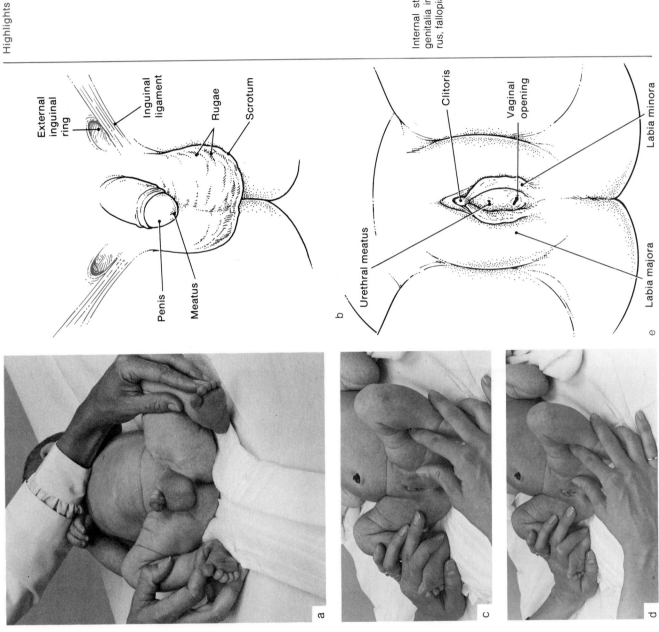

Genitalia

Examination of the genitalia of the neonate includes inspection and palpation of the male penis, testes, scrotum, and external inguinal rings (a and b), and the female clitoris, labia minora and majora, vaginal orifice, urethral orifice, and external inguinal rings.

Inspection

Size, shape, position, and color of the various parts of the male and female genitalia should be noted.

Male The examiner inspects the penis. If the neonate is uncircumcised, the foreskin is usually not retractable.

Following circumcision, the glans penis is exposed and there is a remaining lip of foreskin. The meatus should be centered at the tip of the shaft of the penis.

The scrotum is examined. The color is pink in Caucasians and may be dark brown in dark-skinned babies. In the full-term neonate, rugae are well formed over the scrotum.

Female The examiner inspects the external genitalia and notes the size, color, and condition of the labia majora and minora (c). In the full-term female, the majora usually covers the minora and underlying structures. Transient hypertrophy of the labia majora may be present, along with a white and/or blood-tinged vaginal discharge due to the withdrawal of maternal estrogen.

The vaginal and urethral orifices and the clitoris may be exposed by exerting a gentle downward and lateral traction on each side of the perineum (d). All structures should be present (e). The clitoris is inspected but not palpated due to its sensitivity. It usually appears large in the newborn period.

Highlights

Bartholin's and Skene's glands are not normally visible or palpable in the female neonate.

Pelvic examinations are not routinely performed in the female neonate; therefore, internal structures of the genitalia are not evaluated.

Palpation

Palpation of the testes should begin at the external inguinal ring and proceed downward to the scrotum (a). This technique prevents the testes from retracting into the inguinal canals as a result of the cremasteric reflex. The testes should be descended and approximately equal in size.

The cremasteric reflex can be elicited by stroking the inner thighs of the neonate. Retraction of testes should occur bilaterally.

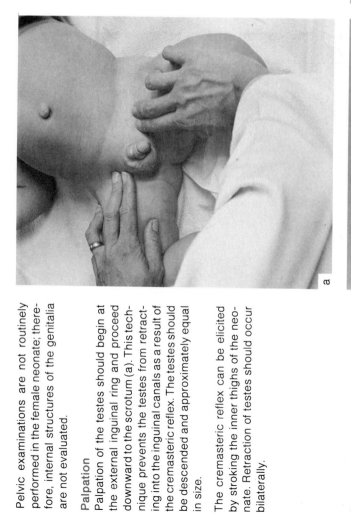

Rectum and Anus
Inspection

The examiner should inspect the neonate to determine the presence of an anus, and its position (b). A patent rectum and anus is verified with the passage of the first meconium stool, 24 to 48 hours past birth. Rectal examination is not usually recommended in the neonate, due to the possibility of traumatizing the baby.

Passage of the first meconium stool verifies patency of the rectum and anus of the neonate.

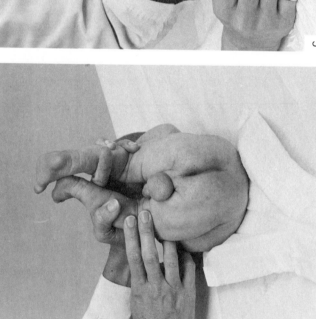

The gluteal reflex is a superficial reflex.

Palpation

The gluteal (or anal) reflex is elicited to evaluate muscular control in this area. By spreading the buttocks of the neonate, the examiner is able to gently scratch the perianal area (c). A quick contraction of the anal sphincter should be noted as the response to the scratch.

Extremities

The examiner inspects and palpates the extremities and peripheral vessels, and elicits certain reflexes to assess the function of the extremities, and the neurologic status of the neonate. The spine should also be evaluated at this time.

Inspection

Begin the inspection by noting the neonate's resting position (a). Normally, all extremities are symmetrically flexed and the legs are externally rotated, and somewhat bowed. Feet are everted. If the neonate was born in a breech rather than vertex presentation, the hips may be markedly flexed and the knees extended.

As the neonate becomes active, spontaneous movements should be observed for symmetry and quality, and for the amount of movement (b). In the early neonatal period movements may be somewhat jerky.

Each part of the upper and lower extremities is inspected for normal structure (c). The number of fingers and toes are counted. It is important to assess the length of the fingers and the creases of the palms. Nailbeds should be pink.

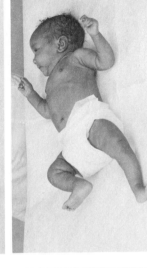
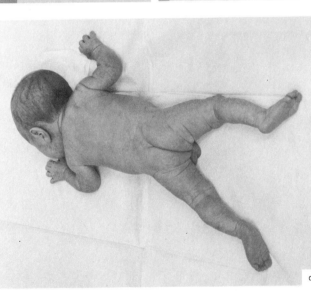

a

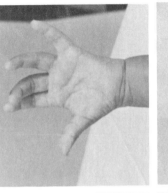
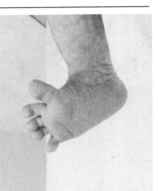

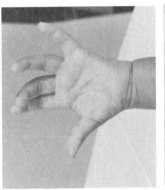
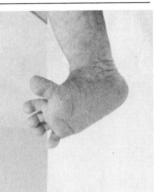

b

c

The position of the neonate's extremities may reflect in utero position.

Symmetry of position and degree of flexion of the extremities are noted.

Occasional tremors may be present in the neonate, and are usually transient.

Dermatoglyphics refers to the study of skin-pattern lines such as palmar creases.

The feet of the neonate often appear flat due to a plantar fat pad.

THE NEONATE

The neonate can normally have tight hip abductors.

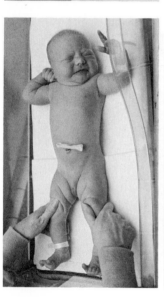
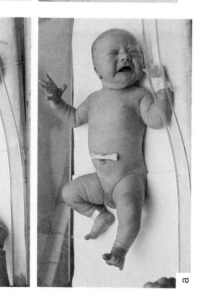
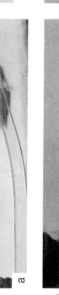

b

a

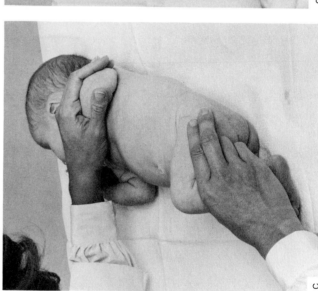

d

c

Palpation

The examiner should palpate all extremities to ascertain the presence of structures, and the degree of muscle tone and resistance demonstrated by the neonate. Alignment and proportion are assessed by passively straightening corresponding extremities. When extremities are released by the examiner, the neonate should resume flexion (a and b).

Joints are put through the full range of passive motion so that the examiner can evaluate the function, muscle tone, and strength of each extremity, and compare corresponding extremities for symmetry.

Peripheral pulses are palpated. The quality, rate, and rhythm of the pulses are noted. If the examiner is unable to palpate any pulses this should also be noted.

An important maneuver performed on the neonate as part of the examination of the lower extremities is Ortolani's maneuver. This will verify the normal movement of the femoral head in the acetabulum. The examiner performs Ortolani's maneuver by placing the hands on and around the neonate's knees and hips, with the index and middle fingers of each hand placed over the greater trochanters (c). The examiner (1) exerts downward pressure on the hips through the flexed knees, (2) abducts the hips at least 70 degrees (d), and (3) adducts the hips, noting smooth movement of the femoral head back into the acetabulum. Any unusual click or clunk heard or felt with this maneuver should be noted, since this may indicate congenital hip dislocation.

The spine is inspected and palpated with the neonate in the prone position (a). The examiner palpates all vertebrae and notes normal curvature of the spine. At birth, only the thoracic and pelvic curves are present, resulting in a C-shaped spine (b). The cervical and lumbar curves develop during the infant and early toddler periods.

Finally, reflex responses in the neonate are evaluated by the examiner. Presence of the reflex, symmetry, and strength are assessed.

The deep tendon reflexes (biceps, triceps, brachioradialus, achilles, and patellar) are elicited in the same manner as in the adult. All other reflexes present in the neonate may be elicited as described below.

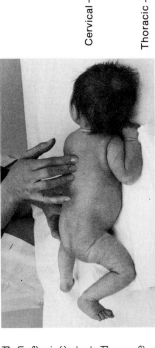
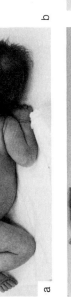
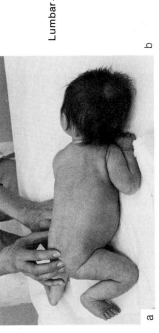

a

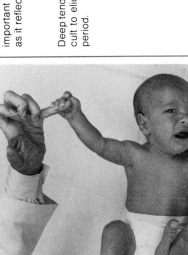

b

Cervical

Thoracic

Lumbar

The Moro reflex is one of the most important to elicit in the neonate, as it reflects neurologic status.

Deep tendon reflexes may be difficult to elicit in the early neonatal period.

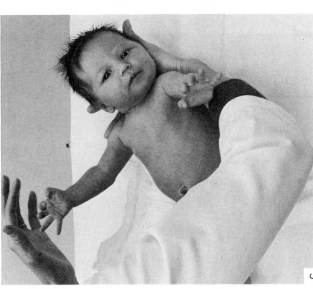

d

c

Moro Reflex Support the neonate's trunk with one hand, and the head and neck with the other hand. When the neck is relaxed, allow the head to drop a few centimeters backward (c). The expected responses include: (1) sudden abduction of the arms and shoulders; (2) extension of the arms at the elbow; (3) extension of the fingers, with the index fingers and thumbs semiflexed, forming the shape of a C; and (4) adduction of the arms at the shoulder.

Palmar grasp Press an index finger into the neonate's palm from the ulnar side and note the neonate's ability to grasp (d). As the examiner's finger is drawn upward, the grip will usually become tighter and the neonate may actually be lifted from a surface.

Photograph c courtesy of Meade Johnson Company

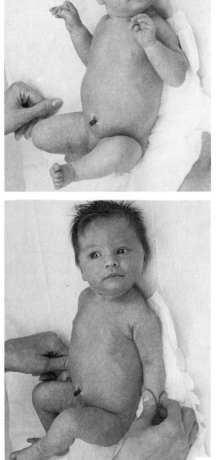

a

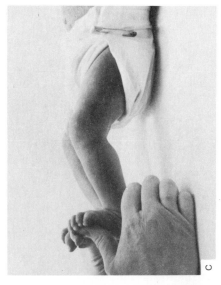

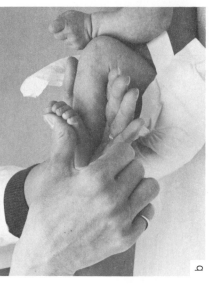

b

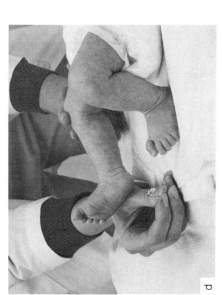

c

d

Arm Recoil Simultaneously extend the neonate's arms by pulling them down at the wrists, and then quickly let go, noting brisk flexion at the elbows (a).

Plantar Grasp Press thumbs against the balls of the feet and note plantar flexion of the feet as the response (b).

Magnet Reflex Apply light pressure to the soles of the feet and observe for extension of the neonate's legs toward the pressure (c).

Withdrawal Reflex Using a sharp object such as a pin, prick the soles of the feet one at a time (d). The response noted is flexion of each leg at the hip, knee, and ankle.

Highlights

Clonus refers to rapid, rhythmic contraction of a muscle occurring in response to maintained passive stretch of the muscle.

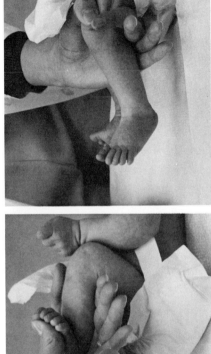

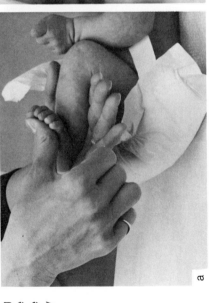

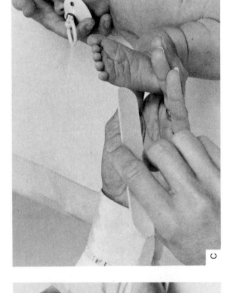

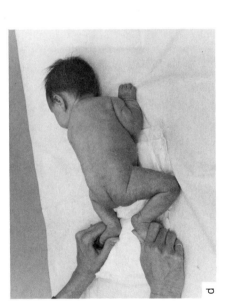

Ankle Clonus Check by pressing thumbs sharply against the soles of the feet, causing dorsiflexion of the entire foot, then quickly release and note any clonus by counting the beats (a).

Crossed Extension Reflex Lie the baby in the supine position. Extend one of the legs and press the knee down. Stimulate the foot of the fixated limb. The free leg should flex, adduct, and extend as if trying to push the stimulating agent away (b).

Babinski Reflex Stroke the lateral aspect of the sole of the foot with a sharp object, beginning at the heel and coming up toward the little toe and across toward the big toe. In the neonate, the normal response is plantar flexion, or incurving of the toes (c).

Bauer's (Crawling) Reflex With the neonate lying prone, the examiner presses on the soles of the feet. The baby should respond by making crawling movements (d).

Highlights

The stepping reflex may fade by 3 to 4 weeks of age.

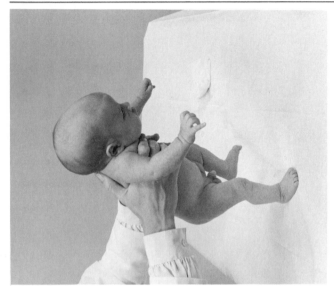

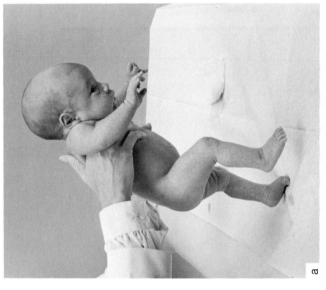

a

Stepping Reflex Holding the baby upright, the examiner touches the soles of the neonate's feet to a table surface, and observes for alternating stepping movements (a).

The stepping and placing reflexes may be difficult to elicit in the first few days of life.

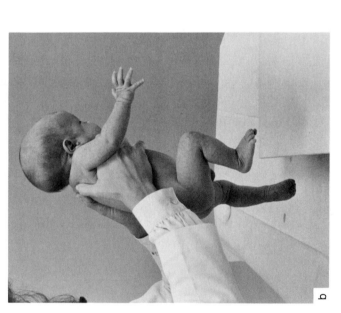

b

Placing Reflex Holding the baby upright, the dorsal side of the neonate's feet are made to touch the edge of a table. The expected response is flexion of the knees and hips, with the feet rising and being placed on the table surface (b).

Galant's Reflex With the neonate in a prone position, the examiner scratches a sharp object along one side of the spinal column from the shoulder to the buttocks (a). In response, the neonate's trunk curves to the side of the scratch (b). The opposite side is also checked.

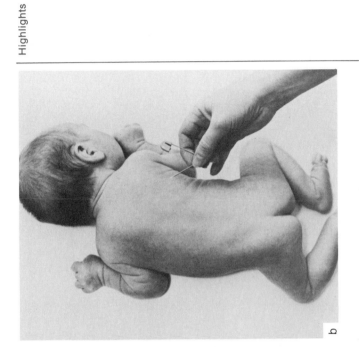

a

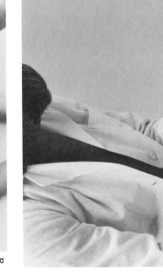

b

Protective Turning Reflex The examiner places the neonate in a prone position with the head midline. Normally the baby will turn the head to one side as a protective response (c).

All of the above reflexes reflect the neurologic state of the healthy neonate. As the neonate matures, certain reflexes will disappear.

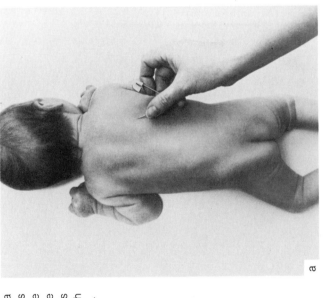

c

Photographs a and b courtesy of Meade Johnson Company.

EXAMINATION AT BIRTH

Apgar Score

The initial physical examination of the neonate takes place after the moment of birth (a) and uses the Apgar score (b). The neonate is evaluated at 1 and 5 minutes of age. The highest score obtainable is 10. Scores from 7 to 10 indicate a good prognosis for the baby regarding mortality and subsequent neurologic sequelae. Low scores of 0 to 3 at 1 minute are associated with high mortality and a high risk of neurologic problems in the survivors.

During the assessment process the examiner should minimize the exposure of the wet neonate to cool ambient air, since a rapid drop in body temperature could compromise the neonate.

The technique for determining the Apgar score is as follows:

1 Measure heart rate by apical auscultation or palpation (c).

2 Measure respiratory effort by observing the neonate's respirations. If the neonate is crying, respiratory effort is usually good (d).

3 Evaluate muscle tone by observing for flexion of all four extremities (e).

4 Evaluate reflex irritability by placing the tip of a catheter or bulb syringe approximately 1 cm into either external naris, and watch the neonate's response (f).

5 Observe the neonate's general body color (g).

If the Apgar score is 8 or more at 5 minutes of age, and the baby's general condition is stable, the nurse then performs an estimation of gestational age.

Refer to Table b for the Apgar scoring system

The Apgar score assesses adequacy of pulmonary ventilation and integrity of the cardiovascular and central nervous systems.

The normal, full-term newborn maintains a flexed position.

It is not uncommon for the extremities of the neonate to be cyanotic (blue) due to sluggish peripheral circulation.

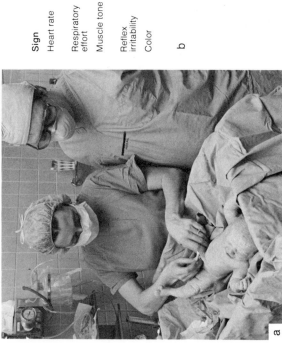

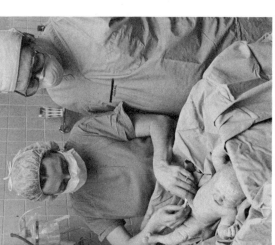

a

Apgar Scoring Method

Sign	Score 0	1	2
Heart rate	Absent	slow, below 100	Above 100
Respiratory effort	Absent	Slow, irregular	Good cry
Muscle tone	Flaccid	Some flexion of extremities	Active motion
Reflex irritability	No response	Grimace	Cry
Color	Blue, pale	Body pink, extremities blue	Completely pink

b

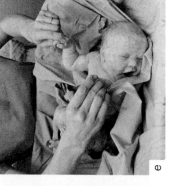

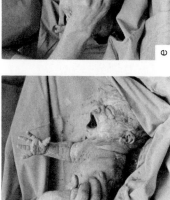

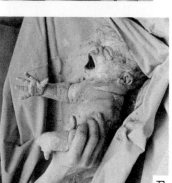

c

d

e

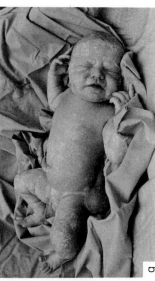

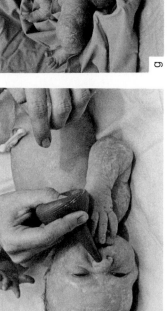

f

g

Highlights

During pregnancy gestational age is determined by calculating from the date of the last menstrual period using Nagele's rule, and measuring the height of the fundus above the symphysis pubis (Mc-Donald's Sign)

Gestational age and birth weight are two important factors affecting the survival of the neonate. Infants born with birth weights small for their gestational ages have greater mortality rates than infants born with weights appropriate for their gestational ages.

Gestational age is a greater indicator of a baby's maturity than is weight.

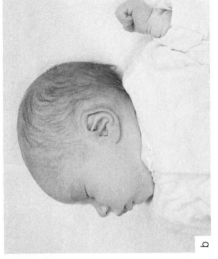

b

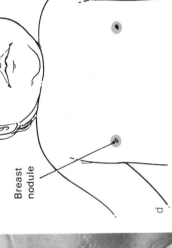

Breast nodule

d

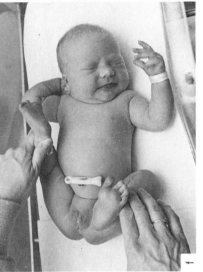

f

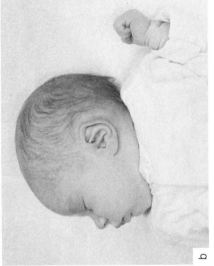

a

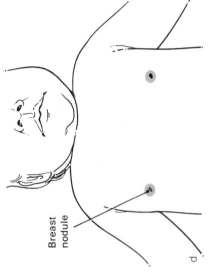

c

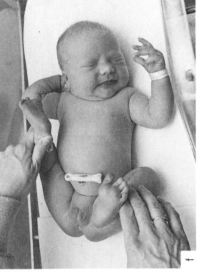

Testicle

Scrotum

e

Gestational Age

When calculating the neonate's gestational age, the examiner evaluates the following signs and notes the findings:

Sole creases: At 36 weeks the infant's foot has deep creases on one-third of the sole; at 38 weeks, the creases extend over two-thirds of the sole; at full term, the infant has full sole creases (a).

Hair texture: At 36 weeks, the head of the infant is covered with fine fuzzy hair; in a full-term infant, the hair has a silky texture (b).

Cartilaginous development of the ear lobe: At 36 weeks the ear has poorly defined structures and little cartilage in the superior portion of the helix. In a full-term infant, the structures are more well defined and the ear is relatively rigid with cartilage (c).

Size of the breast nodule: Before 33 weeks the nodule is less than 0.5 cm; at 37 to 38 weeks, it is 0.5 to 1.0 cm; at term it is over 1.0 cm in diameter (d).

Testicular descent: At 36 weeks the scrotum is small and unfilled; the testes are at the junction of the inguinal canal and the scrotum. At full term, the testes have descended into the scrotal sac (e).

Heel to ear manuever: This manuever is carried out by extending the infant's leg and bringing the heel to the ear without tilting the pelvis or flexing the spine off the examining surface. At 34 weeks this manuever can be performed without difficulty; in a full-term infant, the manuever is impossible (f).

Highlights

With practice, the nurse can complete the Dubowitz examination in 5 to 10 minutes.

Dubowitz Scoring System

In 1967, Dubowitz et al, developed a scoring system for gestational age which provides consistent results during the first 5 days of life and is equally reliable in the first 24 hours of life. The scoring system is based on 10 neurologic and 11 external criteria. The nurse scores the neonate from 0 to 5 for the neurologic criteria, and from 0 to 4 for the external criteria. Not all categories are scored up to 5. The highest score the infant can get for arm recoil is 2. Only for popliteal angle is a score of 5 possible.

Neurological Criteria

The examiner uses the following techniques when assessing *neurologic criteria.*

Posture: Observe with the infant quiet and in supine position (a). Score as follows: arms and legs extended, 0; beginning of flexion of hips and knees, arms extended, 1; stronger flexion of legs, arms extended, 2; arms slightly flexed, legs flexed and abducted, 3; full flexion of arms and legs, 4.

Square window: The hand is flexed on the forearm between the thumb and index finger of the examiner (b). Enough pressure is applied to get as full a flexion as possible, and the angle between the hypothenar eminance and the ventral aspect of the forearm is measured and graded according to diagram. (Care is taken not to rotate the infant's wrist while doing this maneuver.)

Neurological sign	Points						Score
	0	1	2	3	4	5	
Posture							
Square window	90°	60°	45°	30°	0°		
Ankle dorsiflexion	90°	75°	45°	20°	0°		
Arm recoil	180°	90–180°	<90°				
Leg recoil	180°	90–180°	<90°				
Popliteal angle	180°	150°	130°	110°	90°	<90°	
Heel to ear							
Scarf sign							
Head lag							
Ventral suspension							

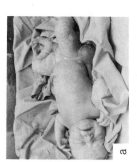

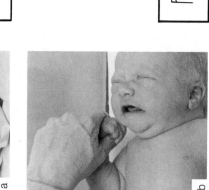

a

b

| 90° | 60° | 45° | 30° | 0° |

Ankle dorsiflexion: The foot is dorsi-flexed onto the anterior aspect of the leg, with the examiner's fingers on the sole of the foot and thumb behind the leg (a). Enough pressure is app-lied to get as full a flexion as possible, and the angle between the dorsum of the foot and the anterior aspect of the leg is measured.

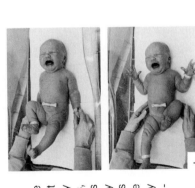

a

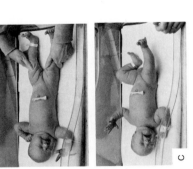

90°	75°	45°	20°	0°

Arm recoil: With the infant in the supine position the forearms are first flexed for 5 seconds, then fully extended by pulling on the hands, and then released (b). The sign is fully positive if the arms return briskly to full flexion; score 2. If the arms return to incomplete flexion or the response is sluggish, score 1. If they remain extended or make only ran-dom movements, the score is 0.

b

180°	90–180°	< 90°

Leg recoil: With the baby supine, the hips and knees are fully flexed for 5 seconds, then extended by traction on the feet, and released (c). A max-imal response is one of full flexion of the hips and knees and scores 2. A partial flexion scores 1, and minimal or no movement scores 0.

c

180°	90–180°	< 90°

Popliteal angle: With the baby supine and the pelvis flat on the examining couch, the thigh is held in the knee-chest position by the examiner. The leg is then extended by gentle pres-sure from the examiner's other hand behind the ankle and the popliteal angle is measured (d).

d

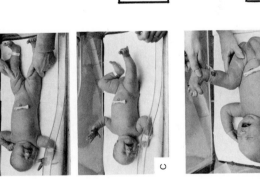

180°	150°	130°	110°	90°	< 90°

Highlights

Heel to ear manuever: With the baby supine, draw the baby's foot as near to the head as it will go without forcing it (a). Observe the distance between the foot and the head as well as the degree of extension at the knee. Grade according to diagram. Note that the knee is left free and may draw down alongside the abdomen.

Scarf sign: With the baby supine, take the infant's hand and try to put it around the neck and as far posteriorly as possible around the opposite shoulder (b). Assist this maneuver by lifting the elbow across the body. See how far the elbow will go across and grade as follows. Score 0 if the elbow reaches the opposite axillary line; 1 if it reaches between midline and opposite axillary line; 2 if the elbow reaches midline; 3 if it will not reach midline.

Head lag: With the baby lying supine, grasp the hands (or the arms of a very small infant) and pull the infant slowly toward the sitting position (c). Observe the position of the head in relation to the trunk and grade accordingly. In a small infant the head may initially be supported by one hand. Score 0 if there is complete lag; 1 if there is partial head control; 2 if the baby is able to maintain head in line with body; 3 if the infant brings the head anterior to the body.

Ventral suspension: The baby is suspended in the prone position, with examiner's hand under the baby's chest (d). Observe the degree of extension of the back and the amount of flexion of the arms and legs. Also note the relation of the head to the trunk. Grade according to diagrams.

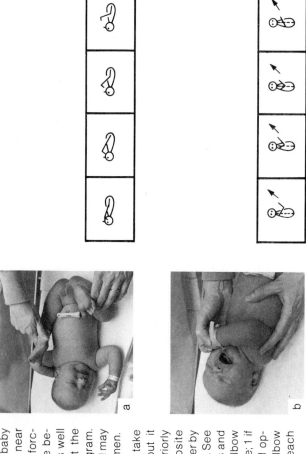

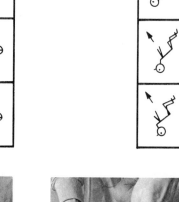

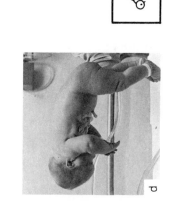

Neurologic Criteria

Criterion	Score
Posture	0–4
Square window	0–4
Ankle dorsiflexion	0–4
Arm recoil	0–2
Leg recoil	0–2
Popliteal angle	0–5
Heel to ear	0–4
Scarf sign	0–3
Head lag	0–3
Ventral suspension	0–4
Total	0–35

If neurologic scores differ on the two sides of the body, the mean score is taken.

External Criteria

The table on this page contains the scoring system for external criteria on the Dubowitz examination. The nurse scores the neonate by comparing findings on each item to this table.

External Criteria

Criterion	Score
Edema	0-2
Skin texture	0-4
Skin color	0-3
Skin opacity	0-4
Lanugo	0-4
Plantar creases	0-4
Nipple formation	0-3
Breast size	0-3
Ear form	0-3
Ear firmness	0-3
Genitals	0-3
Total	0-35

Scoring System for External Criteria

External sign	Score*				
	0	1	2	3	4
Edema	Obvious edema of hands and feet; pitting over tibia	No obvious edema of hands and feet; pitting over tibia	No edema		
Skin texture	Very thin, gelatinous	Thin and smooth	Smooth; medium thickness. Rash or superficial peeling	Slight thickening. Superficial cracking and peeling especially of hands and feet	Thick and parchment-like; superficial or deep cracking
Skin color	Dark red	Uniformly pink	Pale pink; variable over body	Pale; only pink over ears, lips, palms, or soles	
Skin opacity (trunk)	Numerous veins and venules clearly seen, especially over abdomen	Veins and tributaries seen	A few large vessels clearly seen over abdomen	A few large vessels seen indistinctly over abdomen	No blood vessels seen
Lanugo (over back)	No lanugo	Abundant; long and thick over whole back	Hair thinning especially over lower back	Small amount of lanugo and bald areas	At least $\frac{1}{2}$ of back devoid of lanugo
Plantar creases	No skin creases	Faint red marks over anterior half of sole	Definite red marks over > anterior $\frac{1}{2}$; indentations over < anterior $\frac{1}{3}$	Indentations over > anterior $\frac{1}{3}$	Definite deep indentations over > anterior $\frac{1}{3}$
Nipple formation	Nipple barely visible; no areola	Nipple well defined; areola smooth and flat, diameter <0.75 cm.	Areola stippled, edge not raised, diameter <0.75 cm.	Areola stippled, edge raised, diameter >0.75 cm.	
Breast size	No breast tissue palpable	Breast tissue on one or both sides, <0.5 cm. diameter	Breast tissue both sides; one or both 0.5 – 1.0 cm.	Breast tissue both sides; one or both >1 cm.	
Ear form	Pinna flat and shapeless, little or no incurving of edge	Incurving of part of edge of pinna	Partial incurving whole of upper pinna	Well-defined incurving whole of upper pinna	
Ear firmness	Pinna soft, easily folded, no recoil	Pinna soft, easily folded, slow recoil	Cartilage to edge of pinna, but soft in places, ready recoil	Pinna firm, cartilage to edge; instant recoil	
Genitals Male	Neither testis in scrotum	At least one testis high in scrotum	At least one testis right down		
Female (with hips $\frac{1}{2}$ abducted)	Labia majora widely separated, labia minora protruding	Labia majora almost cover labia minora	Labia majora completely cover labia minora		

*If score differs on two sides, take the mean.
Adapted from Farr and associates, *Develop. Med. Child Neurol.* **8**:507, 1966.

The examiner adds the scores obtained for the neurologic criteria and external criteria separately, and then adds the two scores together for a total score.

Finally the total score is placed on the gestational age graph (a). The higher the score, the greater the gestational age of the infant.

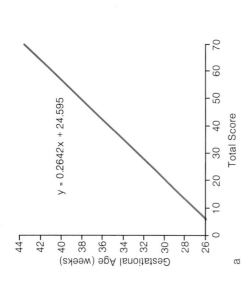

$y = 0.2642x + 24.595$

Gestational Age (weeks)

Total Score

a

Birth Weight

Upon admission to most nurseries, the newborn is weighed. In order to ensure accuracy, the scale is properly balanced ahead of time by the nurse. The baby is completely undressed and placed in the center of the scale (b). The examiner should place one hand lightly over the top of the baby to keep the baby from falling off the scale (c). The baby is promptly removed from the scale and returned to a crib or Isolette for the remainder of the examination.

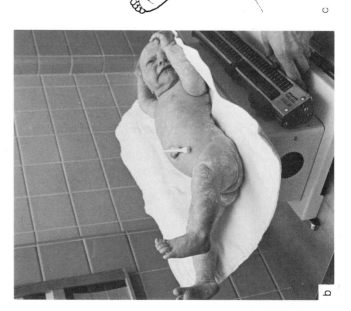

b

c

The weight of most full-term newborns ranges from 2500 to 4300 g (5½ to 9½ pounds), with boys weighing slightly more than girls.

The American Academy of Pediatrics recommends that all newborns be classified by birth weight and gestational age.

Classification by Gestation and Birth Weight

The examiner classifies the neonate according to gestational age and birth weight using the graph at right. Upon determining the appropriate classification, a mortality risk factor is noted for the baby. Results may be used by the nurse to plan for future care of the baby.

1 Neonatal mortality risk (NMR):
There are four colored zones shown:
- White = infants with 4% NMR
- Yellow = infants with 4-25% NMR
- Blue = infants with 25-50% NMR
- Red = infants with 50% NMR

2 Gestational age birthweight distribution:

Gestational age is to be estimated from clinical examination rather than the last menstrual period (see the Dubowitz scoring system).

Gestational age: subdivided along abscissa into three categories:

a Preterm (Pr) = all infants less than 38 weeks gestational age, i.e., 37 weeks + 6 days or less.

b Term (T) = all infants between 38th and 42d weeks gestational age.

c Postterm (Po) = all infants of 42 or more weeks gestational age.

Birthweight: Within *each* gestational age group, there are three sub-groups of infants, defined by birthweight:

a Large for gestational age (LGA) = infants above the 90th percentile.

b Appropriate for gestational age (AGA) = infants between the 90th and 10th percentile.

c Small for gestational age (SGA) = infants below the 10th percentile.

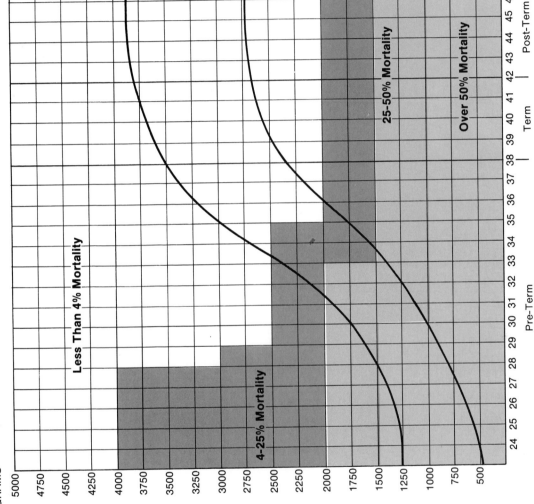

GRAMS

WEEKS OF GESTATION

Less Than 4% Mortality

4-25% Mortality

25-50% Mortality

Over 50% Mortality

Pre-Term · Term · Post-Term

The length of the full-term neonate ranges from 47.5 to 56 cm (19 to 22 inches). The head comprises approximately one-fourth the total length.

The head circumference of the full-term neonate ranges from 33 to 35 cm (13 to 14 inches).

The chest circumference of the full-term neonate ranges from 30 to 33 cm (12 to 13 inches).

The health of the neonate is reflected in somatic growth.

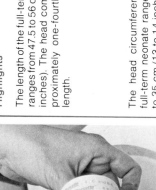

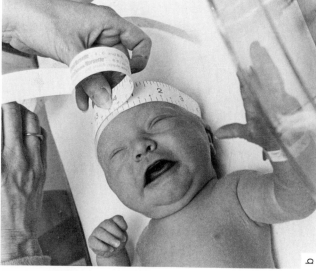

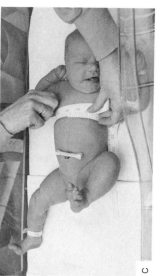

Length

The examiner measures the length of the neonate by placing the baby in a prone position, with the soles of the feet perpendicular to the surface. The measure is taken with an accurate tape from the top of the head to the soles of the feet (a).

Head Circumference

The examiner measures the head circumference of the neonate at the widest area from the occiput to the brow (b). A flexible metal or paper tape should be used for accuracy. Because of molding during the birth process, the head of the newborn may be misshapen. In this case, the head should be measured daily until it returns to a normal shape and size.

Chest Circumference

The examiner measures the chest circumference at the nipple line (c). Normally, the chest circumference of the neonate should not exceed the head circumference, and is usually 1 inch less in size.

Growth Charts

Measurements of weight, length, and head circumference are plotted by the examiner on standardized growth charts (see Appendix). A percentile score is noted for each value. Serial measurements will be done at each subsequent examination; in this way, growth of the neonate can be accurately monitored.

Highlights

Different organ systems mature at different rates throughout the early years of life, accounting for individual variations in growth.

Refer to Chap. 4, Assessing Vital Signs.

The heart beat of the neonate ranges from 100 to 180 beats per minute within 30 minutes of birth, then stabilizes at 120 to 140 beats per minute.

Respirations fluctuate in rate and pattern; periodic breathing is not uncommon. Respirations range from 30 to 80 breaths per minute, with 40 being the norm.

The neonate is an obligatory nose breather.

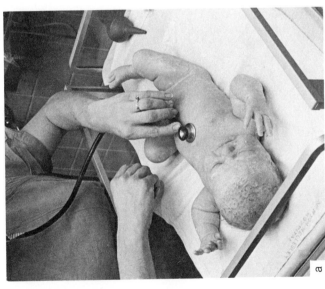

a

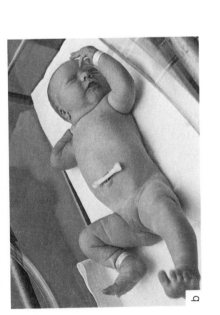

b

Vital Signs

The initial *vital signs* taken after birth provide important data about the neonate's ability to adjust to extrauterine life. Physiologic adjustments are greater in the first hours of life than at any other time. The neonate's survival depends upon making these adaptations.

When assessing vital signs the examiner will:

1 Auscultate and count the apical pulse for 60 seconds, and note the rate and rhythm of the heart beat.

a The diaphragm of the stethoscope is used to assess high-pitched heart sounds (a), and the bell to assess low-pitched sounds.

b Heart sounds resemble a toc-tic sound, and the two sounds should be clearly audible.

2 Observe and count respirations for 60 seconds, noting quality, rate, and rhythm.

a The quality should be noted for several minutes so that variations can be identified; depth of respirations is also noted.

b Rate can be learned by counting abdominal excursions or listening with the bell of the stethoscope in front of the nose; an irregular rate is common.

c Rhythm is noted by observing the respiratory pattern (b); an irregular rhythm is common, reflecting adaptation to air breathing.

d Auscultate breath sounds anteriorly and posteriorly, and note the quality of the sounds.

Highlights

Normal temperatures range from 36.5 to 37°C (97.7 to 98.6°F).

Rectal temperature can be normal during cold stress, and, therefore, may be misleading.

Blood pressures at birth are 60 to 80 mmHg systolic, and 40 to 50 mmHg diastolic.

The blood pressure cuff should cover two-thirds of the upper arm or thigh, or be 20 percent greater than the diameter of the extremity; proper fit results in accurate measurements.

Changes in the neonate's activity can cause fluctuations in blood pressure.

Flush pressure approximates the mean arterial pressure.

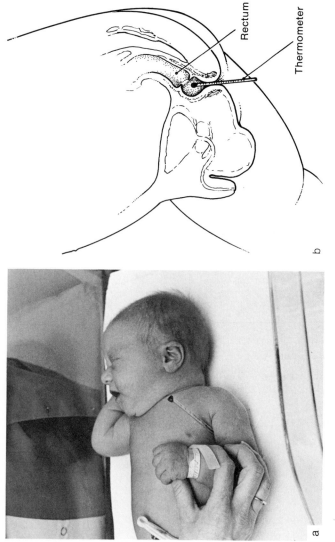

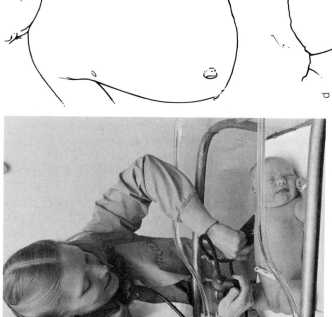

Rectum

Thermometer

3 Measure rectal or axillary temperature using an accurate glass or electronic thermometer.

  a Axillary temperature (a) reflects skin temperature and is more accurate than rectal; the thermometer is placed well into the axilla and held in place by bringing the baby's arm down and close to the body; allow approximately 5 minutes for measurement.

  b Temperature is sometimes taken rectally as the initial method so that the patency of the anus can also be checked (b); the thermometer is lubricated and advanced three-fourths to 1 inch into the rectum, and held in place for 2 or 3 minutes.

4 Measure blood pressure by one of the following methods:

  a Use a Doppler instrument. Blood movement within the artery causes changes in ultrasound frequency which are translated into audible sound by means of a transducer in the cuff.

  b Use the auscultation method, listening for the sound at the brachial artery in the antecubital fossa (c).

  c Use the palpation method. As the cuff is deflated, measure the point at which the arterial pulse reappears.

  d Use the flush method. After applying the cuff, wrap the extremity distal to the cuff snuggly with elastic bandage, beginning from fingers or toes and moving toward the cuff (d); inflate the cuff to 120 mmHg; remove the bandage; gradually deflate the cuff and note the point at which the extremity first becomes pink.

Vital signs should be measured in this manner during the physical examinations at 12 hours and at 4 week of age.

THE INFANT CHAPTER SIX

Arlene Misklow Sperhac

From 1 to 12 months of age the infant changes from a helpless, although sometimes noisy, neonate to a busy, erect child intent on chewing, tasting, fondling, probing, tugging, pushing, and pounding whatever is in reach. More radical changes take place within this relatively brief time than at any other time of life.

The physical changes are numerous. Although infants vary greatly, most babies add about 8 inches (20+ cm) to their length and gain about 15 lb (6+ kg). Their face loses the neonatal look and becomes a chubby, cute baby face surrounded by a full head of hair. Teeth begin to erupt, and the infant advances from a liquid diet to table food.

Socially the infant progresses from staring at faces to smiling, demanding company, and actively participating in games. Vocalization during this period changes from babbling and cooing to the use of some words, many of which can be understood.

Emotionally and intellectually the infant makes great strides. There is progress from a dim awareness of the world in early infancy to an elaborate knowledge of people, surroundings, and objects, of space and spatial relations, of causal sequences, of the workings of the body, and of the many possibilities for action in late infancy. Infants become able to recognize such feelings as pain, aversion, anger, fear, affection, and elation. Emotional attachments are formed with significant others, such as parents, and are crucial for the development of basic attitudes of optimism or pessimism and trust and mistrust.

In this developmental period one must consider the parent or caretaker on whom the infant totally depends. Any infant is the unique child of a unique set of parents. The infant is extremely adaptive and, in order to gain satisfaction, unfolds in the matrix of the parent-infant dual unit.[1] The individual becomes the child of those parents and quickly adjusts and responds to their lifestyle.

Parents are in the best position to assess their children. They observe them more and know them better than anyone else does. They can usually detect subtle changes. Parents have said for centuries that infants could see, hear, and respond. Scientific thinking scoffed and conveyed what neurological evidence told them should be true behaviorally. Frank in 1966 stated that the "human infant at birth and for a varying period of time thereafter has been seen as functionally decorticated . . . therefore the newborn has been considered as largely a reflex organism."[2] Scientists are now saying what parents have always believed: early infant behavior is organized; infants have learning abilities and sensory and perceptual capacities. They are active and interactive relishers and initiators of experience and action.

If the nurse is to provide holistic health care, parental involvement is essential. The nurse must focus on the promotion of health, not just the prevention of illness. Not only must immunizations and assessment of

The infant changes dramatically between 1 and 12 months of age.

The nurse must involve the infant's parents in their child's health care.

The author wishes to thank John J. Harper, M.D., and Margaret B. McFarland, Ph.D., for their advice and support in the preparation of this chapter.

the infant's physical development be provided, but education and anticipatory guidance on the child's and parents' physical, emotional, social, and spiritual growth is vital. Such guidance can help parents to understand holistic health concepts and aid them in their growth toward self-responsibility for their own and their infant's health.

THE HEALTH HISTORY

The health history interview with the parent or caretaker is most valuable when a holistic approach to health care is used. This interview, which may occur in a well baby clinic, home, hospital, or neighborhood health center, usually occurs during the first visit. During each of the health visits made during the first year, cumulative information is gathered. Because of the infant's rapid growth and changes and the immunizations needed during the first year, frequent visits are recommended.

The parents must be interviewed several times by the nurse because of frequent visits during the infant's first year of life.

The nurse begins the health history interview by establishing rapport with the family, which will facilitate working together productively. Verbal and nonverbal assessment of the infant as perceived by the parent is noted by the nurse. The parent relates to the infant in a manner appropriate for how the infant is perceived; therefore, valuable data may be obtained. For instance, if the parent treats the infant as susceptible and weak, the infant will probably be overprotected and treated as vulnerable.

During the interview it may be appropriate to provide the parents with anticipatory guidance, which means telling them what they may expect of the child in the period before their next visit. For example, many infants begin to crawl and are more active in examining things after 6 months of age. The health care worker provides anticipatory guidance by suggesting to the parents that they begin to put dangerous substances such as detergents out of reach before the infant increases exploratory behavior. It is beneficial for parents and their infants when stages of development can be anticipated and preparations made for changes. Table 6-1 outlines the stages of development, general diet, and areas for anticipatory guidance during the first year of life. The nurse may use this table as a tool to enhance data collection during the interview process.

Approach to the Infant

Since the goals of the health interview include an exchange of information, both interviewer's and interviewees' needs must be considered. The nurse should be unhurried and well organized in the approach to the clients. Also, the nurse should be warm, responsive, and relaxed, which will generally help the parents to relax and feel more comfortable. Relaxed parents will find it easier to keep their infant content.

When providing health care, the nurse must give up the role of *doer* and instead involve the parents in the care of the infant.[3] In many instances there is no right or wrong in infant care; therefore, the nurse must be nonjudgmental. The parents need support from the nurse to grow and gain confidence in their abilities to recognize health needs and provide care they feel is appropriate. With anticipatory guidance, the parents will know how the child will progress developmentally and can anticipate and better cope with physical, emotional, and intellectual changes when they occur. During the interview the nurse should approach the parents in a nonthreatening manner and include their observations in the health history, with objective assessments about the infant.

Table 6-1
Health History Data Tool

Name_____

Birth weight_____

Discharge weight_____

Age/Date	Procedures	Head Circumference	Length	Weight	Development	Diet
1 wk	PKU*				V-follows regard	Breast or bottle
2 wk					Head up	
1 mo	Permit				Lifts head Smiles Regards face	60 Cal/lb (120 Cal/kg)
2 mo	Consent Signed Temperature DPT Polio				Oral-sensory Vocalizes Smile social	
3 mo	Hemogloblin				Follows Head turns 90 degrees Laughs	
4 mo	Temperature DPT Polio				Squeals Grasps Head turns 180 degrees	Cereal, fruit
6 mo	Temperature DPT				Rolls Reaches Head-no lag Hand-eye coordination	55 Cal/lb Fluoride Vegetables
9 mo	Hemoglobin				Self-feed Sitting Fallen object	Balanced finger foods, meat
12 mo	Tine test				Walks Cruises Imitates	50 Cal/lb, Table foods

*PKU, phenylketonuria.
Source: Based on a form designed and used by Roy G. Saruer, M.D., John J. Harper, M.D., Edith Sarnesu, R.N., P.N.P., and Rose Kmetz, R.N., P.N.P.

The Szasz model, which depicts possible relationships between health care providers and clients, can be used to understand relationships between parents and the nurse who provides health care for the infant (Fig. 6-1). In A (activity/passivity), the provider makes the child care decisions, and the parent accepts what he or she is told, as in an adult-infant relationship. In B, or guidance/cooperation, the provider perceives the parent as being capable of following directions and exercising some judgment and gives guidance for care while the parent cooperates with what is suggested, as in an adult-adolescent relationship. In C, there is mutual participation with the provider consulting with the parent on concerns and wishes in formulating a plan of care as in an adult-adult relationship with one having specialized knowledge that the other needs. In D, the primary provider for care is the parent who is recognized as the one most aware of the infant's needs and with whom responsibility and decisions rest, while the provider is seen as the assistant, providing counsel and technical assistance. In E, there is self care with the parent as the source. This model can make the nurse more aware of how to function and can help the parents appreciate how varied the nurse's role should be depending on specific parents and infants. For instance, parents may be more comfortable in the guidance and coopera-

See Fig. 6-1 for a model depicting possible nurse–client relationships.

Figure 6-1 Range of provider-client relationships. A, activity and passivity; B, guidance and cooperation; C, mutual participation; D, patient as primary provider; E, self-care. (Adapted from Donald L. Fink, "Holistic Health: Implications for Health Planning," *A J Health Plan,* **1**:23-31 [July 1976].)

Client component

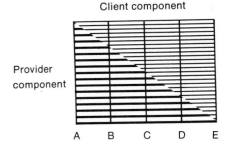

Provider component

A   B   C   D   E

tion relationship initially. As they become more confident they can assume more responsibility for infant care, yet return to the guidance and cooperation or even the activity and passivity relationship with the nurse when necessary. Parents who have several children may be more comfortable in the primary provider role.

It is the nurse's responsibility as a health care professional to assess the needs of the parents and their infants and to help them realize their fullest potential for health and self-responsibility for health care while being available as needed.

Setting

A private, quiet area containing comfortable armchairs should be provided for the parents so that they can relax while cuddling their infant. A nearby carpeted area should be available with safe, age-appropriate toys that older infants may explore while keeping their parents in sight. Infants are often more relaxed if the nurse wears a color other than white.

The Interview

In interviewing the parents, the nurse should follow the communication techniques elaborated in Chap. 3. The tools of communication—language, observation and perception, nonverbal behavior, silence, listening, and watching—are all interrelated and used simultaneously.[5]

See Interviewing Techniques in Chap. 3.

Since this first year is one of rapid physical, emotional, and intellectual growth, the parents may have many concerns and questions. Open-ended and funnel questions may be two of the best interviewing techniques to provide the information the nurse needs and will aid the parents in identifying and exploring their concerns. While the parent is thoughtfully verbalizing the reply, the nurse can use a nonverbal action such as nodding to encourage the parent to continue verbalizing. If the interview is interrupted or must be redirected, this can be done by the nurse's focusing on the infant and restructuring the open-ended question. Such phrases as "Tell me about," "What do you remember about," and "How was" allow the family the freedom to tell the situation from their viewpoint and enable the nurse to identify their concerns.

When interviewing the parents, the nurse will find open-ended questions most useful.

Often there is a need for clarification of words and phrases. Although all present may use clear language, meanings may differ for the participants. For instance, when asked if an infant sleeps through the night, one parent may interpret night as meaning from 1 A.M. to 6 A.M. and another may interpret it as meaning from 9 P.M. to 6 A.M. When a parent describes an infant as "spoiled," what is meant? Reflection is one means of clarification in these instances. Likewise, the parent may not understand a term such as *fever management* or may interpret it differently than the nurse. Therefore, clarification of words and phrases is essential.

Clarification of words and phrases stated by the parents will help promote understanding of data communicated.

The nurse must be sensitive to the often subtle nonverbal cues which may communicate that the parent does not understand statements or questions. Although there may be good rapport, families are often eager to please and will nod and smile appropriately even when they do not understand. Depending on the parents' cues, it may be best to reexplain, using different common terminology, or to ask the parents to repeat what they believe the nurse has said.

The information acquired during the interview should be recorded in a concise, organized manner. It should be written in outline form with headings, short phrases, key words, and standard abbreviations. The record is a legal document, and care should be taken to provide concise yet accurate information.

Client Profile and Biographical Data

To compile a profile of the infant, it is best if biographical data are collected first. Biographical data include name, address, sex, age, date and place of birth, race, nationality, religious affiliation, occupation, and Social Security numbers of the parents.

See Biographical Data in Chap. 3.

Health Status Perception

A question such as "Why is the child attending the clinic today?" will determine the reason for entry into the health care delivery system. Generally the answer is a simple statement such as "well child care," or "a cold."

"Tell me about (infant's name)" will provide the parents' perception of their infant's health. Often terms such as *happy, cranky, fussy,* and *healthy* must be clarified, and time of day and length of time when the concerns occur must be determined by the nurse. Questions presented in Chap. 3 can be used to elicit additional data.

It is important for the nurse to determine the parents' perception of their infant's health state.

Current Health Status and Health Habits

The nurse determines the infant's current health status by asking the parents to elaborate on their perception of the infant's health.

Questions to elicit data

1 How would you describe your infant's health today?

2 Do you think your infant has any health problems?

3 What areas of your infant's health do you feel good about?

Responses to questions should be recorded. Verification of information related will be confirmed through further data collection and nursing assessments.

The infant's health habits will evolve from those of the parents and caretakers. Nutrition, activity, sleep patterns, and personal hygiene will be the most important to the infant during this first year. Therefore, the nurse should determine the family's health habits in these areas.

For example, the parents should be questioned about heavy cigarette smoking, since this could jeopardize the infant's respiratory function. If a child is taught what things can and cannot be explored by putting in the mouth, risk of infection may be decreased.

It is essential to elicit all data so that risks to the infant may be identified and wellness enhanced.

Nutrition, activity, sleep patterns, and personal hygiene are important health habits in the first year.

Past Health Status

The past health history status should begin with the prenatal history.

Questions to elicit data

1 What was the pregnancy like?

2 What was your diet like?

3 Did you have morning sickness that affected your dietary intake?

4 Did you take iron, vitamins, or other medications?

The mother's prenatal history is important data when assessing the infant's past health status.

5 Did you have any illnesses during this pregnancy?

6 How did you feel about this pregnancy?

7 Were you under any stress during this pregnancy?

8 Did you attend any childbirth preparation classes?

Prenatal History The prenatal history should provide information on the intrinsic and extrinsic factors which may affect the infant's physical and emotional development. It can provide insight into the parents' reaction and experience with the pregnancy which could influence their present reaction to the infant and the infant's reaction to the surroundings. It has been found that "the possibility exists that severe emotional stress during pregnancy leaves its mark on the unborn through sympathetic activation of the stress syndrome and migration of hormones across the placental barrier," thus resulting in a fussy infant.[6] Likewise, the parent who describes an easy, uncomplicated, desired pregnancy may have had less stress and have a more content infant. It is also important in the history to identify physical agents such as ionizing radiation, chemical agents such as medications, and biological agents such as infectious agents which can affect prenatal and postnatal development. Prenatal nutrition is also important to determine, since this appears to be a major source of possible brain damage and other pathology.[7] An uncomplicated prenatal history can positively influence an infant's development.

Birth History

Questions to elicit data

1 When was your due date?

2 When was (infant's name) born?

3 What was the total duration of labor?

4 How was the delivery? Was any anesthesia or medication used? Were there any complications? Did the baby breathe right away? Do you know what the Apgar score was?

5 What was the baby's weight?

6 Were any family members present for the delivery?

7 Did you hold the baby after delivery?

8 Where did the delivery take place? If a hospital delivery, did the baby go to the nursery? How long were you both in the hospital?

9 Has the baby been seen by a health care worker since birth? If so, when and why?

Birth and neonatal history may provide important historical data.

The information received from a birth and neonatal history is essential if holistic health care is to be provided. For instance, if the infant was full term, of average weight for gestational age, and had a good Apgar score, the qualities that attract parents and facilitate the establishment of a warm relationship between parents and infant were more likely to have been present.[8] Also, the birth experience should be identified, since effects of specific birth experiences have been seen, especially on the individual infant's in relation to anxiety.[9] The use and depth of obstetrical anesthesia should also be determined, since this may affect the child's behavior. The effects of obstetrical anesthesia appear to be most pronounced in selected areas of cognitive function and gross motor ability, where a lag in the development of the ability to sit, stand, and

Specific birth experiences may affect the infant's behavior.

move about may be seen.[10] Likewise, separation and health problems may affect the mother-infant tie as well as the infant's physiological functioning. Ribble has emphasized the mother's role and the need for her soothing efforts in contributing to the equilibrium that is often hard for a young infant to achieve.[11] In providing the reflex stimulation by contact, she enables the infant to organize respiratory, circulatory, and other functions under the control of the infant's nervous system. Thus, the birth and neonatal history helps the nurse acquire a more complete picture of factors and situations affecting the infant and determine the type, level, and amount of guidance and counseling that the parents may need.

See Past Health Status in Chap. 3.

Depending on the infant's age other pertinent data the nurse may elicit would include history of childhood illnesses, immunizations received, previous hospitalizations, accidents or injuries, and allergies or allergic reactions.

Family History

A family history should begin with each family member's age, sex, and state of health.

Table 3-3 and Fig. 3-2 should be used to complete the family history.

Questions to elicit data

1 What is the mother's age and state of health?

2 What is the father's age and state of health?

3 Are there any siblings? What are their ages, sex, and state of health?

This information can be recorded in a family tree.

Since some diseases and characteristics are transmitted genetically, this information is important to obtain. After asking about illnesses, as explained in Chap. 3, one should ask "Does anyone in the family have a problem which you think is important?" The parent may have a concern which is unfounded, and an explanation to that effect can be given, or there may be a genetic tendency of which one should be aware. Familial characteristics as well as diseases should be explored, since, for example, a particular facies may be a familial characteristic or may indicate the presence of a congenital syndrome.

Life Patterns and Life Styles

Age

During the period between 1 and 12 months there is dramatic change and growth. An infant moves from a helpless little being to an erect child who can communicate and manipulate objects. The infant has achieved physiological equilibrium and is aware of self. Therefore, it is important for the nurse to keep in mind the infant's exact age in months at each health visit so that accurate and appropriate assessments can be made related to a particular stage of development.

With increasing age the infant learns and develops new skills.

Race

The infant's race should be noted. Further, the nurse should determine if any racial characteristics exist which may influence the infant's health status or health care.

See Life Patterns and Life Styles in Chap. 3 for questions to elicit data.

Heredity

The parents should be questioned about hereditary traits, disorders, and diseases which could affect the infant's health. Family history data previously collected can provide the basis for this part of the assessment. It is essential for the nurse to determine the parents' perception of their heredity and how they think it will influence the growth and development of their infant.

Culture

The parents' cultural background and lifestyle must be assessed, since they will affect the nutrition, activity, interaction with, and general care of the infant. Whether the infant is breast- or bottle-fed is sometimes determined by the culture. Expectations of infant activity may vary. American Indian infants spend much time strapped to a backboard on the adult's back, while Greek infants are kept in a straight position. Japanese infants are enveloped by the mother, and black infants are actively encouraged to have early gross motor activity.[12] Evaluation of a parent as rejecting or accepting of an infant cannot be answered by noting the parent's behavior, since rejection or acceptance is not a fixed quality of behavior. Like pleasure, rejection is in the mind of the rejectee. It is a belief held by the child, not an action of the parent, and it is culturally influenced.

The infant's cultural background is greatly influenced by the parents.

Attitudes toward health and illness and the health care system and definitions of health and illness are also largely influenced by culture and lifestyle. An infant with multiple congenital anomalies may be cared for by the parents and valued in one society, while in another the infant may be isolated in the home or institutionalized. Therefore, the nurse must assess both culture and lifestyle and determine attitudes before giving care or offering anticipatory guidance or counseling.

Growth and Development

The infant's growth and development can be determined by observation, talking with the parents, and screening tests. Table 6-2 lists areas of maturation and the average age at which these developments can be seen. Each infant is unique and develops according to an individual schedule. Although the average age for development in the various areas can be cited, the nurse must remember that a wide variation is still within normal range. Parents are often very concerned about development and need calm reassurance about their infant's normality.

The infant's growth and development is unique.

The infant's perceptual system is fairly well developed by 1 month of age. Infants have some astigmatism, which is usually lost by 1 year of age.[13] They can focus on objects which are near but prefer those which are moving, bright, or flashing. The mother's eyes have these qualities and quickly achieve special importance to the infant. Many sounds are just part of the background and are meaningless to the infant. The mother's voice, however, is significant and is associated with food and pleasure. The awareness of tactile and motion perception is acute, and infants respond with pleasure to these when they are gentle. The infant is keenly aware of smells. Infants can distinguish their mothers by smell, and this perception is often an important part of the "image of mother," even into adulthood. By 12 months of age the infant's perceptual system is almost completely developed.

Other areas such as motor development and dentition should be observed, and parents should be questioned regarding these developments if they are not obvious (Table 6-3). It is helpful if the nurse is aware of maturation and the development which might be expected at various ages so that guidance and counseling regarding locomotion, hearing, and vision can be given. A general knowledge of these norms is important if the nurse is to identify developmental lags.

Table 6-2

General Characteristics of Development

Age (mo)	Appearance	Gross Motor	Fine Motor	Speech and Language	Dentition (Eruption)	Hearing	Vision
1	Plump, vigorous, self-absorbed	Marked head lag	Hands fisted	Throaty sounds		Occasional reflex turning of eyes in direction of sound origin (4–5 wk) Responds to loud noise with startle reflex	Able to fix gaze on an object if 12–24 inches in distance and patterned (5–6 wk)
2	Noisy, pleasant	In prone position can push chest up off surface	Hands loosely fisted	Vowel sounds (eh), coos, squeals (2½ mo)		Turns head to side when sound is made at level of ear	Ability to follow objects well established if they are close to eyes (6–8 wk)
3	Chubby, friendly, responds socially	No head lag, head up to 90°	Visual and tactile links developing, sucks hands	Babbles, initial vowels			Visual and tactile links rapidly developing (see, touch, grasp), begins to inspect hands, focusing distance increasing (3–5 mo)
4	Cuddly, happy	Rolls from back to side, kicks	Hands open, searches and "grasps" with eyes	Guttural sounds (ah, goo), vocalizes to toys		Consistent turning of head toward side of sound, widening of eyes, quiet, listening attitude	
5	Drools and sucks on everything	Rolls over completely	Hands clutch each other				
6	Constantly wet around the chin	Bears full weight on feet, crawls	Clings to toys, blanket		Central incisors (mandibular)	Turns toward sound but recognizes it below eye level first, then above eye level	Visual following of an object now present in all directions, depth perception increasing, becoming interested in small objects, visual alertness high but looking may inhibit other responses (6–10 mo)
7	Cheerful in familiar situations	Sits leaning forward on both hands	Palmar grasp, rakes at pellet	Limitation of speech sounds	Lateral incisors (mandibular), central incisors (maxillary)		
8	Wary of strangers	Sits alone	Clinging very prominent			Turns head 45° or more in direction of sound	
9	Mobile on all fours	Pulls self to standing position	Interior pincer grasp		Lateral incisors (maxillary)		
10	Pleasant, busy	Creeps well	Crude release beginning	Says "Dada" or "Mama," non-specifically consonant sounds, imitates sounds		Can locate sounds precisely, responds to own name, comprehends "no"	
11	Investigative	Cruises around furniture	Refined pincer grasp				
12	Busy, cheerful	Walks with someone holding hand	Can release a cube into a cup following demonstration	Says one word other than "Mama" or "Dada" with meaning	First molars	Recognizes objects by name, imitates animal sounds	Visual acuity 20/100, can perform visual function tests at 10 ft (3 m)

Table 6-3
Assessment Questions for 2-Month-Old Infant

Category	Questions
Hearing	Have you had any worry about your infant's hearing?
	If there is a loud sound, does the infant wake and move around?
Vision	Does your baby smile at you when you smile?
	Are you concerned about your infant's vision?
Speech	Does your baby make throaty sounds?
	Does your baby make vowel sounds and coo?
Development	Does your baby move both hands together in the same way?
	Does your infant lift up his or her head when lying prone?

Feeding Skills The infant's feeding skills should be assessed. Most children fill all their nutritional requirements at mealtime. For the infant who wants to suck for long periods and does not want a pacifier but a bottle, water should be given. Liquids containing sugar can have a destructive effect on the child's teeth long after bottle-feeding stops.[14] This is especially true of the infant who wants to take a bottle to bed and has the sweet liquid pooled behind the mandibular incisors.

The infant at 6 to 9 months can drink from a cup held to the lips and will help hold the cup while drinking. By 9 to 12 months the infant can pick up small pieces of food and begin to use a spoon and dish. Infants at this age can use a nonbreakable cup with a wide base and two handles and are usually ready to be weaned. Parents should be encouraged to permit the infant to engage in self-feeding activities when he or she shows interest.

Safety Assessment of and anticipatory guidance regarding safety is essential when providing holistic health care. Parents should be asked about and made aware of safety measures appropriate to various age groups. The greatest dangers to helpless infants are falls, suffocation, and drowning. As infants become more mobile, curiosity develops. As mobility increases, safety problems multiply.

When bathing the infant, the parent must take some precautions. The parent should check the temperature of the water with the elbow. A hand should be kept on the infant at all times during the bath; if the doorbell or phone must be answered, the infant should be wrapped in a towel and taken along.

Travel beds and household infant seats have no safety value in the car, and many car seats on the market provide inadequate protection. The nurse must question the parents to determine if an acceptable, dynamically tested car seat is in use and if installation instructions were carefully followed to provide optimal protection.

Household objects can be dangerous to the infant. Pins, scissors, and other sharp as well as small objects should be kept out of reach. Safety plugs should be placed in wall sockets.

Falls can be avoided by placing the infant in the crib or playpen when no supervision is available. When in a highchair, infant seat, or walker the infant should be strapped in. Gates should be used on stairways.

Poisons and medicines should be kept in a locked cabinet. All painted surfaces which might be chewed should have lead-free paint. The parent should have syrup of ipecac in the home. This is used to induce vomiting in some cases of poisoning. The telephone number of the poison control center should be on every telephone in the home.

To prevent burns, hot water temperatures should be set at less than 52°C (125°F).[15] Guards should be in front of fireplaces and radiators.

Parents must teach feeding skills to infants in order for them to be mastered.

The parents' following of safety precautions is critical to the infant's development.

The nurse must determine how parents have made the home environment safe for the infant.

Pot handles should be turned in toward the range, and hot foods, toasters, coffee pots, and dangling electric cords should be kept out of reach.

Clothing should also be considered. The infant should have clothing which does not restrict movement and flame-retardant sleepwear. Parents may wish to purchase shoes depending on the infant's mobility and the weather. Cloth shoes should be recommended, since these are flexible and allow foot movement. They can be cheaply replaced frequently as the infant's foot grows.

The parents should be asked what they think the infant's safety needs are and how they feel these can best be met. Based on this and the assessment made by the nurse during the visit, anticipatory guidance and counseling can be given.

Screening Tools and Tests The more common developmental screening tools and tests are listed in Table 6-4. Frequently the Prescreening Developmental Questionnaire (PDQ) is used. This is a prescreening tool which consists of 10 questions appropriate to the child's age which the parent answers while waiting for the infant's health care visit. If for two consecutive months the infant is only able to pass eight or fewer items on the questionnaire, further developmental testing is recommended. The PDQ has several advantages: it is inexpensive, demands a minimal amount of time and personnel, demands nothing of the infant, and is based on the parents' observations, the people most familiar with the infant's development.

When considering infant development, the nurse must remember that certain fundamental traits of individuality (constitutional characteristics) exist early, persist late, and assert themselves under varying environmental conditions. Along with the constitutional characteristics of the infant, the environment makes an impression, and individuality in development exists, with a wide variation being normal. It is important

The PDQ is a developmental screening tool.

Table 6-4 lists commonly used developmental screening tools and tests.

Table 6-4
Developmental Screening Tools and Tests

Test	Age	Description
Behavioral Developmental Profile (Marshall town)	Birth to 6 yr	Designed to measure development of handicapped and deprived children
Bayley Mental Scales	1–18 mo	Tests postural development, motor development, perception, attention span, language, object manipulation, understanding of commands, and problem solving
Boyd Developmental Progress Scale	Birth to 8 yr	Measures motor skills, communication skills, and self-sufficiency
Caldwell Home Inventory	Birth to 3 yr	Home observation for measurement of the environment
Cattell Infant Intelligence Test	3 mo to 1½ yr	To determine basal age, mental age, and intelligence quotient (IQ)
DDST	1 mo to 6 yr	Measures personal-social, fine motor—adaptive, language, and gross motor development
Denver Eye Screening Test (DEST)	6 mo and older	Vision screening test
PDQ	1 mo to 6 yr	Prescreening tool for developmental screening

Source: Based on Pamela Roberts, "Use of Screening Tools," in Marilyn Krajicek and Alice Tearney (eds.), *Detection of Developmental Problems in Children,* University Park Press, Baltimore, 1977, pp. 42–43.

for the nurse to remember individuality when determining the infant's overall developmental status.

Behavioral Development

The behavioral assessment of the infant can be done by observing the infant, talking with the parents, and using screening tools and tests. Each infant and mother is unique, and there are wide acceptable variations in behavior. When assessing the infant's behavioral development, the nurse must also consider the mother's parenting tasks and behaviors, since the mother and the infant are a unit.

The developmental schema charts for young and older infants listing the tasks and behavioral characteristics of both infant and mother may help the nurse complete this assessment (Table 6-5). It is important to remember that these developmental periods do not have a beginning or an end; the periods overlap and tasks merely become less critical over time. For example, the question of trust is never fully resolved. The nurse continues to assess and determine whether an infant can or cannot trust, but later it is not as central an issue as it is during this critical stage in infancy.

See Table 6-5 when collecting data about behavioral development.

Table 6-5
The Newborn and Young Infant: Developmental Schema Chart

Infant	Mother
Tasks in Process*	
To adjust physiologically to extrauterine life	To sustain baby and self physically and pleasurably
To develop appropriate psychological response	To give and get emotional gratification from nurturing baby
To assimilate experientially, with increasing capacity to postpone and accept substitutes	To foster and integrate baby's development
Acceptable Behavioral Characteristics*	
Copes with mechanics of life (eating, sleeping, etc.)	Provides favorable feeding and handling, gets to "know" baby
Body needs urgent	Develops good working relationship with baby
Reflexes dominate	Has tolerance for baby
Has biological unity with mother	Promotes sense of trust
Establishes symbiotic relationship to mother	Learns baby's cues
Sucking behavior prominent	Applies learning to management of baby
Cries when distressed	Interacts emotionally with baby
Responds to mouth, skin, sense modalities	Encourages baby's development
Is unstable physiologically	Has reasonable expectations of baby
Functions egocentrically	
Is completely dependent	
Has low patience tolerance	
Is noncognitive, expresses needs instinctually	
Develops trust in ministering adult	
Begins to "expect"	
Minimal Psychopathology*	
Feeding and digestive problems	Indifference to baby
Sleep disturbances	Ambivalence toward baby and its needs
Excessive sucking activity	Self-doubt and anxiety
Excessive motor discharge	Intolerance of baby's characteristics
Excessive crying	Overresponds or underresponds to baby
Excessive irritability	Premature or inappropriate expectations
Hypertonicity	Dissatisfaction with role of motherhood
Difficult to comfort	

Extreme Psychopathology*

Lethargy (depression)
Marasmus
Cannot be comforted
Unresponsive
Infantile autism
Developmental arrest

Alienation from baby
Severe depression
Excessive guilt
Complete inability to function in maternal
  role
Overwhelming and incapacitating anxiety
Denies or tries to control baby's needs
Severe clashes with baby
Vents life's dissatisfactions on baby

Tasks in Process†

To develop more reliance and self-control
To differentiate self from mother
To make developmental progress

To provide a healthy emotional and
  physical climate
To foster weaning, training, habits
To understand, appreciate, and accept
  baby

Acceptable Behavioral Characteristics†

More stable physiologically
Heightened voluntary motor activity and
  exploration
Higher level of patience, tolerance
Instinctual needs in better control
Strong selective tie to mother
Stranger differentiation
Increased verbality, play, and
  sensorimotor behavior
Discernible social responses, joyful in play
Outbursts of negativism and anger
Sensory modalities important
Emergence of idiosyncratic patterns
Demonstrates memory and anticipation
Begins to imitate

Derives satisfaction from serving baby
  well
Responds appropriately to baby's signs of
  distress
Aware of baby's inborn reaction pattern
Has more confidence in own ability
Gives positive psychological reassurance
  (fondling, talking, comforting)
Shows pleasure in baby
Keeps pace with baby's advances
Is accepting of baby's idiosyncracies

Minimal Psychopathology†

Excessive crying, anger, and irritability
Low frustration tolerance
Excessive negativism
Finicky eater, sleep disturbances
Digestive and elimination problems
Noticeable motility patterns (fingering,
  rocking, etc.)
Delayed development

Disappointed in and unaccepting of baby.
Misses baby's cues
Infancy unappealing
Impersonal management
Attempts to coerce to desired behavior
Overanxious or overprotective
Mildly depressed and apathetic

Extreme Psychopathology†

Tantrums and convulsive disorders
Apathy, immobility, and withdrawal
Extreme and obsessive finger-sucking,
  rocking, head-banging
No interest in objects, environment, or
  play
Anorexia
Megacolon
Inexpressive of feeling
No social discrimination
No tie to mother, wary of all adults
Infantile autism
Failure to thrive
Arrested development

Neglect or abuse of baby
Rejection of the maternal role
Severe hostility reactions
No attempt to understand or gratify baby
Deliberately thwarts infant
Complete withdrawal and separation from
  baby

Source: *Problems in Child Behavior and Development,* Milton J. E. Seen and Albert J. Solnit, Lea &
Febiger, Philadelphia, 1968.
*From birth to 6 months.
†From 6 to 18 months.

Stage of Infancy In the period from 1 to 12 months great strides are made in behavioral development. This stage is defined by Freud as the narcissistic-oral stage. Erickson identifies this stage as one of trust and mistrust.[16] The erogenous biological zone is the mouth, and the crises of the stage are weaning and teething. The ego mode of behavior is one of incorporation; the social modality of behavior is receiving and grasping. An important development in this age is separation-individuation. The psychological birth of the infant is discussed using the separation-individuation theoretical framework of Mahler (Fig. 6-2).[17]

Psychological Birth

Autism In autism, which lasts until about 3 to 5 weeks of age, there is no concept or schema of self, no separation or individuation. The infant exists in a closed system similar to that of intrauterine life. There is absolute primary narcissism. This is thought to occur in order to facilitate physiological growth. The mother gradually brings the child out of this state and into an increased sensory awareness of, and contact with, the environment.[18] There seems to be a parallel increase in the periods of infants' alert inactivity and in their awareness of the outside world.[19]

Symbiosis At about 3 to 5 weeks of age the period of symbiosis begins. Unlike the biological concept of symbiosis, this does not describe a mutually beneficial relationship, but rather describes the state of undifferentiation, of fusion with mother when inside and outside are coming to be sensed as different.[20] This awareness of differences between the infant and mother in texture, temperature, and smell is assimilated by the infant's sensorimotor schemata.[21] Attention is paid to the human face, and the face in motion is the first memory engram that elicits a social smile.[22] This increase in attention and in sensitivity to external stimuli can be observed, and this physiological maturational crisis at 3 to 5 weeks has been demonstrated in electroencephalographic (EEG) studies.[23] The infant moves from absolute primary narcissism into a period of primary narcissism as an awareness grows that need-satisfaction comes from outside the self. This growing awareness of differences is obvious at 4 to 5 months, when there is a specific, preferential, smiling response to the mother's face. Bowlby feels that the preferential smile is a crucial sign that a specific bond between mother and infant has been established.[24]

Differentiation At about 4 to 5 months the first subphase of the separation-individuation process occurs—that of differentiation. With differentiation of self and mother from others comes the development of body image. Persistence and goal directedness are seen as the "hatching" process begins and periods of wakefulness and alertness become

Highlights

The infant is in the narcissistic-oral stage according to Freud. Erickson labels the first year as the stage of trust versus mistrust.

Autism refers to no concept or schema of self.

The infant develops an awareness of others outside the self.

The development of body image stems from differentiation of self and mother.

Figure 6-2 Psychological birth of the human infant. Phases are indicated in capital letters. (Adapted from Margaret S. Mahler.)

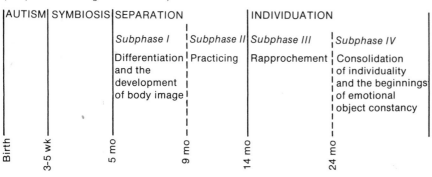

longer.[25] This alertness is most obvious at 6 to 7 months, when the peak of manual, visual, and tactile exploration of the mother's face and body is seen. Infants discriminate between what does and does not belong to the mother's body by pulling hair and pulling off earrings. These explorative patterns develop later into the cognitive function of checking the familiar against the unfamiliar.[26] Infants enjoy a bit of distance from the mother's arms and will play near her while visually "checking back to mother."[27] At about 8 months of age anxiety of strangers is seen, although there are tremendous variations in timing, quality, and quantity. Eye contact is avoided, but as soon as the stranger averts his or her gaze the infant becomes eager to find out about the person. As the infant becomes more comfortable, he or she engages in a visual and tactile exploration of the stranger.[29] There is a comparison and checking of each stranger's image to the mother's image. It is best if this awareness of bodily separation, in terms of differentiation from mother, is parallel with the infant's development of locomotion, cognition, and perception. For example, infants who are walking at 9 months may suddenly find themselves at too great a distance from their mother, and since they are not yet ready emotionally to move that far away, a very intense anxiety can be seen.

Practicing At about 9 months the second subphase of the separation-individuation process, that of practicing, begins. There is a rapid body differentiation from mother, the establishment of a specific bond with her, and the growth of autonomous functions.[30] Transitional objects, those inanimate objects which make separation from mother easier, gain importance.[31] This can be a quilt, blanket, or toy or whatever the infant associates with the mother. These objects are explored by the eyes as well as investigated by the hands and mouth for taste, texture, and smell. The transitional object phenomenon seems related to child-rearing practices; its incidence is lower in a culture or group in which infants receive a greater amount of physical contact and in which the mother is available when the infant goes to sleep.[32]

The infant begins developmental autonomy through "practicing."

The object chosen may help the infant to establish familiarity with a wider segment of the world and to perceive, recognize, and enjoy mother from a distance. The infant can then return to the mother from time to time for emotional refueling. After this emotional refueling, which includes establishment of visual, verbal, or physical contact, energy to practice and explore is restored. During the period when infants are busy exploring the world, weaning can be best accomplished.[33] They will often begin to wean themselves by giving up one feeding at a time. At this period they resent the confinement of breast-feeding or of the held bottle, since they would rather be off exploring and practicing their new locomotor skills as they have what Greenacre calls their "love affair with the world."[34] Exploration increases with the spurt in intellectual development, enhanced by upright locomotion. Anthony recognized Kierkegaard's insights into the infant's need for the mother's emotional support at the point when free walking begins and stated:

Weaning from breast-feeding may best be accomplished when the infant begins exploring.

> The loving mother teaches her child to walk alone. She is far enough from him so that she cannot actually support him, but she holds out her arms to him. She initiates his movements, and if he totters, she swiftly bends as if to seize him so that the child might believe that he is not walking alone . . . and yet, she does more. Her face beckons like a reward, an encouragement. Thus, the child walks alone with his eyes fixed on his mother's face, not on the difficulties in his way. He supports himself by the arms that do not hold him and constantly strives toward refuge in his mother's embrace, little suspecting that in the very same moment that he is emphasizing his need of her, he is proving that he can do without her, because he is walking alone.[35]

As infants learn to walk, there are periods of elation when they are impervious to falls and other, low-keyed periods, which often occur when mother, their source of strength, is absent.[36] Substitute familiar adults are, however, accepted during this period of peak narcissism but they are not accepted during the next period.

Rapprochement Rapprochement occurs at about 14 to 24 months or beyond. During this period the child has a growing realization of separateness and, with it, a vulnerability. The mother can no longer be easily substituted for, even by familiar adults. This culminates in a transient rapprochement crisis often lasting for several weeks, during which time there is an intense separation reaction.[37] The most pronounced separation anxieties are seen at this time.[38]

The fourth subphase, which begins at about 24 months, is the consolidation of individuality and the beginning of emotional object constancy when separation from the mother is established.[39] The child can begin to visualize mother and anticipate her return.

It is helpful if the parents are aware of the infant's behavioral developmental tasks and stages. For example, parents with infants in day care centers may become anxious when a formerly smiling infant now screams when left with the same caretaker. The nurse can assess the infant's stage and prepare the parents for what might be expected. The nurse and parents should view the infant's behavior as signifying growth.

Emotions and Temperament It is difficult to distinguish infants' emotions. Infants seem to have a wide range that they cannot express specifically and that cannot be identified with certainty. Four specific infant cries have been identified: (1) the basic rhythmical cry, often called the *hunger cry*, (2) the mad cry, in which a baby forces excess air through the vocal cords, (3) the pain cry, a sudden onset of a loud long cry followed by an extended period of breath holding, and (4) the cry of frustration, in which the first two or three cries are long and drawn out and there is no breath holding.[40] The mother's personal style (experience) is far more important than the form of crying in determining how she will care for her crying baby.[41] As infants get older, however, emotions differentiate from general to specific and can be readily identified.

Thomas et al. have done extensive longitudinal studies on the temperament, or basic behavioral style of individuals, which they conclude is inborn.[42] Aspects of temperament include activity level, regularity in biological functioning (hunger, sleep, elimination), readiness to accept new people and situations, adaptability to change, sensitivity to noise, light, and other sensory stimuli, mood (cheerfulness or unhappiness), intensity of responses, distractibility, and persistence. Infants vary in these characteristics from birth and have a tendency to continue in one style, although parental handling and experiences may cause change.

Table 6-6 gives some attributes of infants. Generally it can be said that predictable, responsive infants receive more effective parental interactions because they generate parental feelings of efficacy.[43] Infants are instrumental in establishing social conditions which support their own development.

It is important that nurses and parents be aware of the temperament of the infant and aware that it is largely inborn. This can relieve the parents, especially those of difficult infants, from feeling guilty and help them to respond positively to their infant. It also helps parents to adapt to their infant's needs. Parents of an infant with regularity of body function can use a "demand" feeding schedule, while those of a lazy or irregular infant may need to set a flexible schedule based on mutual needs. Recognition of a basic infant temperament can relieve the parents of the

The infant develops a growing realization of separateness.

The nurse must be aware of the infant's behavioral developmental tasks and stages in order to complete the behavioral assessment.

There are four specific infant cries: hunger, pain, mad, frustration.

Temperament is thought to be an inborn characteristic.

Table 6-6
Basic Behavioral Styles of Infants

Easy children: 40%
  Positive mood
  Regularity of body function
  Low or moderate intensity of reaction
  Adaptability
  Positiveness in a new situation

Slow to warm up: 15%
  Low activity level
  Tendency to withdraw from new stimuli
  Slow adaptability
  Somewhat negative mood
  Low intensity of reaction

Difficult: 10%
  Irregularity of body function
  High intensity of reaction
  Withdrawal in face of new stimuli
  Slow adaptability

Mixture of above attributes: 35%

Source: Based on Jeanne B. Brown, "Infant Temperament: A Clue to Childbearing for Parents and Nurses," *Am J Matern Child Nurs,* **2**:231 (July/August 1977).

feeling that they alone are responsible for the infant's behavior. This knowledge may help them to relax, enjoy, and accept their infant.

The infant temperament questionnaire can be used for this assessment with infants between 4 and 9 months of age.[44] This questionnaire consists of 70 statements which give 3 choices for completion. This tool, designed by Carey, covers 9 categories of temperament.

Family Influences on Behavioral Development The family influences the infant's behavioral development. The importance of maternal-infant attachment has been demonstrated. The father has been shown to have a specific role in ego development.[45] Evidence indicates that infants also form various attachment bonds to their fathers, to caregivers in day care situations, and to relative strangers on short acquaintance.[46] These attachments perform functions similar to the attachment to the mother; they serve to promote exploration in a novel environment, and the infant seeks to be near these people in times of stress.[47] Although these other attachments may exist, the family is central to the infant, and the strongest attachment is to the mother.

Birth order and family size have been shown to be factors in intelligence and psychiatric status. In a study of 400,000 Dutch youths aged 19 years who were tested for intelligence, those who were first-born children scored higher than second-born children, who scored higher than third-born children.[48] First-born children also tend to have a lower risk of becoming psychiatrically disabled.[49] Members of smaller families tend to be more capable intellectually and tend to experience less school failure yet have an increased risk of psychiatric disorder.[50] Closeness of children in age may also be a factor in intelligence and psychiatric status. The crucial factor might well be the time that parents have available to give to each child, which is affected by the number of other children close in age who demand their attention.

How the parents perceive and treat the infant is also a factor in behavioral development. The infant may well adapt to a self-fulfilling prophesy. For example, if the family perceives and treats the infant as bright, adaptive, and pleasant, the infant may respond accordingly.

The Broussard Neonatal Perception Index can be used to assess the mother's perception of the infant when the infant is 1 to 2 days or 4 to 6 weeks old.[51] This index compares the mother's perceptions of her infant and the average infant in crying, feeding, spitting, elimination, sleeping, and predictability. Infants who are noted as more desirable than the average infant are considered low risk.

The infant's behavioral development can be assessed using observation, questions, and screening tools and tests. When assessing this development, it is helpful if the nurse considers the infant's stage according to various theorists, the emotions, the temperament, and the family. The interaction between the infant's specific temperament and parental responses or attitudes forms a matrix from which the infant's behavior emerges. The nurse must help parents to understand their infant's behavior and their own reactions to this behavior.

Biological Rhythms

Sleep-Wakefulness Cycle The infant exhibits six states or levels of arousal:[52]

1 *Regular sleep*—muscle tonus is low, eyelids are closed and still, respirations are about 36 breaths per minute, even, and of regular rhythm

The nurse must assess the parents' ability to adapt to and cope with their infant's unique temperament.

The family strongly influences the infant's behavioral development.

Birth order and family size may influence the infant's intellectual development and psychiatric stability.

Infants may adapt behaviorally to the parents' perceptions and expectations.

The six states of arousal in the infant are regular sleep, irregular sleep, periodic sleep, drowsiness, alert inactivity, crying.

2 *Irregular sleep*—muscle tonus is greater, movements follow no sequence, grimaces are frequent, there is intermittent gross mouthing, i.e., chomping, chewing, and licking, respirations are irregular, and the mean rate is greater than during regular sleep

3 *Periodic sleep* (intermediate between regular and irregular sleep)—respiratory rates are *periodic*, i.e., bursts of rapid shallow breathing alternate with bursts of deep, slow respirations similar to Cheyne-Stokes respiration

4 *Drowsiness*—less activity than in irregular or periodic but more activity than in regular sleep, the eyes have a dull glazed appearance, open and close intermittently, and just before closing may roll upward, generally regular respirations may become tachypneic, there may be a high-pitched squeal

5 *Alert inactivity*—the eyes are open and bright and make conjugate movements in the vertical and horizontal plane, the face is relaxed, respirations are more variable and faster than in regular sleep, not seen before $3\frac{1}{2}$ weeks of age

6 *Crying*—vocalization accompanied by gross motor activity, open or closed eyes, tears can be seen as early as 24 hours after birth; characteristic patterns of crying identifiable as early as the first 5 days of life

The state of active wakefulness lengthens with age.

In older infants, a state of active wakefulness is seen, during which they explore their world. This becomes increasingly evident as they mature.

Each infant has a unique sleep pattern. Generally, by 8 to 16 weeks the infant's biological rhythms coincide with daytime and nighttime hours, and he or she will sleep through the night.[53] The younger infant may sleep 17 to 20 hours a day. The 12- to 16-week-old infant will sleep 14 to 18 hours, and by the end of the first year the infant may sleep from 12 to 16 hours a day.

Young infants spend much of their time in irregular or rapid eye movement (REM) sleep. Roffwarg et al. have hypothesized that the REM mechanism serves as an endogenous source of stimulation, an autostimulation, which furnishes great quantities of functional excitation to the higher brain centers.[54] REM sleep might assist in structural maturation and differentiation of key sensory and motor areas within the central nervous system and contribute to their growth. This would explain the rapid decline in REM sleep during growth from 80 percent of the sleep of the 10-week-old premature infant to 50 percent of the sleep of the full-term infant to 35 percent of the sleep of the 1-year-old child.

REM characterizes much of the infant's sleep pattern.

Parents must understand the infant's sleep and wakefulness patterns. The eye movement, groaning, moving, grimacing, and irregular breathing and gasping are normal and require no attention. These normal patterns can be very frightening to an uninitiated parent.

Most infants are content to sleep on their abdomen. This is the preferred position, since it prevents mucus or regurgitated milk from being aspirated. Young infants who oversleep consistently during the day can be helped to establish a better day-night routine by being awakened for daytime feedings. This is especially true with the small infant, who may need more frequent feedings.

During waking hours infants enjoy stimulation and play. They often begin by playing with their bodies. They learn about their capabilities and their separateness from mother and surroundings by examination, movement, and making sounds. Bath time, or when they are not restricted by clothing, is the ideal time for them to explore their bodies and attempt new movements.

The nurse should determine if the parents provide visual, auditory, and tactile stimulation for the infant when the child is awake. By stroking, holding, talking to, and looking at their infant, parents provide this stimulation. The infant can see and touch their faces and hear their voices. By eliciting the stare, the smile, and the grasp reflex, parents can feel some feedback from their infants, which may strengthen their attachment. Older infants also enjoy activities such as peek-a-boo, pat-a-cake, being read colorful infant books, and outdoor excursions. Infants of all ages enjoy interactions with their parents, which are the most rewarding and valuable play opportunities during waking hours.

The sleep-wakefulness cycle should be assessed to determine the parents' perception of the amount of sleep and activity the infant needs and the type of schedule for rest and activity. Guidance and counseling can then be offered if necessary.

Elimination Cycle The characteristics of the infant's stools depend on the type of food ingested. The infant who receives only breast milk will have a yellow-to-golden stool of salvelike consistency, which is faintly acid (pH 4.7 to 5.1) and may contain seedlike particles. Curds and mucus may be found in the stools of both breast- and bottle-fed infants and are of no particular significance. With cow's milk feedings, the stools vary from yellow to light brown, are firmer, less acid and possibly slightly alkaline (pH 6 to 8), and have a stronger fecal odor because of the decomposition of protein. As the infant grows and the amount of milk in the overall diet decreases, the stools become more like those of adults in both color and odor.

The number of stools varies considerably; the infant's comfort and well-being are more important than the number of stools, and parents should be aware of this. Breast-fed infants average 2 to 4 stools a day during the first 3 to 4 months of life, whereas artificially fed infants average 1 or 2 stools. Occasionally the breast-fed infant may comfortably and normally have a bowel movement of usual consistency only once in 4 to 10 days. By the end of the first year the infant may have only 1 stool a day.

The volume of urine the infant produces is 400 to 600 ml per 24 hours. The infant will average from 13 to 20 voidings a day, each with an average quantity of 30 to 45 ml. The infant's kidneys are immature and unable to concentrate urine; therefore, fluid intake should be maintained at an adequate level, especially in warm weather.

Temperature Cycle The infant's temperature is set in a cyclical pattern. The temperature is higher during daytime hours when infants are most active. A normal temperature in infancy may be a degree or more above the adult average.

Parents should be aware of how to take a rectal temperature. The nurse should ask the parents to do this when the infant is brought for a health care visit. This is especially important before immunizations are given, since these may cause a rise in temperature; the parents will feel more comfortable and confident if they can monitor the infant's temperature.

Pharmacological Effectiveness Cycle Active immunization of children provides an effective means of disease prevention and health maintenance. The recommended schedule in Table 6-7 is for normal, healthy infants. If an infant is ill the immunization is postponed, since the fever which sometimes results from the injection may confuse the picture of the illness. Parents should fully understand the immunizations proposed for their infant. They should be assessed for their knowledge about the anti-

The elimination cycle is directly affected by diet.

Table 6-7
Recommended Schedule for Active Immunization of Normal Infants and Children

2 mo	DTP[a]	TOPV[b]
4 mo	DTP	TOPV
6 mo	DTP	[c]
1 yr		Tuberculin test[d]
15 mo	Measles,[e] Rubella[e]	Mumps[e]
1½ yr	DTP	TOPV
4–6 yr	DTP	TOPV
14–16 yr	Td[f]—repeat every 10 yr	

a, DTP—diphtheria and tetanus toxoids combined with pertussis vaccine.
b, TOPV—trivalent oral poliovirus vaccine. This recommendation is suitable for breast-fed as well as bottle-fed infants.
c, A third dose of TOPV is optional but may be given in areas of high endemicity of poliomyelitis.
d, Frequency of repeated tuberculin tests depends on risk of exposure of the child and on the prevalence of tuberculosis in the population group. For the pediatrician's office or outpatient clinic, an annual or biennial tuberculin test, unless local circumstances clearly indicate otherwise, is appropriate. The initial test should be done at the time of, or preceding, the measles immunization.
e, May be given at 15 months as measles-rubella or measles-mumps-rubella combined vaccines.
f, Td—combined tetanus and diphtheria toxoids (adult type) for those more than 6 years of age, in contrast to diphtheria and tetanus (DT) toxoids which contain a larger amount of diphtheria antigen. *Tetanus toxoid at time of injury:* For clean, minor wounds, no booster dose is needed by a fully immunized child unless more than 10 years have elapsed since the last dose. For contaminated wounds, a booster dose should be given if more than 5 years have elapsed since the last dose.

Concentration and Storage of Vaccines
Because the concentration of antigen varies in different products, the manufacturer's package insert should be consulted regarding the volume of individual doses of immunizing agents.

Because biologics are of varying stability, the manufacturer's recommendations for optimal storage conditions (e.g., temperature, light) should be carefully followed. Failure to observe these precautions may significantly reduce the potency and effectiveness of the vaccines.
Source: American Academy of Pediatrics: *Report of the Committee on Infectious Diseases,* The Association, Evanston, Ill., 1977, p. 3.

gens to be administered, the reasons for their use, the associated reactions which might occur, and what they can do to minimize the infant's discomfort from these reactions.

Diphtheria and tetanus toxoids combined with pertussis vaccine (DPT) is given intramuscularly (IM) into the vastus lateralis or the ventrogluteal site. Over 50 percent of infants experience a reaction. There may be an onset of fever within 6 to 12 hours, not exceeding 39.5°C (103°F), which subsides in 48 hours. Parents should know how to take a rectal temperature and how to manage the fever with antipyretics and sponging if needed. Many infants experience a local reaction to the injection, i.e., swelling and/or redness at the site. These symptoms usually peak 48 to 72 hours after the injection and may be partially relieved by a warm, wet washcloth. The parents should be asked if their infant has had a reaction to this injection.

After the trivalent oral polio virus vaccine (TOPV) is given, infants should not be fed for 30 minutes to prevent spitting up of the vaccine. There is some controversy on whether TOPV should be given as scheduled to breast-fed infants or if administration should be deferred until the infant is weaned, since protective antibodies in breast milk may somewhat reduce the effectiveness of the vaccine.[55] Generally, however, TOPV is given with DPT in breast- and formula-fed infants.

The tine or tuberculin test is administered by pressing a single-use tine unit, a disc with four tiny, sharp prongs which contain dried old tuberculin, on the forearm. The parents should be told to contact the health care facility if redness or swelling is present at 48 hours.

Metabolic rhythms By 1 month of age the infant's metabolic rhythms are established. These can be best assessed when the infant is quiet, since stress will cause the blood pressure and respiratory and heart rates to increase.

The average heart rate for the infant aged 1 to 6 months is 120 to 140 beats per minute and for the infant aged 6 to 12 months is 110 to 130 beats per minute. The pulse should be taken apically for a full minute and the rhythm and strength of the pulse assessed. The rate will vary during the time of day, reaching its peak along with the temperature. The pulse is a highly sensitive measure of temperature, increasing about 15 to 20 percent with each degree of rise in temperature.[56]

The average respiratory rate for the infant is 20 to 30 breaths per minute. Respirations should be assessed with regard to rate, quality, and depth. This can be done by observation and palpation. The respiratory rate will also vary according to time of day, since it is also a highly sensitive measure of temperature.

The average blood pressure for the infant is 60 to 90 mmHg systolic and 20 to 40 mmHg diastolic. The systolic is the first sound heard, and the diastolic is the point at which the sounds become muffled. Systolic pressure in the arms is equal to that in the thighs in an infant under 1 year of age.

An infant's blood pressure is often inaudible. To obtain a blood pressure in infants, the Doppler, palpatory, or flush method can be used. The Doppler is the most accurate. This method uses a transducer, which is held over the artery to detect movements of the arterial wall and transmits these as sound. In the palpatory method the systolic pressure is taken to be the point at which the pulse distal to the cuff becomes palpable when the cuff is deflated. In the flush method the arm is elevated, the blood pressure cuff is applied and inflated, and the arm is lowered. The cuff is then deflated, and the point at which flushing appears is recorded as the systolic pressure.

The parents' understanding of immunizations should be assessed.

Blood pressure, heart rate, and respiratory rate should be assessed by the nurse.

See Chap. 5 for the techniques of taking the blood pressure.

The Doppler, palpatory, or flush method can be used to determine blood pressure.

Since biological rhythms are established early in infancy, the infant needs some regularity of experience. By 6 months, the infant is making predictions and altering sleep patterns and eating cycles as a function of the regularities in a day.[57] Parents should be made aware that the infant needs some regularity of experience.

See Table 3-4 and adapt questions to the infant and parents.

Environmental Factors

The infant's environment should be assessed, since it will greatly influence both maturation and sensorimotor development. For instance, if an infant has space and a variety of visual and auditory stimuli such as appropriate toys to explore, books and pictures to study, and a consistent loving caretaker who provides a safe environment with a minimum of frustration, his or her energies may be freer for development than the frustrated infant whose needs are not consistently met and who receives a minimum of stimulation.

Maturation and sensorimotor development are influenced by the environment.

Although maturation proceeds in cephalocaudal sequence and in an orderly, uniform manner, studies of institutionalized infants raise questions on the effect of the environment.[58] Provence and Lipton found retardation in the developmental age and the general maturity level of institutionalized infants as young as 5 months when they were compared with infants living with families.[59] This and other studies show that development in the first year of life not only depends on physiological and maturational factors but also on environmental factors relating to sensory stimulation.

See Environmental Factors in Chap. 3.

Noxious factors in the environment can be potential dangers to the infant's health state. For example, a parent who works in an area with carcinogenic materials may need to shower and change clothes before leaving work, since the carcinogen may or may not be able to be detoxified. A parent working in the health care field who held a child with a communicable disease may want to take special precautions before handling his or her own infant. Parents must be made aware of noxious factors so that they can protect their infant from risk. The nurse should use questions presented in Chap. 3 when collecting data on noxious factors.

Economics

The family's economic status has been shown to be a factor in infant mortality. The following characteristics have been seen as predictive of higher infant mortality: the breadwinner's employment status, mother unwed at infant's birth, mother married but no father in the home, number of children per room, mother under 20 or over 35, and parents' educational level.[60] Infants of parents of a lower economic status may be at higher risk.

See Economics in Chap. 3.

Family economics may also influence ability to purchase health care and items to meet the infant's basic needs. Therefore, the nurse must evaluate economics as it affects the infant's health state.

Community Resources

The health care worker must be aware of community resources that the parents might use for economic assistance, education, guidance, counseling, or support. When there is frequently little or no extended family to whom the new mother can turn for assistance, these resources can be invaluable.

The nurse should determine if the parents are aware of or use various community resources to benefit health.

The new mother sometimes waits for permission to take time for herself.

1 Do you have a babysitter?

2 Is there a babysitting cooperative (often a source of support and information) in the neighborhood?

3 Are there play groups or infant stimulation groups?

4 Are there mother's support groups?

5 Does the local library have study groups, a toy lending library, or selection of good books on child care?

6 For breast-feeding mothers, is there a support group or a La Leche branch?

7 Does the clinic or neighborhood health care center, hospital, or local Red Cross have classes on infant care which would provide information as well as a social situation?

8 Is there a crisis center or hotline or family and children's services?

9 What government agencies are available? If food stamps, welfare, unemployment, or aid to dependent children is needed, who should be contacted?

The nurse must inquire about the use of these resources and determine if parents know how and when to use them. If there is a need, the nurse can be instrumental in meeting that need by making others aware of it and/or beginning to meet this need by organizing forces to deal with it.

Roles and Relationship Patterns

Family Life

The family exerts a tremendous influence on the infant's health, since the infant is totally dependent on family members for care. If a family does not value preventative health measures, the infant may not be provided with immunizations. Likewise, family reactions to difficulties differ; certain types of families tend to aggravate, while others tend to ameliorate, any problem that the infant might have.[61]

Families tend to care for their infant in the manner they learned from their parents. For instance, if parents were abused as children, they are more likely to be abusive parents. Although they may be interested in changing their behavior, this cannot be assumed. The nurse must assess the parents' needs and the infant's health in such situations.

The age of family members must also be considered. If they have several young children, parents may have difficulty caring for the infant. Adolescent parents are more likely to be separated from their infant for periods while they work or finish school, and this might affect their attachment. There may also be a lack of confidence, mood shifts, and changing ideas in young parents which can affect the consistency of care and the patience that the infant needs.[62] On the other hand, older parents may have difficulty adjusting to the new demands and changes in routine imposed by the infant. Since the care of the infant is the responsibility of the parents, the nurse must evaluate parenting behaviors and skills which can affect health. There must be a balanced approach to parenting; it is essential for both parents and infant to grow in an atmosphere of self-regard without infringement of the rights of either parents or infant.[63]

Families tend to care for their infants in the manner they learned from their parents.

Occupation

Howell says that jobs take parents out of the home and demand their time and energy to the extent that it constitutes a major crisis for families and a major impediment to healthy family life.[64] Many jobs do require a time and energy commitment that may leave the worker little to invest in family matters, especially when the family includes an infant who requires much time and energy.

The nurse must assess if different kinds of family schedules interfere with the continuity and regularity in the infant's relationships with parents, since this may affect the child's health, growth, and development. Questions such as "How do you find time for your infant if you work an 8-hour job?" and "How do you spend available time together?" will facilitate data collection. The nurse will also want to know what the parents regard as benefits of their occupation, e.g., health care insurance, vacation time, and services provided.

A certain occupation may expose parents to noxious factors in the environment, as mentioned previously. If dangers can be carried home, such as carcinogenic materials, this poses a health risk. Therefore, the nurse should also explore this area when assessing occupation.

Societal Relationships

In U.S. society the mother is usually responsible for the infant's care. With the frequent withdrawal of social supports, often including the lack of an extended family and little or no neighborhood support, mothers are often isolated. Single mothers are usually in an even more difficult position, since they often have the total responsibility for the child's care and upbringing. Although the nurse can provide some support, parents should be made aware of appropriate community resources.

Cognitive and Perceptual Patterns

The data collected should include information about the infant's sensory perceptions and cognitive abilities based on early education and understanding of early intellectual development. Since the parents are usually the primary informants, questions can be asked of them.

Sensory Perception

It is difficult to accurately determine the infant's sense of smell and taste; therefore, only vision, hearing, and touch are readily assessed. Questions cited in Chap. 5 can be used to elicit data.

Education

The educational level of the infant's caretakers influences the infant care provided. Mothers who have little or no knowledge of child development and little outside support or extended families who can relate some understanding of infants may be at a disadvantage. They may not anticipate areas of growth and development in their infant, and, consequently, not provide needed stimulation and support to foster maturation. The nurse must thus evaluate the educational level of the significant caretakers.

The infant's educational abilities must also be determined. The nurse may use such tools as the Denver Developmental Screening Test (DDST) to assess if the infant's abilities are appropriate for the age. Using knowledge of growth and development, the nurse may also have the infant attempt other tasks to give an indication of current capabilities. For example, most 10-month-old infants should be able to crawl and pull up to a standing position, but the infant cannot learn this skill with-

The parents' occupations can affect the health care provided the infant, and areas of growth and development.

See Noxious Factors.

See Chap. 5 for a description of the DDST.

out the opportunity to try it. Language development, socialization, and motor skills all reflect the infant's educational capabilities; however, these should not be used for predicting future abilities.

Intelligence

The nurse must consider physical, motor, social, and emotional influences on the infant as well as take into account individual differences when looking at an infant's intellectual development. Although various aspects of infant behavior can be studied, all components of development are interrelated and exert mutual influence.

In the sensorimotor stage described by Piaget, which ranges from birth to approximately 24 months, there are 6 substages.[65] The infant changes from a being who responds through reflexes to one who can organize sensorimotor activities in relation to the environment. Each substage serves as a foundation for the next. There are four substages in the period from 1 to 12 months. These correspond to the 3 stages in Décarie's objectal scale (Table 6-8).

In substage 1 of the sensorimotor period from birth to 1 month, reflexes are adaptive in that they enable the infant to survive.

In stage 2, from 1 to 4 months, primary circular reactions (the first acquired adaptations) are seen. Hand-mouth and eye-ear coordination are developing. Beginning intention of behavior is seen. An infant will deliberately try to put a thumb in the mouth, keep it there, and suck it.

Stage 3, that of secondary circular reactions, is seen from 4 to 8 months. The infant repeats an action not for the joy of the action alone but also for the result. For example, an infant will shake a rattle not just for the movement but to hear the noise it produces. Memory traces are being laid down, and the infant begins to anticipate events.

Stage 4, from 8 to 12 months, is one of coordination of secondary schemata and their application to new situations. Infants can solve simple problems by using previously mastered responses. For example, infants will pull off a tablecloth to get a desired toy from the top of a table. The schema of the permanent object is beginning to develop; i.e., if in-

Highlights

As described by Piaget, the infant is in the stage of sensorimotor development.

By 12 months of age, infants can solve simple problems.

Table 6-8
Assessing Intelligence

Piaget Stages		Approximate Age (mo)	(Décarie) Objectal Scale		Approximate Age
Period			Period		
Sensorimotor	**1** Use of reflexes	0–1	Narcissistic	**a** No specific reaction	
	2 First habits and "primary" circular reactions	1–4½		**b 1** Specific reaction to feeding	
	3 Coordination of vision and prehension, "secondary" circular reactions	4½–8 or 9	Intermediate	**2** Automatic smile 2 mos.	0–4 mo.
				3 Negative affect at play interruption	
	4 Coordination of secondary schemas and their application to new situations	8 or 9–11 or 12		**4** Ability to wait	
			Objectal **(a)**	**5** Differentiated smile	
				6 Negative affect at loss of toy	4½–12 mo.
	5 Differentiation of action through "tertiary" circular reactions, discovery of new means	11 or 12–18		**7** Signs of affection	
			Objectal **(b)**	**8** Compliance with requests	
	6 First internalization of schemas and solution of some problems by deduction	18–24		**9** Compliance with prohibitions	12 mo.–2 yrs.
				10 Subtle discrimination of signs of communication	

Source: Thérèse Gouin Décarie, *Intelligence and Affectivity in Early Childhood*, International University Press, New York, 1965.

fants see an object being hidden behind a screen which they then observe being moved to another place, they will look for it in the first hiding place.

The intellectual development of the infant should be considered during the health care visit. For example, from 1 to 12 months there is not a good sense of object permanence; what is out of sight to the infant may be thought not to exist. Thus infants do not have the visual image of the parent.[66] The presence of a calm, reassuring parent may help the infant to remain under control during the health care visit. In addition to providing reassurance to the infant, the parent may benefit by observing the nurse as a role model interacting with the infant. The parent may learn new skills of caretaking and gain confidence in his or her abilities, which directly benefits the infant as well.

Sexuality Patterns

The infant's sex plays a role in development, since male-female infant responses differ. Male infants initially elicit more of a response from mothers, although by 3 months this is reversed. Mothers are generally more successful in calming irritable daughters than irritable sons.[67] By 6 months the female has a longer attention span for visual stimuli, better fixation to a human face, and is more responsive to social stimuli.[68]

Feelings of maleness or femaleness begin during the first year. By 1 year the infant responds to his or her name, which is an important link to gender. Both sexes explore their genitals, although the mouth is the main erogenous zone. Some gender-role behavior is learned as a result of parent-reinforced sex-coded behavior in infancy. In some cultures where males are more highly valued than females, they may receive better care and more attention, hence enhancing their feelings of self-esteem.

The nurse should explore with the parents their feelings about the infant's sex and sexuality and determine how the parents relate to and care for the infant as influenced by the sex.

Nutritional Metabolic Patterns

To the infant, food is more than just a carrier of nutrients to meet the requirements for growth, maintenance, and regulation. It provides oral gratification and pleasure by giving an opportunity for sucking and mouthing. It provides sensory stimulation with its numerous colors, aromas, textures, and consistencies, and a time for socialization, the giving of love. Cicely Williams, in her "cuddling is more important than calories" philosophy, believes that aspects other than *what* to feed an infant are of great importance when the nurse addresses the topic of infant feeding.[69] Cultural differences and parents' individual preferences should also be assessed when discussing this sometimes emotional topic.

For young infants a flexible feeding schedule, rather than a strict 3- or 4-hour schedule, is recommended. Most mothers find that an infant cries from hunger and, if fed until full, will approximate a 4-hour schedule. If the infant does become drowsy after sucking for a few minutes, he or she may need to be burped, since the air in the stomach may have caused feelings of fullness and contentment. To breast- or bottle-feed a baby, mothers should be encouraged to sit in a comfortable chair, relax, and cuddle the baby holding the head in the crook of their arm. This semiupright position prevents air bubbles from forming. The relaxed, unhurried mother who provides rhythmic tactile or auditory stimulation will have a more content infant. Feeding time is the perfect time for strengthening maternal-infant ties when both are alert, in eye contact, and experiencing the closeness and warmth.

Highlights

Parents can greatly influence the infant's later abilities.

See Sex and Sexuality in Chaps. 1, 2, and 5 when assessing this data.

When assessing the nutrition of the infant, the nurse should collect data about intake, scheduling of meals, appetite, and methods of feeding. RDA requirements are given in Table A-12.

See Appendix D for growth percentiles for boys and girls.

Older infants may be content with three meals a day plus two or more snacks. As they graduate to solid foods and can sit in a highchair near the table, meal times can be a delightful time of socialization for the entire family.

For the young infant the diet is usually breast-feeding or formula. Although breast-feeding is the most nutritional choice, it does not necessarily result in optimal closeness of mother and baby.[70] Breast- and bottle-feeding can both elicit positive feelings for mother and infant.

Breast-feeding

If the mother has been breast-feeding, the nurse must have some understanding of the advantages for the mother and the infant and of parental concerns which might be voiced during the interview so that support and encouragement can be given. Human milk is the ideal food for the human infant. It is a convenient fast food which is ready when the infant desires it. If needed, the mother may hand-express breast milk and refrigerate it for up to 24 hours; this is the ideal surrogate method.

Breast milk has many advantages. Its many immune factors protect the infant. Bacterial and viral antibodies are present in human milk, and substances in human milk inhibit the growth of a number of viruses.[71] Leukocytes are also present. Breast milk has more polyunsaturated acids and fat, is better absorbed than cow's milk, and has a low sodium content. The cholesterol content is higher than that of commercial formulas, but there is no evidence that a low cholesterol intake in the first year of life affects the potential for subsequent arteriosclerotic heart disease. It is felt that a safe guide is to pattern dietary cholesterol intake in the early months of life on that found in human milk, since serum lipid and lipoprotein levels change with different ages, and their role is not known.[72] Breast milk contains adequate calories for energy requirements and free water for excretion of solute. Recent studies have shown that although the concentration of iron in human milk is low, the bioavailability is very high (Table 6-9).[73,74] Low serum iron concentration is important because the two proteins in mother's milk, transferrin and lactoferrin, lose their bacteriostatic properties with iron saturation.[75] Overfeeding while breast-feeding is not usually a problem, since the mother does not really know how much the infant has taken; the amount consumed is determined by the infant and modified little by the mother, thus avoiding obesity.

Since potentially harmful substances such as nicotine, drugs, and pesticides pass into the milk and to the infant, mothers should be questioned about use of these substances. Allergic reactions to human milk are nonexistent (Table 6-10).

At the International Symposium on Infant and Child Feeding, it was felt that mothers' failure to breast-feed in industrial countries is directly related to the lack of practical information and personal support from health care professionals.[76] The nurse must provide information on how to avoid sore nipples and how to maintain an adequate milk supply. Mothers must gain confidence and pride in what they are doing for their infants—giving of themselves and providing the very best possible care.

Formula

Infant formula is made to simulate human milk. It does not have the immune factors present in human milk. It does contain the levels of calcium, phosphorous, and other minerals which are in keeping with the infant's needs and physiological capabilities. Formula differs from cow's milk in important ways. The protein has been partially denatured to make it more digestible, avoiding the allergic response of gastroenteric bleeding that some infants' intestinal mucosa have to cow milk proteins.

The nurse must have an understanding of breast-feeding in order to know what questions to ask the mother during the nutrition interview.

Table 6-9
Iron Sources

	Bioavailability	
	Good	Poor
Human milk	✔	
Cow's milk		✔
Regular formula		✔
Iron-fortified formula	✔	
Iron-fortified cereals	✔	
Egg yolk		✔
Infant "dinners"		✔

Source: Based on George Owen, "Iron Deficiency in Infancy," in *Dialogues in Infant Nutrition: A Foundation for Lasting Health*, vol. 1, Health Learning Systems, Bloomfield, N.J., 1978, p. 4.

Noxious substances can pass through breast milk to the infant.

Table 6-10
Food Allergy

Most allergenic
  Cow's milk (whole, 2%, skim)
  Egg white
  Wheat
  Citrus
Less allergenic
  Commercial formula (milk-based)
Least allergenic
  Human milk
  Commercial formula (milk-free)
  Soy
  Casein hydrolysate

Source: Based on Claude Roy, "Food Allergies and Gastrointestinal Disorders," in *Dialogues in Infant Nutrition: A Foundation for Lasting Health*, vol. 1, Health Learning Systems, Bloomfield, N.J., 1979, p. 3.

Because of this allergic response, which results in the loss of red blood cells (RBCs) and serum albumin, many mothers are advised to breast-feed or give formula for at least 6 months and sometimes for the first 12 months of life.

Solid Foods

The types of solid food offered to the infant, and when they are offered, differ greatly based on cultural differences, the infant's neuromuscular maturation, and individual preferences. Some mothers prefer to make their baby food, while others buy commercial products. Some begin solids much earlier than others. There is no set rule. A variety of combinations of foods and milks can be found to be consumed by well-nourished infants at any month during infancy. Recently, however, later introduction of solid foods has been advised by the Committee on Nutrition of the American Academy of Pediatrics. For the parents seeking advice and with no set cultural preferences, introduction of solids can be recommended at 4 to 6 months of age. Parents should be told that when first fed with a spoon, the infant will attempt to suck. Parents may interpret the protrusion of the tongue as a dislike of the food, but it is a result of neuromuscular incoordination and surprise at the taste and feel of the new items in the diet.

If the mother is interested in making baby food, she can be made aware of the advantages to this and of the methods to make it. If she wants to use commercial baby food, she should be encouraged to buy those brands containing no added salt or sugar. The infant does not need the extra calories which added sugar in baby food provides. The acquired taste possibly gained by consuming these sweet foods may result in obesity (Table 6-11). High sodium intake has been shown to accelerate the appearance and severity of high blood pressure in genetically predisposed children.[77] In addition, an infant given excessive amounts of sodium chloride risks hypernatremia.

A general schedule of introducing solids could be recommended to the mother of the infant between 4 and 6 months. Simple foods are introduced singly so that if the infant has an allergic reaction, the offending food can be identified (Table 6-12). Rice cereal could be used for 1 month and then the introduction of other solids could be started at weekly intervals, beginning with bland fruits such as applesauce and bananas and progressing to yellow fruits such as peaches and apricots. These can be followed by carrots, squash, and then beans and peas. Meats are introduced in a similar time sequence: beef for a week, then lamb, and so on. Finger foods can then be introduced (Fig. 6-3).

The nurse must determine when solid foods were introduced and the types and amounts that the infant ingests.

Table 6-11
Infant Obesity: Parent Counseling

Avoid	Encourage
Bottle—last drop	Good feeding
Solids—too early	practices
Food rewards	Physical activity
Clean plate	
Foods with added sugar	

Source: Based on JoAnne Brasel, "Infantile Obesity," in *Dialogues in Infant Nutrition: A Foundation For Lasting Health,* vol. 1, Health Learning Systems, Bloomfield, N.J., 1978, p. 3.

Table 6-12
Food Allergy: Signs and Symptoms

Central Nervous System	Respiratory
Pallor	Rhinitis
Fatigue	Asthma
Irritability	
Gastrointestinal	Dermatological
Abdominal pain	Urticaria
Vomiting	Eczema
Diarrhea	Vascular
Constipation	Shock

Source: Based on Claude Roy, "Food Allergies and Gastrointestinal Disorders," in *Dialogues in Infant Nutrition: A Foundation for Lasting Health,* vol. 1, Health Learning Systems, Bloomfield, N.J., 1979, p. 2.

Figure 6-3 Introduction of solid foods into the infant diet. (Adapted from Lewis Barness, "The Feeding Transitions in the First Year," in *Dialogues in Infant Nutrition: A Foundation for Lasting Health,* vol. 1, Health Learning Systems, Bloomfield, N.J., 1977, p. 4.)

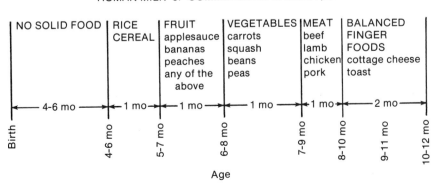

HUMAN MILK or COMMERCIAL FORMULA plus

NO SOLID FOOD	RICE CEREAL	FRUIT applesauce bananas peaches any of the above	VEGETABLES carrots squash beans peas	MEAT beef lamb chicken pork	BALANCED FINGER FOODS cottage cheese toast

←— 4-6 mo —→ ←— 1 mo —→ ←— 1 mo —→ ←— 1 mo —→ ←— 1 mo —→ ←— 2 mo —→

Birth 4-6 mo 5-7 mo 6-8 mo 7-9 mo 8-10 mo 9-11 mo 10-12 mo

Age

Vitamins

Human milk contains most of the vitamins and minerals needed by the infant for the first months of life. Vitamin D may need to be supplemented, since exposure to the sun is unreliable, and fluoride may need to be given, since it is not passed to the infant in human milk. When the mother is not breast-feeding, an iron-fortified commercial formula is recommended. Although this information is generally applicable in most geographical locations, infants should be individually assessed on their need for additional vitamins and minerals.

While taking care to respect individual differences and cultural preferences, nurses should stress that infancy is the ideal time for parents to begin sound nutrition for their children. In no other area is family influence more strong than in food preferences. The association of mother's food and love lasts over the years and may supersede all outside influences.[78]

Exercise and Activity Patterns

The infant depends on adults to permit and direct activity. Studies during the first 2 years of life have shown that infants who were on their mother's bodies for a large part of the day and were nursed on demand but were never spoken to or played with, were intellectually retarded, and were affectively depressed when compared with a group of American children who had received a variety of activities. Physical affection and a variety of stimulation are important for normal growth.

Many kinds of stimulation and opportunities to practice make life interesting to the infant. Excessive homogeneity of experience promotes a listless, nonalert attitude.[80] The first task of development is to understand unusual happenings in the outside world. Mothers should be encouraged to provide infants with this diversity.

The nurse must learn what activities the caretakers and the infant engage in for stimulation, growth, and development. It is important to evaluate if the infant is included in family games, sports, outings, and other activities.

Coping Patterns and Stress Tolerance

Like the neonate, the infant's reactions to stress are related to physical and psychological needs being met. Infants learn to cope with stress through experience. For example, if the infant is temporarily separated from the mother, crying, screams, and other behaviors of protest may ensue until the child is distracted by toys. The infant soon learns that mother will return and eventually deals with the separation by smiling and waving goodbye.

Separation anxiety is most common after 7 months of age but can occur as early as 4 months. If separation is avoided during the early months of life, infants seem to be able to cope with stress more easily. Other behavioral reactions to stress include withdrawal, depression, detachment, and physical resistance caused by such stressors as hunger, wet diapers, tiredness, illness, fear, and rejection.

It is important for the nurse to question the parents about their ability to cope with stress in their infant and to identify stressors and coping abilities in the infant. Data can be collected by adapting questions presented in Chap. 3 to individual interview situations.

Review of Body Components

The review of body components provides a subjective picture of the intactness of the infant. With the young infant, it is best to begin by reviewing

Highlights

The nurse should assess if vitamin or fluoride supplements are being given to the infant.

The infant's food habits are greatly influenced by family food preferences.

Since dramatic changes in growth and development occur in the infant over the first year, activity is an important factor influencing health.

See Exercise and Activity Patterns in Chaps. 3 and 5.

Infants learn to cope with stress through daily experience.

The ability to deal with stress as an adult has its beginnings in the first year of life.

See Behavioral Development when collecting data on stress.

the intrapartal and birth summary sheets and the notes from the last health visit. Copies of this sheet should be given to those providing maternal care and child care and to the parents. The parents should be asked for this sheet and a copy should be made if it is not in the infant's current record. The discharge summary sheet, which is recommended by the American Academy of Pediatrics, provides information on the infant's birth and discharge weights, laboratory studies, diagnosis, and a list of instructions such as bathing, feeding, and cord and circumcision care which were given to, and understood by, the parents.

It is important for the nurse to review the infant's health records for significant past history.

The nurse can begin by following up on concerns or questions which the parent may have regarding the above information. For the older infant, the nurse can follow up on the most recent information in the chart. As the body components are reviewed, attention can be given to any of these past concerns and any current parental concerns. Anticipatory guidance and counseling will be provided verbally, through pamphlets, or at frequent formal child care classes at a later time.

See Chap. 3 for the format used to collect this data on body components.

The nurse should question the parents systematically about each body component until all data are collected. Problems or concerns about the infant should be noted. The infant's diet, including vitamins and medications, and bowel elimination patterns should be discussed. The type and number of wet diapers should be noted. The general activity level, reflexes, developmental level, and behaviors as they relate to each body component should be discussed.

The review of body components provides a picture of the infant as perceived by the parents. The information obtained at this time can also help the nurse determine what areas may need further evaluation during the physical examination.

SUMMARY

The health assessment of the infant allows for thorough data collection of physical, psychological, and sociocultural components and patterns affecting health. Since the parents are the primary caretakers, much of the data will be collected through interviewing of them. The infant is also totally dependent on caretakers for physical care, socialization, education, and enhancement of growth and development. Therefore, it is important that the nurse evaluate the infant-parent relationship and determine if the infant's growth, development, and health are proceeding according to normal parameters as a result of parental care.

REFERENCES

1. M. Mahler, F. Pine, and A. Bergman, *The Psychological Birth of the Human Infant,* Basic Books, New York, 1975, p. 5.

2. L. K. Frank, *On the Importance of Infancy,* Random House, New York, 1966, p. 87.

3. D. L. Fink, "Holistic Health: Implications for Health Planning," *Am J Health Plan,* **1:**24 (July 1976).

4. T. S. Szasz and M. H. Hollender, "A Contribution to the Philosophy of Medicine," *Arch Intern Med,* **94:**585 (1956).

5. R. Murray and J. Zentner, *Nursing Concepts for Health Promotion,* Prentice-Hall, Englewood Cliffs, N. J., 1979, Chap. 3.

6. M. Lieberman, "Early Developmental Stress and Later Behavior," in L. Stone, H. Smith, and L. Murphy (eds.), *The Competent Infant,* Basic Books, New York, 1973, p. 152.

7. R. Maier and W. Brill, "Abnormal Auditory Evoked Potentials in Early Infancy Malnutrition," *Science,* **201:**450 (August 1978).

8. E. Goldson, M. Fitch, T. Wendell, et al., "Child Abuse: Its Relationship to Birth Weight, Apgar Score, and Developmental Testing," *Am J Dis Child,* **132:**793 (1978).

9. P. Greenacre, *Emotional Growth,* International Universities Press, New York, 1971, p. 272.

10. Y. Brackbill and S. Broman, in G. Kolata, "Behavioral Teratology: Birth Defects of the Mind," *Science,* **202:**732 (November 1978).

11. M. Ribble, *The Rights of Infants,* Columbia University Press, New York, 1965, p. 18.

12. R. Murray and J. Zentner, *Nursing Concepts,* p. 396.

13. H. Howland, J. Atkinson, O. Braddick, et al., "Infant Astigmatism Measured by Photorefraction," *Science,* 202:332 (October 1978).

14. R. Knoll and J. Stone, "A Warning to Parents," Paper presented to the American Society of Dentistry for Children, 1977.

15. K. Feldman, R. Schaller, J. Feldman, et al., "Tap Water Scald Burns in Children," *Pediatrics,* **62:**1 (1978).

16. E. Erickson, *Childhood and Society,* Norton, New York, 1964, pp. 247–251.

17. M. Mahler, F. Pine, and A. Bergman, *Psychological Birth,* pp. 39–120.

18. M. Ribble, *Rights,* p. 18.

19. P. Wolff, "The Classification of States," in L. Stone, H. Smith, and L. Murphy (eds.), *Competent Infant,* pp. 269–272.

20. M. Mahler, F. Pine, and A. Bergman, *Psychological Birth,* p. 44.

21. J. Piaget, "The Stages of the Intellectual Development of the Child," *Bull Menninger Clin,* 3:121–122 (1962).

22. M. Mahler, F. Pine, and A. Bergman, *Psychological Birth,* p. 46.

23. Ibid., p. 44.

24. J. Bowlby, "The Nature of the Child's Tie to His Mother," *Int J Psychoanal,* **39:**369 (1958).

25. M. Mahler, F. Pine, and A. Bergman, *Psychological Birth,* p. 53.

26. J. Piaget, "Intellectual Development," p. 122.

27. M. Mahler, F. Pine, and A. Bergman, *Psychological Birth,* p. 55.

28. G. Morgan and H. Riccuitti, "Infants' Responses to Strangers During the First Year," in L. Stone, H. Smith, and L. Murphy (eds.), *Competent Infant,* p. 1128.

29. M. Mahler, F. Pine, and A. Bergman, *Psychological Birth,* p. 56.

30. Ibid., p. 65.

31. D. Winnicott, "Transitional Objects and Transitional Phenomena: A Study of the First Not-Me Possession," *Int J Psychoanal,* **34:**89 (1953).

32. K. Hong and B. Townes, "Infants' Attachment to Inanimate Objects: Cross Cultural Study," *J Am Acad Child Psychiatry,* **15:**49–61 (1976).

33. L. Murphy, "Development in the First Year of Life: Ego and Drive Development in Relation to the Mother-Infant Tie," in L. Stone, H. Smith, and L. Murphy (eds.), *Competent Infant,* p. 477.

34. P. Greenacre, *Emotional Growth,* p. 220.

35. E. Anthony, "Folie à Deux: A Developmental Failure in the Process of Separation-Individuation," in J. McDevitt and C. Settlage (eds.), *Separation-Individuation: Essays in Honor of Margaret S. Mahler,* International Universities Press, New York, 1971, p. 262.

36. M. Mahler, F. Pine, and A. Bergman, *Psychological Birth,* p. 74.

37. Ibid., p. 76.

38. G. Morgan and H. Riccuitti, in L. Stone, H. Smith, and L. Murphy (eds.), *Competent Infant,* p. 1128.

39. M. Mahler, F. Pine, and A. Bergman, *Psychological Birth,* p. 109.

40. P. Wolff, "The Natural History of Crying and Other Vocalizations in Early Infancy," in L. Stone, H. Smith, and L. Murphy (eds.), *Competent Infant,* p. 1185.

41. Ibid.

42. S. Chess and A. Thomas, "Temperamental Individuality from Childhood to Adolescence," in S. Chess and A. Thomas (eds.), *Annual Progress in Child Psychiatry and Child Development,* Brunner/Mazel, New York, 1978, p. 223.

43. S. Goldberg, "Social Competence in Infancy: A Model of Parent-Infant Interaction," in S. Chess, and A. Thomas, (eds.), *Annual Progress,* p. 247.

44. O. Johnson, *Tests and Measurements in Child Development: Handbook,* Jossey-Bass, San Francisco, 1976, p. 426.

45. Margaret B. McFarland, Personal communication.

46. D. Farran and C. Ramey, "Infant Day Care and Attachment Behaviors Toward Mothers and Teachers," in S. Chess and A. Thomas (eds.), *Annual Progress,* p. 311.

47. Ibid.

48. L. Belmont, Z. Stein, and P. Zybert, "Child Spacing and Birth Order: Effect on Intellectual Ability in Two-Child Families," *Science,* 202:995 (December 1978).

49. L. Belmont, "Birth Order, Intellectual Competence and Psychiatric Status," in S. Chess and A. Thomas (eds.), *Annual Progress,* p. 57.

50. Ibid.

51. O. Johnson, *Tests,* pp. 745–746.

52. P. Wolff, "The Classification of States," in L. Stone, H. Smith, and L. Murphy (eds.), *Competent Infant,* pp. 269–272.

53. M. Lewis, *Clinical Aspects of Child Development,* Lea & Febiger, Philadelphia, 1971, p. 20.

54. H. Roffwarg, J. Muzio, and W. Dement, "Ontogenetic Development of the Human Sleep-Dream Cycle," in L. Stone, H. Smith, and L. Murphy (eds.), *Competent Infant,* p. 280.

55. R. Haggerty, "Preventive Pediatrics," in V. Vaughan and R. McKay (eds.), *Nelson Textbook of Pediatrics,* Saunders, Philadelphia, 1975, p. 212.

56. G. Lowrey, "Pediatric Examination," in R. Judge and G. Zuidema, *Methods of Clinical Examination: A Physiologic Approach,* Little, Brown, Boston, 1974, p. 375.

57. J. Kagan, "The Role of the Family During the First Half Decade," in V. Vaughan and T. Brazelton, (eds.), *Nelson Textbook,* p. 167.

58. E. Rexford, L. Sander, and T. Shapiro, *Infant Psychiatry,* Yale University Press, New Haven, 1976, pp. 92–93.

59. S. Provence and R. Lipton, "Institutionalized Infants," in L. Stone, H. Smith, and L. Murphy (eds.), *Competent Infant,* p. 803.

60. U. Bronfenbrenner, "Who Cares for America's Children?" in V. Vaughan and T. Brazelton (eds.), *The Family,* p. 19.

61. E. Rexford, L. Sander, and T. Shapiro, *Infant Psychiatry,* p. 262.

62. M. Howard, "The Young Parent Family," in V. Vaughan and T. Brazelton (eds.), *The Family—Can It Be Saved?* Year Book Medical Publishers, Chicago, 1976, p. 247.

63. K. Colley, "Growing Up Together: The Mutual Respect Balance," in L. Arnold (ed.), *Helping Parents Help Their Children,* Brunner/Mazel, New York, 1978, p. 46.

64. M. Howell, "Families and Work, and Jobs," in V. Vaughan and T. Brazelton (eds.), *The Family,* p. 77.

65. R. Beard, *An Outline of Piaget's Developmental Psychology,* Mentor, New York, 1969, pp. 33–52.

66. P. Wolff, "Developmental and Motivational Concepts in Piaget's Sensorimotor Theory of Intelligence," in E. Rexford, L. Sander, and T. Shapiro (eds.), *Infant Psychiatry,* p. 172.

67. R. Murray and J. Zentner, *Nursing Assessment and Health Promotion Through the Life Span.* Prentice-Hall, Englewood Cliffs, N. J., 1979, p. 72.

68. M. Moss, "Sex, Age and State as Determinants of Mother-Infant Interaction," in L. Stone, H. Smith, and L. Murphy (eds.), *Competent Infant,* p. 1242.

69. C. Lackey, "International Symposium on Infant and Child Feeding," *Nutrition Today,* November-December 1978, p. 12.

70. M. Mahler, F. Pine, and A. Bergman, *Psychological Birth,* p. 49.

71. S. Fomon, *Infant Nutrition,* 2d ed., Saunders, Philadelphia, 1974, p. 366.

72. S. Blumenthal, "Infant Nutrition and Atherosclerosis," *Dial Infant Nutr,* 1:4 (October 1977).

73. C. W. Woodruff, B. A. Latham, and B. A. McDavid, "Iron Nutrition in the Breast Fed Infant," *J Pediatr,* **90:**36–41 (1977).

74. V. Saarinen, M. Siimes, and P. Dallman, "Iron Absorption in Infants: High Bioavailability of Breast Milk Iron as Indicated by the Extrinsic Tag Method of Iron Absorption and by the Concentration of Serum Ferritin," *J Pediatr,* **91:**36–39 (1977).

75. Medical News: "Breast-feeding Lauded by Pediatricians," *JAMA,* **240:**2612 (December 1978).

76. C. Lackey, "International Symposium," p. 14.

77. E. Lieberman, "Hypertension in Childhood and Adolescence," in N. Kaplan (ed.), *Clinical Hypertension,* 2d ed., Williams & Wilkins, Baltimore, pp. 366–384.

78. P. Pipes, *Nutrition in Infancy and Childhood,* Mosby, St. Louis, 1977, p. 100.

79. J. Kagan and R. Klein, "Cross Cultural Perspectives on Early Development," *Am Psychol,* **28:**947–961 (1973).

80. J. Kagan, "The Role of Family During the First Half Decade," in V. Vaughan and T. Brazelton (eds.), *The Family,* p. 167.

81. M. Alexander and M. Brown, *Pediatric History Taking and Physical Diagnosis for Nurses,* McGraw-Hill, New York, 1979, p. 34.

82. G. Owen, "Iron Deficiency in Infancy," *Dial Infant Nutr,* 1:2 (April 1978).

83. L. Filer, "Highlights and Update," *Dial Infant Nutr,* 1:3 (March 1979).

84. C. De Angelis, *Basic Pediatrics for the Primary Health Care Provider,* Little, Brown, Boston, 1975, p. 63.

85. T. Maugh, "Hair: A Diagnostic Tool to Complement Blood Serum and Urine," *Science,* **202:**1271–1273 (December 1978).

86. R. Pihl and M. Parkes, "Hair Element Content in Learning Disabled Children," *Science,* **198:**204–206 (October 1977).

87. F. Rogers, Speech presented to the 2nd National Symposium on Children and Television, October 1971.

88. Margaret B. McFarland, Personal communication.

BIBLIOGRAPHY

Barness, Lewis A.: *Manual of Pediatric Physical Diagnosis,* 4th ed., Year Book Medical Publishers, Chicago, 1972.

Bates, B.: *A Guide to Physical Examination,* 2d ed., Lippincott, Philadelphia, 1979.

Bauman, E., A. Brint, L. Piper, and P. Wright: *The Holistic Health Handbook,* And/Or Press, Berkeley, 1978.

Brown, Marie Scott: *Ambulatory Pediatrics for Nurses,* McGraw-Hill, New York, 1981.

Dickason, E., and M. Schult: *Maternal and Infant Care,* McGraw-Hill, New York, 1979.

Hoekelman, R., S. Blatman, P. Brunell, S. Friedman, and M. Seidel: *Principles of Pediatric Health Care of the Young,* McGraw-Hill, New York, 1978.

Kagan, Jerome: *Infancy: Its Place in Human Development,* Harvard Univ. Press, Cambridge, Mass., 1978.

Knobloch, H. and B. Pasamanick: *Gesell and Amatruda's Developmental Diagnosis,* 3d ed., Harper and Row, New York, 1974.

Krajicek, M. and A. Tearney: *Detection of Developmental Problems in Children,* University Park Press, Baltimore, 1977.

Lewis, Michael I. (ed.): *The Child and Its Family,* Plenum, New York, 1979.

Papalia, D., and S. Olds: *Human Development,* McGraw-Hill, New York, 1978.

Pillitteri, A.: *Nursing Care of the Growing Family: A Child Health Text,* Little, Brown, Boston, 1977.

Scipien, G., M. Barnard, M. Chord, J. Howe, and J. Phillips: *Comprehensive Pediatric Nursing,* 2d ed., McGraw-Hill, New York, 1979.

Shaffer, David I. (ed.): *The First Year of Life: Psychological and Medical Implications of Early Experience,* Wiley, New York, 1979.

Silner, Henry K.: *Handbook of Pediatrics,* 13th ed., Lange Medical Publ., Los Altos, Cal., 1980.

Stone, L., and J. Church: *Childhood and Adolescence,* Random House, New York, 1968.

Thoman, Evelyn B. (ed.): *Origins of the Infant's Social Responsiveness,* L. Erlbaum Assoc., Hillsdale, N.J., 1979.

Vaughan, V., and R. McKay: *Nelson Textbook of Pediatrics,* 10th ed., Saunders, Philadelphia, 1975.

Whaley, L., and D. Wong: *Nursing Care of Infants and Children,* Mosby, St. Louis, 1979.

Personal communication with Margaret B. McFarland, Ph.D.
Personal communication with John J. Harper, M.D.
Taped interviews by Edith Sarneso, R.N., P.N.P.
Taped interviews by Rose Kmetz, R.N., P.N.P.

PHYSICAL EXAMINATION

APPROACH TO THE EXAMINATION

Careful preparation for a physical examination is important if maximum cooperation of the infant is to be gained. After a relationship has been established with the parents, the infant will be more willing to trust, especially if the parents participate during the examination. Infants respond as much to the feeling tone in the examiner's voice as they do to what is said to them. A gentle, friendly, positive, repetitive tone usually gets the best response. A parent's voice may calm the infant. Having brightly colored toys, a pacifier, or a bottle of sugar water available can also be of help (a).

If possible, the parents should undress the infant. The infant needs to be completely undressed, but the diaper may be left in place to avoid accidents. If the room is cool, a blanket, which could be partially removed when various parts are examined, may be used. The infant should be kept warm. The examiner's hands should be washed in warm water. The stethoscope should be warmed by holding it in the palm of the hand before it is used (b).

Refer to Chap. 4 when performing physical examination of the infant, since there are similarities in techniques.

Involve parents in the examination.

Separation from parents may provoke more anxiety than the examination.

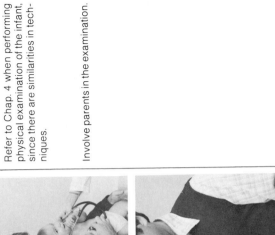
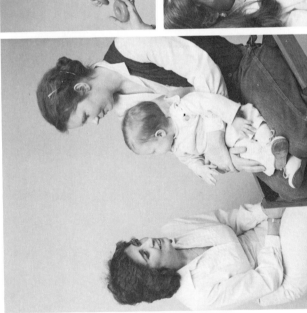
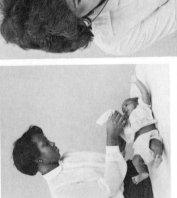
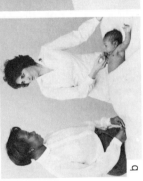
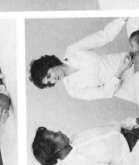
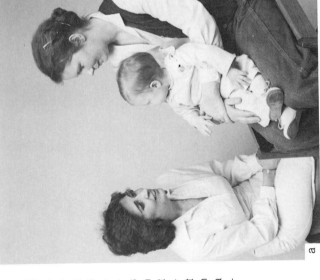
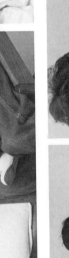
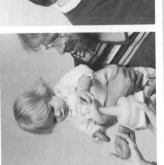

a

b

Immobilization is especially difficult with infants since they do not
like being restrained.

Proper restraint is important for
accurate examination and to avoid
possible injury to the body.

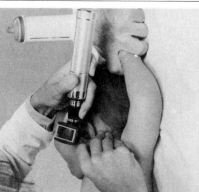
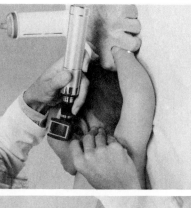
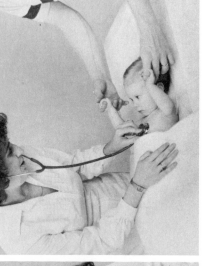
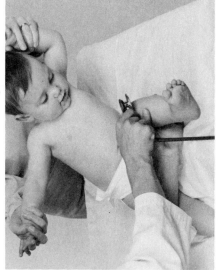
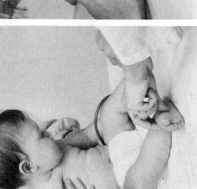
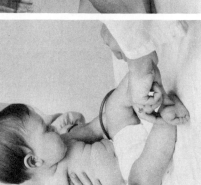
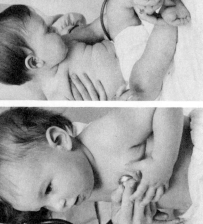
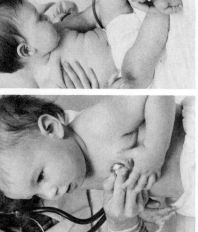
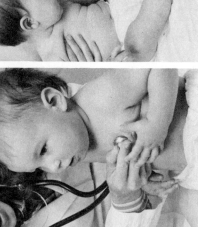
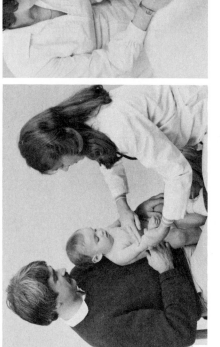

a

b

c

The young infant, up to about 6 months,
may be examined on a padded table with
the parent standing close to the table.
Older infants usually prefer sitting on a
parent's lap (a). A parent can immobilize
the baby's head for the otoscopic, optic,
or oral examination very easily if the infant
is held. To restrain the infant in a supine
position on a table, the arms can be
brought up alongside the infant's head
and a parent may hold them in that position as the examiner turns the head from
side to side to examine the ears (a). Since
the infant is free to kick and a parent is
doing the restraining, there may be little
protest.

The order in which the examination is
done should be determined by the
response of the infant. It is best to take
advantage of the opportunity offered. If
the infant is quiet, the heart, lungs, and
abdomen should be examined first. If the
infant is playful and active, it may be
easier to start with the extremities and
wait for a quieter moment to examine the
chest. The most traumatic procedures,
such as examination of the eyes, ears,
and mouth, should be done last. The
neurological examination can be incorporated into the whole of the physical
examination (b).

One way to organize an examination so
that no part is overlooked is to examine
each adjacent part in sequence. Listening to the chest first, then examining the
feet and proceeding to each adjacent
part; leaving the examination of the
throat and ears until last, may be the
most preferable method for the infant.
Any questionable findings or abnormalities must be promptly referred, since
many problems in infancy can be quickly
and easily corrected if treated early (c).

Highlights
Observation of the behavioral characteristics of infants and mothers as outlined in Table 6-5 can be used.

THE EXAMINATION

General Appearance

The general appearance of the infant should be observed. The state of consciousness as well as posture, symmetry, movements, and reflexes should be noted. Observation of the infant's responsiveness to both the examiner and the parents should also be made (a).

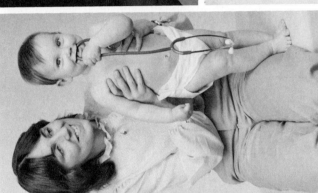
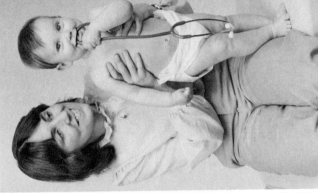
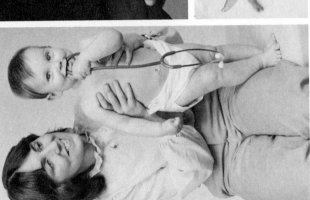
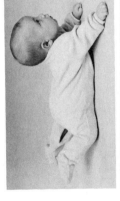
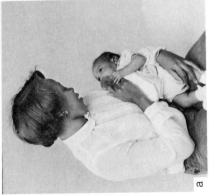

a

The behavioral state, cry, language, cognitive function, and mood should be assessed. General observation of the infant's behavior can give important clues about the infant's general level of functioning. The parent-infant interaction can also be noted.

Measurement of the infant's vital signs are done as described for the neonate in Chap. 5.

Observation of *vital signs* provides the basis for decisions concerning the health of the infant. The temperature, pulse rate and rhythm of respiration, and blood pressure should be determined (b).

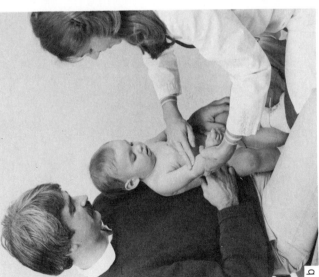

b

In the full-term infant, weight gain averages approximately 20 g per day for the first 5 months of life and approximately 15 g per day for the remainder of the first year. The length of the infant increases during the first year by 25 to 30 cm, or 10 to 12 inches.

Measurement of somatic growth is a crucial part of the assessment, since growth is the central characteristic of normal infants. The measurements are length, weight, and head circumference (c). Chest circumference may also be used. Head and chest circumference measurements are done when those parts are examined. These measurements are then plotted on a standard growth chart (see Appendix). Serial measurements over months or years make up a record of the overall pattern of growth.

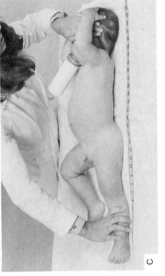
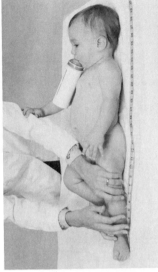

c

The *skin* should be observed for color, consistency and turgor, distribution and

Highlights

Strawberry nevi and Mongolian spots do not disappear until the end of the first or second year. Refer to Chap. 5.

Adipose tissue constitutes 40 to 70 percent of body weight at 4 months of age (it is 28 percent at term).

The brain's maximal postnatal growth is during the first year.

If cloth tape is used it should be checked against wooden or metal standards since it may stretch.

Median Values for Head Circumference

Age, (months)	inches	cm
birth	13.9	35.0
3	15.9	40.4
6	17.1	43.4
9	17.8	45.3
12	18.3	46.6

Source: V.C. Vaugh and R.J. McKay (eds), *Textbook of Pediatrics*, Saunders, Philadelphia, 1975, p. 22.

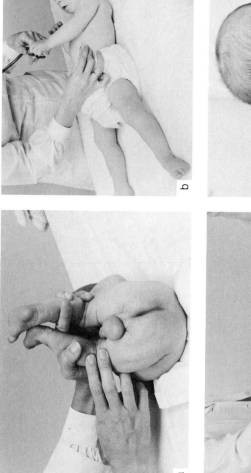

a

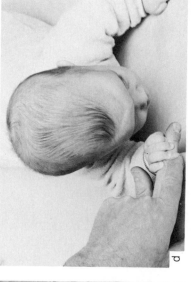

b

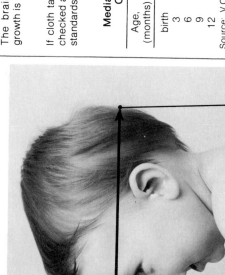

d

c

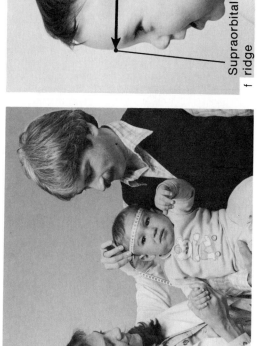

e

f

Supraorbital ridge — Occiput

type of lesions, characteristics of sweat and sebaceous glands, body and scalp hair, and nails. Some of the skin lesions discussed in Chap. 5 may still be present in the infant. Common minor abnormalities such as cradle cap and diaper dermatitis (a) may also be noted.

Skin turgor (b) is observed by grasping the skin on the abdomen with the thumb and forefinger and noting the rate of return to its original position after it is released. The return is immediate if the infant is well hydrated.

The number of fat cells increases very rapidly during the first year of life. Palpation of the skin, preferably over the lateral abdominal wall, allows quantitative measurement of subcutaneous adipose tissue (c).

Sweat glands are active in the infant but do not reach peak activity until 2 years of age. Sebaceous glands are relatively inactive until puberty. The nails of the young infant are soft and pliable (d); by the end of the first year they are more firm.

Head, Face

An examination of the head includes measuring the head circumference and plotting it on a standard growth chart (e). The shape and symmetry of the head should be noted, as should the degree of heal control. The sutures and fontanels should be palpated.

Inspection

To measure head circumference, the measuring tape is applied firmly over the glabella and supraorbital ridges anteriorly and that part of the occiput posteriorly which gives the maximal circumference. By measuring head circumference, normal growth of the brain can be monitored (f).

It is important neurologically for the infant to develop good head control with no head lag when raising from a supine position.

It is important to note when the infant's anterior and posterior fontanels close.

The face should be mobile. The shape of the head should be symmetrical. Flattened areas are sometimes seen in infants who are allowed to lie in one position for a long time (a).

Head control should be noted. By 3 months there should be no head lag. By 4 months of age most infants can hold their heads erect in midline when in a vertical position (b).

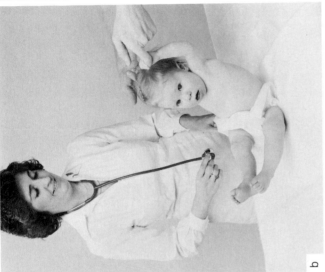

a

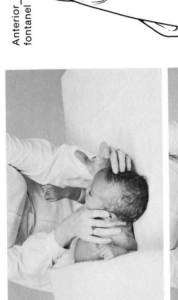

b

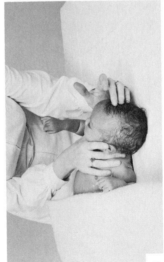

c

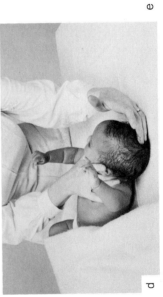

d

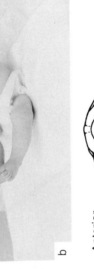

Anterior fontanel

Posterior fontanel

e

Palpation

The sutures are sometimes felt as small ridges until about 6 months of age. There are two fontanels in the young infant, the anterior (c) and the posterior (d). The posterior fontanel is usually less than 0.5 cm and closes at about 2 months of age. The anterior fontanel which is diamond shaped is about 2 cm along the coronal suture by 1.5 cm along the sagittal suture, and closes sometime between 12 and 18 months (e). The fontanels should be palpated with the infant in sitting and lying positions. The fontanels should be firm, never tense or depressed. The pulsating fontanel is normal. Systolic or continuous bruits may be palpated over the temporal areas.

Highlights

The eye's maximal postnatal growth is during the first year.

Thorough eye examination may require restraint of the infant's head by the parent or examiner.

By about 12 months of age visual acuity is approximately 20/100.

Dichromatic color vision and brightness discrimination are present in the 2-month-old.

Alignment of the eyes can be checked by eliciting the pupillary light reflex.

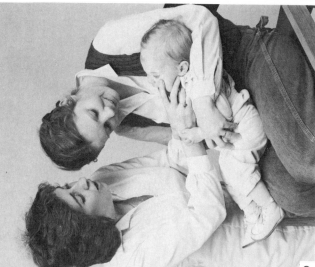
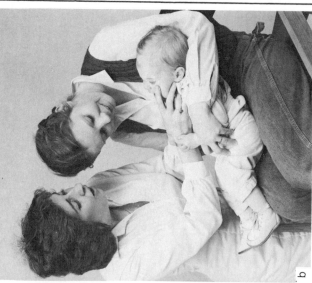

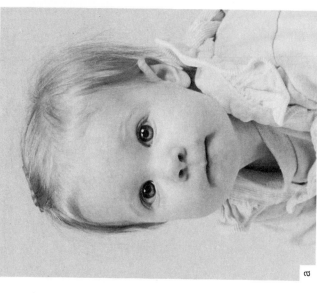
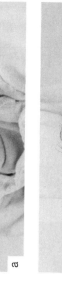

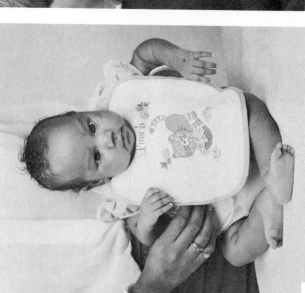

Eyes

Inspection

An examination of the eye includes noting their position, mobility, and symmetry. Observation should be made of the lids, including eyelashes, tear ducts and glands; the conjunctiva; the sclera and cornea; the pupils, including their reaction to light; the lens and the fundus (a,b). Extraocular movements should be tested. Both eyes should be clear and positioned symmetrically. The red reflex should be present on ophthalmoscopic examination, as should other normal findings as described in Chap. 4.

By shining a light directly into the eyes, the examiner can note the pupillary light reflex. The light should fall symmetrically within each pupil in normally aligned eyes.

Transient strabismus a condition in which the eyes are not held in parallel, may normally persist up to 6 months of age (c). If it is observed in infants older than six months this should be noted. With strabismus the light falls off center in one eye (d).

The lids should be clear and have eye lashes. Tears are produced by 4 months of age, but the nasolacrimal sac, on the medial edge of the lower eyelid, will yield mucoid material if there is an obstruction.

The conjunctiva should be pink; the cornea clear. The pupils should react to light equally. The red reflex should be present. The blink reflex is seen when a bright light is introduced into the eye.

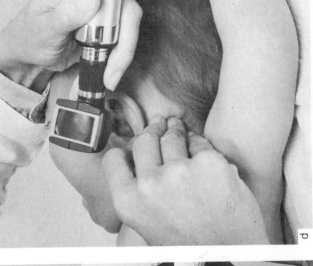

Auditory canal

Infant

Adult

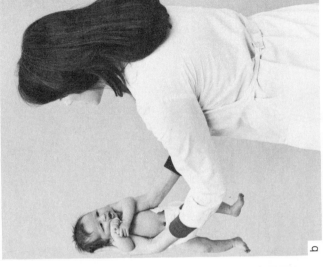

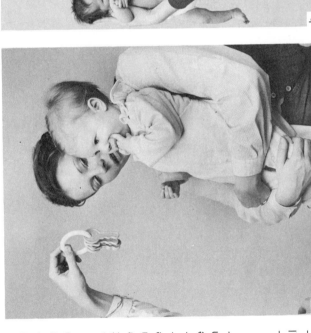

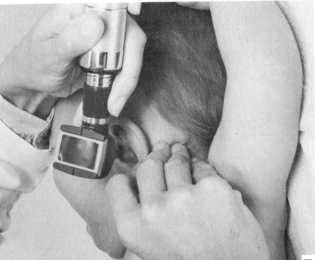

Testing the infant's vision is uncomplicated. Infants at 1 month will fixate and begin to follow a bright toy. At 3 or 4 months, they will fixate, follow, and reach for the toy. By 6 to 10 months, they can fixate and follow in all directions (a).

The vestibular function test is done next. Normally, when the infant is held at arm's length and turned slowly in one direction, the eyes look in the direction to which they are turned (b). When the rotation stops, the eyes look in the opposite direction following a few quick, unsustained nystagmoid movements. The "doll's-eye" movements of the eyes on turning of the body should not be present after 2 months of age.

Ears

An examination of the ear includes noting the characteristics of the external ear, the external canal, and the tympanic membrane and assessing the acuity of hearing.

Inspection

The external ear should be observed for position, size, symmetry, and the presence of preauricular sinuses or tags. The external canal, which can be observed by pulling gently downward on the pinna (c), should be clear. Cerumen, which can be from white to dark brown in color, and soft to dry in texture, may make seeing difficult. The infant's head should be stabilized and the otoscope inserted gently (d). A small 2mm speculum needs to be inserted more deeply into the canal in infants than in older children, since the cartilage and bony structures supporting the ear canal are underdeveloped.

The light reflex on the tympanic membrane is diffuse and does not assume the cone shape until the infant is several months old.

The infant should be observed for responses to sound.

Young infants are obligatory nose breathers.

Assessment of hearing can be done by observing the infant's response to loud noise. Responses may include blinking of the eyes, cessation of body movements, or turning the head toward sound (a). If the infant is less than 3 months of age, a Moro reflex might be seen (b). Noting normal language development (see Table 6-2) is also an indirect method of testing. The parents, however, are the best judges of hearing acuity. If a parent is concerned about a child's hearing, it should be assumed that the infant has hearing difficulty until proven otherwise.

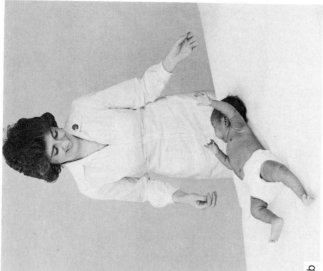

a

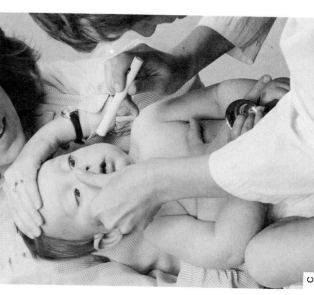

b

Nose

Inspection

An examination of the nose begins with inspection of its shape. The mucous membranes of the septum are checked and the patency of the nares assessed. The turbinates and floor of the nose are examined, and a description of any exudate present is given (d). This examination can be done by pushing the tip of the nose upward with the thumb of the left hand and shining a light into the naris (c). A speculum is usually not necessary.

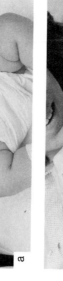

c

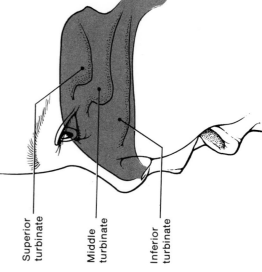

Superior turbinate

Middle turbinate

Inferior turbinate

d

Mouth

The crying infant allows struggle-free glimpses of the mouth and pharynx (a). With the closed-mouthed infant, slipping a tongue depressor between the teeth and onto the tongue while the baby is re-strained by a parent, will permit the ex-aminer to see. Palpation can then be done utilizing the sucking reflex.

Inspection

An examination of the mouth includes inspection of the lips, buccal mucosa, gingiva, hard palate, mandible, tongue, soft palate, posterior pharyngeal wall, and teeth if they are present.

The teeth should be examined for timing and sequence of eruptions, number, character, condition, and position. See Table 6-2 for the period of eruption of deciduous teeth. The frenulum is of adequate length if it allows good mobil-ity of the tongue. No difficulties will be encountered with speech if the tongue can be extended as far as the alveolar ridge.

The pharyngeal tonsils are small in infancy and increase in size during childhood. Little saliva is produced dur-ing the first 3 months of life.

Palpation

The buccal mucosa, gingiva, and hard palate should be palpated for intact-ness.

A sucking reflex can be initiated in the infant until 12 months of age by palpat-ing the palate (b). A rooting response (c) while awake, can be elicited until 3 or 4 months, and a rooting response while asleep can be elicited until 7 or 8 months of age.

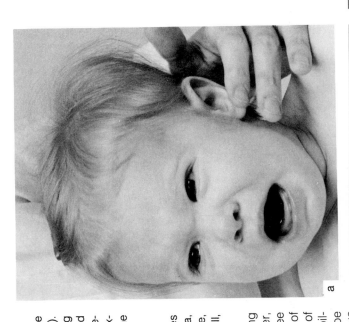

a

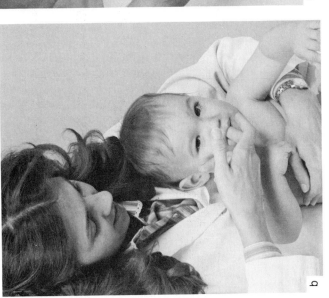

b

c

Highlights

Range of motion and control of movement should be noted when examining the neck.

The thyroid gland is very difficult to palpate in infants.

In the young infant, the chest wall is round. With growth, there is a general flattening of its slope as the lateral diameter exceeds the anteroposterior diameter.

Median Values for Chest Circumference

Age (months)	inches	cm
birth	13.0	33.0
3	15.8	40.2
6	17.1	43.4
9	18.0	45.7
12	18.6	47.3

Source: V.C. Vaugh and R.J. McKay, (eds.), *Textbook of Pediatrics*, Saunders, Philadelphia, 1975, p. 22.

a

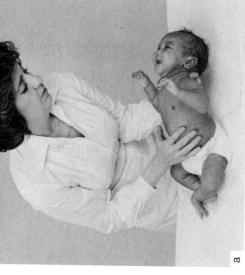

b

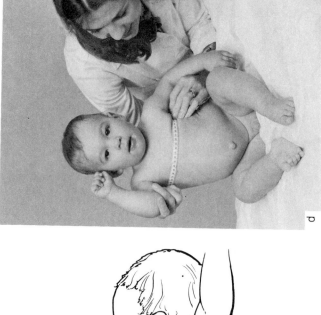

d

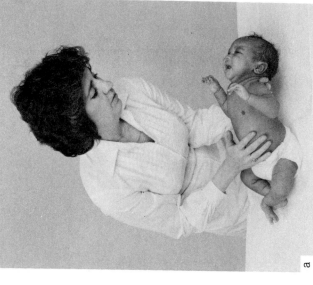

c

Throat/Neck

The neck of a young infant is short, with skin folds between the head and shoulders. A hand can be placed behind the upper back, and the head permitted to fall gently back in order to observe the neck (a).

Inspection

An examination of the neck includes observation of its overall dimensions. The neck should appear symmetrical.

Palpation

Resistance to passive motion (b), size and location of lymph nodes and status of neck vessels should be checked. Palpation of the trachea should be done. Normally, it is midline.

Thorax

Inspection

An examination of the chest includes notation of its size, shape, symmetry, and movement with respirations (c). The examiner should also note the breast characteristics. Movement should be symmetrical and primarily abdominal with no retractions. Respirations are primarily abdominal in the infant because of undeveloped intercostal muscles. The chest circumference is measured by placing the tape around the chest at the nipple line. A measurement on inspiration and one on expiration can be taken and the average recorded (d).

Palpation

The ribs should be palpated to determine whether any are absent and to discover if there is any tenderness (a). Axillary and clavicular areas are palpated to determine any node enlargement (b).

Lungs

Percussion

Percussion of the lungs should be done to determine the adequacy of gas exchange. The percussion note, using the direct or indirect method, is normally hyperresonant throughout; any decrease has the same significance as dullness or flatness in the adult (see Chap. 4) (c).

Auscultation

Auscultation is best accomplished when the infant is content. If the baby is crying, the inspiratory phase can be thoroughly auscultated but predominantly expiratory adventitious sounds can be missed. Inducing forced expiration, by holding the hands on opposing anterior and posterior sides of the chest and, with the stethoscope in one hand, gently squeezing the hands together as expiration is ending, may accentuate these respiratory sounds. All lung fields should be auscultated (d).

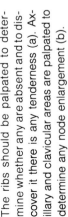
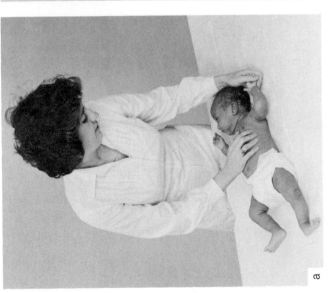
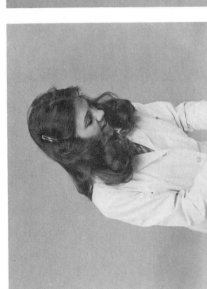
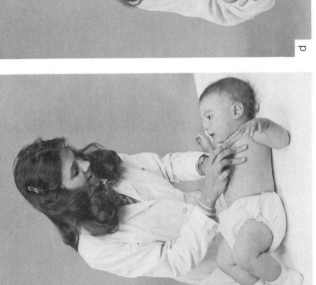

The rate of respiration can be determined by observing abdominal excursions in the sleeping infant and by counting the sounds while holding the bell of the stethoscope in front of the baby's nose.

Because of the thinness of the chest wall, the breath sounds are more clearly heard in the infant.

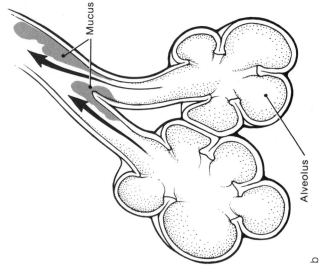

Mucus

Alveolus

b

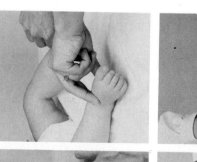

a

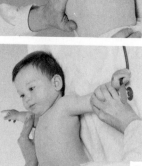
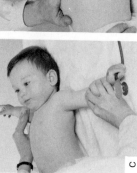
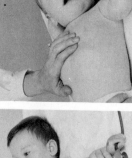
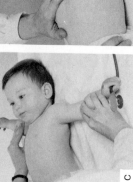
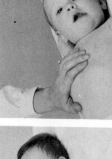

c

Normally, infant breath sounds are bronchovesicular in character. Fine crepitant rales may be normally heard at the end of a deep inspiration (a). Some rhonchi may also be heard in the young infant because of a tiny amount of mucus which may be present in the small lumen of the tracheobronchial tree (b). These usually disappear after coughing. Wheezes, which are normal, palpable, and audible vibrations caused by air, may be heard rushing through the narrow lumen. As the infant gets older, fewer fine rales, little rhonchi, and no wheezing should be heard normally.

Heart

Inspection
The general appearance of the infant is probably the best way to assess the adequacy of the cardiovascular system. Appropriate weight gain, with progressive development, are important findings. No prominent pulsations or veins should normally be seen.

Palpation
The femoral, dorsalis pedis, and brachial pulses should be palpated. Both sides should be palpated at the same time to distinguish fullness and equality. The apical pulse can be palpated in the fourth left interspace just outside the midclavicular line. Determination of blood pressure should be made (c).

Percussion
Percussion, which does have limited value, can be used to outline the cardiac margins. This gives an indication of heart size.

The examiner may be able to percuss' cardiac margins since the heart is in a horizontal position.

Auscultation

Heart sounds can be difficult to differentiate from normal breath sounds, since the pitches and rates can be similar (a). Watching abdominal excursions with respirations and palpating a peripheral pulse while auscultating the chest can help with this differentiation (b). Auscultation is best done while the infant is content. It is performed as in adults (see Chap. 4).

The heart rate and rhythm, and the characteristics of the first and second heart sounds, especially in the second left interspace, should be noted. The timing, grade, quality, duration, point, and transmission of murmurs should be noted. For each heart sound, the intensity, point of maximal intensity (PMI), and degree of splitting should be determined. The PMI is in the fourth left interspace, just outside the midclavicular line (c). S₁ is louder than S₂ at the apex. Splitting of S₂ at the apex, producing an extra heart sound, is common and the split often widens with inspiration. S₂ is louder than S₁ in the pulmonic area (d). Innocent or inorganic murmurs, found in about 50 percent of children, are usually transient in nature. They are soft, blowing, systolic in time, often found along the left sternal border in the pulmonic area, and are less than 3 in grade (moderate but not accompanied by a thrill). If questionable, the murmur should be further evaluated.

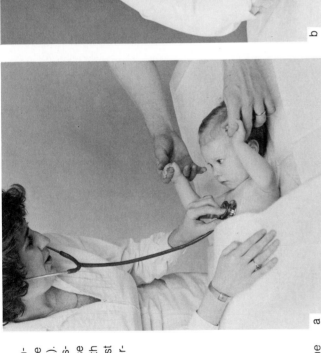

a

b

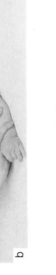

Pulmonary valve sounds

Aortic valve sounds

PMI

Apex and mitral valve sounds

Tricuspid valve sounds (may also radiate to other side of sternum)

c

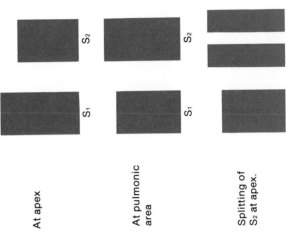

S₁ S₂

At apex

S₁ S₂

At pulmonic area

S₁ split S₂

Splitting of S₂ at apex.

d

The heart rate can be measured by palpation of the peripheral pulses, direct palpation or auscultation, or by observing the anterior fontanelle. Rhythm is more commonly irregular than regular, reflecting sinus arrhythmia and increasing vagal control.

Murmurs are difficult to localize in infants since they are often well transmitted and are heard throughout the chest.

The size and the shape of the abdomen change with age, reflecting changes in intraabdominal and intrathoracic organs.

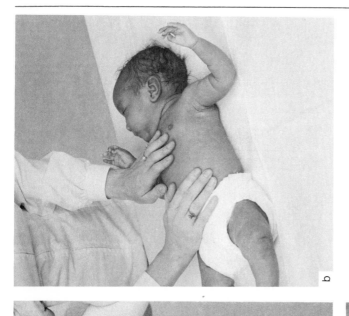

b

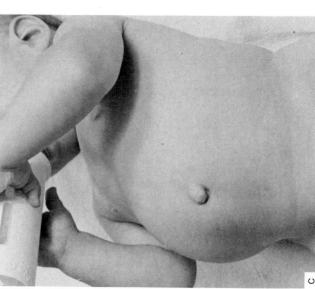

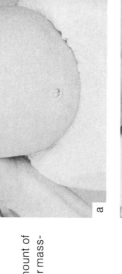

a

c

Breasts

Inspection

The breasts are inspected for position, size and color. The breast enlargement which was present during the neonatal period should resolve by 2 to 3 months of age.

Supernumerary nipples should be noted if present. These are a normal variation (a).

The color of the nipples and areolae should be pink in Caucasians and brownish-pink in dark-skinned babies, such as Blacks.

Palpation

The breasts are palpated for amount of breast tissue. Any enlargement or masses should be noted (b).

Abdomen

Inspection

The abdomen in infants is protruberant due to poorly developed musculature (c). Midline defects such as umbilical hernias and diastasis recti are fairly common and usually disappear by 1 year of age. If a hernia is found, the size should be noted. Subcutaneous abdominal wall blood vessels are often visible in young infants due to the small amount of subcutaneous fat. Abdominal movement, due to breathing and intestinal peristalsis, can be seen.

Normally the liver descends during expiration as the diaphram moves downward; this downward displacement should not be misinterpreted as hepatomegaly, or enlargement.

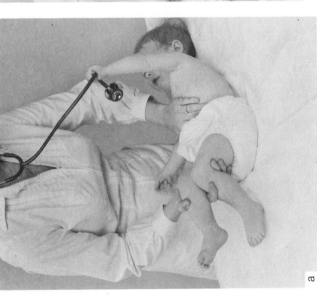

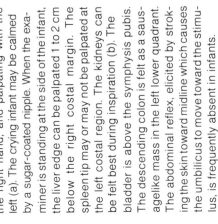

a

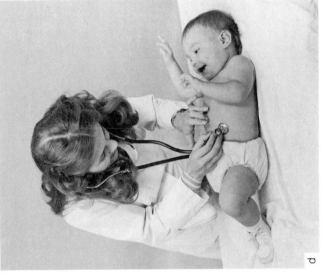

b

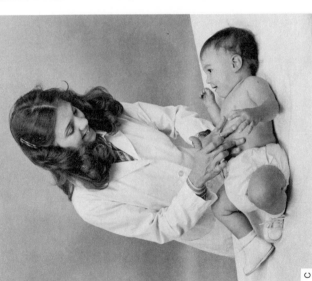

c

d

Palpation

Relaxation of the infant's abdomen for palpation can be done by holding the legs flexed at the knees and hips with the right hand, and palpating with the left (a). The crying infant may be calmed by a sugar-coated nipple. When the examiner is standing at the side of the infant, the liver edge can be palpated 1 to 2 cm below the right costal margin. The spleen tip may or may not be palpated at the left costal region. The kidneys can be felt best during inspiration (b). The bladder is above the symphysis pubis. The descending colon is felt as a sausagelike mass in the left lower quadrant. The abdominal reflex, elicited by stroking the skin toward midline which causes the umbilicus to move toward the stimulus, is frequently absent in infants.

Percussion

Percussion of the abdomen in infants is the same as that in adults. It will outline the relatively large area of the upper abdomen filled by the stomach (c). Lack of tympany may occur normally after a meal.

Auscultation

Auscultation using the diaphragm of the stethoscope should be done after inspection, since palpation and percussion can disturb bowel sounds. This is sometimes best done after listening to the chest. Bowel sounds can be stimulated by stroking the abdominal surface with a fingernail, and their presence should be noted (d).

Ammoniacal dermatitis (diaper rash) is commonly seen during infancy. Proper care of diapers should prevent this condition.

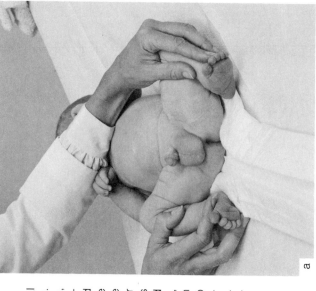

a

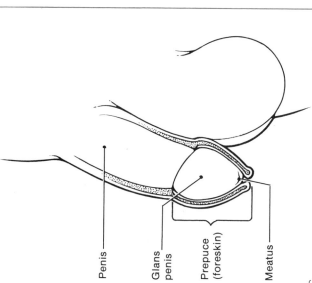

b

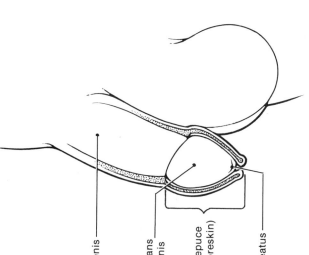

Penis

Glans penis

Prepuce (foreskin)

Meatus

c

Genitalia and Rectum

Inspection

In males, the penis, testes, and external inguinal rings should be examined (a). The clitoris, labia majora and minora, vaginal orifice, urethral orifice, and external inguinal rings should be examined in females. Observations should be made as to the shape and size of the genitals and the orifices, and of the color and condition of the skin. If secretions are present, the amount, color, odor, and type should be noted. In female infants, the perineal structures are easily seen by separating the labia with the thumb and forefinger of one hand (b). Thin vulvar adhesions are sometimes seen. These can sometimes be parted by gentle pressure to the labia majora.

Palpation

In the infant male who is uncircumsized, the prepuce or foreskin of the penis should not be retracted for the first 3 months. It is normally tight, and accidental tearing of the membrane may cause scarring and, later, the formation of adhesions. There is not usually a problem with flow of urine. In older infants and children, the foreskin should be retracted for examination of the glans and the meatus (c).

Highlights

At birth 3 to 4 percent of males have undescended testes; most descend by 3 months of age.

A hydrocele usually disappears spontaneously within the first few months of life.

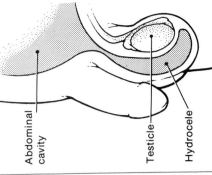

Abdominal cavity

Testicle

Hydrocele

Certain reflexes present only during infancy should be noted during examination of the extremities.

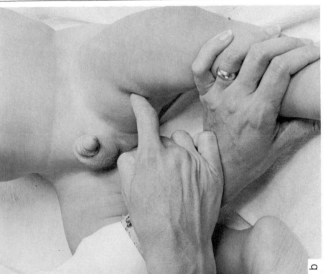

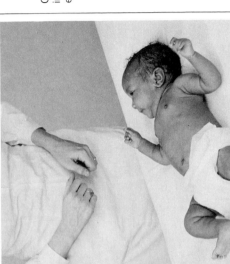

a

b

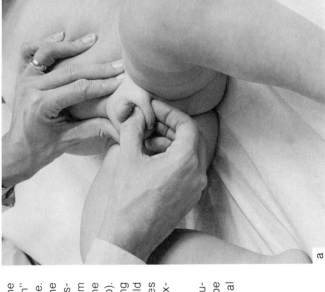

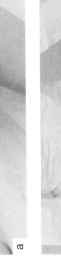

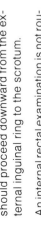

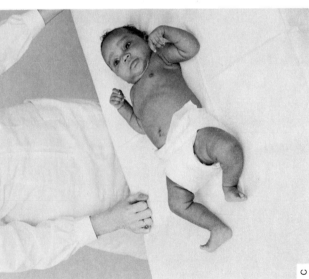

c

d

The testes are sometimes found in the inguinal canal and can be "milked down" (a). They are frequently not equal in size. A hydrocele, a collection of fluid in the scrotum, may be present. The cremasteric reflex, when the skin of the scrotum shrinks, pulling the testes higher into the pelvic cavity, is very active in infants (b). This is stimulated by cold and touching the inner thigh; therefore hands should be warm and palpation of the testes should proceed downward from the external inguinal ring to the scrotum.

An internal rectal examination is not routine for infants. The anal reflex should be elicited and contraction of the anal sphincter noted.

Extremities

Inspection

In the musculoskeletal examination, observation is made of the infant's position, symmetry, and posture, and of skin color, temperature, and sensation (c).

A general assessment can be done even when the infant is asleep. The posture, such as the degree of flexion of the extremities, any hyperextension of the neck, the symmetry of the position of the extremities, and the amount, quality, and symmetry of spontaneous movements, should be noted. Spontaneous assumption of the fencing position through the asymmetric tonic neck reflex (extension of the head to one side) is seen in the infant until approximately 6 months (d).

Highlights

The hand is fisted until about 4 weeks of age; the thumb is normally free.

If the infant wears shoes, they should be investigated. Shoes that are too small or too large can result in foot or gait problems.

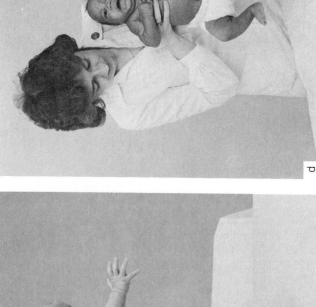

b

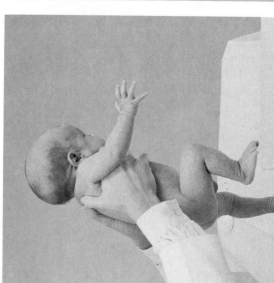

d

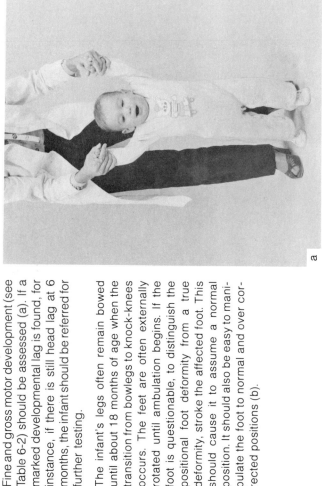

a

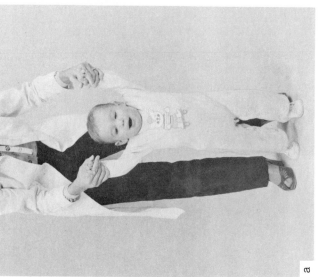

c

Fine and gross motor development (see Table 6-2) should be assessed (a). If a marked developmental lag is found, for instance, if there is still head lag at 6 months, the infant should be referred for further testing.

The infant's legs often remain bowed until about 18 months of age when the transition from bowlegs to knock-knees occurs. The feet are often externally rotated until ambulation begins. If the foot is questionable, to distinguish the positional foot deformity from a true deformity, stroke the affected foot. This should cause it to assume a normal position. It should also be easy to manipulate the foot to normal and over corrected positions (b).

Until approximately 1 year, if the infant is held upright and the dorsal surface of one foot is allowed to touch the under surface of a table top, the infant will place the foot on the table top. This is the placing response (c). Until approximately 3 months of age, the stimulation of the ventral surface of the foot against a table surface will elicit a stepping response. Until approximately 4 months, vertical suspension positioning is seen; that is, while the infant is supported upright with the examiner's hands under the axillae, flexion of the hips and knees should be seen (d). Normally, no adduction or fixed extension of the legs will be seen.

Highlights

Refer to Chapter 5 for a description of the withdrawal reflex.

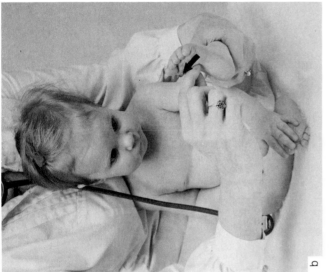

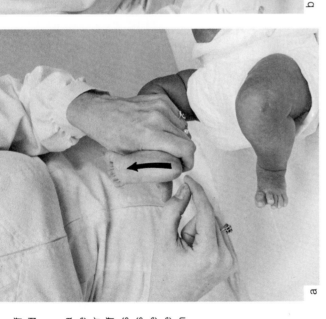

a

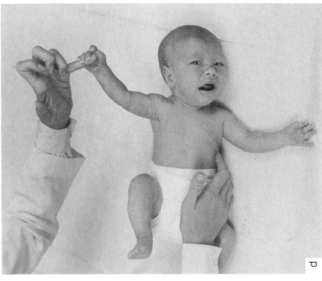

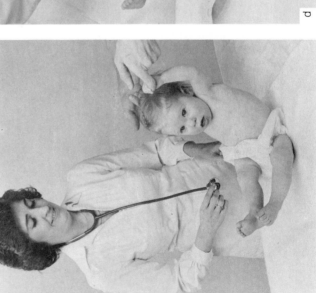

b

c

d

Palpation

The range of joint motion, presence of reflexes, and the size, symmetry, and strength of muscles should be noted.

The infant's feet appear flat, due to a plantar fat pad. If the lateral aspect of the foot is stroked, the Babinski reflex, or dorsiflexion of the big toe and fanning of the smaller toes, is seen (a). This is tested for symmetry in both legs, as is the withdrawal reflex. Stroking from the little toe to the big toe will elicit the plantar reflex, which is normally seen until 8 to 15 months of age (b).

With the young infant, the traction response test is made. The supine infant is pulled into a sitting position and the degree of resistance to extension of the arms at the elbow and the degree to which the head is held in the upright position is observed (c). Some degree of flexion of the elbow should be maintained. The palmar grasp reflex is evident until about 4 months. This is obtained by pressing the palm from the ulnar side when the infant's head is in the midline position (d).

Highlights

Any resistance to passive stretching of the arms and legs should be observed, noting in particular any symmetrical or asymmetrical increase or decrease in movement (a). There should be symmetry of the biceps, patellar, and achilles reflexes (see Chap. 4.). These can be elicited in a young infant by tapping with the index finger. In an older infant, the edge of the diaphragm of a stethoscope can be used to elicit reflexes (b).

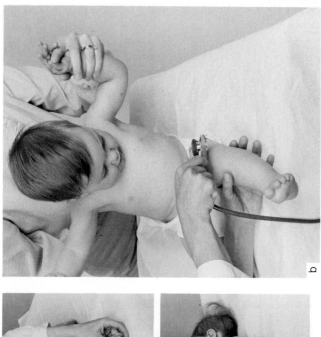

a

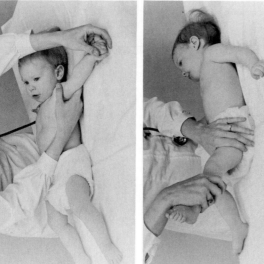

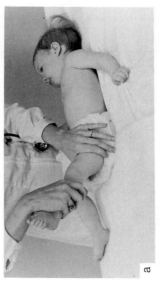

b

It is important to assess normal hip location prior to the time the infant begins to walk using the Ortolani and Barlow maneuvers.

The hips should be checked for normal location at each visit. In Ortolani's test for congenitally dislocated hips, the infant is placed in the supine position with the legs facing the examiner and the hips and knees flexed. The examiner's middle fingers are placed over the greater trochanter (c), a process on the outer side of the femur, and the thumbs, over the lesser trochanter, on the inner side of the thigh (d). The knees are abducted until the lateral aspect of each knee touches the examining table as forward pressure is exerted behind the trochanter. The femoral head should not be felt to slip forward into the acetabulum, and no click should be felt or heard.

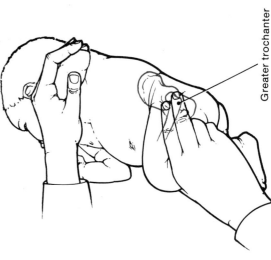

Greater trochanter

Lesser trochanter

c

d

In tests for Barlow's sign, or an unstable hip, the infant's position is the same. One hand of the examiner steadies the pelvis and applies pressure from above downward (a). Backward and outward pressure is applied by the other hand using the thumb placed medially over the lesser trochanter. If the femoral head can be felt slipping into the posterior lip of the acetabulum and slipping back immediately when pressure is released, the hip is said to be unstable or dislocatable and should be closely watched. Normally, there should be no restricted abduction, or shortening of either limb (b).

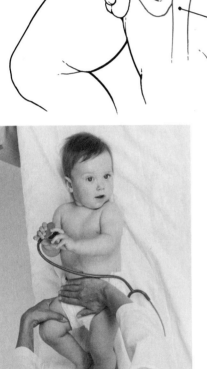

a

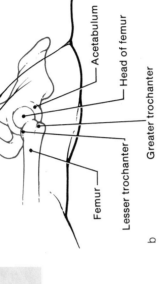

Pelvis

Acetabulum

Head of femur

Greater trochanter

Lesser trochanter

Femur

b

The spine should be checked for flexibility, alignment, and symmetry. Dimples or tufts of hair should be noted. Palpation of the spine should be done to identify each spiny process of the vertebrae (c).

The trunk curvation of Galant's reflex can be elicited with the infant held horizontally and prone in one of the examiner's hands or lying prone on a flat surface (d). The other hand is used to stimulate one side of the infant's back about 3 cm from the midline. A curving of the trunk toward the stimulated side, with shoulders and hips moving in that direction, is seen until the infant is approximately 2 months of age.

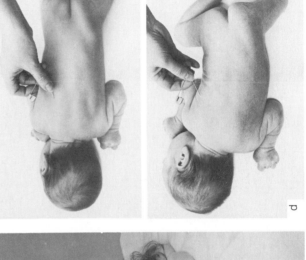

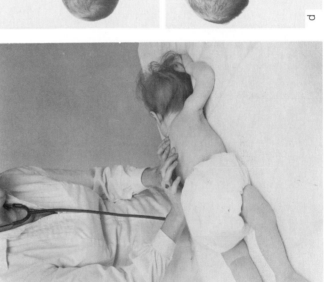

c

d

Movement of the cervical spine is an important normal finding.

Photographs in figure d courtesy of Meade Johnson Company.

465

THE INFANT

THE TODDLER CHAPTER SEVEN

Cheryl A. Olson and Mary Kolassa Lepley

INTRODUCTION

The end of infancy and the beginning of toddlerhood mark what has been described as the "psychological birth of the human infant."[1] Though generally considered to encompass the years 1 through 3, toddlerhood actually begins when the infant takes his or her first halting, independent steps and ends when the child becomes a separate person who has achieved the fundamental cognitive, psychomotor, and social skills which enable one to function in the world.

Erikson has defined the major developmental task of this age group as the establishment of a sense of "autonomy," that is, a sense of one's own individuality and separateness from the environment and the people in it. Failure to establish autonomy leads to a sense of shame and of doubt in one's ability to function effectively in the world.[2]

Assessing the child in this age group requires skill and sensitivity on the part of the health care provider, unlike that needed in any other development period, for this is a particularly turbulent time for parents and toddlers alike. The nurse must be aware of the developmental and emotional needs of the toddler, while at the same time recognize the special needs of the parents and/or caretakers as they attempt to cope with demands made on their time and energy by this active, curious, often ambivalent little person.

> Toddlerhood refers to the years 1 through 3.

> The major developmental task of the toddler is to establish a sense of autonomy.

HEALTH HISTORY

The nurse engaged in collecting the health history of a toddler is confronted immediately with two concerns. First, the nurse must rely on the parent or caretaker for most of the historical data about the child. Therefore, it is important to establish the reliability of the informant. Second, the toddler is generally present at the interview and can be somewhat disruptive to the dialogue between the parent and the nurse. Although there are alternatives to having the toddler present for the interview, in most instances the child should be allowed to remain with the parent.

The toddler's presence during the interview is important for several reasons. The nurse is able to observe firsthand the behavior of the child and the interaction of the parent and the child. The child has an opportunity to become familiar with the nurse in a situation which is relatively nonstressful. Cooperation during the more stressful physical exam is more likely to be achieved if the child has some familiarity with the examiner who will be invading personal territory. And giving the toddler the opportunity to contribute to the health history in a manner appropriate to his or her developmental level conveys the attitude that the child is responsible for the maintenance of his or her own health and well-being.

> Occasionally, toddlers may be disruptive to the data collection process.

> It is important to have the toddler present throughout the health history interview.

Approach

An astute nurse, recognizing the toddler's short attention span, will devise ways to help the child cope with the sometimes lengthy history-taking process. A coloring book and a set of crayons, blank sheets of paper, or a well-chosen storybook may keep the child's attention during part of the interview. In addition, they may provide the nurse an opportunity to observe the child's gross and fine motor skills, note attention span, and assess the child's ability to separate from the caretaker and to work independently. Play of this kind is also helpful in reducing the anxiety attached to what may otherwise be a stressful, unfamiliar situation for the toddler.

It should be kept in mind that the approach to the child in these early encounters will influence not only future relationships with the child but also the child's attitude about health care in general. The child who learns to cope positively with these early health care experiences will be better equipped to deal with future encounters with the health care system.

The nurse's approach to the caretaker must also be given special attention. After introductions, it is important for the nurse to determine whether the caretaker is indeed the child's parent. Frequent errors, misunderstandings, and legal problems can be averted if the nurse does not assume that whoever brings the child to the clinic, hospital, or other facility is the child's parent or legal guardian.

It is also important for the nurse to develop a sensitivity to the parent. This toddler period of development, which follows so closely the more tranquil and settled period of infancy, often leaves parents bewildered, frustrated, and doubtful of their ability to parent effectively. In addition, the problems parents are having frequently do not fall under the traditional category of "medical" problems, and therefore, they may be reluctant to ask for help. A question such as, "Many parents find this particular age a difficult one to cope with. How are you finding it?" may provide an opening to express particular problems or difficulties and to see their concerns as legitimate.

Setting

The health history of the toddler may be collected in a variety of health care settings. The nurse will need to adapt the setting to meet the needs of the toddler and parents. A quiet, private area should be provided so that the toddler has no distractions from other children and adults. A clean, carpeted area is preferable, since the toddler will probably spend some time playing with toys on the floor. Certain components of the physical exam may also require that the toddler be on the floor, such as evaluation of motor skills.

Brightly colored pictures and objects may be used to decorate walls so that the toddler has something to focus attention on, both for fun and for parts of the exam such as vision testing.

The Interview

The communication techniques discussed in Chap. 3 should be used when interviewing the parents of the toddler. Frequently, open-ended questions will elicit the most accurate data and will also allow the parents the chance to verbalize their feelings regarding their child.

Once the parents and nurse have agreed upon what the health history interview is to accomplish, full attention should momentarily be

During the history-taking process, the toddler may need a variety of diversional activities because of a short attention span.

The nurse should establish if the caretaker of the child is actually the parent.

The nurse must be sensitive to the needs of the parents when providing health care to the toddler.

The setting must be adapted to the toddler's stage of development.

Refer to Chap. 3 for a discussion of interviewing techniques.

given to the toddler in an attempt by the nurse to establish contact and rapport. Toddlers will react in a variety of ways to strangers, depending to a large extent on their personality and past experience. Frequently, however, if they are allowed to stay close to the parent initially, they will respond with warmth and curiosity to the nurse. Attempts to separate the toddler from the parent at this time may lead to unnecessary anxiety for the child. The energetic toddler will generally stay with the parent long enough to be assured that the situation is not a threat. Then, the toddler will turn his or her attention to the environment and the objects in it. The nurse may then proceed with the interview.

If the child does become disruptive to the history-taking process, the nurse should provide the child with play materials or books to occupy him or her during the remainder of the interview. Also, the nurse should enlist the help of the parent to set appropriate limits with the child. Parents often have unique and specific ways of eliciting cooperation from their children, and the nurse should take advantage of such situations.

During the interview it is also important for the nurse to determine the nature of the relationship between a child and parent. For example, the nurse should watch interactions between the child and parent throughout the history-taking process.

Does the parent appear to be concerned about or indifferent to the toddler?

How does the parent express concern?

How does the toddler react to the parent?

What kind of physical contact is there between the two?

Does the child sit quietly on the parent's lap or does he or she move about the room exploring, returning to the caretaker only to "touch base"?

Is the caretaker overly permissive or overly restrictive of the child's behavior?

Does the parent demonstrate affection for the child verbally or non-verbally?

If limit setting with the child is necessary, how does the parent set limits?

How does the child respond to the limit setting?

The answers to questions such as these can help the nurse identify strengths and weaknesses in the interactional system which may affect the toddler's health. In addition, exploring with the parents their memories of their own upbringing may provide insights into the toddler-parent relationship.

When the data obtained during the interview are recorded, the nurse must be certain that the information is thorough and concise. Particularly important in this age group are accurate recordings of length (or height if the child is walking), weight, head circumference, vital signs, immunization status, and achievement of development milestones. A complete written assessment of the toddler is essential in order to provide for the continuity of health care.

Client Profile and Biographical Data

Record the name (including nickname) of the child, address, sex, age in months, race, nationality, date and place of birth, and religious affiliation. In addition to the biographical data listed above, the name, ad-

Since many toddlers fear strangers, the child must be allowed time to become comfortable in the nurse's presence.

The nurse should determine the nature of the toddler-parent relationship.

Data must be recorded in a thorough and concise manner.

dress, phone number, occupation, and social security number of the informant (parent or caretaker) must be recorded, as well as the informant's relationship to the child (e.g., mother, baby-sitter, or teacher).

Health Status Perception

The reason for entry into the health care system should be recorded next. If this is a well-child visit, the nurse should ask if there are any particular concerns regarding the toddler. This information will most likely be provided by the parent, but an effort should be made to assess the child's perception of the purpose of the health visit. Also, include why the parent has chosen to bring the child *today*. This will help clarify the parent's perception of his or her toddler's health state.

Current Health Status and Health Habits

To determine the toddler's current health status the nurse should first ask the toddler, "How are you feeling today?" or "Can you tell me why you came to see me today?" Then the parent should be asked to describe his or her perception of the toddler's health. Important data should then be recorded. Additional questions that can be used to elicit greater detail on the subject are listed below.

Questions to elicit data:

What does health mean to you (toddler) and to you (parent)?

How often do you (parent) utilize the established health-care system for your toddler?

What determines whether you (parent) use the system or not?

Where does your child usually receive health care?

Are you (parent) aware of the health hazards common to children in this age group? (For example, accidents claim more lives in this age group than any other cause.)

What other sources of health care information are available to you (parent)?

Also determine if the parent holds different standards for health care for the toddler than for himself or herself. For example, does the parent make sure that the child's immunizations are up to date but disregards his or her own need for immunization?

Next, the nurse should determine how the parent views the role of the recipient of health care.

Questions to elicit data:

Do you feel comfortable seeking health care for yourself? For your child?

Have you talked to your child about coming to the clinic or hospital?

What have you told your child about the visit?

How does your child usually respond to clinic or hospital visits and to the nurses and doctors?

What are your child's expectations of the nurse?

What are your (parent) expectations of the nurse?

When the client profile is being completed, the nurse should include biographical data, the parent's reason for bringing the child for a health visit, and both the parent's and the child's perception of the child's health.

Although the toddler is quite young, he or she should be asked about his or her current health status.

Since the toddler is dependent on the parent for entry into the health care system, the parent's views about health should be determined.

The answers to the above questions will help the nurse establish the toddler's current health status, as well as the probability of the parent's seeking future health care for the child.

Health habits that are important both to the toddler's general well-being and to his or her achievement of age-specific developmental tasks include brushing the teeth, dressing oneself, washing and drying the hands, drinking from a cup, feeding oneself finger foods, developing a sleep routine, and mastering toilet training. Each of these habits is learned through role modeling by parents, siblings, or others in the child's environment.

The nurse should inquire as to which health habits the toddler can perform and as to whether these various tasks are done routinely. Often the one most difficult for the child to achieve is toilet training. This may begin around the age of 2, but mastery may not occur until the early preschool years.

If the nurse identifies that the parents have not instructed the toddler regarding health habits, or that the toddler has difficulty carrying out daily health habits, this should be noted as well.

Past Health Status

When collecting data about the toddler's past health status, the nurse should include the following:

1 Birth history
2 Growth and development status
3 Common childhood illnesses
4 Immunizations
5 Any previous hospitalization
6 Accidents or injuries
7 Allergies or allergic reactions

The toddler's prenatal, natal, and postnatal history should be noted, since medical or health-threatening occurrences at any of these times can have an impact on the child's future well-being. For example, if the child had a natal history of asphyxia, this could possibly result in developmental delays which may not be manifested until the toddler years.

Growth and development should be assessed by noting the toddler's pattern of physical growth measurements and developmental achievements. By referring to growth charts the nurse can determine if the child's pattern of growth has been progressive and appropriate for a given age.

The age at which various developmental achievements occurred should be evaluated. The nurse should note motor skills, language development, and social abilities. Examples of motor skills to inquire about include when the child began to sit, crawl, walk alone, run, pick up objects, throw toys, and self-feed. Language development is noted by determining when the child began to understand words, imitate sounds, and speak actual words and sentences. Social abilities include interactions with his or her family and other persons, the ability to perform tasks such as dressing and toileting, and the capacity to play alone or with other children.

Common childhood illnesses are noted, along with the date and age of the child at the time each occurred. Some of the more common ill-

Early mastery of simple health habits can facilitate the toddler's feelings of independence.

See Behavioral Development for examples of behaviors which may influence the toddler's cooperation in learning health habits.

See Past Health Status in Chaps. 3 and 6 when collecting this data.

If previous client records are available, the nurse should refer to them for details about the toddler's past health status.

See Appendix for growth charts.

The rate of development varies in children as a result of individual uniqueness.

Refer to the Denver Developmental Screening Test (DDST) for norms of certain developmental achievements.

nesses in the toddler years include pertussis, roseola-type viruses, and rubella.

By the age of 1 the child should have received a series (3) of diphtheria-pertussis-tetanus (DPT) immunizations; by 12 months, a tuberculin test and by 15 months, a measles-mumps-rubella (MMR) immunization. The nurse should ask the parent for the child's record of immunizations received, or ask the parent to recall the dates of each immunization and the age of the child at the time of immunization. Adverse reactions or side effects from any immunization should also be noted.

Previous hospitalizations, accidents or injuries, and allergies or allergic reactions should be identified and recorded as described in Chap. 3. It is important to be thorough when recording data, since this may have an impact on the toddler's current health status.

Highlights

Immunization schedules may be altered because of individual characteristics and advances in technology and research.

Family History

The family history of the toddler is collected as described in Chap. 3. The nurse must ask the parent to recall relevant information about both maternal and paternal relatives.

Table 3-3 and Fig. 3-2 should be used to complete the family history.

Life Patterns and Lifestyles

Age

Because of age and immaturity the toddler has little control over what is or is not done for him or her. Therefore, the toddler is dependent on others for meeting basic needs and health care needs. For example, the language skills of the toddler are primitive, which results in the frequent inability to communicate verbally when he or she is hungry, tired, or ill or is in need of holding and cuddling.

The age of the toddler can have a significant influence on how needs are met or provided for.

The toddler's natural curiosity and drive to explore the world, combined with rapidly developing motor skills, make the child particularly prone to accidents, poisonings, and burns. Traffic and water are also hazardous. The toddler has not had the experiences necessary to learn and understand appropriate fear of such hazards. Thus, the parents and caretakers must protect the child and make his or her environment safe.

The toddler may induce considerable stress on parents, family members, and other caretakers. Temper tantrums, demanding behavior, outbursts of crying, and contrariness may be so stress-inducing that some caregivers may be unable to cope with their toddler. Child abuse, which occurs in all age groups, may present itself for the first time during toddlerhood. Symptoms of potential stress in the family must be recognized by the nurse so that appropriate intervention can be provided and trauma to the toddler averted.

See Coping Patterns and Stress Tolerance for additional discussion of this factor.

To assess age-related variables, parents may be asked questions such as those listed below.

Questions to elicit data:

1 How do you know when your child is ill?
2 What do you think are the most likely causes of injury or illness for your toddler?
3 Are there behaviors in your child that annoy or irritate you? How do you handle or cope with these?

Such questions may open new avenues for discussion or exploration by the nurse.

Race

The child's race must be considered in the health history, since specific health problems, such as sickle-cell anemia, are related to race. In addition, growth and development charts are frequently based on norms derived from children with western European and Nordic backgrounds.[3] This could result in inaccurate assessments if race was not taken into consideration by the nurse. Questions such as "What is your ancestral background?" or "With what racial group do you identify yourself or your child?" will help elicit information about the race of the toddler.

Heredity

The nurse should review the data collected about the toddler's family history, since the family history provides a basis for assessment of hereditary factors affecting the toddler. Any hereditary traits, disorders, or diseases should be noted.

Behavior, like physical health, is thought to be influenced by heredity to a certain extent. However, it is often difficult to separate out the influence of the environment and the influence of heredity on the child. The nurse may inquire if the parents recognize any behaviors in the toddler that seem to be familial. Both desirable and undesirable behaviors should be noted.

The nurse should further determine how the parents perceive their heredity and how they think it may affect the growth and development of the toddler.

Culture

The nurse should explore the cultural background of the parents in order to determine how the toddler's health state may be affected by their attitudes and patterns of behavior. Cultural influences will be most pronounced with regard to child-rearing practices.

Since the toddler years are characterized by intense exploration, the parents are frequently challenged by the untiring energy and inquisitiveness of the toddler. Parents must set limits and discipline the toddler so that self-control will be learned. They must also cope with the negativism, obstinacy, and ritualistic behaviors displayed by the toddler. Understanding these characteristics helps the parents realize the importance of these behaviors in relation to the toddler's achievement of developmental tasks.

Thus it is important for the nurse to determine specific cultural patterns which facilitate or deter the toddler's growth and development.

Questions to elicit data:

1 How do you discipline your child?

2 Do you use physical punishment?

3 Do you restrict your child's play area?

4 Do you think your toddler is demanding? Describe.

5 How do you cope with your toddler when he or she displays negative and obstinate behavior?

6 What method have you used to toilet train your child?

7 Do older children get along well with your toddler? How do they treat him or her?

The parents' ability to provide for the toddler's physical welfare is also culturally determined to a certain extent. The nurse should inquire if the parents are able to provide adequate food, clothing, shelter, and health care for their child. Priorities for each may vary depending on economic status as well as culture.

Growth and Development

The physical, cognitive, social, and emotional aspects of growth and development of the toddler should be assessed. Each can be determined by observation, by talking with the parents, and by use of appropriate screening tools.

Refer to Table 6-4 for age-appropriate screening tools and tests.

The nurse must be aware of the changes in the pattern of physical growth, of maturation of motor skills, and of language and social development when assessing toddlers. Physical growth during toddlerhood slows from the rapid growth rate of infancy. There is a sharp decline in the normal rate of weight gain during the second year of life from approximately 7 oz (200 g) per week in infancy to 7 oz (200 g) per month for the toddler. Growth in height continues at a much steadier rate, as a result mainly of the growth of the long bones of the legs. The average child grows about 4 inches (10 cm) and gains 4 to 5 lb (approximately 2 kg) during the second year, and by the age of 2 is approximately 32 inches (80 cm) tall and weighs about 28 lb (13 kg).[4]

The rate of growth and development varies widely as a result of the individual uniqueness of each child.

By the age of 2 years the average toddler is 32 inches tall and weighs 28 lb.

Gross and fine motor skills increase during the years from 1 to 3 as a result of the myelinization of immature nerve fibers. Neuromuscular maturation contributes to locomotor abilities such as sitting, crawling, standing, and walking and to more refined skills such as scribbling and using a pincer grasp. Toilet training, a major developmental milestone, is also dependent upon neuromuscular maturation.

Refer to the DDST for a timetable of average development of motor skills, language, and social abilities.

Language development increases rapidly during the second and third years. By 10 months the infant can respond to simple commands. First words are generally spoken at around 1 year of age, and approximately three words can be understood by this time. By a child's second birthday, effective vocabulary has increased to 272 words. (Effective vocabulary includes words both spoken and understood.) In addition, a child can now put words together in sentences and has mastered some basic grammatical rules. By the third birthday the average child has an effective vocabulary of 896 words.[5]

By the age of 3 the average toddler has a vocabulary of 896 words.

The toddler's social capabilities have their foundation in infancy. Relationships in the second and third year of life still revolve mainly around parents or significant caretakers, but the toddler is now ready to expand his or her social life to include siblings, peers, older and younger children, relatives, and neighbors. Through social relationships the toddler learns the principles of cooperation, sharing, waiting one's turn, and respecting the feelings and possessions of others. In peer relationships, the toddler is able to play with children his or her own age who also have similar abilities. Thus the toddler can gain a realistic sense of self and of his or her own skills.

Peer relationships are particularly important to the toddler's development of a sense of self.

Emotional feelings and reactions are varied in toddlers depending on their basic personalities and age and on how others, both children and adults, react to them. Frequently, emotions will be manifested in one or all of the following behaviors: temper tantrums, dawdling, timidity, contrariness, imitating, acting selfish or aggressive or playing cooperatively, sharing, and showing love. It is important for parents, as well as the nurse, to be sensitive to the toddler's changing emotions and to provide love, support, and guidance in helping the toddler to learn how to deal with various emotions.

See Behavioral Development for clues to assessing emotions.

When assessing growth and development in each of the above areas the nurse can use the Denver Developmental Screening Test (DDST) to gather certain data. Additional questions not covered by the DDST may also be asked.

Highlights

The DDST is not an intelligence test, and this should be made clear to the parents.

Questions to elicit data:

1 Do you think your child's weight and height are appropriate for age? Why?

2 Does your child have good coordination?

3 In what areas of gross and fine motor development do you think your child needs practice?

4 Is your child toilet trained? At what age did this occur? Was this easy to accomplish?

5 At what age did your child learn to feed himself or herself? Can your child drink from a cup well and use utensils?

6 Does your child participate in putting on clothes and shoes? At what age did this occur?

7 Does your child play with other children his or her same age (peers) and with younger and older children? How would you describe these play relationships?

8 Do you think your child is cooperative? Why? Does your child share toys with others?

9 Does your child have temper tantrums? Describe these. How do you handle them?

10 Is your child timid in new situations? Does your child overcome timidity as familiarity develops?

11 How do you differentiate between your toddler's treating others aggressively and his or her treating objects aggressively? Do you handle these behaviors differently?

12 How do you handle your child's contrariness (refusal to be controlled)? Do you allow your child to make some of his or her own decisions?

13 Does your toddler's dawdling bother you? How do you deal with this behavior?

When assessing the toddler's growth and development the nurse can use the DDST, as well as ask specific questions about specific areas.

Answers to the above questions, plus results from the DDST, will provide the nurse with a fairly thorough assessment of the toddler's growth and development.

Behavioral Development

Toddlerhood bridges the gap between infancy and childhood. The role changes which must take place in both the child and the caretakers are, to a great extent, responsible for the turbulence of this period. The relative tranquility of the infant is now replaced by the disconcerting behaviors of the toddler. The mother and father must assume the additional roles of teacher, socializer, and disciplinarian. The toddler, who during infancy had relatively few, if any, expectations or restrictions placed upon him or her and who until now has had no responsibilities with regard to control of behavior, must assume new role responsibilities and a new relationship with the world and the people in it. The rules he or she is expected to follow are changing, and the toddler must learn the new rules for successful adaptation. The nurse who is working with toddlers and their families must recognize the great amount of energy it takes for both parents and toddlers to adjust and should provide needed support and understanding.

The toddler years are turbulent for both the child and the parent as a result of dramatic strivings for autonomy and control by the toddler.

THE TODDLER **475**

Socialization and Behavioral Characteristics of the Toddler *Socialization* is "the process by which the individual becomes a member of a social group through acquisition of the group's values, motives, and behaviors."[6] Socialization is an important aspect of the child's development during toddlerhood. In the United States, socialization during this period focuses on such things as control of bowel and bladder habits, cleanliness, control of anger and of aggressive behaviors, restriction of excessive motor activities, acquisition of language skills, and monitoring of egocentric or antisocial behaviors. Since socialization is closely linked with the behavioral characteristics of the toddler, the two are discussed together.

As the toddler begins to walk upright and takes on more of the characteristics of a child, adults will no longer view the toddler as an infant. For this reason, behaviors such as soiling of diapers or playing with food that were acceptable for the infant come to be viewed as unacceptable for the toddler. The pressure from external forces to behave in new and different ways is complemented by the toddler's own developing psychomotor skills, cognitive abilities, and language skills which drive the toddler to seek greater control over self and environment.

Ambivalence At the same time that internal factors are driving the child to assert more autonomy and independence, the child's awareness of dependence on his or her mother and/or significant others increases. The ambivalence the toddler feels as a result of these conflicting drives expresses itself in sudden shifts of mood and in increased physical activity. One observes this frequently in the toddler who struggles frantically to be free from his or her mother's lap but who only a few minutes later struggles just as determinedly to return to her lap.

Ritualism Routines and habits are especially important to the toddler. Being able to predict what will happen or what a person's response will be in a certain situation gives the toddler a sense of control over his or her life. Thus, one frequently sees toddlers insisting on certain rituals or predictable nap or mealtime routines. Deviations from such routines are upsetting to the toddler and are frequently brought to the caretaker's attention.

> Three-year-old Christopher was being cared for by his father while his mother was away on a short trip. In the rush of dressing Christopher and taking him to the baby-sitter in the morning, his father forgot to feed him breakfast. Although he said nothing at the time and even though the baby-sitter gave him breakfast, Christopher, much to his father's dismay, reported to his mother when she called that evening, "Daddy forgets to feed me!"

His routine had been broken, and this, along with the absence of his mother, left him feeling out of control and powerless. He sought to remedy this by "telling" on his father.

Negativism The word "no" appears in the toddler's vocabulary with increasing frequency throughout the second and third year, though parents soon learn that the word need not always be taken at face value. Indeed, the toddler may be crying, "no, no" at the same time he is complying with the parent's wishes. Negativism, however, is essential in the child's efforts to learn self-control and mastery of the environment. Erikson writes:

> It is necessary that he [the toddler] experiences over and over again that he is a person who is permitted to make choices. He has to have the right to

Parenting and child-rearing practices will have a great impact on the toddler's socialization process.

Parental expectations of the toddler increase as he or she matures.

The toddler's own feelings of uncertainty in a given situation may cause ambivalent responses.

The toddler requires definite order in daily life patterns in order to feel a "sense of control."

When using the word no in response to a situation, the toddler may be testing the extent of new-found independence.

choose, for example, whether to sit or whether to stand, whether to approach a visitor or to lean against his mother's knee, whether to accept offered food or whether to reject it, whether to use the toilet or wet his pants. At the same time he must learn some of the boundaries of self-determination. He inevitably finds that there are walls he cannot climb, that there are objects out of reach, that, above all, there are innumerable commands enforced by powerful adults.[7]

A child who is given the opportunity to make reasonable choices regarding his or her life and activities and who is given freedom to explore the world and practice newly developed motor skills will develop a sense of self-assurance and spontaneity. The child will be able to approach new situations without undue anxiety and will enjoy new and challenging situations. On the other hand, children who are overprotected and not allowed to explore and problem-solve for themselves may lack self-confidence and may learn to doubt their ability to meet new challenges. The ways in which parents deal with the child's negativism and attempts at self-assertion are therefore important components to consider in health assessment of the toddler.

Separation Anxiety During toddlerhood, the child is learning to cope with brief separations from the mother or mother surrogate. Fear of separation, which begins around 7 months of age and peaks at approximately 10 months of age, reaches another peak at 18 months.[8] Lengthy separations during toddlerhood are tolerated poorly and are potentially damaging to the child, who can neither understand them nor express effectively the emotion which surrounds his or her sense of loss and fear of abandonment.

John Bowlby, with an English research team, studied the reactions of healthy children aged 15 to 30 months who were separated from their mothers for a period of time. He discovered that these children passed through three stages in responding to the perceived loss of their mother: (1) protest, (2) despair, and (3) denial.

In the first stage, the child reacted by crying, calling out for mother, banging against the crib, and watching eagerly for her appearance at the door. According to Bowlby, the length of the protest phase was directly related to the warmth of the mother-child relationship. In other words, the protest phase was longer in those children who had experienced warm, intimate relationships with their mothers than in those whose relationships had been unsatisfactory.

During the second stage of despair the overt protesting stopped and the child began to respond to others in the immediate environment. However, if the child's mother should visit during this stage, the child would ignore her and respond more to the gifts or food she brought. The child appeared to have lost all interest in his or her mother.

In the third stage, denial, the child formed only superficial attachments to many adults in the environment. Eventually the child's detachment gave the impression that neither mothering nor any other human contact was important.[9]

Learning to tolerate separations for short periods is an important developmental task for the toddler to master. Once the child has learned from experience that parents will return after brief separations, adaptation will become easier.

Fears and Fantasies Closely related to separation anxiety are the fears and fantasies so commonly found in toddlers. Selma H. Fraiberg writes in her book *The Magic Years:*

It is important for caretakers to be consistent in their discipline of the toddler.

Separation from parents is one of the most significant stressors in the toddler's daily life.

Toddlers may respond to a loss through protest, despair, and denial.

Learning to tolerate short separations is an important developmental task for the toddler.

A toddler's fears depend on the general level of one's anxiety and imagination.

These [years of early childhood] are "magic years" because the child in his early years is a magician—in the psychological sense. His earliest conception of the world is a magical one; he believes that his actions and thoughts can bring about events. . . . But a magic world is an unstable world, at times a spooky world, and as the child gropes his way toward reason and an objective world he must wrestle with the dangerous creatures of his imagination and the real and imagined dangers of the outer world. . . .[10]

Toddlers' fears are many, and all toddlers experience them to a greater or lesser extent. Fears may manifest themselves as nightmares, in which unresolved anxieties from the day present themselves in dreams at night. They may also manifest themselves in behavioral changes, such as the sudden development of fear of taking a bath or of flushing the toilet. The child may watch the water running down the drain or watch feces disappear down the toilet and believe that the same thing could happen to him or her. Sense of self and the limits of one's body are not clearly defined during these years.

At this age the toddler's aggressive and omnipotent feelings may contribute to fears. The child believes that by wishing, things can be made to happen. If harm to another is wished, for example, the child believes that it may indeed occur. Inability to come to grips with one's own aggressiveness and angry feelings may cause projection of these feelings to an imaginary being or animal, such as a "dragon" who "lives in my closet."

Ferocious beasts are common in the imaginations of toddlers. How they cope with such "beasts" is important. While fears and fantasies are common and normal phenomena in toddlerhood, consistent fearfulness which cannot be controlled or alleviated by parental understanding and "protection" should be thoroughly investigated. An understanding of these fears and fantasies will help parents deal more sympathetically with bedtime separation problems as well as with the many other types of separation that must occur in the daily life of the toddler.

Temper Tantrums Frequently the toddler attempts to do things that are just beyond his or her abilities. This results in feelings of frustration. When the amount of frustration becomes too great for the toddler to handle, physical and emotional exhaustion can result in temper tantrums. The toddler seems to lose all control over himself or herself, and sometimes parents lose control as well, since they are uncertain about how to deal with these outbursts.

Even the slightest issue can set off a temper tantrum. For example, if mom is getting ready to go out and is in a hurry to get Tommy dressed, interrupting his play activities to dress him may result in resistance. The child's anger may be so great because of his loss of control over the situation that he may begin kicking, screaming, and resisting any attempts by his mother to dress him. A calm voice of reassurance and patience on the mother's part often can help the child return to stability. Or, in some instances, ignoring the outburst and leaving the room until the tantrum subsides may be the best approach that the parent can take to deal with the tantrum. Since physical injury to the toddler rarely occurs during a temper tantrum, the parent need not feel guilty taking this latter approach. It is important that toddlers learn that overwhelming feelings are understandable but that they cannot be used to manipulate parents into giving in to all wants and desires.

Since temper tantrums are a part of the toddler's normal developmental process, it is realistic to expect that they will occur at least

The toddler may come to fear persons and pets that once were not feared.

Past experiences may precipitate fears and fantasies in the toddler.

Caretakers must provide the toddler with love, understanding, and a sense of control, so that fears may be overcome.

Overwhelming feelings of frustration are the frequent cause of temper tantrums in the toddler.

Behavioral reactions which the toddler manifests during tantrums include crying, screaming, biting, kicking, and resisting contact.

Temper tantrums become less frequent as the toddler matures physically and learns to talk.

weekly. Incentives to go on trying and learning can help the toddler overcome daily frustrations and can foster progression through this difficult stage.

The toddler's behavioral development can be assessed by collecting detailed data about the child's social and behavioral characteristics. The nurse should specifically question the parents about the child's ability to relate to family members, peers, and other adults, and about ambivalence, ritualism, negativism, separation anxiety, fears and fantasies, and temper tantrums.

Questions to elicit data:

1 Does your child exhibit frequent mood change or ambivalence in reactions?

2 What rituals or routines have you followed with your child (for example, as regards meals, bathing, or preparation for bed)?

3 Does your child respond with "no" when given directions? How do you deal with this?

4 How does your child respond to separation from you? Who are the other caretakers in his or her life?

5 Do you think your child has any fears? What are these?

6 Does your child fantasize? How do you respond to this?

7 How often does your child have temper tantrums? What behaviors are manifested? How do you handle these?

8 Do you find it difficult sometimes to deal with any of your child's behaviors? Describe.

Thorough assessment of the above areas will provide the nurse with important information that impacts on all areas of the toddler's health state.

Biological Rhythms

Sleep-Wakefulness Cycle The toddler averages from 10 to 15 hours of sleep in a 24-hour period. Two naps per day are more common in the early toddler period, and the number and length of naps generally decline as the child approaches the preschool years.[11]

Most toddlers sleep a total of 10 to 15 hours per 24 hours.

Awaking two or three times during the night occurs with most toddlers. This may be due to separation anxiety, loneliness, teething pains, illness, nightmares, or a stressful family situation. Often the toddler is able to fall back to sleep, but some may need attention and comfort from a parent.

Establishing a regular bedtime routine with the toddler will facilitate sleep. Routines can include a parent reciting or reading a story, singing a lullaby, rocking the child, or giving the child a bottle of water to suck on. Such activities provide the toddler with love and security and a time to settle down after a busy day.

A bedtime routine established by the parents may facilitate sleep for the toddler.

A circadian sleep-wakefulness rhythm can be identified by the age of 3 months, and a gradual maturation of this cycle occurs between the ages of 2 and 10 years in children.[12] Thus, the toddler should manifest an individual pattern of night sleep, naps, and awake time in a 24-hour period. In order to avoid behavioral or emotional disruptions caused by alterations in the toddler's cycle, it is important that parents allow the child to follow a routine sleep pattern, with only occasional interruptions in the pattern.

See Chaps. 1 and 3 for information on circadian rhythms.

1 What time does your child go to bed at night and get up in the morning? At what times does your child nap during the day?

2 Do you try to follow any routine when putting your child down at night and during the day for naps?

3 Where does your child sleep?

4 Can you identify any sleep problems in your child, such as significant crying at bedtime?

5 Can you identify if your child is overtired? How?

6 Do you feel that it is important that your child get the same number of hours of sleep at the same times each day? Why?

It is important for the nurse to identify the toddler's sleep-wakefulness cycle.

Additional questions that will assist the nurse in data collection are contained in Chap. 3, Table 3-4.

Elimination Cycle During the toddler years the elimination cycle becomes a focus of attention as a result of the parents' efforts to toilet train their child. Research indicates that reliable daytime control of elimination occurs between the ages of $2\frac{1}{2}$ and 3 years, while nighttime control is usually complete by the age of 4 to 5 in most children. The keys to successful toilet training of the toddler are readiness and the ability and willingness to perform the act. A mother who reports that her child was trained by the age of 14 months really is saying that she has trained herself to anticipate the elimination need of the child.

Most toddlers complete daytime toilet training by the age of 3.

It is easier to predict defecation in the normal toddler than urination, since defecation occurs at about the same time each day and is accompanied by a definite urge to eliminate. Therefore, toilet-training for defecation usually takes place first. This excretory pattern can be determined by the parent by keeping track of output over several days. It is important for parents to also understand that voluntary defecation requires intact muscular, sensory, and nervous structures.

The excretory cycle is predictable in the normal toddler.

Most urine is excreted during the waking hours, and thus, a circadian pattern can be noted in most toddlers. The peak of the excretory rhythm is between 8 A.M. and 12 noon, and the trough is between 12 midnight and 4 A.M.[13] However, this elimination cycle can be influenced by age, volume and time of fluid intake, and certain medications. Again, the parents can keep track of intake and output to determine the urination pattern of their child. Also, when the toddler is able to recognize the sensation or urge to "let go" and can verbalize this, voluntary control of the urethral sphincter can occur and will usually be communicated to the parent. This latter occurrence facilitates the determination of the urination pattern.

The urination cycle shows a circadian pattern.

Maturational maturity of muscular, sensory, and nervous structures in the toddler is necessary for successful training.

When assessing the toddler's elimination cycle the nurse should incorporate the above knowledge with information about the parents' attitude about and approach to toilet training. The parents' attitude about toilet training and their understanding of the physiological maturity of the toddler are important to the parent-child relationship and will influence the success of the toilet-training sessions. A parent who methodically instructs the toddler about the process in a nonthreatening and supportive manner and rewards successes with praise will assist the child in accomplishing this major developmental task in a positive manner. A child should never be punished or shamed for elimination accidents or for lack of readiness to become toilet trained.

See Behavioral Development for additional data.

Refer to pediatric texts for more specific details about toilet training the toddler.

Questions to elicit data:

1 Can you recognize your child's need to defecate or urinate? How?

2 When do you think a child should be toilet trained?

3 Is your child now toilet trained at night and during the day? Explain and discuss.

4 Does your child have any problems or difficulties with elimination?

5 Do you expect your child to eliminate on his or her own or with your help?

6 What have you done to support your child in learning to be toilet trained?

7 Does your child have a potty chair that he or she is able to sit on without help?

Additional questions can be developed by the nurse to further assess the elimination cycle based on answers to the above questions.

Temperature Cycle As with the infant and adult, the toddler's body temperature follows a circadian rhythm. Temperature is lowest at nighttime and during early morning hours, rises during the day, and peaks in the late afternoon in a day-active child. One study indicates the lowest value in 2- to 5-year-olds occurs at 3 A.M.[14] Stressors, such as disrupted sleep patterns and illness, may alter the cycle.

In a day-active toddler, the body temperature is lowest in the early morning hours and peaks in late afternoon.

It is important that parents are aware of this data, since they frequently are asked by health professionals to monitor their toddler's temperature. For example, a temperature above 99°F (37.2°C) in the early morning hours may be indicative of an abnormal physiological response and requires further investigation by the nurse.

Teething (eruption of primary teeth) is occasionally cited as a cause of increased body temperature in the toddler. However, teething per se does not usually cause body temperature to rise, and a febrile condition should not be attributed to teething.

Pharmacological Effectiveness Cycle Immunization schedules during the toddler years include (1) a tuberculin test at the age of 1 year, (2) a MMR vaccine at 15 months, and (3) a DPT vaccine and an oral polio vaccine at the age of 1½ years. This schedule is based on the completion of recommended schedules during infancy.

See Table 6-7 for immunization schedules during childhood.

Metabolic Rhythms Physiological functions of the toddler demonstrate a circadian rhythm but deviate from the normal adult values until later in childhood. Metabolic rhythms are best assessed when the toddler is quiet, since stress and physical activity can cause increases in the heart rate, respiratory rate, temperature, and blood pressure.

Refer to the physical examination of the toddler for normal values of metabolic rhythms.

Environmental Factors

Where the child lives and plays is important to the child's health. The high incidence of death among toddlers from falls, poisonings, drownings, burnings, and motor vehicle accidents makes environmental assessment particularly important. Safety in the home should be carefully explored with the parents or other caregivers. Poisons found in household products, insect sprays, and lead paint, for example, pose potential dangers for the inquisitive toddler.

The toddler's home environment should be assessed for safety.

Parents should be asked how they have "child-proofed" their home.

Questions to elicit data:

1 Do you have medicines locked up?
2 Do you have poisons, detergents, and other household chemicals stored out of reach?
3 Do you have covers placed over electrical outlets?
4 Do you have electrical cords to items such as lamps placed out of reach?
5 Do you have gates closing off stairways or decks to prevent falls?
6 Do you maintain your water heater at a safe temperature?
7 When the stove is in use, are you cautious about placement of pots and pans?

The environment should be conducive to learning and to growth and development.

The following questions can be used to assess areas of the child's environment outside the home.

Ideally, the nurse should make a home visit to thoroughly assess the toddler's environment.

Questions to elicit data:

1 Do you use a car seat for your child at all times when riding?
2 Is outdoor play supervised by an adult?
3 Does your child play in a fenced-in backyard?
4 Does your child wear a life jacket when near lakes or swimming pools?

The nurse should also explore with the parents how the toddler's environment is conducive to learning and to promotion of growth and development. There should be adequate and age-specific toys to enhance fine and gross motor skills and books to facilitate reading and language development. It is also desirable to expose the toddler to other children the same age so that social skills can be learned through play.

One screening tool that can be used to systematically assess environmental factors that influence the child's health are the responses to a survey called the Home Observation for Measurement of the Environment (HOME) for children from birth to the age of 3 years.[15] (See Fig. 7-1.) The items covered by the survey require direct observation in the home by the nurse and questioning of the parents or other caregiver.

The "HOME" survey is a screening tool that can be used to assess systematically the social, emotional, and cognitive support the toddler receives from his or her environment.

If the toddler attends preschool or spends time at a day care center, these environments should also be evaluated by the nurse. Besides the parents, teachers and other caregivers exert a significant influence on the toddler's growth and development in physical, psychological, emotional, and behavioral areas. Visiting the location or phone contact with the teacher or caregiver may be necessary for a thorough nursing assessment.

Since the toddler is extremely curious and adventuresome, he or she will be exploring the environment, frequently unaware of potential dangers. Therefore, parents and caretakers must make every effort to secure a safe environment in which the child can learn and play. Also, the child must be taught the concept of safety. By the age of 12 months the child can learn the meaning of single-word phrases such as "no-no," "hot," and "hurt" if they are repeated each time the appropriate situation arises.

See Environmental Factors for a previous discussion of safety.

The nurse should question the parents about specific methods that were used in "baby-proofing" their home and about what aspects of safety the child has been taught. Also, questions presented in Chap. 3 should be used to supplement the data-gathering process.

Economics

As with the infant, the toddler is dependent upon the parents for economic security. Food, shelter, clothing, and health care are provided to the toddler within the financial budget of the family.

The nurse must assess the economic factors existing in the parents' lives that will impact on the toddler. See Economics in Chap. 3 for questions that can be used to collect data from the caretaker.

Community Resources

The nurse should explore with the parents which community resources have been used, if any, to benefit the toddler's health state. These may be resources which help the parents to learn about aspects of child rearing, which provide emotional support to parents of toddlers, or which are used directly by the toddler, such as day care centers.

Since parents or families may be unfamiliar with community resources which might be of benefit to them and their toddler, it is crucial that the nurse develop an awareness of resources in the area so that information can be shared.

Roles and Relationship Patterns

Family Life

The role of the family, especially the parents, is critical in promoting the toddler's development of autonomy and a positive self-concept and provides the foundation for all future interactions. The toddler learns and masters activities of daily living and learns to cope with limit setting, discipline, and anxiety-producing situations through family experiences. Besides the parents, siblings, age-mates, and grandparents offer special opportunities for interpersonal relationships.

Family life carries over into every variable factor that the nurse will assess.

Using the questions identified in Chap. 3, the nurse can begin assessing the toddler's family life and its impact on the child's health state. Additional questions that can be used to collect data should focus on such areas as (1) the effect of the toddler's personality on family functioning, (2) the toddler's ability to relate to and interact with siblings and age-mates, (3) the grandparent's roles as they affect the developing child, (4) the family's expectations of the toddler for achieving age-appropriate growth and development, and (5) the approach parents or caretakers use to instill values in the toddler and the disciplinary measures used to maintain acceptable behavior.

The toddler's development of autonomy depends on family interactions.

See the discussion of the family in Chaps. 2 and 3.

Occupation

The occupations of the parents of the toddler will determine the time available for interaction, the income of the family and their ability to purchase goods and health care, and the parents' methods of child rearing. As for other ages, the nurse should assess occupation as it influences growth, development, and health.

The parent's occupation can affect the toddler's health and entry into the health care system.

Since the toddler can be excessively demanding at times, or stubborn, aggressive, and ritualistic as well as cooperative and playful, parents are challenged to deal with these varying behaviors and characteristics on a daily basis. If both parents, for example, work full time, when they come home at the end of the day they may lack the energy to deal with the child in a healthy and growth-promoting way. Thus, family interactions may become stressed. On the other hand, many parents may find the toddler an enjoyable and refreshing change from a routine workday. The nurse must determine the effect of occupation on the toddler. Questions presented in Chap. 3 can be used to collect data.

Home Observation For Measurement of the Environment (Birth to Three)

Date of interview _____

Child designee _____
                      Name   Age   Sex   Ethnicity

Child's birthday _____   Birth order _____

Mother's name _____   Father's name _____

Address _____
_____

Categories	Raw scores	Percentile scores
I Emotional and verbal responsivity of parent	_____	_____
II Avoidance of restriction and punishment	_____	_____
III Organization of physical and temporal environment	_____	_____
IV Provision of appropriate play materials	_____	_____
V Parental involvement with child	_____	_____
VI Opportunities for variety in daily stimulation	_____	_____
Totals	_____	_____

I Emotional and verbal responsivity of parent

Yes   No

1 Parent spontaneously vocalizes to child at least twice during visit (excluding scolding).
2 Parent responds to child's vocalizations with a verbal response.
3 Parent tells child the name of some object during visit or says name of person or object in a "teaching" style.
4 Parent's speech is distinct, clear, and audible.
5 Parent initiates verbal interchanges with observer - asks questions and makes spontaneous comments.
6 Parent expresses ideas freely and easily and uses statements of appropriate length for conversation (e.g., gives more than brief answers).
7 Parent permits child occasionally to engage in "messy" type of play.
8 Parent spontaneously praises child's qualities or behavior twice during visit.
9 When speaking of or to child, parent's voice conveys positive feeling.
10 Parent caresses or kisses child at least once during visit.
11 Parent shows some positive emotional responses to praise of child offered by visitor.

Subscore

II Avoidance of restriction and punishment

Yes   No

12 Parent does not shout at child during visit.
13 Parent does not express overt annoyance with or hostility toward child.
14 Parent neither slaps nor spanks child during visit.
15 Parent reports that no more than one instance of physical punishment occurred during the past week.
16 Parent does not scold or derogate child during visit.
17 Parent does not interfere with child's actions or restrict child's movements more than three times during visit.
18 At least 10 books are present and visible.
19 Family has a pet.

Subscore

Societal Relationships

The child-rearing practices of the parents or caretakers of the toddler are frequently influenced by societal values and expectations, and subsequently these influences can be seen reflected in the child. Moral development, values, attitudes, and associated roles learned by the toddler must coincide with the expectations of society as the child matures, or stressful situations will occur. If the toddler has developed a high self-

The toddler learns to function within society through role modeling and learning experiences provided by the parents.

III Organization of physical and temporal environment

	Yes	No
20 When parent is away, care is provided by one of three regular substitutes.		
21 Someone takes child into grocery store at least once a week.		
22 Child gets out of house at least four times a week.		
23 Child is taken regularly to doctor's office or clinic.		
24 Child has a special place in which to keep his or her toys and "treasures."		
25 Child's play environment appears safe and free of hazards.		
Subscore		

IV Provision of appropriate play materials

	Yes	No
26 Child has some muscle activity toys or equipment.		
27 Child has a push or pull toy.		
28 Child has a stroller or walker, kiddie car, scooter, or tricycle.		
29 Parent provides toys or interesting activities for child during interview.		
30 Child has learning equipment appropriate to age - cuddly toy or role-playing toys.		
31 Child has learning equipment appropriate to age - mobile, table and chairs, high chair, play pen.		
32 Child has eye-hand coordination toys - items to go in and out of receptacle, fit-together toys, beads.		
33 Child has eye-hand coordination toys that permit combinations - stacking or nesting toys, blocks, or building toys.		
34 Child has toys or materials for literature and music.		
Subscore		

V Parental involvement with child

	Yes	No
35 Parent tends to keep child within visual range and to look at him or her often.		
36 Parent talks to child while doing his or her work.		
37 Parent consciously encourages developmental advance.		
38 Parent invests "maturing" toys with value via his or her attention.		
39 Parent structures child's play periods.		
40 Parent provides toys that challenge child to develop new skills.		
Subscore		

VI Opportunities for variety in daily stimulation

	Yes	No
41 Parents alternate in providing caretaking every day.		
42 Child is read stories by either parent at least three times weekly.		
43 Child eats at least one meal per day with mother and father.		
44 Family visits or receives visits from relatives.		
45 Child has three or more books of his or her own.		
Subscore		

Figure 7-1 Home observation form for measurement of the environment, birth to 3 years of age. Items that may require direct questions are marked with an asterisk. (Adapted from Bettye M. Caldwell, *Instruction Manual Inventory for Infants [Home Observation for Measurement of the Environment]*, Little Rock, Ark., 1970.)

esteem through good parenting, the child will be able to adapt to functioning within society in a healthy way.

When assessing this factor, the nurse should focus on the parents' role in society and their ability to meet societal expectations, as well as the influence that the parents directly exert on the toddler. For example, an acceptable social role for a father may be major financial supporter of the family. Social behaviors related to this role could include maintaining a full-time job outside the home, which directly affects not only available time for father-child interaction but also available money for support of the family. Thus, societal characteristics impact on the general health of the toddler.

Self-Perception and Self-Concept Patterns

By the time the child has entered the toddler years, he or she has formed a self-concept and perceives him- or herself either positively or negatively. Through parental and peer contacts, and other environmental interactions, the child will have formulated a personal sense of worth. Supportive reinforcement of good feelings about oneself is necessary for continuous fostering of positive patterns.

It is very important to question the child about his or her self-perception, if possible, with parents not present. If parents are not present, the nurse will be more likely to actually elicit the child's own perceptions. The questions presented in Chap. 3 can be adapted for the collection of data from the toddler.

If responses cannot be gotten from the child, then parents' impressions about their child's self-perception and conceptions should be identified and noted.

Data collected about life patterns may reinforce data about self-perception and conception patterns.

The toddler may be able to verbalize some feelings about his or her self-perception.

Cognitive and Perceptual Patterns

The cognitive and perceptual patterns that should be explored include the toddler's sensory perceptions and his or her cognitive abilities, which are reflected in the child's education and intelligence.

Sensory Perceptions

The toddler's vision, hearing, taste, smell, and touch perceptions should be assessed as accurately as possible, supplemented if necessary by the parents' knowledge of their toddler's perceptions.

The questions formulated in Chap. 3 can be adapted for the toddler. When it is possible, the nurse should use aids to accurately elicit data. For example, the child can be asked to taste something such as sugar and then asked to describe the taste. As a way of assessing the child's sense of smell, the nurse could ask the child to describe how flowers, peanut butter, or strawberries smell. In other words, familiar things in the child's environment can be used to help make the data collected more accurate.

Education

The education of the child during the toddler years is, to a great extent, dependent upon interactions which occur with parents, caretakers, siblings, significant others, and the environment. Genetic endowment will also greatly influence the toddler's learning and progressive intellectual development.

Since most early learning occurs in the home, the nurse should assess the parents' involvement in directing their child's education. Learning to walk, talk, play, and interact with people and objects in the environment requires that the child be exposed to a variety of experiences. Parents need to create a rich verbal environment by talking with their toddlers. They need to help them learn to use their large and small muscles for walking, climbing, jumping, drawing, throwing an object, and the like. Through verbal directions, demonstrations, and the repetition of speech and actions by the parents, the toddler becomes capable of integrating new experiences that will be put into practice as new skills.

The play environment must also be designed to foster the education

See Intelligence and Chap. 2 for additional discussion of intellectual development.

Parents and caretakers must provide the toddler with an environment which fosters the early education of the child.

of the child. There should be roomy play areas indoors and outdoors with safety features such as gates, fences, screens on windows, and locks on doors. All objects which pose a threat to the child should be removed from the area. A parent or other adult should be present so that the toddler can be supervised during play. Toys or other equipment should be safe and in good repair, as well as suitable for the age of the child. If the toddler is in a day care situation part of the time, the parent should evaluate the facility for safety and fostering of growth and development, using the same standards that apply to the home.

Questions to elicit data:

1 Do you make a conscious effort to talk with your toddler and teach him or her new words?

2 Do you read to your toddler? What types of books do you use?

3 What types of toys or play equipment do you have at home?

4 Do you have a swing set, a sandbox, or other equipment in your backyard?

5 Does your toddler have an opportunity to play with other toddlers of the same age?

6 Does your toddler play with siblings or older children?

7 Does your toddler use pencils or crayons to learn to scribble, color, or draw?

8 Have you taught your toddler to identify and name his or her own body parts?

Additional questions may be asked of the toddler in order to determine the child's reasoning powers and abilities.

See Environmental Factors and Exercise-Activity Patterns when assessing the toddler's education.

Intelligence

The increasing intellectual development of the toddler is apparent in the child's thinking and reasoning processes and in the ability to use language to represent mental symbolism. Although this development is in its early formative stage, dramatic advances can be recognized over a short time.

From about the age of 12 to 18 months the toddler is in Piaget's stage 5 of intellectual development. The child is building upon concepts of object permanence and substance. The toddler becomes curious about objects and seems desirous to learn as much as possible about the nature of objects. In Piaget's theoretical framework, this is called *tertiary circular reaction*.[16]

Piaget's theory of intellectual development can be used by the nurse as a guide when assessing the toddler's educational abilities.

Experimentation with manipulating objects in the environment will eventually lead the toddler to discover new ways of playing with objects or a new means for attaining a goal. For example, the toddler may try to move a toy or change its position through trial and error of various sorts. The child will accommodate (adapt) behaviors until the desirable goal is reached, thus inventing ways to deal with objects in the world. Past experiences assist the child in "understanding" the meaning of these actions.

Also during stage 5, the toddler becomes capable of systematic imitation of new actions or models (such as people). For example, the toddler will begin to imitate specific behaviors of a parent or sibling, such as touching the nose or eyes. Visible movements of objects in the environment will also be understood by the child. For example, if a ball rolls under a chair, the child will search for the ball under the place where it was seen to disappear. Thus, the toddler believes in the permanence or continued existence of an object.[17]

At about the age of 18 months the child enters Piaget's stage 6 and develops the capability of thought and language. This period of symbolic thought, which develops through the age of 2, enables the toddler to use mental symbols and words to refer to objects both present and absent from the visual field. In other words, the toddler develops the ability to "think things out." As a result, the child becomes more efficient at what appears to be an immediate imitation of models and is even capable of imitating a model that is absent. Finally, at stage 6 the child is able to form a mental image of an object and can mentally follow that object through a series of complex changes.[18]

From the age of 18 months through 2 years the toddler develops the capability of thought and language.

Between the age of 2 and 4 the child's cognitive processes expand to include the use of symbols to represent something which is not present and to recall an object from the past. This symbolic function (Piaget) is further reflected in the child's use of symbolic play and use of words to identify or represent an object.[19]

Symbolic function as described by Piaget expands the toddler's cognitive processes.

Reasoning also develops during this time period, and the child shows three different kinds of reasoning, according to Piaget. By using the first type of reasoning the child may reason out an event based on past experiences. By using the second type, the child attempts to reason to achieve a certain goal but distorts the reasoning or thought process so that the goal may be attained. For example, a little girl who sees another child's doll may reason that the doll is just like her own doll, and thus it must be her doll. She then desires to have the doll and takes it for her own.

The toddler begins to use reasoning when dealing with objects and persons in the environment.

The third type of reasoning is called *transducive* by Piaget. The child does not use inductive or deductive reasoning but reasons from the particular to the particular. In other words, if two things are alike in one aspect, the child reasons that they are alike in all aspects. For example, if mom puts on her apron when cooking dinner, the child will reason that mom is going to cook dinner the next time she puts on her apron.[20]

During the toddler years, the child reasons from the particular to the particular (transducive reasoning).

Other aspects of Piaget's theory of intellectual development include concepts of space, chance, movement, geometry, and number. The examiner should refer to Piaget's actual writings or interpretations of these writings for additional depth in understanding intellectual development during the toddler years.[21,22,23]

When assessing the toddler's intellectual development the nurse must bear in mind the stages of cognitive development and attempt to identify each child's capabilities at that point in time. Standard intelligence tests, such as the Stanford Binet Test or the Wechsler Intelligence Scale for Children, are unnecessary for routine evaluation, since the resultant IQ (intelligence quotient) can be influenced by environment and personality as well as heredity and can be improved with education.

Standard intelligence tests are not used for routine examination of the toddler.

One screening tool that can be used by the nurse is the DDST. It is not an intelligence test but will alert the nurse to possible delays in the toddler's language development and personal-social abilities, and thus is a reflection of intellectual development.

The DDST can be used as a screening tool when assessing intellectual development.

When specifically assessing language development, the nurse should evaluate the child's ability to use one- or two-syllable words, nouns, verbs, and adjectives. Nouns and single words characterize early verbal communication between the age of 12 and 18 months. Gradually the child attaches verbs to the nouns, for example, "truck go," "mama sleep," and "baby cry." Through practice with using words appropriately, the toddler then combines a noun or one-word subject, a verb, and another noun or one-word object. For example, the three-year-old may use such phrases as "mama do work," "daddy go bye-bye," or "baby go bed." Adjectives may be used with nouns without the child actually understanding the total concept of the spoken phrase, for example, combinations such as "big dog," "small shoe," or "two socks."

The toddler learns language skills through hearing spoken words, imitating sounds, and practicing word usage.

Additional screening tests to assess language development are the Denver Articulation Screening Exam, the Vineland Social Maturity Scale, and the Peabody Picture Vocabulary Test. These tests may be used by the nurse if data are needed over and above that provided by the DDST.

Muscle coordination of the throat, tongue, and lips is required for speaking.

Sexuality Patterns

See Sexuality Patterns in Chaps. 5 and 6 for age-related details.

Socialization as male or female begins in infancy. It is during toddlerhood that the child develops a beginning awareness of sexual differences and sexual roles, as certain behaviors and activities are inhibited or reinforced by caregivers. For example, a little boy may be told not to cry when he is hurt, while crying is tolerated or even reinforced in a little girl. The boy may then grow up believing that it is wrong to cry or show such an emotion.

Parental attitudes may greatly influence their toddler's sexual identity.

Studies have shown that there are important differences in the way parents behave with girls and boys, based on their own attitudes. Girls are generally given less freedom to be assertive, to explore, and to participate in play activities that are rough or dirty, while boys often are encouraged in these areas. The way parents set up the toddler's room and play environment often emphasizes the parents' belief that girls and boys are different. For example, the girl may be provided with dolls, stuffed animals, and books, while the boy is provided with trucks, cars, and building blocks. Frequently, the differences are created unconsciously on the parents' part, but they can create sex-role stereotypes very early in the child's development. These attitudes and differences must be assessed by the nurse.

Girls and boys are socialized during the toddler years to behave according to certain sexual norms.

There are also differences in the development of boys and girls. Scientists have shown that on the average girls develop faster than boys. For instance, girls talk, walk, and are toilet trained a month or two before boys. Also, by the age of 2, girls are more sociable, more talkative, and more compliant with adult demands than boys, while boys this age are more aggressive. Certainly the parents' cultural background and child-rearing practices can alter these findings and do account for individual differences in each child.

Sex Sexuality Patterns in Chap. 3 for questions used to elicit data.

Also during the toddler years, children begin exploration of body parts, both one's own and those of others. This is a normal and vital way for the toddler to learn about the differences between males and females. Again, parental attitudes can have a great impact on how the child learns and what impressions the child gains about sex and sexuality.

The nurse should explore all of the above areas with parents or caretakers when assessing this factor in the toddler.

Nutritional Patterns

The toddler's dietary intake may be minimal because of a slower growth rate and a disinterest in some foods.

Healthy growth and development of the toddler depend on good nutrition. However, during this time period, the growth rate of the child is slower than in infancy and appetite levels frequently decrease. The toddler may even go on food "jags," refusing to eat certain foods or groups of foods. Parents may complain that their child does not eat well at mealtime but "picks at food" or that their child only wants to snack through the day. The parent, in frustration, may attempt to force or bribe the toddler to eat, thus establishing unhealthy mealtime conflict. By determining whether the toddler's weight gain is appropriate for age and body build (see Appendix tables) and if foods are taken from the four basic food groups daily, the nurse can assess the toddler's nutritional status and often can provide the parents with reassuring information about their child's eating habits.

The toddler needs approximately 1300 kilocalories to meet daily energy needs. Requirements may range from 900 to 1800 kilocalories, depending on age, activity, and basal metabolism. Of the total calorie intake, a suggested proportion is 10 to 15 percent protein, 25 to 35 percent fats, and 50 to 60 percent carbohydrates. The total daily fluid requirement for the toddler is four to six glasses or 1000 to 1500 ml (1 to 1.6 quarts). (See Table 7-1.)

By asking the parent to keep a 7-day record of food intake, including all meals and snacks eaten by the toddler, the nurse can determine eating habits, actual intake, and values the parents place on the foods they feed their child. In addition to the food intake record, other data which are significant to the assessment process include notations of height and weight, a description of the child's general appearance and posture, and an evaluation of muscle coordination, which can be observed during play.

The nurse should also inquire as to whether vitamin supplementation is given to the toddler. Opinions seem to vary, but some health professionals recommend the intake of a daily multivitamin for the active toddler. This may be essential if the toddler's diet is consistently deficient in vital minerals and vitamins.

Exercise-Activity Patterns

During the toddler years the level of the child's activity will fluctuate. With the advent of upright locomotion, the child more actively explores the expanding environment. A deceleration in the rate of physical growth is seen, which is partly related to a loss of appetite and secondarily to increased activity. A variety of activities can be performed smoothly and easily as refinement in gross motor and fine motor skills occurs.

The toddler's growing sense of self-identity allows the child to play and explore without a parent's immediate presence. The development of language in terms of making wants and desires known and expressing

Highlights

Refer to Table A-15 when assessing the basic four food groups.

Refer to Table A-12 when assessing the adequacy of the diet.

Each toddler's diet must be assessed individually, since heredity, age, activity level, metabolism, and family eating habits influence the diet and dietary requirements.

Refer to Behavioral Development when exploring toddler activity.

Table 7-1

An Adequate Daily Diet for a Toddler

Milk and dairy products	
Milk	16 oz (range 12–24 oz)
Cheese	$\frac{1}{2}$–$\frac{3}{4}$ oz (as substitute for 4 oz milk)
Yogurt	$\frac{1}{4}$–$\frac{1}{2}$ c (as substitute for 4 oz milk)
Meat and meat equivalents	
Meat, fish, poultry	Two 2-oz servings
Egg	1 (limit 3 per week)
Peanut butter	1–2 T
Legumes	$\frac{1}{4}$–$\frac{1}{3}$ c cooked
Vegetables	4–5 including green leafy and yellow
Fruits and fruit juices	1 citrus plus 1 or more at other meals
Bread and cereal grains	
Whole-grain or enriched	
white bread	$1\frac{1}{2}$ to 3 slices
Cooked cereal	$\frac{1}{4}$–$\frac{1}{2}$ c (as substitute for 1 slice bread)
Noodles or rice	$\frac{1}{4}$–$\frac{1}{2}$ c
Crackers	1–3
Butter or margarine	Three 1-t servings
Sweets	$\frac{1}{4}$–$\frac{1}{2}$ c simple dessert

Source: Adapted from P. L. Pipes, *Nutrition in Infancy and Childhood*, Mosby, St. Louis, 1977.

learned vocabulary as it relates to objects in the environment facilitates the toddler's activity level and use of play.

The toddler learns to perform self-help skills such as feeding, dressing, toilet training, and bathing. These encourage the toddler's development of independence and competence and enhance the child's self-concept.

If the toddler is not allowed to explore in a safe, "child-proof" environment and activities are curtailed by constant limit setting, the child may begin to doubt his or her ability to accomplish tasks and may even withdraw from human interactions. Therefore parents need to understand this important period of growth and development.

It is the nurse's responsibility to assess how much freedom the parents allow their toddler in activities of learning and play, as well as to assess the toddler's activities for their effect on growth, development, and general health. Data collected about environmental factors may provide additional information.

Coping Patterns and Stress Tolerance Patterns

Situations which threaten the toddler's autonomy and sense of control may frequently result in a stress response which can be manifested in a variety of behavioral reactions. Separation anxiety is the most common stressor for the toddler and begins at about the age of 18 months. When a parent leaves the toddler with a baby-sitter, for example, there may be protests of verbal crying, fighting to escape, and even kicking and biting by some children. Such reactions indicate the toddler's continued attachment and dependence on the parents.

Physical restriction of the toddler, such as during an exam by the nurse, and the loss of accustomed routines and rituals can cause the toddler to feel a loss of control over given situations. The toddler may react to such stresses by verbal uncooperativeness, physical aggression, regression, negativism, and temper tantrums. Parents and nurses need to be aware that such reactions by the toddler are normal, and they also must be able to help the toddler cope with the stressor as well as the behavioral reaction.

During the health history taking, the nurse should question the parents regarding (1) the types of stressors the toddler is exposed to, (2) the child's behavioral reaction to the stressor, (3) the ability of the child to adapt to the stressor, and (4) the parents' reactions to the child's behavior. When possible, the home environment should be conducive to allowing the toddler maximum independence and emotional support. Realistically, however, this is not always possible, so parents must not be made to feel guilty when situational circumstances are beyond their control.

During the physical examination of the toddler, it is important for the parent to remain present so that maximum support and comfort are available to the child. Allowing the toddler to sit or partially recline on the parent's lap will make the examination more manageable. The toddler's cooperation during certain procedures can be gained by allowing the child to handle equipment and practice with it on the parent or a doll. Painful procedures should be performed quickly at the end of the exam, and lengthy discussion or explanations prior to the actual procedure should be avoided.

Stress can be a healthy factor in the toddler's daily experiences if the child is given enough love and support by parents and caretakers to overcome feelings of despair, shame, and doubt. As the child matures and

The major activities of the toddler involve upright locomotion and exploration of the environment.

Independence in the toddler is fostered by encouraging performance of skills such as self-feeding, dressing, and toilet training.

Responses to stress are manifested in a variety of behavioral reactions.

See Behavioral Development for additional discussion of the toddler's responses to stress.

Parents should be present with the toddler during the history taking and physical exam.

gains greater control over the environment, many situations will become less stressful and better tolerated by the toddler.

Review of Body Components

A review of body components should be done at least yearly on the toddler. The format described in Chap. 3 can be used for collecting and recording data. If deviations from normal are found in any area, the nurse should obtain details about such deviations from the parents.

The following sample questions, which are specific to body components, may be helpful to the nurse in obtaining information from parents about their toddler.

Questions to elicit data:

Head

1 Does your toddler complain of headaches?

2 Has your child ever sustained a head injury?

Eyes

1 Do you think your child has good vision?

2 Does he or she squint or rub either eye?

3 Does he or she sit too close to the TV?

Ears

1 Does your child pull at his or her ears?

2 Do you think your child hears well?

Heart

1 Does your child have any history of a heart murmur or heart disease?

2 Does he or she tire easily?

3 Does he or she eat well?

4 Can he or she keep up with children of the same age during play activities?

Extremities

1 Can your toddler walk well, run, and jump?

2 Does he or she have good hand coordination?

3 Have you noticed if his or her shoes wear down unequally?

Similar questions can be developed for each body component being reviewed by nurses. A detailed assessment should be made at the time of the physical examination of the child.

Summary

The health assessment of the toddler is a multifaceted endeavor. The age and developmental stage of the toddler make this assessment a challenge to the most experienced of health care providers. Understanding the toddler's needs and uniqueness will enable the nurse to collect the essential data and process them appropriately. Many of the basic attitudes about health and its meaning are being formed in the years of early childhood, and the nurse can contribute positively to the formation of such attitudes by being sensitive to the needs of the toddler and the parents or caretakers.

REFERENCES

1. Mahler, Margaret: "Symbioses and Individuation: The Psychological Birth of the Human Infant," *Psychoanal Study Child,* **29**:89–106 (1974).

2. Erikson, Erik H.: *Childhood and Society,* 2d ed., Norton, New York, 1963, pp. 51–53.

3. Scipien, Gladys M., Martha U. Barnard, Marilyn A. Chard, Jean Howe, and Patricia J. Phillips: *Comprehensive Pediatric Nursing,* 2d ed., McGraw-Hill, New York, 1979, p. 75.

4. Mussen, Paul Henry, John Janeway Conger, and Jerome Kagan: *Child Development and Personality,* 3d ed., Harper & Row, New York, 1969, pp. 242–243.

5. Ibid., pp. 247–249, 295.

6. Ibid., pp. 242–243.

7. Erikson, E. H.: "A Healthy Personality for Every Child—A Fact Finding Report. Midcentury White House Conference on Children and Youth," in J. Seidman (ed.), *The Adolescent: A Book of Readings,* New York: Dryden and Holt, New York, 1953, p. 208.

8. Mussen, Conger, and Kagan, *Child Development and Personality,* pp. 265–266.

9. Ibid., p. 266.

10. Fraiberg, Selma H.: *The Magic Years,* Scribner, New York, 1959, p. ix.

11. Barnard, Kathryn E., and Marcene L. Erickson: *Teaching Children with Development Problems: A Family Care Approach,* 2d ed., Mosby, St. Louis, 1976, pp. 80–81.

12. Sternian, M. B., and Toke Hoppenbrouwers, "The Development of Sleep-Waking and Rest-Activity Patterns from Fetus to Adult in Man," in M. B. Sternian, Dennis J. McGinty, and Anthony M. Adinolfi (eds.), *Brain Development and Behavior,* Academic, New York, 1971.

13. Tooraen, S. Lynda Ann: "Physiological Effects of Shift Rotation on ICU Nurses," *Nurs Res,* **21**:398–405 (September-October 1972).

14. Hellbrügge, Theodor: "The Development of Circadian Rhythms in Infants," in *Cold Spring Harbor Symposia on Quantitative Biology,* vol. 25, The Biological Laboratory, New York, 1960.

15. Caldwell, Bettye M.: *Instruction Manual Inventory for Infants (Home Observation for Measurement of the Environment),* Little Rock, Arkansas, 1970.

16. Ginsburg, Herbert, and Sylvia Opper: *Piaget's Theory of Intellectual Development: An Introduction,* Prentice-Hall, Englewood Cliffs, New Jersey, 1969, pp 58–60.

17. Ibid., pp. 60–63.

18. Ibid., pp. 63–66.

19. Ibid., pp. 72–83.

20. Ibid., pp. 83–85.

21. *The Growth of Logical Thinking,* A. Parsons and S. Seagrin (trans.), Basic Books, New York, 1958.

22. *The Origins of Intelligence in Children,* M. Cook (trans.), International Universities Press, New York, 1952.

23. *Play, Dreams and Imitation in Children,* C. Gattegue and F. M. Hodgson (trans.), Norton, New York, 1951, 1962.

BIBLIOGRAPHY

Alexander, Mary M., and Marie Scott Brown: *Pediatric History Taking and Physical Diagnosis for Nurses,* 2d ed., McGraw-Hill, New York, 1979.

Barness, Lewis A.: *The Manual of Pediatric Physical Diagnosis,* 4th ed., Year Book Medical Publishers, Chicago, 1972.

Baumrind, Diana: "The Contributions of the Family to the Development of Competence in Children," *Schizophrenia Bul,* 14 (Fall 1975).

Beardslee, Clarissa: "Acquisition of Appropriate Sex Role Behavior: A Review of the Literature," *Maternal-Child Nurs J* (Summer 1974).

Birns, Beverly: "The Emergence and Socialization of Sex Differences in the Earliest Years," *Merritt-Palmer Q* (July 1976).

Bishop, B.: "The What, Why, When and Where of Home Management of Common Childhood Illnesses, Part 1," *Pediatr Nurs,* 4 (Jan.-Feb. 1978).

Bowlby, John: *Attachment and Loss,* vols. I and II, Basic Books, New York, 1969.

Bradley, Robert H., and Bettye M. Caldwell: "Early Home Environment and Changes in Mental Test Performance in Children from 6–36 Months," *Devel Psych,* 12 (March 1976).

Caufield, Colleen: "A Developmental Approach to Hearing Screening in Children," *Pediatr Nurs,* 4 (March/April 1978).

Chinn, Peggy, and Cynthia Leitch: *Child Health Maintenance,* 2d ed., Mosby, St. Louis, 1979.

Dunn, Barbara H.: "Common Orthopedic Problems of Children," *Pediatr Nurs,* (Nov.–Dec. 1975).

Gentry, W. Doyle: "Aggression in Fairy Tales: Comparison of Three Cultures (American, Japanese and Middle Eastern Indian)," *Psychol Rep,* 37 (Dec. 1975).

Fakouri, M. E.: "Some Clinical Implications of Piaget's Theory," *Psych,* 13 (Feb. 1976).

Ferholt, Judith D. Lott: *Clinical Assessment of Children: A Comprehensive Approach to Primary Pediatric Care,* Lippincott, Philadelphia, 1980.

Fox, Jane A. (ed.): *Primary Health Care of the Young,* McGraw-Hill, New York, 1981.

Huber, H., et al.: "Teaching Behavioral Skills to Parents: A Preventative Role for Mental Health," *Children Today,* 7 (Jan./Feb. 1978).

Hughes, James Gilliam (ed.): *Synopsis of Pediatrics,* 5th ed., Mosby, St. Louis, 1980.

Katz, S.: "Is Your Toddler 'Language Delayed'?" *Am Baby,* 39 (August 1977).

Koenigknecht, Roy A., and Phillip Friedman: "Syntax Development in Boys and Girls," *Child Devel* (Dec. 1976).

Maguire, Maureen: Lecture notes, University of Maryland (Feb. 1978).

Mahler, Margaret S.: "Symbiosis and Individuation: The Psychological Birth of the Human Infant," *Psycho-analytic Study of the Child,* 29 (1974).

Malasanos, Lois, Violet Barkauskos, Muriel Moss, and Kathryn Stoltenberg-Allen: *Health Assessment,* Mosby, St. Louis, 1977.

McArthur, Leslie Z., and Susan V. Eisen: "Television and Sex-role Stereotyping," *J Applied Soc Psych* (Oct.–Dec. 1976).

Moore, Shirley, and K. Naomi: "The Effects of Contrasting Styles of Adult-Child Interaction on Children's Curiosity," *Devel Psych* (March 1976).

Owen, G. M.: "The Assessment and Recording of Measurements of Growth of Children," *Pediatrics,* 51 (1973).

Passman, Richard H.: "Providing Attachment Objects to Facilitate Learning and Reduce Distress: Effects of Mothers and Security Blankets," *Devel Psych* (Jan. 1977).

Pipes, Peggy L.: *Nutrition in Infancy and Childhood,* 2d ed., Mosby, St. Louis, 1981.

Rakel, Robert E., and Howard F. Conn: *Family Practice,* 2d ed., Saunders, Philadelphia, 1978.

Rheingold, Harriet L., Gale F. Hag, and Meredith West: "Sharing in the Second Year of Life," *Child Devel* (Dec. 1976).

Scipien, Gladys M., et al.: *Comprehensive Pediatric Nursing,* 2d ed., McGraw-Hill, New York, 1979.

Steele, Shirley M.: *Child Health and Family: Nursing Concepts and Management,* Masson, New York, 1981.

Vital Statistics of the United States Vol. II, *Mortality,* Part B, Section 7, Table 7-5. "Leading Causes of Death in Childhood, U.S., 1967."

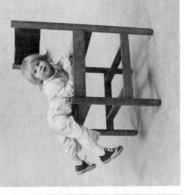
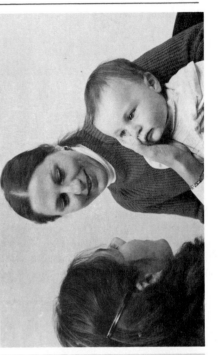
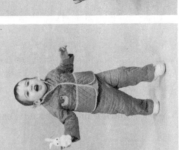
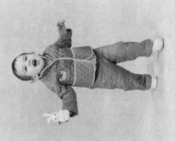
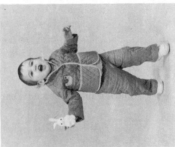
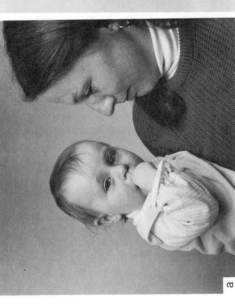

THE PHYSICAL EXAMINATION

APPROACH TO THE EXAMINATION

The physical examination of the toddler can be difficult. Because of uncertainty about body limits, and fear of intrusive procedures, the toddler is reluctant to allow anyone to invade personal space or impose restraint. This, coupled with emergent negativism, can make procedures which are relatively simple to perform on older children and adults difficult to perform on toddlers (a).

There are certain practices which may facilitate the examination and decrease the stress experienced by the toddler and the parents in the process. First, establish contact with the toddler during the less stressful history-taking period. Second, carefully observe the toddler during that time.

Much of the information needed to complete the physical examination can be obtained during history taking. The child's gait, muscle strength, and gross and fine motor control can be assessed while watching the child play (b). Hearing and vision can be roughly assessed in the same way. For example, you can learn whether or not the child responds to commands given from behind, and if visual stimuli elicit a response.

A third practice for the nurse to follow in examining the toddler is to allow the child to sit on a parent's lap for most, if not all, of the examination (c). This will alleviate some of the fear of the various procedures and provide for a calmer child and more accurate assessment. A parent can hold the child on the lap with the child's legs between the parent's legs so that the child can be restrained if necessary. One arm and hand can be used to restrain the child's arms and the other can hold the head, if necessary, for the ear or eye examination.

Highlights

There are five practices for the nurse to follow when examining the toddler:

1 Establish contact during history taking.
2 Observe carefully.
3 Have a parent hold the toddler.
4 Perform intrusive procedures last.
5 Demonstrate frightening procedures.

It is important for the nurse to develop a systematic and thorough approach to physical examination.

Refer to Chap. 4, since there are many similarities between the adult examination and that of the toddler.

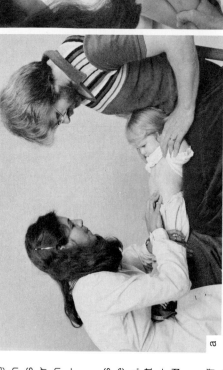
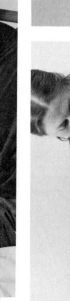

a

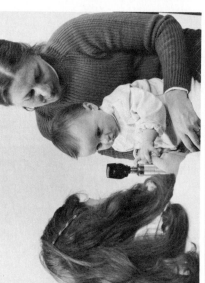

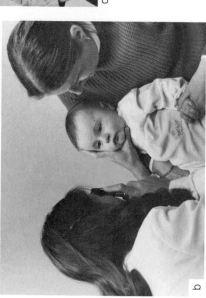

c

b

A variation of this approach is to have the nurse sit in front of the parent with the child's upper torso on the parent's lap, and his or her buttocks and lower extremities on the lap of the examiner. In this position, the abdomen and extremities can be examined (a).

Saving the more intrusive procedures until the end of the examination is the fourth practice (b). In this approach, such areas as the ears, nose, and throat are avoided until the end, since examination of these areas is poorly tolerated by the child.

The fifth practice is the demonstration of frightening procedures on a parent or a toy before performing the procedure on the toddler (c). This will alleviate much apprehension and enable the child to cope more effectively with the examination. For example, using the otoscope to look into the ears of the parent before looking into the toddler's ears will make that procedure much more acceptable to the child.

In general, the physical examination of the toddler follows closely the format discussed in Chapter 4. Differences between the adult examination and that of the toddler are mainly in the sequence of procedures and the emphasis placed on the various parts of the examination. The following discussion highlights certain areas of the examination of the toddler which differ from or receive greater emphasis than those discussed in Chap. 4.

Highlights

Vital signs are noted at the beginning of the physical examination.

Refer to Chap. 5, page 412, for various techniques for measuring the blood pressure of small children.

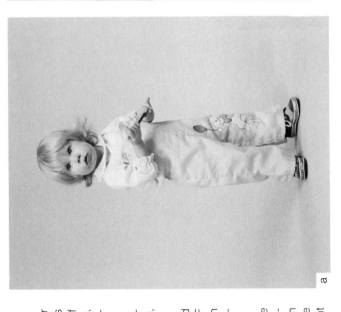

a

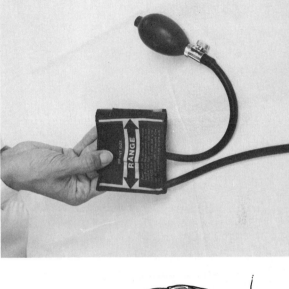

b

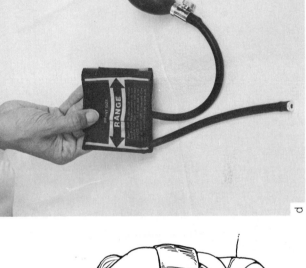

c

d

THE EXAMINATION
General Appearance

The general appearance of the toddler should be observed (a), vital signs should be noted, and measurement of growth recorded. Facial expressions, state of consciousness, and motor abilities should be observed.

Vital signs evaluated by the nurse include temperature, pulse, respiration, and blood pressure.

The *temperature* of the toddler should be taken rectally. It averages over 99°F (37.2°C). The toddler with an infection will frequently show a higher temperature than will older children or adults.

At 1 year of age, the average *pulse rate* is between 110 and 120 beats per minute. Generally, an apical pulse is taken in the toddler, though femoral pulses are important to the complete assessment (b).

The rate of *respiration* in the 1 year-old is between 30 and 40 breaths per minute. By age 2, the rate has decreased to 20 to 30 breaths per minute.

Measuring the *blood pressure* is essential to a complete examination of the toddler. Pediatric cuffs of the proper size are available and should be used (c and d). The proper size of the cuff for the toddler is no less than one-half and no more than two-thirds the length of the upper arm, or the thigh if the leg is used. The average systolic pressure is 96 at 1 year of age, and 99 at 2 years of age. Measurements may be taken using the Doppler, auscultation, palpation, or flush methods.

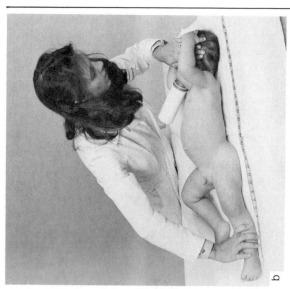

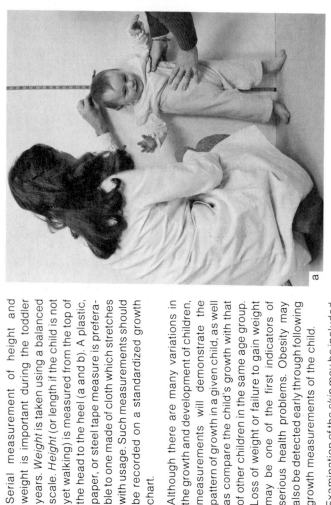

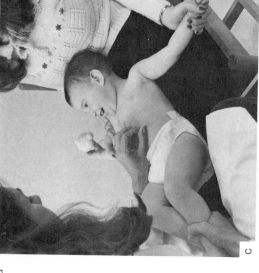

Serial measurement of height and weight is important during the toddler years. *Weight* is taken using a balanced scale. *Height* (or length if the child is not yet walking) is measured from the top of the head to the heel (a and b). A plastic, paper, or steel tape measure is preferable to one made of cloth which stretches with usage. Such measurements should be recorded on a standardized growth chart.

Although there are many variations in the growth and development of children, measurements will demonstrate the pattern of growth in a given child, as well as compare the child's growth with that of other children in the same age group. Loss of weight or failure to gain weight may be one of the first indicators of serious health problems. Obesity may also be detected early through following growth measurements of the child.

Examination of the *skin* may be included during assessment of general appearance. The nurse should carefully observe the scalp, chest, groin, axillae, ears, eyebrows, and nasal crease for color, consistency, and turgor (c), and for the distribution of any skin lesions.

Skin condition may also be noted during the examination of each body component.

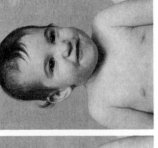
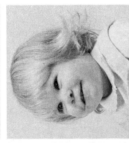
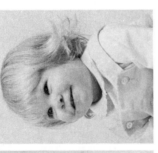
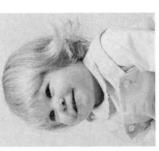
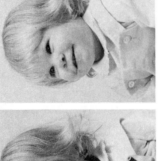
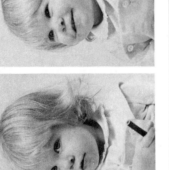
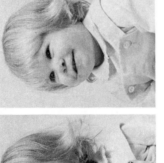
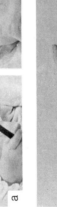

a

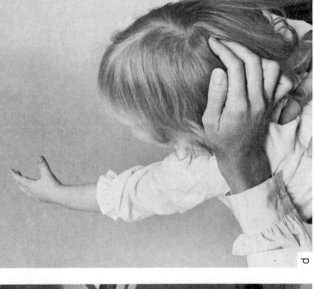

b

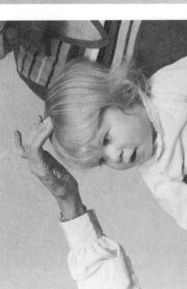

c

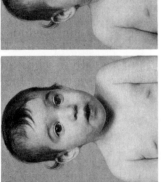

d

Head, Face and Hair
Inspection

The face should be examined for symmetry and mobility. Facial expressions such as alertness and dullness should be noted (a).

The hair should be fine, smooth, and shiny. It should be observed for dryness, scaliness, or patches. If the toddler lies with the head always turned to the same side during sleep, there may be a hairless patch and, in some cases, an asymmetrical flatness of the cranial bones. This can be corrected if it is recognized early and the child is put to sleep with the head turned to a different side each night.

Head circumference (b) should be taken through toddlerhood or at least until all fontanelles are closed. This generally occurs by the nineteenth month.

Palpation

The fontanelles should be palpated to assess for closure, tenseness, and pulsations (c and d). Ninety-seven percent of the time the anterior fontanelle will be closed by 19 months of age. Late closure should be noted and may indeed be a normal finding.

The Ist, Vth, and VIIth cranial nerves should be checked as thoroughly as possible within the limits of the toddler's ability to cooperate.

The anterior fontanelle is usually closed by 19 months of age.

Refer to Chap. 4 for the techniques for examining the cranial nerves.

Highlights

Highlights

Early identification of visual impairment is crucial to successful correction of problems.

The examiner can use parts of the Denver Eye Screening Test (Appendix B) during physical exam of the eye.

Strabismus is incoordination of extraocular muscles, resulting in crosseye.

Two important screening tests to use during the eye examination are Hirschberg's test and the cover test.

These are extremely important tests, since early detection of visual problems can lead to successful treatment, and prevention of further difficulties.

The ophthalmoscopic examination may be done (see Chap. 4) if the nurse believes additional data can be gathered. However, the toddler is usually very resistant to this procedure.

Eyes

It is difficult to assess visual acuity of the toddler without special equipment. Nevertheless, it is important to verify normal vision and identify visual problems at an early age. Qualitative observations made by the parents should be noted. The examiner may also note the toddler's response to and use of colored objects and toys, and his or her ability to move about in the examining room. Normally, the toddler will fixate, follow objects, and search for objects (a).

Inspection

Two techniques which may be useful in screening children of from 1 to 3 years old are Hirschberg's test and the cover test. In Hirschberg's test, or the light reflex test, the examiner shines a penlight into the eye of the toddler in a semi-darkened room. The light should reflect on exactly the same spot on each pupil (b).

For the cover test, one of the child's eyes is covered by the examiner while the child is encouraged to focus his or her eyes on an object about 12 inches from the face. The examiner's hand or a small card is used to occlude the vision of one eye but does not touch it (c). The child is instructed to keep both eyes open during the test. The card is held for several seconds and then quickly removed, and the covered eye is carefully observed. Normally, there should be no movement of this eye. The opposite eye should be tested using the same procedure.

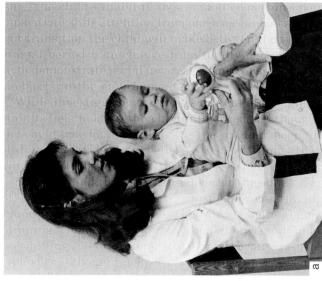

a

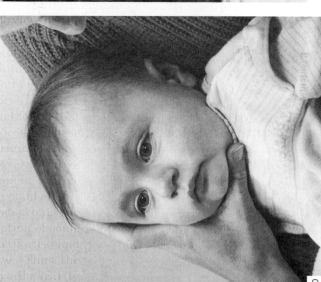

c

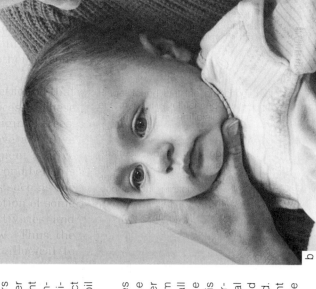

b

Highlights

The otoscopic examination is part of the ear examination for all toddlers.

Normal hearing is necessary for language development.

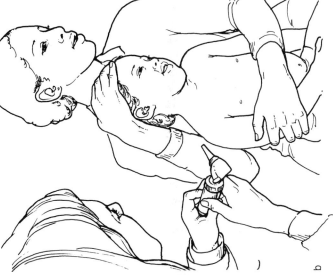

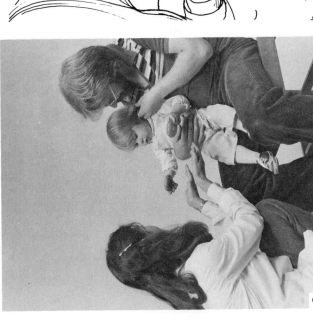

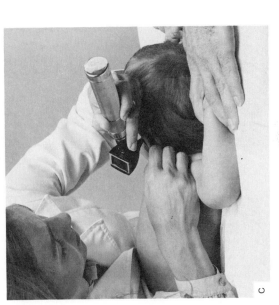

Ears

Rough estimates of auditory acuity can be made by noting the way the child responds to a command (a), or repeats simple sounds upon request. The parents should also be questioned about their toddler's ability to respond to sounds at home.

Inspection

The ear examination is probably least upsetting if the child is allowed to rest in a parent's lap with the head tilted slightly away from the examiner (b). The examiner should rest the hand holding the otoscope against the side of the child's face so that if the child moves the head quickly, the otoscope will also move and not injure the ear.

If the toddler is unable to cooperate, he or she can be placed in a prone position and restrained on the examining table, with the face turned to one side so that the ears can be seen (c). The child can also be placed supine with the arms drawn up on either side of the head by the parent. The examiner can further stabilize the child by leaning across the chest and abdomen. The speculum of the otoscope is then introduced gently into the external canal, and cautiously advanced to the point where the bony portion of the canal prevents further entry.

When performing the otoscopic examination of the toddler it is important to remember that in infancy and early toddlerhood the external ear canal tends to be perpendicular to the temporal bone with a slight upward angle. The direction of the canal changes with growth and becomes more anterior and points downward. Therefore, the pinna must be pulled downward and backward in order to straighten the canal and allow entrance of the otoscope and observation of the tympanic membrane.

Highlights

If foreign bodies are present in the nasal canals, other symptoms may be present.

The examination of the mouth, neck, and throat is usually performed toward the end of the examination because of the intrusiveness of procedures.

Nose and Sinus

Inspection

The nose of the toddler is examined in much the same way as is that of the adult (a). Special consideration, however, must be given to the possibility of foreign bodies in the nasal canals, since this is a fairly common occurrence in toddlers.

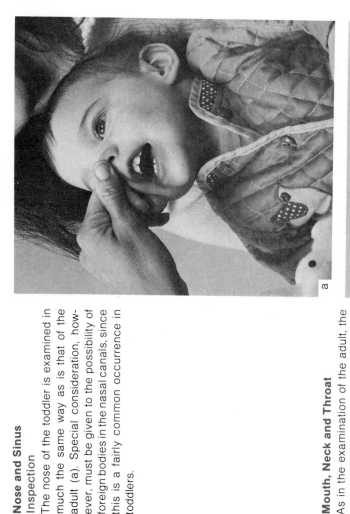

a

Mouth, Neck and Throat

As in the examination of the adult, the nurse will assess all structures from the front to the back of the oral cavity, and the neck will be checked for muscle tone, range of motion, and presence of any lymph nodes. The thyroid gland and trachea should be palpated.

Inspection

Examining the mouth, neck, and throat of a toddler is usually difficult (b). The examiner may wish to have a parent hold the child on his or her lap so that the child faces the examiner. Parental knees can restrain the toddler's legs, one arm of the parent can hold both of the child's arms while the other arm is used to tip the child's head back against the parent's chest. If cooperative, the child should be asked to pant like a puppy, while a tongue blade is used to depress the tongue and expose the posterior pharnyx. A flashlight may be used to improve vision.

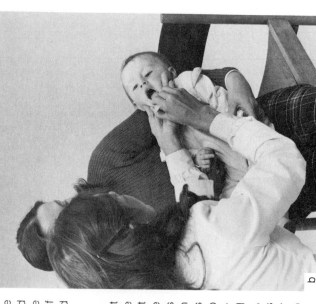

b

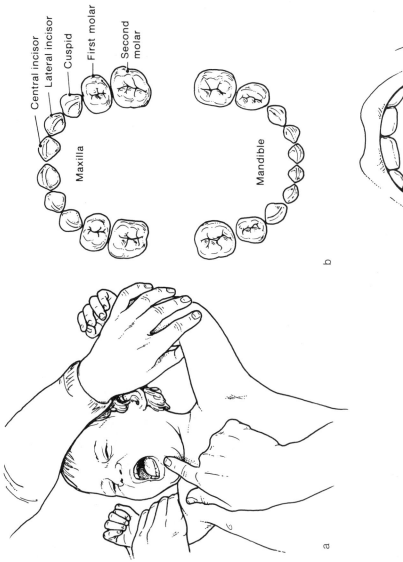

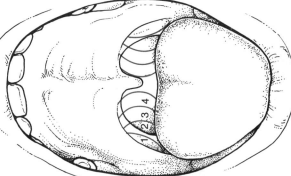

An alternative to this method would be to have the child lie supine on the examining table with a parent holding the child's arms over the head and restraining the toddler's head at the same time (a).

If the toddler refuses to open the mouth, the examiner should insert the tongue blade into the child's mouth toward the back teeth until the gag reflex is elicited. At this time, the child's mouth will open and the posterior pharnyx can be seen. The examiner must gain skill in observing quickly and thoroughly to accurately complete the throat examination of the toddler.

The number, spacing, and condition of any teeth should be noted. By 2½ all 20 deciduous teeth should be present (b). The teeth and gums should be examined for color and condition. In black or dark-skinned children there may be a black line along the gums. This is a normal finding.

The palatine tonsils are proportionately larger in the toddler than in adults, and will appear more prominent during gagging and crying. Tonsillar size can be noted on a scale of 1 to 4+, with 1+ indicating easy visibility and 4+ indicating that the tonsils meet in the midline (c).

Central incisor
Lateral incisor
Cuspid
First molar
Second molar
Maxilla
Mandible

Highlights

Refer to Chap. 6, page 448, for the techniques used in measuring head and chest circumference.

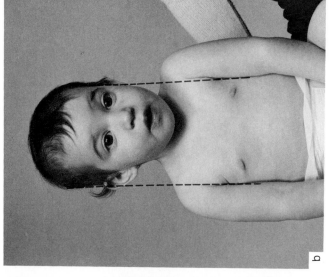

a

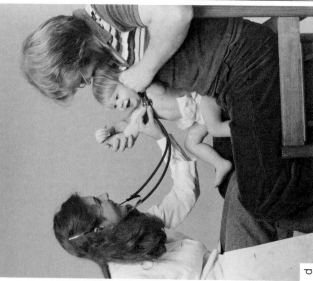

b

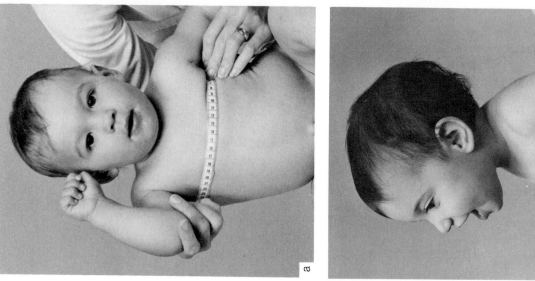

c

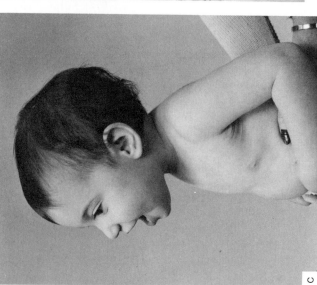

d

Thorax

Examination of the chest of the toddler includes assessment of the lungs, heart, and breasts. The techniques of observation, palpation, auscultation, and percussion are used by the nurse as described in Chap. 4. Chest circumference, measured at the nipple line, should be recorded throughout the second year of life (a). In general, it will be approximately the same circumference as the head throughout the first 2 years of life (b). After this, the chest circumference will increase in size very rapidly while the growth of the head circumference will slow down considerably.

Lungs

Inspection

The examiner should attempt to observe respiratory efforts with the toddler at rest (c). If the child is crying, the inspiratory phase can be observed and auscultated, but the expiratory phase may be more difficult to assess. The rate, depth, and ease of respirations should be noted, and this may be done at any time during the physical examination. In white clients, a normal pink body color will usually reflect adequate gas exchange. In black or dark-skinned clients, color changes may be more difficult to assess, but the lips, earlobes, or nail beds may be gently pinched to check capillary refill. There should be no delay in return to normal color.

Auscultation

Breath sounds are easily heard in toddlers (d), and are usually bronchovesicular, or audible during both inspiration and expiration. Respirations tend to be abdominal, reflecting the greater use of the diaphragm over the thoracic musculature in normal breathing.

Heart

A complete examination of the heart should be performed on the toddler. It should include notation of rate, rhythm, size, and characteristics of the first and second heart sounds. The peripheral pulses should be palpated (a).

The procedures for examining the heart described in Chap. 4 should be followed when assessing the toddler.

Auscultation

The presence of murmurs, soft blowing or rasping sounds, should be noted. As many as 50 percent of normal children have "innocent" murmurs.

Over 90 percent of these murmurs are systolic. They are usually louder with the child in a lying rather than sitting position.

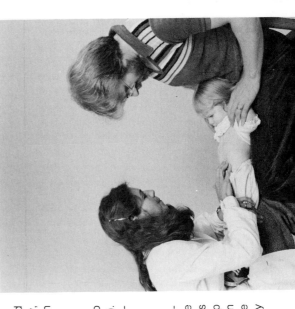

a

b

Breasts

The breasts are inspected and palpated for position, color, and size. Normally, findings are similar to those described in Chap. 4.

Abdomen

The abdominal examination is similar to that performed on adults (see Chap. 4). All abdominal organs should be evaluated by the nurse.

Palpation

Frequently, the abdomen is most relaxed at the end of expiration, and the nurse can quickly palpate organs at this time (b). The liver edge and spleen tip may be normally palpable, especially on deep inspiration. Umbilical hernias are frequently found in toddlers, and usually resolve spontaneously.

Genitalia

Inspection

The examination of the female genitalia in the toddler is generally limited to the external genitalia (a). Care must be taken to note any unusual discharge or irritation in the perineal area which might suggest pinworms, foreign bodies, or infection.

Palpation

The examination of the male genitalia is similar to that of the adult male. Special attention is given to determining if the testes are descended (b), and if a good stream of urine passes from the urethral meatus. If the male is uncircumcised, the foreskin of the penis should be checked for easy retractability.

Rectum and Anus

Palpation

If it is necessary, the nurse can gently prepare the toddler by telling the child that this is "like having your temperature taken." The procedure should then be done as quickly as possible using the technique described in Chap. 4.

A rectal examination is usually not performed in toddlers unless there is parental concern or specific indication.

Extremities

Inspection

The examiner should note the child's use of extremities during play, and observe walking and turning (c). The full range of active motion of hands, arms, feet, legs, and hips should be assessed, and position and posture noted.

Note the undressed child's gait (d). The gait will be wide-based with prominent lumbar lordosis when the child is first learning to walk. Later, as the toddler becomes more sure of foot, the base of the gait will narrow. Also note how the child walks with and without shoes, and how the bottoms of the shoes are worn.

The toddler has a wide-based gait when first learning to walk.

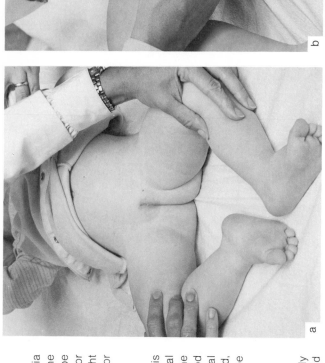

a

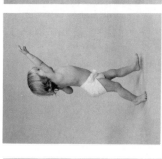

b

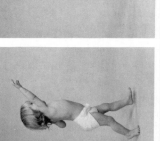
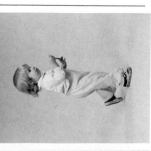
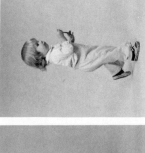

d

c

Because of hyperplasia of muscle cells, there is an increased growth spurt at 2 years of age.

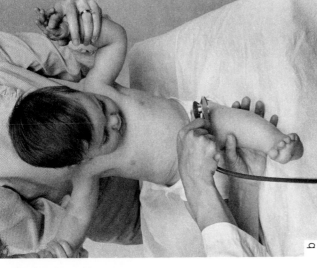

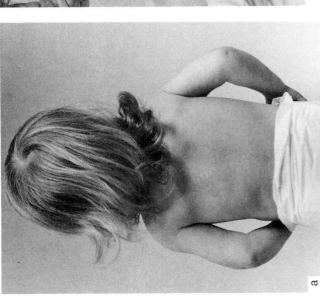

Physiological bowlegs with externally rotated feet and "toeing in" are common findings in the toddler under 2 years old. Although a normal finding, both should disappear by the time the child is about 2½ years old.

The spine should be relatively straight; therefore, any curvatures should be noted (a).

Palpation
Muscle size, symmetry, and strength, and deep tendon reflexes (b) are evaluated in the same way as with an adult. Note any reluctance of the child to use any of the extremities. The full range of passive motion should be performed with all the extremities.

DIAGNOSTIC TESTS

In addition to the physical examination the nurse may obtain certain laboratory test data on the toddler. A hemoglobin and hematocrit determination are useful for ruling out anemia in the healthy child. Blood lead levels are also important in this age group, since lead poisoning is still a common problem in this country. Stool for ova and parasites may be ordered if the child is a recent immigrant or is suspected of having pinworms. The tuberculin skin test is administered every 6 months on children from populations at risk for tuberculosis. Routine urinalysis and culture of a clean voided specimen should also be performed on all toddlers.

THE PRESCHOOLER

Nancy Kay Olson Hester and Mary Kolassa Lepley

INTRODUCTION

Preschool children, ages three through five years, are emerging from toddlerhood and becoming social beings. Increased language skills and gross motor abilities enable the preschooler to move away from the parent-centered environment. Three tasks in which the preschooler is involved are increasing independence, refining basic developmental skills, and developing socialization skills.

In order to correctly assess the health of the preschooler, it is essential that the nurse become familiar with the range of normalcy for the 3-year-old, the 4-year-old, and the 5-year-old.[1,2,3]

The preschooler offers the nurse a unique opportunity to assess a child that is in transition from infant-type behaviors to more adult-type behaviors. While continuing to exhibit fragments of dependent behaviors, the preschooler also is beginning to act and think independently. The cognitive level of the preschooler offers the nurse a chance to be creative in approaching the child, in communicating with the child, and in teaching the child. The emergence of the preschooler is an exciting stage of development. It is also a stage in which the physiological system is still fluid enough to effect changes in certain conditions. A good example of this type of condition is amblyopia (reduced visual acuity); it can be prevented during this stage but beyond this time is generally considered irreversible.

This is a time when the child is also developing many values relating to health. These values will, in part, influence the child's future ideas about health, as well as his or her preventive health behaviors. Thus, it is important that the child's encounters with the health care system are positive, self-satisfying, and beneficial so as to encourage a high level of wellness.

> During the preschool years, the child strives for increased independence, refinement of developmental skills, and increased social skills with peers and adults.

THE HEALTH HISTORY

Approach

The interview with a preschooler most often is not with the preschooler but rather with the child's parent or caretaker. This can present some problems in that the response given by the parent is the parent's perception and may not reflect the child's perception. Hence, it is important to involve the child in the interview. Validation of the parent's responses by the child as well as validation of the child's responses by the parent will help the nurse gain a more realistic picture of the situation. It will also aid the nurse in depicting areas of conflict between the parent and the child. At times, separate child and parent interviews are helpful to establish good baseline data. Of course, to do this successfully, the pre-

> Health history data must be collected from the preschooler and his or her parents.

> The nurse must gain both the preschooler's and the parents' trust for a successful interview to result.

schooler must be willing to cooperate and must see the nurse as someone who can be trusted.

Setting

The parent and child interview(s) can occur in a number of settings including the home, a clinic, an office, and/or a hospital. Each setting has its strengths and limitations. If there is a choice, the nurse will need to weigh these factors to determine where the interview can best be conducted. For the parent and the preschooler it is important that the setting have a minimal number of distractions. A room with ringing telephones or a multitude of visible gadgets can interfere not only with the interviewing process but also with the child's attention and rapport, especially during screening tests. It is essential that the room allow for privacy of conversation.

The Interview

Perhaps two of the best types of interviewing questions are the open-ended question and the funnel question. Both types of questions allow the parent to respond with answers other than "yes" and "no." For example, instead of asking "Did Johnny eat breakfast today?" which requires either "yes" or "no," the nurse asks "What did Johnny eat for breakfast today?" This open-ended question lets the parent and/or child respond in more depth and affords the nurse the opportunity to explore Johnny's nutritional status with subsequent open-ended questions.

Open-ended questions and funnel questions can be used effectively during the interview.

In the funnel question a situation is posed but no value judgment on the issue is offered. The following is an example:

> There are many ways to handle a child who doesn't want to eat meals. Some parents force the child to eat, some offer rewards, and some choose to ignore the behavior. What do you do when your child refuses to eat his or her meal?

This type of question allows the parent to respond freely without knowing the nurse's bias and/or expected answer.

In communicating with the preschool child, it is important that the nurse understand the child's level of cognitive functioning. The child's ability to answer questions is directly related to the abstractness or concreteness of the question. The more abstract the question, the less the child will comprehend. (See Intelligence for a complete discussion.)

The preschooler's cognitive ability should be considered when questioning the child.

Listening is perhaps the most important part of the interview. What is the child and/or the parent really saying? A part of listening involves the nurse reflecting back to the parent or child what was thought to be heard and clarifying any misunderstandings or miscommunications.

Refer to Chap. 3 for a discussion of interviewing techniques.

Patience is another interviewing technique that should be used by the nurse. The preschooler needs time to feel comfortable with the nurse, time to formulate thoughts, and time to respond to questions from the nurse. Therefore, the interview should not be rushed.

The nature of the parent-child relationship should be determined during the interview as it was with the toddler. Observations made by the nurse of interactions between the dyad can provide insight into the strengths and weaknesses of the relationship. Such factors may ultimately affect the child's health state.

See The Interview in Chap. 7 for questions regarding the parent-child relationship.

Recording of data obtained during the interview should be thorough and concise. Growth measurements, vital signs, immunization status, and achievement of developmental milestones must be recorded accurately so that ongoing assessments can be made.

Client Profile and Biographical Data

All of the biographical information needed on the client has previously been discussed in Chap. 3. For the preschooler, it is also important to ask if the child has a nickname and then to use it. For example, if Rochelle is called Shelly, she might not respond to the nurse if called Rochelle.

When completing the client profile, include biographical data.

Health Status Perception

As a health care advocate for the child, the nurse needs to involve the child in the interview. When determining the reason for entry into the health care system, the child as well as the parent should be addressed. The nurse might say to the child: "Tell me why you think you came here today." If the child does not know why, the nurse can then discuss this with the child. If the child came because of a referral from another health professional or organization, the nurse should explore the parent's and child's interpretation and feelings surrounding the referral.

Because of age, the preschooler is dependent upon the parent for entry into the health care system. It is essential that the nurse stress the importance of health maintenance, promotion, and prevention to the parents and to the child. Usually the preschool-age child enters the health care system for either of the following reasons: a normal well-child evaluation (this may be either parent-initiated or preschool-initiated) or a minor acute illness such as a cold or the flu.

Preschoolers are most often dependent upon parents for entry into the health care system.

The nurse should emphasize the relevance of monitoring the child's health status at least yearly to provide for prevention and early detection of health-related problems (such as nutritional deficiencies, anemia, obesity, chronic otitis media, or amblyopia) that could affect school performance, social functioning, and overall happiness.

In order to understand the preschool-age child's perception of health, the nurse should ask the child specific questions. Two examples are "What does it mean to 'feel good'?" and "What does it mean to 'feel sick'?" The child, however, may have difficulty in understanding these abstract concepts and may give little or no response to the nurse. Since the child's perception of health is influenced by the parent's definition of health, it is important that the nurse explore the parent's perceptions also.

Some preschoolers may not be able to accurately verbalize their perceptions of health.

Current Health Status and Health Habits

At this time the nurse should explore what the child's current health status is. If the child has been ill, the nurse should note when the illness began, what the course of the illness was, what treatment was instituted, and what the effect of the treatment was. If the child is ill at the time of this visit, it is important to find out what the parent thinks will help the child to recover.

See Current Health Status in Chap. 7 for sample questions to use when collecting these data.

The nurse should explore the health behaviors and practices of the child and the family. What do the parents think contributes to the child being healthy or not healthy at this time? This is a prime time to let the parent and the child discuss the importance of good nutrition, exercise, rest, and the like.

The preschooler continues to refine health habits that were learned as a toddler. By now the child should be able to brush the teeth and should also be seen by a dentist for routine care. At the age of 3, the preschooler can dress with supervision, and by the age of 5 the child can choose clothes, match colors fairly well, and dress unsupervised.

Toilet training is usually completed by the age of 4, allowing for occasional accidents. Since it may be a requirement for entry into a preschool, parents may have been pressured to teach toilet training by the age of 2½ or 3. Once this developmental task is accomplished, regression may occur as a result of stress in the preschooler, such as the arrival of a new sibling. With the understanding and support of the parents, the child will eventually resume the previously learned task.

Feeding skills have improved over the toddler years; however, the preschooler still enjoys finger foods. Utensils are used with better coordination and dexterity with practice. Role modeling by parents and older siblings can be helpful. By now the child should also have been weaned from a bottle and should use a cup or glass without spilling.

Cleanliness is still not a great concern for the preschooler, with the exception of soiled underpants. Toileting accidents can be very embarrassing for the child, and, therefore, the child should not be punished. Bathing is usually done with some supervision; however, the preschooler may enjoy doing this independently.

The nurse should inquire as to the preschooler's adeptness at performing the above health habits routinely. If parents have not allowed the child the opportunity to learn such skills, this should also be noted. Sociocultural factors may influence the preschooler's learning of certain health habits, and this must be taken into consideration during the assessment process.

Past Health Status

The nurse needs to explore the preschooler's past experiences with health professionals. For example, if the child equates coming to the nurse with "getting a shot," it is likely that he or she will be frightened and uncooperative during the assessment. It is equally important that the nurse take the opportunity and time to clarify any misconceptions that the child may have. Examples would be the child who believes that if he cries, he will get a shot, or a child who thinks she is coming to the nurse because she has been bad.

In exploring the past health history, the nurse should obtain a good baseline history. This is needed to determine if the child is at high risk for any problems, particularly developmental. The prenatal, neonatal, infant, and toddler histories should be complete on the preschool child. Some important factors the nurse should assess the history for are (1) diseases in the family history which are genetically transmitted and those which tend to be familial, (2) prenatal complications and health practices of the mother (i.e., smoking, alcohol consumption, etc.), (3) labor and delivery complications, (4) neonatal problems such as respiratory distress, jaundice, low birth weight, and feeding problems, and (5) infant and toddler developmental lags, illnesses, injuries, and ingestions of chemicals and drugs. The immunization status of the child should also be determined.

The preschool-age child will probably be of little help in gathering the above information. Birth and hospital records, the child's baby book, and the parents are sources for obtaining the needed information.

Family History

As mentioned previously, the family history is important in providing baseline information. It can alert the nurse to look for possible conditions that might otherwise be overlooked. (For further information see Heredity and also Chap. 3.)

Highlights

Brushing teeth, feeding and dressing self, toileting, and bathing are health habits performed by the preschooler.

Toileting accidents can occur if the child is stressed or forgetful during play.

See Behavioral Development for a discussion of behaviors which may influence the learning of health habits.

See Past Health Status in Chaps. 3 and 7 when collecting these data.

Table 3-3 and Fig. 3-2 should be used to complete the family history.

Age

The preschooler's age dictates continued dependence on the parents for fulfillment of basic needs, affection, and structuring of safe, educational experiences. The child strives for independence as the toddler does but is more capable of attaining set goals because of increasing motor, language, and personal-social skills. The preschooler's central task is to develop a sense of initiative, and the child is able to do this with guidance and support from parents as well as from others who play a significant role in the child's life (teachers, caretakers, etc.). The great strivings made during the preschool years prepare the child for entering school and competing with peers for recognition. The child must relinquish explorations of fantasy and focus on the reality of the situation at hand.

Significant advances in growth and development occur between the ages of 3 and 5.

Despite these significant advances in maturation and development, the advancing age of the child may be somewhat traumatic for the parents. The preschooler reaches a point at which he or she begins questioning previous teachings, and sometimes prefers the companionship of peers or others. The parents must realize that a certain degree of separation from their child is inevitable and that the outside social environment has begun to take over some of the previous parenting tasks. Thus, the nurse may need to support the parents in these adjustments and provide reassurance with regard to the ongoing importance of their parenting roles.

Parents may have difficulty accepting their preschooler's increasing independence and socialization.

Age also influences the amount of time the child spends in play. As attention span increases and other interests and responsibilities take over, less time is spent in play and the number and variety of play activities diminish. The preschooler's play is oriented to imitation of persons (especially the parent of the same sex) and to use of favorite toys and rhythmical games. Imaginary play also is important, since make-believe is reality for the preschooler. The child acts out feelings and experiences through play.

Play activities are influenced by age.

The preschooler is more prone to certain accidents because of age. With increased locomotion, independence, and refinement of gross and fine motor skills, the child is more capable of getting into trouble. Accidents which predominate in the preschool years are pedestrian traffic accidents, drownings, burns, and poisonings. Thus, safety continues to be of major importance in early childhood.

The preschooler is prone to certain accidents because of age.

Questions to elicit data:

1 How do you think your child's age has influenced his or her development?

2 How would you describe your child's behavior in attempting to complete a task (initiative)?

3 How do you think your role as a parent has changed with your child's increasing age?

4 How do you think your child's age influences his or her play activities?

5 What types of play does your child most often engage in?

6 What types of accidents do you see as potential threats because of your child's age and capabilities?

Race

Racial characteristics of the preschooler can have an effect on the child's health state. For example, blood pressure varies with race; in the United States, blacks have higher blood pressure readings than whites of the

The preschooler's race may predispose him or her to certain health conditions.

same age. Also, sickle-cell anemia is more prevalent in blacks than in other races.

Growth and development charts are frequently based on the norms of one race. Thus, if such charts are used for a child of a different race, they may give inaccurate data regarding the child's placement within the norm. Other data, such as familial characteristics, must also be considered during assessment.

Heredity

The heredity of the preschooler is extremely important in determining the overall health status. The nurse should carefully examine the family history for any serious, chronic, or recurrent illnesses or abnormalities, such as birth defects, genetic diseases, and neuromuscular disorders. Data included in the family tree may alert the nurse to areas requiring early preventive care or screening for detection of developmental problems and/or diseases.

Data collected about the preschooler's family history provide the basis for assessment.

An example of the role of heredity is a child who has a positive family history for a hearing loss. It would be important to routinely monitor the child's hearing ability to detect any early losses. Another example is the child who is below average for his or her age in both height and weight. If the parents are also small, the child's small stature is probably related to heredity rather than nutritional, metabolic, or physiological reasons.

Culture

Culture and lifestyle play important roles in the preschooler's health status. A child whose parents are vegetarians, for example, may become anemic if he or she is not receiving iron-enriched vegetarian foods. Subsequently, the parents may become defensive and anxious about the child's diet when asked for a diet history. Another example of the interplay of culture and health is the child who is taught not to cry even if something hurts. This child becomes stoic when facing pain and stress. This often occurs in American Indian and Oriental cultures and in white male offspring. Hence, a child who is taught not to show pain or cry may deny that he or she has had any pain when being seen by the nurse.

Culturally determined child-rearing practices can affect the preschooler directly.

When assessing culture as a factor affecting the preschooler, it is important to identify aspects which enhance or inhibit the child's growth and development. There will obviously be interplay between culture and various other factors in the child's environment, such as social characteristics, family life, activity, and education.

See Family Life, Nutritional Patterns, and Behavioral Development for additional information on cultural influences.

Questions to elicit data:

1 How would you describe your methods of disciplining your preschooler?

2 How much freedom do you allow your child in exploring new experiences or trying new skills?

3 What restrictions do you place on your child?

4 What self-caring skills (e.g., toileting, dressing, and feeding self) does your child perform independently?

5 How do you think your own upbringing has influenced your child-rearing practices with your preschooler?

Additional data collected during the rest of the health history taking will add clarity to this particular area of the preschooler's history.

Growth and Development

Physical, cognitive, social, and emotional characteristics of the pre-schooler should be assessed by the nurse. Data may be collected through direct observation of the child, by talking with parents, and by use of appropriate screening tools. A basic understanding of general norms for each characteristic is essential to the assessment process. (See Table 8-1.)

The physical growth of the preschooler continues at a slow rate. Weight gain averages 3 lb (1.5 kg) to 5 lb (2.5 kg) per year. Height gradually increases with growth of the long bones and adds 2 inches (5 cm). By age 5, the average child weighs 40 lb (18 kg) and measures 42 inches

Highlights

The preschool era is a crucial time to assess the child's developmental status.

Weight and height increase steadily between the ages of 3 and 5.

Table 8-1
Normative Achievements of the Preschooler's Adaptive Development

Area of development	Age 3 years	Age 4 years	Age 5 years
Motor achievements	Tries to draw a picture; may add an eye or leg when asked to draw a complete person Helps dry dishes Unbuttons front and side of clothes Undresses and helps dress self Uses toilet; stays dry at night Washes hands Feeds self May brush teeth	Makes drawings with form and meaning but rarely detailed Represents person by head and eyes Adds two parts to complete drawing of a person Buttons front and side of clothes Laces shoes Brushes teeth May bathe self with direction Takes partial responsibility for toileting May attempt to print letters	Makes drawing of person including body, arms, legs, feet Adds about seven parts to complete drawing of person Puts three or more details in drawings Prints first name and maybe other words; forms small letters well Dresses self except for tying shoes Washes self without wetting clothes
Verbal abilities	Has 900-word vocabulary Uses plurals Creates a phrase and repeats it Repeats six-syllable sentences Uses language more fluently and with confidence (whether or not anyone listens) Sings simple songs	Has 1500-word vocabulary Uses mild profanities and name-calling Uses language aggressively Asks many questions Uses phrases and exclamations	Has 2100-word vocabulary Talks constantly Uses adult speech forms Finds speech more important in peer relationships Participates in conversation without monopolizing it Asks for definitions Asks fewer but more relevant questions Laughs frequently during conversation
Perceptual and conceptual characteristics	Has beginning understanding of past and future—*tomorrow* and *yesterday* still confusing	Learning number concepts—counts to 3, repeats four numbers, counts four coins Names one or more colors well Has poor space perception	Specifies what he or she will draw or paint Copies a triangle Constructs a rectangle from two right triangles Does not fully understand time gradations Knows weeks as units of time; names weekdays Knows four or more colors Knows his or her age and residence Determines the heavier of two objects Beginning to understand kinship relations, such as uncle, grandmother, etc. Beginning to develop power of reasoning
Cognitive characteristics	Shifts frequently between intelligent adaptation and play or imitation In the symbolic or preconceptual period of cognition Shows persistence of realism, irreversibility, concreteness, and animism	In Piaget's period of intuitive thought—egocentrism and centering Focuses on present state of displayed objects rather than on process of change	Continues period of intuitive thought—egocentrism and centering

Source: From E. Nahigian, "The Preschooler—3 to 5 Years," *Comprehensive Pediatric Nursing*, 2d ed., G. Scipien et al. (eds.), McGraw-Hill, New York, 1979, p. 248.

(108 cm). Motor development continues to advance with age, resulting in dexterity, increased strength, and refinement of activities and previously learned skills. At about the age of 5, the child also begins to lose the temporary teeth that erupted during infancy and toddlerhood.

Cognitive development is manifested in symbolic or preconceptual thinking whereby the child acts out thoughts. The child tends to be very egocentric with minimal social awareness or regard for others. This egocentrism also permeates language, so that the child assumes that others think as he or she does and that others understand all communications. When assessing the preschooler, the nurse may need to use nonverbal approaches, such as play or drawing, in order to more clearly understand the child's thoughts.

Socially the child's encounters extend from the family to include other adult and peer relationships. The preschooler now separates well from parents and can interact more easily with unfamiliar people. With practice, the child takes on new roles and responsibilities which help build feelings of independence and self-satisfaction. These roles may include mom's helper around the house or playmate or sex-identifying (male and female) roles based on imitation of a parent. Thus, it is important that the preschooler be allowed to experience a variety of social encounters with appropriate guidance and reinforcement so that personal-social behaviors develop normally.

Emotional feelings and reactions frequently are patterned after the child's parents unless there are other adults more significant to the child. A nurturant and loving parent-child relationship will foster security, trust, independence, and positive self-esteem, since these give the preschooler strength to achieve autonomy and initiative. Thus, child-rearing practices, as well as supportive experiences outside the home, teach the child certain emotional characteristics. Frustration, anger, selfishness, and dissatisfaction will occur infrequently if the preschooler is given adequate support and the opportunities for achievement and mastery of skills and new experiences.

When assessing growth and development in each of the above areas, the nurse may use a variety of standardized screening tests. Table 8-2 outlines some of these tests.

Highlights

See Intelligence for a more complete discussion of cognitive development.

Social development includes opportunities to interact with persons outside the family and the taking on of new roles.

Emotional characteristics seen during the toddler years, such as temper tantrums, are now infrequent.

Refer to Table 8-1 for normative achievements of the preschooler's development.

Refer to Table 8-2 for an outline of screening tests.

Table 8-2
Developmental Screening Tools and Tests

Tools and Tests	Age	Description
Denver Developmental Screening Test (DDST)	0–6 yr	Gross and fine motor skills, personal–social, language
Pediatric Developmental Questionnaire (PDQ)	1 mo to 6 yr	Prescreening tool for developmental screening
Denver Articulation Screening Exam (DASE)	2½–6 yr	Assess acquisition of speech sounds
Denver Eye-Screening Test (DEST)	6 mo and older	Vision-screening test in four parts
Slosson Intelligence Test (SIT)	Birth to adulthood	Gross and fine motor skills, language, cognitive development, mental age, IQ
Developmental Test of Visual-Motor Integration (VMI)	2–15 yr	Gross and fine motor skills, cognitive development
Goodenough-Harris Drawing Test	3–15 yr	Gross and fine motor skills, cognitive development
Peabody Picture Vocabulary Test (PPVT)	2 yr to adulthood	Language, cognitive development, mental age, IQ

Source: Adapted from Pamela Roberts, "Use of Screening Tools," in Marilyn Krajicek, and Alice Tearney (eds.) *Detection of Developmental Problems in Children,* University Park Press, Baltimore, 1977, pp. 42–43.

For an objective measure of four areas of development (gross motor, fine motor, language, and personal-social), the nurse can use the Denver Developmental Screening Test (DDST). The items in this test need to be administered in the designated manner or the results of the test may be erroneous. It is equally important that the interpretation of the results follows the criteria listed in the manual. If the child fails the test with either an abnormal or a questionable result, the child should be re-screened in about 7 days.

Other developmental screening tools include the following:

Developmental Test of Visual-Motor Integration by Keith Berry

Peabody Picture Vocabulary Test by Lloyd Dunn

Vineland Social Maturity Scale by Edgar Doll

Thorpe Developmental Inventory by Helen S. Thorpe

Goodenough-Harris Draw-a-Man Test

The nurse should be proficient in the use of any test and should administer the items accordingly.

Besides the preschooler's overall development, the nurse should assess vision, hearing, and speech. The child's visual acuity should be checked to test for any decrease in vision. The Snellen E can be used and is an easy tool for the nurse to administer. The best approach is to involve the child in a game of pointing which way the "legs of the table" point. Since the tool requires no verbalizations from the child, preschool children usually will cooperate provided that the "game" does not take too long. Parents can be involved in helping to administer the test to increase the child's cooperation. The Denver Eye-Screening Test (DEST) is another test suitable for the preschooler that also tests visual acuity.

It is important that the child's hearing be assessed during the pre-school era. An impairment in the child's hearing can adversely affect the child's speech, as well as social and emotional development. A child who has had more than six bouts of otitis media is at risk for a hearing loss. Pure-tone audiometric screening can be used. Often, however, the younger preschool-age child is frightened by the earphones. The nurse may need to have the parent assist in order to gain the child's trust.

Speech can be assessed by using the Denver Articulation Screening Exam (DASE), which assesses the child's articulation skills, or how well the child says the sounds in words, and the Peabody Picture Vocabulary Test (PPVT), which assesses the child's receptive language and overall verbal intelligence and thus the child's understanding of words that are heard. The use of both of these screening tests should provide the nurse with adequate data concerning language development.

One speech concern parents often have is stuttering. When the child is about 4 years old, speech may be disfluent, with the breaking up of sentences and words. Many parents interpret this as stuttering, but it is not. It is normal for a child to exhibit some disfluency, and the parents should be encouraged to be patient with the child and let him or her say the words and sentences without help.

After completing the assessment of growth and development using appropriate screening tools and tests, the nurse should try to analyze the data and summarize both the strong and weak points of the individual child. Observations of the child during the entire health history-taking and physical examination process will also provide significant data to supplement this particular assessment.

Behavioral Development

Assessing behavioral development is essential in the health assessment of the preschooler. It will give the nurse insight into how the child copes with stress, how he or she adapts to change, and how stress and change affect the child's day-to-day behaviors and health.

The behavioral repertoire of the preschooler is a composite of many factors including heredity, developmental level, the environment, and sociocultural factors. The child has learned certain behaviors and is continually experimenting with new behaviors. As the child moves from a parent-centered environment, a vast number of experiences which affect behavior will be encountered. It is important that the nurse explore the child's capabilities in each of the areas discussed below so that appropriate behavioral responses can be verified and any potential or real problems recognized. An early assessment of the child's capabilities in these areas can facilitate health maintenance or restoration.

Feeding The child should be self-feeding and should be using utensils with little difficulty. This process of development can be interrupted, however, if the parent does not allow the child the needed independence or expects too much of the child. Hence, it is important to discover the parent's philosophy regarding mealtimes and the expectations the parent has for a preschooler. The preschooler is also beginning to make decisions and develop ideas about likes and dislikes. The nurse should determine if the parents allow the child to make food choices and should discuss the child's likes and dislikes with both the parent and the child. A nutritional assessment in the form of a 24-hour recall can be used by the nurse to look for nutritional strengths and weaknesses. The nurse should inquire whether the child is given vitamins and nutritional supplements. Since pica can affect the child's nutritional well-being, the nurse should discuss with the parent any unusual substance the child eats.

The preschooler should be allowed to self-feed and make food choices.

Toileting As stated before, the child should be completing the task of being daytime toilet-trained. The child, however, may still not be night trained. The nurse should explore with the parent how the toilet-training was accomplished, when it was started, and when it was completed. The elimination pattern should be reviewed.

The number of accidents the child has (both wet and soiling) along with the circumstances of the accidents should be explored, including how the parent handles them. Some children get involved in outdoor play and don't take time to go in the house for toileting activities.

See Growth and Development and Elimination Cycle for more information about toileting.

Sleeping The nurse should determine the child's sleeping patterns. By now the child should be out of the crib and in a youth or regular bed. It is preferable that the preschooler sleep alone and in his or her own room to foster privacy and independence. Since this is not possible for some families, the nurse should inquire as to who the child sleeps with, the age of the person, the size of the bed, etc. The child definitely should not be sleeping with the parents.

See Sleep-Wakefulness Cycle for additional information on sleeping.

Dressing The preschool-age child is able to dress and undress. The 3-year-old may still need some assistance with which is the front and which is the back and with buttons and other fasteners. The preschooler likes to select his or her own clothes but needs help in selections appropriate for the weather and activities. The child is learning to match colors but needs help in matching types of clothes, e.g., shirts and jeans. The nurse should determine who dresses the child, which dressing tasks the

The preschooler enjoys picking out clothes and dressing without help.

child does alone, and with which ones the child needs help. As in the other areas, the nurse should explore what expectations the parents have for the child.

Play A preschool-age child has evolved from parallel play to interactive play. The nurse should determine what the parents' philosophy of play is, what type of play they prefer that the child engage in, what types of play are harmonious with the functioning of the household, and what play is disharmonious. For example, loud, boisterous play may create friction between parent and child in a small-size apartment. It is important that the nurse know if particular types of play are encouraged and examine the effect on the child's psychosocial development. For example, a child who is encouraged to play alone quietly will not be learning how to socialize with peers. This could affect the child's ability to adjust to kindergarten where interactive play is necessary. Hence, the nurse should look at where the child plays and how much time is spent in various play activities and determine if there is a balance between quiet and boisterous play and indoor and outdoor play and playing alone and playing interactively with others. Watching television is not an appropriate type of play unless the parents have supervised the selection of programs and limited the time spent in front of the television.

It is also important to explore how many and what types of toys, games, and books are available in the home. Are they age-appropriate? Are they safe? Do the parents teach the child how to play with toys? How much time does the parent spend playing with and/or reading to the child? The list of questions to aid the nurse's assessment is virtually endless. It is, however, essential that the nurse determine how the child's play affects personal-social, fine and gross motor, and language development, as well as the child's overall happiness.

Loss and Separation The preschool child tends to interpret loss and separation as he or she does death—something that disappears. The finality of death, an abstract concept, is not well understood by the preschooler. Perhaps the most important aspect of dealing with a loss or death is for the parents to be honest with the child. The parents should be prepared for the preschooler to ask many questions and should respond with concise and honest answers. The parents should also acknowledge the child's sadness and hurt. Since a preschooler experiences loss and separation in various ways, including the death of a significant person, death of a pet, or the loss of a favorite toy, the parents should help the child by keeping the communication channels open for the child to discuss these losses.

If the parent has unresolved attitudes toward death, he or she will be unable to explain this concept to the child. The parent may try to hide the death from the child to "protect" him or her. If a pet has died, the parent may hasten to substitute another pet. These actions should be avoided, since they will prevent the child from learning about death and experiencing the grief process.

Grief and Mourning A child who experiences a loss will need support with the grief process. The child will first deny the loss and ask many questions about the loss. The child may look for the lost object or the person. Sadness and crying may be followed by loss of interest in eating and playing and finally by withdrawal. The preschooler needs a lot of support, touching, patience, and understanding from the parents and significant other persons.

Interactive play helps the preschooler develop socialization skills.

It is important to determine the types of play the preschooler engages in.

Loss and death are difficult concepts for the preschooler to understand.

Various behaviors are manifested in the child who is grieving or mourning.

If the parent is emotionally unable to help the child in the grief process, the child will need help from another source. A good friend or a relative such as a grandparent may be able to fill this need. At times, however, professional help may be required. Depending on the severity of the child's reaction, the appropriate person should be consulted, such as a nurse, a psychologist, or a social worker.

Behaviors and Discipline The normal development of the preschooler will, in part, determine the child's behavior. As the child refines gross and fine motor skills and language performance, the child also moves into a wider circle of socialization. The preschooler enlarges his or her behavioral repertoire and experiments with new behaviors. Many of these new behaviors will become behavior problems if they are not curtailed. Thus, discipline plays an important role in the preschooler's development and in preparing the child for easier adaptation to school.

Some of the common behavior problems of the preschool child include (1) negative use of language in the form of whining, baby talk, back talk, and nagging, (2) inappropriate facial gestures such as grimaces, spitting, or sticking out the tongue, (3) aggressive behaviors, i.e., hitting, teasing, bossing, and boisterous play, (4) dependency, and (5) noncompliance. Behaviors such as these occur normally. The child needs to learn the social appropriateness of these behaviors. The longer the parents wait before teaching the child what behaviors are appropriate, the harder the change in behavior will be for the child. However, in order to do this parents need to be made aware of which behaviors are appropriate and normal for the child's development and age. Whatever discipline regimen the parents choose to use, it should positively reinforce the "good" behaviors and negatively reinforce the "bad" behaviors.

Some behavior problems are situational, for example, those which occur at mealtime, at bedtime, during toileting, and during dressing. Again the child needs to learn both appropriate and healthful behaviors. For example, if Johnny refuses to eat at meals except for dessert, it will affect him socially and nutritionally. Hence Johnny needs to learn that eating only desserts is not an acceptable behavior.

Behavior problems may center around mealtime, bedtime, toileting, and dressing.

There is a third group of behaviors that needs to be considered. These are behaviors that were condoned in infancy and toddlerhood but are inappropriate for the preschooler. Perhaps the most common behavior in this category is thumb-sucking. With the thumb in the mouth, the preschooler will have increasing difficulty with social skills such as language and fine motor skills. Consequently, a socialization problem may occur which could cause difficulties in school performance.

The assessment of behavior problems and discipline regimen is essential for a holistic health approach. There are several questions that the nurse can use to elicit information about the child's behavior and about the parents' way of handling it.

Questions to elicit data:

Mealtime: Describe your child's behavior at dinner. What do you do when he or she spills? refuses to eat? etc.

Bedtime: Many preschool-age children fight going to bed. How often does your child refuse to go or fight going to bed? What do you do?

Aggressive behavior: Preschool children often engage in aggressive behaviors such as teasing, hitting, and noisy play. What aggressive behaviors does your child engage in? Which ones bother you the most? What do you do about them?

Overall behaviors: Which of your child's behaviors bother you? Which behaviors do you want to change?

The nurse can elicit specific data about behaviors and discipline by designing questions to address common preschooler situations.

In these examples the nurse is gaining information not only about the child's behavior but also about the parents' methods of discipline in specific instances. If the nurse then explores the parents' discipline regimen, a total picture of the discipline in the home can be obtained. The nurse should also explore how the parents handle "good" behaviors and "bad" behaviors. The nurse should determine the parents' philosophy of discipline, since to many parents, discipline means punishment only.

Questions to elicit data:

What behaviors does your child most often get rewarded for? What kinds of rewards does he or she get?

What behaviors does your child most often get punished for? In what ways do you punish him or her? Do you think this punishment works?

In summary, the role of the child's development in the creation of behavior problems cannot be underestimated. The child's behavior affects his or her personality, the ability to interact with others, and development of a positive self-image.

Biological Rhythms

Sleep-Wakefulness Cycle Most authorities agree that by the age of 2 to 3, the child's sleep-wakefulness cycle, physiological rhythms, and hormonal cycles are established. The sleep-wakefulness cycle is fully developed by age 2.[4,5,6] The REM pattern (rapid eye movement) of sleep is like an adult pattern by the preschool era. Colquhoun has investigated patterns of sleep behavior and has reported that in children, naps represent 12 percent of the sleep for toddlers, 5 percent for 4-year-olds, and 0 percent for 5-year-olds. It is estimated that children from 2 to 5 need about 9 to 16 hours of sleep per day, which decreases as the child gets older.

When assessing the sleep-wakefulness cycle it is essential that the nurse explore the parents' perception of the amount of sleep the child needs and elicit information regarding the schedule the parents use for the child's sleep and rest times. Also, the sleeping patterns of the family should be determined so that congruency or conflict with the preschooler's pattern can be identified. The following is an example of how conflict in family sleep patterns can be a potential stressor for all concerned.

Mary and John have two children, Jimmy, who is 3 years old, and Susie, who is 9 weeks old. On exploring Jimmy's sleep pattern, the nurse discovered that he needs about 13 hours of sleep—daytime naps from 1 P.M. to 4 P.M. and nighttime sleep from 8 P.M. to 6 A.M. Susie, an active infant who is described by her mother as "not sleeping a lot," sleeps from 9 A.M. to 11:30 A.M., 7 P.M. to 11:30 P.M., and 2:30 A.M. to 6:30 A.M. John and Mary go to bed around 10:30 P.M. and wake around 6 A.M. However, since Susie arrived, Mary is now awake from 11:30 P.M. to 2:30 A.M. every night and gets only $4\frac{1}{2}$ hours of sleep per night! Since Susie naps in the morning and Jimmy in the afternoon, Mary is unable to nap and is exhausted.

In this situation, the infant's sleep cycle is out of synchrony with the rest of the family's, but, most important, with the mother's. In order to help resolve the situation, the nurse needs to explore alternative ways for Mary to get more rest so that her health and caretaking responsibilities are not jeopardized.

While further assessing the child's sleep-wakefulness cycle, the nurse should determine if there are any external factors that might interfere with the child's sleep. Some significant factors include noise, heat,

See Chaps. 1 and 3 for more detailed information on circadian rhythms.

Preschoolers average 9 to 16 hours of sleep per 24 hours.

Synchronous sleep patterns in family members is important to health.

The child's sleep environment should be assessed for potential stressors.

light, and disturbances from siblings. The nurse should offer the parents suggestions on how to change or eliminate any problematic environmental conditions.

Upon completion of this assessment, the nurse should have a clear idea of the child's sleep and awake pattern. If the parent is unable to give the nurse an adequate description of the sleep-wakefulness cycle, the parent can be asked to keep track of the child's nap times and bedtimes, wake times, and temperament before and after sleeping. The nurse can then use these data to assess the child's need for sleep.

Questions to elicit data:

1 How much sleep do you think your child needs in 24 hours?
2 What time does your child go to bed at night and get up in the morning? At what time does your child nap?
3 How long does it take for your child to fall asleep?
4 What does your child do before going to sleep?
5 Do you follow any bedtime rituals (e.g., reading a story)?
6 Does your child awaken during sleep? Does he or she have nightmares?
7 How would you describe your child upon awakening (e.g., happy, irritable, or crying)?
8 Do you ever have to wake your child to get him or her ready for preschool or a baby-sitter? Does this ever present a problem?
9 Do you think your child gets enough rest?
10 How does your child's pattern of sleeping fit into the family's daily schedule?

Elimination Cycle Children are usually toilet trained by or during the preschool years. A circadian pattern can be noted in most preschoolers for urination, with 600 to 750 ml being excreted in a 24-hour period. Defecation patterns vary in rhythmicity, since it is normal for the child not to have a daily bowel movement.

When assessing the preschooler's elimination cycle, it is important to question both the parents and the child. Parents may not be able to give some information, since the child (particularly by age 4) is independently handling this task. It is also pertinent to determine the parents' perceptions of normal elimination patterns, since these may influence their training of the child.

Questions to elicit data:

1 How often do you think your child should eliminate (urinate and defecate)?
2 How often does your child eliminate? What amount (small or large) is eliminated?
3 Is your child toilet trained? How well does your child handle this task?
4 How would you describe the color and odor of your child's urine and stool? What consistency is the stool?
5 Does your child awaken during the night to eliminate? Do you restrict fluids at bedtime?
6 Does your child have any problems or difficulties with elimination?

The temperament of the preschooler may determine the pattern of the sleep-wakefulness cycle.

Allowing the preschooler to wake naturally will allow for a more complete rest cycle.

It is important to determine the parents' perceptions regarding their child's sleep-wakefulness cycle.

See Elimination Cycle in Chap. 7 for information regarding toilet training.

Preschoolers show a circadian pattern in urination.

Defecation may not occur daily in the preschooler.

In order to get more objective data regarding the elimination cycle, the nurse should have the parent keep a daily record for 1 week. The record should include the time the elimination occurred and the amount of urine and/or stool eliminated. The nurse can then assess this pattern more accurately.

Temperature Cycle The preschooler's temperature tends to follow a circadian pattern. In a day-active child, the temperature is lowest in early morning hours and peaks in the late afternoon. Stressors, such as illness or overdressing, can alter the cycle.[7]

The best way to assess the child's temperature cycle would be to set up a time chart and have the parent take the child's axillary or oral temperature and record it. The nurse can then assess the child's individual cycle. However, this should be done only when there is a significant rationale for doing it. Many preschool children do not like to have their temperatures taken. The preschool child may internalize this activity and, perhaps, may be fearful of a thermometer when he or she is ill and needs the temperature taken.

Pharmacological Effectiveness Cycle By the age of 3, the child should have had DPT (diphtheria, pertussis, and tetanus) immunizations, three doses of TOPV (trivalent oral polio vaccine), and one measles, mumps, and rubella vaccine (singularly or in a multiple vaccine combination). At age 5 the child will get one more DPT immunization and one TOPV. This timetable has been set up to maximize the effectiveness of the immunizations. For example, when the measles (rubeola) vaccine first was administered, children as young as 9 months received it. Now, after much research, it has been determined that the measles vaccine will result in a significantly higher antibody level if given at 15 months, thus affording better protection to the child. Hence, it is of importance for the nurse to assess when the child received the immunizations and to determine if the time intervals are appropriate.

It is also important for the nurse to assess what side effects the child has had from the vaccines. Pertussis vaccine can cause a wide range of side effects from none to severe, including high fevers. It may be necessary to consider not giving pertussis vaccine to a child who has had a severe reaction.

The possibility exists that the side effects of immunizations could be minimized if they were synchronized with the body rhythms. However, specific information regarding this issue is presently not available.

Metabolic Rhythms By the age of 3 the metabolic rhythms are established. Table 8-3 identifies the metabolic norms for preschool children. When assessing the child's heart rate, the nurse should be aware of the stressed or relaxed state of the child. A child who is stressed either by exercise or by emotions will probably have a higher heart rate than a

Highlights

The elimination cycle can be influenced by age, volume and time of fluid intake, and certain medications.

The preschooler's temperature tends to follow a circadian rhythm.

See Table 6-7 for immunizations during childhood.

Side effects to any immunizations should be noted.

See Table 8-3 for metabolic norms of the preschooler.

Heart rate, respirations, and blood pressure readings can be affected by stress.

Table 8-3
Metabolic Norms of the Preschooler

Age	Mean heart rate ± 2 S.D.	Mean blood pressure, mmHg	Respiration, rate/min
3	105 ± 35	100/60	20–30
4	105 ± 35	100/60	20–30
5	105 ± 35	100/60	20–25

Source: Adapted from T. Johnson, "Development of the Lungs" and "Changes in the Developing Cardiovascular System in Relation to Age," in *Children Are Different: Developmental Physiology*, 2d ed., Ross Laboratories, Columbus, Ohio, 1978, pp. 127–141.

child who is relaxed. The rate will also vary during different times of the day, reaching its peak along with the temperature. Besides the rate, the nurse should assess the rhythm and the strength of the pulses (apical, carotid, femoral, and peripheral).

The blood pressure, like the heart rate, can be affected by stress in the child. The preschooler may be fearful of the blood pressure cuff; therefore, it is helpful if the nurse demonstrates use of the cuff prior to the test. The width of the blood pressure cuff should be one-half to two-thirds the length of the upper arm, since erroneous readings can be obtained using an improper width. In preschoolers a blood pressure greater than 110/70 is suspect. The nurse should also assess discrepancies between left and right arm readings.

Respirations are diaphragmatic in the preschooler.

The respiration rate can be assessed primarily by observation and palpation. Respirations continue to be diaphragmatic in character until about the age of 5 to 7, when the costal elements are more prominent. The nurse should observe the respirations for rate, including rhythmicity, for symmetry of chest movements, and for the character, noting any retractions. The nurse can also explore with the parent what has been noticed about the child's breathing, both during activity and rest periods.

Venipuncture to determine serum levels is not a routine procedure.

The serum levels of electrolytes vary according to the child's body rhythms. Since the only way the nurse can accurately assess the serum levels is through venipuncture, it is suggested that this not be done for preschool children unless it is absolutely warranted. Pain research done by Hester et al. has shown that children tend to recall invasive procedures as "hurting a lot."[8] Therefore, such procedures should be done only if necessary and not on a routine basis.

Urine can be collected from the preschooler to be analyzed for electrolytes. It is important that the nurse record the time the specimens are obtained in order to determine the child's biorhythm. As was previously discussed, the elimination cycle follows a circadian rhythm.

Environmental Factors

The home environment and day care or preschool centers can have an impact on the preschooler's growth and development in all areas. Like the toddler's environment, safety and educational stimulation are prime considerations with the preschooler as well.

The preschooler's environment should be safe and educationally stimulating.

Parents should be questioned by the nurse about the safety of environments in which the child lives and plays. It should be determined if medications, insecticides, weed killers, fertilizers, paint, cleaning items, and the like are stored properly in the home. Precautions taken to prevent accidents such as falls and drownings should be discussed. If the child attends a day care center or a preschool, parents should be aware of precautions for safety taken by the facility.

With the preschooler's increasing independence and beginning attempts to separate from parents and caretakers, safety may be overlooked. Some parents may expect the child to automatically respect poisons, power tools, and the like and, therefore, may fail to protect their child from such items. The preschool child also engages in imitative play. If daddy is seen working with the power saw, the child may try using it the next day. Thus, the nurse needs to assess the safety of the child's play areas both indoors and outdoors. A home visit is the ideal way to assess the environment, but it is not always practical. Therefore, the nurse should explore what the parents think the child's safety needs are and should have them describe play areas and discuss any concerns they might have about possible hazards to the child. For example, parents who live in a high-traffic area may be concerned about the lack of fences around the public playground. The nurse should also review with the parents poisonous substances found in the home such as cleaning

The safety of the environment is a prime concern with the preschooler.

Imitative play may lead the preschooler into unsafe situations.

agents, plants, insect and yard sprays, and the like. These should be kept well out of the child's reach.

It is also important to consider the child's safety while traveling in a car. What is the parent's philosophy toward car seats and seat belts? How often does the child use a car seat or a seat belt? Does the child stay in the car seat or leave the seat belt on? Parents should understand that restraining the child not only protects but also controls the child's behavior such that he or she cannot run around in the car or bother the driver.

Since the preschooler is very impressionable and likes to learn rules, this is a good time for the child to learn some simple safety rules. For example, it is important to look both ways before crossing a street or it is important not to play with matches. The child also needs to learn about strangers, that is, not to accept candy or leave in a car with them. The nurse should assess the child's knowledge about safety and the source of the knowledge to determine whether the child is safe from physical and emotional harm.

The preschooler's environment should be educationally stimulating. Books, toys, records, and games should be age-specific and appropriately challenging for the child in order to promote cognitive, motor, and language development. Parents should inquire into learning activities available to their child in day care and preschool facilities. Social encounters in all environments in which the child lives and plays should encourage cooperativeness and interaction with peers and other adults.

The nurse may find it necessary to make a home visit in order to more thoroughly assess the child's environment. If a visit is made, the Home Observation for Measurement of the Environment (HOME) for children 3 to 6 years can be used as a screening tool. (See Fig. 8-1.) It is a reliable and valid way of observing and assessing the positive and negative aspects of the environment from the child's point of view. Findings can also be used by the nurse to instruct parents regarding changes or improvements that can be made to enhance the preschooler's growth and development.

Economics

The preschooler continues to be dependent upon the parents for economic security. Housing, goods, health care, and education will be provided within the family's budget. If the family is unable to purchase items to meet the child's basic needs, then community resources or governmental support may provide supplements to the parents' financial income.

The nurse must assess all factors in the family's life that directly effect economic status and that will impact on the preschooler's health. Questions cited in Economics in Chap. 3 can be used to collect data from the parents.

Community Resources

It will aid the nurse in coordination of the preschooler's health care if past and current resources used by the family are identified. The nurse can use this information to help determine which of the child's needs are being followed adequately and, hopefully, prevent the duplication of services. Some common resources used by the preschooler include a dentist, social services, neighborhood health clinics, a community health nurse, and day care settings or preschools.

Roles and Relationship Patterns

Family Life

During the preschool years, the family plays an important role in the child's health and development. The parents must learn to foster the

Car safety should include use of car seats designed for children, and use of seat belts.

See Environmental Factors in Chap. 7 for questions to ask when assessing the preschooler's environment.

The preschooler's environment can be assessed using the "HOME" as a screening tool.

See both Occupation and Education for data related to economics.

See Community Resources in Chap. 3 for questions used to elicit data.

Date of interview _____

Child designee _____
                    Name   Age   Sex   Ethnic group

Child's birthday _____ Birth order _____

Mother's name _____ Father's name _____

Address _____

Categories	Raw scores	Percentile scores
I Provision of stimulation through equipment, toys, and experiences	_____	_____
II Stimulation of mature behavior	_____	_____
III Provision of stimulating physical and language environment	_____	_____
IV Avoidance of restriction and punishment	_____	_____
V Pride, affection, and thoughtfulness	_____	_____
VI Masculine stimulation	_____	_____
VII Independence from parental control	_____	_____
Totals	_____	_____

I Provision of stimulation through equipment, toys, and experiences

1-15 The following are present in the home and either belong to child or child is allowed to play with them:

	Yes	No
1 Toys for learning colors, sizes, shapes (typewriter, pressouts, play school, pegboards, etc.).		
2 Toy or game for facilitating learning of letters (blocks with letters, toy typewriter, letter sticks, books about letters, etc.).		
3 Three or more puzzles.		
4 Two toys necessitating some finger and whole-hand movements (crayons and coloring books, paper dolls, etc.).		
5 Record player and at least five children's records.		
6 Real or toy musical instrument (piano, drum, toy xylophone or guitar, etc.).		
7 Toy or game permitting free expression (finger paints, play dough, crayons or paint and paper, etc.).		
8 Toys or game necessitating refined movements (paint by number, dot book, paper dolls, crayons and coloring books).		
9 Toys to learn names of animals (books about animals, circus games, animal puzzles, etc.).		
10 Toy or game for facilitating the learning of numbers (blocks with numbers, books about numbers, games with numbers, etc.).		
11 Building toys (blocks, tinker toys, Lincoln logs, etc.).		
12 Ride toy (tricycle, scooter, wagon, bike with or without training wheels).		
13 Medium wheel toys (trucks, trains, doll carriage, etc.).		
14 Large muscle toy (jump rope, swing, ball, climbing object, etc.).		
15 Ten children's books.		
16 At least 10 books are present and visible in the apartment.		
17 Family buys a newspaper daily and reads it.		
18 Family subscribes to at least one magazine.		
19 Family member has taken child in one outing (picnic, shopping excursion) at least every other week.		
20 Child has been taken out to eat in some kind of restaurant three to four times in the past year.		
21 Child is taken to grocery store at least once a week.		

22-24 Child has been taken by a family member to the following within the past year:

	Yes	No
22 Airport.		
23 A trip more than 50 miles from the child's home (50 miles radial distance, not total distance).		
24 A scientific, historical, or art museum.		
Subscore		

II Stimulation of mature behavior

	Yes	No

25-32 Child is encouraged to learn the following:

25 Colors.

26 Shapes.

27 Patterned speech (nursery rhymes, prayers, songs, TV commercials, etc.).

28 The alphabet.

29 The telling of time.

30 Spatial relationships (up, down, under, big, little, etc.).

31 Numbers.

32 The reading of a few words.

33 Parent tries to get child to pick up and put away toys after play session — without help.

34 Child is taught rules of social behavior which involve recognition of rights of others.

35 Parent teaches child some simple manners—to say, "Please," "Thank you," "I'm sorry."

36 Some delay of food gratification is demanded of the child, e.g., not to whine or demand food unless within ½ hour of mealtime.

Subscore

III Provision of a stimulating physical and language environment

	Yes	No

*37 Building has no potentially dangerous structural or health defect (e.g., plaster coming down from ceiling, stairway with boards missing, rodents, etc.).

*38 Child's outside play environment appears safe and free of hazards (no outside play area requires an automatic "No").

*39 The interior of the apartment is not dark or perceptibly monotonous.

*40 House is not overly noisy (television, shouts of children, radio, etc.).

*41 Neighborhood has trees, grass, birds—is aesthetically pleasing.

*42 There is at least 100 square feet of living space per person in the house.

*43 In terms of available floor space, the rooms are not overcrowded with furniture.

*44 All visible rooms of the house are reasonably clean and minimally cluttered.

*45 Parent uses complex sentence structure and some long words in conversing

*46 Parent uses correct grammar and pronunciation.

*47 Parent's speech is distinct, clear, and audible.

48 Family has TV, and it is used judiciously, not left on continuously (no TV requires an automatic "No"—any scheduling scores "Yes").

Subscore

IV Avoidance of restriction and punishment

	Yes	No

*49 Parent does not scold or derogate child more than once during visit.

*50 Parent does not use physical restraint or shake, grab, or pinch child during visit.

*51 Parent neither slaps nor spanks child during visit.

*52 Parent does not express overannoyance with or hostility toward child—complain, say child is "bad" or won't mind.

*53 Child is not punished or ridiculed for speech.

54 No more than one instance of physical punishment occurred during the past week (accept parent report).

55 Child does not get slapped or spanked for spilling food or drink.

Subscore

Highlights

* Observation item

Note: Parent refers to mother, father, or other caregiver who is present for interview.

V Pride, affection, and thoughtfulness

	Yes	No
56 Parent turns on special TV program regarded as "good" for children (*Captain Kangaroo, Magic Toy Shop, Walt Disney, Flipper, Lassie,* educational TV, etc.).		
57 Someone reads stories to child or shows and comments on pictures in magazines five times weekly.		
58 Parent encourages child to relate experiences or takes time to listen to child relate experiences.		
59 Parent holds child close 10 to 15 minutes per day (e.g., during TV, story time, visiting).		
60 Parent occasionally sings to child or sings in presence of child.		
61 Child has a special place in which to keep his or her toys and "treasures."		
62 Child's artwork is displayed some place in house (anything that child makes).		
★63 Parent introduces interviewer to child.		
★64 Parent converses with child at least twice during visit (scolding and suspicious comments not counted).		
★65 Parent answers child's questions or requests verbally.		
★66 Parent usually responds verbally to child's talking.		
★67 Parent provides toys or interesting activities or in other ways structures situation for child during visit when his or her attention will be elsewhere. (In order to score "Yes," parent must make an active guiding gesture or suggestion to structure child's play.)		
★68 Parent spontaneously praises child's qualities or behavior twice during visit.		
★69 When parent speaks of or to child, parent's voice conveys positive feeling.		
★70 Parent caresses, kisses, or cuddles child at least once during visit.		
★71 Parent sets up situation that allows child to show off during visit.		
Subscore		

VI Masculine stimulation

	Yes	No
72 Child sees and spends some time with father or father figure 4 days a week.		
73 Child eats at least one meal per day, on most days, with mother (or mother figure) and father (or father figure). (One-parent families get an automatic "No.")		
Subscore		

VII Independence from parental control

	Yes	No
74 Child is encouraged to try to dress himself or herself.		
75 Child is permitted to choose some of his or her clothing to be worn except on very special occasions.		
76 Child is permitted some choice in lunch or breakfast menu.		
77 Parent lets child choose certain favorite food products or brands at grocery store.		
78 Child is permitted to go to another house to play without having the caregiver accompany him or her.		
79 Child can express negative feeling without harsh reprisal.		
80 Child is permitted to hit parent without harsh reprisal.		
Subscore		
Total Score		

★Observation item

Figure 8-1 Home observation form for measurement of the environment, 3 to 6 years of age. "Parent" refers to mother, father, *or* other caregiver who is present for interview. Observation items are marked with an asterisk. (Adapted from Bettye M. Caldwell, *Instruction Manual Inventory for Infants [Home Observation for Measurement of the Environment]*, Little Rock, Ark., 1970.)

child's achievement of the major developmental task of initiative. By parents setting realistic standards, maintaining consistent measures of discipline, and allowing freedom to test abilities, the preschooler will develop self-reliance and a healthy degree of assertiveness and inquisitiveness. If parents are overly domineering, set rigid rules for conduct, or prevent exploration of mental and physical abilities, the preschooler may grow up lacking self-confidence, maturity, and the inner drive to master new and challenging skills.

Highlights

Parents, siblings, and grandparents have a significant influence over the preschooler's thinking and behavior.

Siblings and grandparents who interact with the preschooler may also have a significant influence on the preschooler. Siblings will often teach the younger child through play. For example, the preschooler will learn how personal property such as toys can be shared during play and will begin to understand concepts of ownership and acceptable social behavior. Loving grandparents can provide security, as well as opportunities for educational interchange. For example, a grandparent may have more time to read to the preschooler or teach language skills than a parent who is working all day. Times together can become very special for both the child and the adult.

Caretakers must allow the preschooler the freedom to test abilities and learn from mistakes.

Preschoolers become aware of their position and role in the family.

During the preschool years, the child's world expands to include peer and school relationships.

Also during this time period, the preschooler's world expands outward from the family to include relationships with peers in the neighborhood and in school and with other adults such as teachers and day care supervisors. At this time the parents must learn to separate from the preschooler and accept the fact that their child's thinking and behavior will be greatly influenced by others. Parents need "to allow independent development while modeling necessary standards."[9]

The nurse can begin the assessment of family life by asking the parents the questions identified in Family Life in Chap. 3 as well as the following additional questions.

Questions to elicit data:

1. What kinds of decisions do you let your child make?
2. How do you help your child in making decisions?
3. How often does your child help with household chores?
4. How do you feel about leaving your child with a baby-sitter or relative for more than a day or evening?
5. How would you describe your family relationships?

Refer to Family Life in Chap. 3 for questions for collection of data.

Further assessment of family life will occur during the remainder of the history-taking process.

Occupation

The preschool child needs time with family members. The occupation(s) of the parent(s) should be assessed to determine the number of hours the parents are gone from the home and how the parents coordinate shift work with family time, if this is the case. The amount of time for family activities should be determined, as well as the type of activities in which the family engages.

It is important for the preschool child to have opportunities to talk with the family and to be held and cuddled, as well as to have time in which the child can learn how to interrelate with parents, siblings, and other relatives. One experience the family can engage in to foster this interrelationship is the following: At dinner time each family member can share what happened to him or her on that day. The child then gets to practice communication skills and also learns what the other family members do during the day, how they express their feelings, and how they deal with situations that are humorous, frustrating, and/or static.

The parent's occupation will determine available time to be spent with the preschooler and the ability to purchase food, goods, housing and health care.

A working mother can affect a preschooler in various ways. If the mother views her work as a positive stress and continues to take time to spend with her preschooler, the child will probably adapt positively to the mother's working. However, if the mother views her work negatively and is frequently tired and irritable, the preschooler may have problems in adapting to the situation. For example, the child may become irritable or moody, become clingy, whiny and demanding, or regress in developmental tasks such as toileting. An important variable in the child's successful adaptation will be the day care or preschool setting the child is in during the day. Valuable educational experiences can expand the child's resources for coping with the stress in the home.

The occupations of the parents will also determine the income of the family and the amount of money available for purchasing food, goods, housing, and health care. Therefore, the nurse should inquire as to the adequacy of financial income. If a parent is forced to work two jobs, for example, in order to support a family, this could have unfortunate effects on the mental and physical health of the parent and the child as a result of stress and lack of contact.

Societal Relationships

Once the preschooler moves from being in the home full time, societal influences greatly increase. Baby-sitters in the neighborhood and teachers or supervisors in day care centers and preschools will have a direct effect on the child. Values and attitudes learned from the parents will often be tested when the child is faced with new and challenging situations. The child may have the self-confidence and independent strength to adapt to change or may become frustrated and withdrawn if the demands are too great. Gradual introduction of the child to encounters within various societal areas will ease this transition.

The preschooler moves from the home into societal settings which can influence behavior and mastery of one's environment.

Social behaviors are learned by the preschooler from persons other than the parents. The preschool teacher, for example, may gently demand cooperation from a child with success, even when such behavior is not manifested in the home. As the child becomes more self-assured and comfortable within society, additional behaviors will be acquired. This is especially important in preparing the child for entry into regular school.

Data collection should attempt to identify areas of societal impact on the preschooler's health, growth, and development.

Questions to elicit data:

1 Do you like going to the day care center (or preschool)? What do you do there?

2 What kinds of games or play can you do at the day care center (or preschool)?

3 Do you like your teacher? Why?

If the preschooler is unable to answer the nurse's questions, then data must be obtained from the parents regarding the effect of societal influences on their child.

Self-Perception and Self-Concept Patterns

By the age of 3 the child has a concept of self-identity and understands the concepts of good and bad. Too often when a child engages in an unacceptable behavior, the child is labeled as "bad" rather than the behavior labeled as "bad." This will affect the child's self-image if the child is told repeatedly that he or she is bad. A similar situation occurs with the use of the word "good." A child who has been repeatedly told that he or she is

The child's self-image can be affected by labeling such as "bad boy."

good may develop a conflict when engaged in bad behaviors such as hitting a sibling. Hence, it is important to explore the child's own understanding of self-image and the parent's perception of the child's self-image.

The preschool-age child is beginning to assert independence and alliance with peers in decision making. The child may develop a conflict over what he or she wants, what parents want, and what peers want. If the preschooler feels his or her parents' love is contingent on certain behaviors or decisions, self-image may be affected by how the child reacts behaviorally. The nurse needs to explore how the parents are handling the child's independence and decision-making abilities. A description of the child's relationships with peers can give the nurse clues to the child's self-image and ability to interact with others.

The questions presented in Chap. 3 can be adapted for the collection of data regarding the preschooler's self-image and conception patterns.

Cognitive and Perceptual Patterns

The components of this pattern area are the preschooler's sensory perceptions and cognitive abilities, which are based on the child's education and intelligence.

Sensory Perception

The preschooler's vision, hearing, taste, smell, and touch perceptions should be assessed by questioning the child as well as the parents.

Questions formulated in Chap. 3 can be adapted for the preschooler. Citing examples of familiar things in the preschooler's environment may help in data collection about taste, smell, and touch.

Education The assessment of this factor is quite similar to that for the toddler. Interactions with parents, siblings, relatives, and other caretakers are important to the child's educational process and socialization. Also, the availability of a stimulating and safe environment is a necessary variable for enhancing opportunities to practice new skills and reapply and extend experiences.

The 3-year-old has an increased sense of balance, a flourishing vocabulary, and a strong desire to imitate and please others, especially parents. The child enjoys gross and fine motor activities such as sedentary play with toys and use of crayons. Motor discrimination play, as building a tower with blocks, teaches eye-hand coordination and depth perception and is fun for the child.

Four- and five-year-olds have increasing control over their bodies, which results in better equilibrium, spatial orientation, and precision of movement. Refinement of gross and fine motor skills can thus be observed. The preschooler can draw crude pictures of objects important in the environment with a pencil or paints. When the child is asked to hop, jump, or catch a ball, he or she can perform with good neuromuscular maturity. Language development includes use of a large number of words, articulation, use of a basic grammatical structure, and categorization of the environment using abstract words (e.g., "animals" instead of "dog").

Intellectual growth of the preschooler is also characterized by an increasing memory ability, the learning of rules of logic, and the reasoning out of problems using logic. When the child is encouraged to apply concepts and language to familiar and enjoyable situations, learning progresses more readily. Thus, it is important for parents and caretakers to be aware of their child's particular level of development and provide opportunities for intellectual growth.

During the assessment of the preschooler's education, the nurse should direct questions to parents which will elicit specific data concerning the child's physical, intellectual, and social development. The nurse should also explore the parents' satisfaction with outside environments, since many preschoolers are in day care settings or preschools. How the child has adjusted to a new setting, to educational aspects, and to socialization with teachers and peers is important to overall health. A qualified teacher, for example, can engage the child in learning to refine gross and fine motor skills through activities such as running, jumping, hopping, pasting, cutting, coloring, and painting. Speech and language development can be enhanced by teaching the child to listen to stories and songs and to other children and by letting the child express thoughts, frustrations, and feelings. One of the most important aspects of preschool is teaching the child to become socialized. The child needs to learn how to be part of a group and how to play with peers and share objects such as toys and books.

At the end of the preschool era, the child will be entering kindergarten. The nurse should assess both the child's and the parents' readiness for school entry, their expectations, and their fears. Knowledge of the parents' previous experience with the school system will be helpful in the nurse's assessment.

Intelligence The preschooler's cognitive level of functioning has been described by Piaget as preoperational. This period of intellectual development (ages 2 to 7 years) builds on the sensorimotor period (birth to 2 years) and the acquisition of symbolic function seen in the toddler (ages 2 to 4 years). It is divided into the preconceptual stage, ages 2 to 4, and perceptual or intuitive stage, ages 4 to 7. A major characteristic of this period which permeates language, thought, and reasoning is egocentrism—the child's inability to see another person's point of view or the incapacity to shift attention from one aspect of a situation to another. A major transition the child will make between the two stages of the preoperational period is to change from totally egocentric thinking to being able to demonstrate social awareness and consideration for other persons and objects in the environment.

While investigating the child's content of thought, Piaget found that certain beliefs held by the child influenced the thought process. These beliefs held true for such things as the sun and moon, the origin of trees, and dreams.[10] The first belief is that all things that move are alive (animism). Thus, an object such as a tree or piece of equipment is alive like a person, and this may cause fear for the child. The second belief is that some person or being is responsible for creating things such as the sun and moon (artificialism). The third belief is the perception of some continuing connection (participation) between human activities and those of things. For example, trees grow because people grow. Thus, the preschooler's thought patterns may, at times, seem very illogical to adults. When working with the preschooler, the nurse must be cognizant of these beliefs and adapt situations to the child.

The preschooler's reasoning capabilities also reveal some illogical characteristics due to the child's inability to think simultaneously about several aspects of a situation. The child has a tendency to group together several ideas or events into a confusing whole (syncretism), he or she cannot see a relationship among separate events (juxtaposition), ordinal relations cannot be understood, and the child does not believe that a part belongs to a whole but instead thinks each are separate entities.[11]

Another concept that the preschooler cannot understand is conservation, or the idea that two equal amounts of something can be changed in

Preschools and day care settings can be helpful in preparing a child for kindergarten.

See Intelligence in Chap. 7 for foundational information.

The preschooler is egocentric and often unaware of other points of view.

Intellectual development is based on heredity, environmental interplay, and the personality of the child.

Piaget found that the preschooler's thought is influenced by beliefs in animism, artificialism, and participation.

Abstract words and concepts such as health, pain, tomorrow, and dangerous are not understood by the preschooler.

The preschooler can focus on only a limited aspect of a problem or situation.

An example of the child's inability to conserve is seen with math problems; he or she can count to 10 but without comprehending the meaning.

size, shape, volume, or length and still remain equal. This inability affects the child's understanding of relationships between events, objects, and things in the process of transition. The inability to conserve can be tested using the clay test. Two balls of clay, equal in size, are shown to the child. The child is asked if they are the same. Upon agreement that they are the same, one of the balls is rolled into a hot dog shape and the child is asked if they are the same. The preoperational child will say the hot dog shape has more clay.

With regard to language, the preschooler demonstrates both communicative and noncommunicative speech.[12] During socialized or communicative speech, the child attempts to transmit a message to the listener. However, there usually is no attempt made to give details or justify statements, and, therefore, he or she does not assume the listener's point of view. This behavior stems from the child's egocentrism.

The preschooler's language is egocentric and repetitious and lacks consideration for another's ideas or feelings.

Noncommunicative or "egocentric" speech is characterized by repetition of another's statement, by monologue in which the child converses out loud to himself or herself, and by collective monologue in which the child speaks to others who do not listen because they cannot understand the egocentric communication. Most often the child will talk of himself, to himself, or by himself. As the child gets older, egocentrism decreases and communication becomes effective and purposeful. The child eventually learns proper grammar and sentence structure, ordering of events, causality, and significant features to include in speech. Until the child learns these, the nurse may need to use alternative methods or nonverbal approaches. Play can be one of the most effective methods, since the child tends to express feelings, emotions, and ideas through imitation or through objects such as dolls.

Play can be used to assist the child in communicating during the health interview.

With exposure to new and varied experiences, persons, and environments, the child's thinking goes through a process of "decentration." Thinking no longer focuses on one aspect (centering), but the child is able to consider the complexities of a situation, the other person's point of view, and the intent and outcome of one's behavior (moral judgment). This process of centering and decentering may occur in a varied sequence of stages for different areas of cognitive development. Also the ages at which stages of substantive development occur vary considerably in different cultures, according to Piaget's findings. Thus, the individuality of each child must be considered when assessing intelligence.

Centering and decentering are processes of thought which occur in the preoperative period.

Many other aspects of intellectual development have been studied and interpreted by Piaget. These include moral behavior, classification of objects or events, mental imagery, the concept of number, and the concepts of chance and space. It is necessary to review translations of his original works in order to gain an indepth understanding of these extensive studies.

Refer to translations of Piaget's original works for a more detailed account of intellectual development.

In summary, when assessing the intelligence of the preschooler, the nurse must have a good understanding of theories of cognitive development and their application to the health interview and physical examination. Also, the nurse must determine through data collection if the child's thought processes fall within developmental norms. This determination will possibly clarify if the child is ready for school entry and scholastic learning. The DDST can be used to verify normative development and rule out possible developmental delays.

The child's understanding of abstract concepts can be aided through concrete representations.

The DDST can be used for screening purposes during the preschool years.

As was discussed with the toddler, routine intelligence tests are not performed. The Stanford Binet Test or The Wechsler Intelligence Scale for Children can be used to further assess children who present with potential intellectual or developmental delays. These tests must be conducted by a qualified person, such as a psychologist. Thus, referral by the nurse may be necessary. Furthermore, results of such tests must be

Results of standardized intelligence tests may provide the nurse with more specific data concerning a particular child.

used with caution, since it is believed that IQ (intelligence quotient) tests may be predictive of future achievements only past the age of 6. Even after this time, the child's IQ can be improved with education and inherent motivation.

Sexuality Patterns

The preschooler is very interested in his or her own body and its intactness and how it compares with other children. This sexual curiosity is an important developmental phase and helps the child gain an understanding of sexual identity. The child's curiosity may be manifested in direct questions to parents about sex, such as "Where do babies come from?" "Why doesn't Mommy have a penis?" "How does the baby get born?" Such questions are an attempt to understand how the body functions and why girls and boys are different. Curiosity may also be seen in overt behaviors such as actual visual exploration of self or of the opposite sex. For example, a parent may discover a little boy and girl looking at and fondling one another's genitals in an attempt to understand why they are different. Parents' reactions to such discoveries must not be guilt provoking for the child, but instead the parent should attempt to satisfy the child's inquisitiveness through verbal explanation. In such a situation, children are not really interested in the actual manipulation of the sex organs but in gaining an understanding of "why" and "how" they are different. Thus, emphasis should not be placed on the actual behaviors of the child but on providing accurate information whereby the child can learn about sexual identity and basic bodily functions. Since the preschooler begins developing a conscience (superego), any behavior that provokes a negative reaction by the parent will be guilt-producing for the child and may affect the child emotionally over time.

The sexual development of the preschooler also centers around resolution of the Oedipal complex for boys and the Electra complex for girls. According to Freud's psychoanalytical theory, a boy wishes to possess his mother solely and, thus, competes with his father for her affection. Similarly, the girl becomes coy and seductive toward her father in order to win his affections from her mother. The child imitates the behaviors of the same-sex parent closely in an attempt to replace the opposite-sex parent, thus taking on characteristics of masculinity or femininity and resolving the complex. By the end of the preschool period, the child begins to realize that such a sexual relationship is not possible and instead expresses interest in the same-sex peer group. Nevertheless, child-rearing practices and imitation of the same-sex parent influence the specific sex typing of the child. For example, girls will dress in a feminine way and play with "girl" toys such as dolls, while boys will do the opposite. Attitudes and beliefs about sexual identity subsequently are formed. Whether biological or environmental influences have the greatest effect on sexual identity is an unresolved issue. Nonetheless, both do influence to some degree the formation of a male, or masculine, or female, or feminine, identity in the child.

One activity related to sexuality that tends to confuse or disturb parents is the preschooler's interest in masturbation, or self-stimulation of the genitals. If this behavior is not excessive, it is both normal and healthy, since it is part of a child's bodily exploration and helps satisfy sexual curiosity. If parents' beliefs about masturbation are that it is dirty or unhealthy, then this behavior in the child may be reprimanded. Thus, it is important for the nurse to determine parental feelings and then provide accurate information regarding masturbation. This will help relieve the parents of anxiety and provide an opportunity for open discussion of sexuality and sexual needs of the developing child.

The preschooler possesses a strong sexual curiosity.

It is common for the preschooler to want to visually and tactilely explore the genitals of self and of the opposite sex.

The child wants to know "how" and "why" the sexes are different.

The preschooler imitates the parent of the same sex in an attempt to win the total affection of the opposite-sex parent.

Children learn masculinity and femininity from parental role modeling of sexual behaviors.

Masturbation is common in young children and is considered normal bodily exploration.

Parental attitudes about sex will influence the content and depth of information that is given to the child.

When assessing sex and sexuality holistically, it is important for the nurse to also determine the parents' perceptions of sex roles for both male and female, their understanding of sexual development in the preschooler, and any biases they may have due to certain attitudes or beliefs. Since preschoolers rely on parental information or misinformation regarding sexuality and acceptable sexual behavior, it is critical that parents feel comfortable discussing the topic. Parents may need assistance from the nurse in how to approach sex education. By using the parents' philosophy and accurate facts, the nurse can help the parents decide when sex education should begin, where and how it should be taught, and how much role modeling is appropriate. Initially finding out what the child thinks or understands will guide the content and depth of teaching. Maintaining an honest approach to the subject is also important. The preschooler will comprehend only a certain amount, but correct information lays the foundation for future learning. Honesty also tells the child that parents can be trusted, and this will carry over into other areas of the child's education and development.

It is important that the nurse determine the parents' understanding and philosophy of sexual identity and sexuality.

The preschooler should be provided with accurate information regarding sex.

Questions to elicit data:

1 What questions has your child asked about sex or sexual identity?

2 How do you answer your child's questions?

3 Has your child engaged in any sexual activities? Describe.

4 What interest has your child shown in his or her body and in that of the opposite sex?

5 Does your child play with boys and girls? Have you noticed any differences in behaviors during play with boys and with girls? What were the differences?

6 Does your child masturbate? How do you feel about this?

7 What information have you given your child about his or her sex and bodily functions related to sex?

Additional questions can be formulated according to the depth of data the nurse needs to thoroughly assess this factor.

Nutritional Patterns

The preschooler is dependent on parents and caretakers for exposure to nutritious foods, and the family's preferences for certain foods will certainly influence the child's nutritional status. Culture and lifestyles will also play significant roles in the family's food selections.

Many 3-year-olds may still be in the stage of decreased appetite, a carry-over from the toddler years. Some children will go for months without gaining any weight and yet remain healthy. This may alarm parents, who then attempt to bribe the child to eat. The nurse's assessment of the child's daily food intake, activity levels, and growth measurements will provide data which often reassure parents that the child is doing well despite limited caloric intake.

Usually by the age of 5 the child is ready to enjoy meals with the family and looks forward to this "social event." New food items and varied menus become more acceptable, since the child is now greatly influenced by the food habits of others. Therefore, parents can take advantage of this change and introduce additional well-balanced foods to the diet. If the preschooler still has a few favorite foods, these items should still be allowed as part of the meal plan.

For some children there may be the concern of overeating or intake of too many calories, which can lead to excessive weight gain. Studies have

Finger foods are still enjoyed by the preschooler.

See growth charts in the Appendix for determining the percentile measurement of growth for the child.

Food items should be colorful and attractive in order to appeal to the child.

Impeccable table manners cannot be expected of the preschool child.

shown that obese preschoolers do become obese adults. Therefore, the nurse should not overlook the presence of obesity in all or most family members of the preschooler. Thorough assessment of the diet can provide information that may alert the nurse to the threat of obesity while there is still time for preventative intervention with the child.

Simple rules about diet, eating habits, and the components of the *basic four food groups* (milk and dairy, meats, vegetables and fruits, bread and cereal) should be taught to the preschooler at a beginning level. Since the child enjoys the challenge of learning and practicing rules, this is an opportune time for parents to begin this task. For example, while pouring a glass of milk, the mother can say, "It is good to drink four glasses of milk each day." Through role modeling and repetition, the child will soon incorporate healthy eating behaviors into the daily diet.

The preschooler's diet is considered to be adequate if approximately 40 kilocalories per pound (90 kilocalories per kilogram) is consumed per day. The protein, fat, and carbohydrate proportions are the same as for the toddler: 10 to 15 percent of protein, 25 to 35 percent of fats, and 50 to 60 percent of carbohydrates. Total daily fluid requirements also continue to be four to six glasses or 1000 to 1500 ml per day. Table 8-4 contains a sample diet for a normal preschooler.

The nurse can determine the adequacy of the preschooler's daily diet by asking the parents to keep a 7-day record of food intake, including all meals and snacks. If vitamin and/or mineral supplementation is given, the types and amounts should be recorded. The nurse should also attempt to identify parental values and practices regarding foods, since these impact on the child. Once the preschooler's diet pattern has been assessed, the nurse can then judge if growth measurements and development truly reflect a well-balanced diet.

Exercise and Activity Patterns

Major activities of the preschooler include play and mastering of self-help skills that were learned at a beginning level as a toddler. With movement from the home into other environments, the child frequently ac-

Highlights

Food attitudes learned in childhood will usually remain with the child into adulthood.

Activity level and metabolism can affect caloric and fluid needs.

See Table 8-4 for a sample diet for the preschooler.

A 24-hour recall or 7-day record of the preschooler's intake can assist the nurse's assessment of diet.

See Behavioral Development for an assessment of activities of daily living, including play.

Table 8-4
An Adequate Daily Diet for a Preschooler

Milk and dairy products	
Milk	16 oz
Cheese	$\frac{1}{2}$–$\frac{3}{4}$ oz (as substitute for 4 oz milk)
Yogurt or ice cream	$\frac{1}{4}$–$\frac{1}{2}$ c (as substitute for 4 oz milk)
Meat and meat equivalents	
Meat, fish, poultry	2 oz ($\frac{1}{4}$ c)
Egg	1 (limit 3–4 per week)
Dried beans, peas	3–4 T (occasional replacement for meat)
Peanut butter	1–2 T
Vegetables	
Cooked green leafy or deep yellow	3–4 T at 1 or more meals
Raw (carrots, lettuce, etc.)	2 or more pieces
Fruits	
Vitamin C source (citrus, tomatoes, etc.)	1 medium-sized orange or equivalent
Other fruits	$\frac{1}{3}$ c at 1 or more meals
Bread and cereal grains	
Whole-grain or enriched bread	2 or more slices
Whole-grain restored or enriched cereal	$\frac{1}{2}$ c or more
Potatoes, noodles, or rice	3–4 T
Crackers	1–3
Butter or margarine	1 T
Sweets	$\frac{1}{3}$ c simple dessert at 1 or 2 meals
Vitamin D source	400 IU

Source: Adapted from M. V. Krause and L. K. Mahan, *Food, Nutrition and Diet Therapy*, Saunders, Philadelphia, 1979, p. 327.

quires other new skills that will further enhance the child's sense of self and mastery of previous levels of growth and development.

Rituals are still an important part of the child's daily patterns. For example, bedtime stories that were enjoyed as a toddler continue to entertain the preschooler. Toilet training and self-help skills such as feeding oneself are accomplished with more consistency and accuracy.

Imaginary playmates are very real for the preschooler. The family must remember to incorporate these "playmates" into activities such as the evening meal. Dreams and fantasies will carry over into other activities of the preschooler, such as play. A little girl, for example, may enjoy imitating her mother's bridge group by setting one up herself with all her imaginary friends present.

Motor activities are more purposeful for 3- through 5-year-olds. The child doesn't just play with blocks, for example, but will build structures of his or her own design. Many preschoolers become quite adept with pencils, crayons, and scissors as well. Gross motor skills include riding a tricycle, jumping, throwing and catching a ball, and even skating.

When assessing the preschooler's activity level, the nurse should try to gain data from observation of the child as well as verbally from the parents. Specific questions can be asked regarding (1) types and frequency of play, (2) mastery of self-help skills, (3) gross motor and fine motor skills, (4) language development, and (5) the ability to interact with peers, older children, and adults.

Coping Patterns and Stress Tolerance Patterns

The preschool child reacts to stress in much the same variety of ways as adults. Children experience anger, fear, jealousy, curiosity, envy, joy, grief, and affection. These emotions are normal. Too often, however, the child is not allowed to express these emotions nor is he or she helped in identifying what these emotions are. The nurse should assess how the child handles various emotions and how the parent helps the child in dealing with them.

Funnel questions can be a good interviewing technique for exploring emotions. Examples include "Some people think young children never get angry; some think they get angry just like adults do. What do you think? Does your child ever get angry? How does he or she handle anger?" Answers to such questions will provide data so that further assessment can be structured by the nurse.

There are many changes that can cause stress in the child. Any change in lifestyle can be significant, such as parental role changes (mother begins working outside the home), a change in a parent's job, the relocation of the family, the hospitalization of a significant person in the child's life, a divorce, or a death in the family. Stress can adversely affect the child's health if the stressor is not identified and the emotion handled. The child may complain of headaches and stomachaches or become irritable or withdraw. Thus, the nurse should assess if there are presently any stressors in the child's life and if there are any potential stressors. The parent and the child should be asked how the stress was handled, what emotions the child experienced, and how the parent assisted the child. The nurse should also assess the parent's capability to help the child with the stress reaction or behavioral response.

Review of Body Components

A review of body components should be done at least yearly on the preschooler. The format identified in Chap. 3 can be used for collecting and recording data. It should be completed prior to the actual physical exam-

Fantasies, dreams, and rituals are important components of the preschooler's activities.

Data collected on the DDST can be used to assess the preschooler's activity.

Stress is manifested in a variety of behavioral responses.

The nurse should identify stressors that the child is exposed to.

Parents need to assist the child in learning to cope with stress.

ination. The data will provide the nurse with a subjective picture of the intactness of the child's body components and should include specific notations regarding past and present insults to the individual. Special attention should be given to any of the areas that are current concerns. If deviations from normal are found, the nurse should obtain details of such deviations.

Highlights

The nurse can use the format for data collection described in Chap. 3 as a guide for the review of body components.

Questions to elicit data:

Throat

1 Does your child complain of sore throats or that "it hurts when I swallow"?

2 Has your child ever had a strep throat?

Lungs

1 Has your child ever had an upper respiratory infection? How often?

2 Have your ever noticed that your child has difficulty breathing?

3 Does your child become easily exhausted during play?

4 How well does your child tolerate exercise? Describe.

Bladder

1 When was your child toilet trained?

2 Has your child ever had urinary tract infections?

Similar questions can be developed for each body component being reviewed by the nurse. A more detailed assessment is subsequently made at the time of the physical examination.

Table 8-5
Diagnostic Tests

Type of screening	Rationale	Significant health history	Standardized test	Interpretation of results

Blood
  Hematocrit and
    hemoglobin
	Anemia may not be identified except through lab tests.	Lack of iron sources in diet
		Fatigue
		Frequent infections
			Capillary tube
			Cyanmethemoglobin
				<34 indicates anemia
				<11.0 g/dL indicates anemia

Sickle cell	Presence significant for future genetic counseling.	Positive family history Black race	Hemoglobin Electrophoresis	If hemoglobin S abnormality is homozygous, then sickle-cell disease; if it is heterozygous, then sickle-cell trait
Urine pH	High pH can indicate urinary tract infection, alkalosis, and potassium depletion. Low pH can indicate metabolic or respiratory acidosis, pyrexia, or metabolic disorders.	Too numerous to cite	Dipsticx or Combistix	Normal: 4.5–7.5
Specific gravity	Test reveals the ability of the kidney to concentrate or dilute urine.	Less than or greater than 600–750 mL of urine output per day	Hydrometer or urinometer	Normal: 1.002–1.030
Protein	Protein in urine can indicate renal damage or urinary infection.	Complaints of itching and burning on urination	Combistix or Urostix	Normal: none to trace
Glucose	Glucose in urine ordinarily indicates diabetes mellitus.	Excessive thirst Weight loss Fatigue	Urostix Clinistix Combistix Tes-Tape	Normal: none

Table 8-6
Normal Urinalysis Results

Color	Clear, yellow, or straw-colored
Odor	Mild if fresh specimen Ammoniacal at room temperature
pH	Slightly acidic (varies according to time of day and freshness of urine)
Specific gravity (concentration)	1.002–1.030
Protein	Negative
Ketones	Negative
Glucose	Negative
White blood cells and casts	Negative (may be present if specimen contaminated)
Red blood cells	Absent
Bacteria	Absent or few

Summary

The health history of the preschooler provides a thorough assessment of areas of growth and development and of the many variables and patterns which impact on the child's health state. The assessment of behavioral development provides the nurse with insight into characteristic responses of the preschooler to stress, change, and maturation. If the findings are normal, the nurse is able to reassure parents of the well-being of their child.

REFERENCES

1. Tudor, Mary (ed.): *Child Development,* McGraw-Hill, New York, 1981.

2. Murray, R., and J. Zentner: *Nursing Assessment and Health Promotion Through the Life Span,* Prentice-Hall, Englewood Cliffs, New Jersey, 1979.

3. Hurlock, E.: *Developmental Psychology,* 4th ed., McGraw-Hill, New York, 1975.

4. Conroy, R., and J. Mills: *Human Circadian Rhythms,* J. and A. Churchill, London, 1970, pp. 115, 118.

5. Colquhoun, W. (ed.): *Aspects of Human Efficiency,* English Universities Press, London, 1972, pp. 31–46.

6. Bassler, S.: "The Origins and Development of Biological Rhythms," *Nursing Clinics of North America,* **11**(4):575–582 (December 1976).

7. Hellbrügge, Theodor: "The Development of Circadian Rhythms in Infants," in *Cold Spring Harbor Symposia on Quantitative Biology,* vol. 25, The Biological Laboratory, New York, 1960.

8. Hester, N., R. Davis, S. Hanson, and R. Hassenein: "The Hospitalized Child's Subjective Rating of Pain," Unpublished research, University of Kansas, 1978.

9. Friedman, A., and D. Friedman: "Parenting: A Developmental Process," *Pediatric Annals,* **6**(9):13 (September 1977).

10. Ginsburg, Herbert, and Sylvia Opper: *Piaget's Theory of Intellectual Development: An Introduction,* Prentice-Hall, Englewood Cliffs, New Jersey, 1969, pp. 98–99.

11. Ibid., pp. 109–113.

12. Ibid., pp. 86–93.

BIBLIOGRAPHY

Alexander, Mary, and Marie Brown: *Pediatric History Taking and Physical Diagnosis for Nurses,* 2d ed., McGraw-Hill, New York, 1979.

Barness, Lewis: *Manual of Pediatric Physical Diagnosis,* 4th ed., Year Book Medical Publishers, Chicago, 1972.

Bassler, Sanda: "The Origins and Development of Biological Rhythms," *NCNA* **11**(4):575–582 (Dec. 1976).

Chinn, Peggy, and Cynthia Leitch: *Child Health Maintenance,* 2d ed., Mosby, St. Louis, 1979.

Colquhoun, W. P.: *Aspects of Human Efficiency,* English Universities Press, London, 1972.

Conroy, Robert W., and J. N. Mills: *Human Circadian Rhythms,* J. and A. Churchill, London, 1970.

Crowell, Carol: "Pediatric Gynecology" Symposium, University of Kansas Medical Center, Kansas City, Kan., Jan. 1977.

Dunn, L. M.: *Peabody Picture Vocabulary Test,* American Guidance, Circle Pines, Minn., 1965.

Ferholt, Judith D. Lott: *Clinical Assessment of Children: A Comprehensive Approach to Primary Pediatric Care,* Lippincott, Philadelphia, 1980.

Fomon, Samuel: *Nutritional Disorders of Children Prevention Screening, and Followup,* DHEW Publication No. (HSA) 77–5104, U.S. Government Printing Office, Washington, D.C., 1977.

Fox, Jane (ed.): *Primary Health Care of the Young,* McGraw-Hill, New York, 1981.

French, Ruth: *The Nurse's Guide to Diagnostic Procedures,* 3d ed., McGraw-Hill, New York, 1971.

Friedman, Alma, and David Friedman: "Parenting: A Developmental Process," *Pediatr Ann,* 6(9):10–22 (September 1977).

Friedman, Stanford B., and Robert A. Hoekelman: *Behavioral Pediatrics: Psychosocial Aspects of Child Health Care,* McGraw-Hill, New York, 1980.

G. I. Series: *The Infant and Child,* A. H. Robbins, Richmond, Va., March 1974.

A Guide for Eye Inspection and Testing Visual Acuity of Preschool Age Children: A Screening Process, National Society for the Prevention of Blindness, New York, no date.

"Guidelines for Identification, Audiometry," *ASHA,* Feb. 1975, pp. 94–99.

Hester, Nancy: "Discipline and the Nurse Clinician's Role," *Issues in Comprehensive Pediatr Nurs,* 1(4):11–18.

Hester, N., R. Davis, S. Hanson, and R. Hassenein: "The hospitalized child's subjective rating of pain," unpublished research, University of Kansas, 1978.

Hurlock, Elizabeth: *Developmental Psychology,* 4th ed., McGraw-Hill, New York, 1975.

Johnson, Thomas, William Moore, and James Jeffries (eds.): *Children Are Different: Developmental Physiology,* 2d ed., Ross Laboratories, Columbus, Ohio, 1978.

Kerlinger, F.: *Foundations of Behavioral Research,* 2d ed., Holt, Rinehart, and Winston, New York, 1973.

Knight, Jane: "Fair play for children," seminar presentation, Association for Care of Children in Hospitals, Washington, D.C., June 1978.

Krajicek, Marilyn, and Alice Tearney (eds.): *Detection of Developmental Problems in Children,* University Park Press, Baltimore, 1977.

Maier, Henry W.: *Three Theories of Child Development,* revised ed., Harper & Row, New York, 1969.

Murray, Ruth, and Judith Zentner: *Nursing Assessment and Health Promotion through the Life Span,* 2d ed., Prentice-Hall, Englewood Cliffs, N.J., 1979.

Nahigian, Eileen: "The Preschooler—3–5 Years," in *Comprehensive Pediatric Nursing,* 2d ed., ed. by G. Scipien et al., McGraw-Hill, New York, 1979.

Natalini, John: "The Human Body as a Biological Clock," *AJN* 77:1130–1132 (July 1977).

Northern, Jerry, and Marion Downs: *Hearing in Children,* Williams and Wilkins, Baltimore, 1975.

Peterson, Robert: "Vision Screening and the Detection of Amblyopia in Children," *Sight-Saving Rev,* Summer-Fall 1974, 85–88.

Sauvé, Mary, and Angela Pecheret: *Concepts and Skills in Physical Assessment,* Saunders, Philadelphia, 1977.

Scipien, Gladys, et al.: *Comprehensive Pediatric Nursing,* 2d ed., McGraw-Hill, New York, 1979.

Slattery, Jill: "Dental Health in Children," *AJN* **76**(7):1159–1161, 1976.

Smith, Jane: "Promoting Childhood Dental Health," *Pediatr Nurs,* May/June 1976, 16–19.

Steele, Shirley M.: *Child Health and Family-Nursing Concepts and Management,* Masson, New York, 1981.

Tom, Cheryl: "Nursing Assessment of Biological Rhythms," *NCNA,* **11**(4):621–630 (Dec. 1976).

Tudor, Mary (ed.): *Child Development,* McGraw-Hill, New York, 1981.

Turnbull, Sister Joyce: "Shifting the Focus to Health," *AJN,* Dec. 1976, 1985–7.

Webb, Wilse B.: "Patterns of Sleep Behavior," in *Aspects of Human Efficiency,* ed. by W. P. Colquhoun, English Universities Press, London, 1972.

Whaley, Lucille, and Donna L. Wong: *Nursing Care of Infants and Children,* Mosby, St. Louis, 1979.

PHYSICAL EXAMINATION

APPROACH TO THE EXAMINATION

With the preschooler, the completion of the physical examination will be largely dependent on the nurse's ability to get the child involved. The nurse needs to elicit the child's cooperation. The preschool child will be more comfortable if the parents are allowed to remain in the room. (The 3-year-old may still need to be held by the parent during most of the examination.) Following are some simple guidelines which will help the nurse gain the child's confidence and cooperation:

1 Talk to the preschooler; tell the child exactly what you intend to do (a).

2 Let the preschooler help with the examination (b).

3 Let the preschooler play with some of the examining equipment, such as the stethescope and tongue blade. This will decrease fears.

4 Make a game out of the examination whenever possible (c).

5 Be firm but gentle with the child when giving directions and performing procedures.

6 Make positive statements to the child. If the child has no choice, don't allow a choice by asking a question rather than making a statement.

7 Be patient and unhurried.

8 Compliment the child on his or her cooperativeness.

Although the preschooler usually will be willing to undress for the examination, the nurse should avoid having the child undress too soon. The child's underpants should be left on for the child's privacy until the genital exam is done. A gown may be worn if the room is cold.

The nurse needs to involve the preschooler in the physical examination process.

Refer to Chap. 4, "Physical Examination," for specific techniques and procedures of examination.

The less upsetting procedures of the physical examination should be performed first.

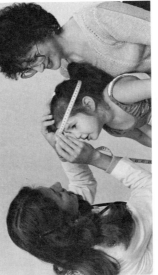
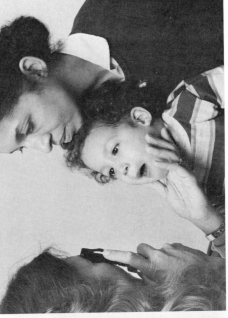

a

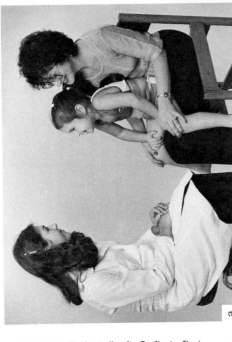
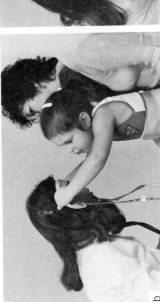
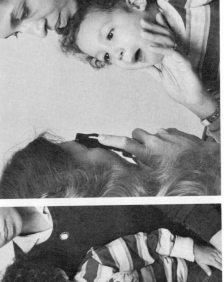

b

c

When assessing general appearance of the preschooler, the nurse should also note vital signs and body measurements.

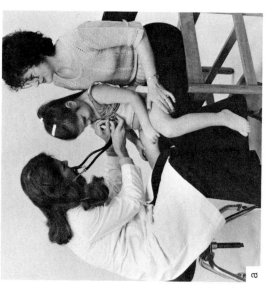

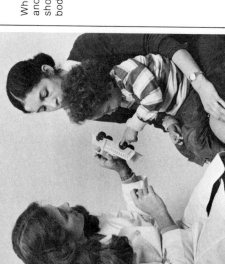

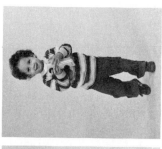

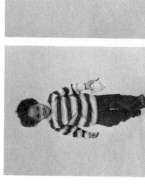

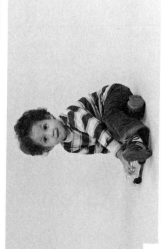

The order of the examination of a child will be slightly different from that of an adult. The thorax, abdomen, and genitals, of the preschooler will be examined before the head, eyes, ears, nose, mouth, and throat. The rationale for this change in order is that the preschooler may be frightened by the ophthalmic and otoscopic examinations; hence, if the nurse begins with the less upsetting portions of the examination, the child and the nurse may develop a better rapport (a).

THE EXAMINATION
General Appearance

The child's overall appearance should be observed by the nurse (b). Note how the child stands, and if the child has an erect posture. Also observe symmetry as the child stands, sits, and moves.

The skin should be observed for intactness, color and texture. The nurse should note any birthmarks or skin discolorations.

The child's behavior, facial expression, and emotional status should be assessed. Significant indicators of the preschooler's emotional status are mood fluctuations, and the congruity of the child's verbal and nonverbal communication (c).

The child's height (a) and weight (b) should be obtained. These measures should be plotted on growth charts and the nurse should observe the growth pattern of the child as well as whether or not the height and weight are proportional.

The child's vital signs including temperature, pulse, respirations, and blood pressure are taken. When taking the preschooler's temperature, the nurse should ask the parent if the child is capable of holding a thermometer in the mouth. If he or she is not, a rectal or axillary temperature should be obtained. The preschooler may need to be held by a parent during the procedure.

The pulses are obtained in the same manner as are an adult's. Usually this presents no problem for the preschooler.

The skin should be checked for turgor (c). To do this the nurse takes a large pinch of skin on the lower abdomen (see Chap. 4). If the skin is normally hydrated, it will return to normal position when released. Also, the nurse should measure the size of any birthmarks.

Taking the blood pressure may be upsetting for the preschooler. The nurse needs to use a child's cuff (which is one-half to two-thirds the width of the child's upper arm) to obtain an accurate reading. The child will probably be frightened and will need to be prepared by the nurse for the procedure. The nurse should explain that the cuff will get tight on the child's arm (d). Demonstrating the technique on the parent or on a toy may be helpful. Letting the child pump the bulb may help alleviate the child's anxiety. (The normal values for the vital signs are presented in Highlights column.)

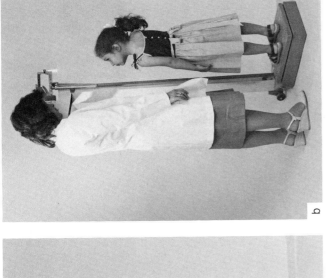

a

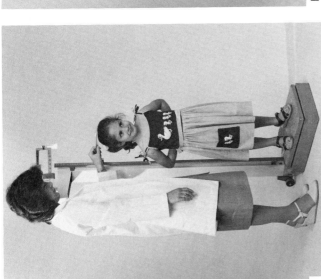

b

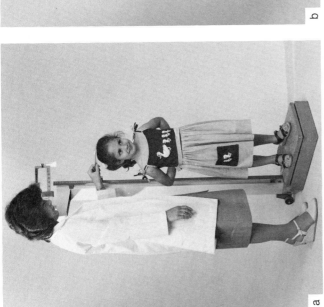

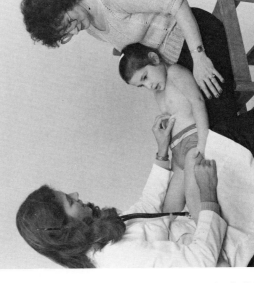

c

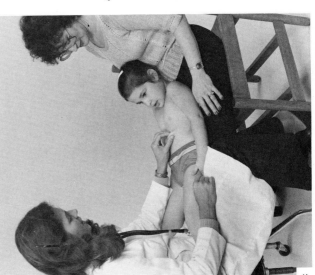

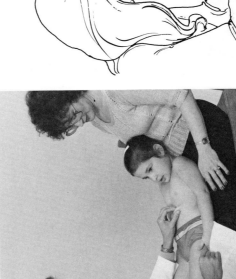

d

A rectal or axillary temperature should be taken if the child cannot hold an oral thermometer in the mouth.

Preschoolers are often frightened by the procedure of blood pressure measurement.

The preschooler's cerebral function should be assessed throughout the examination.

Age	Mean Heart Rate ± 2 S.D.	Mean Blood Pressure (mmHg)	Respiration (Rate/Min)
3	105±35	100/60	20-30
4	105±35	100/60	20-30
5	105±35	100/60	20-25

Adapted from Johnson, T. "Development of the Lungs" and "Changes in the Developing Cardiovascular System in Relation to Age" in *Children Are Different: Developmental Physiology* (2nd edition) Columbus: Ross Laboratories, 1978, pp. 127-141.

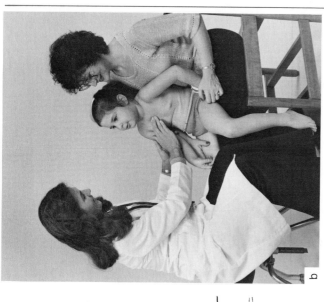

b

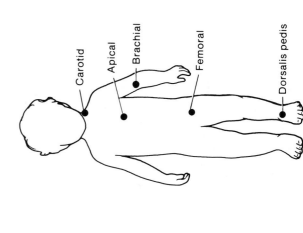

Carotid

Apical

Brachial

Femoral

Dorsalis pedis

c

a

Thorax

Along with the general structure of the thorax, the heart, lungs, and breasts are examined.

Inspection

The nurse should inspect the anterior portion of the thorax for shape and structure. This is best done with the child supine and with the chest elevated 45 degrees by raising the examining table or using a pillow or parent for support (a). The chest should be observed for symmetry and shape. Abnormal shapes can be related to heart problems.

Palpation

The anterior thorax should be palpated for normal placement of underlying structures, ie., ribs, sternum (b), and xiphoid process. The clavicles should be intact.

Heart

Palpation

The apical, brachial, femoral, carotid, and dorsalis pedis pulses should be palpated (c). Rate, rhythm, quality, and symmetry of corresponding pulses should be noted.

Percussion

Percussion is of little help in the examination of the heart except to determine the size of the heart.

The nurse should allow the child to listen to his or her heartbeat with the stethoscope.

The examiner may auscultate other areas of the chest for ectopic sounds.

Often a third heart sound may be heard in the preschooler.

Innocent murmurs are heard in 50 percent of normal children.

Preschoolers' respirations may be changing from abdominal as seen during toddler years, to costal or thoracic.

Auscultation

The next procedure is to auscultate for heart sounds. This is an ideal time to elicit the preschooler's cooperation by letting the child listen to the beating of the heart (a). In the nurse's examination of the heart, seven areas should be auscultated in both the recumbent and sitting positions: the sternoclavicular, aortic, pulmonic, anterior precordial, apical and epigastric (b). Perhaps the major difference from the heart sounds in adults is that a third heart sound may be heard in the preschooler (see Chap. 4). This is normal in children and is best heard at the apex of the heart. Innocent murmurs usually will be located in the pulmonic area and occur in as many as 50 percent of normal children. The innocent heart murmur is best heard with the bell of the stethoscope when the child is sitting. It is usually low pitched, either musical or vibratory, and occurs early in systole. It should be no greater than grades I or II and should be of short duration. It does not affect the child's growth and development. It may be more audible when the child has a high fever.

Lungs
Inspection

Respirations in the preschooler are usually in the transition phase, changing gradually from abdominal to costal or thoracic. This transition will be completed by 7 years of age. The nurse should first observe the thorax (c) and look for symmetry of the chest movements. Any intracostal, subcostal, or suprasternal retractions should be noted as these are usually not normal.

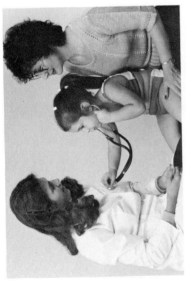
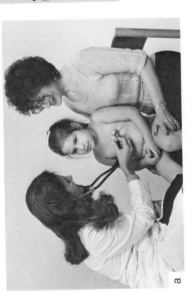

a

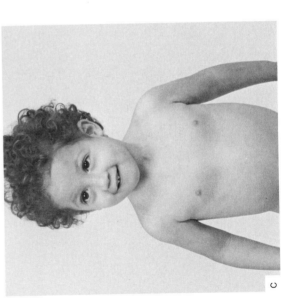

b

Sternoclavicular
Pulmonic
Apical
Epigastric
Aortic
Anterior precordial

c

Palpation

Palpation of the thorax will help the examiner evaluate the evenness of the chest movement and determine the respiratory rate. Palpation can also be used to test for fremitus. In this procedure the child should say "ninety-nine" repeatedly while the nurse palpates the child's chest (a). The vibrations of the child's vocalizations will be felt. As in adults, the nurse should detect any changes in sensation which could indicate areas of consolidation.

Percussion

Percussion techniques are the same as in adults. Children usually do not object to this technique especially if they are told to "listen for the sound of a drum."

Auscultation

On auscultation, breath sounds are usually louder in young children due to the thinness of the chest wall. The quality of the sound offers little help to the nurse in that the sounds tend to be bronchovesicular or bronchial; however, the nurse should evaluate the symmetry of the breath sounds (b and c). The rate of respiration decreases with age because the number of alveoli increases until the child is about 8 years of age. This results in an increase in lung capacity and facilitates adequate gas exchange.

Breasts

Inspection

The nipples and surrounding tissue in both male and female preschoolers should be examined for position, size, and color. Auxiliary nipples should be noted.

Percussion techniques on the pre-schooler are performed the same as on adults.

The rate of respirations decreases with age because of the increasing number of alveoli.

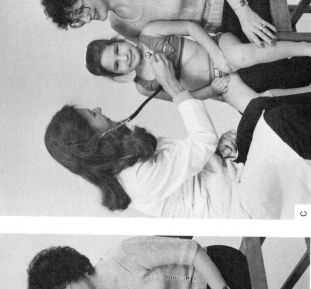

c

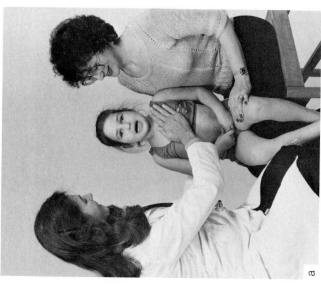

a

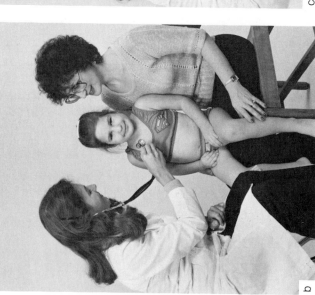

b

A "pot belly" can be observed when the preschooler is standing.

The stomach, liver, spleen, kidneys, bladder, and bowel are palpated during the abdominal examination.

Abdomen

Inspection

When observing the child's abdomen, the nurse should be aware that the "pot belly" is normal for the preschooler in the standing position (a). This is due to the lumbar lordosis normally present in preschoolers. However, when the child is lying on the back, it is normal only up to the age of 4. The nurse may note an umbilical hernia, commonly found in black children.

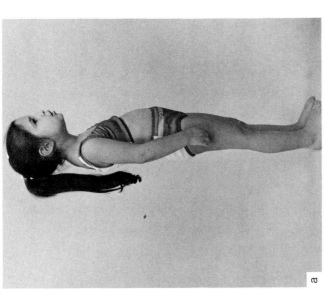

a

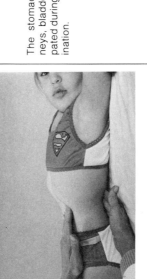

c

Palpation

For the palpation of the abdomen, the child should be in a supine position, with knees drawn up, and head slightly elevated. The nurse should have the child pant "like a puppy." This position and activity help to relax the abdominal wall. Palpation should be performed to determine areas of tenderness, locate masses, and determine organ size. A ticklish child can be helped to overcome laughing if his or her hand is placed under the nurse's hand during the palpation. The liver may be palpable 1 to 2 cm below the right costal margin, while the tip of the spleen may be palpated normally (b), especially on deep inspiration or in thin children. Stool in the intestines may be felt, as may a distended bladder.

The kidneys of the young child can be palpated by using the ballottement technique (described in Chap. 4). Usually 1 to 2 cm of the right kidney and the tip of the left kidney can be felt (c).

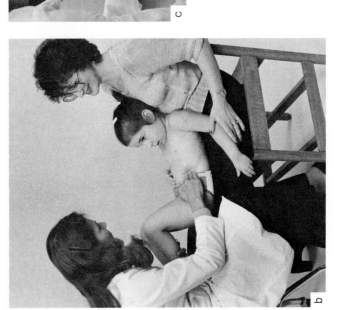

b

A rectal examination is usually not performed in preschoolers.

Internal vaginal examinations are not routinely done on preschoolers.

The nurse should wash his or her hands after touching the genitalia.

Auscultation

The nurse should auscultate the abdomen for bowel sounds prior to palpation (a). Bowel sounds should be heard in all four quadrants.

Rectum and Anus

Palpation

Usually in young children a rectal examination is not performed, unless there is a parental concern, or specific indication. It is a source of discomfort and may result in an upset child. The anus can be observed while examining the genitalia.

Genitalia

If the bladder was palpated in the abdominal examination, the nurse should allow the child time to go to the bathroom prior to the genital examination. This will help the child to be more relaxed. The genitals of both males and females should be examined in a matter-of-fact way, but rapidly.

Inspection

In female preschoolers the external genital area, including the clitoris, the labia minora and majora, the vaginal and urethral orifices, and the external inguinal rings, should be examined primarily by observation (b). The labia should be spread apart and the nurse should observe the color, condition, and size of structures. Adhesions, discharges, skin discoloration, and signs of irritation should be noted. The child may assist by using her finger to spread the labia. No internal vaginal examination is done on a preschool female. The vaginal opening should be observed without the use of instruments. Occasionally, due to poor hygiene or falls, the vaginal opening may be adhered shut. This condition requires referral, preferably to a pediatric gynecologist.

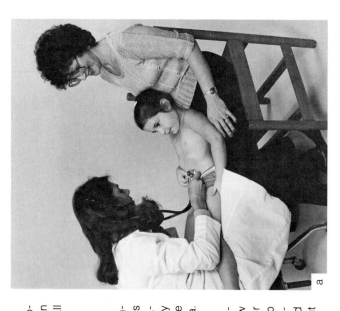

a

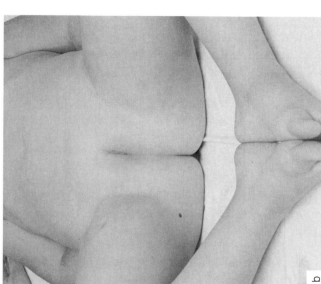

b

Hydroceles, or the accumulation of serous fluid in the testes, often occurs suddenly between 2 and 5 years old.

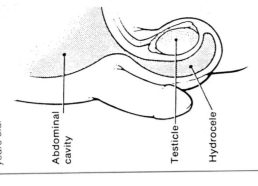

Abdominal cavity

Testicle

Hydrocele

In male preschoolers the external genital area, including the penis, testes, and external rings, should be examined carefully and the condition of structures noted (a). Hydroceles and testicular descent should be checked for and noted.

Head, Hair, and Face

Inspection

By now the child should be comfortable with the nurse, and the examination of the head, hair, and face will be less upsetting. Fortunately, the preschool child is usually very cooperative.

The hair on the head should be shiny and clean, not dry and brittle (b and c). It should cover the entire head. Hair is present on the rest of the body in varying amounts. The hair on the legs and the arms will become more obvious during the preschool years. It should be evenly distributed. Excessive hair and tufts of hair on the spinal or sacral areas should be noted.

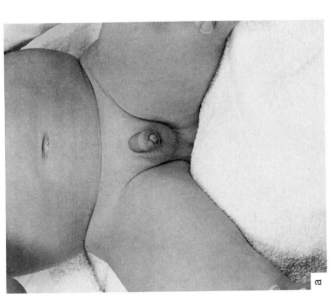

a

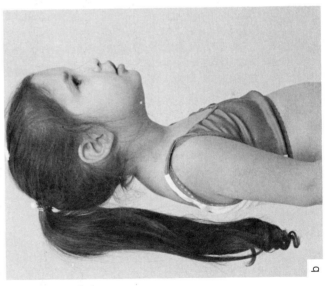

b

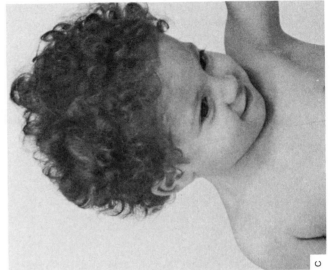

c

Some minor facial anomalies may be noted in normal children.

Growth of the head and brain is monitored by measuring head circumference.

Bruits are adventitious sounds of venous or arterial origin.

The scalp should be examined closely for condition and cleanliness. Note any discolorations or scars.

The general appearance of the face should be noted (for example, bright, alert, happy) as well as the symmetry of the facial features (a). The face should be observed for any minor anomalies such as hypertelorism (wide-set eyes), hypotelorism (close-set eyes), synophrys (fusing of eyebrows), and low-set ears. Minor anomalies can be found in normal children, and are often familial.

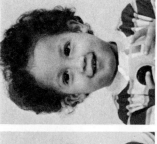
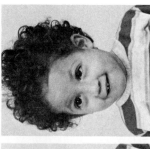
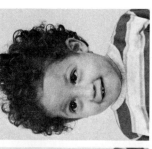
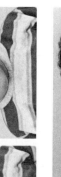
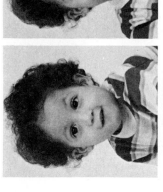
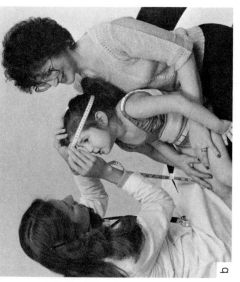

Palpation
The nurse should monitor the growth of the head by measuring its circumference. The tape should be placed around the occipital area and the glabella. This size in centimeters should be plotted on a growth chart (b).

Percussion
If the head is percussed, the sound will be flat.

Auscultation
Systolic or continuous bruits may be auscultated over the temporal areas in normal children.

Eyes

Inspection

Both the structural components and the functional capacity of the eyes should be examined. The structural components include the lids, eyelashes, tear ducts and glands, conjunctiva, sclera, cornea, pupil, and lens (a). The examination of the external structures (the iris, pupil, conjunctiva, etc.) is like that of an adult. Epicanthal folds may be present and be normal.

The examination of the internal eye, the funduscopic examination, may be difficult to accomplish in the preschooler. The red reflex should first be observed. Then, depending on the child's ability to hold the eyes still and the nurse's skill with the ophthalmoscope, the fundus should be observed (b). To facilitate this portion of the examination, the room should be darkened. The door to the room can be open slightly for both the child's and the nurse's benefit. The nurse should have the child look at a picture, perhaps of an animal, across the room. The funduscopic examination, otherwise, is like that of an adult. It should be noted, however, that the funduscopic examination of the young child may require dilation of the pupils.

To examine the functional capacity of the eyes, the nurse should assess visual acuity with the Snellen E test (c). The pupillary light reflex test, Hirschberg's test, and the cover test should be used to assess the eyes for strabismus. Cranial nerves IV and VI are assessed in the child as in the adult (see Chap. 4).

Refer to Chap. 4, for the examination of the eyes.

A funduscopic examination should be done on the preschooler.

The examiner can use parts of the Denver Eye Screening Test (in the Appendix) during physcial examination of the eye.

Dilation of the pupils is usually done by an ophthalmologist.

Refer to Chap. 7, for a description of Hirschberg's test and the cover test.

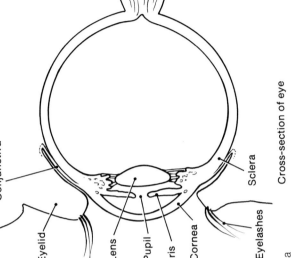

Conjunctiva

Eyelid

Lens

Pupil

Iris

Cornea

Sclera

Eyelashes

Cross-section of eye

a

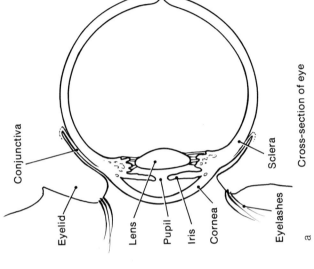

b

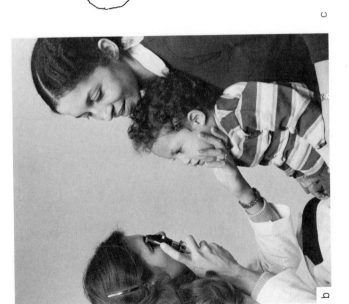

c

The preschooler may resist the otoscopic exam, therefore, positioning is important.

For the otoscopic examination, the nurse should use the largest speculum possible, to improve vision.

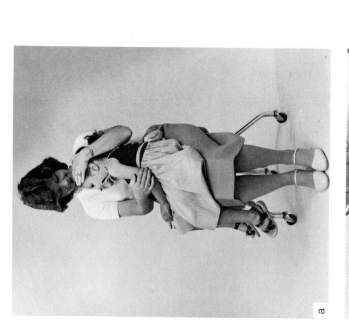

a

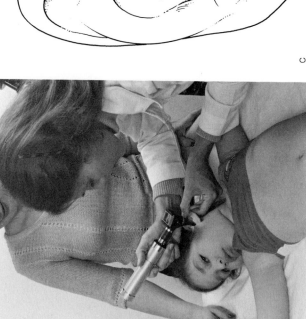

b

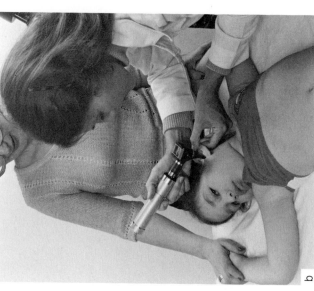

External auditory canal

c

Ears

Inspection

The nurse should examine the ear for structure and for functional capacity. The external ear should be observed for location and intactness. To examine the internal ear the nurse needs the cooperation of the child. Preschool children may react with fear to this portion of the examination and need reassurance. The parent may be able to assist in holding the child. A good position is to have the parent sit on a chair and hold the child with one side of his head against the parent's chest (a). The parent should hold the head in place while the nurse examines one ear. This prevents trauma from the speculum. If the child still resists, the nurse may need to use a more involved restraining procedure than is usually needed for preschoolers (see Chap. 7).

The nurse should use the largest speculum possible and enter the canal to a depth of one-fourth to one-half inch. Since the canal faces down and forward, the auricle should be pulled up and back so that the canal can be seen (b). This movement should be painless. The tympanic membrane in the preschooler, unlike in the infant, is vertical and slanted away from the examiner (c). The mobility of the tympanic membrane can be checked by insufflation. If the membrane does not move, there is probably fluid behind it. White opacities on the tympanic membrane may be a result of old infections.

A curette or irrigation can be used to remove cerumen from the ear canal.

The procedure for irrigating the ear canal must be carefully followed.

If there is cerumen blocking the ear canal, the examiner should remove it by using a curette or by irrigation. These methods should be used only if necessary. When the curette is used, the child must be restrained on the table. The curette is inserted through the head of the otoscope and then into the ear (a). Since the blood vessels and nerves are close to the surface of the skin in the canal, it is likely that blood and pain will accompany this procedure.

Irrigation of the ear canal should only be used if the nurse is sure the tympanic membrane is intact. The nurse will need the child's cooperation for this procedure. A syringe is used to squirt warm water slowly into the ear canal. The water should be directed toward the superoposterior wall of the canal (b). The nurse should be aware that this procedure can cause the child to become dizzy, especially if the water is not warm enough. A kidney basin should be used to collect the water that drains out of the ear. This procedure is time-consuming (about 20 minutes per ear) and it is messy. The nurse should remember to drape the child with towels to prevent the child from getting wet.

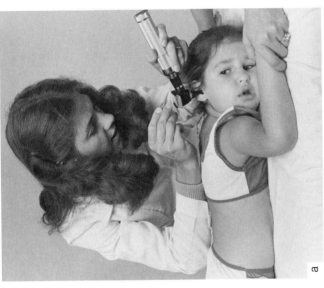

a

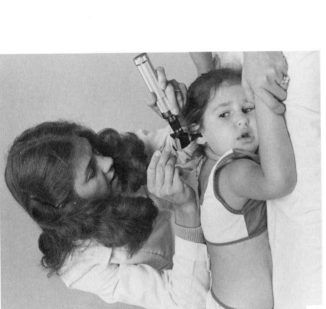

Cerumen

Syringe

b

Palpation

The nurse should palpate behind the ear for the postauricular nodes (a). Nodes 1 to 2 mm in diameter are normal.

The nurse should consider vestibular function testing only if nystagmus (oscillating movements of the eyes) or an unsteady gait are found.

Nose and Sinus

Inspection

The nose should be observed for both structure and function. A speculum is not usually necessary for this part of the examination but can be used. The nurse should gently push up and back on the tip of the nose to expose the nares. A short, broad speculum should be inserted into the rim of the nares (b) so that the nurse can view the septum, mucosa, turbinates, vestibule, and the meatuses. The examination is similar to the adult's (see Chap. 4).

A common problem in this age group is foreign bodies, such as crayons, beads, etc., in the nose. The nurse should carefully observe the nose for such objects.

Percussion

As in adults, percussion of the child's maxillary (c) and ethmoid sinuses should not cause pain. The frontal sinuses, however, are not usually developed in the child until 5 to 8 years of age.

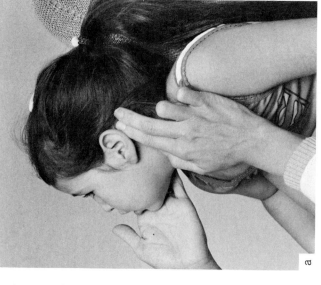

a

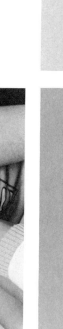

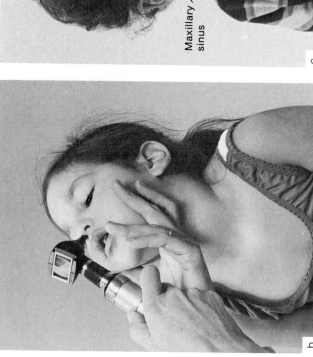

Maxillary sinus

b

c

A common problem among preschoolers is the placement of foreign bodies into the nares.

A short broad speculum can be placed on the otoscope for visualization of the nares.

Mouth

Inspection

When examining the mouth of a preschooler, the nurse should avoid using a tongue blade, if at all possible. The child should be sitting with the head slightly tilted back, mouth open, and tongue slightly protruding. If the child will say "Aaah," the pharynx will be more visible (a). If the nurse is unable to see the posterior portion of the mouth, a tongue blade may be needed to hold the tongue down. An uncooperative child will need to be restrained. It may be helpful if the nurse demonstrates this procedure on a parent or on a toy before attempting it on the preschooler.

The nurse should evaluate the condition and number of teeth, as well as the occlusion of and spacing between the teeth (b). The child should have a complete set of 20 primary teeth (c). At the end of the preschool era, the child will begin to lose the primary teeth. The nurse should observe for caries and the cleanliness of the child's teeth. Normally, the teeth should be white.

A preschool child should be brushing all the teeth every day, and this should be apparent on examination.

Highlights

When examining the mouth, the use of a tongue blade should be avoided if possible.

The preschooler should have a complete set of 20 primary teeth.

The nurse should assess the preschooler's ability to clean the teeth by brushing. The child's teeth should be flossed by a parent.

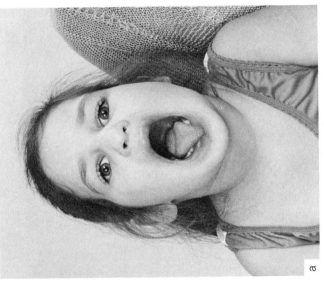

a

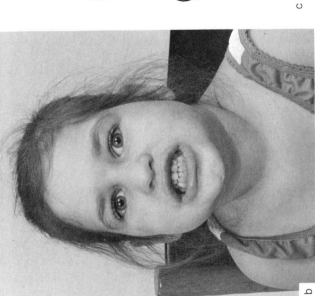

b

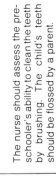

Central incisor
Lateral incisor
Cuspid
First molar
Second molar

Maxilla

Mandible

c

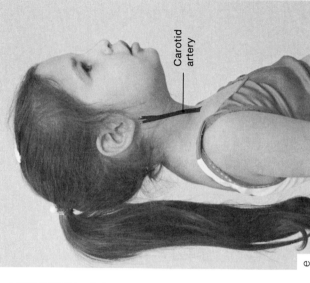

Examination of the thyroid gland may be completed by using one of two methods described here.

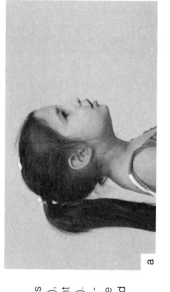

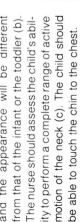

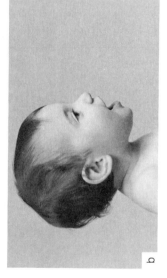

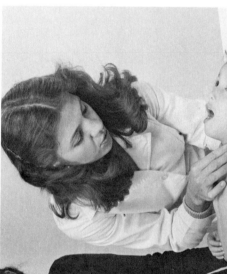

Neck and Throat

Inspection

The neck lengthens around 3 to 4 years of age as a result of vertebral growth (a), and the appearance will be different from that of the infant or the toddler (b). The nurse should assess the child's ability to perform a complete range of active motion of the neck (c). The child should be able to touch the chin to the chest.

Palpation

Lymph nodes in the cervical area may be palpable but should not be greater than 1 cm in diameter.

The trachea should palpated and will be slightly to the right of the midline.

Although difficult to palpate in children in this age group, the thyroid can be assessed in one of two ways. The child can be supine and the nurse can palpate the thyroid with the thumb and first two fingers (d). The second alternative is to have the child sitting, and to examine the thyroid from behind as in the adult (see Chap. 4).

Auscultation

The nurse should auscultate for murmurs over the carotid area and assess the status of all the neck vessels (e).

Extremities

Inspection

This part of the examination is usually fun for the preschooler, and most children will be very cooperative. First, the child's posture should be observed (a). Pay special attention to the configuration and mobility of the back. The extremities should be observed for structure, alignment, and condition.

The child's gait should be observed carefully, as this is a good indicator of cerebellar function (b). For further assessment of cerebellar function the nurse can observe the child's tandem walking, running, walking on toes and heels, and hopping. Rapid movement and point-to-point tasks, also indicative of cerebellar function, are performed by the preschooler in an awkward manner.

Knock-knee, or genu valgum, can occur between 2 and 6 years of age. The nurse should pay special attention to this on the preschool examination, and note its presence.

Palpation

The bones should be palpated for tenderness and nodules. The joints should be assessed for mobility, and the muscles for mass, tone, and strength.

Perhaps the most important reflex to test is the knee jerk or patellar reflex (c). This will give a good indication of the child's reflex function. Although the upper extremity reflexes should also be tested, the reflex response is often difficult to assess. Thus, it is not always a reliable index.

By preschool age the Babinski reflex should no longer be elicited; the flaring of the toes is replaced by the grasping motion of the toes (d).

The preschooler enjoys demonstrating strength in the use of the extremities.

Cerebellar function is assessed when examining the extremities.

The motor examination is like that of the adult.

The patellar reflex is the most important reflex to elicit in the preschooler.

See Tables 8-5 and 8-6 for Diagnostic Tests.

THE PRESCHOOLER

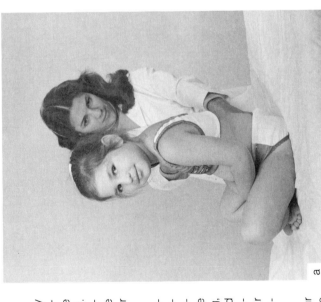

a

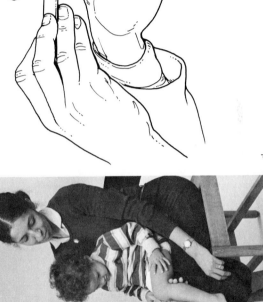

b

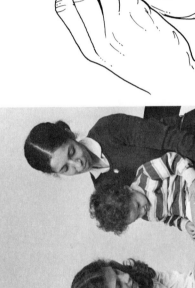

c

d

THE SCHOOL-AGED CHILD CHAPTER NINE

Gladys M. Scipien, Marilyn A. Chard, and Dorothy A. Jones*

THE HEALTH HISTORY

The school-age years, or middle childhood (ages 6 to 12), is a critical stage in psychosocial, cognitive, and physical development. It is a period of time often ignored or overlooked by adults in general and health care providers in particular. Perhaps the reason for this neglect can be found in the fact that the school-aged child is becoming more self-sufficient and requires less time and attention than were necessary during the preschool years.

However, the school-aged child is entering a crucial period of growth and development. While the family is being pushed away, the child is busy cultivating friendships and nurturing loyalties. Life is exciting, and personal experiences can promote self-esteem, provide innumerable opportunities for healthy and successful peer-adult interactions, and encourage participation in a myriad of new learning activities. The importance of middle childhood cannot be minimized, because the adjustments a child makes during this time will have a lifelong effect on his or her performance and perception of self.

The school-aged child (ages 6 to 12) is involved in a highly active period of psychosocial, physical, and emotional growth.

Setting

Data gathering from the school-aged child may take place in a variety of settings: home, hospital in-patient unit, hospital out-patient department, neighborhood health clinic, health maintenance organization, private office, or school. Regardless of the setting, the same components that make up the client-nurse dialogue described in Chap. 3 play a part here.

Approach to the Client

By age 7, the child begins to engage in logical thinking and can focus on a particular topic. These skills increase with age. Therefore, the child can be asked to express personal thoughts and opinions about a particular issue or health problem during the interview. Subjective information may be obtained from both parent and child, but it is the child who can best express his or her own perceptions of the reason for coming to the health care facility.

Establishing a data base for the school-aged child is made easier by the individual's improved cognitive skills and use of language.

Questions to elicit data

1 What did your mother (father) tell you about coming here?
2 How do you feel about being here?
3 Some boys (girls) who have this problem think .... Does that make sense to you?

*Contribution to Chapter Nine made by Dorothy A. Jones, R.N., M.S.N., F.A.A.N.

A particular experience and the nature of symptoms can be explained by the child, who can be asked to identify possible causes of the symptoms or worries. He or she can also judge the extent to which a problem has interfered with school attendance or other activities. Whatever information is elicited from the child should be taken seriously, so that trust can be built and maintained.

Because the child may be fearful of the encounter with the nurse, it is important to create an environment in which the child feels safe. Use of a preferred name or nickname may help to diminish tension. Also helpful to the child at this time is the assurance that his or her emotions and feelings are normal. A comment such as "Many boys and girls find coming to the hospital a little frightening. What about you?" from the examiner, will allow the child an opportunity to react honestly without fear of criticism.

Creating a secure environment for the child will improve the quality of the nurse-client interaction.

While the child should be encouraged to verbalize, the parents will also continue to provide information. When interviewing the child in the parent's presence, the nurse can also assess parent-child interactions. Some indications of parent-child conflicts can be ascertained through noting whether or not the parent allows the child to speak without additions, interruptions, or correction of the narrative.

When possible, the child should be asked to respond to questions. Parental responses are also important during this age period.

Entry into the Health Care System

There are approximately 55 million school-aged children in the United States, and 7 million of them have never visited a health care facility (office, clinic, or hospital), except on an emergency basis.[1] That is an astounding statistic, and it graphically points to the great need for determining the overall health of many children whose status is otherwise unassessed.

While health promotion is important for the school-aged child, over 7 million children in the United States have never visited a health care facility.

For the school-aged child who does receive such attention, entry into the health care system may occur through a routine physical, a camp or school physical, or during treatment for an accident or for more acute health problems.

School Health Care

Collecting initial baseline data concerning physical, developmental, and emotional growth for appraisal of the school-aged child is important. All children may not be brought to health care facilities, but all do attend school and hence are available there for health assessments, screening programs, and health education. Thus the needed population is most readily available through school health care facilities. All data should be collected annually so that the individual's progress can be monitored and actual or potential health problems can be identified. The nurse can also consult with parents as needed. Such information sharing can enhance a child's potential, facilitate adjustment to school, and permit optimal functioning within the prescribed health parameters.

Entrance to the health care system for the school-aged child occurs for a variety of reasons, including annual physicals, camp physicals, and acute or chronic problems.

School health records become very important for the child, in that they permit progress through the school years to be carefully monitored, and actual or potential problems quickly identified.

Special attention can also be directed through these appraisals to children with handicaps and chronic illnesses. In addition, school health maintenance offers the nurse opportunities to teach health principles which can foster the child's proper development and help him or her to formulate a concept of health which can have a lifelong influence. Instruction in personal and dental hygiene, nutritional practices, and accident prevention, as well as in strategies to optimize wellness, can have far-reaching effects on the impressionable school-aged child.

Client Profile and Biographical Data

There are various methods available for recording demographic data regarding the child's overall health profile. These methods provide the

Figure 9-1 Essential components of the school-age child profile.

Client Profile and Biographical Data

Date of interview _____

Name _____ Nickname _____

Date of Birth _____ Place of birth _____

Age _____ Sex M F Race/Nationality _____ Religion _____

Parents' names _____

Address _____

_____

Telephone number _____

Current Health Status

_____

_____

Past Health Status

Prenatal (list trimester)

_____ bleeding _____ illness _____ injury _____ infection _____ hypertension

_____ toxemia _____ medication _____ drugs (including alcohol) _____ smoking habits

Intrapartum

Length of labor _____ Type of delivery _____

Birth experience _____

Birth weight _____ Birth length _____

Birth head circumference _____ Apgar score _____

Neonatal

_____ jaundice _____ cyanosis _____ infection _____ respiratory difficulty

Developmental milestones (list age)

sitting alone _____ walking alone _____ first word _____

use of complete sentences _____ use of tricycle _____

List parental concerns _____

_____

Serious illness and hospitalization (age, place, healthcare provider)

_____

Accidents and/or injuries (what and when)

_____

Allergies (what and reaction)

_____

Travel (where and when)

_____

Immunizations (date or age)

DPT _____ 1 _____ 2 _____ 3 _____ B _____ B

Polio _____ 1 _____ 2 _____ 3 _____ B _____ B

dT _____   _____

MMR _____

Other

Childhood diseases (state age)

measles _____   mumps _____   hepatitis _____   strep. throat _____

German measles _____   chicken pox _____   scarlet fever _____

Screening tests	Dates	Results
Vision	_____	_____
Hearing	_____	_____
Urinalysis	_____	_____
Testuria	_____	_____
CBC	_____	_____
Reticulocyte count	_____	_____
Developmental tests	_____	_____
Last tuberculin test	_____	_____

Family history

	Age	Height	Weight	Education	Occupation	Health	If deceased, age and cause
Mother	—	—	—	—	—	—	—
Father	—	—	—	—	—	—	—
Siblings	—	—	—	—	—	—	—
MGM	—	—	—	—	—	—	—
MGF	—	—	—	—	—	—	—
Maternal aunts	—	—	—	—	—	—	—
Maternal uncles	—	—	—	—	—	—	—
PGM	—	—	—	—	—	—	—
PGF	—	—	—	—	—	—	—
Paternal aunts	—	—	—	—	—	—	—
Paternal uncles	—	—	—	—	—	—	—

Social history

Grade in school _____ School performance _____

Temperament _____

Friends _____

Interests _____

Typical day (include eating, elimination, and sleeping patterns; hobbies; TV viewing; school; play)

_____

_____

Discipline _____

Support systems _____

Family interactions _____

Culture _____

Religion _____

Review of components (same as in adults)

_____

_____

nurse with an opportunity to establish a data base that can be added to, transferred, and easily summarized throughout the individual's life. Use of the computerized record will facilitate this process. Reference to Fig. 9-1 and Chap. 3 will help to provide the reader with guidelines for data collection about the client profile and biographical data.

Figure 9-1 provides an overview of the components of the client profile of the school-aged child.

Health Perception/Health Management

The child's process of socialization gains momentum at the time he or she enters school. Generally, a child's health attitudes and health-seeking behaviors are formed before adolescence (refer to Fig. 9-1).

Current Health Status

Values and beliefs which influence a child's health habits are largely determined by the family. Parents' attitudes toward health are observed by the child. What parents do when they are ill, the use of home remedies and folk medicines, nutritional practices in the home, frequency of exercise and planned activity, and other such health behaviors significantly influence the school-aged child. Habits established during these years will often affect the level of wellness achieved as the individual moves toward adulthood.

Parents' attitudes toward health and wellness influence how the child will value health.

The early school years furnish the nurse with a prime opportunity to influence health-seeking behaviors and to assist the child in formulating and internalizing a personal concept of wellness.

Past Health Status

The child's prenatal, intrapartum, and neonatal history, as well as all developmental milestones, are of particular importance in assessing the school-aged client. Health problems already identified, as well as potential ones, can often be isolated in this way. Such problems can be of particular significance in growth and development during the middle childhood and adolescent years. (See Fig. 9-1 for identification of components to consider when reviewing the past history of the school-aged child.)

Birth history should be included when assessing the school-aged child.

Screening

Screening is a basic ingredient of prevention. Testing at school-entry level makes it possible to identify previously unknown physical problems, and it is therefore imperative to establish screening programs for the detection and confirmation of such problems. In certain situations, a health problem which could result in a permanent impairment (e.g., deafness) can be identified. Screening procedures also allow for early discov-

Screening is the basic ingredient for promoting wellness in the school-aged child.

Table 9-1
Methods of Tuberculin Skin Testing

Test	Method of administration	Reading time interval	Results
Heaf gun	Heaf gun injects concentrated purified protein derivative (PPD) with 6 simultaneous punctures, 1 mm in depth	3–7 days	Presence of 4 or more papules, positive
Tine test	Four tines predipped in old tuberculin (OT) are pressed into the skin	48–72 hours	One or more papules 2 mm or larger, positive

ery of other conditions which can be treated effectively or stabilized (e.g., impaired vision). Although some health problems may not be present during one examination, they can emerge at a later time.

Both time and cost should be primary considerations in setting up screening programs, and testing procedures which are inexpensive and easy to perform should be used. The programs should be devised so as to allow large numbers of children to be tested, yet yield very few false positive results, which would necessitate additional examinations.

Procedures used to detect active tuberculosis such as the Heaf gun and Tine tests are simple to use, relatively inexpensive, and reliable. They should be performed on all children during the first year of school and annually thereafter on those children who come from a community whose population has a positive reaction rate in excess of 1 percent; otherwise, tuberculin tests should be done every 3 years.[2]

Some states require skin testing of all children in certain grades. Surely the prevalence of tuberculosis is incentive enough for rigidly adhering to such screening policies. (See Table 9-1 for a more detailed presentation of testing procedures.)

Visual and hearing screening should also be conducted during the early school years. These tests are discussed later in this chapter in relation to cognitive-perceptual pattern assessment.

Immunization Schedule Normally, immunizations of children are begun in infancy and continued during toddlerhood and the preschool period, with boosters for polio, diphtheria, tetanus, and pertussis given at the time a child starts school. However, in 1976 it was estimated that about 20 million American children, 6 to 14 years of age, were either partially or completely unprotected against these common communicable diseases. This statistic is staggering because 45 states,[3,4] have laws which stipulate that immunizations must be up to date and current when a child enters school. However, school and health officials have been lax, indeed negligent, in enforcing this regulation, and high numbers of immigrants in certain areas of the country make the problem even greater.

Noncompliance has reached incredible proportions, and several factors have contributed to this. One is that there is minimal parental concern regarding these "harmless" diseases, an attitude which may stem from ineffective parent education as well as from a societal consensus that the potent antibiotics currently available are effective in inhibiting serious complications. Another factor in noncompliance is the generally poor record of follow-up visits to physicians' offices and clinics. Regardless of the reasons for the widespread neglect, efforts need to be directed toward enforcing state health regulations concerning immunizations now and in the future.

Tuberculin testing should be conducted during the first year of school, annually thereafter in children living in areas where incidence of tuberculosis is high, and every 3 years in the remaining population.

Refer to Table 9-1 for methods of tuberculin testing.

Careful evaluation of a child's immunization record is important prior to entry into school.

Today there is a high incidence of noncompliance in meeting immunization schedules.

Table 9-2
Primary Immunization Schedule

Highlights

First visit	Td*, TOPV†, tuberculin test
Intervals after initial visit	
1 month	Measles, mumps, rubella
2 months	Td*, TOPV†
8–14 months	Td*, TOPV†

*Tetanus and diphtheria toxoid (adult type)—After the age of 14, Td should be repeated every 10 years. If an injury which is minor and clean should occur, no booster is needed by a child whose immunization schedule is complete, unless more than 10 years have passed. If the wound is contaminated and 5 years have passed since the child's last dose, then a booster should be administered.
†Trivalent oral polio vaccine
Source: Adapted from Jarvis, L.: "Childhood Immunizations," *School Age Child, Issues in Comprehensive Pediatric Nursing,* **3**(3):50 (September 1978). Used with permission.

Children 6 years old or over who were not immunized in infancy, or whose programs were interrupted, must begin new schedules. The modified primary immunization schedule devised by the American Academy of Pediatrics is found in Table 9-2. But immunization practices change, and the schedule requires frequent evaluation. The continued monitoring of children is crucial in providing the protection that is available to them. Such protection is assured when the nurse assumes responsibility for diligently assessing every child's immunization record annually.

Refer to Table 9-2 for a list of required immunizations.

Family History

The family history of the school-age child is collected as described in Chapter 3. The nurse must ask the parent(s) to recall relevant information about both maternal and paternal relatives.

Life Patterns and Life Styles

The school-aged child is experiencing part of a life process which supports growth and contributes to the evolution of life patterns. Life for the school-aged child follows a pattern of freedom and exploration. For many, it is a time of minimal responsibility and demand. Activities that contribute to the process of development vary from year to year and ultimately affect the adolescent and adulthood years.

For many, middle childhood is a time for freedom and exploration.

Age

The school-age period is for many, a time of great change. Children in this age group encounter many experiences that affect their physical, emotional, and social growth. While the physical changes are slower and are more gradual than in preschool years, they are still affecting body size as well as facial contour. Great strides are evident in cognitive development and the emergence of conceptual thought.

Certain developmental tasks are mastered between ages 6 to 9. There are specific characteristics that typify each year, and these observed behaviors confirm the rapid developmental changes.

At *6 years of age,* for example, boys and girls play together. Children engage in loud, boisterous activity, and they appear to be in constant motion. Gross motor skills (running, jumping, hopping, etc.) are refined; fine motor abilities lag behind but will improve in the classroom setting. Children of this age start projects enthusiastically and almost never finish them. Egocentrism is evident in all their interactions, but they possess very positive attitudes toward the world and the people in it. Six-year-olds are lovable, charming, and innocent.

Table 3-3 and Fig. 3-2 should be used to complete the family history.

Six-year-olds are loud, energetic, active. They are refining gross motor skills as well as fine motor abilities.

At *age 7,* an assimilation and internalization of prior experiences result in the child's growing quieter, and activities, which reflect a year spent in school, are more cognitive in nature. While 7-year-olds are polite, courteous, and sensitive to others, they tolerate criticism and teasing poorly. They develop more persistent work habits in the classroom setting; they become aware of the fact that they are being evaluated. They are now anxious to please, and they exhibit a more cooperative spirit in activities with their peers.

Eight-year-olds are active and gregarious children who have thoughts on everything and advice for everyone. The question "Why?" characterizes this insatiably curious year. Collecting all sorts of items occupies their time, and friends who are of the same sex are now becoming more important. It is a year when children begin to realize their parents are not perfect, and school takes on a social focus.

With the *9-year-old,* there is increasing refinement of behavior. The self-confidence which began to emerge in the previous year continues to increase as a result of sustained involvement with peers in a variety of organizational activities. This year is full of group endeavors such as Scouting and Little League. Maturity allows children to recognize their own faults and weaknesses now, and they begin to accept responsibility as well as blame for their actions. There is a "best friend" by this time, and while the peer group remains important, the child realizes that the group evaluates him or her as a person. Typically, the 9-year-old is more independent, more self-directed, and more highly motivated by self-interest than by a sense of obligation.

The *10-year-old* reaches a period of calm which often brings contentment with the world. This peace is reflected in a personal sense of well-being and self-confidence. This age group is peer-oriented, and group norms take on great importance. Secret codes and "private" clubs are formed, and admission to the group is selective. The individual tends to be curious, cooperative, and loyal to peers. The ability to reason is increased, and communication between the child and parent is positive.

The *11- to 12-year-old* is reaching adolescence. During this period the individual becomes more critical of authority, and conflicts with parent figures are not uncommon. The child is often moody, at times unreasonable, loyal to peers, and often struggling with sexual identity. It is a time of physical growth, bringing greater need for independence and a new sense of self-identity.

Race and Heredity

The importance of a child's race and genetic endowments cannot be overlooked. Specific health practices, as well as predisposition to particular health problems, can be influenced by racial inheritance. Other genetic factors (discussed in Chaps. 5 and 6) can also influence the school-aged child's development. Much of the discussion that follows will reflect the unique contributions of race and inheritance to the general health status of the school-aged child. Specific questions used to elicit data in this pattern area can be found in Chaps. 3, 5, and 6.

Culture

For the school-aged child, cultural background and family social position can dramatically affect lifestyle. The school one attends, peer group selection, club membership, and social status are influenced by one's cultural background. Because parents are often the child's role model, cultural practices, customs, rituals, and beliefs are valued and continued. Often, these practices are rejected during the adolescent period as the child begins to sort out and clarify values.

The 7-year-old is quiet in activities, courteous, sensitive to others, and anxious to please.

The 8-year-old is active and gregarious and questions everything. Collecting items is important, as is affiliation with children of the same sex.

The 9-year-old child becomes more self-confident, participates more actively in groups, and is more highly motivated by self-interest.

The 10-year-old is peaceful and content with self. He or she is peer-oriented and group norms take on importance.

The 11 to 12 year-old child becomes more critical of authority, and conflicts with parents arise.

Reference to genetic endowment is an important part of a data base. Frequently, genetic alterations may manifest themselves during the early school years.

Culture can affect the child's lifestyle and can influence peer group selections, social status, and opportunities for future development.

Culture also has a significant impact on the parenting practices that influence the growth and development of children. Frequently, the degree to which a child achieves certain goals is seen by the cultural group as a reflection of "good" or "bad" parenting. For example, in some cultures stoutness in a child is valued, and a youngster's sturdy build reflects to the credit of the parents who provide so well, even though the child's nutritional habits may be directed toward overeating patterns which will be difficult to break as he or she ages.

The importance of one's cultural background, therefore, cannot be underestimated. Questions presented in Chap. 3 under this pattern area should be included and elaborated upon in building the school-aged child's data base. Of particular importance to histories of children in this age group are questions which will evoke from the parents their individual parenting practices.

Highlights

Culture has an important influence on child-rearing practices. Within many cultures judgments as to whether the parents are "good" or "bad" are based on the child's physical and emotional growth patterns.

Questions to elicit data

1 Are there any particular customs that you routinely utilize to maintain your own health?
2 What do you do when your child becomes ill?
3 Are there particular child-rearing practices unique to your culture?
4 How do you discipline your children?

Growth and Development

A developmental assessment is critical in determining whether a child is able to perform a variety of tasks which he or she is expected to master at a specific age. Testing in these tasks takes a very different form when the nurse works with a school-aged child. For instance, assessing the ability of a 6-month-old infant to sit without assistance is easily accomplished. However, there are many variables which affect the performance of a child between 6 and 12 years of age. In testing children of this age group, it is important to remember that (1) no single testing tool is an adequate measurement and (2) the test score reflects a child's performance of specific skills and tasks on one specific day.

In assessing a child's growth and development it is important to remember that (1) no single testing tool is an adequate measurement and (2) the test score reflects a child's performance of specific skills and tasks on one specific day.

Physical and Mental Development In examining Table 9-3 it will become apparent that while gross and fine motor skills are being assessed, language and cognition, which should advance at a rapid rate after 2 years of age, are also being evaluated. These motor skills tests serve several purposes. For example, while the Goodenough-Harris Drawing Test assesses overall development, it also provides an index of self- and social awareness. The Peabody Picture Vocabulary Test (PPVI), the Developmental Test of Visual-Motor Integration (VMI), and the Wide Range Achievement Test (WRAT) can identify sensory problems and perceptual or learning disabilities, while the Denver Developmental Screening Test (DDST), and the Slosson Intelligence Test (SIT) are useful in documenting delays in development. In addition, it is important for the nurse examiner to recognize that physical growth occurs in spurts, with the most pronounced period of growth coming toward the end of middle childhood (10 to 12 years of age). See Table 9-4 for normative growth rates.

Refer to Table 9-3 for a list of developmental tests used with the school-aged child. Examples of these tests included in the appendices.

Table 9-4 presents physical growth norms.

Behavioral Development

There are major developmental changes which occur in children between the ages of 6 and 12 years, and all of them influence and affect subsequent development. The theme of this period is mastery. Prime inter-

Table 9-3
Selected Instruments Used To Test Development

Instrument	Age/Years	Areas sampled	Administration time
Denver Developmental Screening Test (DDST)	0–6	Gross and fine motor skills; personal/social; language	10–25 minutes
Slosson Intelligence Test (SIT)	0–adult	Gross and fine motor skills; language; cognitive development; mental age; IQ	15–30 minutes
Peabody Picture Vocabulary Test (PPVT)	2–adult	Language; cognitive development; mental age; IQ	10–15 minutes
Developmental Test of Visual-Motor Integration (VMI)	2–15	Gross and fine motor skills; cognitive development	1–10 minutes
Goodenough-Harris Drawing Test	3–15	Gross and fine motor skills; cognitive development	5 minutes
Verbal Language Development Scale (VLDS)	0–15	Language and language age	5–10 minutes
Wide Range Achievement Test (WRAT)	5–adult	Gross and fine motor skills; achievement readiness	10–20 minutes

Source: Adapted from Robert A. Hoekelman *et al., Principles of Pediatrics,* McGraw-Hill, 1978, p. 205. Used with permission.

Table 9-4
Normative, Heights and Weights for Boys and Girls at Ages 6 through 12

	Age 6	Age 7	Age 8	Age 9	Age 10	Age 11	Age 12
Male height (mean cm)	110.4	115.5	120.0	124.5	129.4	134.6	138.0
Female height (mean cm)	108.3	113.5	119.2	124.2	129.6	135.1	139.6
Male weight (mean kg)	17.4	19.4	21.3	23.5	25.5	28.8	31.7
Female weight (mean kg)	16.4	18.7	20.8	22.8	24.8	28.6	31.2

Source: Adapted from G. M. Scipien *et al.* (eds.), *Comprehensive Pediatric Nursing,* McGraw Hill 1979, p. 262. Used with permission.

ests turn from the family to peers and teachers; this maturational process widens experimental horizons and increases social contacts. Conflicts arise because the child wishes to remain in the childhood period while seeking adult status.

School is an exciting adventure, but it also precipitates fear in some children. Adjusting to new authority figures, participating in large groups, establishing new routines, and accepting restrictions on activities can create tension for the child. Parental separation of major proportion is another crisis for some children. Leaving the familiar and secure environment of the home can have a substantial impact on a 6-year-old child; however, the process can be facilitated through a parent's understanding and encouragement.

Learning, which had its beginning within the home, now continues on a much grander scale for the child. Attending school enhances the child's acquisition of more independence, which is essential for coping with the world at large. In essence, it is in the school environment that the child learns to reconcile innermost needs with the situations of life.

According to Erickson, middle childhood is the period of *industry* vs. *inferiority,* a stage when it is essential for the child to develop a sense of industriousness rather than of inadequacy. Obviously, it is necessary for children to master certain competencies and skills which will subsequently influence their overall development. It is essential for all children to conscientiously explore new aspects of life, especially school-related endeavors, in order to gain the mastery and enjoy the success of such pursuits. Yet, in pursuing each opportunity for success the child also risks discouragement and failure. These experiences with success and failure influence a child's level of aspiration and also affect the sense of self-esteem. For this reason it is important for the parents or other support groups to provide encouragement for the child, even when performance is not perfect. If the child's motivation is to be sustained, it is important for the adult to realize that it may take some children more time to succeed than others.

Social Capabilities Contact with other children enables the school-aged child to meet many new friends, and these playmates will have a profound effect on growth through the middle years of childhood. Initially, peers serve only as partners in play, with boys and girls participating together; however, during ages 8 and 9, the child generally selects a best friend and moves toward group activities with friends of the same sex. As the child continues to grow, it is the peer group which reinforces appropriate sex-role behaviors; teaches fair play, cooperation, and compromise; facilitates the acquisition of values and attitudes different from those of the family; molds leadership potential; and aids in the development of a self-concept which enhances autonomy. Therefore, acceptance by the group is imperative for healthy growth. Unsuccessful social interactions at this level have further implications. Children who have difficulty in forming peer relationships during this period will no doubt have problems in cultivating future relationships.

Values and Beliefs Development of the superego (consciousness) is a part of social, cognitive, and psychological development of the school-aged child. The younger child is somewhat rigid in following rules, viewing only a "right" and "wrong" way of behaving. The child is somewhat moralistic and quick to condemn the supposed wrong actions of another. Piaget describes this action in terms of moral realism, pointing out that, for them, misdeeds have built-in punishment.

As children age, they become less harsh in their views of their own actions and those of others. Adults can enhance this growth by helping the child view punishment as an action taken because of a deed, not as a judgment of the child's worth per se. Providing the child with fair rules, a good role model, and every opportunity to advance his or her self-concept is important in formulating a child's superego.

Lying According to Prazar,[5] by 6 or 7 years of age "children are aware of the morality of lying and stealing. Although they are quick to accuse peers of cheating and lying, they continue to cheat seemingly guiltlessly in game situations.". The school-aged child may lie in an attempt to test the moral codes imposed by adults. Or the lie can become the child's means of protection if parents place unrealistic expectations on him or her.

Highlights

Erickson describes the stage of development for a school-aged child as *industry* vs. *inferiority.*

Parental support for the child's performance, even when it is not perfect, is essential to sustained motivation and to the child's self-esteem.

Important relationships evolve from "playmate" to "best friend" during the school-age years.

As the child continues to grow, the peer group becomes increasingly important.

Moral realism is the assumption that moral rules exist in their own right.

The younger school-aged child follows rules rigidly. As the individual nears adolescence he or she becomes more lenient.

The school-aged child may lie in order to test moral codes imposed by adults.

Parents are important role models for children. Thus, if parents do not find value in telling the truth, then their children may not value truthfulness. Parental values and expectations, then, as understood by both parents and child, must be elicited before intervention is attempted. Once this information is ascertained, the health care provider can discuss with the parents age-appropriate behaviors and their own importance as role models.

Biological Rhythms

As the child's physical, emotional, and social development progresses, biological rhythms begin to emerge. The patterns established will continue to be refined. Reference to the discussion of biological rhythms found in Chap. 3 will provide additional questions to identify these evolving patterns.

Sleep-Wakefulness Pattern Normally children require an average of 8 to 10 hours of sleep, but this will vary with each individual. During periods of increased physical growth, the need for sleep may increase.

It is not uncommon for interruptions in sleep/rest patterns to occur at this age. Frequently, sleep disturbances are the result of increasing awareness of the concept of death. This knowledge, usually gained through television and books, can be frightening to the child, who views himself or herself as powerless in face of the perceived danger. Preparing the child for sleep in a relaxed manner (e. g., through quiet talking or reading sessions) and establishing bedtime routines (e. g., prayers) may help diminish anxiety. Adults, through their presence and support, can increase the child's own coping resources and help alleviate fears.

Sleep patterns may become disrupted as the child becomes more aware of death and of his or her powerlessness in its presence.

A nightlight may be used to reduce anxiety related to sleep disturbance.

Elimination Patterns Assessment of the school-aged child's elimination patterns is similar to that for the young adult (refer to discussion of elimination patterns in Chap. 3). Suffice it to say that the school-aged child will experience minimal problems with this pattern area, provided there are no health problems, structural defects, or poor self-care habits. Good health habits, including proper hygiene, proper nutrition, and adequate fluid intake, along with the establishment of regular elimination patterns, will help limit health problems for the child.

Refer to Chap. 3 for a complete discussion of elimination patterns.

A midstream, clean-catch urine specimen should be obtained from the child during the yearly examination. The nurse can use a test such as the Bili-Labstix to test for urine pH, protein, glucose, ketones, bilirubin, and blood by dipping a reagent strip, which has a standardized color code, into the urine sample. Readings for the above can be taken within 30 seconds, abnormal values noted, and the child referred to the physician immediately.

School-aged girls have very short urethras and are 10 times more prone to urinary tract infections than males. Testuria, Bac-U-Dip, and Uricult are examples of bactiuric screening measures which should be used to test the urine of school-aged girls at periodic intervals. In addition, teaching the child good hygiene habits, including proper wiping, may help eliminate this specific health problem.

School-aged females have a short urethra and are prone to urinary tract infections. As a result, good hygiene is essential for this age and sex group.

Nocturnal Enuresis The involuntary discharge of urine after age 5 in girls and 6 in boys is termed *enuresis.* Such urination during nighttime sleep is known as *nocturnal enuresis,* while that which occurs in the daytime is called *diurnal enuresis.*[6]

Recent statistics regarding incidence relate to nocturnal enuresis. Cohen[7] reports that "approximately 15 percent of all 5-year-olds, 7 percent of 8-year-olds, and 3 percent of 12-year-olds" are afflicted, while Bindelglass[8] found that 22 percent of 5-year-olds, 10 percent of 10-year-

Involuntary discharge of urine is termed *nocturnal* and *diurnal enuresis.*

olds, and 1 to 2 percent of 20-year-olds have nocturnal enuresis. Both reports support the premise that incidence is age-related. In the absence of urinary tract infection and/or obstructive lesions of the distal outflow in the urinary tract, the assumption is made that children with this problem have a smaller bladder capacity than nonenuretics; that is, adequate neuromuscular control is delayed. A family history of enuresis is a common finding.

A family history of enuresis is a common finding in enuretics.

Subjective data elicited during assessment should include the frequency of the enuresis (e. g., 5 wet nights out of 7); the presence of primary enuresis (the child has never experienced consistent dryness) or secondary enuresis (the child has no enuresis for 3 to 6 months and then relapses); environmental factors affecting the frequency; past and present management techniques and response; effect of enuresis on the child's relationships with family members and peers; past history of neurologic trauma, growth failure, or developmental delays; and a history of toilet-training efforts. A thorough physical examination should be conducted.

For those children whose enuresis is assumed to be associated with delayed neuromuscular control, three modes of treatment are available: drug therapy, conditioning, and bladder training. Imipramine is the most commonly used drug but is only temporary in effect. The urine-alarm apparatus has a higher success rate than imipramine, but initial treatment may take as long as 6 weeks. To date, the most successful modality is the "dry-bed" training reported by Azrin and associates.[9] This treatment[10] involves the use of the urine alarm plus "increased social motivation to be nonenuretic, self-correction of accidents, positive reinforcement for correct toileting, increased intake of fluids, urine inhibition training, training in rapid awakening, and practice in nighttime toileting."[11]

Environmental Factors

The school-aged child can be at risk for all the same environmental health hazards that affect adults. Therefore, questions identified in Chap. 3 in the discussion of environmental factors may be used to assess this area.

Environmental hazards can be particularly noxious to the school-aged child.

In addition, the media have identified several geographic areas of the country (e. g., Love Canal, New York) where environmental hazards have had an especially serious effect on children. The use of specific materials (e. g., lead paints, asbestos) in the home and school has also created problems for the child of school age. Smoking in the home and pollutants in the outside air pose added dangers. It is of critical importance to carefully identify potential or actual environmental sources that can have a serious effect on a child's health and level of wellness and eliminate such hazards where possible.

Economics

The child's economic status has an effect on his or her growth and development. Middle-class and more affluent children are provided with an environment that relieves them of responsibilities and permits them to expand and explore their world freely. They likely have the means to buy needed supplies, to attend social functions, to take advantage of community and cultural resources, and to travel. They also have the luxury to "think about" what they want to be when they grow up and the means to obtain their goals more easily than less privileged children.

Availability of economic resources within the home environment can provide the child with additional opportunities for learning and social interaction.

On the other hand, children from a low socioeconomic background have a greater potential for "delayed language development, and inadequate socialization experiences to facilitate the school-age child's moving into the 'foreign' culture of middle-class schools."[12]

Children from a low socio-economic background may have (1) delayed language development, (2) fewer preschool learning experiences, and (3) inadequate social experiences.

Even when money is available to children from less privileged backgrounds, it is generally used to purchase materials needed immediately. Luxury items and cultural activities are not a financial priority. Frequently, some crisis (e. g., illness) can sabotage any plans for the future and force the family of lower economic status to focus on the "here and now." The children may even be forced to give up school time to help support the family in time of need.

Economics influences the growth and development of the school-aged child in other ways. Children of low income status who are not able to gain approval of accomplishments from adults (who may be out working) may seek the needed approval from peer groups. This can result in negative experiences for the child. The economics of the situation can enhance or detract from the total growth of the child at this period in time. Even opportunities for growth that are available to low-income children thus can remain unused simply because the children are unaware of their existence.

Lack of available resources may mean the child must leave school to help in family support.

Community Resources

Many communities have a number of resources that can be used by the school-aged child. Community agencies such as the YMCA and YWCA offer swimming lessons, courses in safety, and other such activities. Scouts, parent groups, religious groups, boys' and girls' clubs and activities (e. g., Little League baseball), and other community projects (e. g., Head Start) provide opportunities for children regardless of race, color, creed, and economic status.

Numerous community resources can contribute to a child's development through the school years.

Parents as well as children need to be made aware of the resources within their community, for such resources can provide opportunities for the child to increase knowledge, social skills, and language ability, while developing fine motor movements and muscle strength.

Utilization of community resources provides the school-aged child with many opportunities for physical and psychosocial growth.

Roles and Relationship Patterns

As school-aged children develop, they become increasingly aware of the various roles people play. For this age group, the parents remain the source of security and support. However, as children pass into the tenth and eleventh years, peer groups take on greater significance in their development.

The family is a continued source of stability for the child through the school years.

Family Life

The family is the young child's source of strength and support. Through the family, children learn acceptable behavior, interpersonal skills, and values. Children who are exposed to older adults (e. g., through extended families) have an opportunity for much enrichment. Aunts, uncles, grandparents, and close family friends all become involved in child rearing and participate in nurturing functions. This is of particular importance if the child's parents are frequently out of the home. Siblings of similar age serve as playmates; older siblings serve as role models.

Children exposed to older adults have much opportunity for enrichment and growth.

Siblings of similar age serve as playmates. Siblings who are older serve as role models for the child.

The increasing divorce rate, the more frequently made choice to raise a family outside of marriage, and single-parent adoptions have all contributed to a rise in the number of single-parent families. According to statistics, one child in 15 now lives with one parent. While the development of the school-aged child is not limited by having one parent, problems can occur. For all children the support of a second parent can be a valuable asset and can help balance decisions. In addition, the child nearing 10 begins to identify closely with the parent of the same sex. In the single-parent family this tendency can be inhibited. However, when children are exposed to extended families, role identity may be ascribed to an adult other than a parent figure.

One in 15 children lives within a single-parent family.

As the child nears 10, he or she begins to identify with the parent of the same sex.

Throughout the interview, the nurse examiner should note the interactions between parent(s) and child. Questions relating to family dynamics, including interaction with siblings, should be asked in order to determine the child's perception of his or her role within the family structure. (Refer to Chap. 3).

Parent-Child Relationships At times the parents may view the child as an ego extension. Such an attitude can cause problems if the child beginning school is confronted with parental goals. The child can also be seen by the parent as someone to contribute to the income of the family, serve as messenger, or complete the daily chores at home. While such role assignments may have positive effects, they may also be a source of tension between the child and parent. During the assessment period the nurse should determine the responsibilities of the child to the family at large.

Younger children tend to view their parents idealistically. As the child begins to near adolescence (9 to 10 years of age), the parents are no longer seen as infallible. Because the child may have difficulty accepting parental imperfections, this new awareness can create a strain between the child and parents.

The parents need to respond to the changing needs of the child. Their role becomes one of emotional supporter and guide. Reassurance and reinforcement help to strengthen the child's sense of self and prepare him or her for the future. Parental structuring of experiences that ensure success helps strengthen relationships as well as the child's sense of self-worth.

When parents have difficulty letting go of the child, especially when it appears that peer values are in the ascendance, problems can occur. These tensions precipitate crises and lead to frequent arguments. Parents should begin to allow the school-aged child greater independence as he or she begins to mature. Allowing the child to go on campouts, overnight trips, and slumber parties can be a way for the parent to foster greater independence while still providing guidance.

Peer Group Relationships As the child begins to gain a greater independence from the parent(s), peer groups become increasingly important. They provide a significant part of social development and help prepare the child for adulthood. The group experience allows the child to begin to formulate a picture of how others see him or her. This can impact on the child's self-perception and on the role he or she can safely assume within a group.

Peer group acceptance is often based on somewhat superficial competencies. The child who is intelligent, athletic, and creative tends to gain quicker access to the group. While peer groups appear cohesive, they can change without notice, and rejection from the group can cause the child to become withdrawn and feel a sense of failure.

Questions to elicit data

1 Do you belong to a group or club?
2 Why do you belong to this particular group?
3 Who are your best friends?
4 Do you go away with your friends (e.g., on camping trips, slumber parties, etc.)?
5 What do you think your parents' opinion of your friend(s) is?
6 Have you ever been rejected by a group?
7 How did this make you feel?

Parent-child relationships are affected as the child enters school and as the peer group begins to offer important resources and alternate role models for the child.

As the child nears adolescence, parents are no longer seen as infallible.

During the school years, the parent's role focuses on reassuring and reinforcing the child in the search for greater independence and autonomy.

As the child gains greater independence from parents, peer groups become increasingly important.

Children who are athletic, intelligent, and creative have greater acceptance in peer groups.

Self-Perception and Self-Concept Patterns

As the school-aged child begins to gain independence and increased knowledge about his or her body and physical needs, a sense of self-esteem and personal worth begins to emerge. "The primary ingredients for fostering self-esteem seem to be (1) a high degree of acceptance by parents and other (e.g., peer groups); and (2) clear and consistent limit; and (3) flexibility within these limits to permit individual actions."[13]

Self-esteem is affected by (1) acceptance by (2) clear, consistent limits, (3) flexibility.

Parents need to support children during this period of searching. Increasing amounts of praise and support from authority figures (e.g., parents) help to enhance the sense of self-worth. Conversely, if inconsistent limits are set for the child, problems in identifying self-worth arise. "Parents who encourage autonomy in their children within defined and enforced boundaries seem to foster higher self-esteem than parents who set few limits on behavior or whose strict limit setting allows for no questioning."[14]

Increasing amounts of praise and support from authority figures (e.g., parents) help to increase the child's sense of self-worth.

Again, peer groups serve to foster self-esteem and social identity. High status within a group helps to promote a better self-concept. Lack of encouragement and praise can lead to a poor self-concept and withdrawal from the group. Lack of group status or membership tends to make the child dissatisfied with himself or herself and can contribute to a lack of self-esteem. Children will need assistance from adults in fostering their own sense of well-being if they are rejected by "the group."

High status within a group helps promote self-esteem.

To assess this area, questions suggested in the discussion of self-perception and self-concept patterns in Chap. 3 should be used.

Questions to elicit data

1 How do you think your parents feel about your accomplishments?

2 Can you identify some successful experiences?

3 How do you feel about yourself?

4 Do you think it's harder for you to accomplish certain skills than for other children? If so, why? Answers to these questions and others will reveal the child's self-opinion.

Cognitive and Perceptual Patterns

As the school-aged child undergoes development, several changes occur which relate to increased cognitive maturity. According to Piagetian theory, these changes are characterized by several stages. The school-aged child is said to be in the period of *concrete operations*. During this time the individual can understand principles and the relationships between events and objects (syncretic thinking); can operate with symbols; can classify information; can *decenter*, or focus on more than one thing at a time; and can apply logic to solve a problem. During this developmental period, memory increases and language competence is more extensive. The individual tends to think in concrete rather than abstract terms and is reflective when presented with a problem.

According to Piaget, the school-aged child enters a cognitive period of *concrete operations*; in this period the child has the ability to understand principles and relationships between things, to focus on more than one thing at a time, and to apply logic when solving a problem.

The 6-year-old is in a stage of preconcrete thinking. The child has a command of language and uses it to share in the experience of others. He or she is not yet capable of understanding fundamental relationships between and among phenomena. The child's egocentricism hinders his or her ability to see another person's point of view. Centering, which causes a child to focus, or center, on one aspect of something, may impair an understanding of all other aspects. As movement occurs from one stage of development to another, a disequilibrium is created, enabling the child to integrate, to accommodate, and to assimilate experiences and, hence, to learn.

The 6-year-old child is in a period of preconcrete thinking.

By the time they reach 7, children can recognize time and are more tolerant of a delayed response while alternatives are considered. The child's verbal communication has increased substantially; memory has improved and there is a greater understanding of past, present, and future.

Children from the eighth through the twelfth years are in the stage of concrete operations. Egocentrism and centering are overcome. Classification, which involves placing objects in groups according to attributes such as color or size, is mastered. Proficiency in seriating objects according to characteristics such as length and weight is also demonstrated. Capable of using certain principles of relationships between events and objects, these children understand the concept of conservation of mass, which stipulates that something remains the same despite a different arrangement or shape, provided nothing is added or taken away. This understanding is a form of conceptual thinking. During this period children also master the concept of reversibility, which means they understand that a process can be performed in a reverse order so that the materials involved can be returned to their original condition.

Occasionally the school-aged child uses hypotheses and carries out abstract operations from the concrete. Logical though processes, however, develop slowly, and children in this stage of cognition can be contradictory in some of their comments. Adult thinking becomes evident in formal operations with 11- to 15-year-olds, when capabilities of solving more complex problems emerge.

Assessment of this pattern area can be made by asking the questions identified in Chap. 3 in the discussion of cognitive-perceptual patterns. In addition, evaluation of cognitive abilities as measured by developmental test scores (refer to Table 9-3) may help to facilitate assessment of this pattern area. Data can also be gathered from parent and teacher perceptions of the child's Sensory Motor performance and abilities at home and in the classroom.

School Readiness

Social, cognitive, and physical skills which were developed in the preschool period continue to be used and further refined as the child enters a period of more formalized learning. Entry into school enables the developing child to function at an optimal level of potential and helps in the acquisition of skills essential to successful daily living. Cooperation with peers, increased socialization, critical thinking, acceptance of evaluations and criticisms, making judgments based on logic and reasoning, and increasing industry are some of the developmental goals to be mastered in the classroom setting. To facilitate this the classroom environment needs to be a flexible place where the child can explore new horizons and acquire information to deal successfully with the realistic demands of the adult world.

Children who receive encouragement and support from parents as they explore their surroundings are eager to continue their learning, to receive praise, and to enjoy their success. However, there are some 6-year-olds who find the classroom experience a threatening one. These feelings can be attributed to a basic insecurity or a perceived loss of personal identity. While there are some children who demonstrate regressive tendencies, others are simply emotionally unprepared for the start of school.

Children who are ready for school demonstrate certain characteristics; i.e., they are usually able to make friends easily, are outgoing in their social interactions, and tend to exhibit emotional stability. In addition, they have a degree of self-confidence and a certain basic body of knowledge which they have acquired as a result of adult and peer interaction and through television and storytelling.

Although a battery of tests such as DDST and PPVT allows an examiner to acquire a profile of the total child, none of them evaluates the academic preparedness of a 6-year-old. Yet each child needs to be assessed for school readiness. This can be determined only by analyzing a variety of factors, and since there are no fixed criteria available, it behooves the health care provider to examine childhood physical development patterns, cognitive and emotional patterns, and familial variables critically. In addition, the profile of the child as a learner should be evaluated in the context of a particular school, for it is the interface of these elements which determines whether a child is ready to start formal learning.

In queries to parents, the nurse should elicit information about the child's problem-solving abilities and his or her responses to frustration and failure. Evaluation of the child's levels of curiosity and imagination is important, too. It is also essential in talking with parents to evaluate their own preparedness for having the child start school.

Independence in self-care activities, a relatively easy separation from the mother, and experiences with peers in group settings all tend to increase a child's readiness. The ability to communicate is crucial when one considers that reading, writing, and arithmetic are complex communicative modalities which are usually introduced during the first grade. Therefore, it is necessary for a child to be able to use the language and to have understandable speech, enabling him or her to convey wants, needs, and desires. Again, the Sensory Motor Skills should also be evaluated at this time.

School Performance Performance in the classroom reflects the child's ability to sustain an effective attention span, absorb information of an auditory and visual nature, and assimilate and remember what is seen, heard, and touched. Success in these areas increases self-confidence and self-esteem, while frustration and failure can lead to withdrawal and a lowered self-concept.

Oftentimes perceptual and cognitive deficits are identified as the child begins school. These dysfunctions can cause problems in academic performance and in a child's ability to relate to and play with peers. Sometimes a child is unable to associate visual information with auditory input, and the disparity in processing can be the factor precipitating learning difficulties.

When problems in performance arise, it is necessary to identify causative factors. It is important to rule out a possible physical basis for such problems before evaluating other causes. Neurological and motor assessments may reveal an underlying physical problem. Lacking physical causation, the problem should then be assessed in light of whether the child has the intellectual ability and the emotional maturity to function at an acceptable level. The use of achievement and psychoeducational workups may be necessary to resolve the issue and allow the child to achieve maximum potential.

Learning Problems Children who have learning disabilities demonstrate a variety of characteristics, which include short attention spans, hyperactivity, poor muscular coordination, perceptual deficits, labile emotions, difficulties with expressive or receptive language, and poor peer relationships. As one might expect, children who have difficulty learning demonstrate their frustrations through a variety of disruptive behaviors such as passiveness, impulsiveness, withdrawal, or pugnaciousness.

Sensory Motor Competence enhances the child's ability to adjust to school.

It is important for the child starting school to have an understandable language pattern.

School performance is dependent upon a child's ability to sustain an effective attention span, absorb auditory and visual data, and remember what has been seen, touched, and heard.

When problems arise in school performance, it is important to determine the cause as soon as possible.

Visual Impairment Approximately 30 percent of the school-age population has some visual impairment, and screening these children is essential if further deterioration is to be prevented.[15] Good vision is most important to the child who is just beginning school. If vision is poor, important components of the educational process can be missed.

Although visual changes are present in $7\frac{1}{2}$ million children, only about one-fourth of them demonstrate any symptoms of impaired vision.[16] Certain behaviors can indicate a problem. Typically, children with impaired vision rub their eyes, cover an eye when reading, tilt their heads when reading or coloring, sit up close to the TV set, hold objects close to their eyes, blink frequently, squint, and frown. Often, they complain of not being able to see a blackboard and have trouble reading or doing close work.

Assessment should focus on determining the behaviors noted above. Giving the child a book to read will provide the nurse with information about vision. Parents and teachers should be questioned about the child's visual competence. Screening the school-aged child for visual acuity, color vision, and visual fields is critical. (Refer to the discussion of the physical examination of the eye in Chap. 4.)

If they know the letters, young children can be tested for visual acuity using the Snellen alphabet chart. Adequate light is absolutely essential during this test, because visual acuity increases with the intensity of the light. Visual acuity is determined by using a standardized symbol at a standardized distance and recording it as a fraction. For example, 20/40 is an illustration of one result in which the numerator is the distance between the client and the chart, while the denominator is the distance at which a normal eye can read the specific line. In essence, 20/40 means that a child sees at 20 feet what someone with normal vision sees at 40 feet. A 20/30 visual acuity is adequate for a school-aged child up to 8 years. Beyond that age it should be 20/20.

Normally children are farsighted, or *hyperopic*. This condition decreases as they advance through the lower grades. School-aged children must be able to use both eyes together in order to have coordinated binocular vision. *Heterotropia* is a defect in focusing eyes together. Nonbinocularity causes double vision, suppressed vision in the affected eye, and eventually loss of sight. The child does not appear to demonstrate an eye problem, and parents are normally unaware of any difficulty. Ideally this condition should be discovered early; it is invariably noted in the course of a screening.

Color blindness is extremely rare in girls, and so it is not necessary to test them. However, all males should be tested with the Ishihara plates or the Hardy-Rand-Rittler pseudoisochromatic plates (HRR). Because color perception does not change with time, boys need be tested only once. If test results indicate a problem, the child should be retested before a referral is made.

There are two types of color vision deficiencies: (1) red, or protan type (browns, reds, and black are confused) and (2) green, or deutan (greens, browns, purples, and gray are involved). There is no treatment for these deficiencies, and the focus is on educating parents, teachers, and children. It is especially important to identify color blindness early since color-coded tests are becoming increasingly popular in many school systems.

Hearing Problems A child's ability to hear is critical to language development. Physical growth of the lower part of the face during the early school years results in proportional changes in the eustachian tube, making it longer, narrower, and more slanted. These changes make it more difficult for microbial organisms to invade the middle ear. The most frequent hearing loss in grades K to 2 is conductive peripheral loss

Approximately 30 percent of the school-age population has some visual impairment.

Children who indicate problems in visual ability should be examined carefully.

20/30 visual acuity is adequate for a school-aged child up to 8 years of age. Beyond age 8, visual acuity should be 20/20.

Normally, children are hyperopic (farsighted) in the early school years, a problem which decreases as the child advances through the grades.

Color blindness is rare in girls.

caused by eustachian tube obstruction related to the development of serous otitis media. Poor management and treatment can result in a permanent hearing loss because of a ruptured, scarred, or stiff tympanic membrane.

Auditory screening tests conducted during the school years are effective, not only for identifying intermittent or permanent losses, but also for preventing further hearing loss. Hearing is considered normal when frequencies, or wave lengths, of 500 to 8000 cycles per second are heard at 25 decibels (dB). Hearing should be tested every other year (i.e., in 6-, 8-, and 10-year olds); however, children with protracted illnesses, hearing deficits, and ear problems and students in speech therapy need this examination annually. About 5 percent of the children who participate in this procedure need follow-up examinations.

Refer to Chap. 4 for a discussion of the Rinne and Weber tests.

The Weber and Rinne tuning-fork tests should be incorporated into any auditory assessment. Audiometers with air conduction capabilities are used to test the entire auditory system. Children who fail this examination should be referred to audiologists who can perform more definitive testing, including threshold audiograms.

Hyperactivity According to Binder and Butler[17] "hyperactivity, associated with attentional deficits, impulsiveness, and distractability" is the most common manifestation of a learning disability in children who are in primary grades. Approximately 5 percent of primary schoolchildren are hyperactive.[18]

The child so affected is generally of average intelligence but fails to meet the predicted potential for academic performance. Although central nervous system involvement is implied, the etiology remains obscure. The child's attentional deficits, impulsiveness, and distractability lead to frustration, temper tantrums, and restlessness. Such behavior interferes with peer and adult interactions. The child becomes increasingly friendless and unhappy, does poorly in school, and develops a poor self-concept. Without interruption of this cycle, the child may become a school dropout.

In assessing hyperactivity, the most important elements are a thorough history and observation of behavior. Parents, teachers, and school nurses are invaluable sources of subjective data based on their observations of the child's behavior in different settings. Tests should be made to rule out vision and hearing deficits as etiologic factors. A thorough physical examination and appropriate diagnostic tests will differentiate other causes for the child's learning disability. A psychologist's evaluation is important in determining the child's self-image and coping mechanisms, family dynamics, perceptual learning skills, cognitive skills, and academic skills. Once the diagnosis of hyperactivity is made, intervention revolves around family counseling and behavioral, psychological, medical, and educational therapy for the child.

Sexuality and Reproductive Patterns

For the school-aged child, especially in the early years (ages 6 to 9), there is a strong interest in and identification with the parent or adult figure of the same sex. This is carried into social activities and play. Identification with the adult of the same sex seems to reinforce the individual's sexual identity and sense of self as male or female.

Stereotypes which have affected sex roles in the past are less obvious today, but they do exist. For there are little girls who strongly identify with mother's role (cooking, playing with dolls, etc.). Yet there are others who prefer to play sports. Conversely, boys may enjoy cooking or even playing house as much as they enjoy baseball. The more liberated

Highlights

Hearing tests are frequently conducted during the school years in order to determine auditory problems early and limit impairment in learning.

Hearing tests should be done when the child enters school and, if the results are normal, every 2 years thereafter.

Approximately 5 percent of children in the primary grades are hyperactive.

Hyperactivity is characterized by attentional deficits, impulsiveness, distractability, temper tantrums, and restlessness.

Children 6 to 9 years of age strongly identify with a parent of the same sex.

Today sex roles are less stereotyped, and as a result boys can cook and girls can play sports traditionally reserved to males.

the role identification, the better able the child is to cope with sexual maturation.

Girls begin to mature sexually about 2 to 3 years before boys. The onset of this maturity is associated with menarche and the development of secondary sex characteristics. This usually occurs between the ages of 10 and 12 or in early adolescence. Often menarche is preceded by a growth period. Sexual maturity begins in males several years later than in females. Increase in the size of the penis and testes are two confirming signs. Voice changes may also be noted.

During the early school years, recognition of the opposite sex in a more sexual way is submerged. The child is free of any conflict and able to invest energies in exploring life. Sexual curiosity in young children takes the form of physical exploration of their bodies. They are interested in knowing physical function and will ask questions of adults. These questions should be answered honestly and directly.

An adult's reluctance to explore these issues is confusing to the child and often causes him or her to turn to the peer group for information. This will quite likely cause further confusion for the child and increase the risk of misinformation. For the information related to sexual issues that a growing child shares with friends of the same sex is too often obtained from media (e.g., television, books, etc.) and communicated in secret conversations with one another. School sex-education programs, although controversial, can be a source of support in this area of development.

The nurse examiner may need to explore the child's perception of his or her own sexuality and should provide time to answer the child's questions, if appropriate to do so. Data can be elicited by the nurse through questions similar to those presented in the discussion of sexuality and reproductive patterns in Chap. 3.

Nutritional Metabolic Patterns

Nutrition is an important component of the school-aged child's growth and development. The preadolescent stage (about age 10 for girls, 12 for boys) is a time of significant physical growth (refer to Table 9-4). During this period there is generally an increase in the child's appetite. The foods ingested at this time are especially important to the child's overall health state.

In this school-age period children need a balanced diet, with increased amounts of calories, proteins, vitamin A, and calcium. Their calorie needs are double those of an adult. High energy output and growth account for this need. "Physical activity uses about twenty-five percent of calories ingested; twelve percent is used for growing; five percent for dynamic food action; and eight percent is lost in feces."[19]

Good nutrition is often influenced by many external factors. Economics, food fads, cultural and religious customs all play a part in our diet. Health problems associated with nutritional intake may have their origin in these factors. While children need a balanced diet, peer pressure can affect food intake. If the food is not "in," it may be unacceptable to the child. Rushing to school or other activities may cause the child to skip breakfast, eat hurried lunches, or choose foods that are quick and available. Soft drinks replace water, potato chips replace fruit, and other convenience foods replace a good, nutritious meal.[20]

But mealtimes can provide an opportunity for family members to share time as a group, and for the school-aged child, involvement in food preparation can be a positive experience. This age group thrives on mastery of skills, and cooking, setting the table, and washing the dishes may

Highlights

Girls begin to mature 2 to 3 years before boys.

Sexual maturity begins in girls with the onset of menarche and the development of secondary sex characteristics.

The male's sexual maturity begins with an increase in the size of the penis and testes.

Sexual curiosity of school-aged children takes the form of exploration of their bodies.

Reluctance to discuss sexual issues may be confusing to the child and may force the individual to seek out the peer group for information.

Nutrition is an important component of a child's growth and development.

The school-aged child needs twice as many calories as an adult.

About 25 percent of a child's caloric intake is used for physical activity.

Economy, food fads, cultural and religious influences all contribute to a child's nutritional status.

Mealtime should be an opportunity for family members to share time as a group.

be enjoyable activities for the child. It is important to assess the atmosphere surrounding mealtime because it may affect the child's eating patterns.

During the assessment, it is important for the nurse examiner to evaluate the child's eating patterns. Questions suggested in the discussion of nutritional patterns in Chap. 3 would be helpful. When evaluating this pattern area, the nurse can also evaluate hygiene practices. Care of the body, including skin, should be considered. Dental caries is a problem for this particular age group; since the younger school-aged child carefully carries out tasks, rituals such as frequent brushing and tooth care may be easy to teach. A high number of children may also need orthodontic work (i.e., braces). This may subject the child to teasing, and support will be needed, along with a clear explanation of the need for such work. In cultures where good parenting is reflected in an obese child, weight control will be problematic for the nurse.

Exercise and Activity Patterns

During the school-age years, a child's muscular strength doubles and endurance grows. While the child may not yet have the endurance of an adult, overall stamina is increasing.

Planned regular activity (exercise) becomes important for the child. Not only does it help to set a pattern for life, it also refines present skills and helps in the development of various muscle groups. Activities such as running, climbing, and bike riding help improve coordination and smoothness of movement. On the other hand, baseball and rope jumping help to develop large muscle groups. Fine motor skills are also increased during this period. School and community activities which focus on art, ceramics, and other crafts help refine these movements.

All exercise and activities help to promote the child's sense of self and of accomplishment. Praising accomplishments and creating experiences that will be successful can help to ensure this goal. Too much emphasis on winning and competition can destroy the child's interest in activities and affect the self-concept. Attention must therefore be shifted to the benefits of activity for the child.

When assessing this pattern area, questions suggested in Chap. 3 in the discussion of exercise and activity patterns may be appropriate. In addition, the use of leisure time should be considered when assessing a child's activities. Attention should be paid to the time a child spends in relaxation. It is important for the nurse to help the child see the value of quiet time, however that may be spent. Bedtime reading and storytelling often provide a source of relaxation for both the parent and child.

Prevention of Sports-Related Injuries

Over the past few years, health care providers have developed an increased interest in the prevention of sports-related injuries. Although the preseason examination (sports physical) has done little or nothing to prevent injuries, it does offer an opportunity to screen school-aged children.

Garrick[21] describes a preseason screening program which has been tested and found to be effective. A complete history and a thorough physical examination are required. Following the screening process, the decision regarding the child's participation in athletics is made. Possible responses include "no participation," "partial," "full," or "no decision until further testing."

Two sports in which school-aged children should not compete are wrestling and weight lifting. Wrestling is contraindicated for young ath-

Dental caries is a particular problem for the school-aged child.

During the school-age years, a child's strength doubles and endurance increases.

Regular activity and exercise is important for the school-aged child, for it helps in acquisition of new muscle groups and the refinement of physical skills.

Praise for accomplishments helps to improve the child's sense of self.

Leisure time is as important an experience for the child as for the adult.

Over the past few years much emphasis has been placed on prevention of sports-related injuries.

Wrestling and weight lifting are two sports to be avoided by the school-aged child.

letes who cannot pull up on a bar seven times in succession. Weight lifting is dangerous. Prior to Tanner's third stage of sexual development, no weights should be lifted above the head. If a weight-lifting exercise cannot be done 12 times in succession, then it should not be included in the young athlete's weight-lifting repertoire.

Throughout the school years, the nurse can be instrumental in guiding the child toward participation in age-appropriate athletics. Through careful observation and education, the incidence of sports injuries can be decreased, if not completely eliminated. Use of protective devices (e.g., kneepads) should be stressed when a particular activity could result in an injury. Supervision of athletic activities and the use of strict safety rules may also decrease injuries. Swimming competence and the use of life jackets, along with knowledge in resuscitation, may also reduce accidents and even deaths related to swimming programs.

Coping and Stress Tolerance Patterns

The ability of the school-aged child to cope with stress is dependent upon many factors. These include personality and temperament, responses to and memories of previous stress experiences, level of physical and emotional development, as well as the child's ability to cope with life's stressors.

A child's ability to cope is often influenced by such things as previous experiences with a particular stressor, the child's personality, and his or her physical and emotional development.

Much of the child's response to stressful situations seems to be determined by how he or she takes on new situations and his or her expectation of failure or success. In adopting successful coping strategies, the child relies upon the parent or adult figure for security and support. When the child is not successful, he or she must be helped to cope with the situation. Parents can help the child look at the reasons for disappointment and encourage the child to try again.

Responses to stressful situations depend upon the child's expectation of success or failure in new situations. The child relies upon parents for support during times of stress.

For some children, successful coping can be achieved "by suppressing the stimuli which are threatening and focusing on the experiences to be mastered."[22] It is only through experience with stress that the child begins to gain strategies needed to deal with life's crises. The child learns early to use strategies that result in a response to his or her need. Crying and sulking, as well as being extremely cooperative and helpful, can all be successful tactics. These reactions, however, may become less effective as the child grows and begins to interact with groups outside the family.

Experience with stress helps the child perfect strategies to deal with stress.

Assessment of this pattern area (refer to the discussion of coping and stress tolerance patterns in Chap. 3) is of critical importance. Some behavioral responses of this age group may be manifestations of stress responses.

Reactions to Death

Felice and Friedman[23] note that 6- to 8-year-old children view death as a prolongation of sleep, while 8- to 10-year-olds may personify death. The 6- to 8-year-old child asks what it is like to be buried in the ground, if the person is cold and needs to eat, and with whom he can play. The 9- to 10-year-old child may see death "as a monster who sneaks in during the night and kills the living."[24]

Children between 6 and 8 years of age see death as a prolongation of sleep.

The school-aged child's reaction to the death of a family member takes many forms. The child may release feelings by fighting with friends, trying to hurt playmates physically. Other grief reactions include "regression, enuresis, nightmares, sullenness, somatic complaints, school phobia, withdrawal, hyperactivity, whining, crying, anorexia, or assuming the mannerisms of the dead sibling."[25]

Children may release feelings about the death of a family member by starting a fight, withdrawing, crying, or experiencing somatic complaints.

Many behavioral problems may occur later because of unresolved grief. If a family member has died, the nurse should assess the child's perception of death and analyze the child's reaction to the loss. Whatever form the reaction takes, the child must first be helped to deal with grief before any behavior problems can be dissipated.

Nailbiting

According to Sarles and Heisler,[26] 40 percent of school-aged children have, at one time or another, engaged in nailbiting. This self-stimulating behavior may be a manifestation of stress, and it can become a habit.

Nailbiting in children may be a manifestation of stress.

In gathering subjective data the nurse should attempt to determine the relationship between nailbiting and underlying tension. Data should also include present management techniques and response. During physical appraisal, the child's fingers should be carefully inspected for infection and hangnails. Since nailbiting may be an extension of thumb-sucking, the presence of dental malocclusion should be determined. In discussion with the parents the nurse should warn them against any display of anger or threat of punishment when the child engages in this activity. Behavioral reinforcement or a combination of reinforcement techniques and the application of a bitter-tasting commercial preparation to the child's fingers can be effective in correcting this behavior.

Stealing

Developmentally, the school-aged child's sense of property rights is not completely mature. Thus, "an 8-year-old may pick up loose change from a table in an unsupervised situation. However, after age 9 respect for property should be well integrated into the child."[27] Children who have poor self-esteem may steal as a means to achieve parental notice, buy friendship, or attain peer approval.

Children who steal may have poor self-esteem and see this action as a way of gaining parental attention.

When parents present their child's stealing as a concern, the health care provider must elicit from parents and child their perceptions of parent-child relationships, their values regarding intra- and extrafamilial stealing, the child's self-image, and child-peer relationships. Once this information has been ascertained, discussion of age-appropriate behavior and methods of improving parent-child and child-peer relationships can ensue.

School Phobia

In this instance, phobia does not mean fear of school, but the resistance of a child to going to school. It is a symptom of anxiety within the school-aged child and very different from the truancy which occurs in adolescence. About 1.7 percent of the school-age population is affected,[28] most of them children between 6 and 8 years of age. Invariably, these children are obsessive, perfectionistic, anxious students who simply elect to remain at home rather than to attend school. Academically, they are average to superior in their performance. Often they have demonstrated some difficulty coping in prior situations.

About 1.7 percent of school-aged children are affected by school phobia.

A phenomenon which is present in all socioeconomic strata, school phobia can develop in either sex as a result of any number of life situations which propel the child into an anxious state. Death, divorce, parental illness, overprotectiveness of a mother, and hospitalization have all been implicated. The problem is considered to be a parental one as much as it is a child's with mutual dependency contributing to the dilemma.

Somatic complaints that the troubled child verbalizes include headache, stomach aches, and diarrhea, as well as a variety of other symp-

School phobia can be reflected by somatic complaints.

toms, none of which suggests a physiologic basis. First- and second-graders who were ill prior to the phobic episode may utilize those earlier complaints to prolong their confinement.

Since the etiology is complex and varies among individuals, there is no single treatment plan. It is important that parents, child, teacher, nurse, and school officials cooperate in efforts directed toward reducing the anxiety-provoking situation, improving the child's self-image, promoting satisfying parent-child interactions, and resolving the family crisis if one is present. Usually the young child can return to school without great difficulty or any residual sequelae. The same is not true of the adolescent truant.

Review of Body Components

Review of body components follows the taking of the health history and includes growth measurements, vital signs, and physical appraisal of each body system. Generally, the child is first weighed and measured. Then the temperature and blood pressure are taken. Palpation of the pulses and observation of respirations are incorporated in examination of the body systems.

Summary

Assessment of the school-aged child is both challenging and exciting. The information collected at this time can significantly impact on the overall health and wellness of the child as he or she progresses toward preadolescence. In addition, data assessed during the taking of the health history form the basis for the physical examination to follow. The format for recording this data is similar to that outlined in Chap. 3.

REFERENCES

1. National Center for Health Statistics, Health Resources Administration, U.S. Department of Health and Human Services, Hyattsville, Md.

2. Ciro Sumaya, "Tuberculin Skin Testing" in Robert A. Hoekelman *et al.* (eds.), *Principles of Pediatrics: Health Care of the Young,* New York, McGraw-Hill Book Company, 1978, p. 190.

3. "Fact Sheet on Immunization Initiative," Department of Health, Education and Welfare, Public Health Service, Center for Disease Control, Spring 1977, p. 1.

4. Linda Jarvis, "Childhood Immunizations," *The School Age Child: Issues in Comprehensive Pediatric Nursing* 3(3):36 (Sept. 1978).

5. G. Prazar, "Lying and Stealing" in R. A. Hoekelman et al. (eds.), *Principles of Pediatrics,* p. 607.

6. M. Cohen, "Enuresis" in R. A. Hoekelman et al. (eds.), *Principles of Pediatrics,* p. 595.

7. Ibid.

8. P. M. Bindelglas, "The Enuretic Child," *Fam Prac* 2(5):375–380 (1975).

9. N. H. Azrin, T. J. Sneed, and R. M. Foxx, "Dry-Bed Training: Rapid Elimination of Childhood Enuresis," *Behavior Research and Therapy* 12:147–156 (1974).

10. Ibid.; E. R. Christophersen and M. A. Rapoff, "Enuresis Treatment," *Issues in Comprehensive Pediatric Nursing* 2(6):34–52 (March-Apr., 1978).

11. Christophersen and Rapoff, "Behavioral Problems in Children" in G. M. Scipien et al. (eds.), *Comprehensive Pediatric Nursing,* 2nd ed., New York, McGraw-Hill Book Company 1979, p. 361.

12. J. Triplett, "The Role of Experience in Child Development" in G. M. Scipien et al. (eds.), *Comprehensive Pediatric Nursing,* p. 102.

13. M. Sieman, "Mental Health in School Aged Children," *Amer J of Maternal Child Nurs* 3(4):215 (July-Aug. 1978).

14. J. Triplett, "Role," p. 96.

15. Robert J. Haggerty, "Preventive Pediatrics" in V. C. Vaughan and R. J. McKay (eds.), *Nelson's Textbook of Pediatrics,* Philadelphia, W. B. Saunders Co., 1975, p. 209.

16. Otto Lippman, "Vision Screening of Young Children," *Amer J of Pub Health* **61**(8):1598–1601, (Aug. 1971).

17. F. Z. Binder and J. E. Butler, "Children with Learning Disabilities," *Issues in Comprehensive Pediatric Nursing,* **3**(3):3 (Sept. 1978).

18. T. J. Long, "Dealing with Common Classroom Behavior Problems" in R. A. Hoekelman et al. (eds.), *Principles of Pediatrics,* p. 550.

19. J. L. Wilde, "The School Aged Child" in M. J. Smith et al., *Child and Family, Concepts of Nursing Practice,* New York, McGraw-Hill Book Company, 1982, p. 270.

20. Ibid., p. 270–271.

21. J. C. Garrick, "Sports Medicine," *Pediatr Clin North Am* **24**(4):737–747 (Nov. 1977).

22. J. Triplett, "The Role of Experience . . . ," p. 92.

23. M. Felice and S. B. Friedman, "The Dying Child" in R. A. Hoekelman et al. (eds.), *Principles of Pediatrics,* p. 231.

24. Ibid., p. 231.

25. J. Gyulay, *The Dying Child,* New York, McGraw-Hill Book Company, 1978, p. 46.

26. R. M. Sarles and A. B. Heisler, "Self Stimulating Behaviors" in R. A. Hoekelman et al. (eds.), *Principles of Pediatrics,* p. 591.

27. Ibid., p. 608.

28. Christophersen and Rapoff, "Behavioral Problems . . . ," p. 375.

BIBLIOGRAPHY

Bindelglas, P. M.: "The Enuretic Child," *Fam Prac* **2**(5):375–380 (1975).

Cohen, M.: "Enuresis," in R. A. Hoekelman et al. (eds.): *Principles of Pediatrics: Health Care of the Young,* New York, McGraw-Hill Book Co., 1978.

"Fact Sheet on Immunization Initiative," Department of Health, Education and Welfare, Public Health Service, Center for Disease Control, 1977.

Igoe, Judith Bellaire: "The School Nurse Practitioner Program," in Joanne E. Hall and Barbara R. Weaver (eds.): *Distributive Nursing Practice: A Systems Approach to Community Health,* Philadelphia, J. Lippincott, 1977.

Jarvis, Linda: "Childhood Immunizations," *The School Age Child: Issues in Comprehensive Pediatric Nursing* **3**(3):36 (September 1978).

Nemir, A., and W. Schaller: *The School Health Program,* Philadelphia, W. B. Saunders, 1975.

Scipien, G., et al.: *Comprehensive Pediatric Nursing,* 2d ed., New York, McGraw-Hill Book Co., 1979.

Sieman, Mari: "Mental Health in School Aged Children," *Amer J Maternal Child Nurs* **3**(4):215 (July–August 1978).

Smith, M., et al.: *Child and Family Concepts of Nursing Practice,* New York, McGraw-Hill Book Co., 1982.

Refer to Chap. 4 for complete details of the physical examination.

The child's growing sense of modesty must be considered when preparing him or her for the physical examination.

The child should be allowed to choose the stage of undress for the examination.

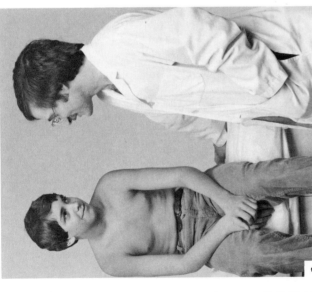

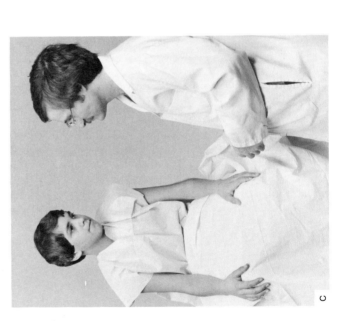

PHYSICAL EXAMINATION

The physical examination of the school-age child is similar to that described in Chap. 4. Findings unique to this age group are presented in the following discussion.

APPROACH TO THE EXAMINATION

At approximately 5 years of age, a child's sense of modesty becomes apparent. This developmental milestone should be considered by the examiner during the physical examination. The child should be allowed to decide whether parent(s) and/or siblings are to be present and the state of dress to be used for the examination. Three alternative states of undress are acceptable:

a Strip to the waist for examination of the upper body. Then clothe the upper body and strip from the waist down except for the underpants; drape the lower body for removal of the underpants.

b Strip to the underpants and use a simple drape.

c Strip to the underpants, put on a gown, and use a simple drape.

Each alternative should be explained to allow the child to make his or her preferred choice. The examiner should be aware that girls may object, even before breast development, to baring their chests.

Because the school-age child is curious about the how and why of a situation, the examiner should explain the purpose of the instruments to be used: such as the stethoscope, the otoscope, and the ophthalmoscope (a). Removing some of the mystery surrounding the examination and initiating a relaxed conversation about school, hobbies, pets, and friends encourages a child's cooperation.

Explanatory comments should continue throughout the examination (b). For example, by drawing a picture of the structures seen through the otoscope and explaining them, the examiner is often able to reduce a child's anxiety regarding the procedures to be undertaken. In addition, admiring a child's muscles during a test for muscle strength gives him or her a sense of personal pride.

Many children of this age group like to handle the instruments and are curious about what they experience. Many will listen to their heartbeats through the stethoscope, look in the examiner's ears and eyes with the otoscope and the ophthalmoscope, and place a tongue depressor in the examiner's mouth (c). If the child's parent is present, the child may use the instruments on the parent in order to obtain an idea of what the examiner will see and hear during the examination. Unlike the preschooler who may have a similar request, the school-age child is interested not in playing with the instruments but in understanding the mechanics and technology of the procedures. The older child who has learned some anatomy in school may become rather excited about actually seeing structures that he or she has seen only in textbook photographs.

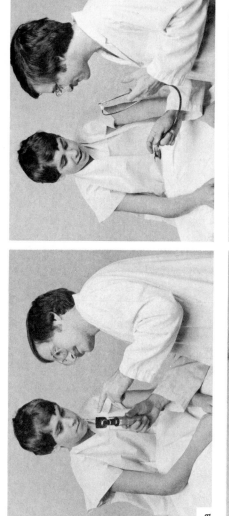

a

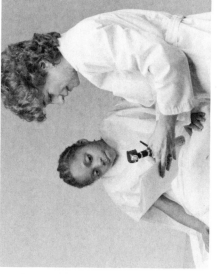

b

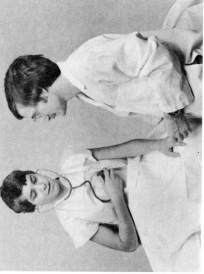

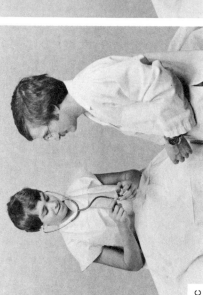

c

Highlights

Explaining the use of various medical instruments used during the physical examination reduces the anxiety and often increases cooperation.

Allowing a child to handle the instruments to be used during the examination satisfies his or her need to understand the mechanics and technology of the procedures.

THE EXAMINATION

General Appearance

The school-age child appears better coordinated and more in control of body movements than during the preschool years. Posture tends to improve, and the child is often slimmer and more graceful (a).

Although growth patterns vary according to sex and cultural group, in general, "baby fat" has disappeared, the legs are longer, and the individual seems to have more control of his or her movements.

Measurement

The physical examination includes the measurement of growth and vital signs. After being weighed (b) and measured (c), the child's temperature and blood pressure are taken. Palpation of the pulse and observation of respiration are incorporated in the examination of the body systems.

Weight and Height To ensure accuracy, the child is measured in underclothes and stocking feet. Average weight gain and height increase during the school-age period are 6.5 lbs (3 kg) and 2.5 inches (6 cm) per year, respectively. The preadolescent growth spurt occurs at about 10 years of age in girls and 12 years in boys. The weight and height charts for boys and girls aged 2 to 18 years, developed by the National Center for Health Statistics (NCHS), are arranged according to seven percentiles (5th, 10th, 25th, 50th, 75th, 90th, and 95th). Approximate weights and heights of school-age boys and girls are shown in the table at the right (d).

Highlights

Unlike the preschooler, the school-age child appears slimmer, better coordinated, and more in control of body movements.

Growth spurts in the school-age child are cyclic.

Weight increases are often observed in late summer and fall.

The height of the school-age child increases 2.5 to 3 inches (6 to 7 cm) per year. Boys are taller than girls until age 10. Between the ages of 10 and 14, girls are usually taller than boys.

Table source: National Center for Health Statistics, Health Resources Administration, U.S. Department of Health, Education and Welfare.

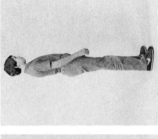
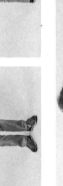
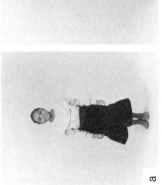

a

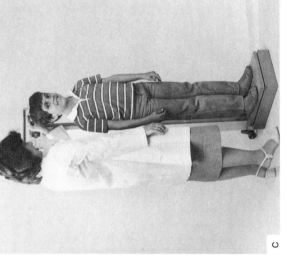

b

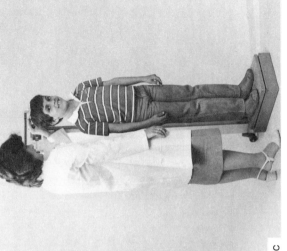

c

Table d - Approximate Body Weights and Heights of School-Age Children

Age, years	6	7	8	9	10
Body weight, lb (kg in parenthesis)					
Boys	37.5—58.5 (17.0—26.5)	42.0—66.0 (19.0—30.0)	45.0—77.0 (20.5—35.0)	49.5—88.0 (22.5—40.0)	54.0—99.0 (24.5—45.0)
Girls	35.5—57.5 (16.0—26.0)	39.5—66.0 (18.0—30.0)	43.0—77.0 (19.5—35.0)	48.5—89.5 (22.0—40.5)	53.0—103.5 (24.0—47.0)
Height, inches (cm in parenthesis)					
Boys	42.5—49.0 (108.0—124.0)	44.5—51.0 (113.0—130.0)	46.5—53.5 (118.0—136.0)	48.5—56.0 (123.0—142.0)	50.5—58.5 (128.0—148.0)
Girls	42.0—48.5 (107.0—123.0)	44.0—52.0 (112.0—129.5)	46.0—53.5 (117.0—136.0)	48.0—56.5 (122.0—143.0)	50.0—58.5 (127.0—149.0)

Note: The lower numbers represent the 5th percentile; the higher numbers, the 95th percentile.

Temperature, Pulse, and Respiration

The school-age child's temperature is 97 to 99°F (36 to 37°C). The average pulse rate for a 6-year-old is 80 to 90 beats per minute with a range from 75 to 115 beats per minute, and the average respiratory rate is 24 to 26 breaths per minute.

In children from 8 to 10 years of age, these rates diminish slightly to a pulse of 80 to 84 beats per minute with a range from 70 to 110 beats per minute, and to 22 to 24 breaths per minute, respectively. The heart rate changes with respirations, accelerating in inspiration and slowing on expiration.

Respirations are both abdominal and costal until 7 years of age, when they become predominantly costal (a).

Blood Pressure

Percentile charts for both systolic and diastolic pressures according to sex, developed by the Task Force on Blood Pressure Control in Children, are reported in the table at right (b).

Normal *pulse pressure* is 20 to 50 mmHg. By using blood pressure percentile charts, the health care provider can follow a pattern of pulse pressure over time.

Pulse pressure is the difference obtained between the measured diastolic and systolic blood pressure readings.

Table source: "Report of the Task Force on Blood Pressure Control in Children," *Pediatrics* 59 (suppl): 803 (May 1977).

a

Table b - Approximate Blood Pressure Readings of School-Age Children

Age, years	6	7	8	9	10
Blood Pressure Readings (systolic/diastolic), mmHg.					
Boys	78—114/46—78	80—118/50—80	84—122/52—82	86—126/53—84	90—130/56—86
Girls	80—113/46—79	82—117/49—80	85—121/52—82	88—124/54—82	91—128/56—84

Note: The lower numbers represent the 5th percentile; the higher numbers, the 95th percentile.

Highlights

By the end of the school-age period, the skull has reached adult size.

*Smith, M., et al. (eds.): *Child and Family*, New York, McGraw-Hill Book Company, 1982, p. 268.

During the school-age years the face becomes more conspicuous and angular often due to the fact that the skull is growing slower than the face and related structures.

Head

In general, examination of the head and of the hair and scalp reflects findings similar to those described in Chap. 4.

Inspection

Although the skull measures about 20 to 21 inches (51 to 54 cm) in circumference in the school-age child (a), it grows slowly, reaching adult size by the end of this age period.* Growth may be reflected in changes in facial structures. (See also Face.)

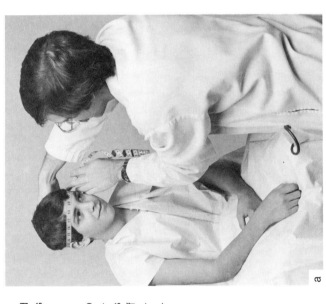

Face

Inspection

Because facial structures may grow faster than the skull, the facial appearance of the school-age child may become more conspicuous and take on a more angular look. Near the end of this period, the "babyish" appearance of the child has disappeared (b).

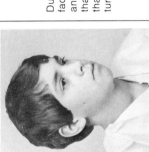

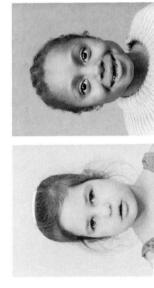

Mouth

Inspection

Particular attention should be paid to the jaw size, as it affects both the spacing of the teeth and appearance.

Permanent teeth begin to erupt when a child is approximately 6 years of age (a). Girls usually experience the trauma of losing "baby" teeth about six months earlier than do boys. The first teeth to erupt are the central incisors (b). Sometime during the sixth year, the first molars appear.

When the child is about 7 years of age, the lateral incisors make their debut. During the child's ninth year, the roots of the lower central and lateral incisors and the first molars complete their growth. The lower cuspids erupt at the age of 10. Other teeth that erupt during the school-age period complete their root growth in preadolescence or adolescence. Consequently, fluoride should be given until the age of 17 to fully provide protection. In general, black children tend to develop permanent teeth earlier than do white children.

Nose and Sinuses

Inspection

Inspection of the nose and sinuses is similar to that described in Chap. 4.

Although sinus development is variable, it is usually completed between the ages of 8 and 10 (c). Transillumination of the sinuses prior to complete development would not be valuable.

Permanent teeth continue to erupt during the school-age years. Consequently, braces should not be considered until the growth of the 6-year molars is complete.

Permanent teeth erupt earlier in girls than in boys, and in general, black children develop permanent teeth earlier than do white children.

Figure b from Mary Tudor, Child Development, McGraw-Hill, 1981, p. 73.

Sinus development is usually completed between the ages of 8 and 10.

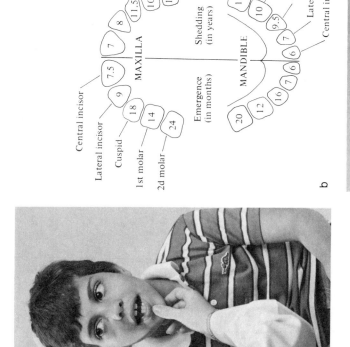

a

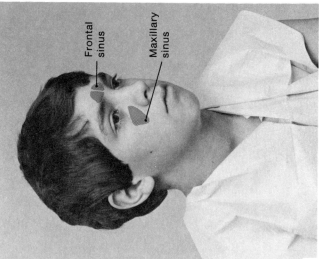

Central incisor — 7.5
Lateral incisor — 9
Cuspid — 18
1st molar — 14
2d molar — 24

7
8
11.5
10.5
11.5

MAXILLA

Shedding (in years)

Emergence (in months)

MANDIBLE

20
12
16
7
6
6
7
9.5
10
11

2d molar
1st molar
Cuspid
Lateral incisor
Central incisor

b

Frontal sinus

Maxillary sinus

c

Although 20/20 vision is sometimes achieved as early as age 6, it is more often reached by age 11. Similarly, *binocular vision* is sometimes fully developed by age 6 but more often by age 11.

Binocular vision is the ability to use both eyes in a coordinated way.

Hearing should be tested every other year in the school-age child.

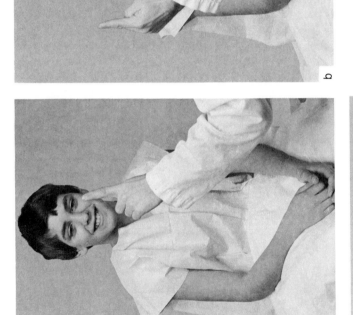

b

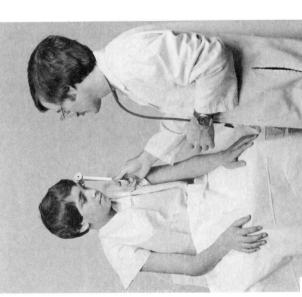

a

c

Eyes

Inspection

Examination of the external eye often reveals changes in the shape of the eyes. This variability results from the growth of facial bone structure and inherited familial and cultural traits.

Visual acuity, 20/20 or better, is usually reached by age 11. However, some children achieve 20/20 vision by age 6. The *hyperopia*, or farsightedness, that is usual in children decreases with age.

Binocular vision, the ability to use both eyes in a coordinated manner, is usually fully developed by age 11, although some studies indicate that 51 percent of the children have binocular vision by age 6 (a).

Visual fields and eye-muscle coordination should be tested to observe visual competence (b). Normally, the examination should reveal findings similar to those described in Chap. 4.

Ears

Inspection

Special attention should be paid to *auditory acuity*. Normally, the child should be able to detect frequencies, or sound waves, from 500 to 8000 cycles per second (Hz) at 25 decibels (dB), the "threshold" of sound.

The remainder of the ear examination is similar to that described in Chap. 4 (c).

592

Highlights

Refer to Chap. 4 for a complete discussion of the neck.

Palpation of the neck muscles may show increased but not optimal strength.

Lymph nodes in the neck may be palpable until age 12.

Neck

Inspection

the neck should develop in proportion to other body structures.

Palpation

Palpation of the sternocleidomastoid muscle may reveal increased strength in the school-age child (a). However, the strength of this muscle has not yet reached its optimal level. Also, lymph nodes in the neck of the school-age child may be palpable until approximately 12 years of age (b).

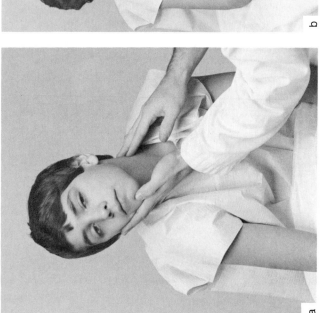

a

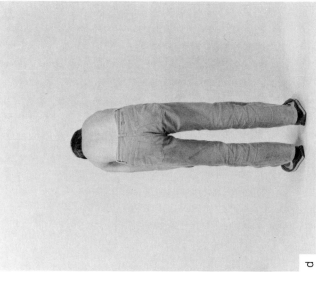

b

Thorax

Inspection

Normally, the shape of the thorax will be similar to that described in Chap. 4. Size will of course be dependent on the child's rate of overall growth and development.

The shape and diameter of the thorax may be altered by the presence of *scoliosis* (lateral curvature of the spine), which has a high incidence in the school-age group.

To inspect for these changes, have the client stand erect with the feet together and back towards the examiner (c). The client should then bend forward at the waist until the back is parallel with the floor (d).

In normal children both sides of the back are on the same level. When scoliosis is present, one shoulder blade is more prominent than the other, the thoracic cavity appears slanted, and a contralateral tilt of the pelvis may occur.

Scoliosis - lateral curvature of the spine.

Scoliosis is frequently seen in school-age children as early as age 7.

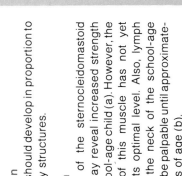

c

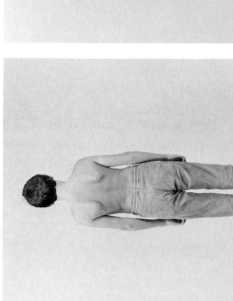

d

Lungs

Examination of the lungs in the school-age child is similar to the findings described in Chap. 4.

Heart

Inspection

The heart of the school-age child is small in relation to body size (a). It grows slowly with development often accompanying physical growth spurts. Regardless of size, however, the heart is able to supply the resources needed to perform physical and metabolic activities. Excessive, sustained athletic activity may increase fatigue during this age period.

Because the size of the heart of the school-age child is small in relation to body size, sustained activity may decrease stamina and increase fatigue.

Palpation

During this age period heart rate will begin to slow down in comparison with the rate in earlier stages of development (average of 70 to 110 beats per minute).

The pulse rate begins to slow down during this age period.

Auscultation

Auscultation for heart sounds should be performed and may reveal innocent murmurs in the early school-age child (see Chap. 8).

Breasts

Inspection

Breast development in girls, which begins between the ages of 8 and 13, is evidenced by an increase in the diameter of the areolar area of the breast (b). Completed breast development usually coincides with menarche.

Breast development begins in girls between the ages of 8 and 13.

Palpation

Self-examination of the breast should begin with the onset of menarche. (Refer to the examination presented in Chap. 4.)

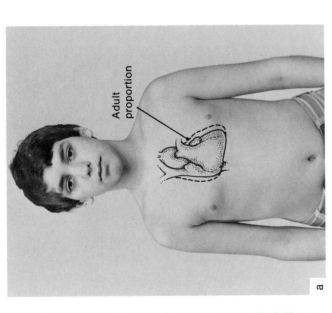

Adult proportion

a

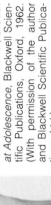
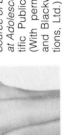
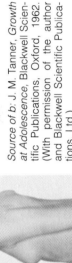
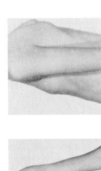
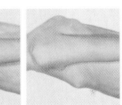
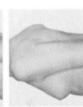

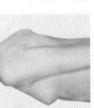
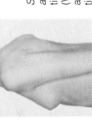
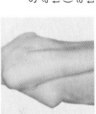
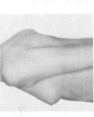
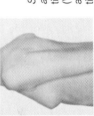
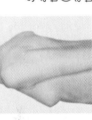

b

Source of b: J. M. Tanner, *Growth at Adolescence*, Blackwell Scientific Publications, Oxford, 1962. (With permission of the author and Blackwell Scientific Publications, Ltd.)

Highlights

The shape of the abdomen becomes more scaphoid as the potbelly of early childhood disappears.

Bladder capacity increases and kidney function improves during this age period.

Girls usually mature sexually earlier than do boys.

The development of secondary sexual characteristics begins in both boys and girls during the school-age years.

Source of b and c: J. M. Tanner, *Growth at Adolescence,* Blackwell Scientific Publications, Oxford, 1962. (With permission of the author and Blackwell Scientific Publications, Ltd.)

Abdomen

Inspection

The shape of the abdomen of the school-age child becomes increasingly scaphoid as the potbelly of early childhood is lost (a). In general, there is a slimming of the body. As girls approach adolescence, the appearance of secondary sexual characteristics give rise to a more rounded physical shape.

As the gastrointestinal system develops, its stability increases, and the child is able to tolerate longer periods without food. Episodes of nausea and diarrhea decrease.

Along with an increase in bladder capacity, kidney filtration and concentration improve. The myelinization of the central nervous system helps to stabilize physiological responses, and improved muscle control helps to increase bladder and bowel efficiency.

Genitalia

Inspection

In girls, pubic hair appears between the ages of 8 and 13 (b). The preadolescent growth spurt follows in about 1 year and menarche in 2 years.

In boys, pubic hair appears and testicular enlargement begins between the ages of 9½ and 13½ (c). The penis starts to increase in size shortly thereafter. Although the penis may appear small or practically nonexistent in boys who suffer from exogenous obesity, it is actually quite normal in size.

Parental guidance regarding the onset of menarche and nocturnal emissions and their significance to the child's development should begin when secondary sexual characteristics begin to develop.

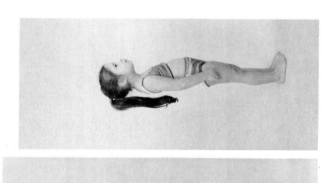

a

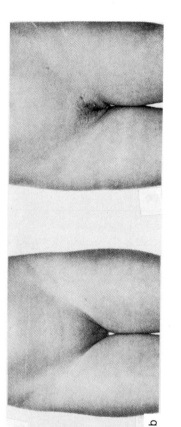

b

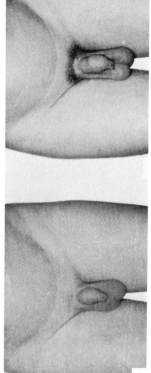

c

Palpation

In the male, the testes are sometimes normally retracted (a). To "milk" the testes into the scrotum, the child should assume a squatting position. Frequently the pressure thus exerted by this action is often sufficient to force the testes into the sac. If not, the examiner should palpate the testes in the inguinal canal and then "milk" them into the scrotum.

Rectum

Inspection

The size of the rectum varies with age. To facilitate the child's cooperation during a rectal examination, the examiner should carefully explain the procedure to be followed.

The actual procedure is similar to that described in Chap. 4.

Extremities

Inspection

Because various parts of the body grow at different rates and because the lower extremities experience their most rapid growth during this age period, both boys and girls are often long-legged (b). This phenomenon, evidenced by the steady lowering of the midpoint of height from the umbilicus to halfway between it and the symphysis pubis, allows an improvement in general movement and a more coordinated and controlled gait.

As growth progresses, the cartilaginous (soft) bone structure of boys and girls in the early school years is gradually replaced by bone (ossification) (c). Bone growth often parallels sexual maturity. Advanced bone development suggests the onset of early puberty.

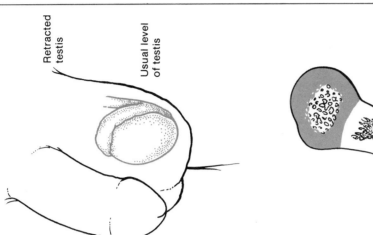

a

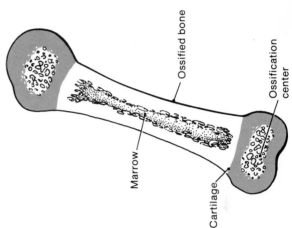

c

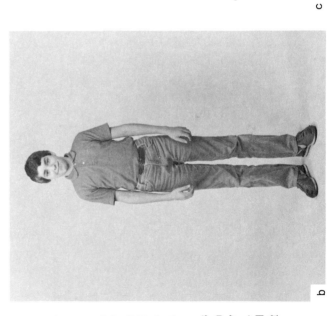

b

Highlights

Palpation of the testes is an important part of the male genital examination.

When the testes are retracted they should be "milked" into the scrotum.

The rectal examination is similar to the findings described in Chap. 4.

The rectal examination should be carefully described to the child to insure cooperation.

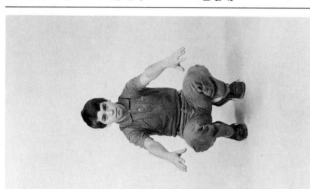
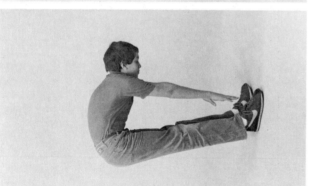
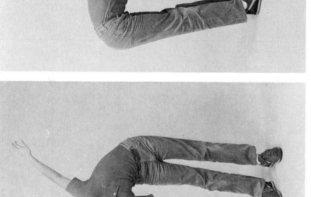

a

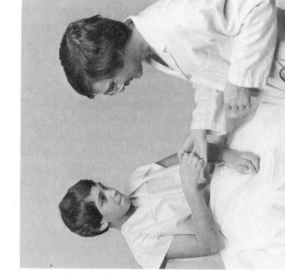

b

Strength and muscle flexibility improve as muscle fibers lengthen. As the myelinization of the central nervous system stabilizes body responses, the coordination of fine and gross motor skills generally begins to improve and the child has more control of his or her body (a).

Early mild scoliosis (lateral curvature of the spine) may be suggested during the examination of gait (see Thorax).

Palpation
Although muscle strength doubles during this age period, as revealed in the palpation and testing of muscle grip (b), resistance, and so on, it is not equal to that of an adult.

ADOLESCENCE CHAPTER TEN

Karen L. Miller

Adolescence is the transitional stage of life that begins at pubescence and continues to the onset of adulthood. In the continuum of growth and development, adolescence has been recognized as an important period of physiological and psychological change and adjustment. Until recently, there has been little research of adolescent physical and psychological development or emotional response to health and illness. Adolescents have been considered either children to pediatric practitioners or immature adults to specialists in internal medicine or surgery.

> Adolescence is the transitional stage of life during which a child becomes an adult.

Today, the unique needs of adolescents are beginning to be identified by health care providers. This care has been facilitated by laws which permit diagnosis and management of some conditions of minors without the approval of their parents. In addition, psychologists have made it known that adolescents should interact directly with health providers, without parental intervention, and finally, newer technical advances, particularly radioimmunoassay, allow measurement of very small amounts of hormones and earlier detection of pubescent endocrine change.[1]

> Health care for adolescents has recently been seen as a separate entity, requiring special services to this population.

The practice of adolescent health care is branching out into all segments of the health care system, including outpatient and inpatient facilities, community health centers, private physicians' offices, college-based health clinics, and school health programs.

The trend toward adolescent health screening and outpatient health care will involve nurses more than ever before with the adolescent population. The nurse's special skills in observation, assessment, and planning for health care are needed to help keep this "essentially healthy" client population in contact with health professionals. When the adolescent client is found to have a personal, social, or health problem, the holistic approach and caring aspects of nursing will help meet this young client's total needs.

> The role of the nurse in adolescent health care is expanding.

HEALTH HISTORY

The holistic approach to health history is especially suited to meet the health needs of adolescents. Certain variables may affect a health assessment of an adolescent client. One important factor is recognition of the client as an individual. Each adolescent has certain expectations of the interview and a unique response to health history questions. In addition, failure to consider developmental aspects of adolescence almost guarantees that the interviewer will fail to accurately assess the client.

> Refer to Chap. 3 when completing the health history of the adolescent.
>
> The approach used by the nurse in completing the health history must incorporate developmental aspects of adolescence.

Knowledge of the client's age is a useful indicator of developmental stage, but the chronological age of an adolescent frequently bears little relationship to the behavior of an individual client who acts and reacts according to feelings and not to what is expected of that particular age group.[2] The wide range of psychological development and behavior seen among adolescent clients from preadolescents to young adults also makes it difficult for the nurse to gather reliable health history information.

> Knowledge of the client's age is helpful in determining the individual's health status.
>
> The chronological age of an adolescent may not always correspond to the developmental stage of the adolescent.

Frequently, it is necessary for the nurse to make an appraisal of the adolescent client's thought process or thinking ability. This kind of information helps the interviewer to better understand what the client is trying to say and vice versa.

In addition to appraising the pattern of logical thinking used by the adolescent client, the nurse should be aware of the client's nonverbal communication patterns. Adolescents tend to use a variety of physical means to communicate, including body position, arm and hand waving, eye rolling, and facial expression. Since adolescents are frequently uncomfortable in a dialogue situation with adults, they will express themselves through physical rather than verbal communication. It is helpful for the nurse to learn to interpret the nonverbal communication patterns of adolescent clients and to be aware of each client's own physical communication patterns.

Young clients are particularly sensitive to the reactions of others. Therefore, the nurse must take care not to alienate an adolescent client through "negative" nonverbal communication.

When planning the setting for the interview, consideration should be given to environmental factors. Careful planning of the environment can minimize stress for the client and enhance nurse-client interaction. The adolescent client must be assured of privacy and that the interview will be uninterrupted. Full attention of the nurse during the time of the conversation is another important factor related to data collection.

Since teenagers are less cognizant of time than are adults, it is important to establish the time limitations at the beginning of the dialogue.

Take time to explain to the adolescent client your role as a nurse in providing care.

A flexible approach to adolescent clients is needed until it is possible to appraise the client's maturational level. Frequently it is useful to perform a few parts of the physical examination, such as the vital signs, to allow the client time to relax before health history questions are asked.

A flexible attitude toward client interaction is important to data collection.

Data Collection

When interviewing adolescents, it is important to approach the individual honestly since teenagers can be distrustful of adults. Honesty requires a clear elucidation of the role the health care provider will play and the responsibility the teenager will assume for personal health care management. Questioning should allow the client opportunities to express feelings. When direct questioning is used, its use should be carefully explained. For example, the nurse might say, "I'm going to ask a lot of questions now that will help me get to know you better. With the information we get, we can plan together what is best for you."

Privacy and honesty are important attributes to a successful health history.

Another important consideration during the data collection phase is the role of parents. Often it is the parents who bring the teenager to the hospital or clinic and are concerned about the outcome of the examination. However, regardless of whether the parents are present at the time of the admission and examination, they should not be present in the room when the adolescent client is being interviewed and examined. The nurse should make it clear to the client that information gained during the history taking is confidential. There are exceptions to this general rule, which include a client's plans for suicide, injury to others, or plans to run away from home. When the nurse's confidentiality with the client is to be broken, it should be explained carefully.

The role of parents is important, yet the adolescent generally requests parents to be excluded from the interview.

The issue of client confidentiality is of particular concern to adolescents.

Recording the Data

The data gathered during the interview should be recorded in a logical manner in a permanent record accessible to all members of the health care team as discussed in Chap. 3. When recording information about the preadolescent or adolescent client, it is important to consider the laws of consent and confidentiality which may apply to these particular clients.

There has been growing concern among health professionals in the last decade about the rights and privileges of minors. Recent legislation has supported the rights of minors in health care matters in what is coming to be collectively termed the *mature minor rule*. This principle gives minors who have achieved sufficient maturity or are able to understand the risks and benefits of treatments they are to receive, the right to give valid informed consent. This principle applies to treatments of various sorts and includes confidentiality of health care records. It is important that the nurse become aware of the legal status of adolescents in their particular state. Since the mature minor rule is inconsistently applied, the problem of minors being able to obtain confidential health care information on their own consent still exists.

Of further consideration is the issue of the availability of a minor's recorded health care information from the perspective of present and future interests.[3] It is possible for health history information to be available on request to some agencies, such as insurance companies and statistical bureaus. When making entries into any client's permanent health record, it is important for the nurse to keep in mind the ramifications of the availability of information. Care should be taken in what is recorded and what words are used. Adolescents frequently request that certain information be kept from family members. Also, the youth may be justifiably concerned about certain information becoming available to the public and decreasing chances for future education, work opportunities, personal relationships, and so on.

Entry into the Health Care System

When an adolescent seeks health care, it is generally because of a specific problem or because of school, camp, or athletic physical examination requirements. For some adolescents, introduction to the health care system may follow a major illness or catastrophic injury. Rarely is a complete health history taken for the adolescent client. For these reasons many health needs of adolescents are left unmet.

Client Profile

It is important to emphasize to the adolescent client the need for biographical information. The client should understand that health history questions are modified in accordance with this information. Biographical data or client profile information should include the following:

1 Name, address, sex, marital status, race, nationality, religion, and date and place of birth
2 Blood type (if available) (Refer to Chap. 3 for further discussion of this category.)

Health Status—Health Perception

The client's reason for entry into the health care system should be identified. The nurse should ascertain whether the adolescent client has initiated contact with a health professional independently or whether a parent or guardian initiated this contact.

Current Health Status The current health status gives important information to the nurse concerning the client's perception of his or her present health. This is particularly important in adolescence as there is much misinformation as to what is "normal" in the areas of growth and development, especially as it relates to sexual development and activity.

Health Perception The client should be encouraged to describe his or her general health status at the time of the interview. Recording of this response should be in the client's own words. In addition, the client's perception of health and health-related values should be elicited at this time. It is important to use language that is easily understandable to the adolescent client for questions about health and health values. Clarification of the meaning of health and illness may provide the nurse with insight into the adolescent understandings and values related to health and wellness.

Client perception of the "client" role can also be generated at this time. The nurse should explain the term "client" to the adolescent before proceeding with questions in this area. Refer to Client Profile in Chap. 3 for suggested questions.

Past Health Status   The adolescent should understand the reason for health professionals' need to be familiar with past health information. The nurse should emphasize the intention of providing good health care and of working with the client to plan for total health needs. Birth history, growth and development from birth to the present, childhood diseases, immunizations, allergies, and previous hospitalizations can all be discussed at this time.

Family History   The need for a family history is essential to providing an adolescent with a comprehensive plan for care. The nurse needs to take time to explain to the adolescent the need for the family history, especially as it relates to prevention of familial tendencies or inherited disorders. By giving a rationale, the nurse avoids being perceived as inappropriately prying into the teenager's background.

Many teenagers will not know about the medical histories of other family members. If more information is needed, the nurse should explain this to the individual and request permission to seek additional data from the parent or guardian.

Health Habits   It can be said that adolescents generally tend to view health care, hospitals, physicians, nurses, and other health care professionals as part of the adult "culture" or environment. For this reason there are occasions when some adolescents will intentionally choose to engage in unhealthy habits as an indication of their independence from adults. This phenomenon has been shown in a variety of studies of adolescents with chronic illnesses.

The most significant unhealthy habit that is rapidly increasing in the healthy adolescent population is cigarette smoking. Despite media advertisement and physician emphasis on the proven dangers of smoking, some people still begin this habit as teenagers. Many choose cigarette smoking because of a desire for independence or rebellion rather than for enjoyment. All health professionals should work toward educating young people about the hazards of smoking and should set a healthy example by not smoking themselves. Adolescents respond much better to example than to admonishment.

Established activities, engaged in regularly should be elicited to estimate the client's commitment to health optimization (refer to Chap. 3).

Life Patterns and Lifestyles

Discussion of life patterns include those factors that make up one's lifestyle. These include age, race, heredity, culture, growth and development, biological rhythms, and environmental and economic factors as well as community resources.

Highlights

It is important to use language that is understandable to the adolescent client when eliciting data.

Refer to Chap. 3 for suggested questions on past health status.

A brief explanation about the need for the family history will prevent the adolescent client from feeling as if the nurse is inappropriately prying.

When the nurse gathers information about the family history, many feelings about the family members can also be elicited.

Adolescents sometimes choose to express their independence by engaging in habits that are considered unhealthy by most adults.

The problems of cigarette smoking and substance abuse are two unhealthy habits found among teenagers.

The nurse must evaluate the adolescent client's health state as it is influenced by ethnic background, lifestyle, and family customs.

Age   Age can play a part in the way an adolescent responds to health care and health needs, but it does not specifically determine maturational level. Adolescents vary greatly in maturity at any given age. Older or more mature adolescent clients will often be able to make responsible decisions about health care without parental or adult intervention. Younger or immature adolescents tend to rely heavily on adult guidance in making decisions about themselves, especially regarding health needs. Adolescents of any age generally must be prompted to seek health care. For this reason health professionals should educate the adolescent client in the importance of regular health care and activities of health promotion whenever the opportunity arrives.

Race   Adolescents are subject to the same influences as adults in the way that race influences their susceptibility to certain disease processes. Race can affect the lifestyle patterns, including nutrition and health perception and activity. The adolescent is particularly vulnerable to the standards set by the peer group with whom they associate. Certain racial groups may condone practices and hold beliefs not prevalent within other groups. The nurse should be familiar with the unique characteristics of the different racial groups within the client population.

Heredity   When talking to adolescent clients about family inheritance or predisposition to a health problem it is important to explain why the information is necessary. Often adolescents will not immediately understand that they may be affected by the health or illness of relatives. It is important to assess the clients' perceptions of their families, health and attitudes toward health and illness. In addition to asking the usual information about the clients' close relatives, it is useful to ask clients whether they feel affected by illnesses of family members or if they believe family members "passed on" any illnesses to the client. If possible, the nurse should verify specific information regarding genetic history with adults, since adolescents may be unreliable sources of this kind of information.

Culture   Despite the variety of cultural influences on any particular client, there are several universal "tasks" of adolescence that will affect personal physical and emotional well-being. Each adolescent, regardless of cultural differences, must learn to make significant changes in life patterns and lifestyle from preadolescent years to young adulthood. The teenager must learn to change from being cared for by others to taking care of others and to sever close ties with the nuclear family and establish them with unfamiliar people. Intimate love occurs outside family relationships in most cultures. Adolescents are expected to learn to love and care for others and to work to provide for their loved ones. Cultural influence on an adolescent begins with these basic tasks. Should an adolescent be unable to meet them, physical or emotional health may be compromised.

Cultures also differ considerably in the way they support the achievement of maturity. These differences can produce a variety of attitudes toward health and illness among adolescents. Biological, social, and psychological development and achievement may each proceed at a different pace, with these differences providing major stresses to the adolescents of each society. Norm of adult status in most of the world is socioeconomic responsibility, rather than sexual reproduction.[4] In order to understand the differences among the adolescent clients' attitudes toward health and illness, it is essential for the nurse to be familiar with

Age does not determine maturational level, but it does provide some guideline for assessing the developmental level of an adolescent.

Adolescents vary greatly in maturity at any given age

Maturity is measured differently within various cultural groups. The nurse must learn what criteria are used to evaluate physical and social maturity within a particular ethnic group.

Refer to Chap. 3 for additional questions concerning race.

Regardless of cultural differences, each teenager must learn to make changes in lifestyle during adolescence.

Cultures differ considerably in the way the achievement of maturity is supported.

western culture's definition of adulthood. At age 12, during very early adolescence, an individual is regarded as an "adult" by owners of movie theaters, airlines, and amusement parks. This change of status does not include any privileges; rather, it requires the penalty of higher admission prices for entertainment and travel. At age 16 in most states, an adolescent is considered an "adult" for the purpose of driving a car. In addition, the teenager is no longer subject to child labor laws. This does confer some adult privileges along with responsibilities associated with legal issues.

Another important change occurs for adolescents at age 18. At this age people may marry without parental consent and may vote, and males become subjected to the military draft in times of national need. In most states alcoholic beverages are prohibited at this age, and adolescent females may legally consent to sexual intercourse. (Prior to age 18 any sexual intercourse is legally considered to be rape, regardless of the feelings of the couple involved.)

At age 21 the adolescent attains most adult privileges and responsibilities conferred by society. At this time an individual is allowed to drink all alcoholic beverages, sign a binding financial document, and accept full legal penalties for crimes.

Attainment of maturity will vary in our culture, especially when considering societal allowances made for some adolescents and young adults relative to their economic and educational situations. Many American youths are permitted to depend on parents for financial and emotional support while they are in college (18 to 22 years or older); however, peers who are not pursuing higher education are expected to be independent from parental support. (Refer to Chap. 12 for a further elaboration.)

The nurse can establish functional maturity of adolescent clients by asking questions related to financial support and legal responsibilities. It is most useful to elicit the clients' perception of their own situations and then to verify the responses through questioning of parents or guardians when possible.

Societal Characteristics Societal stereotyping of adolescents occurs in any given culture and during any given span of years. Adolescents are continually regarded as a group by adults for many reasons. There are few clear guidelines for the adolescent to meet the challenges of society for independence, vocational decisions, legal responsibilities, marriage, and family. This problem has worsened in recent years as a result of rapid social changes, including the decline of the extended family, increasing segregation by age, and polarization of adults into groups of social class, political philosophy, and cultural belief.[5]

As independence from parents and family begins to occur in early adolescence, the influence of other adolescents on an individual's lifestyle and behavior increases. The peer group can provide the adolescent with a sense of belonging and power that otherwise cannot be obtained. To become a part of this adolescent group, the individual tends to conform in lifestyle, behavior, appearance, musical taste, and so on. Adolescents form their own "culture" with its own social obligations, language, customs, and philosophies.

Because of the vulnerability of young teenagers, the pressures of peer group conformity may also be harmful. Individual judgment may often be forfeited to the desires of the group as a whole, creating great stress and anxiety in some adolescents. It is the rare adolescent who has developed enough ego strength to stand alone against the crowd. It should be remembered that teenagers will perceive their behavior as

Highlights

Within western culture there are various indicators that mark the progression toward adulthood.

Age 18 is an important milestone within western culture.

At age 21, an adolescent is allowed adult status and the privileges and responsibilities conferred by our society.

Today, adult responsibility may be delayed because of the prolonged dependence on parents as individuals complete their schooling.

The nurse must establish the functional maturity of the adolescent client.

Independence from family and parents begins to occur in early adolescence.

Peer influences and pressures can affect behavior and create an adolescent culture with set rules for dress, language, and so on, thereby increasing stress for the adolescent.

highly individualistic or original, because it is different from that of adults.

Another important characteristic to consider is the relationship between the parents of an adolescent and his or her peer group or friends. Frequently, values and beliefs of parents will be dramatically different from those of the adolescent's friends. This can potentially result in friction between these two influential factions and can be a source of stress, especially if the teenager feels that a choice must be made between loved family members and friends.

Adolescents can experience conflict between the values of their peers and those of their parents.

The interview provides an excellent opportunity for the health professional to determine the reaction of the adolescent client to societal stereotyping and peer group pressure. Questions about friends should be nonthreatening and nonjudgmental. The nurse should emphasize the need for data about normal daily activities and social contacts because there are times when health can be affected by these factors. The client must not feel that the nurse is prying or curious about his or her life. If the interview is going well, how the client feels about being a teenager should be evident from responses to various questions.

The nurse should always explain the need for information about family and friends in a nonthreatening and nonjudgmental manner.

Growth and Development The transitional period of adolescence includes the years from pubescence to the onset of adulthood. These years contain a variety of functional physiological and psychoemotional changes. To assess these changes, it is necessary for the nurse to be familiar with the definitions of the states of adolescence.

The stages of growth and development provide only general guidelines as all individuals mature at varying rates.

Preadolescence The school-age child of 8 or 9 years begins to experience progressive endocrine changes which are emotionally unsettling and result in vague physical sensations. At this time the child enters the stage of preadolescence, which includes the years 10 to 12 for girls and somewhat later, 10 or 11 to 13 years, for boys. The preadolescent stage is characterized by increases in physical activity and energy which are related to hormonal changes but do not seem to be associated with any significant changes in sexual drive.[6]

Adolescent girls generally mature slightly earlier than adolescent boys.

Early Adolescence Pubescence is the time during which reproductive functions begin to actively mature and is associated with the stage of early adolescence. This phase extends from ages 12 to 14 years for girls and from 13 to 15 years for boys. Early adolescence usually coincides with the advent of menarche in females and active spermatogenesis in males. Estrogen, testosterone, and allied hormones are at levels close to those of adults.[7]

Midadolescence The stage of midadolescence begins when the teenager starts to relate to the opposite sex. The midadolescent gradually becomes more self-assured and able to make some independent decisions. For these reasons the youth at this stage has particular difficulty in adjusting to controlling or confining situations, such as illness or hospitalization. This period extends between the ages of 14 to 15 years and 17 to 18 years.[8] During midadolescence there is a wide range of psychological and physiological changes occurring among individuals of the same age. Societal privileges and responsibilities are increased. Family harmony and communication may be disrupted as the midadolescent's activity outside the home is increased. Until the individual can overcome feelings of insecurity and inadequacy which mark the end of this stage, support and patient guidance by adults, including health professionals, must be given.

The stage of midadolescence marks a period of disruption in the home as teenagers feel the conflicts of increased responsibility and privileges that take them away from home for increased activity.

Late Adolescence Late adolescence is the last stage before adulthood. This stage usually includes the ages between 17 to 18 years. During this period the older teenager moves into more intense personal relationships with the opposite sex. Often a relationship with a particu-

Late adolescence is marked by the development of more intense personal relationships.

lar person will become the focal point for social activity. Activities with family members tend to decrease during late adolescence, and relationships with parents move toward adult friendships. The thought process of the adolescent becomes more logical. There is an increasing ability to utilize abstract ideas. The end of the stage of late adolescence is marked by planning for the future. The older adolescent will concentrate on personal plans for higher education, occupation, marriage, and family. Illness or hospitalization can be stressful at this period if plans for the future are interrupted or made impossible. The status of young adulthood is reached when the adolescent begins to adjust to full societal responsibilities and personal life goals.

At each stage of adolescence the expectations, perceptions, and behaviors of adolescent clients differ. A varying focus of strengths and areas of concern accompanies each phase. It is important that the nurse recognize the growth stages of adolescence so that the needs of the adolescent client can be better assessed.

Biological Rhythms Sleep patterns and elimination patterns can occur as measurable examples of biological rhythms in adolescents.

Sleep-Wakefulness Cycle Adolescent clients may have an unusual sleep-wakefulness cycle, especially if they live outside the family. Older adolescents tend to prefer sleeping late in the morning and going to bed late at night whenever possible. It is important to assess the amount of sleep that the teenager needs and is able to obtain during each 24-hour period. Because adolescents are sensitive about their personal habits, the nurse should always be careful to ask questions about these subjects in a nonjudgmental manner. Questions such as, "Do you feel rested when you wake after sleeping?" or "Do you feel you get enough sleep?" or "How would you describe the way you sleep?" allow the client to describe personal perceptions (questions about dreams and waking during the sleep period should be included). A teenager may often have complaints about fatigue or inability to do well in school because of poor sleeping patterns.

Elimination Patterns Many adolescents do not eat regular, nutritional meals for a variety of reasons. Changes in elimination patterns can also be due to school stressors, dating, etc. This common occurrence may lead to poor urinary and bowel habits. Although adolescent clients may be embarrassed to discuss this subject, assessment of elimination patterns is important. The nurse should explain why this kind of information is needed. To help the client relax, it is sometimes useful to explain to the client that some health problems are related to urination and bowel movements before proceeding with specific questions.

Environmental Factors The environment includes factors such as the home, neighborhood, national and state boundaries, climate, and surroundings that must be assessed during a health history. It is impossible to adequately evaluate the adolescent client without knowing the person's external environment. Because of developmental changes and psychoemotional vulnerability, adolescents are particularly affected by their immediate environment.

Recent studies indicate that neighborhoods seem to affect the behavior of adolescent individuals. For instance, large urban areas produce more juvenile delinquents than do small towns or rural areas. Although delinquents tend to come from backgrounds of socioeconomic deprivation, a teenager who is poor but lives in an upper-middle-class neighborhood has less chance of becoming delinquent than do peers living in deprived areas.[9]

Since "environment" is a term with both broad and varied meaning, it is difficult to elicit information about environment from adolescent clients. The nurse must make astute observations as well as ask questions which will lead clients to talk about their surroundings.

Questions to elicit data

1 "What kind of neighborhood did you live in as a small child?"
2 "Do you still live there?"
3 "Have you lived in the same house all of your life?" (Refer to Chap. 3 for Additional Questions).

Many adolescents today are justifiably concerned with the potentially noxious forces including environmental pollution, nuclear energy, and political unrest in the world. These subjects are frequently discussed by teenagers. The nurse should be sensitive to the possible effect of these issues on the adolescent population. This discussion may stimulate the adolescent client to ask questions or voice concerns about the personal hazards of environmental and world conditions and identify ways to optimize health care in view of these concerns.

Threats to personal survival because of potentially noxious environmental factors can be distressful to the adolescent.

During the 1960s, many adolescents found the Vietnam War to be "unhealthy" and protested against U.S. involvement. Today many adolescents are concerned about issues such as conservation of natural resources and air pollution, etc.

Economic Status Until the age of 15 to 16 years most adolescents must rely on parents for financial support. Many young teenagers supplement their "spending money" through various odd jobs, such as baby-sitting, newspaper delivery, lawn mowing, and errand running. Some of these jobs, although low-paying, require maturity and responsibility. When legally permissible, some adolescents will drop out of high school in favor of working for economic gain. This decision is, by and large, a poor choice for most teenagers because they are usually unskilled and unable to find good jobs. An unemployed adolescent may experience unusual stress as a result of frustration, dependence on others, and continual rejection by the working society, as discussed in the behavioral assessment.

Until the age of 15 or 16, most teenagers earn money from various odd jobs.

Adolescents frequently drop out of school because of the desire for economic independence.

Older adolescents who choose to stay in school and to pursue higher education are often forced to find employment to help support themselves or their family or to help pay for school. These jobs may cause undue stress to the individual as many are low-paying and require long hours of work, thus taking away from social interactions and study responsibilities. The nurse may interview young clients who express feelings of being overwhelmed because of economic pressures.

It is important to evaluate the adolescent client's economic status by asking questions that will specifically summarize a client's financial situation.

Questions to elicit data

1 How would you describe your financial status?
2 Are you financially dependent on anyone?
3 How do you earn spending money?

When the client expresses concern about his or her economic situation, further exploration into the specific concerns are indicated. (Refer to the discussion in Chap. 3 for added Questions.)

Community Resources Many communities devote much time and energy to the development of resources directed toward the needs of adolescents. These range from programs emphasizing prevention and detection of drug and alcohol abuse to athletic programs to providing places and programs for teenagers to socialize. Both the client and the parents should be asked about their knowledge of the availability of such resources in their community. In addition, the schools often prove a valuable resource for adolescent clients and their families.

Roles and Relationship Patterns

The adolescent is struggling with transition from the role of a child to a role that allows for greater independence and personal freedom to make decisions. During this time the nurse must become a good listener, facilitating discussion rather than judging activities and thoughts. Since role changes occur most dramatically at this time, support and counseling become important nursing interventions.

Family Life Recent declarations by the media imply that the American family is "dying" and is no longer the most important extrinsic factor in the life of an individual family member. Despite those statements, the impact of family background on childhood and adolescence is still of central importance in evaluating an adolescent client's values, intelligence, aspirations, and lifestyle. "Especially important predictors are the educational attainment of the parent(s), their occupation(s), socioeconomic status as reflected in the physical environment of the home, and the quality of parent-child relationships."[10]

Since adolescence is a transition period covering several years, there are usually marked differences between the adolescent and the family depending on the developmental stage of the teenager. For instance, early adolescence is the time for increasing peer group interactions. At this time there is a low point in family relationships. As the adolescent matures and adapts to societal demands for outside relationships, there is a more positive parent-child interaction. This occurs regardless of whether the "family" means the traditional nuclear family, single-parent family, extended family, or communal kind of family.[11]

Parenting Behaviors and Adolescence The style of parenting to which adolescents are accustomed will often dictate their behavior and relationships with others. Ideally, adolescents need parents who are neither dictators nor totally lenient toward the teenager. Most adjusted adolescents have parents who are good role models, respected by the teenager, and honest in their own personal relationships.

To elicit information about the family and its influence on the adolescent client, the nurse should allow the client room for expression of perceptions without having to respond to many structured questions. The client should be asked open-ended questions.

Questions to elicit data

1 Tell me about your family.
2 What kind of parents do you have?
3 Does your family get along together?
4 What kind of restrictions do you have at home?
5 How does your family feel about your friends?

Occupation Studies indicate that most adolescents progress through predictable stages in developing vocational goals. The first period is called the *fantasy period* and occurs in early and middle childhood when occupations are likely to be selected that seem adventurous and exciting, such as astronaut, firefighter, explorer, or ranch hand. These are emotional and at times unrealistic choices, come from child's play and televi-

Recreational groups for teenagers have declined in popularity in recent years. Many communities lack organized, supervised activities for adolescents.

The family is still a major influence on the adolescent client.

The impact of the family changes as the adolescent moves through the various developmental stages is critical.

Parenting styles influence a teenager's behavior and self-perception.

Always try to be nonjudgmental in facial expression and verbal response to the teenage client's remarks about parents and family and avoid taking sides in family disagreements if possible.

Adolescents progress through stages in developing vocational goals. These stages are:
1. Fantasy period
2. Tentative period
3. Realistic period

sion suggestion. The next period is the *tentative period,* which begins with preadolescence and extends to middle or late adolescence. During this stage individual interests, capabilities, and values merge to guide the adolescent toward choices of occupation which may be actually performed. The final or *realistic period* of adolescence is established as teenagers mature and can better assess their motivation and abilities. Most adolescents are 17 to 19 years old when they enter into this last stage of realistic vocational plans.[12]

Because of the ever-increasing demands of society for financial success as a measure of personal worth, adolescents are usually well aware of the need to choose a job or career. Traditionally, boys have been more occupied with a career decision than have girls. However, recent developments in women's rights have increased the motivation for girls to aspire to life careers outside marriage and child-raising. Occupational planning may cause great stress for adolescents of either sex regardless of background. Therefore, it is important to evaluate the client's thinking about future occupational plans.

Societies often measure personal worth by financial success. As a result, adolescents are forced to choose a job or career.

Cognitive-Perceptual Patterns

Reassessment of the individual's ability to perceive through the senses is often accomplished through the physical examination. In addition, developmental growth is determined through use of language, cognitive skills, and perception of personal assets. For the adolescent, much of this self-perception is in an evolving state, influenced by the level of education as well as the development of cognitive functions.

Education The process of education in the United States affects the life of every adolescent. This is true even if the individual has chosen to leave school at a young age, as minimum educational requirements are legally imposed by state regulations. School remains the center of everyday activity for most adolescents who physically occupy the classroom for 6 to 8 hours each day. Within this age group there are increasing problems of truancy and lack of classroom discipline.

School is the center of activity for most adolescents.

Each grade level within many schools includes students from different cultural, economic, and academic backgrounds. Given the current emphasis on decreased spending for education and increased pay for qualified teachers, the school systems are faced with the impossible tasks of responding to each student's needs without adequate support and resources.

Studies indicate that many of the most serious developmental problems of preadolescents and young teenagers are related to junior high schools or middle schools. The developmental tasks of exploring, decisionmaking, and autonomy are often thwarted by the controlling environment of most school systems. Parents, teachers, and guidance counselors may unknowingly create great anxiety in the adolescent by expecting too much educational, athletic, and social achievement.[13]

The tasks of adolescence are frequently thwarted in the controlling environment of most junior high or middle schools.

In caring for all adolescents involved with the school and college system in our country, the health practitioner must recognize the value of working closely with educational institutions to meet a client's total health needs. It is important to communicate with schools and to initiate integrated services between educational professionals, school health nurses, and outside health professionals.

The nurse must recognize the value of working with educational institutions if one is to impact effectively with the adolescent client.

The health history allows time for the nurse to discuss with the adolescent the impact of the educational process on personal and life goals. Questions should relate the developmental tasks of the individual to school activities so that the nurse can determine the integration of education into the adolescent's lifestyle.

Refer to Chap. 3 for additional questions concerning education.

1 What kind of school do you go to?

2 Is your school large or small?

3 Are you satisfied with your education up to now?

4 What are your main interests in school?

5 Does your school allow you to make decisions about what courses to take? Do you like this?

6 Do you have any choice in extracurricular activities?

7 Do your friends like school? And teachers?

8 Have you ever thought about dropping out of school?

Because the subject of school is likely to cause both positive and negative responses in clients, the nurse must be prepared to listen carefully to a client's complaints and discussion about school. The individual should be directed to answer the questions without using the time for venting only negative feelings about school. Astute interviewing will elicit extrinsic educational factors that may affect the client's health.

Many adolescents feel negatively about their educational experiences. The nurse must allow the client to vent some of these feelings without letting them predominate the interview.

Intelligence During the years from preadolescence to young adulthood, there are both qualitative and quantitative changes in the intelligence of an individual. These changes are predictable within the range of adolescence but cannot be pinpointed at a specific age. While taking the history the nurse should assess the adolescent client's cognitive ability in order to ask appropriate questions and to adequately evaluate responses.

Between preadolescence and young adulthood both qualitative and quantitative changes occur in the intelligence of an individual.

There has been an inability of scientists, psychologists, and educators to agree on the best method of measuring intelligence. However, it is generally accepted that an adolescent progresses through several stages of cognitive development. According to Piaget,[14] the major stage of cognitive development in adolescence is the stage of formal operational thinking. It is during this stage that the individual learns to formulate hypotheses, becomes capable of deductive reasoning, and can provide scientific explanations for events. The preadolescent tends to view problems in the context of the present, while the adolescent can begin to conceptualize abstract components of a problem. In talking to older teenagers, this difference becomes evident when they attempt to explain actions in terms of hypotheses, such as "perhaps it was due to the weather" or "maybe you were too angry to respond." Typically, adolescents are willing to change their hypothesis or opinion if data support the change. Preadolescents usually will choose one hypothesis and will not modify it even if presented with negative data.

Along with physical and social changes, the adolescent also moves through various stages of intellectual development. Although there has been no consensus as to the methods of measuring intelligence, there is an acceptance of the differing phases of cognitive development.

According to Piaget, formal operational thinking is the major stage of cognitive development.

Preadolescents tend to view problems in the context of the present, while the adolescent begins to conceptualize abstract components of a problem.

Because of the uncertainty regarding exactly when formal operational logic occurs, it is essential for health professionals to ask questions that will stimulate an adolescent's thinking process.

Questions to elicit data

1 Why do you feel that you were a healthy child?

2 Why do you suppose you have been depressed or 'down in the dumps' recently?

It is also important to keep in mind that the situation of the interview itself may cause a client to be anxious and to revert to less mature logic patterns. This same response may result when the adolescent is fatigued or ill.

Refer to Chap. 3 for additional questions concerning intelligence.

Sexuality and Reproductive Patterns

In the holistic sense, human sexuality encompasses all aspects of femininity and masculinity. Sexuality involves the need to love and be loved by another, the ability to give and receive tenderness and affection and the desire for sexual pleasure. As emphasized in Chaps. 2 and 3, human sexuality does not begin at adolescence; rather, it is at this point in the life cycle that sexuality and sexual needs are brought into focus. The developmental task of coming to some understanding of one's sexuality is most significant during adolescence because of the physiological maturing process of adolescence and because adolescence is a period of self-review and identity formation.

The young adolescent becomes increasingly concerned with issues of body image and self-image in the struggle to establish self-identity. Concerns about physical size, bodily functions, and performance begin to raise questions and doubts about sexuality that require answers. The health professional caring for adolescent clients must be aware of this normal developmental process involving body image and sexuality since many of the psychosomatic and physical complaints seen in adolescents relate to dysfunction or to anxious concerns about this developmental task.[15]

Part of the reason that sexuality becomes an area of conflict during adolescence is the attitude of adults toward overt sexual activity during this time. It is acceptable for a child to hug and kiss others during preadolescence, but this same behavior may be unacceptable once the person reaches adolescence. Overt sexuality by teenagers is considered provocative and dangerous and makes some adults uncomfortable, particularly the teenager's parents.

Adolescents are unable to understand the arbitrary attitudes of many adults regarding sexual behavior. The same adults who may have influenced the teenager's sexuality since childhood are now often unable or unwilling to answer questions about sexuality honestly. At this point many teenagers turn away from parents as models for sexual behavior and turn to friends and adults outside the family.

Sexual Role Development

Development of masculinity or femininity is influenced not only by other people, but also by social and cultural constraints. The concept of "the sexual revolution" or an abrupt change in social behavior and attitudes toward sex has been the topic of many recent empirical studies. There is a prevalent belief that such a revolution has occurred within the last decade and that promiscuous adolescent sexual behavior is part of the result. Studies have indicated that no such physical, sexual, or behavioral changes have occurred. Instead, there has been a rethinking of traditional values and moral systems with emphasis on meaningful relationships. "The past decade has brought about change in the motivation, need for affection, consideration of consequences, and desire for commitment by adolescent or young adult sexual partners."[16]

Traditional patriarchal sexual values are still dominant in American cultural systems. For adolescents, there are confusing messages about acceptable and unacceptable sexual behavior. Boys are still allowed more freedom than girls in experimenting with sex; however, recent studies of adolescents have indicated that virginity is not as important to either sex as it has been in the past.[17] The influence of commercial advertising's attitudes toward sex and sexual behavior is probably another significant variable regarding an individual's opinions toward sexuality. Sexual allure is freely exposed in magazines and on television, but restrictions are still enforced for many teenagers at a time when curiosity is greatest.

Intellectual curiosity about sexuality and the act of sexual intercourse is a major component in adolescent sexual development. Frustration at this age results from a general lack of sufficient information about sex in a culture where sexual innuendos are associated with almost every facet of daily adult life. In addition, many adolescents sense that there is more to sexuality than the sexual act. Since feelings are difficult to describe, adults are often unable to discuss with teenagers the importance of masculine or feminine issues and the relationship between sexual partners.[18]

Sociocultural changes in American life include better birth control methods, availability of safe abortion, availability of sex literature, and decreased need for parental consent related to health care. It is unclear how these changes will affect present-day adolescents and their sexual role development. Surveys show that many midadolescents and late adolescents refuse to believe that sexual associations should be limited to married couples and that sexual feelings and desires are isolated from other feelings within the individual.[19]

Traditional attitudes and values regarding sexuality are changing. Because of the dichotomy of American values relating to sexual behavior and rules for sexual identity, the present-day adolescents are left to search for their own sexual identity and moral code with very few parental or societal guidelines. It is easy to understand why many teenagers have difficulty establishing a consistent sexual identity.

Sexual Health The relationship of adolescent male or female sexual identity to health and illness attitudes varies among individual clients. Generally, females tend to be more concerned with themselves as physical beings in terms of outward appearance. They are more aware of health as it relates to their concept of beauty. It is usually easier to interest teenage girls in physical examination for the purpose of avoiding or alleviating illness than it is to interest adolescent boys in health issues. In addition, the onset of menstruation is a major physical and emotional time for girls which increases their concern for normal or "good" health.

Despite the fact that boys may not be as interested in health matters as are girls, it is important to remember that societal values prohibit males from expressing themselves as dependent in many situations, including illness. The nurse should explore health concerns with adolescents of both sexes. An adolescent's perception of personal physical self and body image may be influenced by prior experiences that led to self-recognition as attractive or unattractive, strong or weak, or masculine or feminine, regardless of the reality of physical appearance and capabilities.[20]

Menstruation One of the most important parts of a health history relates to information about sexual maturity and menstruation. Most adolescent females view the menarche or the onset of menstruation as a normal developmental milestone separating them from childhood.

There are many societal notions concerning the shamefulness or even danger of menstruation. As a result, there are individuals who fear or deny the process. In a study of the emotional reactions of 475 girls to the onset of menstruation, it was found that half reacted with indifference, a significant minority were chagrined or anxious, and a few were terrified. Only 10 percent were curious, interested, delighted, or proud.[21]

Highlights

Adult guidance is needed to help adolescents explore the facets of sexual development.

If parents can maintain an open communication system with their adolescents during early adolescence and midadolescence, late adolescence usually provides few conflicts.

An adolescent girl tends to be more concerned about her outward appearance and thus may seek out a health care service if it promises to help her appearance.

Adolescents of both sexes are concerned about self-identity, and the nurse needs to explore this body-image concept. (Refer to the section on self-perception/conception in Chap. 10 for more information concerning body image.)

Physical and emotional maturation do not necessarily coincide. A good measure of emotional maturation is how the adolescent deals with challenge and conflict.

The onset of menstruation is an important milestone for adolescent girls.

Physical discomfort may also lead to a negative reaction to menstruation. Commonly, females will complain of headaches, backaches, cramps, and abdominal pain. Usually the younger adolescent or preadolescent will complain more of physical discomfort than will older adolescents. As puberty progresses and menstruation becomes more regular, physical discomfort should decrease. During a health history the nurse should determine any problems associated with menstruation and emphasize that information about the normal menstrual process is needed to facilitate adjustment to the process.

In addition, the nurse should ask the client about specific moods before, during, and after menstruation to better understand the level of hormonal changes for a particular individual. The period beginning on about day 22 of the menstrual cycle is referred to as the *period of premenstrual tension* and is characterized by depression, irritability, anxiety, and feelings of low self-esteem.[22] Because these changes may accompany normal menstruation during adolescence, premenstrual tension may be prolonged and erratic, causing emotional instability and concern for some females.

At this time the learning needs of a client regarding sexual development and menstruation should be assessed. Planned teaching about sex, sexuality, and menstruation can occur following the examination period with follow-up as needed.

Nocturnal Emission About 1 to 2 years after the onset of puberty, nocturnal emission or the release of seminal fluid during sleep will occur in adolescent males. Just as the onset of menstruation can be of concern to females, nocturnal emissions may be accompanied by erotic dreams, and some males will feel guilt or fear about this normal occurrence. During the health history the nurse should assess the occurrence of and the client's coping with nocturnal emissions. The nurse should evaluate the need for further teaching or discussion of sexuality and normal adolescent physical maturity.

Adolescent Pregnancy For many young adolescents, sexual relationships may take the place of parental neglect or lack of affection. For others, overt sexual behavior may be the method used to deal with the stress and anxiety of normal maturation. This is not to imply that sexual relationships among adolescents are inherently "wrong" or morally promiscuous, although this is a belief of many adults in our society. What is unfortunate about teenage sexual liaisons is that society has not dealt effectively with the problem of educating young people about birth control and the responsibilities of parenthood. Often teenagers are unable to deal with their own sexuality and the emotional bonds that sexual overtures may bring. The facts about adolescent pregnancy make this problem a frightening one to health professionals, one that is reaching "epidemic" proportions.

Today, teenage pregnancy is an increasing phenomenon. The problems of the pregnant adolescents are of special concern to health professionals. For many reasons teenagers have more problems during pregnancy than do older women. Statistics clearly show that there is an association between infant low birth weight and teenage mothers. Infants born weighing 2500 grams (g) or less [5 pounds (lb) 8 ounces (oz) or less] have higher rates of infant mortality, mental retardation, and birth defects. Babies born to teenage mothers are more likely to be of low birth weight than are infants born to mothers in their twenties; thus there is an inverse relationship between birth weight and age of the mother (the lower the age of the mother, the higher the incidence of low birth rate).

Highlights

Complaints of physical discomfort frequently accompany the younger adolescent's onset of menstruation. The nurse must assess the nature of the complaint in light of a girl's reaction to the process of menstruation.

Emotional reactions to the menstrual period are related to hormonal changes and learned responses.

The nurse should provide an opportunity for the adolescent to learn more about physical functioning and sexuality. The nurse can offer information through reading material, classes, films, etc.

Nocturnal emissions occur in males at the onset of puberty.

According to the U.S. Department of Health, Education, and Welfare National Center for Health Statistics, nearly 600,000 births in 1975 were to mothers under 20 years of age. Of these, 38.2 percent were to girls 15 to 17 years of age, and 59.7 percent were to those aged 18 to 19 years.

Births to teenagers comprised 19 percent of all U.S. births in 1975, in contrast to 17 percent in 1966.

The rate of childbearing for young teenagers has not followed the general decline noted for older women.

During 1966 to 1975 there was an 18.3 percent decline in the birthrate of older teenagers, as compared to 15- to 17-year olds, who have experienced a 21.7 percent increase in birthrate.

Teenage pregnancy is becoming a major national health concern. Statistics show that babies born to teenagers have a greater risk of health problems.

There is an association between low infant birth weight and teenage pregnancy.

This inverse relationship is seen regardless of race or legitimacy status.

Pregnant teenagers come from all cultures and socioeconomic levels. The fact that many of these adolescents are unmarried complicates the already difficult situation since close psychoemotional support of the pregnant woman by the father of the baby may be lacking.

Because of the many psychoemotional and physiological developments in normal adolescence, the teenager who is faced with pregnancy must take on an enormous extra burden during her transition to adulthood. When the nurse is interviewing or examining a pregnant adolescent client, it is essential to keep in mind the numerous threats to normal adolescent development, including body image changes, independence, rapid physical growth, and identity formation. Behaviors and attitudes of this client may be greatly affected by the conflicts she is experiencing with these development tasks and the tasks of pregnancy. (Refer to Chap. 12, for a complete discussion of pregnancy.)

Nutritional Metabolic Patterns

The adolescent years are full of changes, especially in the area of physical growth and development. With the transition to adolescence comes alteration in nutritional needs. Additionally, the adolescent's eating patterns are reflective of concerns about body image and peer acceptance. Many adolescents socialize at fast-food restaurants, where the staple food item consists of "empty calorie" foods such as carbonated beverages and potato chips. Others choose diets that emphasize increasing awareness and identification with ecological and alternative lifestyle concerns (vegetarian, fruitarian, macrobiotic, etc. diets).

Regardless of the diet the adolescent may choose, it is important that the nurse evaluate the total dietary intake thoroughly before attempting to alter or supplement the client's eating style. The adolescent is generally more receptive to information on how to incorporate appropriate nutrients into the existing diet than to suggestions that the lifestyle be changed in order to obtain the needed nutrients.[23]

The nurse should recognize the interplay between drug use and nutritional status when assessing the adolescent client. Different drugs can have a marked effect on the nutrition of the adolescent. These effects can be produced directly by altering metabolism or indirectly by producing changes in appetite. The nurse needs to question the adolescent about what is eaten daily and whether there have been any change in the diet. If there are changes, the nurse should explore the reasons behind them.

Many adolescents experience a change in eating that results from being overly conscious of weight. In teenage girls the normal physiological fat deposition around the abdomen and pelvic girdle raises concerns about being overweight.[24] In pursuit of thinness, the female adolescent, in particular, might seriously jeopardize her health (e.g., anorexia nervosa).

Use of oral contraceptives can also influence the nutritional needs. It is not uncommon for adolescents to attribute weight gain to use of the birth control pill. Since many find any weight gain unacceptable, the tendency is to stop taking the contraceptive, which will most likely put the individual at greater risk of pregnancy. A pregnancy places added nutritional demands on the still-developing adolescent.

Adolescent females and males alike are concerned about diet when they are engaged in a serious athletic program. The usual emphasis is in increasing endurance and muscle building. The teenager engaged regularly in sports may be on a diet to gain or lose weight. The desired

Highlights

When the nurse is interviewing or examining a pregnant adolescent client it is essential to keep in mind the numerous threats to normal adolescent development, such as body image changes, independence, rapid physical growth, and identity formation.

Refer to Chap. 12 for a more complete discussion of pregnancy.

With the onset of adolescence comes differing nutritional needs and tastes.

See Chap. 3 for further information on assessment of dietary intake.

Drug use can have a marked effect on the nutritional status of adolescents.

During the training period an athlete's diet should be well-balanced and prudent, with sufficient energy to meet athletic needs, which typically range as much as 5000 to 6000 calories a day.

outcome is usually a reduction in body fat and an increase in muscle. The appropriate regime consists of an increase in exercise supported by controlled increment in food intake. The typical diet should range from 5000 to 6000 calories per day.[25]

The nurse must question the teenager about diet and activity. Of importance to note is whether the family can financially support the diet of the young athlete. It is not uncommon for the economically disadvantaged family to be unable to provide the needed foods for the athlete.

Adolescent males and females alike are prone to many influences that can shape and alter their eating patterns. It is essential that the nurse be aware of the potential dietary variations as well as the attendant risks and benefits that accompany a particular diet or eating style. Effective nutritional education needs to take a dual approach. The teenager must be recognized as an individual who has made some personal choices concerning diet. Additionally, the nurse must also take a family approach as the family's eating styles greatly impact on the adolescent.

Activity and Exercise Patterns

Statistics show that organized recreational activities and clubs are currently declining in their appeal to teenagers. Enrollments in most large youth organizations such as the Boy Scouts, the Girl Scouts, the YWCA, the YMCA, and Jewish youth organizations are decreasing each year. For some adolescents in rural America, 4-H clubs are still active. Religious youth groups meet the needs of a growing number of teenagers, especially those from the white middle class. But for the majority of adolescents from all types of cultural and socioeconomic backgrounds, there is a lack of opportunity to become involved with the community or with peers in an organized, supervised way.

Because of the lack of adequate recreational activities, most adolescents are left to organize their own forms of "action." What is most commonly seen in adolescent group activity is the unorganized congregation of teenagers at shopping centers and fast-food restaurants. Here adolescents can meet freely and participate in their own social environment. Another form of recreational activity that can be detrimental to the individual is the youth "gang" which often turns its activity and energy to antisocial behavior.

In order to assess an adolescent client's various means of psychoemotional support, the nurse should ask the individual to briefly explain what he or she does for recreation or relaxation and where the client meets with friends and what activities they do together. Establishment of a regular activity pattern is important, for nutritional as well as cardiovascular health. Physical fitness helps to ensure soundness of mind, body, and spirit in the individual. Incorporating a regular plan of activity or exercise during adolescence may help ensure adherence as the person ages. School sports continue to occupy much of the adolescent's time and should be encouraged by the nurse.

Coping and Stress Tolerence Patterns

Stress is a part of everyone's life, and adolescents are no exception. Much of their stress relates to the increased emphasis on peer approval and conformity that is characteristic of the adolescent period. As explained in Chap. 3, not all stress is harmful, but adolescents are particularly vulnerable to stress as they have not developed sufficient coping mechanisms to effectively deal with negative stress. As our society grows in complexity, the potential stress factors to which adolescents are subject increase. There are many millions of troubled adolescents who are unable to deal with stress in its various forms, including difficulties arising from drug use, sex, and conflicts with parents.

It is vital that the nurse determine major stressors impacting on the adolescent client's life and how the adolescent is presently dealing with the stress. If the coping mechanism used is ineffective or harmful, the nurse can help the adolescent client to explore resolution or at least provide a way of coping more productively with the problem. Questions presented in Chap. 3 may help to develop this area further.

Adolescence and Stress Assessment of the psychoemotional development of an adolescent includes evaluation of the personal, social, and health history of the individual client. There are no specific developmental assessment tools for the adolescent population. Most problems of psychoemotional development are discovered as the adolescent interacts within society. Professionals in the school or vocational areas may be the first to detect trouble in an adolescent.

During the adolescent process of physical maturation there may be numerous inhibiting factors that prevent simultaneous psychological development. Overwhelming anxiety may cause an adolescent to remain fixed within childhood behavioral patterns and to adhere to emotional responses that protect the youth from the difficulties of physical maturation. Anxiety and stress are associated with the behavioral patterns of "abnormal" adolescent development. Kugelmass has stated, "The ultimate measure of youth is not where he stands in moments of comfort and convenience, but where he stands in moments of challenge and conflict."[26]

Most adolescents develop a tough core of security and an anchorage in reality that permits them to withstand the various stresses of this stage of development. However, the excesses of normal adolescence often reach emotional extremes which may lead to disruptive behavior patterns.[27]

Responses To Stress Adolescent reactions to stress and anxiety may assume a variety of behavioral manifestations, from the extreme of severe psychiatric illness to delinquent behavior to self-destructive actions such as alcohol and drug abuse. Lack of maturity and logical thought process may contribute to the severity of adolescent response to stress. Many teenagers do not intend to behave in an unacceptable or deviant manner but are unable to control themselves or to think logically about the consequences of their behavior.

It is possible that health professionals who care for clients in the adolescent population will find indications of severe stress and anxiety during the holistic health history and physical examination. Specific behavioral deviations may be recognized that are threatening to the health or life of the teenage client. For this reason it is important for nurses and other health professionals to be aware of some of the most common types of unhealthy adolescent behavior patterns. Because of the high statistical incidence of these behavior patterns, it is thought that some adolescent actions are probably normal behaviors taken in excess or to extremes. In either case the adolescent client may be using the unacceptable behavior as an escape from reality and the stress of normal development in our "high-tension" society.

Adolescent Delinquency The lessons learned from authority figures about right and wrong during childhood will largely determine the person's lifelong code of ethics.[28]

Conflicts related to personal identity, sex, drug use, and parental influences increase the stress of adolescence.

Overwhelming anxiety may cause an adolescent to remain fixed within childhood behavioral patterns.

Adolescents react to stress in a variety of different ways. Many adolescents act impulsively and are not aware of the potential consequences of their acts.

Some teens use unacceptable behavior as a way to escape from stress.

Adolescents are frequently involved in offenses which are not considered crimes in the adult sense. These include truancy, running away from home, gambling, and certain types of sexual activity performed for money. Juvenile crime is defined as that behavior which is criminal specifically for minors. Since the definition of juvenile crime varies among states and at different times, it reflects adult attitudes toward and fears of adolescents.[29]

The health status of a young client is rarely considered by professionals who deal with adolescents in the juvenile justice system or juvenile rehabilitation programs. It is difficult to determine exactly to what extent poor health and poor health habits influence adolescents involved in criminal behaviors. A recent study indicates that the health status of delinquents either in institutions or on probation is poor. Poor health may not be a direct cause of delinquency or improved health a way of changing deviant behavior; however, it is unlikely that the nature of adolescent delinquency or its control can be clearly understood without taking health status into account.[30]

Adolescence and Drugs Since the early 1960s there has been great emphasis on drug use and abuse in this country. Health professions have been involved in attempts to study types and effects of unprescribed pharmacological products available to adolescents and young adults. Because of the strong emotional feelings that are usually part of any discussion of drug use by teenagers, it is difficult to deal effectively with this growing phenomenon.

When teenagers are questioned about why they abuse drugs, the answers are often vague and uncertain. Professionals who deal with adolescents have attempted to define the reasons for drug use by this age group. Drug use and abuse is dependent on several factors, including current emotional needs, the effect of particular drugs; peer group drug use; and availability, price, and quality of drugs. One pharmacologist, T. G. Hofmann,[31] relates drug use to the need of the user to alter his or her mood, produce a "new" experience, change self-perception, or enhance daily function.

Psychiatrists believe that drugs may be used to help the individual deal with stressful situations and to reduce normal anxiety levels. The natural curiosity of the adolescent makes the "experimental" quality of unprescribed drugs desirable to this age group. Teenagers may also use drugs as a way to impress peers or to rebel against the family and parental rules.[32]

Adolescent drug use usually takes two distinct forms: the frequent daily user and the occasional user. The adolescent who is a frequent daily user may constantly be "high" as a result of taking a single drug or a variety of drugs. These are the teenagers who generally have trouble with the law or with school because of their chronic intoxication. Many of these teenagers will admit to using drugs immediately on getting up in the morning and then to stay "high" throughout the day.

The occasional drug user is the teenager whose primary reason for using one or a variety of drugs is to enhance weekend recreational activities. This adolescent will refrain from drug use during the week or whenever academic or vocational responsibilities preclude intoxication. Often occasional drug users combine drug use with alcohol as a social means of relaxation, much as older adults use alcohol for "social drinking" purposes.

Age seems to be a factor in teenage drug use. Older adolescents tend to be more selective in their use of certain drugs for certain purposes. Experience with drugs allows more discriminating use. Younger teen-

Highlights

Arrests of youths begin to steadily increase after age 10 years, peak at age 16 years, and significantly decrease after age 17 years.

Juvenile crime is behavior prohibited in minors and may include acts not considered criminal if done by an adult.

Health professionals need to work with legal authorities as certain types of deviant behavior can be caused or influenced by poor health.

Drug use is prevalent in our society, particularly among adolescents.

Drug use and abuse is dependent on several factors, including current emotional needs, the effect of particular drugs, peer group drug use, availability, and price and quality of drugs.

Just as adolescents have a natural curiosity about sex, they also have curiosity about certain drugs.

In the holistic health history it is important for the nurse to determine whether the teenager is a frequent or occasional drug user.

Drugs may be used by the adolescent to relieve stress.

As adolescents mature, their use of drugs becomes less erratic.

Table 10-1
Commonly Abused Drugs Which Can Cause Physical Dependence

Narcotics	Barbiturates	Sedative-Hypnotics (Nonbarbiturate)
Morphine	Amytal	Placidyl
Heroin	Hexobarbital	Doriden
Codeine	Nembutal (Pentobarbital Sodium)	Quaalude (Methaqualone)
Methadone	Seconal (Secobarbital)	Librium (Chlordiazepoxide Hydrochloride)
Demerol (Meperidine)	Phenobarbital	Valium (Diazepam)

agers may use drugs more erratically and use a greater variety of drugs. As late adolescents become young adults, drug use generally decreases and as work and family responsibilities increase.

Statistics are not conclusive, but the incidence and frequency of drug use by teenagers and young adults remains higher now than during the explosive surge of the 1960s.[33] Studies indicate that 80 percent of adolescents in the United States have used alcohol or drugs. Some view this as part of normal adolescence because of its prevalence.

Drug abuse by adolescents is often associated with stress and anxiety. Drug abusers use the effects of drugs as an escape from the responsibilities of reality. It is appropriate to place the phenomenon of compulsive drug use in the same category as other "escapist" or anxiety-reducing compulsive activities, such as food addiction, gambling, smoking, and alcoholism. All these compulsive habits provide a degree of external relief from internal conflicts.[34]

It is important to distinguish between the experimental or recreational drug user and the compulsive drug user. The compulsive drug user is the client who is or will become the drug abuser. Drug abuse by this client is essentially unrelated to the type of drug that is used. Physical dependence (i.e., regular drug use) may not be a factor in compulsive drug use. However, psychological dependence is always a contributing factor in drug abuse.

Psychological drug dependence has been difficult to describe. It implies a compulsive, driving need to find and use drugs consistently. Drug abusers cannot seem to face their normal lives without the effects of drugs. Despite this compulsive need, there is no one psychiatric syndrome that leads to drug abuse.[35] Unless a drug abuser is physically addicted to drugs, physical signs and symptoms of abuse may be difficult to detect. Often psychological drug dependence is manifest by difficulty in coping with activities of living, such as school, work, family and peer interaction, and sexual interaction. (Refer to Table 10-1.)

Assessment of drug use should be a routine part of the holistic health history. Information concerning drug use and its effects should be evaluated along with other psychosocial data collected during the holistic health history, such as family relationships, peer interactions, sexuality, educational progress, and social activities.

Self-Perception—Self-Concept Pattern

Although the study of human nature and development has been included in our earliest historical recordings, consideration was not given to the specific period termed *adolescence* until the early twentieth century.

Many theories have been suggested to explain the process of adolescent growth and development. Until recent years most conceptions of this stage of life were viewed from personal or spiritual experiences and

Studies indicate that 80 percent of adolescents in the United States will have tried alcohol or smoked marijuana before graduation from high school.

Experimentation with drugs is so prevalent that it may be considered a normal part of adolescent development.

Drug abuse is more likely to occur in the compulsive drug user.

Drug abuse is difficult to assess. Often a clue to possible abuse is seen in the adolescent who is having problems in school or with socializing.

Adolescence was not considered a separate stage of growth and development until the early twentieth century.

from philosophical beliefs. Scientific methods of experimental research have eliminated earlier misconceptions about adolescent development, but many issues still remain unresolved.

G. Stanley Hall wrote the famous volume *Adolescence* in 1916 and is still considered the father of "psychology of adolescence." Hall based his theory of adolescence on the premise that development was influenced by physiological factors. He assumed that these physiological factors were genetically predetermined and that growth, development, and behavior were internal maturational forces, unaffected by environmental factors.

As discussed in Chap. 2, there are several theoretical approaches to human growth and development which are used to help explain contemporary human behavior. Of particular importance are recent studies which utilize theories advanced by Piaget, Gesell, Erikson, and Havighurst.

The primary focus of *Piaget's theory of development* is the cognitive ability of the individual. As cognitive ability progresses, the complexity of problems that can be handled effectively increases. Development may then be measured by an adolescent's ability to formalize operational thinking. The teenager's capacity for abstract thought influences his or her behavior and response.[36]

According to *Gesell's concept of growth,* maturation is a process that produces changes in individual form and function. Gesell writes that "mental growth is a patterning process; a progressive morphogenesis of patterns of behavior."[37] The process of maturation is an intrinsic component of growth that is substantially affected by extrinsic (environmental) factors. Gesell uses the term "maturation" to include both biological development and behavioral changes.

Erik Erikson's theory of ego identity is clearly linked with modern evaluation and exploration of adolescent development and behavior. According to Erikson,[38] "The growing and developing youth is faced with a physiological revolution within himself and with tangible adult tasks ahead . . . is now primarily concerned with what he appears to be in the eyes of others as compared with what he feels he is . . . ." The adolescent must reestablish ego identity in light of childhood experiences and accept physical and sexual changes as an integral part of self-development.

Robert Havighurst[39] has drawn upon several theories of adolescence to compile an all-encompassing list of *developmental tasks of adolescence*. Other theorists have concentrated on one or more of these tasks as the basis for explanations of adolescent psychoemotional behavior. The Havighurst list indicates the broad range of societal and personal expectations for the adolescent period of life. (Refer to Highlights column.)

The recurrent theme of all theorists concerned with the period of adolescence is that the primary developmental task of adolescence is the formation of a self-identity. Adolescents spend the majority of their teenage years in the search for personal identity. This is a process which begins in infancy and will continue throughout adulthood. Part of the need to identify the self as a separate person is the need to establish independence from parents. "Seeking freedom and assuming self-responsibility manifest themselves differently as adolescents mature from early to late stages of growth."[40]

Independence During early adolescence physical and cognitive changes result in a change in the need for the family. The young teenager feels the need for separation from the close emotional bonds of the family. Although this tendency toward independence may cause disturbing changes for both the teenager and the parents, this shift in adolescent behavior patterns is a necessary part of the developmental proc-

Since Hall's initial survey of the adolescent period, cultural anthropologists and psychoanalytic theorists have successfully challenged his biogenetic theory.

Piaget's focus on the cognitive and intellectual development of adolescents.

Gesell's theory emphasizes changing form and societal functioning.

Erikson's theory is concerned with ego development.

Havighurst's theory emphasized developmental tasks:
1. Achieving a sense of independence from parents
2. Acquiring the social skills required of a young adult
3. Achieving a sense of oneself as a worthwhile person
4. Developing the necessary academic and vocational skills
5. Adjusting to a rapidly changing physique and sexual development
6. Achieving an internalized set of guiding norms and values

All theorists seem to emphasize the formation of self-identity as being the primary developmental task of adolescence.

Breaking away from the nuclear family is an often painful but necessary task of adolescence.

ess. The early adolescent becomes less influenced by parental attitudes and values and makes beginning attempts to establish an independent system of values.

Withdrawal from adult guidance in early adolescence may cause a kind of "mourning reaction" or episodes of depression in the teenager. Since the cause of the depression is obscure to both the adolescent and the parents, the reaction is frequently termed "moodiness" or "growing pains."[41] "In large measure, the mood swings of adolescents are directly related to the making and breaking of relationships, whether in actuality or only in their fantasies."[42]

Adolescent depression often results from the making or breaking of relationships.

Parental trust of the teenager is commonly a problem within the family. Adolescents spend more time away from the home and in the company of peers and frequently will deliberately choose to associate with people who are socially or personally unacceptable to their parents. In this way adolescents can express their independence from the family and freedom of choice in relationships.[43]

Adolescents sometimes choose to express their independence by choosing friends or engaging in relationships not approved of by the family.

At this stage of development, the realization that family ties will soon be physically broken during late adolescence often causes teenagers at this developmental stage to become more satisfied with family life. If communication with parents or other adults has been adequate throughout earlier adolescence, there are generally few conflicts in late adolescence. However, if parents or important adults in the teenager's life have not been supportive, progressive dissatisfaction and conflict can lead to an abrupt severing of family relationships at this developmental stage. By the end of adolescence many teenagers feel a sense of competence and an ability to be responsible for themselves.[44]

Review of Body Components

This general history is followed by a more specific review of body systems. The adolescent should be questioned about present or past problems or concerns that have arisen. If the adolescent client is confused or unable to recall specific information about personal health care in the past, the nurse should request that the information be obtained from the parents or guardian. The general format for obtaining information on the review of body components is similar to that suggessted in Chap. 3. Areas that might be of particular concern to the nurse working with the adolescent client are discussed in the following paragraphs.

Refer to Chap. 3 for a more complete discussion of body system review.

General Appearance. Questions relating to general appearance involve a variety of areas, including the skin, head, face, hair distribution, eyes, ears, nose, throat, mouth, and neck.

Teenagers are prone to skin problems and characteristically are concerned about the prevention and treatment of acne. The nurse will need to question the teenager about the onset of skin problems and what is being done at home to deal with the problem. Frequently over-the-counter antiacne treatments are used, and the nurse needs to know what is being used and how often.

Teenagers are prone to skin disruptions (acne), which may precipitate questions

Adolescent boys are often concerned about hair distribution, especially as it relates to facial hair. Starting to shave is an important milestone in the life of every adolescent boy, and "late developers" are frequently concerned about their lack of facial hair.

Distribution of facial hair in males and pubic hair in females may be of concern to the adolescent.

Both sexes are usually interested in the development of axillary and pubic hair as pubescent secondary sex characteristics develop. Again, within the adolescent population there is much comparison of physical development, and teenagers may have problems with their particular stage of development.

Adolescents are prone to dental cavities and gum disease. The nurse needs to question the adolescent client about dental hygiene and any mouth, gum, or dental problems.

Chest Review of the respiratory status of the adolescent client is not unlike that for an adult. Some teenagers have been told that they have a "heart murmur" or extra heart sound, which may represent a normal finding for this age group. It is important that the nurse question the teen about any discomfort, shortness of breath, or other problem that may accompany normal activities. Adolescents who are engaged in regular athletic programs should also be questioned concerning their activity level and whether this has been altered for any reason.

Many adolescent girls are concerned about breast development. The wearing of a bra and the frequent concern about what is perceived as over- or underdevelopment should be discussed. Obesity in either sex tends to increase the breast area size. Obese teenage boys may have some worries that they are developing "breasts." This topic needs to be discussed with the adolescent client, especially if concern is expressed.

Abdomen The review of this area is similar to that discussed in Chap. 4.

Genitalia

Male Concerns about human male genitalia usually relate to the development and size of the penis. Hopefully, the nurse will be able to elicit any questions the adolescent may have relating to this aspect of physical development and assure him that penis size is not related to sexual ability or interest.

Female Concerns about human female genitalia are usually concurrent with the onset of menstruation. The nurse should question the adolescent about the onset and frequency of menstrual periods. Many teenagers experience menstrual irregularity and/or discomfort with the menses, and the nurse should ask questions about this. In addition, some adolescents will have experienced problems with the use of contraceptive methods. The adolescent client of either sexes should be asked about sexual activity and any problems related to the use of contraceptives

Rectum and Anus The review of body components for the rectum, anus, and extremities are identical to that of the adult as discussed in Chap. 4.

Summary

Adolescence, as a separate stage of growth, was not recognized or studied until the twentieth century. Early theorists emphasized the physiological changes that characterized adolescence. Later theorists came to see the interplay of physical and psychological factors and the search for self-identity as the major theme of adolescence.

One major shift in the adolescent's life comes in relationship to the family. In an attempt to seek independence, family bonds are strained. The strained relationships are a necessary part of the teenager's growth, and there is some ambivalence surrounding the new freedom. This ambivalence can cause the moodiness typically ascribed to adolescents.

Although sexual interests and concerns exist before adolescence, the sexual needs are brought more sharply into focus at this stage of the life cycle. Adolescents struggle with notions of body image and what is "normal" growth and development. At this stage teenagers begin to develop curiosity and interest in sexual relationships. Frequently, formerly supportive adults are confused or uncomfortable with the teenager's sexual curiosity. The changing roles of males and females leave many teenagers with little idea of what is expected from them.

The nurse can be a valuable resource by giving correct information concerning growth and development, sexuality, birth control, and other factors. If a sensitive, trusting relationship can be established between the nurse and the teenager, a wealth of information can be exchanged which can impact not only on an individual, but on a whole community of teenagers.

Adolescents are subject to stresses placed on them by their families, schools, and friends. The reactions to these stresses may result in a teenager who develops an inner core of confidence or one who is vulnerable to less healthy coping patterns. Problems such as delinquency, drug abuse, and pregnancy may result. The nurse who works with adolescents must develop the ability to obtain information about the adolescent's concerns, while maintaining a nonjudgmental attitude.

Termination of the health history should be organized and deliberate. The nurse can summarize by simply reviewing the data briefly and asking the client if anything has been forgotten or confused. The adolescent client will appreciate the chance to clarify information.

It is beneficial for an adolescent client to know whether the nurse can be contacted at a later time if necessary. Such communication should be for the purpose of relating health information. The nurse may wish to give the client a telephone number where he or she can be reached at an office or hospital. The limitations of future contact should be clearly stated to the adolescent, but the availability of this form of professional contact may add to the teenage client's trust of health professionals and adults.

REFERENCES

1. Howard E. Kulin, "The Physiology of Adolescence in Man." *Human Biology,* **46:**133–144 (February 1974).

2. William A. Daniel, *Adolescents in Health and Disease,* C. V. Mosby, St. Louis, 1977, p. 95.

3. Adele Hoffman, R. D. Becker, and H. Paul Gabriel, *The Hospitalized Adolescent,* Free Press, New York, 1976, p. 216.

4. Committee on Adolescence, Group for the Advancement of Psychiatry, *Normal Adolescence: Its Dynamics and Impact,* Scribner, New York, 1968, p. 34.

5. John Janeway Conger, *Adolescence and Youth—Psychological Development in a Changing World,* Harper and Row, New York, 1973, p. 288.

6. Committee on Adolescence, Group for the Advancement of Psychiatry, *Normal Adolescence,* p. 55.

7. Hoffman et al., *Hospitalized Adolescent,* p. 14.

8. Ibid., p. 16.

9. Joan Lipsitz, *Growing Up Forgotten,* Lexington Books, Lexington, Mass., 1977, p. 23.

10. Ibid., p. 24.

11. Ibid., p. 24.

12. Conger, *Adolescence and Youth,* pp. 379–380.

13. Daniel, *Adolescents in Health and Disease,* pp. 20–21.

14. Jean Piaget, *The Psychology of Intelligence,* Routledge and Kegan Paul, London, 1950.

15. Daniel, *Adolescence in Health and Disease,* p. 66.

16. Ibid., p. 67.

17. Ibid., p. 68.

18. Ibid., p. 67.

19. Conger, *Adolescence and Youth,* p. 110.

20. Ibid., p. 111.

21. J. Bardwick, *Psychology of Women: A Study of Bio-Cultural Conflicts,* Harper and Row, New York, 1971, p. 232.

22. Ibid.

23. Susan B. Caghan, "The Adolescent Process and The Problem of Nutrition," *Amer J Nurs,* **75:**1729 (October 1975).

24. U. S. Government Printing Office, *Factors Influencing Adolescent Nutrition,* No. 225–901, 1977.

25. Caghan, "The Adolescent Process," p. 1730.

26. I. Newton Kugelmass, *Adolescent Medicine,* Charles C Thomas, Springfield, Ill., 1975, p. 22.

27. Joseph L. Stone and Joseph Church, *Childhood and Adolescence,* Random House, New York, 1968, pp. 546–547.

28. J. Roswell Gallagher, Felix P. Heald, and Dale C. Garell, *Medical Care of the Adolescent,* Appleton-Century-Croft, New York, 1976.

29. Daniel, *Adolescents in Health and Disease,* pp. 22–23.

30. Harris Chaiklin, Franklin Chesley, and William Littsinger, "Delinquency and Health Status," *Health and Social Work,* August 1977, p. 25.

31. F. G. Hofman, *A Handbook on Drug and Alcohol Abuse,* Oxford University Press, New York, 1975, p. 78.

32. Schonberg, "Drug Abuse Counseling," p. 32.

33. Hofmann et al., *Hospitalized Adolescent,* pp. 79–82.

34. Ibid., p. 79.

35. Ibid.

36. Rolf E. Muuss, *Theories of Adolescence,* Random House, New York, 1962, pp. 1–9.

37. Ibid., p. 151–176.

38. Erik Erikson, *Childhood and Society,* Norton, New York, 1963, p. 67.

39. R. J. Havighurst, *Developmental Tasks and Education,* Longman's–Green, New York, 1953, p. 282.

40. Daniel, *Adolescents in Health and Disease,* p. 61.

41. Schonberg, "Drug Abuse Counseling," pp. 66–67.

42. Ibid., p. 67.

43. Daniel, *Adolescents in Health and Disease,* pp. 60–61.

44. Ibid., p. 63.

BIBLIOGRAPHY

Bower, Fay Louise: *The Process of Planning Nursing Care,* Mosby, St. Louis, 1977.

Bragg, Terry: "Teenage Alcohol Abuse," *JPN and Mental Health Services,* Dec. 1976, 10–17.

Brody, Eugene B.: *Minority Group Adolescents in the United States,* Williams and Wilkins, Baltimore, 1968.

Caghan, Susan: "The Adolescent Process and the Problem of Nutrition," *AJN,* Oct. 1975, 1728–1731.

Campbell, Patricia B.: "Adolescent Intellectual Decline," *Adolescence,* **10**(44):630–634 (Winter, 1976).

Chaiklin, Harris, Franklin Chesley, and William Bittsinger: "Delinquency and Health Status," *Health and Social Work,* Aug. 1977, 25–37.

Cohen, Michael: "The Process of Adolescence—Its Psychologic and Physiologic Basis," *Pediatr Nurs,* July/August, 1978, 27–29.

Daniel, William A.: *Adolescents in Health and Disease,* Mosby, St. Louis, 1977.

Dragastin, Sigmund, and Glen H. Elder, Jr.: *Adolescence In The Life Cycle,* Wiley, New York, 1975.

Ganong, William, F.: *Review of Medical Physiology,* Lang Medical Publications, Los Altos, Cal., 1971.

Giuffra, Mary: "Demystifying Adolescent Behavior," *AJN,* Oct. 1975, 174–1727.

Heald, Felix, and Wellington Hung: *Adolescent Endocrinology,* Appleton-Century-Crofts, New York, 1970.

Hofmann, F. G.: *A Handbook on Drug and Alcohol Abuse,* Oxford University Press, New York, 1975.

Howe, Jeanne: *Adolescence,* McGraw-Hill, New York, 1980.

Kalafatich, Audrey J.: *Approaches to the Care of Adolescents,* Appleton-Century-Crofts, New York, 1975.

Kugelmass, I. Newton: *Adolescent Medicine,* Springfield, Ill.: 1975.

LeBow, Jay A.: "Evaluating the Seriousness of Adolescent Adjustment Reactions," *Primary Care,* **2**(2):281–287 (June, 1975).

Loewendahl, Evelyn: "Therapeutic Approaches to Adolescence," *Amer Corrective Therapy J,* **29**(5):169–172 (Sep.–Oct. 1975)

Lowery, George H.: *Growth and Development of Children,* Year Book Medical Publications, Chicago, 1973.

Marks, Andrea: "Health Screening of the Adolescent," *Pediatr Nurs,* July/August, 1978, 37–41.

McKinney, John Paul, Hiram E. Fitzgerald, and Ellen A. Strommen: *Development Psychology,* The Dorsey Press, Homewood, Ill.

Mercer, Ramona: *Perspectives on Adolescent Health Care,* J. B. Lippincott, New York, 1979.

Muuss, Rolf E.: *Theories of Adolescence,* Random House, New York, 1962.

Presseilin, Barbara: "Adolescents, Nature and Nurture," *Educational Horizons* **61**(4):151–209 (Summer 1983).

Ravenscroft, Kent, Jr.: "Normal Family Regression at Adolescence," *Amer J Psychiatry* **131**(1):31–35 (Jan. 1974).

Rohn, Reuben, and Richard Sarles: "Adolescents Who Attempt Suicide," *J Pediatr,* April 1977, 636–638.

Scipien, G., et. al.: *Comprehensive Pediatric Nursing,* McGraw-Hill, New York, 1979.

Schonberg, Kenneth S.: "Drug Abuse Counseling," *Pediatr Nurs,* July–August 1978, 31–33.

Sider, Roger C., and Sidney D. Kreider: "Coping with Adolescent Patients," *Med Clinics of North Amer* **61**(4):839–854 (July 1977).

Stone, Joseph L., and Joseph Church: *Childhood and Adolescence,* Random House, New York, 1968.

Smith, M., et al.: *Child and Family Concepts and Practice,* McGraw Hill, New York, 1982, especially Chaps. 2, 3, and 15.

Tanner, J. M.: *Growth at Adolescence,* Charles C Thomas Publishers, Springfield, Ill., 1962.

PHYSICAL EXAMINATION

Physical examination of adolescents includes certain areas not relevant to younger children or adults. Most specific are the areas of skeletal growth and sexual development.

APPROACH TO THE EXAMINATION

Most adolescents respond favorably to the physical examination when they understand the reason for it and the procedure that the nurse will use while performing it. Teenagers appreciate being clearly informed of what is expected of them during any interaction with a health professional (a).

Although physical examination of the adolescent client does not differ significantly in techniques used with the adult client, the approach to the client is different. The nurse must be careful to be aware of the emphasis on body image in the teenage years and must strive to make the physical examination as relaxed as possible to alleviate embarassment. The nurse must respect the teenager as a competent person who seeks the explanation for procedures and strike a balance between telling too much and treating the adolescent as a child.

The rate of growth and development vary widely among teenagers, and the nurse must be familiar with the differences that that fall within the range of "normal." The nurse must share knowledge of what is normal with the teenager, as most adolescents have some anxiety over their own body development. In sharing this information the nurse not only reassures a particular client but establishes a rapport with the client (b).

Because of the adolescents' concern with their sexuality, the genitalia will be examined last.

Since body image and privacy are important to adolescents, the physical examination should be conducted in a private and comfortable setting.

To minimize client embarrassment and discomfort, examination gowns should be used whenever possible. It is important to cover those parts of the body not being specifically examined.

It is possible to obtain additional health history information informally during conversation with the adolescent client as routine measurements are taken.

During the physical examination the nurse must be sensitive to the needs of the teenager, including levels of anxiety and body image.

Careful explanation of the genital examination should occur prior to the assessment. For this reason it will be completed at the end of the physical examination.

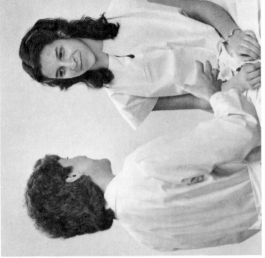

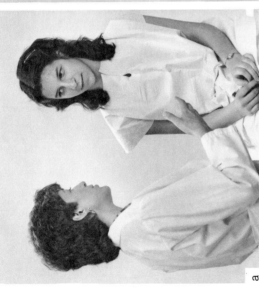

a

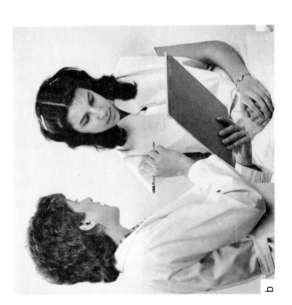

b

THE EXAMINATION
General Appearance

Appraisal of the general appearance of the adolescent client includes observation of body size, weight, bone structure, skin, and facial expression. Normally, there will be great variability with age, genetic inheritance and other factors (a).

Measurements

It is useful to begin the examination with simple procedures that may help the adolescent client to relax, such as vital signs or height and weight measurements.

Blood pressure Blood pressure assessment is a valuable index of the cardiovascular system during adolescence (b). Blood pressure levels for adolescents are somewhat lower than normal levels for adults.

Boys aged 12 to 17 years tend to have higher systolic pressure than do girls of the same age (c). The level increases in boys more rapidly with age than in girls. Diastolic blood pressure tends to be more normally distributed among youths at each year of age than does systolic pressure.

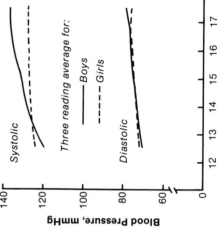

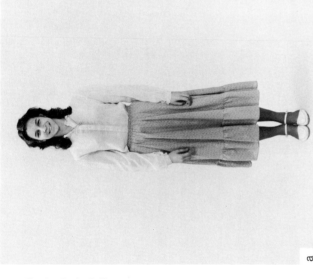

a

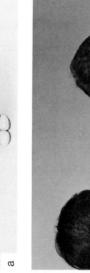

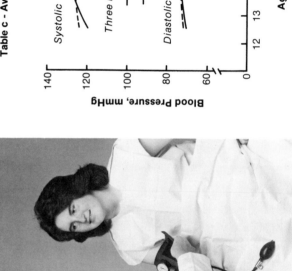

b

Table c - Average Blood Pressure

Systolic

Three reading average for:
—— Boys
- - - - Girls

Diastolic

Blood Pressure, mmHg

140
120
100
80
60
0

Age in Years

12 13 14 15 16 17

c

Refer to Chap. 4 under *General Appearance* for a further discussion of height/weight, vital signs, etc.

Boys between 12 and 17 years tend to have a higher systolic blood pressure than do girls of that age.

Table source: J.M. Tanner, *Growth at Adolescence,* Blackwell Scientific Publications, Oxford, 1962. (With permission of the author and Blackwell Scientific Publications, Ltd.).

The primary reasons for recording height and weight measurements are to assess serial data of individual growth and development and to make predictions of future growth.

Table source: J.M. Tanner, *Growth at Adolescence,* (Blackwell Scientific Publications, Oxford, 1962). With permission of the author and Blackwell Scientific Publications, Ltd.

The thymus is the only organ that does not increase in size during adolescence.

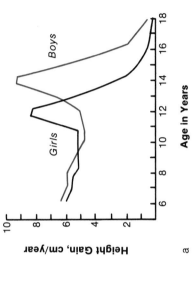

Table a - Adolescent Growth Spurt in Height for Boys and Girls

Boys

Girls

Height Gain, cm/year

Age in Years

a

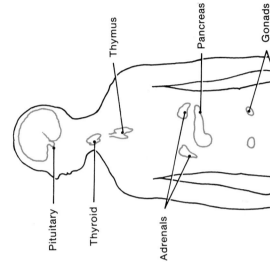

Thymus

Pancreas

Gonads

Pituitary

Thyroid

Adrenals

b

Height and Weight Height and weight measurements are important indicators of adolescent growth and development.

Dr. James M. Tanner, an English physician, has developed a system for staging and observing the physical changes observed during adolescence. As this staging method is appropriate, it will be included in the guidelines for physical examination of adolescents. Tanner has also described the physiological changes of adolescence as the "adolescent growth spurt." This is a universal phenomenon influenced by genetics, nutrition, climate, race, socioeconomic variables and culture. The "growth spurt" is an important variable to explore when considering the adolescent physical examination (a).

Timing of the adolescent growth spurt varies considerably between boys and girls and within each sex. For boys, the "spurt" occurs sometime between 12½ and 15 years of age. Girls experience the growth spurt earlier than boys; however, the peak velocity of growth for girls, which occurs at about 12 years of age, does not reach the same degree of intensity as that for boys, who tend to peak at 14 years of age. Girls tend to reach a growth spurt at around 12 years. Table a compares timing of the growth spurt for boys and girls.

Hormonal Basis of Growth Spurt During the adolescent growth spurt morphological changes occur in the endocrine glands (b). The *anterior pituitary* and the *gonads* influence an adolescent's psychosexual development and physical maturation. The thyroid, adrenals, and pancreas also participate in the growth spurt. The thymus is the only organ which does not increase in size during adolescence and actually decreases in total mass.

626

The pituitary gland or hypophysis is located at the base of the brain (a) and controls the activity of several other glands through stimulation or inhibition of glandular secretion. The pituitary is divided into three sections, the posterior, intermediate, and anterior lobes. The anterior lobe controls the secretion of six hormones, three of which are gonadotropic hormones or those which control the activity of the gonads. It is believed that the onset of puberty begins with secretion of gonadotropins.

Results of height and weight measurements should be compared against recent growth charts. Recent reference standards developed by the National Center for Health Statistics should be used as guidelines for comparing height and weight measurements.

In normal and healthy individuals up to 25 percent of the total mass of the body can consist of fat cells in quantities large enough to form adipose tissue. Some of this fat is located internally, surrounding organs such as the kidney. However, more than half of the fat is found subcutaneously, where it "blankets" the individual.

For accurate measurement of adolescent growth and development, assessment of the composition of the body or the constituents of its mass is essential. Analysis of body mass is measured by determining the skinfold thickness at specific sites (b). This simple method provides an accurate and significant parameter for estimating the percentage of body fat.

Highlights

The onset of puberty is thought to occur with the secretion of gonadotropins.

The reference curves should be not only age- and sex-appropriate, but also race-specific. Unfortunately, data for all ethnic groups are not currently available, therefore, statistics represented should be interpreted with caution.

For growth charts, see Appendix.

See Chap. 4 for the instructions on measuring skinfold thickness and use of calipers.

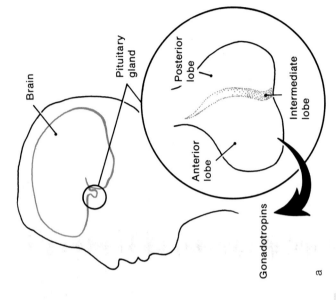

Brain

Pituitary gland

Posterior lobe

Anterior lobe

Intermediate lobe

Gonadotropins

a

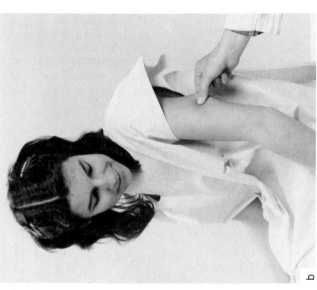

b

Facial hair begins to appear in males during adolescence.

The impact of acne on the life of a teenager may be enormous. Often they feel that blemishes affect their popularity and social interactions as well as physical well-being.

The nose is considered to be a secondary sexual characteristic which begins to develop at age 12 to 13 years. Full growth is usually attained in the female by age 16 and in the male by 18 years.

Adolescents should have a full complement of adult teeth except for the third molars. Physically immature teenagers may have delayed eruption of the canines.

Poor oral hygiene contributes to many periodontal disorders which are common to adolescents. It may be necessary to refer clients to dental professionals if examination of the mouth is not satisfactory.

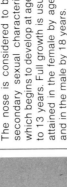

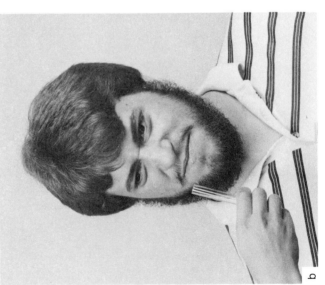

c

Head and Face

Inspection

Physical examination of the head is similar to that described in Chap. 4.

When examining the face of the adolescent clients, particular attention should be paid to examination of the skin and neck (a). Normally the skin color, texture, and pigmentation should be evaluated according to the guidelines presented in Chap. 4. Frequently, skin eruptions in the adolescent (acne) may be noted. Scars or marks should also be noted.

Palpation

Palpation of the face and neck should reveal data similar to that in Chap. 4.

Nose, Sinuses and Mouth

Physical examination of the nose, sinuses, and mouth is completed as described in Chap. 4.

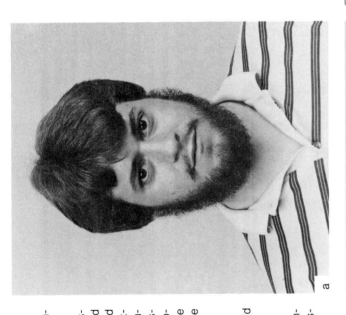

a

Inspection

The examiner should ask the adolescent client about his or her sense of smell to determine any abnormalities in nasal function (b). Because the nose is developing during early adolescence, there is the possibility of occlusion of nasal cavities with some decrease in smelling capacity.

Idiopathic absence of teeth may occur in some adolescents, particularly the superior lateral incisors or the inferior second premolars. Some clients may also have more than the usual number of teeth.

As a result of generally poor eating habits or lack of adult guidance, teenage clients may not yet have established good oral hygiene. Therefore, accurate assessment of teeth and gums should be conducted by a procedure similar to that noted in Chap. 4 (c).

b

Efficient vision and hearing are essential for the adolescent client who may be involved in school, job, or military service.

Decreased achievement in school frequently may be due to poor vision or hearing undetected throughout childhood.

Eyes and Ears

Because many adolescents may not have been previously screened for vision and hearing deficiencies, the physical examination provides a good opportunity for the nurse to perform simple screening tests (a and b). Refer to Chap. 4 for specific methods used to assess the eyes and ears.

Neck and Throat

Physical examination of throat and neck is completed as described in Chap. 4.

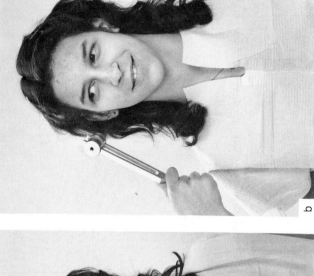

a   b

Thorax

Physical examination of the thorax for the adolescent client is similar to that of the young adult (refer to Chap. 4).

It is important to remember that the anatomy of the chest and the respiratory system will be somewhat smaller than that of the adult client. Anatomically, the growth of the diameter of the tracheo-bronchial tree is proportionately less than body height growth (c).

Lungs

The lungs increase in size during the adolescent growth spurt. The landmarks used to determine the anatomical location of the borders of lungs and lung lobes are the same as those used for adult clients (see Chap. 4).

A chest x-ray may be included in the baseline physical data gathered for every patient. The adolescent client who has never had a chest x-ray may need to be referred for this test.

Table c – Tracheal Diameter vs. Body Length

	Height, cm	Tracheal Diameter (mm)
Birth	51	5.9
1 year	75	8.2
8 year	129	11.0
15 year	164	12.2
Adult	168	15.5

Table source: Polgar, Promadhat: *Pulmonary Function Testing in Children: Techniques and Standards*, Saunders, Philadelphia, 1971. (Courtesy of W.B. Saunders, Inc.)

It is useful to ask minor questions or talk throughout this examination to put the teenager at ease.

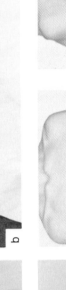

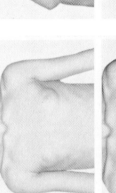

Precordium

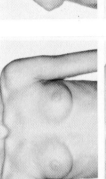

b

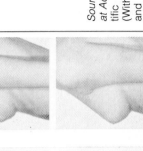

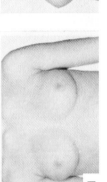

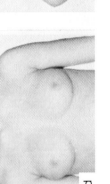

Adolescent clients should be taught to examine their own breasts on a regular basis.

Breast changes progress according to normal development and sex maturity ratings.

d

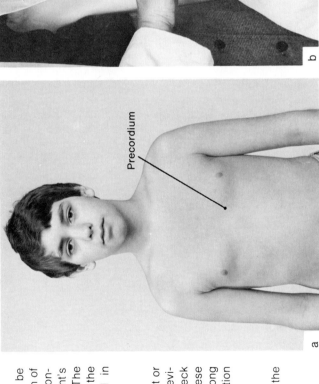

c

Source of d: J. M. Tanner, *Growth at Adolescence,* Blackwell Scientific Publications, Oxford, 1962. (With permission of the author and Blackwell Scientific Publications, Ltd.)

Heart

Because many adolescents may be fearful or anxious about examination of the heart, this procedure should be conducted with consideration for the client's need for modesty and relaxation. The approach for the examination of the heart is completed as described in Chap. 4.

Inspection

On inspection the young adolescent or the underweight client may show evidence of vascular distention of the neck veins, and precordial activity (a). These findings should be considered along with other parts of the examination before they are noted as abnormal.

Palpation

Palpation should include feeling for the quality of all major pulses (b).

Breasts

The breast examination is essentially the same as that for an adult (c). Breast changes progress similarly to normal developmental process noted as sex maturity ratings (d).

From early adolescence through the teenage years, breast tissue increases in the female providing shape and contour to the chest wall. In the male, breast tissue deposition is minimal. Inspection and palpation of breast tissue should be included in the physical examination by a procedure similar to that presented in Chap. 4.

Abdominal organs increase in size as the adolescent continues to grow and develop.

Abdomen

The abdominal examination for the adolescent client is similar to that found in Chap. 4.

Because many adolescent clients may feel embarrassed during palpation of the abdomen, it is generally useful to explain the procedure carefully before starting the examination.

The abdominal organs increase in size as adolescence progresses. The relative size of the abdominal organs should correlate to general body size; examination should not be made more difficult because of normal physical growth.

Proper draping of the adolescent client during the abdominal examination will greatly decrease anxiety and feelings of embarrassment (a). Draping will also help to prevent chilling which may cause tightening of the abdominal muscles, making examination difficult.

Rectum and Anus

Physical examination of the rectum and anus is completed according to the procedure described in Chap. 4.

Extremities

The basic assessment of the extremities is similar to that of adults (refer to Chap. 4).

There are three general elements of total physical fitness: muscular strength (b), flexibility (c), and endurance (d). Each of these elements should be appraised during the physical examination. Although there are several more complex methods of measuring physical fitness capacity, some simple methods can be used as a routine part of the general physical examination.

A healthy person is physically fit to the extent of being able to (1) perform daily work and tasks without undue fatigue, (2) maintain adequate reserves of energy with which to enjoy recreational activities and leisure, and (3) meet and survive unexpected demands such as climbing several flights of stairs quickly.

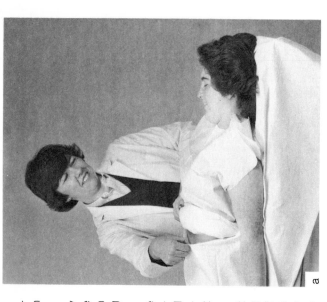

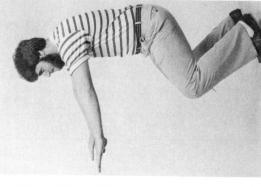

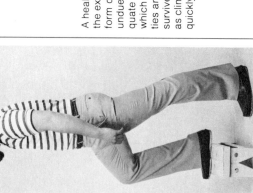

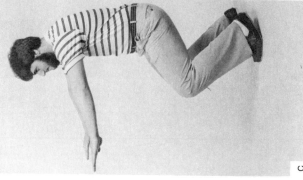

The nurse may incorporate examination of the extremities earlier to relax an adolescent client who seems particularly restless.

Restricted flexibility may frequently be undetected in adolescent clients because of failure to assess physical fitness and muscular and joint flexibility.

The step test permits a determination of the "recovery" or fitness index which is a measure of the rate at which the heart slows down after stressful exercise and is thus an indicator of cardiovascular fitness. Oxygen debt is repaid more rapidly by a good cardiovascular system.

The recovery index is calculated by using resting pulse rates and the following formula:

$$RI = \frac{\text{duration of exercise in seconds}}{\text{sum of 30 second recovery pulses} \times 2} \times 100$$

Should the client become greatly fatigued or express pain during the step test, the test should be stopped immediately and further examination of the symptoms be conducted by the health team.

Inspection

Evaluation of muscular and joint flexibility can be made by observation of full range of motion. The client may be able to release some "nervous" energy and relax for the remainder of the examination if asked to do a few physical exercises and range-of-motion movements of the extremities and joints (a).

Physical endurance may be assessed through the use of a number of stress tests that are designed to measure the amount of available energy for muscular activity. These tests are not routine components of the physical examination. However, there is a simple method that can be used to test endurance during the physical examination period.

Step Test The step test is easy to use since it requires minimal equipment and no special aptitude on the part of the client. To carry out the test, the client should be asked to step up and down on an available step or bench (b) that is set at a height that correlates with the client's height (see the data given in the table on the right [c]).

During the test the client is asked to step up and down the bench 30 times per minute, using the same foot to step up and down each time and rising to his or her full height at the top of the step.

After 4 minutes the client is asked to sit in a chair for pulse recording at specific 30-second intervals. Thus the resting or recovery radial pulse of the client should be taken at 1 to 1½ minutes after the client has been seated, 2 to 2½ minutes and 3 to 3½ minutes. The recovery index can be quickly estimated from the recovery pulse rates by data given in the table on the right (d).

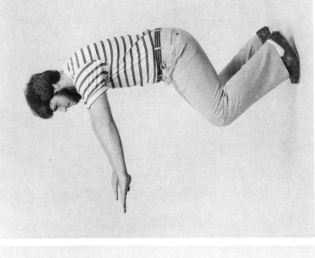

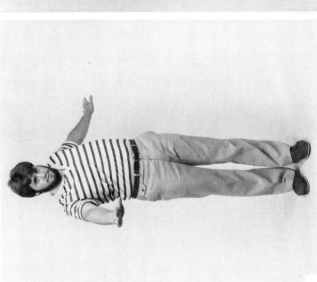

a

b

Table c-Patient Height—Bench Height for Step Test

Patient Height, cm (in.)	Bench Height, cm (in.)
<152.4 (60)	30.48 (12)
152.4-160.02 (60-63)	35.56 (14)
160.02-175.26 (63-69)	40.64 (16)
175.26-182.88 (69-72)	45.72 (18)
>182.88 (72)	50.8 (20)

Table d-Rapid Calculation of Recovery Index

When the Sum of Three 30-Second Recovery Pulse Count Is	The Recovery Index Is	The Fitness Evaluation Test Is
≥199 or More	≤60	Poor
171-198	61-70	Fair
150-170	71-80	Good
133-149	81-90	Very Good
≤132	≥91	Excellent

Hormonal Changes and Sex Characteristics

The hypothalamus stimulates the anterior pituitary to secrete the gonadotropins (a). The reason for this stimulation is unclear. The gonadotropic hormones secreted by the anterior pituitary include the *follicle-stimulating hormone* (FSH), the *leutinizing hormone* (LH), the *leuteotropic hormone* (LTH).

The gonads or sex glands secrete the sex hormones that are primarily responsible for the physiological changes of early adolescence. The male sex hormone androgen is responsible for the development of the penis, the prostate gland, and the seminal vessels. Later, it is responsible for *secondary sex characteristics*, pubic hair, axillary hair, facial hair, and decrease in voice pitch. Along with the development of the penis comes nocturnal emissions with some sperm cells (see discussion under Health History and sleep patterns).

The estrogen or female sex hormones are also secreted by the gonads. These hormones control the development of the female reproductive organs — the ovaries, fallopian tubes, vagina, and uterus. They also influence the development of the menstrual cycle (b) and growth of breast tissue. *Menarche*, or the first menstrual cycle, begins about age 13. There is some evidence that immediately following menarche most girls are sterile and that it is some months after menarche before many girls experience regular periods or become fertile. The secondary sex characteristics of females include pubic and axillary hair, breast enlargement, fat deposits around the hips, widening of the pelvic and hip bone structure, and a broadening of the shoulders.

Highlights

Gonadotropic hormones secreted by the anterior pituitary include FSH, LH, ICSH, and LTH.

The male sex hormone androgen is responsible for the development of the penis, prostate gland, and seminal vessels.

Estrogen is secreted by the gonads.

Adult males tend to be taller than adult females, despite the fact that there are a few years during adolescence when females tend to be taller than males.

Figure b from Dorothy A. Jones et al, Medical-Surgical Nursing, A Conceptual Approach, 2nd ed, New York, 1982, p. 127, fig. 4-2.

Brain

Pituitary gland

Posterior lobe

Anterior lobe

Intermediate lobe

Gonadotropins

a

Puberty

Menopause

Estrogens excreted in urine, mg/24 h

Age, yr

b

Highlights

ACTH is primarily responsible for onset of the growth spurt.

The secretion of adrenocorticotropin (ACTH) is primarily responsible for the onset of the physiological growth spurt. Growth hormone is not secreted continuously but is present in the blood in varying and rapidly fluctuating amounts in response to various stimuli. It has not been shown that secretion rates are altered during adolescence.

The classifications of secondary sex characteristic changes that occur during puberty and define the sex maturity rating of a particular teenage client are listed in the tables on the right (a and b). These classifications or stages should be used as a descriptive method for evaluation of the physical maturity of an adolescent client. The classification can be easily referred to during the physical examination.

In approaching the adolescent client about sexual function and maturity it is important to keep in mind the evaluation of psychoemotional and behavioral characteristics of the individual client assessed during the health history. Each client will respond differently to physical examination of the reproductive system. Be certain to explain clearly the reason for the examination and the method to be used.

Classification of Genitalia Maturity Stages in Boys

Stage	Pubic Hair	Penis	Testes
1	None	Preadolescent	Preadolescent
2	Scanty, Long, Slightly Pigmented	Slight Enlargement	Enlarged Scrotum, Pink, Texture Altered
3	Darker, Starts to Curl, Small Amount	Longer	Larger
4	Resembles Adult type, but Less in Quantity; Coarse, Curly	Larger; glans and Breadth Increase in Size	Larger, Scrotum Dark
5	Adult Distribution, Spread to Medial Surface of Thighs	Adult	Adult

a

Classification of Sex Maturity Stages in Girls

Stage	Pubic Hair	Breasts
1	Preadolescent	Preadolescent
2	Sparse, Lightly Pigmented, Straight, Medial Border of Labia	Breast and Papilla Elevated as Small Mounds; Areolar Diameter Increased
3	Darker, Beginning to Curl, Increased Amount	Breast and Areola Enlarged, No Contour Separation
4	Coarse, Curly, Abundant, but Amount Less Than in Adult	Areola and Papilla Form Secondary Mound
5	Adult Feminine Triangle, Spread to Medial Surface of Thighs	Mature; Nipple Projects Areola Part of General Breast Contour

b

Tables adapted from Tanner, J.M.: Growth at Adolescence. ed. 2, Blackwell Scientific Publications, Oxford Eng., 1962.

Male Genitalia

During physical examination of the genitalia of the adolescent client it is especially important to keep in mind the wide variation in development among teenagers.

Sex maturity ratings (SMR) are used in evaluating the physical development of adolescents.

Adolescent males usually have had previous examinations of the genitalia since pediatricians will routinely check for external genital abnormalities. For this reason, examination of the genitalia is not as traumatic for males as for females. Reassurance during examination of the genitalia is necessary for all teenage boys. The genital examination for male adolescents is similar to that for adults (refer to Chap. 4 [a]).

Inspection

Adolescent male maturational changes include primary and secondary sex characteristics. Males have only external genitalia, which makes examination relatively easy. Male pubertal changes include (b):

1 Enlargement of the testes and scrotum.

2 Change from pale to pink color of the scrotum for Caucasian males.

3 Darkening of the color and roughening of scrotal tissue for all boys as puberty progresses.

4 Increase in penis length and width.

5 Pubic hair growth.

6 Axillary hair growth (change assessed during the examination of the chest and axilla).

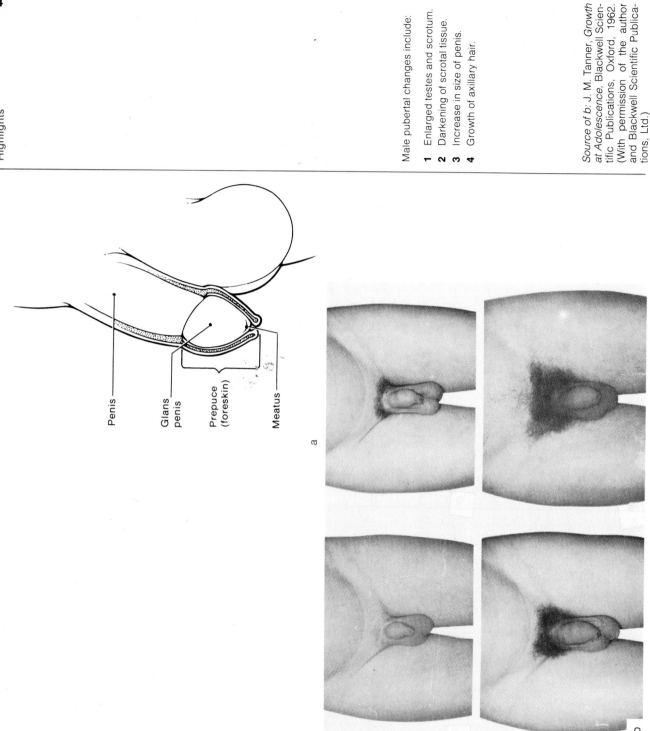

a

b

Male pubertal changes include:

1 Enlarged testes and scrotum.

2 Darkening of scrotal tissue.

3 Increase in size of penis.

4 Growth of axillary hair.

Source of b: J. M. Tanner, *Growth at Adolescence,* Blackwell Scientific Publications, Oxford, 1962. (With permission of the author and Blackwell Scientific Publications, Ltd.)

Penis

Glans penis

Prepuce (foreskin)

Meatus

Genital examination should be carefully explained to the adolescent to help reduce fear and discomfort.

The female adolescent requires more explanation and emotional support prior to the pelvic examination than that necessary for an adult.

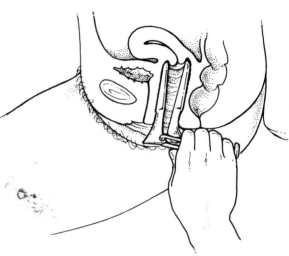

c

Palpation

Palpation of the male genitalia is conducted by a procedure similar to that described in Chap. 4 (a).

If the examiner is female, the young client may feel uncomfortable and fearful that erection may occur. The examiner must have the ability to reassure the client that physical response to palpation is possible and not abnormal. Good rapport and trust between client and examiner will usually decrease the boy's anxiety.

Female Genitalia

Adolescent female maturational changes include primary and secondary sex characteristics (see the second table in the Hormonal Changes and Sex Characteristics section). These include rapid development of internal and external genitalia during puberty.

There is no set age for the first pelvic examination; however, it is certainly performed when there is a gynecologic problem indicated by the client. It is generally agreed that if a client has not had a pelvic examination by the late adolescent period, she should be educated about the procedure and urged to have the examination (b).

Most adolescents regard the pelvic examination as a painful and frightening experience. The approach of the health practitioner is extremely important. Talking to the client throughout the examination is essential. Directions for relaxation and positioning should be detailed and unhurried. The examiner should always use language that is understandable to the client.

Should a pelvic examination be appropriate for the adolescent client, the procedure is similar to that for adult clients (refer to Chap. 4) (c).

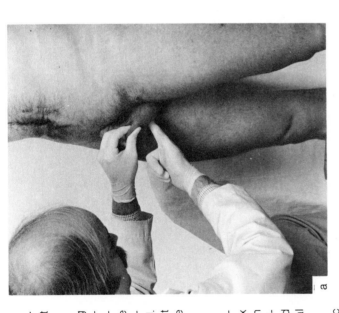

a

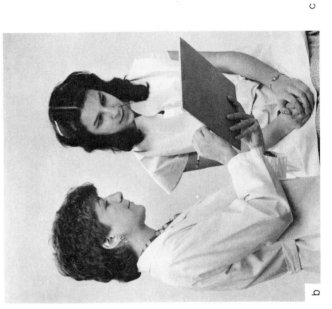

b

Highlights

During maturation of the female genitalia the following changes occur:

1 The labia majora become more prominent and covered with hair.

2 The labia minora become enlarged.

3 The hymen will be intact with an opening of about I cm (0.4 in.).

4 The clitoris varies in size to about 2 cm (0.8 in.).

5 The vagina is usually 8 to 10 cm (3.2 to 4 in.) in depth by the time of menarche.

6 The vagina becomes significantly more elastic in tone.

7 The uterine mucosa undergoes endometrial and endocervical changes.

8 The uterus and ovaries increase in size.

Many teenagers express concern about their physical maturity and are unsure about "normal" growth and development. A discussion of these issues with the client is most appropriate at the conclusion of the physical examination.

Adolescent growth is so variable, especially during early adolescence, that chronological age is a poor standard of reference for health practitioners especially when trying to determine sexual maturity. The SMR is a readily available classification that is easy and inexpensive.

See the tables in the section on hormonal changes and sex characteristics for a review on secondary sex characteristics.

Inspection

During inspection of external genitalia it will be noted that (a):

1 The labia majora become prominent and covered with hair.

2 The labia minora lose their pale appearance and become enlarged.

3 The intact hymen will have an opening of about I cm [0.4 in].

Palpation

Palpation of the female genitalia is similar to that described in Chap. 4.

Diagnostic Tests

Most of the diagnostic tests used when conducting the physical assessment of the adolescent client do not differ from those utilized in the adult examination (refer to Chap. 4).

There are a series of serum and endocrine laboratory values that have been assigned to adolescents according to their SMR. These values enable health professionals to make more accurate diagnoses of physical disorders for their age group. For example, there are wide differences in expected hematocrit levels for adolescent boys with biological development more significant than chronological age. A 12-year-old boy at maturity rating 4 would be expected to have a higher hematocrit value than a 14-year-old boy at SMR 2.

Other methods available for determination of biological maturity are bone age measurements, dentition, and skinfold thickness assessment. The latter has been discussed under the section on physical examination of skin. Bone age determinations are highly accurate but impractical for the routine physical examination and expensive. Dentition is not as accurate as development of secondary sex characteristics for determination of maturity.

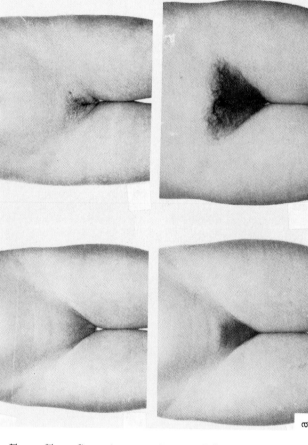

a

Source: J. M. Tanner, *Growth at Adolescence,* Blackwell Scientific Publications, Oxford, 1962. (With permission of the author and Blackwell Scientific Publications, Ltd.)

THE YOUNG ADULT

CHAPTER
ELEVEN

Lynne E. Johnson Phillips

INTRODUCTION

The current literature on adulthood varies in definition of the young adult; ranges from 18 to 24, 25 to 45, 20 to 40, and 20 to 30 years of age have been used to define this group. For the purposes of this chapter the chronological span from 20 to 35 years of age will be considered an acceptable compromise for defining the young adult.

The reader might surmise from the number of definitions cited above that much research on adulthood, particularly the young adult, has been published. Unfortunately, this is a false assumption. As late as 1970, a review of literature on developmental psychology appeared in the *Annual Review of Psychiatry,* with major divisions entitled "Infancy," "Childhood," and "Adolescence." There was no literature cited on adult or geriatric psychological development![1] But as the study of the elderly begins in earnest, gerontological researchers are filling in the void in the data. However, changes in a 75-year-old could not be documented until the developmental aspects of the middle and young adult population were not known.

Another problem arises when one attempts to explain the paucity of data—that is, the validity of conducting developmental research. Consider the following quote from a recent psychology book: "An adult is an individual who has *completed* his growth and is ready for his status in society with other adults."[2] This statement suggests that once physical growth terminates, the individual stagnates. It is a misleading statement. In today's society, individuals can look forward to living into their seventies, a fact that means the young adult can expect to spend many years "growing."

"While we spend about one quarter of our lives growing up and three quarters growing old, it seems strange that psychologists and others have devoted most of their efforts to the study of childhood and adolescence."[3] Young adulthood is a dynamic, energized period of development. The changes occurring may be more subtle than those seen in a child, but, change worthy of further study *is* occurring.

> Young adulthood covers a chronological span anywhere from 18 to 40 years of age.

> Literature written about the young adult is limited.

> Even though physical growth may terminate in the early adult years, the individual continues to grow cognitively, emotionally, socially, and spiritually.

> The young adulthood is a dynamic, energized, fluctuating period of development.

THE HEALTH HISTORY

Health history may be a new experience for the young adult. Parents often assume the role of information giver for the child and adolescent. But as a young adult, the individual assumes personal responsibility for giving accurate information and for actively participating in the promotion of health. Parents are no longer present to depend on. This change may come as a subtle realization to the young adult, and it is an important factor the nurse needs to consider when collecting a health history.

> Participating in the health history may be a new experience for the young adult.

Establishing a Data Base

Because of the newness of the experience, the young adult may need more time to give a health history. Additional reassurance and support will be needed to insure an interdependent relation between client and provider. It is essential that the nurse-client dialogue be clearly established, so that the client will feel free to discuss all parameters of health, without fear of reprisal.

An inherent part of the health history is teaching and counseling the young adult in methods of maintaining and/or gaining optimum health. Much of this information may be shared by the nurse during the health history and physical exam. The nurse must have a grasp of adult development as well as an awareness of the salient issues facing the young adult. Being sensitive to the client's needs and his or her expectation of performance during the history-taking period is critical. Clearly defining the roles of nurse and client will help to enhance the data-collection process.

Lucille Kinlein clearly defines the process:

> The first and perhaps most important difference between the history that I take from a nursing perspective and that which is taken from a medical perspective is that in nursing, the relating of information is not really a history per se. I mean that what has previously happened to, for or with the person is not nearly as important as where the client is now in regard to the past. Whereas in medicine it is impossible to make an accurate diagnosis without a careful history of the patient's past medical events, it is possible to give nursing care without knowledge of the past. . . . The client will communicate to the nurse the points that are important to him, and in the initial stages this is all the nurse should work with.[4]

Role as a Young Adult Client

The client role is a new one for the young adult. While the individual has had health care in the past, the full implication of the word "client" is just becoming clear. There are a number of required tasks that the young adult must accomplish as an active consumer of health care. These include:

1 Conscious acceptance of the necessity of seeking health care

2 Deciding how to enter the health care system

3 Setting up an appointment with a health care provider

4 Arriving at the health care facility at the correct time and date

5 Actively participating in sessions

6 Learning what is necessary to improve health status

7 Carrying out the prescribed health care plan

8 Paying for health care through an established insurance plan or with personal funds

As can be seen in Fig. 11-1, there are many integral components of the client role. The young adult may have difficulty with any or all of these phases. The nurse needs to be sensitive to this fact and carefully determine the client's acceptance of a new role.

Other factors may influence the person's role as client. Since most people of this age group are healthy, there is little focus on appreciation of good health and health care. Frequently, the young adult enters a health care system with the "*you* make it go away—*now*" attitude[5] and demands the impossible. While part of this attitude may be attributed to an inability to assume a "sick role," it also reflects the individual's concept of the health care system and his or her role within it.

Given perception and general ability, the nurse should be able to formulate the role of client and intervene, when necessary, to improve the young adult's knowledge as a consumer of health.

The nurse-client interaction provides the young adult with additional support in taking responsibility for his or her health.

The nurse must have clear expectations of the client and communicate them to the young adult.

Kinlein clearly differentiates the importance of the nursing history vs. the medical history.

Assumption of the client role implies that the young adult has decided to:
1 enter the system;
2 assume responsibility for making and keeping appointments;
3 actively participate in health care;
4 carry out health plans;
5 pay for services.

The young adult's misperception of the health care system ie. immediate relief for a problem—may limit his or her understanding of the agency's role.

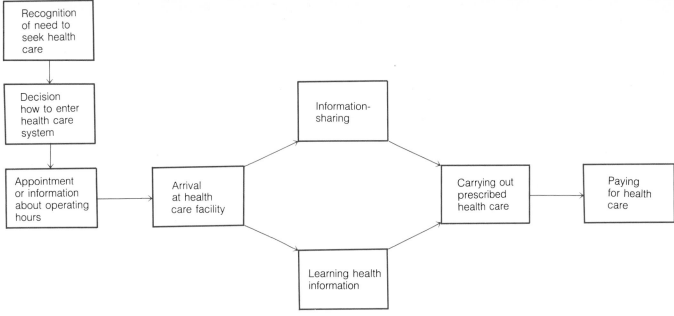

Figure 11-1 Role of the young adult as client.

Entry into the Health Care System

Entry into the health care system may be problematic for the young adult. If the individual grew up under the care of a family physician, an established entry point may be set. However, in today's mobile society this is not often the case.

The young adult, being basically healthy, often seeks drugstore-type remedies or advice from peers for minor health problems. Usually, he or she is unsure as to how or where or when to approach the health care system. However, there generally comes a point when professional help is required, perhaps for a prework or a college physical or when self-remedies are no longer working. The young adult may then be faced with selecting a private physician from the yellow pages or on a friend's recommendation or going to an emergency room or a community clinic.

Choices may also be influenced by the fact that the individual does not have a prepaid insurance plan and lacks money to pay for the services of a private physician. Selection of community resources may be an option in this instance, but often these services have the connotation of being free care (i.e., care of less quality) for the indigent.

The nurse usually has no influence over the young adult until after the decision is made to seek health care services. At this point, the nurse can explore with the client the various health facilities available and can identify which ones have already been tried. Discussion and information sharing about community resources and the different aspects of each is appropriate at this time.

Client Profile

Obviously, the setting for a health interview should be private and conducive to the interchange of information; that is, the site should have a pleasing atmosphere and comfortable chairs. This may appear to be idealistic, but there is no reason why a pleasant atmosphere cannot be created. In the long run it will increase the effectiveness of nurse-client communication.

The initial short-answer biographical data required—name, age, address, sex, race, nationality, religion, marital status, etc.—is straight-

The young adult often seeks drugstore remedies and peer group advice before selecting health care services.

Emergency rooms, free clinics, private physicians, and group insurance plans are some options used by young adults in seeking health care services.

forward and should present no problem to the data-collection process. The demographic data discussed under this category in Chap. 3 is similar to the information that should be collected from the young adult client at this time.

Health Status Perception

A study done in 1975 posed the question: "What do you consider to be the prime of your life and why?" The young adult felt the prime would occur in the future, the middle-aged adult felt the prime time was the present, and the aging adult felt the prime had passed.[6]

Despite the perceptions revealed in this study, the young adult years are in fact characterized by peak physical attractiveness, agility, speed, and strength. Young adult bodies look and perform at their zenith. But during these years of superb physical condition, imperceptible changes are occurring. A person's muscle tone peaks between 20 and 30 years of age. At age 25, height begins to decrease, and the proportion of body fat increases, even though weight may remain stable. Visual acuity and hearing are at their best at age 20 and remain constant until age 40, when a gradual decline begins. Death rates from all causes increase throughout the life span, but a marked increase is noted after age 30.[7] The frequency of illness and disability also increases with age, but the incidence of accidents decreases with age. In the adult years fewer acute illnesses occur, but an increased incidence of chronic disease is noted.

The imperceptible changes and the few gray hairs and wrinkles that begin to appear in the young adult do not seem to cause attitudinal changes. A study done in the United States evaluating attitudes toward one's body showed no significant differences between a group under 25 years old and a group between the ages of 25 and 40.[8] Another study has shown that those young adults who derived their total self-esteem from physical appearance and prowess showed psychological patterns of aging sooner, i.e., when they noticed tangible signs of aging. Those individuals who valued inner qualities felt and functioned young for many years after their physical decline began.[9]

The framework within which young adults view health and important health concepts can vary from one based on conservative, traditional values to one open to experimentation with alternative lifestyles and health practices. In recent years, the literature has often discussed the young adult as a member of a counterculture, a distinct group which seems to have very special ideas of its own, with an underlying focus on the "natural."

This belief in the natural has many implications, all of which influence one's perception of health during the young adult years and thereafter. The natural way often puts to test the established views of health and nutrition. Nontraditional means for dealing with illness—means such as yoga, mind control, or macrobiotic diets—often prevail. "Naturalists" appear to be more flexible in lifestyle. Communal living is a style frequently chosen and may present a variety of health problems related to sanitation, food preparation, water supply, waste disposal, personal hygiene and communicable diseases.[10] Many mental stressors also exist for the young adult of this group. Frequent changes in living situation, economic insecurity, perhaps a lack of sound, intimate, interpersonal relationships can all create potential stress for the young adult.

Another group of young adults may be faced with an entirely different life set. These adults may or may not be under the influence of the counterculture; however, they are married, with children, perhaps, and

Refer to Chap. 3 under components of the health history for a complete discussion.

Young adulthood is characterized by peak physical attractiveness, agility, speed, and strength.

Health perception varies in young adults, ranging from the conservative, traditional values to nontraditional ones.

The nontraditional, "naturalist" view is expressed by many individuals who are flexible, and able to cope with a variety of lifestyles and related changes.

Communal living is an example of nontraditional lifestyle.

The traditional lifestyle for the young adult focuses on marriage, children, and occupational achievement.

The perceptions of the single young adult must also be considered when evaluating health perceptions of this age group.

have not only their own health to consider but the health of their children. They have multiple decisions to make concerning their health practices and child-rearing practices. Single young adults may also be members of the more-or-less traditional group and may also manifest problems related to life stress and to health perception.

It becomes obvious at this point that choices in lifestyle have implications in the client's perception of health. By listening carefully to the young adult's conversation, the nurse can gather information about that lifestyle. Questions suggested in Chap. 3 under this heading can be used to gain added data.

Refer to Chap. 3, under Health Perception/Health Management, for a complete list of questions used to assess this pattern area.

Questions to elicit data

1 Do you have a roommate?
2 What kinds of things do you eat?
3 What do you do when you get sick?
4 Are you interested in or do you have any experience with nontraditional health care, like acupuncture or healing by touch?

Health beliefs of the young adult can be influenced by family friends, by educators, and by past personal experiences with health care systems. Many researchers feel that the *locus of control* also influences one's health perception and values. In general terms, the locus of control defines how an individual regards the events and forces that shape one's life. If one feels a personal responsibility then he or she has an internal locus of control; if one feels that life is shaped by events and people over which he or she has no control then that individual exhibits an external locus of control. Of course, most people have a fluctuating locus of control, dependent upon current stressors; however, the dominance of either internal or external locus of control becomes a factor influencing one's health perception.

Refer to Chap. 1 for discussion of the health belief model.

The health beliefs of the young adult are influenced by locus of control, family, etc.

Current Health Status

The present state of health of the young adult should become apparent during the course of the interview. It is important to note that the young adult may not be adept at expressing thoughts in terms of health. Therefore, the nurse should allow the client to direct the conversation, remaining a nonjudgmental listener. In this way the nurse can make an assessment of the client's perception of health and specific health habits as the client responds to the interaction.

The client's present health state can be determined through direct questioning and observation.

Past Health Status

Eliciting information about the young adult's previous health status is achieved through techniques similar to those described in Chap. 3. Most young adults generally have had good health, experiencing only minor health problems and childhood illnesses. This age group is at risk for car accidents, homicide, suicide, and in some instances, early heart disease and breast cancer.

The health problems of the young adult may be minimal, but screening for those elements that comprise the client's past health is important. Birth history has limited significance, but provides patterns of growth and development, records of immunization, and a record of allergies important to health promotion behaviors.

The nurse needs to know if the client has always been in good health mentally and physically; if that is not the case, more detailed information regarding each problem should be elicited.

The client's past health status may be insignificant, but if health disturbances have occurred, they should be fully described.

Family History

As the client ages, the significance of familial health problems is of increasing importance. Therefore, careful analysis of familial health history, as described under that section in Chap. 3, should be made.

Life Patterns and Lifestyle

The life pattern of the young adult is affected by a multiplicity of factors. These include the client's age, culture, developmental characteristics, the environment and economic variables. A discussion of the unique effect of these factors on the young adult follows.

Age

The concept of holistic health implies that as individuals age, they change. "Age is a useful and powerful index in classifying large amounts of information—knowing an individual's chronological age one can make a number of predictions about his most likely anatomical, physiological, psychological, and social characteristics."[11]

The young adult is in a period of physical and psychosocial growth. In the absence of any significant childhood disease or chronic health problems, the young adult is in an age of optimization of wellness. Questions presented in Chap. 3 in the discussion of age can be used at this time.

Heredity

One of the factors to consider during a holistic health interview is the client's family and the influence it has on the client. Generally, a genetic history is taken, including a family tree. (Refer to Chap. 3 for a complete discussion of the family tree.)

By eliciting information concerning parents, siblings, grandparents, and other family members, the nurse is able to predict potential health problems for the client and to take measures to intervene appropriately. For example, the 20-year-old male with a prominent family history of heart disease needs to be apprised of the potential health alterations that can result from such a history. Measures such as control of cholesterol and unsaturated fat consumption, exercise programs, daily stress-reduction activities, and weight control can be advised to help reduce risk factors associated with coronary disease.

Another aspect of heredity concerns the impact of familial health problems on the client's offspring. As infectious disease in children has steadfastly come under control, the relative importance of congenital concerns has increased. During the 1960s genetics finally became an integral part of health care. With modern scientific advancement, rapid and accurate diagnosis of a possible genetic abnormalitity can more quickly be made. Currently, one out of every eight pediatric beds in the United States is occupied by a child with a congenital disorder in which genetic factors play a part.[12] It is also estimated that 20 percent of the American population has genetic concerns either for their own health or for their progeny.[13]

The nurse, while completing a health interview on a young adult, should explore the individual's understanding of genetically transmitted diseases and answer questions of concern. A history of Tay-Sachs disease, diabetes, phenylketonuria, or hemophilia within a family raises serious concern that the client's offspring may have an increased risk for developing these problems. If these concerns are identified, it is important to refer the client (and his or her spouse) for genetic counseling. The National Foundation March of Dimes (P. O. Box 2000, White Plains,

Family health history should be included in the assessment, as discussed in Chap. 3.

Refer to Chap. 3 in the section on age for questions to utilize when assessing this area.

In the absence of illness, the young adult cycle is an age of self-optimization.

The identification of family tree helps the nurse identify a client's risk factors and familial health problems. (Refer to Chap. 3.)

Identification of inherited predisposition to specific health problems can help the young adult reduce risk factors.

The discussion of genetically transmitted diseases can be important for the young adult considering marriage and children.

If genetic predisposition to a particular problem (e.g., Tay-Sachs) is identified, referral to a counseling center is essential.

N. Y. 10602) publishes a directory of genetic counseling centers and lists the services each center offers.

After the initial referral the nurse still has an important liaison role with the client. The individual will need support at this time, as knowledge about a particular problem may affect self-concept and create barriers in social relationships. In addition, while the client and spouse are receiving long-term counseling, the nurse can help them receive maximum benefits from the counseling service.

Culture

When dealing with clients it is inevitable that the nurse will encounter people of many different cultures. A family's beliefs about causes of illness and cures, the people who are instrumental in care and cure (folk practitioners), family definitions of health and illness, the use of self-medication, and general familial health practices all are influenced by cultural background and all in turn impact on the young adult's response to the health care system.[14]

For the young adult, the importance of culture cannot be negated in the assessment.

Young adults seeking health care from a dominant health care system may come from a wide range of ethnic affiliations. The nurse must recognize the young adult's cultural heritage and be sensitive to the impact it has on the health interaction.

Departure from cultural customs for traditional health care practices may be stressful for the young adult.

When the young adult does approach a system of care outside folk medicine, it may be with fear and trepidation; he or she may perhaps even be ostracized by members of the ethnic group. Therefore, it is vital that the nurse interact with the client in a way that indicates an interest in the cultural group and a recognition of the importance specific cultural values do have in a person's life.

Many of the young adult's health values are influenced by cultural inheritance.

Questions to elicit data

Additional questions regarding culture and its impact on lifestyle are found in Chap. 3.

1 What are your cultural preferences for food? for music? for art? for recreation?

2 What occupations are esteemed by your culture?

3 What types of behaviors are valued?

4 What are your cultural taboos and sanctions?

5 What is your position (in degree of belief and adherence) relative to the overall cultural system?

Such relevant data will help to broaden the nurse's view of the client as well as of the ethnic group as a whole.

Growth and Development

Physical Capabilities "Physical development reaches its peak during the young adult years."[15] By age 20 the genetic determination of one's growth pattern is fully evident. Maximal muscle power, coordination, and physical strength are reached during this time as well. Between 20 and 30 the brain reaches its maximal weight; however, it is thought to continue its cognitive development. In the healthy young adult other bodily processes, e.g., metabolism, cardiac and respiratory functions, cellular growth, and cellular perfusion are working at optimal levels.

Physical development reaches its peak during the early part of the young adult years.

In general, the physical capabilities of the healthy young adult are at their maximum. Therefore, it is a time when the individual has the physical strength and stamina to embark on many activities (e.g., occupational, athletic, sexual) that influence the life patterns which emerge now and develop throughout adulthood.

Physical capabilities are at an optimum during young adulthood.

Normal physical attributes of the young adult are discussed throughout Chap. 4.

Emotional and Social Capabilities The emotional and social developmental process of the young adult is encompassed in the word *maturation*. This term can be a nebulous one, having many interpretations. Maturity can be defined by societal expectations, which equate it with leaving home, working full time, entering marriage and parenthood. As defined legally, maturity is attained from 18 to 21 years of age. In addition, one can examine the physiological status of the body and define maturity using a biological age. However, for the purposes of health care, psychological age seems to be the most helpful determinant of maturity. Table 11-1 presents a comparison of various theorists and their views of maturity.

Refer to Table 11-1 for a further discussion of theories of maturity.

The young adult often appears externally mature but may be filled with internal anxieties and ambivalences. This is particularly true during the very early adult years, when conflicts arise as the individual begins to gain inner behavioral control and forsakes the adolescent ways of externalizing reactions to the environment (e.g., peer conformity, fantasy, overt sexuality, and abandonment of family).

Maturity, then, becomes the time for the young adult to develop capacities and traits that can be integrated for daily use and for achievement of future goals. The mature person can utilize his or her past experiences to maintain stability and identity in the presence of crisis, to handle frustration, and to deal constructively with strain and conflict.[16]

The young adult, particularly in his or her early twenties, is becoming aware of the components of behavior. By the time the individual has reached the thirties there will probably be a sense of comfort with this developmental process.

There are some very specific criteria of maturity which will enhance the ability of the health team to assess a client's maturity level and thus formulate an appropriate plan of care.[17] These criteria include:

1 A determination for independence
2 An ability to apply knowledge and experience
3 An ability to communicate experiences to others
4 A sensitivity to others
5 An ability to deal constructively with frustration
6 An ability to maintain self-control
7 A willingness to assume responsibility

A state of *interdependence*. The young adult needs to learn the delicate balance between the states of dependence and independence. This balanced state is called interdependence, and it has three aspects: emotional, social and economic interdependence.

First is *emotional interdependence*, which is the most difficult to achieve. To accomplish this type of interdependence, the young adult must arrive at the point where emotional needs are best met by peers, particularly of the opposite sex, and not by parents. Having reached this point, the young adult can begin to gratify the emotional needs of others in the family and in other reference groups.

The establishment of healthy emotional ties is a slow process for the young adult. The passive dependence of childhood and independent behavior of adolescence can exist concomitantly with interdependent behavior of young adulthood. However, the latter behavior requires the ability to love and to direct love to a variety of individuals and objects.

At the opposite pole of interdependence is independence, acted out to the point of rejection of intimacy and acceptance of isolation. (This state

Highlights

Maturity can be defined from a sociological, physiological, chronological, or psychological perspective.

The mature person is able to utilize past experience, to communicate concrete and abstract ideas to others, to deal constructively with frustration, and to maintain self-control; he or she is sensitive to others' needs, and is willing to assume responsibility and independence.

Interdependence is that delicate balance between dependence and independence.

The mature individual is able to assume a level of interdependence emotionally, socially and economically.

Table 11-1
Comparison of Theorists on Definition of Maturity*

Sigmund Freud takes the view that mature, adult personality functioning is characterized by patterns of behaving that effectively deal with one's sexual urges and environment. According to Freud, the mature adult has a stabilized self-concept, or ego identity, and has developed a number of adaptive ways of handling his desires, wishes, and fantasies. In Freud's theory, having more or less successfully passed through previous stages of personality development, in the final, genital stage, the person becomes able to love others on a more altruistic basis. In addition to providing love and care, marriage traditionally fulfills a principal biological function of this stage: reproduction. In Freud's view, if an individual has developed into a reality-oriented and socialized adult, he also will have formed social attachments that allow him to enjoy the pleasure and companionship of others in both work and play.

Alfred Adler believes that, in the development of personality, the mature adult is one who becomes able to free himself from self-imposed restrictions and to face reality as necessary. In Adler's view, the individual must develop a style of life that is his own, and this unique identity then unifies his personality and organizes and directs his behavior. According to Adler, the direction of this behavior is ideally toward others, and this social interest shows itself in the desire for interaction and in a concern for others. In this view, marriage and parenthood, the development of interpersonal relationships, and the formation of friendships are all expressions of this social interest.

Harry Stack Sullivan emphasizes that the mature adult is one who can deal effectively with potential sources of anxiety and who engages in satisfying interpersonal relationships. In this view, the individual's self-concept or identity also is seen as organizing and directing his actions, as well as having a stabilizing influence on his interpersonal relationships. According to Sullivan, the ability of the mature adult to be intimate and to have mutually satisfying relationships is usually shown clearly in marriage and parenthood. However, friendship and relationships with others also generally are considered important, because they provide further sources of pleasure as well as additional opportunities for personal growth and change.

Erik Erikson holds that a mature level of personality development depends on successful resolution of the crises of previous stages. In his view, successful resolution results in the formation of a clear sense of identity, which gives the individual a sense of perspective and direction and a feeling of unity and purpose. Erikson's theory emphasizes that development continues during adulthood; it does not stop. Thus, marriage and the formation of an intimate, loving relationship, as well as parenthood and a concern with productivity, involve and are a result of ongoing psychosocial processes of development. At each step, successful psychosocial resolution also contributes to the adult's ability to engage in a widening radius of mutually satisfying and close friendships.

Erich Fromm stresses that the personality development of the mature individual is characterized by his living in harmony with nature and society. According to Fromm, this involves transcending one's limits by creativity and by devoting oneself to society without conforming. Thus, the individual's sense of himself, his identity, is seen as coming from the development of a creative and constructive control over nature and from participation in society. In Fromm's view, marriage and parenthood can be seen as epitomizing the possibility of productive self-realization. In addition, being a creatively active adult, according to Fromm, is likely to lead to the formation of many deep bonds of brotherhood and friendship.

Walter Mischel considers the adult who shows mature ways of behaving to be one who has successfully learned the roles of adulthood and who effectively performs them. In this view, self-esteem during adulthood continues to derive in part from others' praise and acceptance of what one says and does. Marriage and parenthood can in turn be considered two complex roles that build on previous experience but also require learning new behavior. Throughout the adulthood years, according to this view, new friendships and other relationships can also be expected to develop as a result of an individual's continuing participation with others in various social, recreational, and vocational activities.

*From Robert E. Schell (ed.): *Developmental Psychology Today*, 2d ed., Random House, New York, 1975, p. 389.

will be discussed later under behavioral development.) Questions directed toward assessment of client support systems are helpful in evaluation.

Questions to elicit data

1 With whom do you live? (Even married couples may live with a set of parents.)

2 Do you have much contact with your family?

3 Do you have dependent, independent, and interdependent roles in your marriage?

4 Which of these predominates?

Social interdependence is demonstrated when the young adult is accepted into a society possessing those qualities and traits associated with adulthood. While some individuals accept their place within society, others strive for power and prestige in organizations of older adults. For the older adults, a younger person must prove worthy of acceptance by showing competence in a variety of situations. Therefore, the young adult's ability to be self-directed becomes critical.

Self-direction, or the knowledge of one's own goals, and recognition of what membership within certain adult groups means to those goals, are necessary if an individual is to achieve group placement. A few general questions will help the nurse assess development in this area.

Social interdependence is manifested by an individual's ability to participate as a member of an adult group, while retaining his or her own self-orientation.

Questions to elicit data

1 Do you belong to any groups?

2 What contributions do you feel you make to society?

3 Do you feel accepted in the adult world?

4 What things make you feel like an accepted adult?

5 What things make you feel you are not an accepted adult?

While groups serve important purposes (e.g., allowing the individual to have a forum for expressing personal beliefs) they can be problematic as well. If the group begins to serve as a substitute for self-orientation or becomes, as it were, a surrogate parent, the individual becomes dependent on the members and fails to gain independence. Thus, it is important for the individual to retain a healthy balance within various group memberships (e.g., religious, occupational, educational, civic), so that a state of interdependence can be achieved.

The third aspect of balanced independence is *economic interdependence*. Acceptance into the adult world rests on the presupposition of financial autonomy, i.e., freedom from financial support of one's parents. However, many young adults are influenced by the strong emphasis on higher education, making economic interdependence difficult. The cycle of extended education, with its parallel period of parental authority, causes many young adults to postpone intimacy and their own parenting roles. The cycle is reflected in the current trend in our society toward later marriages and older first-time parents.

Economic interdependence can be hampered in young adulthood if parental support is provided for advanced educational pursuits.

It should also be noted that there are still many adults who do pursue intimacy and parenting in their early twenties. Generally, these individuals have been able to establish their economic interdependence with society and are not dependent on family members for financial support.

Questions to elicit data

1 Are you financially independent of your parents?

2 How much longer do you foresee financial dependence?

3 Does the use of parental money have any adverse effects? on you? on your parents? on your family?

Foresightful application of knowledge and experience. The maturing adult needs to learn how to establish a locus of evaluation within himself or herself in order to determine what knowledge is essential and how new information can be used to achieve one's goals in life. Accomplishing

One's ability to apply knowledge and past experience makes dealing with new life situations easier.

this task has relevance to the whole spectrum of client education. The more mature young adult will be able to value health teaching, for example, in a way that will influence the quality, and perhaps the effectiveness, of future plans. It is too simplistic to judge client compliance solely on the basis of this one criterion; however, the ability of the client to recognize and value pertinent information is significant to achieving mature health care.

The ability to communicate experience. The young adult needs to develop the ability to express emotional aspects of his or her experiences and to become more skilled in communicating abstract concepts to others. The nurse may be able to obtain insight into the individual's ability to communicate effectively if, during the client interview, the opportunity to discuss a variety of experiences arises. If this does not occur, the nurse may find this aspect of maturity difficult to evaluate.

The young adult begins to gain experience in communicating abstract concepts to others.

Sensitivity to the needs of others. The adolescent is very ego-oriented, but in the process of maturing the young adult learns to examine and consider the needs of others. This enhanced awareness potentiates the person's ability to communicate with others. The nurse may be able to assess this sensitivity towards others during the interview from direct experience—through the nurse-client interaction.

A concern for the needs of others helps distinguish the young adult from the adolescent.

The ability to deal constructively with frustration. During adolescence the individual has difficulty maintaining a consistent behavior pattern. Changing standards and values and sexual and emotional drives make it difficult. But as a maturing young adult, the individual learns to delay gratification of all needs—physical and psychological—and to tolerate frustration, disappointment, anxiety, and deprivation.

Adequate capacity for self-control. As the adolescent grows, there is an increased ability to *handle* affection and emotional, sexual, and physical impulses. The young adult learns how to direct these life energies toward well-chosen activities and goals and to operate according to appropriate standards of conduct.

Dealing effectively with disappointments and frustration reflects a person's effective coping responses.

Willingness to assume responsibility. The young adult learns to anticipate and set long-term goals. Concomitantly, the individual is better able to overcome fear of failure and to accept disapproval of peers.

The last three criteria of maturity put forth here can be assessed by evaluating the client's finesse in handling new situations.

Knowledge of how the young adult handles new situations helps the nurse to determine the person's maturity.

Questions to elicit data

1 Do you meet new situations by avoiding or accepting the challenge?
2 Do you readily accept life changes and minimize them?
3 Is change such a stress that you belabor frustrations and have difficulty making change?

The maturing young adult should be able to accept new situations and the frustrations that accompany change with minimal difficulty.

There is one further point to be aware of in assessing the clients' ability to deal with new situations. When evaluating a client's response to life changes the nurse should differentiate between verbalization and actual performance. The less mature young adult may be well able to formulate a list of actions needed to handle a new situation, and this is certainly the first step. However, when the client is questioned further about actions specifically taken, the nurse may discover that the change process was arrested at the intellectual level. The mature young adult will be able to formulate *and* initiate action to meet or promote change in an organized manner and with minimal difficulty.

The young adult should not only be able to formulate a list of actions to take when handling a life crisis but should be able to take the actions as well.

The maturing process leads to adequate adjustment to oneself and to others, promotes mental health, and safeguards against prolonged conflicts and anxieties. Maturity is not a static state; it is a lifelong process in which the individual must be sensitive, aware, and realistic in undergoing changes in personal status as well as in the environment and in society.

Behavioral Development

Becoming an adult is an experience in disillusionment. The fantasy world of the adolescent fades as reality testing of the adult state becomes more pressing. The things feared by the adolescent do not seem quite so frightening after they are experienced as a young adult.

There is a normal increase in the tendency toward depression as the young adult leaves adolescence and the disillusionment process begins. The young adult also seems to lose much of the aggression and the hostility that mark the adolescent. While some of these forceful attributes are now directed toward work situations, others become more internally located, causing the young adult to surrender to the "growing-up" process with discouragement and regret.[18]

Growing out of adolescence means growing into a time for freedom that provides the young adult with a chance to make choices among people and experiences, thereby extending the satisfying experiences of childhood, while avoiding the unpleasant ones. Leaving adolescence also requires the eventual separating of oneself from the family and its concomitant financial support. The young adult begins to establish independence by establishing living space, developing his or her own authority, and increasing the differentiation between self and parent along with the psychological distance from family. Quite often, the armed services may offer an institutional milieu to help ease this family transition.

The nurse should be able to assess this transition with minimal difficulty. A few general questions about the living situation and family involvement should elucidate the self–parent differentiation process that is crucial to the young adult's behavioral development.

Questions to elicit data

1 Does your family live in town?
2 How often do you see them?
3 How often do you talk to them by phone?
4 How much influence do you think your family has on your life?

Eric Erikson has identified intimacy vs. isolation as one of the major developmental tasks of the young adult. "In youth you find out what you *care to do* and who you *care to be*—even in changing roles. In young adulthood, you learn whom you *care to be with*—at work and in private life, not only exchanging intimacies, but sharing intimacy. In addition, however, you learn to know what and whom you can *take care of*."[19] Achieving a true sense of intimacy seems an enigma to many young adults, who fear a loss of personal identity in establishing personal relationships.

Many young adults may find discussing this area of their life with a nurse difficult. If the client feels strongly about this, of course, his or her opinions and feelings must be respected. However, the nurse should attempt to impress upon the client the need for data. While doing a health history the nurse can reiterate that health includes more than physical well-being, that there are developmental tasks peculiar to each stage in life, and that it is important to evaluate them for health history. For just

Growth from adolescence to young adulthood may result in disillusionment and depression. That is all quite normal.

The aggression and hostility expressed during adolescence often become internally focused in young adulthood.

The young adult begins to establish separate living space, as well as a sense of authority, a sense of differentiation, and a psychological distance from the family.

Developing a sense of intimacy is an important part of the young adult's development.

Some young adults have difficulty discussing intimacy, while others welcome the chance to do so.

as it is important to evaluate when a baby starts to sit up, it is important to determine how well a young adult is relating to people outside the family unit. Some young adults may be having a lot of difficulty with intimacy and will welcome the chance to discuss their experiences with a professional person; others may not. It is to be hoped that the nurse will be able to assess in some way the adequacy with which intimacy is being achieved.

As the young adult becomes more intimate, emotions and feelings become confused. "Love" is a difficult concept for the young adult. It is a shattering dream to find that one does not "fall in love" but that "love grows into love."

Intimacy implies more than physical genital contact and orgasm. In its fullest sense, intimacy is the ability to share personal identity with another in order to achieve mutual satisfaction and support. Each person does not absorb the other's identity. Intimacy provides periods of meshing personalities which enhance a tender, close, open relationship, a team effort for the mutual benefit of two people. However, while the individual is involved in a relationship, he or she should be able to stand on the strength of his or her separate identity.

The negative pole of intimacy is isolation. In this situation, closeness is perceived as a threat to identity. The individual fears that intimacy will obscure the precise edges of his or her own identity, and isolation is adopted as a barrier to keep the self-identity intact. Quite often the young adult who seems unable to develop intimate relationships has had negative childhood experiences which promoted the development of a rigid or a totally diffuse identity. That person now believes that self-identity cannot stand if an individual loses himself or herself to another, i.e., if he or she experiences the emotion love.[20]

Erickson has identified another task crucial to young adult development—*generativity vs. stagnation.* Generativity implies a productive lifestyle. Work is deemed important for both maturation and mental health.

Job development usually means settling into a work situation, enjoying a financial independence from the primary family, and beginning steps toward achievement of goals. Work has a different meaning for each young adult: it can mean prestige and social recognition; it can be a basis of self-respect and of a sense of worth; it can be a chance for varied interaction, service, and creative self-expression; and it can be a means of earning a living.

As can be seen from Table 11-2 most of the stages of work development occurs during the young adult years. The task consumes probably 40 to 50 percent of the hours in a young adult's day. Generativity may also consume numerous mental hours. These mental hours may be spent

Intimacy implies more than physical contact; in its fullest sense, it implies an ability to share personal identity with another in order to achieve mutual satisfaction and support.

The negative pole of intimacy is isolation.

Refer to the section in this chapter which discusses sexuality and reproductive patterns.

Generativity, or productive lifestyle, is another stage in the young adult's development.

The meaning of work varies with each individual.

Table 11-2 gives a timetable for work development.

Table 11-2
Socialization of Work Development

Step	Age	Process
Crystallization	14–18	Emergence of awareness of career choices
Specification	18–21	Onset of job training
Implementation	21–24	Entry level position
Stabilization	25–33	Establishment in a field
Consolidation	35–	Reweaving and embellishment of vocational direction

Adapted from D. E. Super, *The Psychology of Careers*, Harper & Row, New York, 1957, p. 229.

productively to improve job performance, or they may be spent in hours of anguished indecision about job change, job transfer, a new field, and so forth.

Mentors play a prime role for the young adult. These individuals are usually persons to 8 to 15 years older who possess wisdom and authority. The mentor gives the young adult his or her blessing and teaches him the "ropes" of the job world. Unfortunately, there appear to be fewer of these surrogate-parent role models for females, but this is changing, and increasing numbers of women are benefiting from a mentor's support.

Mentors play a significant role for the young adult in developing a clear working role.

The main value of a mentor is actually received after the relationship ends. The termination generally occurs toward the end of the young adult years and is usually met with a sense of abandonment and loss. However, as the young adult begins to resolve this grief, he or she is left with a sense of rejuvenation and a need to become his or her own person within the work milieu.

The early adult years is a time for much psychosocial growth. The young adult is expected to establish and maintain intimate relationships, obtain an education, develop a trade, find a job and do well at that job, be financially independent, perhaps marry, begin parenting—and still establish self-identity and find self-fulfillment. Perhaps a reason for the near-perfect health that most young adults enjoy is that they have no time or energy for physical illness; all of their strength and concentration must go for the establishment of their future life.

The early adult years is a time for significant psychosocial growth.

The role of the nurse becomes one of assessing how all these psychosocial issues are being met and resolved. Individuals who are unduly stressed or unhappy with aspects of their life, whether personal or professional, can develop an altered health state in response to stress. This makes it critical for the nurse to determine the success with which the behavioral development of the young adult is occurring.

Questions to elicit data

1 Do you like your job?
2 Have you thought about other job/career possibilities?
3 Are you satisfied with your earning potential?
4 Are you satisfied with your present relationships?

Biological Rhythms

As discussed in Chap. 3, biological rhythms have a significant effect on each individual's life cycle. Although human beings have long noted the effects of biological rhythms, from the turning of leaves to the sleep-wake cycle, there was no significant interest in the subject from a scientific viewpoint until 1935, when the International Society for the Study of Biological Rhythms was established. Since 1935 the science of chronobiology has grown by leaps and bounds.

Biological rhythms begin to stabilize and form a pattern during the young adult years.

The capacity for rhythmic change is an inherent characteristic of all living things. In the young adult human many of the individual's biological rhythms begin to stabilize. It is important to see the patterns becoming established so that disturbances can be quickly identified and causes isolated.

Sleep-Wakefulness Patterns Of all the rhythmic patterns, the most important for the young adult is the sleep-wakefulness cycle. Many factors influence the need for rest and sleep, including physical health, type of occupation, and amount of daily exercise. The young adult is generally full of energy and participates in a myriad of activities—among

The young adult may experience altered sleep patterns due to increased tension and responsibility, work-related stress, and lifestyle changes.

them attending school, participating in family responsibilities, and working. All of these activities present new and exciting frontiers to explore as an adult, with minimal or no parental influence.

The young adult often maintains an active lifestyle, interrupting sleep patterns along the way. Traditionally, it has been thought that the young adult requires 7 to 8 hours of sleep per night, but some members of this age group seem to do well with less.[21]

The percentage of time spent in each stage of sleep decreases with age; however, interestingly enough, the percentage of time spent in Stage 1 REM (rapid eye movement) sleep does not change through life, consistently comprising 20 to 25 percent of total sleep time. This particular biological rhythm is thought to be very important for maintaining a stable psychological balance in each individual, no matter what age.

Frequently, the young adult will take medication to alter sleep patterns. Because of significant stress (e.g., trying to achieve, to maintain a family, to establish meaningful relationships, to participate in extracurricular activities), the young adult may have difficulty falling asleep. He or she becomes overtired and increasingly worried about the inability to sleep. Medications may seem a logical way to get some rest quickly. All too often the potential hazards of sleep medications are overlooked, and the young adult may become a prime target for some specific health problems.

Sleep medications significantly decrease REM sleep. If these medications are taken consistently, there is a gradual return to the normal amount of REM sleep. However, when the medication is stopped, the individual may undergo withdrawal symptoms, including insomnia, nightmares, fatigue, and increased sensitivity to pain. These symptoms may last up to 5 weeks.

If there is a problem in sleep habits, the nurse needs to explore the client's current lifestyle to see if adequate time is being allocated for sleep. If stress is hindering sleep, means other than medication should be established for handling and decreasing the problem. The client might be encouraged to take a brief rest period during the day or to participate in stress-reduction exercises. Such activities may prevent sleepless nights. Brief periods of watching television, reading, or sewing may be just enough to bring easy rest at the end of the day.

Whatever the prescription, the young adult needs to know the impact that a sustained, frantic, exhausting schedule will have over time. Good sleep habits established during the young adult years will not only have a significant impact on sustaining current health but on maintaining long-term wellness as the client ages.

Assessment of this pattern area can be made through questions presented in Chap. 3 in the discussion of biological rhythms.

Elimination Patterns Assessment of elimination patterns can be made through responses to questions similar to those discussed under this heading in Chap. 3. Eating habits, stress, and fluid intake and retention can all affect elimination patterns of the young adult.

Environmental Factors

An individual's environment can be considered from several aspects. One of the most obvious is climate. General questions about how the client tolerates present weather conditions may be important. For the young adult, relocating in different parts of the country for employment or schooling may include adjusting to new weather patterns. For example, moving from the east coast to Colorado may result in complaints of fatigue which can be corrected with minor changes in lifestyle (e.g., increased sleep).

The average young adult requires 7 to 8 hours' sleep; however, some persons in this age group do well with less sleep.

The percentage of time spent in stage 1 REM sleep does not change, no matter what the individual's age.

During REM sleep, dreaming occurs. Early in REM sleep (stage 1) dreams are shorter; in other stages dreams are longer and reflect life events.

Young adults may utilize sleeping aids because of difficulty in falling asleep.

Sleep medications decrease REM sleep.

The nurse should help the individual establish alternate means of handling stress so that it does not hinder sleep.

Exercise, yoga, or just watching television may be relaxation techniques used to induce sleep.

Refer to Chap. 3 for a complete discussion of sleep-rest patterns.

Changes in living environment can affect the health of the young adult.

Adjusting to changes in living environment and to proximate social relationships can be stressful to the young adult.

A second vantage point from which to consider environment is the client's actual physical surroundings and the client's level of comfort in those surroundings. Many young adults in college or just starting out on their own may not be able to afford living quarters in the "best" areas. Therefore, questions of safety and space may become issues. To save money many young adults may choose to live in a group or to share their dwelling with others of the same age. This may prove a great experience for some and stressful to others.

In addition, the effects of pollutants and harmful waste products can affect the individual's quality of life. Smoking may be an activity engaged in by many young adults, and the detrimental effects of smoking or of exposure to smoke should be discussed by the nurse.

Questions such as those presented in the discussion of environmental factors in Chap. 3 may help to elicit data.

Questions to elicit data

1 What kind of neighborhood do you live in?

2 Do you live in the city or the suburbs?

3 Do you feel safe in your present living situation?

4 What is the tempo of life around you?

All of these questions give the nurse a sense of the client's living space and provide subtle clues that may aid later on in identifying potential problem areas.

The third, and most obtuse, aspect of environment involves psychological characteristics.

Questions to elicit data

1 Do you like your living arrangements?

2 Is there a supportive peer group?

3 Does this peer group help you become happier, or do they continually pull you down with problems?

4 Whom or what do you seek in times of stress?

Answers to these questions can help the nurse examine the mental environment in which the client has placed himself or herself. This information, in addition to data gained about the mental set of the client, can be significant.

Economics

During the young adult years, the client usually obtains a permanent full-time job and earns economic independence. At first, the individual may feel quite affluent. Often, with increasing experience in self-support, the young adult finds out that money does not go as far as he or she would like.

Some young adults may still be financially dependent on parents, often until their mid-twenties, due to a choice to pursue higher education. Other individuals attending college may be independent of parents by virtue of loans and part-time employment. But for both of these groups, financial income is limited, and there is a struggle to meet basic needs.

Young adults who marry face other financial concerns. If both partners are working, they may have a very comfortable income, often generating more income than either one has ever seen before. Other married couples, choosing to have a family, may have to rely on a single salary, with added financial demands made by the increasing family size. Therefore, the economic status of the young adult can vary immensely.

The young adult may be faced with many stressors, including a strong competitive desire for rapid escalation into affluence. This may place the young adult in jeopardy, with too many bills from too easily obtainable credit cards, and increased work loads to pay the bills. Another stressor may be simply keeping up with the bills that come with the presence of children while attempting to buy a house.

Neugarten has done studies on young adults based on economic parameters and has been able to establish some general characteristics, both quantitative and qualitative. Young adulthood seems to last longer for the upper middle class. People of this economic stratum regard these years as a time for exploration of relationships, jobs, and lifestyles. The working class does not view young adulthood as a time of experimentation. For them issues are defined and settled early in life and then preserved accordingly. The serious reality of life is readily accepted. Upper-middle-class men tend to marry between the ages of 25 and 35, while working-class men marry much younger. One final conclusion was that the young adult in the higher socioeconomic class is likely to be older when he or she finishes school, gets a job, marries, and has children.[22]

The nurse may not elicit much information in this area, particularly because many clients will be sensitive to issues of money.

The client's economic status varies with lifestyle.

According to Neugarten, young adulthood lasts longer for the upper middle class. Persons within this group spend more time experimenting with life styles, relationships, and occupations.

Adults of the working class tend to define issues early in life and settle into routine more quickly.

Questions to elicit data

1 Is your income satisfactory for your lifestyle? Are you having any financial difficulties?

2 If so, how are you reacting to this problem? Any difficulty sleeping? Do you feel anxious or worried?

3 Do you have any plans for handling this situation?

The focus here should be on assessing physical and psychosocial problems that result from economic problems. (Refer to Chapter 3 for additional questions.)

Community Resources

The young adult may utilize community resources in a variety of ways. The client may use them (emergency rooms, free clinics, etc.) as a mechanism for entry into the health care system and follow-up services. Secondly, the young adult may contribute time and volunteer services to community agencies. He or she may be a Scout leader, a counselor, or a resource person for others in the community. The individual may also use services such as continuing education programs offered by schools or other facilities to develop skills in crafts, to learn cardiopulmonary resuscitation techniques, or to participate in other and varied training programs.

Reference to the section on community resources in Chap. 3 may generate questions to evaluate the young adult's participation in community resources.

Roles and Relationship Patterns

The expansion of relationships and the potential for involvement in many new roles is an important part of the young adult's developmental growth. Departure from the primary family unit, entering the work

The young adult experiences the development of a variety of new roles and relationships.

force, choosing to develop an intimate relationship with another individual, to marry, or to start a family all present new roles and/or relationships in which the young adult may participate. Effective handling of these new roles will positively affect all aspects of the individual's lifestyle. It is therefore important to carefully assess the young adult's ability to cope with the many changes of this period.

Family Life

For the young adult, separation from the primary family and establishment of a more independent lifestyle occurs. An interdependent relationship with the family unit also exists.

Marriage The decision to marry is one that seems to take longer for young adults today. Marriage is a definite statement, one that identifies a new way of living and a new status in society. Society's expectation is that young adults will marry, and statistics show that 90 percent of males and 86 percent of females do.[23] Individuals tend to choose partners who share similar beliefs, values, and goals. The selection of a partner is seen as an appropriate way to secure intimacy and evolve a mutually satisfying relationship.[24]

Young couples who have traditional expectations of marriage express greater happiness than those couples who are seeking more expressive roles, for example, self-actualization or romantic love. It seems that in traditional roles the rules for behavior are more clearly delineated and other options are limited; thus stress and anxiety are decreased.[25]

The desire for the matrimonial state is higher in females than males, but marriage seems to be more beneficial for males.[26] Men are happier with marriage although when the male partner is unhappy the couple is unhappy. Conversely, it is found that when the female partner is unhappy this feeling does not seem to transfer in the same way to the couple as a dyad.[27] Married men have better mental health than married females or single men. Single females are much better off in terms of psychological stress than married women. More married females feel that they are close to nervous breakdowns than do single females; they also exhibit more phobias, depressions, and passivity.[28]

The average age for a female to marry is 20; for a male it is 23, although the trend toward later marriages may alter these statistics. Men with only a basic education try very hard to achieve in their occupation and tend not to be involved in their marriage. Their basic philosophy is to provide for their family and look elsewhere for a sense of accomplishment and self-esteem. College-educated men, in contrast, seem to have more inner conflicts and are ambivalent about their roles. They feel that they are expected to be successful providers and still participate in an active manner with housework and child rearing.[29]

The young adult planning marriage should be certain in his or her own goals and should discuss plans carefully with the intended partner. Both individuals should be able to identify their expectations and the lifetime goals they are interested in achieving. Each partner should also be able to isolate some personal goals so that conflicts are reduced if, after marriage, one partner returns to school or expands career opportunities.

If the client is soon to be married, a few general questions about readiness are appropriate.

Questions to elicit data

1 Are you ready to be with only one person?

2 Are you ready, in an emotional sense, to leave your family?

During the young adult period, the individual establishes a more interdependent relationship with the primary family.

Most young adults (90 percent of males and 86 percent of females) will marry.

Marriage is a more highly desired goal for females but more beneficial for males.

Married men seem to have better mental health than married females and single men.

The average age for marriage for females is 20 and for males 23. These statistics will be affected by the increasing trend toward later first-time marriages.

For the young adult, marriage is an opportunity for intimacy and security.

3 Why are you getting married?

4 Have you thought about what the future might bring?

5 Have you thought about failure and divorce?[30]

This line of questioning should allow the nurse to assess the preparedness of the client for marriage.

If the client is married, the nurse will need to know in general terms how the marriage is working.

Each partner must have a sense of personal identity as well as a shared relationship with the other.

Questions to elicit data

1 How long have you been married?

2 What does your spouse do?

3 Do you spend a lot of your free time with your spouse?

4 What kinds of things do both of you enjoy doing together? alone?

5 Have you delineated chores?

6 Are you happy with your marriage?

7 What are strengths and weaknesses of your marriage?

8 Have you ever considered divorce?

Divorce A discussion of marriage must include the topic of divorce. Five to seven percent of young adult marriages are terminated by divorce.[31] If the young adult has been unable to achieve a sense of identity and independence before entering marriage, intimacy cannot be achieved and divorce seems more likely. Most divorces for young adults under 29 years of age occur during the first 3 to 5 years of marriage.[32] Divorce in young adults is more prevalent in couples from lower socioeconomic groups, couples who have less education, less financial security, fewer personal resources, and who married at an earlier age.[33]

Marriage is increasingly viewed today as a loving, sharing relationship between two people rather than as a social institution for procreation. This view helps to explain the increased divorce rate. When couples are no longer mutually satisfied with their lifestyle, a decision is made to dissolve the marriage. Today, this decision is supported by more liberal societal and even religious views about divorce.

The dissolving of a marriage, however, is accompanied by much stress and disillusionment. Divorce will result in a change in role and status and force the individual to reexamine personal identity, goals, and future plans. Divorce is particularly traumatic for the young woman whose self-definition depended upon the role of wife, and even mother, and who now finds herself on her own. In addition, many females measure success by, and derive feelings of worth from, "capturing" and "holding on to" a man. The women's liberation movement has been somewhat successful in changing this societal attitude, but still women in particular feel the acute sting of failure with divorce.

If divorce is a reality or has already occurred, it is important for the nurse to help the client deal with the change in role. What seems essential is a clear assessment of why the marriage didn't work and the client's response to the loss of a spouse. Physical and emotional reactions to this loss must be evaluated, and when necessary, referral for counseling made to help the client (1) deal with the current crisis, (2) plan for reentry into a "single's" lifestyle and (3) define future plans and revise goals.

If the client is divorced, the nurse may want to obtain a brief background history.

Lack of self-identity and independence before marriage makes it difficult for the adult to achieve intimacy in marriage.

Divorce is more prevalent in couples from a lower socioeconomic group, couples who have less education and financial security and fewer personal resources to cope with the stress of marriage.

Dissolving of a marriage, regardless of the reason, can be traumatic for the individual.

Questions to elicit data

1 How long were you married?
2 How long have you been divorced?
3 What happened to your marriage?
4 Was the divorce a mutual decision?
5 How did you handle this difficult time?
6 Would you like to get married again?
7 Do you have any children?
8 What kind of legal arrangements were made for the children?

Parenting Generally, the decision to have or not have a child occurs within the first few years of marriage.[34] If young adult couples wait too long they usually begin to feel pressure from parents and others to start a family. The interdependence of generations is the strongest societal force that encourages young adults to have children.

The active decision to have children is a sign that the couple feel they can take care of others as well as themselves. However, the arrival of the first child often brings stress to the marriage. Tension exists between husband and wife because of new responsibilities. Feelings of inadequacy in caring for a new baby, new division of chores, new schedules, jealousy, and competition all combine to create a change in both roles and relationships.

American mothers seem to have a unique responsibility in child rearing. This is brought about by such things as:

1 The strong child orientation of American society
2 The need to learn and carry out complex child-rearing practices without benefit of handed-down traditional practices, preparental education, or societal support
3 Almost total maternal responsibility for child rearing
4 The modern view that if mothering is superior, the child will grow up to be superior
5 Society's mandate that all problems be handled in a systematic, rational, and calm manner, a difficult feat when dealing with the emotional nature of child rearing
6 Rapid societal changes and societal heterogeneity[35]

Many young women become mothers before they have matured. Even so, it is found that women younger than 24 years of age adjust to their new role more easily than do males, who may not have reached an appropriate level of emotional maturity. These males can develop role-strain and discomfort. Couples less than 24 years old may see their marriage affected by the "20-year disenchantment" 18 months after the baby is born. Their parenting is affected by social immaturity. Often the prebirth expectations for the child are unrealistic, and after the baby is born problems occur. The immature male usually feels little commitment to his wife or child and spends much time away from home.[36]

However, for young adults who have reached a level of emotional maturity, parenting is less stressful. Many individuals from large families have been previously involved with child rearing and are less threatened by the prospect of children.

Again, the maturity of the couple and their ability to discuss children prior to marriage may help to reduce anxiety when the decision to have a

The decision to have or not to have children usually occurs within the first few years of marriage.

Children can bring stress to the marriage and affect the relationship of husband and wife.

In the United States, child-rearing responsibilities frequently fall on the mother, although this trend is changing.

child is reached. If role conflicts between parenting and career advancement exist, then children can present even more problems for the couple.

The nurse can help to identify the couple's concept of the family. If the client has children, some brief information is desirable.

Questions to elicit data

1 How many children have you? (names and ages)
2 How do you and your spouse handle the division of labor in caring for the children?
3 Do you have any particular philosophy of child rearing?
4 Are you having problems with any of your children?
5 How often do you and your spouse go away or go out without the children?
6 Do you plan to have additional children?
7 Are you satisfied with your present role as mother?   father?
8 Would you like a change in roles?

Single-Parent Families Within this country, individuals may choose to have a child but remain unmarried. Other adults are forced to rear children alone as a result of divorce or of the death of a spouse, while adoption by a single person is another option.

Single parenting due to divorce, death of a spouse, or choosing to raise a child alone, is another lifestyle frequently seen today.

The single-parent lifestyle is another area to consider when evaluating parenting patterns. In addition to the questions above, the nurse will need to explore the parent's role in child rearing and the source of support in coping with problems.

Any or all of the information elicited about family patterns may have a bearing on the young adult's physical or mental health. As indicated, there may be times when the nurse feels the client needs counseling from a different health professional; in this case, appropriate referrals are made.

Occupation Many psychologists have realized the important contribution of work to the development of mental health and maturity. A job offers the young adult security, enjoyment, and the promise of goal achievement. The first year of employment is a critical period for the individual. It is a time of initiation and excitement and a time of fears about competence and self-worth. For many, the relationship with the mentor (see earlier discussion in this chapter under behavioral development) may help to reduce the stress of this period of initiation.

Work can be a time of excitement as well as of fear for the young adult.

Refer to earlier discussion under Behavioral Development for an understanding of mentorship roles.

Most of the research done in this area has been based on men in industrial settings; minimal research has been done on men in nonbusiness careers or on working women. Data available, however, seem to suggest that people with lower job status (i.e., skilled manual labor) are motivated primarily by extrinsic factors such as pay and job security. Conversely, professional white-collar workers receive job satisfaction from more intrinsic rewards, such as achievement, responsibility, self-fulfillment.[37] Interestingly, 84 percent of all workers state they are satisfied with their jobs, but 90 percent of workers over 30 and 75 percent of workers under 21 give that answer.[38]

Persons with positions of low status are motivated to work for pay and security.

White-collar workers are motivated by intrinsic rewards, such as self-fulfillment and achievement, as well as by extrinsic rewards.

Initially, just having a job can be satisfying for the young adult, whether the individual likes the job or not. A job gives the young adult independence and hope for a promotion or a better job in the near future. Job satisfaction among minority groups is consistently lower, but their jobs are generally lower paying and less rewarding. Increased education

A job gives the young adult independence.

and increased opportunities seems to correlate with increased job satisfaction.

Some differences in pursuing work have been noted between the young adults of today and those of previous decades. The majority of today's young adults still continue to have a true desire to produce good work; however, they no longer see a job solely as a means to earn a living. They are seeking power and are trying to do so in a way that will further self-actualization. The youngest segment of the labor force is seeking work that will also satisfy a desire for community, fellowship, participation, challenge, self-fulfillment, freedom, and equality.[39]

A prevalent attitude among young adults is that one's own needs are equally, if not more, important than those of family, community, and employer. Three out of four young adults, with or without college education, verbalize the need for self-expression and self-fulfillment as a personal value.[40]

Young adults today seems less fearful of economic insecurity and are thus able to demand the potential of self-fulfillment in job situations. They also tend to have a pessimistic outlook on the ability of an employer to provide them interesting and challenging work. This attitude may be one reason so many young adults have their own independent businesses in the arts and trades, opportunities that, while economically risky, allow the individual freedom and complete autonomy.

Today's young adults are also not so awed by authority and are not typically subservient. Even without going to college, they are better educated than their parents.

The nurse will want to have work history from the client, including the young adult's current work, the type of work completed in the past, and present job satisfaction. The client's attitude toward work in general, along with the perceived pressures associated with his or her position, should be elicited. These questions, along with those provided in Chap. 3, offer the nurse an opportunity to see how well an individual is assuming his or her occupational role. As the client discusses plans for occupational advancement, the nurse can also evaluate future life goals.

Societal Relationships The young-adult stage of life can be divided into two phases: entry years and developmental years. The *entry years* are characterized by preparation for a career, development of interpersonal relationships, and establishment of self-concept. The *developmental years* are characterized by career commitment, establishment of significant relationships, and the beginning of parenthood. It is difficult to assign age ranges for these two phases because of variance of time schedules for completion of high-school, college, graduate school, and marriage for each young adult.[41]

Research done by Keniston has shown that the majority of society is conformist-oriented in interpersonal relationships and in gaining approval for its own sake. However young adults are increasingly expressing more autonomous values, and these values are oriented more toward universal ethical principles.[42] Young adulthood is a time for commitment, for tempering ideas and ideals.

A prominent societal characteristic of young adulthood is its variety of lifestyle options. This chapter has already discussed marriage, divorce, and parenting roles of the young adult. It has also touched on premarital cohabitation, an increasing trend in young adults.

Singlehood is another viable option for the young adult. There is an increasing number of single young adults in the 20 to 34 age group.[43] Unmarried young adults may be treated as immature, nonconformists who cannot or will not assume life responsibilities, i.e., marriage and

Young adults seeking work today are more concerned with job satisfaction and opportunities for self-expression.

Self-employment is one opportunity for the adult to achieve greater job satisfaction.

Occupational stressors can affect the young adult's health.

The young-adult stage of life can be divided into two stages: the entry years and the developmental years.

The entry years are characterized by preparation for a life career, development of self-concept, and establishing relationships.

The developmental years are characterized by commitment, parenthood, and intimacy.

The prominent societal characteristic of young adulthood is a variety of lifestyles.

Singlehood is a viable option for the young adult today.

children. Pressure from families to marry may be experienced by the individual and can produce unnecessary stress.

Singlehood may meet many needs of the young adult who does not feel ready to marry or who has not found a suitable spouse. However, the single young adult plays the role of sole financial support and house manager and may face special problems of aloneness in lack of companionship, in maintenance of emotional balance, and in feeling out of place in social gatherings. Generally, singlehood increases the chances for education, personal advancement, and community service.[44] The young adult needs to be aware and reassured that marriage and parenthood are not the only means to demonstrate emotional maturity.

Because of an openness not previously experienced by society as a whole, homosexual relationships are more prominently apparent in the young adult society. Communal living, mate swapping, contract marriages are all newer phenomena characteristic of the young-adult years. The impact of these phenomena on society as a whole has not been fully analyzed.

The science and technology boom after World War II has undermined the traditional institutions of religion for many young adults. Others of this age group still adhere to formal religion. Regardless of religious preference, young adults generally have established some code of moral-ethical behavior, some sort of philosophy on which to base their lives. This follows from the concern and commitment to mankind as a whole that they generally evidence.

At this point in the health interview assessment the societal characteristics of the young adult should be evident. The practitioner has probably been able to determine already whether the client is in the entry or developmental years of this stage of life. Information has most likely already been elicited about lifestyle in terms of significant relationships.

The nurse may now want to explore specific values and beliefs.

Questions to elicit data

1 Do you belong to a specific religion?
2 Do you go to church regularly?
3 Do you have a philosophy of life which guides your actions?
4 What do you value in life?
5 How do your values influence your present lifestyle?

Self-Perception and Self-Concept Patterns

During the young adult period, the individual has the opportunity to gain greater independence and develop a stronger self-concept. Living away from the family unit, the individual has an opportunity to observe others as they act upon personal values and beliefs. Naturally, positive reinforcement will help strengthen the individual's confidence. However, negative reactions may force the individual to take a look at other people's views. This can be threatening, but as the person matures, he or she begins to gain a greater sense of self-confidence.

The work situation, while new and exciting, may also affect one's self-confidence. Entering the work force challenges the individual to verbalize his or her points of view and to take stands on issues without the benefit of family or even faculty support. The person is forced to stand on his or her own, take risks, and accept the consequences for personal actions.

Interpersonal relationships, particularly intimate relationships, can also be challenging to one's self-concept. As the individual begins to consider marriage or a close relationship with another individual, it becomes critical to establish independence and self-identity not related to direct parental influence. Failure to achieve this may seriously jeopardize future relationships and limit the young adult's development.

Attitudes developed during adolescence, along with parental support and confidence in the individual, help to promote the sense of self-responsibility and self-worth needed to survive the young adult years. The young adult must have a strong sense of his or her own strengths and weaknesses. Recognition of attitudes and other factors that may limit personal growth is critical if the individual is to successfully survive the crisis of adulthood. If such recognition is not achieved, some crisis such as loss of a position, failure to receive a promotion, divorce, or loss of a relationship may severely threaten a person's self-concept and interfere with achievement of life goals.

Questions set forth in Chap. 3 under discussion of this pattern area can be used to assess the young adult client. In addition, information presented under the section on life patterns and lifestyles within this chapter is important reference.

Cognitive and Perceptual Patterns

The young-adult years are a time of optimal cognitive and perceptual functioning. During this time, sensory perception is heightened, the individual is engaged in mastery of new skills and new knowledge, and the intellect is stimulated by these exciting and challenging events. Assessment of this pattern area will provide the nurse with some insight into the individual's cognitive and intellectual development. The following paragraphs discuss the characteristics of this pattern area that are unique to the young adult.

Sensory Perception

The young adult's sensory perception is at peak capability. Muscular-skeletal development and power is reached by the early twenties. Visual and auditory acuity are said to reach their maximum at 10 years of age. The viewing range lengthens gradually thereafter until about age 50.[45] Peripheral perception is optimally effective.

Questions presented in this pattern area in Chap. 3 can be used to adequately evaluate young-adult sensory perception.

Education

Educational background varies, of course, with each young adult. For some individuals, completion of high school and the learning of a trade may be the goal. Other young adults pursue higher education through community college, a baccalaureate education, or graduate study. Individuals who choose professions (e.g., physicians and lawyers) may be in school for a prolonged period of time.

While individuals in every cultural group have lengthened the time spent in academic pursuit, there are still many individuals who do not have the opportunity, because of financial considerations or family responsibilities, to pursue advanced education. The present economy has increased the number of young adults enrolled in part-time study.

Careful analysis of the individual's long-term goals are critical to making decisions regarding education. If the individual plans to be, or is, married, both partners should be encouraged to clarify how personal goals will affect their relationship. In addition, knowledge of the client's educational achievement will help to direct the nurse in plans for teaching health promotion and preventive behavior.

The young adult must be aware of personal strengths and weaknesses in order to direct his or her growth.

Refer to Chap. 3 under Self Perception/Self-Concept Patterns for further discussion.

During the young adult years, sensory perception is heightened mastery of knowledge and skills increases, and the intellect is stimulated.

Visual acuity reaches maximum at age 10 and lengthens gradually until about age 50.

Educational levels vary with each young adult, depending upon personal goals.

Determination of the educational level of the client is important for the nurse in terms of planning health teaching.

Intelligence

The first edition of the Stanford-Binet intelligence test (1917) indicated that intellectual growth stopped at age 12. In successive revisions this estimate was put at between 16 and 21 years of age.[46] In 1930 Jones and Conrad found peak test performance to occur in the twenties, but more recent cross-sectional studies have reported peaks at 30 and 50.[47] However, an important factor in intelligence testing is that, after a certain point, speed performance tends to decrease with age. Ghiselli found that there was no age effect in intelligence performance of 1400 well-educated subjects between the ages of 20 and 65, when time units were removed from the tests given.[48] Generally, longitudinal studies have shown that intelligence either remains the same or slightly increases during the adult years.

Many studies have been done comparing male and female intelligence. One study did retests of the Stanford-Binet on 48 men and women between the ages of 12 and 50—a span of 38 years. Men who had higher intelligence quotes (IQs) at age 12 had gained more in IQ by their mid twenties than had those males who started with a lower IQ. Women who had higher IQs at age 12 had gained less by their mid twenties than had those women who started with lower IQs.[49] Another study found that women's early intellectual characteristics correlated more with their intelligence at age 40, whereas men's occupational experiences tended to produce more changes in their behavior, thus causing more fluctuation in their IQs.[50] Shaie et al. found significant sex differences in the Primary Mental Abilities test. Females tended to be superior in verbal meaning, reasoning, and word fluency. Males were superior in spatial and number relationships and general intellectual ability.[51]

Consideration of intelligence has significance for the health history in terms of assessment of the client. The nurse needs to be able to make a judgment about the client's level of intelligence, since this assessment will affect the depth of any teaching to follow. A young adult with a college education may well understand the physiological intricacies of gastric ulcer development and its relation to hydrochloric acid, whereas a young adult from a rural community who lacks the same education (but not necessarily having a lower intelligence) may need a less complex explanation of ulcer development.

The nurse should be alert for clues about intelligence. Judgments can be based on responses to questions. Factors such as word usage, ability to do abstract thinking, and appropriateness of questions asked by the client can be used to establish intellectual level. The astute assessment of intelligence will, in the long run, enhance the efficacy of the nurse in caring for clients.

Sexuality and Reproductive Patterns

The young adult years are a time of optimal physical competence. Sexual maturity is a part of this development. The capacity of both sexes to respond quickly and repeatedly to sexual stimuli is common in the sexually active individual.

While physical development is at its peak, issues related to sexual maturity become matters of concern. These include (1) exploration of traditional as well as nontraditional roles; (2) establishment of sexual identity; (3) selection of contraceptives, and (4) childbearing.

Exploration of various sexual roles has been influenced by relaxation of societal values. The feminist movement and changing roles for men and women have resulted in a breakdown of stereotyped roles and of the impact of that stereotyping on sexual development. Changing adult

Longitudinal studies have demonstrated that intelligence either remains the same or slightly increases during the adult years.

One study has attributed fluctuations in IQ to occupational experiences.

Use of terminology during the nurse-client encounter or health teaching experience should be appropriate to the client's level of education and intelligence.

Sentence structure, evidence of abstract thinking, and appropriateness of questions asked can give the nurse a sense of the client's intellectual ability.

While physical sexual development is at its peak, issues related to sexual maturity (e.g., exploration of traditional and nontraditional lifestyles and sexual identity) are matters of concern to the young adult.

Exploration of sexual roles has been influenced by a relaxation in societal values and diminished stereotyping of male and female roles.

roles, increasing divorce rates, the singles lifestyle, as well as the gay liberation movement, have all contributed to allowing the person time to explore roles and establish a sense of identity in and satisfaction with a selected role. Many young adults become hurt, dismayed, or disappointed by various sexual encounters because their identity of self is not defined and they have not been able to achieve intimacy in these varied experiences.

Young, unmarried, male adults have traditionally been more sexually active than unmarried women; however, that trend is slowly changing. In 1968, 23 percent of college women reported having premarital coitus, compared with 10 percent in 1958.[52] Middle-class and working-class men report the same amount of premarital activity, whereas middle-class women report a significantly lower frequency of premarital sex than working-class women—31 vs. 82 percent.[53] Two-thirds of college students today believe that their sex standards are the same as those of their parents.[54] All of these statistics seem to indicate that unmarried young adults are not that much different sexually from what their parents were. The freedom felt today to speak of sexuality seems to make premarital sexual exploration more explosive than ever before; in fact, the openness with which we address this topic has also enabled young adults to be more honest and forthright about their relationships.

Use of contraceptives has increased freedom for sexual exploration and has allowed couples to postpone decisions in planning a family. The choices of whether to have children, when to begin a family, how to integrate family and a career, and which parenting patterns to adopt are all part of the young adult's concept of sexuality. By having a clear choice in sexual identity, the individual can make the subsequent decisions to share life with another individual, to remain single, or to have children.

The young adult will often request information about contraception from the nurse, and counseling can be provided as needed. The female young adult also has some very specific health care needs. Pregnancy is almost exclusively a phenomenon of young adults. The other realm of health care specific to the female relates to routine gynecological exams and issues of birth control and sexual behavior. Specifics about female health can be found in Chap. 12.

Many of the young adult males (and females) of the 70s and 80s have a unique health care characteristic; they are veterans of the Vietnam war. The injuries in this war were more extensive than in previous wars because of increased weapon technology. And, because of increasingly sophisticated medical care, many of the wounded soldiers who would have died in other wars lived. Of wounded army personnel separated for disability, 54 percent were separated for amputation or paralysis of extremities as compared with 28 percent from the Korean war and 21 percent from World War II.[55]

The devastating effects of war on these young men ranged from actual physical pain, handicap, and paralysis to psychoemotional problems such as loss of identity and sense of self, apathy, cynicism, guilt, and depression. Hopefully, many of these problems were worked out during the late 60s and early 70s at the time of injury or war exposure; however, when interviewing veterans, the nurse must not forget to consider these factors in the total concept of health, particularly in relation to sexuality and self identity. The war experience may have very definite influences on present health and health perceptions. The nurse should ascertain if, indeed, the client was in Vietnam. If so, then a few general questions related to such are warranted.

Highlights

A poorly defined self-identity can result in disappointing sexual encounters.

Premarital sexual activity seems to be a common component of young adult relationships today.

Open discussion of sexual concerns has enabled young adults to be more honest about sexual relationships.

Use of a variety of contraceptive devices has increased freedom for sexual development and allows postponement of the decision to have children or not.

Clarification of sexual identity can facilitate decisions involved in a relationship with another individual.

Refer to Chap. 12 for further discussion of pregnancy and childbearing.

The effect of the Vietnam war continues to affect the health and self identity of many veterans.

1 Were you injured?

2 Do you have any health problems today which stem from Vietnam?

3 Have you been able to come to terms with yourself about this war and your participation in it?

The nurse needs to assess the intimacy achievement of the young adult, if it seems appropriate. In addition to the questions suggested under this pattern area in Chap. 3, there are other areas to consider.

Refer to the discussion of sexuality and reproductive patterns in Chap. 3.

Questions to elicit data

1 Are you experimenting with premarital sex? If so, do you have adequate birth control information and equipment?

2 Have you had some difficult experiences with close relationships?

3 What has been the long-term effect on you?

4 Have you felt yourself gravitating toward isolation-type behavior?

5 Have you experienced some mutual satisfaction in the pursuit of intimacy?

6 Are you generally successful in the achievement of intimacy?

Nutritional Patterns

Adequate nutrition is often a nemesis for the young adult. Many members of this age group, particularly those in their early twenties, do not know how to prepare food and place no importance on these skills. All too often, adolescents are not taught the basis of adequate nutrition and the art of preparing food; they, therefore, are at a loss to plan and prepare nutritious meals on their own. The use of "junk" foods and "fast" foods, particularly in the early adult years, can be problematic. Junk food is easier to prepare and often has more appeal than meat, fish, vegetables, grains, and so forth. Fast foods may become a habit for the people of this age group, who are, as a rule, active and busy. Eating at a fast-foods place is easier than planning and preparing meals at home and perhaps eating alone.

Young adults generally have healthy bodies which can endure much abuse, whether lack of sleep, alcohol and drug abuse, lack of exercise, or poor nutrition. The ability of the body to withstand poor eating habits does the young adult a disservice, however, and leads to a lack of appreciation for the effects of poor nutrition on future health status.

Another problem for the young adult may include fad weight-reduction diets or other types of fad diets (e.g., some vegetarian diets) which are deficient in essential elements for adequate nutrition. Physical appearance is often considered more important than a balanced diet, especially during the early adult years, and problems such as anorexia nervosa are common in this age group.

The young adult has increased needs for vitamins C, E, B_6, and riboflavin. Females have increased need of vitamins A and B_{12}. Anemia may be an added problem for the menstruating adult. Increased amounts of iron should be encouraged in this age group.

The nurse should elicit from the client a diet history similar to that presented in Chap. 3 under nutritional patterns.

Nutritional deficits can occur in the young adult because of an increase in junk food intake, an inability to prepare foods, and lack of interest in eating.

Young adults can endure poor nutrition for a short period. However, disturbances in other pattern areas may be due to nutritional alterations.

Poor nutrition can affect the individual's future health status.

The importance given to physical appearance by the young adult often affects eating patterns.

The young adult needs increased amounts of vitamins C, E, B_6, A, B_{12}, iron, and riboflavin.

Refer to discussion of nutritional patterns in Chap. 3 for a complete listing of questions used to assess this area.

Questions to elicit data

1 Are you happy with your present weight?

2 Do you understand the four basic food groups and how to construct a proper balanced diet?

3 Do you know how to cook?

4 Have you ever been on a fad diet?

5 What type of food do you feed your children?

6 Do you have any particular views about nutrition?

These questions should allow the nurse an opportunity to assess the nutritional habits of the young adult and the need for teaching in this area. Nutrition is often a sensitive area for the young adult; therefore, it is important that the nurse not lecture but rather have a nonthreatening discussion with the client about these concerns.

Exercise and Activity Patterns

From the preceding discussions in this chapter it is very evident that the young-adult years are active ones. Major decisions about marriage, children, career, and lifestyle are made. It is a time for dating and for experimentation with all of life's options in food, people, clothes, hobbies, and so forth. Young adult years bring the peak in human physical condition, so individuals of this age group have much energy and a flair for life.

Single young adults generally have a varied circle of friends. After marriage, patterns of friendships may change. Some couples may have only a few close friends; others may have a wide circle of acquaintances. Problems can result if husband and wife differ in their selection of friends. Of course, the presence of children will give young adults less time and freedom to pursue many activities.

The importance of a regular activity plan should be stressed. Regular physical exercise has been shown to have a significant effect on reducing some of the physiological changes associated with aging.[56] In addition, regular activity can impact upon sleep-rest patterns and on nutrition, and can serve as a mechanism for helping to reduce stress in the young-adult years. It is not surprising that many large corporations provide tennis courts, tracks, swimming pools, and the like for their employees.

> It is important for the young adult to establish a regular activity pattern.
>
> Regular activity reduces some of the physiological changes associated with aging.
>
> Exercise can help to reduce stress in the young adult.

For the young adults, exercises which stimulate aerobic activity, decrease the heart rate, and stimulate respirations should be encouraged. Running, jogging, bike riding, swimming and outdoor activities may be included in this list.

The type of information the nurse needs for assessment is similar to that presented in Chap. 3.

> Social networks established by the young adult may be a way to increase leisure time.

Questions to elicit data

1 Do you date much?

2 How many friends do you have?

3 What do you do with your friends?

4 Do you and your spouse have different groups of friends? a mutual group?

5 How much exercise are you able to fit in around your children's schedule?

6 Do you spend much time alone?

These questions may give the nurse insight into the client's use of leisure time. Frequency of vacations should be considered as well. For the single, working young adult there may be more time and money available for vacations. However, individuals should be asked to describe their leisure activities also. Painting, sewing, or reading may not be very strenuous, but they do provide relaxation. For the young adult on a hectic schedule, this time can be invaluable.

Highlights

Lifestyle significantly influences a person's ability to vacation and to participate frequently in leisure time activities.

Coping Patterns and Stress Tolerance Patterns

The young adult is faced with many complex issues that affect personal and professional growth. The nurse should have an appreciation for the stressors of the young adult. The years between 20 and 30 are a time of exploration and some quasi commitment to adult roles, memberships, responsibilities, and relationships. It is a time for sexual exploration and for exploration of intimacy. During this time the young adult should be able to arrive at some self-definition and a sense of what his or her relationship is to the world. It is a time of choice: job, career, mate, lifestyle, children, morals, ethics—provisional as these choices may be.

Young adults are faced with many stressors.

Between the ages of 28 and 32, the individual begins to question whether he or she should make a stable life structure based on choices already made. At this point drastic changes may be made. (Refer to the discussion of stress and change in Chap. 2.) The commitments are deeper, and there is more interest in work and family. Long-range goals and plans are developed, and life is characterized by order, stability, security, and control. The individual at this age is concerned about being a success by age 40.

Multiple changes in the young adult's life can increase tension and result in disturbance of health patterns.

The 30s are considered a stabilizing period for the young adult.

These changes can increase tension and interrupt health habits. Each of the issues facing the adult client can, in and of itself, be stressful. However, multiple stressors or a growing number of unresolved stressors can be demanding on the individual and may result in tension, interrupted sleep, and poor nutrition.

Multiple stressors in the young adult years can alter eating patterns, interrupt sleep, and lead to depression.

During adolescence, the individual had an opportunity to develop strategies for handling disappointments, frustrations, and crises. These coping mechanisms will be challenged and expanded during the young adult years, as the individual assumes more responsibility for choices and actions.

Coping strategies will be challenged and expanded during the adult years.

The way an individual handles stress during the young adult years can influence future life experiences. At times, substance abuse increases in an attempt to relieve physical and emotional responses to stress. When needed, appropriate referral for counseling can be made by the nurse. However, with a little discussion, some introspection, and some distance from the situation the client can be helped to employ personal resources to manage a situation. The most important factor is knowing when coping mechanisms are becoming ineffective and utilizing resources appropriately.

Substance abuse can increase in the young adult's attempts to cope with the effects of stress.

Questions presented in Chap. 3 will be appropriate to use when discussing this pattern area. Issues unique to the individual (e.g., stress of marriage, of parenting, etc.) can be explored in greater depth as the need arises.

Refer to discussion in Chap. 3, under coping patterns and stress tolerance.

Review of Body Components

Review of body systems of the young adult is similar to the review presented in Chap. 3. The reader is referred to that discussion at this time.

Recording the Health History Data

Data collected about each young adult is recorded in a manner similar to that presented in Chap. 3.

REFERENCES

1. F. Merrill Elias, Penelope Kelley Elias, and Jeffery W. Elias, *Basic Processes in Adult Developmental Psychology,* St. Louis, C. V. Mosby Co., 1977, p. vii.

2. D. B. Bromley, *The Psychology of Human Aging,* Baltimore, Penguin, 1966.

3. E. B. Hurlock, *Developmental Psychology,* 3d ed., New York, McGraw-Hill, 1968.

4. M. Lucille Kinlein, *Independent Nursing Practice With Clients,* Philadelphia, J. B. Lippincott, 1977, p. 52.

5. Suzanne Brodnax, "The Health of Young Adults in the Counterculture," *Nurs Clinics North Amer* 8:15–23 (March 1973).

6. Daniel Yankelovich, *The New Morality: A Profile of American Youth in the 1970s,* New York, McGraw-Hill, 1974, p. 29.

7. P. Daniel and M. Lachman, "The Prime of Life" in Rebelsky (ed.), *Life: The Continuous Process,* New York, Knopf, 1975.

8. E. Berscheid, E. Walster, and G. Buhrnstedt, "The Happy American Body: A Survey Report," *Psychology Today,* **7**(6):119–131.

9. C. Binder, "The Course of Human Life as a Psychological Problem" in W. R. Looft (ed.), *Developmental Psychology, A Book of Readings,* Hinsdale, Ill., Dryden, 1972, pp. 68–84.

10. Brodnax, "The Health of Young Adults. . .," pp. 18–19.

11. J. E. Birren, *The Psychology of Aging,* Englewood Cliffs, N.J., Prentice-Hall, 1964.

12. Kay Corman Kintzell, *Advanced Concepts in Clinical Nursing,* 2d ed., Philadelphia, J. B. Lippincott, 1977, p. 110.

13. Ibid., p. 110.

14. Marie Foster Branch and Phyliss Perry Paxton (eds.), *Providing Safe Nursing Care for Ethnic People of Color,* New York, Appleton-Century-Crofts, 1976, p. 159.

15. D. Jones *et al., Medical-Surgical Nursing: A Conceptual Approach,* New York, McGraw-Hill, 1982, p. 64.

16. Douglas H. Heath, *Explorations of Maturity: Studies of Mature and Immature College Men,* New York, Appleton-Century-Crofts, 1965.

17. Justin Pikunas, *Human Development: A Science of Growth,* New York, McGraw-Hill, 1969, chap. 19.

18. J. E. Birren, *Psychology of Aging.*

19. Eric Erickson, *Dimensions of a New Identity,* New York, Norton, 1974, p. 129.

20. Barbara M. Neuman and Phillip R. Neuman, *Development Through Life,* Homewood, Ill., Dorsey Press, 1975, p. 273.

21. Nathaniel Kleitman, *Sleep Wakefulness,* (rev. ed.), Chicago, University of Chicago Press, 1963.

22. B. L. Neugarten, "Adult Personality: Towards a Psychology of Life Cycle" in B. L. Neugarten (ed.), *Middle Age and Aging: A Reader in Social Psychology,* Chicago, University of Chicago Press, 1968, pp. 137–147.

23. Lillian E. Troll, *Early and Middle Adulthood—The Best is Yet to Be—Maybe,* Monterey, Calif., Brooks/Cole Publishing Co., 1975, p. 81.

24. H. Carter and P. C. Glick, *Marriage and Divorce: A Social and Economic Study,* Cambridge, Mass., Harvard University Press, 1970.

25. B. R. Cutter and W. G. Dyer, "Initial Adjustment Processes in Young Married Couples," *Social Forces* **44**:195–201 (1965).

26. Jessie Bernard, *The Future of Marriage,* New York, World (Bantam Press), 1973.

27. R. G. Tharp, "Psychological Partnering in Marriage," *Psychological Bulletin* **60**(2):91–117 (1963).

28. Ibid.

29. J. Veroff and S. Feld, *Marriage and Work in America,* New York, Van Nostrand Reinhold, 1970.

30. R. B. Murray and J. P. Zentner, *Nursing Assessment and Health Promotion Through The Life Span,* 2d ed., Englewood Cliffs, N.J., Prentice-Hall, 1979, p. 283.

31. Troll, *Early and Middle Adulthood,* p. 93.

32. Murray and Zentner, *Nursing Assessment,* p. 308.

33. Ibid., p. 308.

34. O. Brim, "Adult Socialization" in J. Clousen (ed.), *Socialization and Society,* Boston, Little, Brown, 1968.

35. H. A. Lopata, *Occupation: Housewife,* London, Oxford University Press, 1971.

36. V. DeLissovay, "High School Marriage—A Longitudinal Study," *Marriage and Family* 35:245–255 (1973).

37. J. Crites, *Vocational Psychology,* New York, McGraw-Hill, 1969.

38. R. Quinn, G. Staines, and M. McCullough, *Job Satisfaction: Is There A Trend?,* U. S. Department of Labor, Manpower Research Monograph No. 30, Washington, D.C., U. S. Government Printing Office, 1977.

39. Troll, *Early and Middle Adulthood,* p. 115.

40. Yankelovich, *New Morality,* p. 37.

41. Carroll E. Kennedy, *Human Development: The Adult Years and Aging,* New York, Macmillan Company, 1978, p. 210.

42. K. Keniston, "Youth: A New Stage of Life," *American Scholar,* autumn 1970, pp. 631–654.

43. Murray and Zentner, *Nursing Assessment,* p. 294.

44. Pikunas, *Human Development.*

45. Jones *et al., Medical-Surgical Nursing,* p. 64.

46. Troll, *Early and Middle Adulthood,* p. 31.

47. J. Botivinick, Learning "Children and Older Adults" in L. R. Gaull and P. B. Bates (eds.), *Life Span Developmental Psychology,* New York, Academic, 1970, pp. 258–284.

48. E. E. Ghiselli, "The Relationship Between Intelligence and Age Among Superior Adults," *J Genetic Psych* 90:131–142 (1957).

49. J. Kangas and K. Bradway, "Intelligence at Middle Age: A 38 Year Follow-Up," *Developmental Psychology* 5:333–337 (1971).

50. M. P. Honzik and J. W. Macfarlane, "Personality Development and Intellectual Functioning From 21 Months to 40 Years," paper presented at the American Psychological Association Symposium on Maintenance of Intellectual Functioning With Advancing Years, Miami Beach, Fla., 1970.

51. W. Shaie, G. Laborivie, and B. Buesch, "Generational and Cohort—Specific Differences in Adult Cognitive Functioning," 9(2):151–166 (1973).

52. R. R. Bell and J. B. Chaskes, "Premarital Sex Experience among Coeds 1958 and 1968," *J Marriage and Family* 32:81–84 (1970).

53. E. J. Kanin, "Premarital Sex Adjustments, Social Class and Associated Behaviors," *Marriage and Family Living* 22:258–262 (1960).

54. I. L. Reiss, "The Sexual Renaissance: A Summary and Analysis," *J Soc Issues* 22:123–137 (1966).

55. Alan Cranston, cited in J. B. Gerald, "In Praise of Wounded Men," *Harper's* 242:98–103 (April 1971).

56. Jones, *Medical-Surgical Nursing,* p. 65.

BIBLIOGRAPHY

Bischof, Ledford J.: *Adult Psychology,* 2d ed., New York, Harper & Row, 1976.

Brackbill, Y. (ed.): *Division of Developmental Psychology* (Division 7) *Newsletter,* Winter 1971.

Branch, Marie Foster and Phyliss Perry Paxton (eds.): *Providing Safe Nursing Care for Ethnic People of Color,* New York, Appleton-Century-Crofts, 1976.

Compton, Carol Yauk: "War Injury: Identity Crisis for Young Men," *Nurs Clin of North Amer* 8:53–66 (March 1973).

Elias, Merrill F., Penelope Kelly Elias, and Jeffrey W. Elias: *Basic Processes in Adult Developmental Psychology,* St. Louis, C. V. Mosby Co., 1977.

Goldberg, Stella R. and Francine Deutsch: *Life Span—Individual and Family Development,* Monterey, Calif., Brooks/Cole Publishing Co., 1977.

Hehler, Bill: "Wellness Promotion and Risk Reduction on University Campus," in Donna Aguilla (ed.), *Family and Community Health, J Health Promotion and Maintenance,* 3:1 (May 1980), p. 25.

Hurlock, Elizabeth B.: *Developmental Psychology: A Life Span Approach,* 5th ed., New York, McGraw-Hill Book Co., 1980.

Lugo, James O. and Gerald L. Hershey: *Human Development,* Macmillan, 1974.

Pederson, Paul and Walter J. Lonner (eds.): *Counseling Across Cultures,* Honolulu, The University Press of Hawaii, 1976.

"Post-traumatic Stress Disorder in Vietnam Veterans," series, *AJN,* **82**:1694–1704 (1982).

Schell, Robert E. (ed.): *Developmental Psychology Today,* 2d ed., New York, Random House, 1975.

Schlossberg, Nancy K. and Alan D. Entine (eds.): *Counseling Adults,* Monterey, Calif., Brooks/Cole Publishing Co., 1977.

Schlossberg, Nancy K. *et al.: Perspectives on Counseling Adults,* Monterey, Calif., Brooks/Cole Publishing Co., 1978.

Schuster, Clara Shaw and Shirley Smith Ashburn: *The Process of Human Development,* Little, Brown and Co., 1980.

Sexsmith, Donna G.: "Stressors in Early Adulthood," in Donna Aguilla (ed.), *Family and Community Health, J Health Promotion and Maintenance,* **2**:4 (Feb. 1980), pp. 43–52.

Troll, Lillian: *Early & Middle Adulthood—The Best is Yet to Be—Maybe,* Monterey, Calif., Brooks/Cole Publishing Co., 1975.

Maureen Jane Guarino McRae and Mary Kolassa Lepley

INTRODUCTION

In the United States another baby begins its development about every three
seconds. Each second ticked off by a watch represents an average of 3¾
babies conceived around the world. A day of a child's birth is shared by
16,000 other American babies. Three and a half million of them are born
each year, out of four and a quarter million pregnancies [82 percent suc-
cess].[1]

According to the National Center for Health Statistics, U.S. Department of Health, Education, and Welfare, the number of births in the
United States rose in 1977. The birth rate rose from 14.8 births per 1000
population in 1976 to 15.3 in 1977. Birth statistics for the first half of
1978, 1,595,000 live births, were lower than comparable data for 1977,
1,610,000. However, the estimated number of births for 1978 was
3,298,000, again a rate of 15.2 per 1000 population.[2]

Statistics such as these focus attention on the magnitude of nursing
responsibility for the pregnant female.

Expectations of this responsibility are explicit in standards of maternal child nursing practice.

Maternal and Child Health Nursing Practice is based upon knowledge of the
biophysical development of individuals from conception through the child-
rearing phase of development and upon knowledge of the basic needs for
optimum development.[3]

Present-day maternity care demands that the nurse be equipped
with the academic and clinical expertise required to assess, plan, intervene, and evaluate the client via the nursing process.

The holistic approach further demands an understanding of and an
appreciation for the inseparable relationship of the "soma" and the "psy-
che." As it relates to the pregnant female, this approach necessitates
knowledge of the biological, social, cultural, and environmental variables
that influence the pregnant female's concept of "wellness."

An appreciation of the various factors that influence the childbearing experience must be incorporated into the assessment of each individual pregnant woman.

The nurse's role in caring for the pregnant female has been influenced by many factors. These include the trend toward a more "natural"
approach toward childbearing, the home birth options, the nurse midwife's growing acceptance and recent legalization in many states in this
country, the education of nurses as "practitioners" and "clinical specialists" prepared for primary health care delivery, the accessibility of family
planning services and contraceptive counseling, the legalization and
availability of abortion services, and most important, the education of the
consumer and her expectations of health care.

While the holistic approach to the pregnant female is fascinating and
challenging, it requires a high level of nursing knowledge.

The pregnant female represents a
large portion of the clients seen in
the health care system.

The natural and physical sciences provide information that acts as the rationale for care of a biologic nature and as such forms a critical basis for the selection and practice of much of maternity care, the behavioral sciences provide knowledge basic to understanding the *Holistic* [emphasis added] and dynamic nature of maternity nursing, the cultural and social context of patient-nurse interactions, and the psychologic responses of both to the reproductive process.[4]

Highlights

Many recent changes in society and in health care delivery have impacted on the role of the nurse.

In order for the nurse to perform a holistic assessment she must appreciate the individuality of each woman.

The initial prenatal assessment consists of the following:

1 The health history

2 The physical examination

3 Diagnostic tests

THE HEALTH HISTORY

In gathering health history data from the pregnant female the nurse must realize that pregnancy affects virtually every organ system in the female. The information must be carefully gathered and succinctly recorded. It must include an assessment of the many factors that may potentially alter, deter, or enhance the progress and the outcome of pregnancy. These factors include physiological and behavioral variables, as well as extrinsic influences in the woman's environment. For example, a history of compromised cardiac status prior to pregnancy is a physiological factor that may potentially influence the prenatal course; ambivalence and depression are behavioral factors that exert an influence over the prenatal period; and cultural belief and behavior are extrinsic factors that must be considered in health teaching.

The nurse is the ideal person to assess the physiological and emotional components of pregnancy.

While a complete and concise health history early in pregnancy provides basic information for assessment and intervention, it must be ongoing throughout the prenatal course as body responses to the stress of pregnancy occur.

Approach

Although the nurse may be knowledgeable regarding the concerns that commonly are expressed by the pregnant female, each woman must be allowed to express her perception of how this pregnancy may influence her as a unique person.

The nurse should possess interviewing skills which will facilitate the woman's participation rather than the nurse's oratory. Leading phrases and open-ended questions will facilitate this flow of communication. See Table 12-1.

The nurse must be aware that no two pregnancies are alike, and that even a second or third pregnancy in the same woman may evoke different feelings and concerns than previous pregnancies. So many factors surround a pregnancy that each one is assessed on an individual basis with empathy and understanding.

For example, while some women perceive pregnancy as a healthy, happy condition, there are others who may describe the physical alterations in their bodies as troublesome, unexplainable, and worrisome. Still others may see the altered behavioral and emotional changes as frustrating and disconcerting. The nurse must be aware that there is a wide range of normal responses, and no two women will present the health care provider with an identical range of needs and concerns.

Table 12-1
Sample Questions When Interviewing

Incorrect	Correct
Have you been feeling well during the pregnancy?	Tell me how you have been feeling since you found out that you were pregnant.
Are other people in the family happy that you are pregnant?	What is the reaction of family members to this pregnancy?
Have you had any nausea or vomiting?	How does it feel to be pregnant?
Will you have help at home after you deliver?	What kind of help will you have at home after you deliver?
Are other members of the family excited about this pregnancy?	What does this pregnancy mean to other family members?

Setting the climate for a comfortable, empathetic, sincere, and trusting relationship may promote a significant series of prenatal visits which allow for interaction, education, understanding, and growth.

The Interview

A thorough health history, psychosocial history, and physical exam early in pregnancy provide the foundation for successful assessment, intervention, education, and evaluation of the many factors that may be active during the prenatal period and will continue long after delivery. Good antenatal care is preventive care.

See Chap. 3 for a discussion of the interview.

The information gathered in the interview should be recorded so that it is readily accessible to all health care providers who will come in contact with the woman during her pregnancy. Depending on the health care system, the prenatal course could include many providers. In private practice, the woman may be seen by only her primary physician and the nurse. In a clinic facility or in a large teaching hospital, she may see many health professionals. If it is indicated, she may also meet the nutritionist, the social worker, and a number of others. The written record is essential for optimum continuity of care, as well as for assurance that services are not duplicated. Data should be recorded completely and concisely, as this record will follow the woman into the labor and delivery and postpartum experience, and therefore can provide valuable information to another series of health providers.

The pregnant female may be seen by various health care providers in different settings.

Client Profile and Biographical Data

The client profile should be concise and should be recorded in such a way that the health providers have a sense of the client, her physical and emotional status, her environment, and reason for entering the health care system. If the woman is of a different (foreign) ethnic origin or if there is a language barrier, this should be documented in the profile. In addition to information outlined in Chap. 3, the nurse must include gravida, parity, history of abortions (spontaneous or induced), date of LMP (last menstrual period), weeks of gestation by dates, and the client's perception of her pregnant status.

See Chap. 3 for a discussion of how to collect biographical data.

Questions to elicit data:

What made you first think you were pregnant?

When were you sure that you were pregnant?

Did you perform your own pregnancy test at home?

It is important to obtain information relative to marital status and occupation. The marital status may alert the nurse to the need for supports, as well as to the attitude toward the pregnancy. Information concerning the client's occupation may be helpful in interpreting symptoms due to fatigue, environmental hazards, or occupational tensions.

Health Status Perception

Ideally prenatal care should begin as soon as the woman suspects she is pregnant, however there may be clients who enter the system earlier or later than optimal for diagnosis and evaluation.

Clients may enter the health care system early or late in their pregnancy.

While a very early entry may represent anxiety, excitement, or concern, it may also indicate the need for educating the client about her reproductive functioning. On the other hand, a woman who comes for prenatal care late in pregnancy may be indicating the following:

Various attitudes, feelings or beliefs may be reflected in the client's timing of her entry into the health care system.

1 Early ambivalence regarding pregnancy
2 Ignorance regarding the significance of amenorrhea
3 Lack of knowledge regarding her own reproductive functioning
4 Lack of understanding of the importance of health care and assessment during pregnancy
5 Cultural attitudes
6 Lack of information regarding availability of appropriate health care systems.

While the reason for entry into the health care system is usually obvious in the pregnant female, the time of entry must be assessed.

Perception of Pregnancy

The nurse must also assess the client's perception of the pregnancy including alterations in the emotional or behavioral feelings of the woman.

See Behavioral Development for additional information.

Questions to elicit data:

How did you feel when pregnancy was confirmed?

How do you feel now about being pregnant?

Further, the nurse must assess the client's perception of how this pregnancy may alter her lifestyle, self-image, femininity, sexuality, career goals, economic status, and family and social relationships. The nurse may ask, "Will this pregnancy affect your career?"

Clients perceive their pregnancies according to their own personal life situation.

A teenage girl, single and deserted by the father of her child, who is developmentally stressed may expect that the pregnancy will make up for the loss of a loved one or will prove her independence in her capacity to reproduce. The 34-year-old mother of four who is economically stressed may expect that her pregnancy will add increased financial burdens to her family. The nurse should obtain information regarding these alterations.

Questions to elicit data:

Have there been any changes in your life since you discovered you were pregnant?

How do you think this pregnancy will affect your family?

A woman who has planned her pregnancy after the achievement of her educational goals and at a time when she would financially be able to provide for a new family member may see her pregnancy as a significant event in her accomplishment of individual and family goals.

Current Health Status and Health Habits

Since pregnancy causes alterations in virtually every organ system of the body, the current health status provides information which may influence the maternal physiological response to the added stress of pregnancy.

For example, a woman whose physical or psychological health is already compromised by a condition such as diabetes or a history of depression will respond differently to the added stress of pregnancy than will the woman who is in optimal health. The diabetic woman may find that pregnancy alters her well-established insulin schedule. A woman with a history of depression may find that her condition is exacerbated by the feelings of fatigue that accompany early gestation.

The nurse must also include information regarding the use of medication which may be taken for physical or emotional health conditions, since drugs such as aspirin and the antidepressants have been shown to have teratogenic effects.

The nurse should include the following information about the present pregnancy:

Client's age

Gravida and para

Spontaneous abortion

Induced abortion

Last Menstrual Period (LMP)

Weeks of gestation by dates

Weeks of gestation by uterine size

Client's physical and emotional perceptions

This information will provide the necessary history to assess the progress of fetal growth and will give some indication of the outcome that can be anticipated during this pregnancy based on past obstetrical history.

For example, a woman with a history of repeated spontaneous abortions is at risk for repeated problems with abortion. A present pregnancy may arouse emotions from past history if a previous pregnancy ended in demise. Since an induced abortion in the past may have been related to physical, social, emotional, or economic issues, any history of abortion should be explored with the woman.

The nurse should also include information such as the following that may indicate pathology, and will alert health care providers to the need for further evaluation of the status of the pregnancy:

Gastrointestinal symptoms

Headaches and dizziness

Edema

Pain

Urinary tract symptoms

Bleeding

Fatigue

Immunizations

Medications

Allergies

For example, a negative rubella titer in a woman indicates that she has no immunity against rubella. This should be included in the immunization history.

The nurse should question the woman about the use of tobacco, alcohol, and drugs, since education and intervention may be necessary, based on our present knowledge regarding the noxious potential of these factors.

See Physical Examination for normal changes of pregnancy.

Pregnancy, for many women, represents the only time that they present for formal health care. Women are "tuned-in" to their bodies during pregnancy, and may be most receptive to womens' health issues at this time. Therefore it is a fruitful time for health teaching, and the nurse should use this opportunity to the fullest. The nurse should determine if the client has Pap smears between pregnancies, and if she does not, the nurse should try to assess the reason for this health habit. Also it is important to know if the client practices self-breast examination.

See Chap. 3 when assessing the past health status.

Past Health Status

The nurse should include in the past health history the client's health history, previous hospitalizations, menstrual history, and obstetrical history.

The health history will alert the nurse to conditions that may affect the pregnancy or conditions that may be exacerbated by the pregnancy.

A woman who is taking medication for a medical condition may need counseling as to the potential noxious affects of her medication. A woman who became pregnant while using oral contraceptives may be at risk for fetal abnormalities. A woman with a history of hypertension, heart disease, or urinary disease may need to be observed for complications of pregnancy secondary to these physical conditions.

The nurse should include the following in the past history:

Heart disease

Urinary disease

Hypertension

Rheumatic fever

Asthma

Tuberculosis

Venereal diseases

Diabetes

Varicose veins

Thyroid dysfunctions

Epilepsy

Allergies

Blood dyscrasia

Blood transfusions

Gallbladder disease

Endocrine disturbances

All body components are stressed during pregnancy. The past history provides a baseline for assessment.

Previous Hospitalizations The nurse should list with dates all operations and serious injuries, particularly injuries to the pelvis, urinary tract, bowel, or abdominal wall. Because of the anatomical relationship of these structures to the reproductive organs, damage or weakness in any of these body components may alter or impede the normal course of pregnancy in childbirth.

Menstrual History The nurse should include the following in the menstrual history:

Age at menarche

Average interval between periods

Duration and amount of flow

Thoroughness in collecting data about the menstrual history is essential when assessing the pregnant female.

Pain in relation to flow

Date of onset and character of LMP

Date of previous menstrual period

Date of quickening in relation to LMP

Expected date of confinement (EDC)

Menstrual disorders

Contraceptive methods

The nurse should also ascertain whether the woman had increased nervousness or depression around the time of her period. This information may help to anticipate emotional fluctuations in response to pregnancy, since both are directly related to hormonal alterations in the female. Further, the history should include whether the woman had any difficulty becoming pregnant.

Use of contraceptive methods prior to pregnancy or at the time the pregnancy occurred must be included, since these may have a significant influence on the calculation of gestational age. Some contraceptive methods alter the menstrual cycle and the time of ovulation.

The date of the last normal menstrual period is needed. Since quasi-period, painless bleeding can occur during pregnancy, the EDC must be determined by the last normal menstrual period rather than the last sign or episode of bleeding.

The menstrual cycle and pregnancy are influenced by hormones.

Obstetrical For each previous pregnancy, whether completed successfully or not, the nurse should record the following information:

Past reproductive history will provide clues to the areas of concern to be addressed during the present pregnancy.

1 Date (month and year of termination)

2 Complications of pregnancy

3 Labor
   a Spontaneous or induced—reason for induction
   b Duration of each pregnancy in comparison with its EDC—the presence of a pattern of early or late delivery
   c Length of labor—length of "strong labor" or occurrence of brief or precipitate labors

4 Delivery
   a Method
      (1) Vaginal or cesarean
      (2) Vertex or breech presentation
      (3) Spontaneous or assisted—forceps or version
   b Anesthesia—type used if any
   c Complications of previous deliveries
   d Patient's perception of previous deliveries

5 Previous children at birth
   a Birth weight
   b Condition—Developmental or congenital anomolies
   c Sex-linked disorders

See Heredity for further discussion of sex-linked disorders.

6 Breast-feeding
   a Success or failure and duration with previous children
   b Woman's perception of success or failure

7 Present health of other children

Past reproductive history will provide clues to the areas of concern to be addressed during the present pregnancy. The birth weight of previous children is important for determining a weight pattern, the maturity of the newborn, and possible maternal disease such as diabetes. The presence of sex-linked disorders in previous children raises the possibility of their presence in the expected infant if the infant is the same sex. For example, hemophilia, which is a hereditary hemorrhagic diatheses due to deficiency of the coagulation factor VIII, affects males and is transmitted as an X-linked recessive trait. A stillbirth or death of a previous child under the age of 1 is significant obstetrically.

Family History

It is important for the nurse to be aware of diseases in which heredity may be a contributing factor, such as diabetes mellitus. The nurse should include in the family history:

> Heart disease
> Diabetes
> Multiple pregnancies
> Epilepsy
> Congenital abnormalities
> High blood pressure
> Bleeding disorders
> Emotional problems

The presence of any familial or inherited disorders should be noted. Table 3-3 and Fig. 3-2 can be used to elicit family history data.

Life Patterns and Life Styles

Age

Age is a very significant factor when discussing the pregnant female. The reproductive capacity of a woman runs on a biological clock, and the pregnant female represents a woman whose biological clock is still ticking. On the other hand, a woman may develop heart disease at any age, malignancy has no respect for age, and many clients who enter the health care system for specific disease or illness represent a variety of age groups.

The capacity to reproduce is present in women between puberty and menopause, a period spanning approximately 30 years of a woman's life. If puberty at ages 10 to 16 and menopause at ages 45 to 55 represent the parameters of reproductive capacity, the female may become pregnant for perhaps a very limited period of her entire life span. The age of the father does not affect reproductive functioning, since males maintain reproductive capacity sometimes beyond age 70.

The importance of assessing this factor in the health history is the following:

1 Extremes of age place women in a "high risk" category.
2 The perception of the pregnancy as the woman relates it to her age is important.

The very young are at high risk, since they may not be nutritionally ready (as in the adolescent on food fads) and they are still developing physically and emotionally. At the other extreme, the incidence of Downs syndrome increases 100-fold in women 45 years and older. A woman who feels the need to get pregnant before age 30 for fear of growing "too old" has a real concern for running out of reproductive capacity.

The nurse needs to facilitate the expression of any concerns related to age.

Questions to elicit data:

How does it feel to be pregnant?

How will this pregnancy change your life?

As previously discussed, no matter what the age at which a woman conceives, the pregnancy is always superimposed on the developmental tasks peculiar to that age.

See Behavioral Development for additional information.

Race

As discussed previously, race may influence the outcome of pregnancy in that some diseases are more common among persons of certain races or national origins than in the general population. Sickle-cell disease is one such inherited disease in black Americans, Tay-Sachs disease in Jews of eastern European origin, Thalasemia in Asians and southern Europeans, and cystic fibrosis in whites.[5]

Heredity

Heredity is a very significant factor in assessing the pregnant client. The pregnant female must be seen as a member of a family that itself may have a history of hereditary traits such as hypertension or hereditary anomalies. Both the father and the mother contribute their own heredity to the fetus.

Hereditary defects include changes in chromosome number, structural anomalies in chromosomes, and gene mutation.

Hemophilia and color blindness are examples of sex-linked traits in men. Turners syndrome and Downs syndrome are chromosomal defects. Sickle-cell disease is caused by a mutant gene. Tay-Sachs disease and phenylketonuria (PKU) are inherited enzyme deficiencies. Cystic fibrosis is an inherited metabolic disorder.

Although chromosomal defects can be diagnosed prenatally, others such as PKU can only be diagnosed after birth.

The nurse needs to be aware of the potential for hereditary disorders by carefully obtaining and recording information in past health history, family history, and past obstetrical and neonatal history, keeping in mind that race is another important factor in disorders of heredity. Pregnancy is probably the most important time for the nurse to thoroughly investigate this factor, since heredity implies transmission of a trait to an offspring—something which can occur only by reproduction.

Culture

In gathering information about the pregnant female, the nurse needs to realize that language, tradition, religion, and the ethnic origin of the client all exert an influence over one's perception of health and illness. In addition, culture dictates childbearing and child-rearing practices.

Culture dictates childbearing and child-rearing practices.

In our present-day society, the concern with overpopulation, as well as religious beliefs, also must be considered as having an influence on reproductive functioning. Religious beliefs that frown on artificial methods of contraception will affect the client's perception of health teaching. That is, if the client believes in religious teachings, then the nurse must respect these and should provide education and health teaching that are consistent with these beliefs.

Language is another cultural variable that the nurse must respond to.

In order to work with the culturally different, one must reach out, be sensitive to his differences, and understand his reticence in accepting new and foreign ideas. What may be good for the majority may not necessarily be good for all.[6]

Although trends in childbirth have been influenced by a modern trend toward a more natural experience, studies document that women of different cultures deliver their children in hospitals. American Indians, while having traditional religious and ceremonial practices for childbearing, have 99 out of 100 of their women deliver their children in a hospital.[7]

The nurse must be aware that what is perceived as a deviation from the "normal" pattern of behavior in a client may represent a very comfortable milieu for a pregnant woman of a different culture.

> Noncompliance by the pregnant woman may result from the nurse's inability to assess cultural attitudes and beliefs.

Some Chinese women, for example, refuse to take iron supplements during pregnancy, fearful that iron will harden bones and make delivery difficult.[8] While maintaining respect for these beliefs, the nurse could suggest a diet high in iron. In doing so the nurse not only recognizes the need for maintaining respect for individual beliefs but also at the same time promotes acceptable ways to include optimal health care during pregnancy.

A combination of a high-calorie diet and lack of exercise added to the cultural preference of American Indian men for heavy women, can all add up to produce grossly overweight females.[9] During the prenatal period these cultural patterns may make nutritional needs and weight gain in the American Indian woman a real concern for the nurse.

Another example of the influence of culture on the pregnant female and her comfort with the health care system is the Puerto Rican woman. In her culture, excessive modesty and submissiveness to males are cultural patterns which may influence the woman's use of the health care team.[10] A female health care provider may be needed for the physical assessment of this client in order to provide an atmosphere which is conducive to her cultural beliefs.

> Culture will influence the outcome of pregnancy for many clients.

These are but a few examples of the influence of culture on the pregnant female's acceptance of the health care system. There is no excuse for ignoring this influence, since it exerts a profound effect on the outcome of pregnancy. The nurse must be sensitive to this factor and respond in ways that will promote the client's acceptance of health teaching.

Growth and Development

The physical, cognitive, social, and emotional capabilities of the pregnant female should be assessed by the nurse. The level of growth and development attained by the woman in each of these areas will reflect on her childbearing and child-rearing abilities and practices.

Currently, there are no developmental assessment tools to assist the nurse in this evaluation of the pregnant female. Therefore, the nurse must try to elicit information that will be pertinent to pregnancy and to the client's potential for mothering by exploring individual capabilities.

The discussion of growth and development, and questions used to elicit this data included in Chap. 3 should be used by the nurse when assessing the client. The client's emotional capabilities can be explored by asking the following questions.

Questions to elicit data:

Do you feel that you are emotionally ready for this baby?

How do you think you will be able to cope with the demands of a new baby?

Do crying babies bother you?

Have you ever cared for small babies or children?

Do you associate with other pregnant women?

What have you done to prepare yourself for labor and delivery and the new baby?

Do you think that your own parents did a good job in raising you? How would you have wanted to change their parenting practices?

Does the father of this baby share your ideas about childbearing and child-rearing?

The nurse should keep in mind that pregnancy is a maturational crisis which may alter, interfere with, or enhance the already existing psychological status of the woman. Answers to the above questions will assist the nurse in determining the client's emotional sense of well-being.

See Pregnancy as a Developmental Task for further discussion of growth and development during pregnancy.

Behavioral Development

A knowledge and understanding of the principles and normal ranges of human growth, development, and behavior are essential to Maternal and Child Health Nursing Practice. Concomitant with this knowledge is the recognition and consideration of the psychosocial, environmental, nutritional, spiritual and cognitive factors that enhance or deter the biophysical and psychological maturation of the individual and his family. [American Nurses Association Standard II Rationale][11]

Behavioral changes during pregnancy not only are normal but also are predictable.

The holistic health assessment of the pregnant female is mandated by standards of maternal and child health nursing practice. Inherent in an understanding of the behavioral components that may accompany the biological, physiological, and endocrine alterations of pregnancy is the ability to identify the "normal" course of events to which the pregnant female is most susceptible.

It is apparent that our rapidly changing society and increased mobility often destroy the intimacy and socialization afforded by the extended family. The ever-present economic flux, the women's movement, and the increasing single parent population have impacted on both the pregnant female and her offspring.

There are however predictable behavioral changes that have long been identified as characteristic of the pregnant female.

Behavioral Components of Pregnancy

Pregnancy is a time of changing feelings, of sensitivity, and of increased susceptibility to any crisis, and moreover there are characteristic changes in early, middle, and late pregnancy.[12]

See Table 12-2 for the physical and behavioral changes of pregnancy.

The physical and behavioral changes of pregnancy are listed in Table 12-2.

Early Pregnancy (First Trimester) "The first trimester is characterized by ambivalence, no matter how planned and desired the conception was."[13] The need to mother and the wish to be mothered are feelings which women often experience, as well as the wish to be taken care of and the reassurance of the love and care of the person close to her.

Feelings of ambivalence characterize the first trimester of pregnancy.

Physical symptoms common to the first trimester of pregnancy cause uncertainty and instability. Amenorrhea is the only evidence of a situational change in early pregnancy. Symptoms such as breast changes, gastric awareness (nausea and vomiting), urinary frequency, and amenorrhea lie only in the realm of presumptive signs of pregnancy, and nothing

Table 12-2
Physical and Behavioral Changes of Pregnancy

Physical changes	Behavioral changes
First trimester	
Amenorrhea	Uncertainty
Breast changes	Ambivalence
Fatigue	Instability
Urinary frequency	The questions "Now?" and "Who Me?"
Gastric awareness	Need for reassurance and love
Second trimester	
"Quickening"	The question "Now?"
Braxton Hicks contractions	Sense of well-being
Pregnancy beginning to "show"	Increased dependency
	Desire to be passive and alone
	Revision and reassessment of plans
	Pregnancy a reality
	Image of child primary focus
Third trimester	
Increased Braxton Hicks contractions	Fantasy, introjection, and projection used to establish role as mother
Increased bulk and displacement after "lightening"	Anxiety about labor and delivery
Urinary frequency	Concern with EDC
Fatigue	Feelings of vulnerability to damage or loss
Constipation from decreased motility of GI tract	Protectiveness toward infant
Fatigue	Increased need for seclusion
Thoracic breathing before lightening	Concern with health and sex of infant

demonstrable can be seen, heard, or felt. A lack of criteria to test reality leads to the feelings which Reva Rubin describes as "cognitive style" for early pregnancy.[14]

Rubin has written that for the greater majority of women who become pregnant, whether for the first or subsequent pregnancy, the issue to work on during the first 3 to 4 months is the question "Now?".

The questions "Now?" and "Who, me?" are dominant stimuli for behavior in the early stage, or first trimester, of pregnancy. They recede to quiescence during the middle stage, or second trimester, and become dominant again in the last stage, or third trimester.

Middle Pregnancy (Second Trimester) The physical signs of the second trimester include perceptible Braxton Hicks contractions, feeling of fetal life or movement, and changes in the female contour. The woman begins to "show" that she is pregnant.

"Quickening" ushers a sense of well-being related to the reality of the pregnancy. Late in the second trimester there is an increased dependency, passivity, and desire to be alone. These feelings peak in the third trimester and last until after birth.

During this trimester, plans for the household and for careers must be reviewed, reassessed, and adapted to the reality of the pregnancy. The middle stage of pregnancy has as its primary focus the condition of the child. The mother wants a visual image of her child and is concerned with the sex.

Late Pregnancy (Third Trimester) In the third trimester the woman uses *introjection* and *projection* to establish her identity and role as a mother.[15] Awareness of a threat to the mother's existence physically appears to be aroused by anticipation of the oncoming trauma of labor and delivery. For the multigravida, adding a new sibling to the family may be anxiety-provoking.

See Reva Rubin's article "Cognitive Style in Pregnancy"[14] for a discussion of early pregnancy.

Physical signs in the pregnant female during the second trimester make pregnancy a reality.

Introjection and projection are used by the woman during the third trimester.

During this time the woman is concerned with her EDC. She becomes extremely protective of her baby and withdraws to quiet and seclusion.

The seventh month is probably the most difficult, for it is during this time that the woman feels most vulnerable to damage or loss. This explains the need for protectiveness and seclusion.

Near term, increased fear and anxieties surface. There are concerns about motherhood, concerns about changes in family and marital relationships, and concerns about labor. The sex and health of the infant are also foremost in the mind of the woman at this time.

It is these "normal" predictable behavioral changes that the nurse must concentrate on in the behavioral assessment of the pregnant female.

According to Abraham Maslow's theory, when one moves through an anxiety-provoking experience, one achieves growth.[16] To the extent that persons seek to avoid anxiety and responsibility by refusing to avail themselves of their new possibilities and by refusing to move from the familiar to the unfamiliar, they sacrifice their freedom and constrict their autonomy and self-awareness.

Many of the behavioral changes of pregnancy are anxiety-provoking. Nevertheless, pregnancy offers an opportunity for the woman to grow and develop new roles and a new sense of developmental uniqueness. The nurse can enhance this growth by understanding the dynamics of pregnancy and the behaviors that accompany it. On the basis of Maslow's theory, growth in the pregnant female may be fostered by increasing her understanding of the changes occurring in her body and by educating her so that she will become aware of the "normalcy" of these changes.

Growth occurs when the attractions of growth are enhanced and the dangers are minimized.

Maslow's theory[17] can be expressed diagrammatically as follows:

enhance dangers   enhance attractions

SAFETY ————————— GROWTH

minimize attractions   minimize dangers

While the feelings and fears experienced during pregnancy may be intense and varied, the nurse can use Maslow's theory to foster growth in the following ways: Safety is felt in familiar feelings and in a familiar environment; therefore, a woman who is fearful of her changing emotions during pregnancy or a woman who is unsure of the reasons for these altered emotions felt safer in her prepregnant status, and is fearful of the changing feelings. By assessing these individual feelings in the pregnant female and understanding the factors that cause them (physiological and hormonal alterations), the nurse can intervene to enhance the attractions and minimize the dangers in the new status of pregnancy and thus foster growth.

Pregnancy as a Developmental Task

Pregnancy is a developmental task superimposed on a preexisting stage of development.

Pregnancy can be compared to other critical life periods which Erikson calls developmental crises.[18]

Greta Bibring regards pregnancy as:

a step in the development of the individual.[19]

Ringquist notes:

As a crisis, pregnancy is a turning point from being a separate person to becoming a parent for the primigravida and involves solutions not previously required in her life.[20]

Pregnancy is viewed as a developmental milestone similar to puberty, menarche, and menopause. Its manner of resolution deeply affects the emotional maturation of the woman.

The developmental task of pregnancy is superimposed on the preexisting stage of development. For example, the adolescent who is struggling with the conflict of independence vs. dependence discovers she is pregnant. She must confront the need for independence felt from within and yet face the reality that this pregnancy may thrust her back into reliance (dependence) on others (parents) for emotional, financial, and situational support. Thus pregnancy produces not only stress but also further developmental struggles. The altered physical, behavioral, social, and environmental climate produces challenges which must be confronted in order for growth to occur.

Biological Rhythms

An assessment of biological rhythms is a major component in the care of the female client. Understanding these rhythms and the sequelae from alterations or deviations in them helps the nurse appreciate the biological significance of human reproduction. Biological rhythms are used in the assessment, diagnosis, and treatment of clients throughout their reproductive years.

Reproductive capacity runs on a biological clock.

The biological rhythms which affect pregnancy include those cycles which are ever-present in the normal female's reproductive years.

Menstrual Cycle The menstrual cycle is an endogenous cycle occurring in the female. This cycle must function in order for pregnancy to occur. Hormonal deficits that cause alterations in this cycle may also cause complications of pregnancy.

It is important to gather information related to infertility problems and previous spontaneous abortions, which may indicate a deficient luteal phase. A pregnant woman may have a history of infertility even though she is seen after she has achieved a pregnancy. Prenatal management may need to be altered in response to a history of such difficulties.

Temperature Cycle The temperature cycle in a female with a normal menstrual cycle can be used to predict ovulation and conception. The effect of progesterone in the luteal phase of the menstrual cycle (progesterone is only present after ovulation) is to raise the basal body temperature (BBT) by 0.5°F (0.3°C). A prolonged rise in basal temperature is considered in the diagnosis of pregnancy.

Lunar Cycle About 280 days, or 40 weeks, elapse, on the average, between the first day of the last menstrual period and delivery of the infant. Two hundred eighty days correspond to $9\frac{1}{3}$ calendar months, or 10 units of 28 days each. The unit of 28 days has been commonly but imprecisely referred to as a lunar month of pregnancy, since the time from one new moon to the next is actually $29\frac{1}{2}$ days.

The duration of pregnancy is 10 lunar months, 9 calendar months, or 280 days.

Metabolic Rhythms Heart rate, respiration, and blood pressure are all altered in response to pregnancy. For a detailed explanation of the metabolic changes see the physical examination section on maternal physiological changes of pregnancy.

Maturation Pregnancy is a maturational crisis. The nurse's interventions must be based on the degree to which pregnancy alters, interferes with, or enhances the already existing psychological status of the woman.

Environmental Factors

For the pregnant female, the environment includes not only the external physical environment (residence, population density, and pollutants) but also the intrauterine environment. So many factors from the environment contribute to the well-being of mother and fetus that every day research studies add to data supporting the hazards from the surroundings. In addition to the already known noxious potential of drugs, chemicals, and radiation to fetal growth and development, there are recent studies and reports of the dangers of hair sprays, hair dryers, cleaning fluids, and chemicals that are in everyday use by many pregnant women.

In assessing environmental factors, the nurse should be aware of the most updated literature reporting potential dangers to women of childbearing age and should counsel women accordingly.

While there are many factors over which the nurse has no control, such as population density, it should be kept in mind that where population density is a concern, the danger of contacting harmful viruses in the environment increases. The client's immunization history thus becomes a priority at this time.

The development of the fetus is the result of a complex interplay among genetic factors and environmental influences.

> The etiology of birth defects is not completely understood, but it is recognized that most birth defects have an environmental component in their multifactorial etiology. Wilson attributed 5 to 9 percent of developmental defects in man to environmental factors, 25 percent to genetic factors, and over 65 percent to unknown factors.[21]

Past history of congenital defects should alert the nurse to possible problems. The nurse needs to be aware of the potential teratogens (agents which cause damage to the embryo or fetus) in the environment, and through education and counseling the nurse should make an effort to see that the potential noxious factors in the external physical environment do not become part of the intrauterine environment.

The most sensitive time for developmental disturbances is between day 13 and day 60 of gestation, since this is the time of major embryonic differentiation and organogenesis. However, the fetus is susceptible to teratogenic effects throughout gestation. Prenatal diagnosis of some defects can be done with use of amniocentesis. For example, Down's syndrome can be diagnosed by amniocentesis. However, there is no control presently over its occurrence, except to be aware that the potential for Down's Syndrome increases with maternal age.

Causes of human developmental defects include genetic factors, radiation, fetal infections, drugs, and chemical and mechanical factors (see Table 12-3).[22]

> Qualitatively speaking, the placenta does not act as a barrier to noxious materials except under rare circumstances; when we speak of the environment, we refer to the chemical milieu surrounding embryonic cells during the period of organogenesis.[23]

Included in the factors over which the nurse may have some influence through health education of the pregnant female are those environmental agents over which some control is possible.

Viruses Although at the present time there is no control over cytomegalovirus (a virus which causes fetal anomalies), the nurse does have access to a history of contact or immunization for rubella which is the other virus known to cause fetal anomalies.

See Physical Examination for further discussion about fetal development.

Table 12-3
Causes of Human Developmental Defects

Categories	Known causes	Suspected causes
Genetic factors	Changes in chromosome number Structural abnormalities in chromosomes Gene mutation	
Radiation	Therapeutic use of radiation Exposure to nuclear radiation	Diagnostic use of radiation (during early development)
Fetal infections	Rubella virus Cytomegalovirus Herpes virus *Treponema pallidum* (syphilis) *Toxoplasma gondii* Leptospires	Mumps Echovirus Influenza Varicella Vaccinia Coxsackie viruses Hepatitis
Drugs and chemicals	Thalidomide Aminopterin Progestogens, estrogens, androgens Diethylstilbestrol Methylmercury	Steroids (cortisone acetate and those used in pregnancy tests) Methotrexate Some antibiotics (streptomycin, tetracyclines) Antithyroid drugs Barbiturates LSD Marijuana Aspirin Phenytoin Dexamphetamine Excessive vitamins Reserpine Tricyclic antidepressants Nicotine (tobacco)
Mechanical factors	Intrauterine fetal compression	

Source: T. V. N. Persaud and K. L. Moore, "Causes and Prenatal Diagnosis of Congenital Abnormalities," *J Ob Gyn Neon Nur,* 1974. Used by permission.

A rubella titer is a part of every prenatal workup. A titer of < 8 tells the nurse that the woman is not immune to the rubella virus and that she is at risk for grave fetal anomalies if she contacts the virus during early pregnancy.

The incidence of malformation in the fetus if the mother contacts rubella is 50 percent if infection occurs in the first 4 weeks, 40 percent if infection occurs during the second 4 weeks, 30 percent during the third 4 weeks, and 10 to 20 percent between 12 and 16 weeks of gestation. Anomalies in the fetus include microcephaly, mental retardation, corneal clouding, eye lesions, liver malfunction, nephritis, patent ductus arteriosus, cardiac defects, maldeveloped bone growth, and inner ear damage. Rubella is also associated with spontaneous abortion and premature labor. Women who contact rubella during early pregnancy should be counselled and given the opportunity for elective termination of the pregnancy.

Cytomegaloviruses may cause microcephaly, chorioretinitis, cerebral calcification and seizures, progressive anemia, and hepatomegaly. Cytomegalovirus cannot be diagnosed prenatally. Twenty to eighty percent of all pregnant women had exposure to Cytomegalovirus in a 1974 British study.[24]

The viruses of smallpox, herpes simplex, mumps, rubeola, and hepatitis may infect the fetus and cause serious disease or death.

Active vulvovaginal herpes at the time of labor is an indication for cesarean section within 4 hours of ruptured membranes. Hepatitis in the mother may produce a toxic infant who may or may not have hepatitis.

Drugs Prescription drugs and addictive drugs, as well as over-the-counter drugs, may be hazardous to the fetus. Pregnant women must be educated as to the risks involved in taking any medication (prescribed or not) during pregnancy.

Aspirin may interfere with neonatal platelet aggregation.[25]

Since the horrors of thalidomide and more recently the DES (diethylstilbestrol) issue, the nurse should be even more aware that clients must be cautioned about the use of any drug during pregnancy. Thalidomide causes limb defects, absence of ears, deafness, and heart anomalies. Vaginal adenocarcinoma has developed in young women many years after their mothers were given stilbestrol during pregnancy.

Even drugs prescribed for a maternal condition may be teratogenic. The risks and benefits of the following drugs and their teratogenic effects should be explored with the pregnant female:

Antithyroids can cause congenital goiter.

Quinine can cause deafness.

Synthetic vitamin K and sulfonamides can cause hyperbilirubinemia.

Tetracycline can stain fetal bones and deciduous teeth.

Warfarin can cause hemorrhagic disease of the fetus.

In addition to the potential noxious effects of drugs, there is increasing evidence to substantiate the potential hazards of alcohol and smoking during pregnancy on fetal development.

Alcohol In 1973, Jones et al. coined the term *fetal alcohol syndrome* (FAS) after studying the offspring of chronic alcoholic mothers.[26] This study showed that alcohol causes devastating effects in the offspring and that the related growth deficiency is irreversible. Some common abnormalities identified by Jones[27] in his study of infants born to severe chronic alcoholic mothers are listed in Table 12-4.

It is known that alcohol crosses the placenta; it is not known whether it is the alcohol or the breakdown products of the alcohol that cause the damage.

Prior to the identification of this syndrome, health professionals had attributed the learning and developmental problems in children of alcoholics to disruptive homes or poor caretaking. However, the work on FAS suggests that the damage to these children occurs in utero; therefore, the time for prevention is before the fact. Research indicates that physical and mental deficiencies can result in the offspring of alcoholic mothers who drink heavily during pregnancy and that even social drinking may have detrimental effects on the birth weight and behavior of infants.[28]

Furthermore, while studies suggest that structural damage occurs during the first trimester, pilot observations[29] from a 1974 study carried out by Rosett et al. showed that a decrease in alcohol consumption during the third trimester of pregnancy lowers the risk to the offspring, suggesting that "since late gestation is the period when adverse factors have the

Mental and physical deficiencies can result in the offspring of women who consume large amounts of alcohol.

Table 12-4
Abnormalities Associated with Fetal Alcohol Syndrome

Growth and performance abnormalities
    Prenatal growth deficiency
    Postnatal growth deficiency
    Microcephaly
    Developmental delay or mental deficiency

Craniofacial abnormalities
    Short palpebral fissures
    Midfacial hypoplasia
    Epicanthal folds

Limb abnormalities
    Abnormal palmar creases
    Joint anomalies

Other abnormalities
    Cardiac defect
    External genital anomalies
    Hemangiomas
    Ear anomalies

Source: K. Jones and D. Smith, "Recognition of Fetal Alcohol Syndrome in Early Infancy," Lancet, 2:999 (1973). Used by permission.

greatest effect on fetal growth, cessation or marked reduction of alcohol consumption may facilitate growth and functional development."[30]

The Department of Health, Education, and Welfare recommends that women consume no more than 1 ounce of absolute alcohol per day (2 social drinks).[31] The nurse should assess alcohol consumption in women with these recommendations in mind until more research data are available to guide assessments.

Smoking Thirty-three percent of women of childbearing age are smokers.[32] Recent research, however, supports the fact that smoking during pregnancy affects fetal growth. Evidence suggests that maternal smoking interferes in some way with fetal weight gain, and this is thought to be related to the hypoxia caused by carbon monoxide in cigarette smoke.[33]

A study by Murphy et al.[34] showed that when women were controlled for age, parity, socioeconomic status, and length of gestation, there was a significant difference in the birth weight of children born to women who smoked and to women who did not. Comstock et al.[35] claim that decreased birth weight in offspring of women who smoke is directly related to the number of cigarettes smoked by the mother, and Bangai[36] notes that the mean birth weight in infants of mothers who smoke may be 6 to 8 ounces less than that of infants born to nonsmokers.

Further, Butler et al. found that children at ages 7 and 11 years manifest a deficit due to smoking.[37] Those born to mothers who smoked 10 or more cigarettes per day were retarded in reading, mathematics, and general ability as compared to progenies of nonsmokers.

Davies et al. report observations of shorter lengths and smaller heads in the infants of heavy smokers, confirming that smoking in pregnancy causes general retardation of uterine growth.[38]

In view of the evidence presented here it is obvious that pregnant women need to be evaluated, and counseled as to the potential risks they impose on the intrauterine environment during gestation. The nurse needs to reinforce the potential hazards to the woman by sharing the information that is available at the present time.

Although the decision to abstain from smoking ultimately rests with the woman herself, the responsibility for health education rests with the

The nurse should assess the amount of smoking done daily by the client.

See Health Habits in Chap. 3 for questions about smoking.

The nurse should evaluate the client's understanding of risks to her fetus due to smoking.

nurse. By providing the education the nurse ensures that the client makes an informed choice.

Radiation

The fetus appears to be most susceptible to radiation induced deformity or death between the 30th and the 60th day after the first day of last menstrual period.[39]

Radiological procedures in a woman of childbearing age should be done in the first 14 days of the menstrual cycle or prior to ovulation. Women need to be questioned about their understanding of the effects of radiation on the fetus. Any exposure to radiation during the pregnancy should be noted so that follow-up evaluation can be done.

Economics

The nurse needs to evaluate the client's capacity to provide for the new family member and to ensure adequate health care for herself and her family. Pregnancy adds expenses that may stress a financially burdened family or a family who must rely on the woman's salary to live comfortably. The nurse should ask the client how the pregnancy will influence her ability to provide for herself and other members of her family economically, and assistance from community resources should be offered when necessary. Economic status is no reason for compromising health. Questions included in Chap. 3 can also be used when collecting data.

Community Resources

In addition to the services usually provided in the prenatal setting by primary physicians, nurses, nutritionists, and social services, there are other sources of assistance available to the pregnant woman which may help her in preparation for the task of childbearing and child rearing.

The prenatal period is the ideal time for preparation, and the nurse should evaluate the client's ability to utilize the community resources.

On the basis of the assessment of the woman's (couple's) expectations for the childbearing experience, the nurse can help the woman prepare for the fulfillment of these expectations by using appropriate resources. For example, a woman who is planning to have prepared childbirth should be told about parent education classes that are available in the community.

Lamaze, LaLeche League, and Planned Parenthood, as well as individual private hospitals, provide a series of formal classes to teach the physiology of labor and childbirth and teach psychoprophylactic techniques to prepare a woman for labor and delivery. Use of these resources should be noted.

In assessing the woman's plans for infant feeding, the nurse may find that the client plans to breast-feed. Along with evaluating her preparation for breast-feeding, the nurse may suggest that she establish communication with a community resource such as LaLeche League, which is an organization which provides a 24-hour communications system for breast-feeding mothers.

Women should also be encouraged to select a source of infant care during the prenatal period. If a source has been chosen, this should be noted. During this time the client should also be asked to discuss her plans for follow-up for her infant. Communication with a health provider prior to delivery is important. The nurse should be familiar with the community resources available for pediatric care so that assessments and referrals can be completed.

Many community resources are available to pregnant clients, and use of various resources can often enhance the childbearing experience.

Many of the requests for services made during the prenatal period may be a reflection of current trends. The return to more "normal" processes during labor and birth is allowing women the freedom to choose the type of labor, anesthesia, analgesia, position for delivery, and childbirth experience that best accomodates to their expectations for a gratifying experience.

The home birth movement, the request for alternative birthing rooms and centers, and requests for "birth under water" are a few examples of current trends.

All requests should be explored and discussed prenatally so that the advantages and disadvantages of such alternatives are fully understood by the client. Any involvement by the woman with childbearing and birthing resources and plans for use during the childbearing process should be noted.

Roles and Relationship Patterns

Family Life

Because it is the family that has the potential to offer the greatest support to the pregnant female, the nurse has a responsibility to evaluate the availability of this support as well as the lack of it.

Family support is important for the pregnant female.

In assessing the family structure the nurse needs to know if the family composition is an extended family, generations living together or in close proximity; a nuclear family, including husband, wife and children; or a single-parent family, in which the client and her offspring will be the family members. The single-parent family is becoming more accepted in today's society, but still represents a variety of emotional issues. The nurse is in a unique position to assess the needs of the single parent.

The importance of understanding the family structure, especially in the case of the pregnant client, is that pregnancy, being a time of crisis and vulnerability, is a time when support from those who care is much needed.

Family constellation and relationships provide information to help the nurse assess the need for physical, emotional, and economic assistance.

In addition to evaluating family structure it is also important to determine the perception of the pregnancy by other family members.

How the woman's family perceives the pregnancy may have implications for support provided to the woman.

Questions to elicit data:

What is the client's home life like?

Where is her home?

Does she have a place to call home?

Who does she call her family?

If her family includes her parents and she is unwed, do her parents accept this pregnancy?

Who are the other family members, their ages, and their role in the family?

What is the health of family members?

Who can the client count on for support?

It is important to keep in mind that pregnancy is a time of physical and emotional changes and that pregnant women have an increased need to feel cared for and loved during this time in their lives. If these needs cannot be fulfilled, the nurse should be aware of the need to assess the

Many physical and emotional changes occur with pregnancy, so it is important to identify if the family acts as a support system for the woman.

client's reaction to this deficit. Most importantly, the nurse needs to be sensitive to the client's perception of the family.

The nurse also needs to explore with each woman what the new baby means to the family. Will an additional family member add stress to an already overextended economic struggle? Will the family suffer from a loss of maternal income? What are the family goals?

Whether a pregnancy is planned or unplanned, a new member will alter family structure. The single-parent family may face social and financial burdens. The absence of the extended family may be seen as detrimental in that supports from extended family members may be needed.

The nurse must explore the family constellation with the woman and explore her perception of the effect of the pregnancy on her family.

Occupation

It is important to evaluate the stressors that may be imposed during pregnancy by the client's occupation. The physical changes that accompany pregnancy (the fatigue so common in the first trimester) may transform a previously comfortable work environment into an exhausting one.

An important consideration in assessing the occupation of a pregnant woman is to evaluate the potential risks involved. For example, does the client have a job in which she is exposed to chemicals, radiation, or high-level noise? Does her occupation include homemaker and mother of active toddlers in which the stress is produced in a different way? A woman does not have to be employed out of the home to perform work that is tiring and stressful.

Occupation means many different things to pregnant women. While some women would be bored not working during the 9 months of pregnancy, others work out of economic necessity during pregnancy.

The nurse should assess the client's occupation, her motivation, and her perception of the work environment. Generally, pregnant women should be encouraged to continue to work if fatigue is not a problem, if the environment is not considered potentially harmful, and if the pregnancy is progressing normally.

Societal Relationships

The nurse needs to assess the client as a person and as a member of a peer group and/or family and then as a member of a society. In the social structure, as in the cultural structure, the pregnant woman is under the influence of traditions, customs, and values.

Self-Perception and Self-Concept Patterns

One of the most obvious tasks which must be attended to is that of coming to grips with the effect of pregnancy on self-image. The nurse could ask, "How does it feel being pregnant?" The nurse should listen to the woman's response, assess her nonverbal expressions, and validate the woman's feelings with her.

Pregnancy involves a tremendous role change for the woman. The rapid changes which occur in a woman's body may alter her perception of herself and may represent a real crisis. The nurse needs to assess the woman's perception (in her own words) of what these changes mean for her individually in order to collect data and intervene in a therapeutic manner.

The increased need for love and security during pregnancy, alterations in the feminine contour which in our society is regarded highly, and alterations that result from a growing pregnancy in this feminine identity may all threaten a woman's self-image.[40]

Pregnancy-induced fatigue may influence the pregnant female's ability to work.

Potential risks for the woman and her fetus may exist as a result of her occupation.

See Chap. 3 for questions to elicit data about societal characteristics.

Physical changes and emotional feelings during pregnancy may alter the woman's self-perception patterns.

Pregnancy has different meanings for each woman.

On the other hand, a woman may see pregnancy as proof of feminity and an opportunity to prove her identity.

The amount of stress a pregnant woman experiences in altering her body image to fit her changing body depends on the degree to which her usual patterns of responses, behaviors, and coping mechanisms are inadequate to handle her feelings resulting from the pregnancy.[41]

Cognitive and Perceptual Patterns

Sensory Perception

The woman's sensory perceptions may be altered during pregnancy as a result of the normal physiological changes which occur in her body. Some women experience temporary changes in vision or hearing, while others become more sensitive to certain tastes and smells. Many women become much more sensitive to touch and actually enjoy stroking (effleurage) their pregnant abdomen. Therefore, it is important to determine the current status of the client's sensory perceptions through questioning.

See Chap. 3 for questions used to elicit data about sensory perception.

Education

Pregnancy is a time of increased awareness of the need to learn about the process of reproduction, labor, delivery, breast-feeding, and preparation for childbirth.

In order to provide for the educational needs of the pregnant female, an assessment of her plans for childbirth and infant feeding and of her specific goals for her pregnancy experience needs to be completed so that education can be planned based on her individual needs.

A woman who is planning on natural childbirth should be encouraged to attend prenatal childbirth classes. It is essential to assess the client's motivation for these plans. Does she want natural childbirth because she wants to witness the birth experience or does she want natural childbirth to please her partner? There is a great deal of difference in the motivational factors surrounding the pregnancy, since pregnancy and childbirth involve many people. The nurse must also discuss with the client what her husband's or partner's wishes are.

In planning education based on individual needs, the nurse must evaluate the level of understanding and capacity to return information that has been learned. Does the client understand that natural childbirth is *not* painless childbirth and is she capable of understanding the stages of labor. If not, then all information should be simplified in such a way that she comprehends what is being taught. Pictures and return demonstration are excellent means of teaching and ensuring that the client understands what has been taught.

Some women believe that prenatal childbirth classes guarantee painless labor.

Return demonstrations show the nurse that the client understands. This technique should be used to reinforce teaching.

On the other hand, a very knowledgeable client may not need visual aids and may be more interested in and capable of understanding the physiology of birth and the mechanisms involved in psychoprophylaxis, for example, that psychoprophylaxis teaches a conditional response to pain.

Intelligence

The nurse must be sensitive to the capacity of the woman to comprehend information, teaching, and important needs in order to potentiate an optimal outcome of pregnancy. The nurse should clarify with the client her perceptions of information exchanged during the interview.

For example, does she understand the significance of prenatal care and the importance of nutrition? If behaviors appear to be inconsistent with expectations of care, the nurse needs to assess whether this is non-compliance or lack of understanding on the part of the woman. The nurse may need to simplify interactions to the level of understanding that the woman can comprehend.

The nurse should keep in mind that culture and economic status may also affect the extent to which a woman cooperates, or utilizes the health care regimen recommended for her.

Sexuality and Reproductive Patterns

Pregnancy provides many women with the fulfillment of their sexual role, identity, and femininity. For others, a pregnancy is proof that someone else finds them sexually attractive. Despite growing scientific interest in sexuality, the influence of pregnancy on this variable aspect of human behavior is not well understood.

It was found in a study of 260 women interviewed in the postpartum period that for most women coital activity declines in a linear fashion once pregnancy is discovered.[42] Orgasmic activity, sexual interest, and noncoital behavior are similarly affected.

The decrease or increase in sexual activity is not predictable by socio-economic or other demographic factors (See Table 12-5).

"Pregnancy is a unique event in terms of a woman's sexuality and should be treated as such."[43] The complicated series of physical, hormonal, and psychological changes during pregnancy produce variable and individualistic responses, in that the nature of human sexuality is, by itself, highly individualistic.

Some of the physiological alterations of pregnancy that may affect sexual arousal include nausea and vomiting, disturbance of metabolism, and breast tenderness. Alterations that may increase libido may be engorgement and sensitivity of the genitals. Masters and Johnson found an increase in sexual tension and performance in the second trimester that they associated with increased congestion of the pelvic vasculature.[44] Letting the woman know that changes in sexual behavior occur during pregnancy and that these changes are normal will enhance her ability and willingness to discuss this very personal issue.

The concept of self-image plays a major role in sexuality during pregnancy. Some women think of themselves as more feminine, while others consider themselves unattractive. Also, the need to feel nurtured and cared for may be fulfilled sexually.

Masters and Johnson have shown that pregnancy does not seriously alter a woman's basic sexual response. Much that occurs between two people during pregnancy depends on what has gone on before between them.

Table 12-5
Reasons for Changes in Sexual Feelings and Performance

Physical discomforts	40%
Fear of injury to baby	27%
Loss of interest	23%
Awkwardness having coitus	17%
Recommendation of physician	8%
Reasons extraneous to pregnancy	6%
Loss of attractiveness in woman's own mind	4%
Recommendation of person other than physician	1%
Other reasons	15%

Source: Don A. Solberg, Julius Butter, and Nathaniel Wagner, "Sexual Behavior in Pregnancy," *N Engl J Med*, 288:1098 (1973). Used by permission.

In order to assess the influence of pregnancy on sexuality, the nurse must use a holistic approach. In other words:

> To understand what is happening, we must look at the entire woman, not just her pregnancy.[45]

The behavioral assessment of the pregnant female of necessity must include a sexual history. The nurse must be aware that what is considered "normal" and "comfortable" for one woman may be troublesome for another. Furthermore, the nurse must have a sense of the prepregnant sexual relationship in order to assess the changes that can realistically be attributed to the pregnancy. Pregnancy is not a cure for preexisting conflict. As was discussed in Pregnancy as a Developmental Task, pregnancy adds stress. The nurse's role is to assess the "normal" responses and to have the ability to explore these feelings with the woman.

Nutritional Patterns

The increased demands placed on the maternal organism during pregnancy require adequate nutrition.

> The evidence that reasonably high maternal weight gain bears a definite direct relation to increased birth weight and lowered incidence of prematurity has led to lessening emphasis on strict regulation of caloric intake during pregnancy.[46]

The best diet for the pregnant woman consists of simple well-balanced meals in which she increases her caloric intake an average daily increment of 300 kilocalories above the normal diet. The nurse should educate pregnant women to avoid food fads, and dieting during pregnancy should be discouraged. The nurse should also stress that the old-fashioned notion that pregnant women must "eat for two" can lead to excessive weight gain.

The recommended daily dietary requirements for the pregnant woman are included in Table 12-6.

Highlights

The ability of the woman to freely discuss sexual concerns will depend to a great extent on the nurse-patient relationship.

Table 12-6
Recommended Daily Dietary Allowances for Selected Nutrients for Pregnancy and Lactation

Nutrients	Nonpregnant girl or woman				Pregnant girl or woman				Lactation (850 mL daily)		
	11–14 yr	15–18 yr	19+ yr	Added need	11–14 yr	15–18 yr	19+ yr	Added need	11–14 yr	15–18 yr	19+ yr
Calories, kcal	2200	2100	2000	300	2500	2400	2300	500	2700	2600	2500
Protein, g	46	46	44	30	76	78	76	20	64	68	66
Calcium, g	1.2	1.2	0.8	0.4	1.6	1.6	1.2	0.4	1.6	1.6	1.2
Iron, mg	18	18	18	*	*	*	*	*	*	*	*
Vitamin A, µg RE†	800	800	800	200	1000	1000	1000	400	1200	1200	1200
Thiamine, mg	1.2	1.1	1.0	0.4	1.6	1.5	1.7	0.5	1.7	1.6	1.5
Riboflavin, mg	1.3	1.3	1.2	0.3	1.6	1.6	1.5	0.5	1.8	1.8	1.7
Niacin equivalent, mg	15	14	13	2	17	16	15	5	20	19	18
Ascorbic acid, mg	50	60	60	20	70	80	80	40	90	100	100
Vitamin D, µg	10	10	5	5	15	15	15	5	15	15	15

*The increased requirement during pregnancy cannot be met by the iron content of habitual American diets nor by the existing iron stores of many women; therefore the use of 30 to 60 mg of supplemental iron is recommended. Iron needs during lactation are not substantially different from those of nonpregnant women, but continued supplementation of the mother for 2 to 3 mo after parturition is advisable to replenish stores depleted by pregnancy.
†Retinol equivalent (RE) replaces international unit (IU) as the standard measure of vitamin A activity.
Source: From Food and Nutrition Board, *Recommended Dietary Allowance,* rev. ed., National Academy of Sciences, National Research Council, Washington, 1979.

In evaluating the nutritional status of the pregnant female, the nurse should gather information about the customary diet, remembering that culture and religion can exert an influence over dietary habits. The nurse should provide nutritional information which will be accepted and which accommodates to the financial capacity of the client. The nurse should keep in mind that a woman whose budget is severely stressed will be unable to afford expensive foods.

Exercise and Activity Patterns

As was discussed under Occupation, the physical changes of pregnancy may decrease a woman's tolerance to the routines that were quite comfortable prior to the pregnancy.[47] It is important for the nurse to discuss the changes in the activity tolerance level and educate the woman so that she understands that these physical feelings will be most pronounced during the first trimester and again during the third trimester. For example, during the third trimester of pregnancy, the weight of the growing uterus can become a burden which may be exhausting.

Reinforcing with the client that these alterations are perfectly normal may decrease any anxiety related to these changes in her activity or tolerance level. The nurse should also point out that activity tolerance is even more diminished during the summer months when weather becomes an aggravating factor to the already stressed pregnant woman. However, it should be kept in mind that dramatic changes may need further evaluation. For example, if the fatigue is accompanied by symptoms such as weakness, dizziness, or fainting, pathology such as anemia must be ruled out.

Coping Patterns and Stress Tolerance Patterns

It has long been recognized that pregnancy may be a source of anxiety. Alteration in body image, anticipated changes in life style, concern over having a normal baby, family and financial stresses may all be anxiety-provoking.[48]

Further, pregnancy requires adaptation of various kinds. It may revive the psychic conflicts of previous developmental phases; i.e., old, unresolved conflicts with the woman's own mother arise as motherhood approaches for the woman herself. However, it may also offer opportunities for finding new solutions.[49] Meeting the challenges of pregnancy and the subsequent transition to motherhood may be stressful for a woman.

Pregnancy is a "naturally" stressful event.

The role of the nurse in facilitating this transition is to understand and appreciate the individuality of stress-provoking events for each woman and to evaluate her responses to these stressors. A woman under the stress of economic difficulty who becomes unexpectedly pregnant will have to deal with the crisis of both events.

Appreciation for the individuality of each woman is an essential component of the nursing assessment.

First and foremost, the nurse must help the woman understand that a major change, such as pregnancy, affecting her physical and emotional well-being is naturally a stressful event. The nurse may ask the woman, "What kind of changes have taken place in your life since you found out that you were pregnant?"

See Chap. 3 for questions used to elicit data about coping with stress.

Review of Body Components

When gathering data related to body components, the nurse must phrase questions in a way that can be clearly understood by the client so that specific information is obtained. If the nurse were to ask a woman if she

See Chaps. 3 and 4 when completing data collection on the review of body components.

has ever had cardiorespiratory disease, the question might not be understood. Rather, the nurse must ask specific questions to gather the data. For example, the nurse might ask a question such as "Have you ever been told you had a heart murmur?"

A careful review verifies normal findings or provides clues to the existence of significant diseases omitted from the past history. Symptoms or signs should be recorded in all the categories described in Chap. 3. All body components will respond in some form or other to the physiological stress of pregnancy. When gathering this information, the nurse must address each component separately.

Summary

Health assessment of the pregnant client must include data about the adolescent or adult woman as well as normal physiological, psychological, behavioral, and sociocultural changes that occur as a result of the pregnant state. Variations in all pattern areas are likely during pregnancy, and it is important to be able to document that a healthy state of being exists to assure normal outcome of pregnancy for both the woman and her baby.

REFERENCES

1. Rugh, R., and L. Shettles: *From Conception to Birth,* Harper & Row, New York, 1971, p. 18.

2. National Center for Health Statistics, U.S. Department of Commerce, Bureau of the Census, Washington.

3. American Nurses' Association Standards of Maternal and Child Health Nursing Practice, American Nurses' Association, Missouri, 1973.

4. Ibid.

5. Rugg, Coralese C.: "Childbearing in Sickle Cell Anemia: A Nursing Approach," *J Ob Gyn Neon Nurs.* **6**(3):23–25 (1977).

6. Farris, Lorene Sanders: "Approaches to Caring for the American Indian Maternity Patient," *Maternal Child Nursing,* **1**(2):82–87(1976).

7. Ibid.

8. Mead, M.: "Understanding Cultural Patterns," *Nurs Outlook,* **4**:260(1956).

9. Farris, "Approaches to Caring for the American Indian Maternity Patient," p. 83.

10. Parken, Marguerite: "Culture and Preventive Health Care," *J Ob Gyn Neon Nurs,* **7**:40–46 (1978).

11. American Nurses' Association Standards of Maternal and Child Health Practice.

12. Horsley, J. Stephen: "The Psychology of Normal Pregnancy," *Nurs Times* **66**:401(1966).

13. Rubin, Reva: "Cognitive Style in Pregnancy," *Am J Nurs,* **70**:502(1970).

14. Ibid., p. 502.

15. Ibid., p. 508.

16. Maslow, Abraham H.: *Toward a Psychology of Being,* 2d ed. Van Nostrand, New York, 1968, p. 47.

17. Ibid.

18. Erikson, Erik: "Identity as the Life Cycle," *Psychol Issues* **1**:1–171(1959).

19. Bibring, Grete L.: "Some Considerations of Psychological Processes in Pregnancy," in *Psychoanalytic Study of the Child,* International Universities Press, New York, 1959, p. 114.

20. Ringquist, Mary Ann: "Psychologic Stress in the Last Three Months of Pregnancy," in Leota Kester McNall and Janet Trask Galeener (eds.), *Current Practice in Obstetrics and Gynecologic Nursing,* vol I, Mosby, St. Louis, 1976, p. 71.

21. Persaud, T. V. N., and K. L. Moore: "Causes and Prenatal Diagnosis of Congenital Abnormalities," *J Ob Gyn Neon Nurs,* **3**:50–55 (1974).

22. Ibid., p. 52.

23. Page, Ernest W., Claude A. Villee, and Dorothy B. Villee: *Human Reproduction: The Core Content of Obstetrics, Gynecology & Perinatal Medicine,* 2d ed., Saunders, Philadelphia, 1976, p. 201.

Highlights

The nurse should collect data by phrasing questions in a way that can be understood by the woman.

24. Walker, James, Ian MacGillivray, and Malcolm C. MacNaughton (eds.), *Combined Textbook of Obstetrics and Gynecology,* 9th ed. Churchill Livingstone, New York, 1976, p. 497.

25. Ibid., p. 500.

26. Jones, K., and D. Smith: "Recognition of Fetal Alcohol Syndrome in Early Infancy," *Lancet* 2:999–1001(1973).

27. Ibid.

28. Streissguth, A. P.: "Maternal Drinking and the Outcome of Pregnancy: Implications for Child Mental Health," *Am J Orthopsychiatry,* **47**:422–31 (1977).

29. Rosett, H. L., E. M. Ouellette, L. Weiner, and E. Owens: "Therapy of Heavy Drinking During Pregnancy," *Obstet Gynecol,* **51**:45(1978).

30. Ibid., p. 45.

31. *Alcohol and Your Unborn Baby,* Department of Health, Education, and Welfare, Alcohol, Drug Abuse, and Mental Health Administration, DHEW Publication no. (ADM) 78—521, Rockville, Maryland, 1978.

32. Bangai, Andrew L.: "Smoking. Some of Its Less Publicized Sequels," *Chest,* **69**(1):55(1976).

33. Comstock, G. W., F. K. Shah, M. B. Meyer, and H. Abbey: "Low Birth Weight and Neonatal Mortality Rate Related to Maternal Smoking and Socioeconomic Status,"*Am Obstet Gynecol,* **111**(1):53–59(1971).

34. Murphy, John F., Melcahy Riesteard, and John E. Drumm: "Smoking and the Fetus," *Lancet,* **2**:35(1977).

35. Comstock et al., "Low Birth Weight and Neonatal Mortality Rate Related to Maternal Smoking and Socioeconomic Status."

36. Bangai, "Smoking. Some of Its Less Publicized Sequels."

37. Butler, N. R., H. Goldstein, and E. M. Ross: "Cigarette Smoking in Pregnancy: Its Influence on Birthweight and Perinatal Mortality," *Brit Med J,* **2**:127 (1972).

38. Davies, D. P., O. P. Gray, P. C. Ellwood, and M. Abernethy: "Cigarette Smoking in Pregnancy: Associations with Maternal Weight Gain and Fetal Growth," *Lancet,* **1(7956):**385–7(1976).

39. Danforth, David N. (ed.): *Obstetrics and Gynecology,* 3d ed., Harper & Row, New York, 1977, p. 502.

40. Caplan, G.: *An Approach to Community Mental Health,* Grune & Stratton, New York, 1961.

41. Weinberg, Janie Spelton: "Body Image Disturbance as a Factor in the Crisis Situation of Pregnancy," *J Ob Gyn Neon Nurs,* **7**:19(1978).

42. Solberg, Don A., Julius Butler, and Nathaniel N. Wagner: "Sexual Behavior in Pregnancy," *N Engl J Med,* **288**:1098–1103(1973).

43. Ibid., p. 1102.

44. Masters, W. H., and V. E. Johnson: *Human Sexual Response,* Little, Brown, Boston, 1966, pp. 141–168.

45. Clark, Ann L., and Ralph W. Hale: "Sex During and After Pregnancy," *Am J Nurs,* **74**:1430–1431 (1974).

46. Danforth, *Obstetrics and Gynecology,* p. 313.

47. Walker, MacGillivray, and MacNaughton, *Combined Textbook of Obstetrics and Gynecology,* p. 94.

48. Ascher, Barbara H. CNM, MS, "Maternal Anxiety in Pregnancy and Fetal Homeratasis" *J Ob Gyn Neon Nurs,* **7**:18(1978).

49. Nadelson, Carol: "'Normal' and 'Special' Aspects of Pregnancy," *Obstet Gynecol,* **41**(4):611(1973).

BIBLIOGRAPHY

Alvear, J. Brooke: "Effect of Smoking on Fetal Growth," *Lancet,* **1**(8022):1158(1977).

Benedek, T.: "Sexual Function in Women," in *American Handbook of Psychiatry,* vol. I, Basic Books, New York, 1959.

Benson, Ralph C.: *Handbook of Obstetrics and Gynecology,* 6th ed., Lange Medical Publishers, California, 1974.

Burch, P. R.: "Effects of Cigarette Smoking on the Fetus and Child," *Pediatrics,* **60**(5):766–767(1977).

Caplan, G.: "Psychological Aspects of Maternity Care," *Am Public Health,* **47**:25(1957).

Clark, A. L., and R. W. Hale: "Sex During and After Pregnancy," *Am J Nurs,* **74**(8):1430–1431(1974).

Colman, A. D., and L. L. Colman: "Pregnancy as an Altered State of Consciousness," *J Birth Fam,* **1**(1):7(1974).

Duvall, E: *Family Development,* 5th ed., Lippincott, Philadelphia, 1977.

Erikson, E.: *Identity, Youth, & Crises,* Norton, New York, 1968.

——: "Identity and the Life Cycle," *Psychol Issues,* **1**:1–171(1959).

Haire, P. B.: "The Pregnant Patient's Bill of Rights," *J Nurse Midwifery,* **20**:29(Winter 1975).

Hanson, J. W., K. L. Jones, and D. W. Smith: "Fetal Alcohol Syndrome: Experience with 41 Patients," *J Am Med Assoc* **235**:1458–1460(1976).

Hellman, L. M., and J. A. Pritchard: *Williams Obstetrics,* 14th ed., Appleton-Century-Crofts, New York, 1971.

Ibid. 15th ed., 1975.

Jensen, Margaret Duncan, Ralph C. Benson, and Irene Bobak: *Maternity Care the Nurse and the Family,* Mosby, St. Louis, 1977.

Jones, K., D. Smith, C. Alleland, and A. Streissguth: "Patterns of Malformation in Offspring of Chronic Alcoholic Mothers," *Lancet,* **1**:1267–1271(1973).

Kynderly, Katie: "The Sexuality of Women in Pregnancy and Postpartum: A Review," *J Ob Gyn Neon Nurs,* **7**:28–32(1978).

Martin, Leonide L.: *Health Care of Women,* Lippincott, Philadelphia, 1978.

Maslow, Abraham H.: *Motivation and Personality,* Harper & Row, New York, 1954.
——: *Toward a Psychology of Being,* 2d ed., Van Nostrand, New York, 1968.

Masters, W. H., and V. E. Johnson: *Human Sexual Response,* Little, Brown, Boston, 1966, pp. 141–168.

Mead, M.: "Determinants of Health Beliefs and Behavior," *Am Public Health,* **51**:1552(1961).

McNall, Leota Kester, and Janet Trask Galeener: *Current Practice in Obstetric & Gynecologic Nursing,* vol. I, Mosby, St. Louis, 1976.

Milo, N.: "Values, Social Class and Community Health Services," *Nurs Res,* **16**:26(Winter 1967).

Nadelson, Carol: "'Normal' and 'Special' Aspects of Pregnancy," *Obstet Gynecol,* **41**(4):611(1973).

Niswander, Kenneth R.: *Obstetrics, Essentials of Clinical Practice,* Little, Brown, Boston, 1976.

Notman, Malkah T., and Carol C. Nadelson (eds.), *The Woman Patient: Medical and Psychological Interfaces,* vol. I, Plenum, New York, 1978.

Paynick, M. L.: "Cultural Barriers to Nurse Communication," *Am J Nurs,* **64**:87(1964).

Perkins, M. R.: "Does Availability of Health Services Ensure Their Use," *Nurs Outlook,* **22**:496(1974).

Poland, Betty J., and Katherine Ash: "The Influence of Recent Use of an Oral Contraceptive on Early Uterine Development," *Obstet Gynecol,* **116**:1138–42(1973).

Raid, Duncan E., Kenneth J. Ryan, and Kurt Benirschke: *Principles and Management of Human Reproduction,* Saunders, Philadelphia, 1972.

Rubin, Reva: "Attainment of the Maternal Role. I. Processes," *Nurs Research,* **16**:237–245(Summer 1967).
——: "Attainment of the Maternal Role. II. Models and Referrants," *Nurs Research,* **16**:342–346(Fall 1967).

Simmons, J. P.: "Female Sexuality and Life Situations: An Etiological Psycho-Social-Sexual Profile of Weight Gain and Nausea and Vomiting in Pregnancy," *Obstet Gynecol,* **38**(4):555–563(1971).

Smoyah, S.: "Cultural Incongruence and the Effect on Nurses' Perception," *Nurs Forum,* **7**:234(1968).

Solberg, D., J. Butler, and N. Wagner: "Sexual Behavior in Pregnancy," *N Engl J Med,* **288**:1098–1103(1973).

Strickland, E. H., et al. (eds.): "Environmental Influences on the Fetus," in *Current Concepts in Clinical Nursing,* vol. 4, Mosby, St. Louis, 1973.

Zabriskie, J. R.: "Effects of Cigarette Smoking during Pregnancy," *Obstet Gynecol,* **21**:405(1963).

Highlights

This section describes unique changes seen in the physical examination during pregnancy.

Special attention is given to the examination of the breasts, abdomen, and pelvis throughout pregnancy.

Until 32 weeks gestation, the woman is examined once a month; from 32 to 36 weeks she is seen every 2 weeks; and from 36 weeks until term she is examined weekly.

See Chap. 4 for a detailed discussion of each body component covered during the physical examination.

In a very obese woman, change in body contour may not be obvious while the woman is in a sitting position.

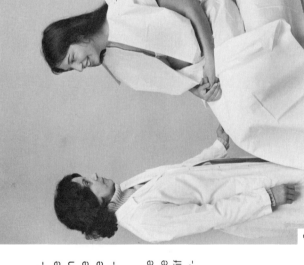

a

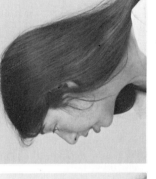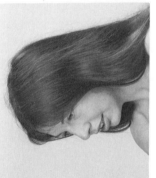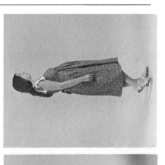

b

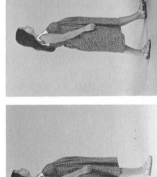

c

PHYSICAL EXAMINATION
APPROACH TO THE PHYSICAL EXAMINATION

The woman should be in a sitting position on the examining table, facing the examiner, draped or clothed in a gown (a). She should be instructed to put the gown on so that it ties or opens in the front to facilitate the later breast, abdominal, and pelvic exams.

The client may keep her bra on until the time of the breast examination—some women will feel more comfortable if allowed to do so. All other undergarments must be removed.

THE EXAMINATION
General Appearance
Inspection

Initial observation begins when the pregnant female is first seen for prenatal care. The examiner must focus on the changes in body components that occur in pregnancy.

The examiner, while talking to the woman, should note the skin color, appearance, facial expression, and state of nutrition (b). Also note whether there are obvious signs of pregnancy, such as increased abdominal size.

Symmetry, posture, and body build are assessed.

Gait (c) and range of active motion are observed.

Composure, mental status, speech, and disposition are assessed and noted throughout the examination.

Highlights

Not all pregnant clients will present with the skin changes described here.

Skin changes peculiar to pregnancy begin to appear about the 16th week.

During inspection, the examiner may find the following pigmentation changes which have occurred in response to the melanocyte stimulating hormone.

1 Hyperpigmentation of the abdominal midline called *linea nigra* (a)

2 Pigmented nipple and areola of breasts (a)

3 *Spider angiomas*, which are cutaneous vascular changes due to increased amounts of circulating estrogen and to vasodilation and stasis of blood flow

4 Mottling of cheeks and forehead called *chloasma* or "mask of pregnancy" (b)

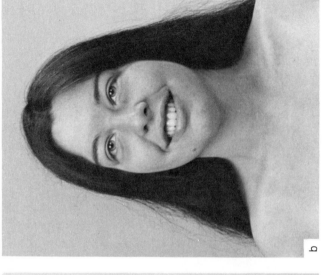

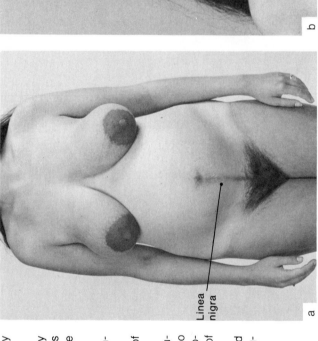

Linea nigra

a

b

Localized areas of erythema over the fingers, fingertips, and palms may occur, due to vascular changes (c).

Any of the following changes may also be noted during examination of the skin:

1 Hyperpigmentation may cause skin to darken over bony prominences (d), the labia majora, perineum and perianal area.

2 Increased sweating from exocrine glands is common, and usually occurs in the first trimester.

3 Pruritis may be localized or widespread, perhaps due to estrogens.

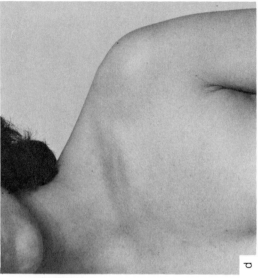

c

d

Head

Palpation

Cervical and other lymph nodes are palpated for disorders of the lymphatic system (a). Normally none are present.

Note the texture, color, and general hair distribution of the head and body.

Hair tends to straighten, and there is occasional hair loss over frontal and parietal regions. Facial and body hair may increase. This is thought to be due to an increase in androgens and corticotrophic hormones. These findings should be noted.

An increase in facial and body hair may occur during pregnancy.

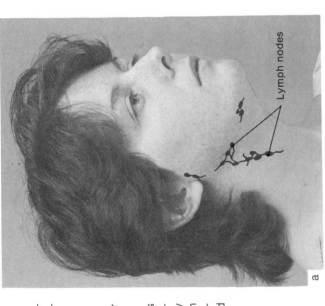

Lymph nodes

a

Eyes

Inspection

Changes which the examiner may note during the eye examination include:

1 An increase in pigmentation of the eyelids and periorbital regions (b)

2 Conjunctival vascular changes consisting primarily of some degree of vasoconstriction. Minimal stress may cause conjunctival hemorrhages (c). Normally, there are no retinal changes

Refer to eye section in Chap. 4.

An ophthalmoscopic examination is not done at each prenatal visit, unless indicated.

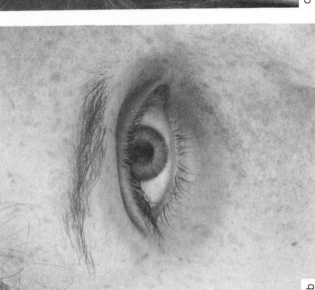

b

c

Ears

Inspection

There are no documented changes in the external, middle, or inner ear. Some women complain of mild hearing loss due to blocked Eustachian tubes.

Nose

Inspection

The examiner inspects for changes in the nose.

Nasal mucosa is responsive to estrogen, and becomes hyperemic and edematous.

Generalized hyperemia with engorgement of the turbinates (a) is a well-documented change, and can be noted on inspection.

Nasal and sinus secretion is increased.

Epistaxis, or nosebleeds, rhinitis, which causes nasal stuffiness and discharge, and mouth breathing are frequent problems for the pregnant female.

Mouth

Inspection

The examiner inspects for changes in the mouth (b).

Tissues of the mouth may exhibit hyperemia and edema.

Excessive salivation (ptyalism) may develop in early pregnancy.

Hypertrophy of the gums, called *pregnancy epulis,* may occur due to proliferation of interdental papillary blood vessels, which results in local inflammation and hyperplasia (c). Symptoms include gingival swelling and bleeding which may interfere with mastication.

Special attention must be given to symptoms such as nosebleeds which occur in response to hormonal changes.

Hyperemia is an excess accumulation of blood in the extremities due to relaxation of the arterioles.

Appetite patterns change during pregnancy.

Ptyalism (excessive salivation) may be very annoying to the pregnant woman.

Encourage good dental hygiene and dental care during pregnancy.

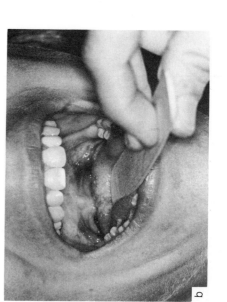

Epulis

c

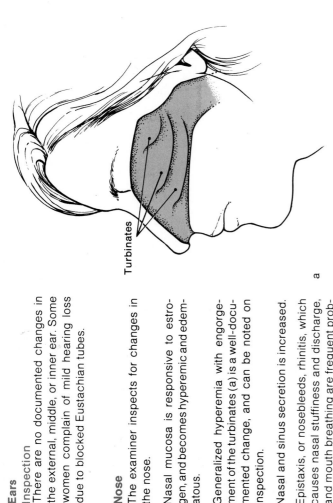

Turbinates

a

b

Neck and Throat

Inspection

Tissues of the posterior pharynx may exhibit hyperemia and edema, and this should be noted.

Palpation

Upon palpation (a), women may have an enlarged thyroid, or *goiter of pregnancy*. This corresponds to increases in radioactive iodine uptake.

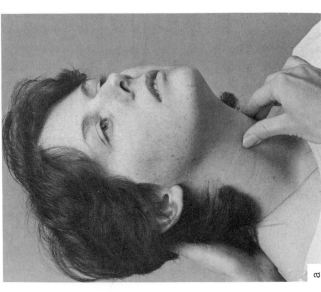

a

Lungs

Inspection

Respiratory rate is counted by the examiner.

Tissues of the respiratory tract exhibit hyperemia and edema. Oxygen consumption increases by almost 20 percent between the 16th and 40th week of pregnancy. This is accomplished by a rise in tidal volume (of 45 percent) and a rise in respiratory rate (b).

There is an expansion of the thoracic cavity, permitted by relaxation of costosternal and costovertebral ligaments (c).

Upward displacement of the diaphragm (estimated to be 4 cm in a primigravida) occurs to accommodate the enlarging uterus.

After 24 weeks gestation, thoracic breathing replaces abdominal breathing.

Dyspnea (shortness of breath) may occur late in pregnancy, and should be noted and explained to the client.

Costosternal ligaments

Costovertebral ligaments

Diaphragm

c

Tidal volume

Respiration rate

Pregnant

Non-pregnant

b

Heart

Percussion

The enlarging uterus elevates the dia-phragm causing a counterclockwise rotation and a lateral upward displace-ment of the heart (a). This movement increases the transverse diameter of the heart. Percussion of the heart borders should be done to detect these changes in position.

Cardiac output increases by about 30 percent during the first and second tri-mester and remains elevated until delivery.

Auscultation

Auscultation of heart sounds is done, and rate and rhythm noted.

Physiological cardiac murmurs may be heard. They are generally soft, systolic, and blowing in quality, and are usually localized in the pulmonic area and at the apex. Murmurs should be noted.

Breasts

Inspection

The epidermis of the nipples and areola should be examined for fissures, and nipple inversion (b).

Palpation

Hyperplasia of breast tissue begins early in pregnancy due to gradual development of glandular tissue. Breasts are palpated and any changes noted (c).

Cardiac displacement can cause an increase in pulse rate and palpi-tations in the pregnant female.

Blood flow increases most pre-dominantly in the uterus, kidneys, and skin, with slight increases to the breasts and intestines.

The increase in plasma volume may cause a pseudo anemia dur-ing pregnancy at the time of maxi-mum volume expansion. There-fore, hematocrits may be done periodically.

Dramatic changes in the blood pressure (greater than 10 mmHg) are suspect, and should be noted.

Refer to Chap. 4 for complete dis-cussion of heart sounds.

A good, well-fitting bra should be worn for support during pregnancy. Bra size will change progressively throughout pregnancy.

Wet, soapy hands should be used to ensure accurate examination of breasts.

Preparation for breast feeding in the third trimester includes tough-ening of the nipples and areola, and correction of nipple inversion through nipple rolling.

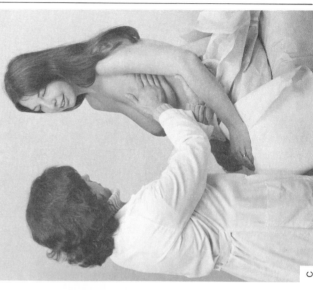

Non-pregnant

Pregnant

Heart

Diaphragm

a

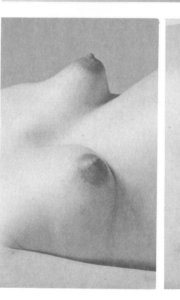

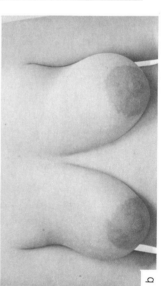

b

c

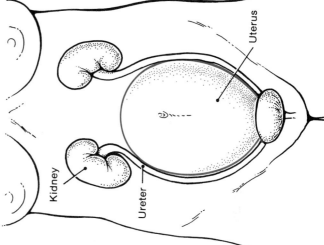

b

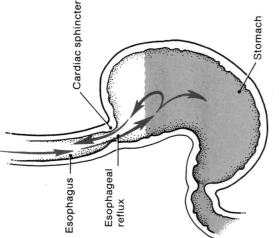

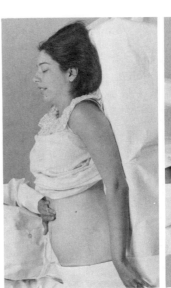

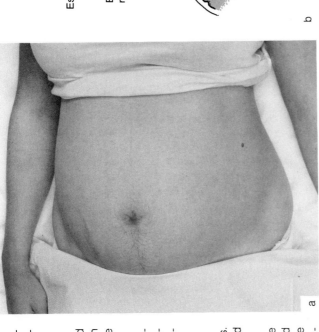

a

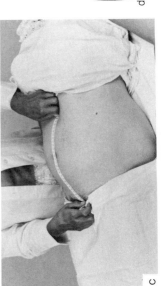

c

d

Abdomen

Inspection and palpation of the abdomen are essential to the initial and successive prenatal examinations.

Inspection

Inspect for scars, and striations, and note contour (a). These will vary with client's past history, and present stage of gestation.

Acid indigestion (heartburn) is commonly caused by hypochlorhydria, decreased gastric motility, and esophageal reflux (b).

Palpation

Palpate for height of the uterine fundus. Before 13 weeks gestation it is palpated bimanually.

After 13 weeks fundal palpation is done abdominally with the flat of fingers and palms. To measure fundal height, a tape is placed on top of fundus to the symphysis pubis. As gestation continues, the measurement will increase. Fundal height may vary with a woman's height. The progression of growth is more important than the exact location (c).

Liver Liver function seems unchanged during pregnancy. The examiner should note the size and position of the liver.

Spleen Spleen function also seems unchanged during pregnancy. The examiner should attempt to palpate the spleen.

Kidneys The kidneys are palpated and size is noted. Renal blood flow increases 25 percent during the first and second trimester, returning to prepregnant levels by the third trimester. The ureters become dilated and elongated, and are displaced in later pregnancy by the uterus (d).

Percussion

Bladder The bladder is percussed. Tympany is usually noted.

Bladder mucosa increases in vascularity and there is a decrease in bladder tone as a response to the influence of hormones on smooth muscle.

Frequency of urination due to increased bladder sensitivity and from compression of the bladder by the uterus occurs during the first and third trimesters of pregnancy (a).

Genitalia
Inspection

The examiner inspects the vulva, vagina, mucosa, cervix, and uterus. Pelvic inspection is performed using a speculum with the client positioned in stirrups (b).

On speculum examination, a characteristic bluish discoloration of the cervical and vaginal mucosa is noted at 6 to 8 weeks gestation (*Chadwick's sign*).

The vagina is long and congested due to increased vascularity; rugae are increased.

Vaginal discharge is usually profuse, causing a leukorrhea high in glycogen.

On speculum examination of the cervix, thickening of the mucous layer, increased blood supply, and proliferation of glands near the external os are prominent.

There is a constant flow of relatively thick, clear, odorless mucus produced by hypertrophied endocervical glands and everted endocervical columnar epithelia.

Highlights

Pregnant women are prone to urinary retention and thus to increased susceptibility to infection.

The pelvic examination confirms pregnancy.

The examiner's gloves and instruments for speculum examination must be clean, but need not be sterile. The speculum should be warmed prior to insertion. Never use lubricant on the speculum.

Vulvar or perineal varicosities may become more pronounced as pressure from the uterus increases.

Leukorrhea stimulates the growth of vaginal bacilli, leading to an increase in lactic acid content that reduces the vaginal Ph to between 4.0 and 6.0. This discharge is often a concern, and may be described by some women as uncomfortable or annoying.

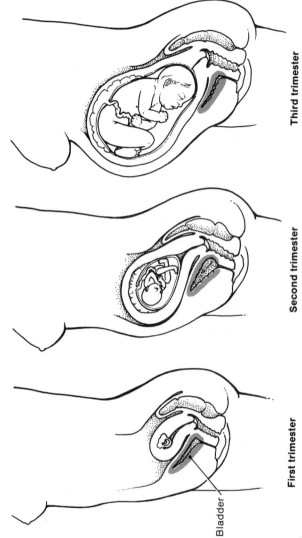

First trimester Second trimester Third trimester

Bladder

a

b

Palpation

On bimanual examination the cervix feels soft and may admit a fingertip.

The uterus is bimanually palpated and fundal size noted (a). This is especially important during the first trimester, when the uterus is a pelvic organ.

Uterine shape is globular by 10 to 12 weeks gestation, and becomes progressively more ovoid (b).

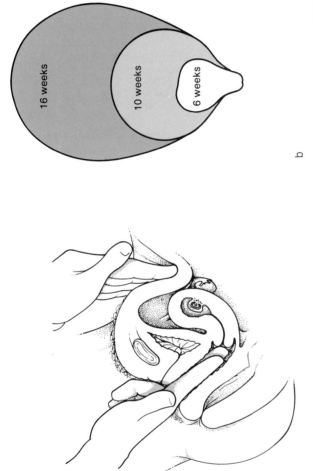

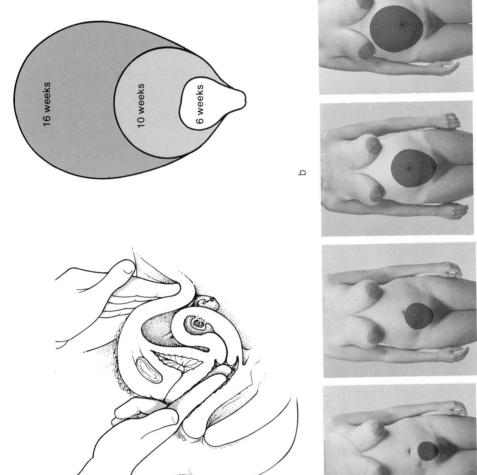

Enlargement of the uterus is most pronounced on the fundus, and at each month of pregnancy the examiner will find the fundus at different heights (c):

1 9 weeks — symphysis

2 12 weeks — intraabdominal organ

3 16 weeks — between symphysis and umbilicus

4 20-22 weeks — at umbilicus

5 36 weeks — at xiphoid

Fundal height is noted at each prenatal visit.

Highlights

See Chap. 4, physical examination of the female pelvis for the technique of bimanual examination.

The woman should be offered a mirror so that she also can see her cervix. This will help the woman understand changes in her body.

During examination, a Papanicolaou smear, gonococcus smear, and a Trichomonas smear may be taken for routine lab work.

The uterus is converted from an organ weighing 60 g (2 ounces) prepregnancy, into one weighing about 1000 g (2 pounds) at term.

Fundal height is an objective criteria for evaluation of fetal growth and gestational age.

Figure a adapted from Dorothy A. Jones et al., Medical-Surgical Nursing, A Conceptual Approach, McGraw-Hill, 1982, p. 13, fig. 5-1. Used with permission of McGraw-Hill Book Company.

The **adnexa uteri** is the term used to denote the area of the ovaries and the fallopian tubes.

During vaginal exam the ischial spines are easily felt to estimate their prominence. Midpelvic contraction is suspected if spines are prominent.

Pelvic measurements may be done in early or late pregnancy. It is easier in late gestation when pelvic tissues are relaxed.

Anteroposterior diameter is the shortest inlet measurement and the most important.

Diameters of the inlet, midpelvis, and outlet are only estimates, and x-ray pelvimetry is necessary for an accurate determination of pelvic configuration.

Obstetric conjugate is a few millimeters shorter than the true conjugate. It is the shortest inlet diameter through which the baby's head must pass as it descends into the birth canal.

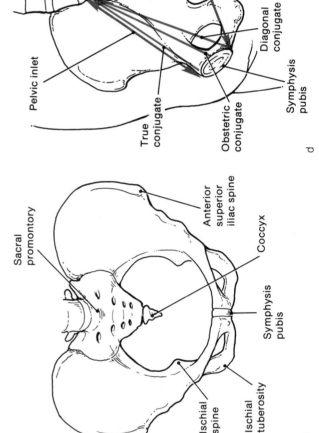

Corpus luteum

Progesterone

Estrogen

Vessels

Ovary

b

Sacral promontory

Pelvic inlet

True conjugate

Obstetric conjugate

Symphysis pubis

Diagonal conjugate

Pelvic outlet

d

Ovaries and fallopian tubes

a

Sacral promontory

Anterior superior iliac spine

Coccyx

Symphysis pubis

Ischial spine

Ischial tuberosity

c

On bimanual examination, normal-sized ovaries are not usually palpable.

The ovaries and fallopian tubes are carried up from the pelvis into the abdominal cavity by the enlarging uterus (a).

Ovarian vasculature undergoes marked hypertrophy.

The corpus luteum of gestation remains 3 to 4 cm in diameter until approximately midpregnancy (b).

Examination of the *bony pelvis* (c) is a part of the pelvic examination done only during pregnancy. The purpose of obtaining pelvic measurements is to evaluate the maternal pelvis and its ability to accommodate to the fetus at delivery.

The client remains in stirrups.

The anteroposterior, transverse, and right to left oblique diameters of the plane of the *pelvic inlet* are measured to estimate inlet capacity. **Anteroposterior** diameter is the distance from the symphysis pubis to the sacrum.

There are three measurements of the anteroposterior diameter (d).

1 **True conjugate** - distance from the top of the symphysis pubis to the middle of the promontory of the sacrum.

2 **Obstetric conjugate** - distance between posterior surface of the symphysis and sacral promontory.

3 **Diagonal conjugate** - distance from the inferior border of the symphysis to the sacral promontory.

Highlights

Measurement of the diagonal conjugate is somewhat uncomfortable for the client.

True evaluation of the adequacy of the pelvis always awaits labor.

It may be difficult to reach the promontory of the sacrum during the early months of pregnancy because the vaginal tissues are tight and the perineum is rigid.

At mid-pregnancy these tissues stretch more easily and thus the diagonal conjugate measurement is sometimes deferred until mid-pregnancy.

The diagonal conjugate is the only diameter of the inlet that can be measured without the use of x-ray and is measured clinically.

To measure the diagonal conjugate, the first two fingers of the examining hand are introduced into the vagina until the tip of the second finger touches the promontory of the sacrum (a). The point at which the lower margin of the symphysis pubis rests on the forefinger is then marked by the nail of the index finger of the other hand and the fingers in the vagina are withdrawn. The nail of the index finger, which is used as the marker, is held firmly in place until the distance between it and the tip of the second finger is measured (b). The distance is the length of the diagonal conjugate.

The **transverse diameter** is the greatest width of the inlet (c).

The **right to left oblique** measurements are the two diagonal diameters from each sacroiliac joint to a point on the pelvic inlet diagonally across from the joint (c).

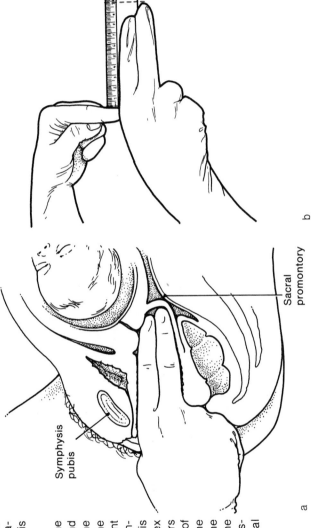

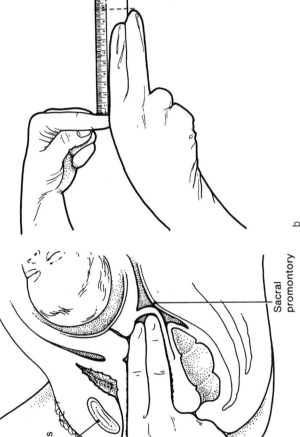

a

Symphysis pubis

Sacral promontory

b

c

Sacral promontory

Sacroiliac joint

Transverse diameter

Ischial spine

Ischial tuberosity

Symphysis pubis

Oblique diameter

Anterior superior iliac spine

Highlights

Numbers given in parentheses are approximations of an adequate pelvic configuration.

The midpelvis cannot be measured precisely by physical examination. However, flat, dull, or blunt ischial spines contribute to a greater diameter.

The transverse diameter is the most important measurement of the outlet because it is the shortest diameter through which the baby must pass as it emerges from the birth canal.

Refer to Chap. 4 for further discussion of the rectovaginal examination.

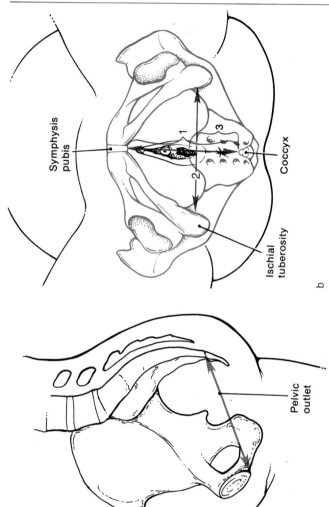

The measurements used to estimate diameters of the plane of the *pelvic outlet* (a) include:

1 Anteroposterior diameter - (b) extends from the middle of the lower margin of the symphysis to the tip of the sacrum (9.5 to 11.5 cm or more).

2 Transverse (intertuberous, bi-ischial) diameter - (b) distance between the inner edges of the ischial tuberosities. This measurement is performed with a pelvimeter (greater than 8 to 10.5 cm)

3 Posterior sagittal diameter - (b) distance between the intertuberous diameter and the tip of the sacrum (7.5 cm). Measured with a pelvimeter.

The examiner now performs a rectovaginal examination. This is done to locate the coccyx and determine its degree of movement (c). Mobility of the coccyx permits its backward displacement during labor, which increases the anteroposterior diameter of the outlet by about 2 cm.

The woman should lie on her left side to relieve pressure on vital organs and the inferior vena cava.

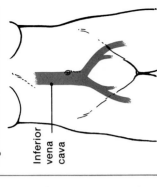

Inferior vena cava

Swelling and pain in the rectal area, and rectal bleeding are common symptoms in pregnancy.

Hemorrhoids may become more pronounced as pregnancy progresses.

Constipation is a common complaint during pregnancy due to hypoperistalsis, abdominal distension, and displacement of the intestines.

Blood volume begins to increase after about 8 to 10 weeks gestation, averaging a peak of about 1,500 ml of which 450 ml are red cells and 1000 ml is plasma. This represents a rise of from 40 to 50 percent over prepregnant levels. Maximum volume expansion of from 25 to 60 percent is reached by 35 to 36 weeks gestation, where it remains constant until after delivery.

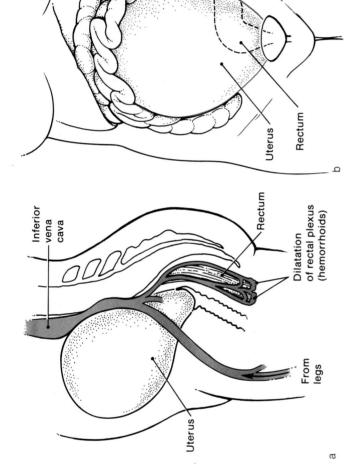

Sigmoid colon

Uterus

Rectum

b

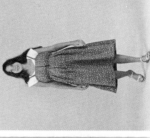
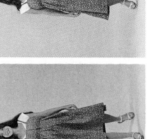
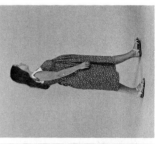
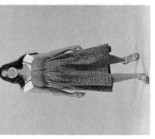

d

Inferior vena cava

Rectum

Dilatation of rectal plexus (hemorrhoids)

Uterus

From legs

a

Cervical lordosis

Dorsal kyphosis

Lumbar lordosis

c

Rectum and Anus

Inspection

The anus should be inspected for presence of hemorrhoids or fissures.

Hemorrhoids can frequently occur in pregnancy due to pressure from the uterus on the venous return from the lower extremities (a). The problem can intensify as pregnancy progresses.

The smooth muscles of the large intestine are more relaxed, causing decreased motility and possibly resulting in constipation.

Palpation

An attempt is made to palpate the rectum. The rectosigmoid colon occupies a large part of the pelvis causing the enlarging uterus to be displaced laterally, rotating to the right on its longitudinal axis. Also, displacement of the intestines by the uterus is common (b).

The smooth muscles of the bowel are more relaxed due to the hormone, progesterone.

Extremities

Physical examination includes peripheral-vascular components, musculoskeletal components, and neurological reflexes.

Inspection

The examiner should observe and assess posture and spinal curvature. Common changes to be noted include lumbar lordosis compensated by accentuation of dorsal kyphosis and cervical lordosis (c).

The examiner may note a waddling gait due to pelvic and postural changes (d).

Highlights

Venous pressure may rise as much as 10 to 30 cm of water during pregnancy.

Musculoskeletal changes result from the enlarged uterus pressing forward and causing muscular distention and forward tilting of the pelvis.

Pain in the buttocks and lower back is a frequent complaint due to hypermobility of pelvic joints.

A brachial plexus traction syndrome may cause numbness in the upper extremities. This is more common in early morning and at night.

Hyperreflexia may be an ominous sign during pregnancy.

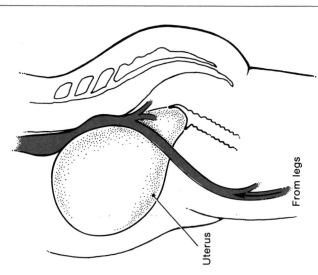

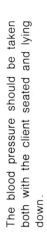

From legs

Uterus

b

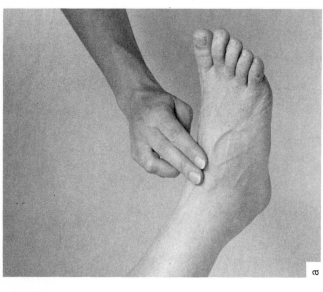

a

Palpation

The examiner should palpate the lower extremities (a). Edema in the lower extremities, a common finding, is not an ominous sign unless it occurs with headache, increased blood pressure, and albuminuria.

Numbness and tingling of the hands and fingers, which can progress to partial anesthesia, may be noted in the upper extremities. Leg cramps and numbness in the lateral femoral area may be due to a calcium-phosphorous imbalance or to nerve compression.

The examiner should check reflexes early in pregnancy to establish a baseline. Reflexes should remain unchanged as gestation progresses.

The blood pressure should be taken both with the client seated and lying down.

The systolic blood pressure is usually unchanged. The diastolic blood pressure is slightly decreased due to a decrease in peripheral resistance.

Venous pressure seems to increase significantly in the lower extremities when the client assumes a supine, sitting, or standing position. This is due to pressure on pelvic veins and the inferior vena cava by the enlarging uterus (b). The examiner should look for a fall in blood pressure, and edema, especially in the feet and legs.

PHYSICAL CHANGES DURING EACH MONTH OF PREGNANCY —MATERNAL, EMBRYOLOGICAL, AND FETAL

The format of this section varies from the rest of the physical examination section; maternal changes can be noted on the left, and embryological or fetal changes on the right of each page.

Physical examination up to this point has focused on changes occurring in the anatomical structures of the pregnant female. To assess the client more thoroughly during prenatal examinations, it is necessary for the examiner to also focus on unique physical changes which occur progressively in the client and embryo-fetus during each month of pregnancy. There are 10 lunar months (28 days each) in pregnancy. Gestational weeks of the embryo-fetus begin at the time of conception, or the second week of the first lunar month. Therefore, using conceptual age, the actual length of gestation is 38 weeks, or 9.5 lunar months.

First Month

The physical examination during the first month of pregnancy reveals no objective criteria with which to diagnose pregnancy, because physical changes do not appear as early as hormonal changes.

The diagnosis of pregnancy is difficult to make before the second missed period.

Positive biologic tests for pregnancy are accurate in 95 to 98 percent of cases, when they are taken about 2 weeks after the first missed period. At this time, the trophoblast begins to elaborate large quantities of HCG (human chorionic gonadotropin).

The pregnant female usually suspects pregnancy after the first missed menstrual period. She may come to the examiner for care at any time after this (a).

Conception to Embryo
Embryo (1 to 4 weeks gestation).

Fertilization initiates the first of three stages of human prenatal development: zygote, embryo, and fetus.

At ovulation the *ovum* is shed. Once the ovum is fertilized by a sperm the chromosomes intermingle (1). The ovum is now a single-cell *zygote*. By about 3 days a solid ball of about 16 cells is present called the *morula* (2). On the fourth day the morula is transformed into a *blastocyst* (3). Fertilization fluid from the uterus has entered the cavity. The blastocyst has an *outer cell mass* of trophoblastic tissue and an *inner cell mass* which eventually becomes the embryo, amnion, and yolk sac.

On the sixth day the blastocyst attaches to the endometrium of the uterus (4). After implantation, *trophoblastic* proliferation continues, and by 11 days a sluggish placental circulation is established on the maternal side.

During the second week the inner cell mass differentiates further into the bilaminar *embryonic disk* which consists of the ectoderm and endoderm. These germ layers give rise to the embryo; the embryonic disk lies between the amnion and the primitive yolk sac (5).

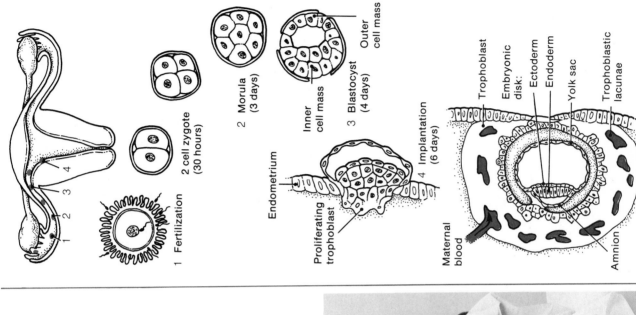

1 Fertilization

2 cell zygote
(30 hours)

2 Morula
(3 days)

Inner cell mass

3 Blastocyst
(4 days)

Outer cell mass

Endometrium

Proliferating trophoblast

4 Implantation
(6 days)

Maternal blood

Amnion

Trophoblast

Embryonic disk:
Ectoderm
Endoderm

Yolk sac

Trophoblastic lacunae

a

Embryo

The third week of life is significant in the transformation of the disk into a trilaminar embryonic disk with the development of the mesoderm (1). This begins the *period of organogenesis* which lasts through the eighth week. Primary germ layers evolve and the embryo gradually changes to human form.

By the end of the third week the *syncytiotrophoblast* gives rise to the primitive utero-placental circulation (2).

Nervous system and vital organs develop. Liver cells aggregate. The thyroid gland begins forming. Stomach, liver, and pancreas are defined. Lung buds may be seen. Building blocks for muscles form. Heart and blood vessels form. Kidney structure develops. The gallbladder appears.

By the end of the first month the embryo is about ¼ inch long. The embryo has curved forward on its long axis so that the head and tail almost meet. Anatomical structures and systems are in rudimentary form (3).

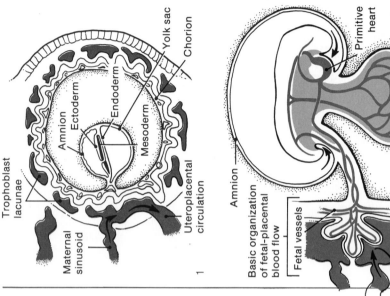

Trophoblast lacunae

Amnion
Ectoderm
Endoderm
Mesoderm

Yolk sac

Chorion

Maternal sinusoid

Uteroplacental circulation

1

Amnion

Primitive heart

Yolk sac

Basic organization of fetal-placental blood flow

Fetal vessels

Chorion

Maternal vessel

2

Lung bud

Heart

Gut

To placenta

3

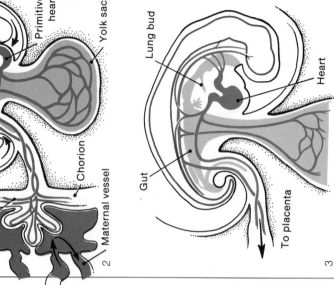

Spiral arteries

Uterine gland

a

During the first month of pregnancy women may have "subjective" signs such as:

1 Amenorrhea at 2 weeks

2 Morning sickness (nausea and vomiting at 3 to 5 weeks

3 Early breast changes at 3 to 4 weeks (heaviness, soreness, tingling)

These are considered "presumptive" signs of pregnancy.

Positive lab tests are considered *probable signs* of pregnancy.

There are no objective findings apparent on physical examination at this time to confirm the diagnosis of pregnancy, but tremendous growth changes are occurring in the embryo.

The uterus is already beginning to enlarge due to hypertrophy and hyperplasia of its muscle fibers, together with an increase in its elastic tissue. Blood vessels are also enlarging and engorging (a).

Embryo (4 to 8 weeks gestation)

During the second month the embryo grows by hyperplasia, differentiation, and specialization. All major organ systems will be formed.

There are no objective criteria to evaluate the well-being of the embryo at this stage.

Significant changes in development occur day-to-day (1 and 2).

Day 31
Muscles appear in pelvic region. Arms and legs form as protruding buds. Spinal cord nerve roots form. Optic stalk appears in brain. Stomach and esophagus begin. Cardiac valves appear. Germ cells move toward genital ridges.

Day 32
More pelvic muscle blocks appear.

Day 33
The brain is a series of fine cavities lined with embryonic nerve tissue. The cerebral cortex can be seen. Ear pits can be seen on the side of the head.

Day 34
More tail muscles form.

Day 35
Germ cells arrive along the embryonic kidney ridge. The olfactory lobe is present. Jaws are forming. The pituitary gland is forming. Spleen and liver ducts form. Intestines elongate. Cavities form for heart, brain, and viscera.

Day 36
All muscle blocks have appeared. Arm and leg buds are formed. There are fetal movements, but they are imperceptible by the woman.

Day 37
Intestines begin to bend. Outer ear chamber closes. Brain stem recognizable.

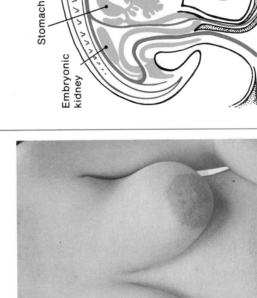

External view — Limb buds, Optic cup, Amnion, Yolk sac, Umbilical cord

Internal view — Spinal cord, Brain, Liver, Stomach, Heart, Embryonic kidney

Second Month

During the second month of pregnancy the number of presumptive and probable signs increase.

If the client has come to the examiner for prenatal examination, the following should be noted:

1 During the first 8 weeks of pregnancy the uterus remains a pelvic organ.

2 Urinary frequency occurs due to increased bladder sensitivity and to pressure on the bladder from the enlarging uterus (a).

3 Breast symptoms include progressive fullness and sensitivity. Striations may appear, glands of Montgomery enlarge, and the nipple and areola pigment (b).

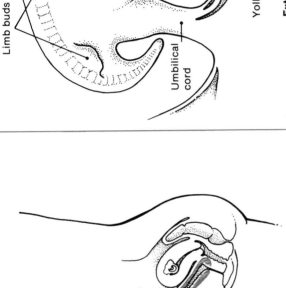

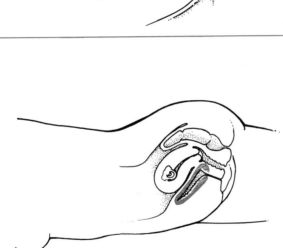

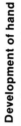

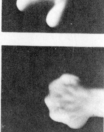

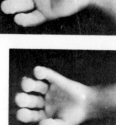

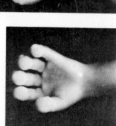

Day 38

Upper and lower jaw parts begin to fuse. Eye muscles begin to form. Rudiments of hands develop (1).

Day 39

Nerve fibers connect with olfactory lobe and lay the groundwork for sensation of smell.

Day 40

Eyes become pigmented. Teeth and facial muscles begin to form. Diaphragm forms. Limbs, back, and abdominal muscles form. Heart begins partitioning into chambers. Liver takes over red blood cell manufacturing from the yolk sac.

Day 42

Early reflexes begin. Rudiments of fingers and toes become evident (2). First traces of undifferentiated gonads appear. In the male, the penis begins to form.

The *seven-week* embryo is 4/5 inch long.

All fingers are present (2). Ears and eyes develop rapidly. Body muscles organize.

Source: J. Dickason and M. Schult, *Maternal and Infant Care*, 2d ed., McGraw-Hill, New York, 1979.

Ear

Eye

Nose

Limbs

1

Development of hand

5 weeks

6 weeks

7 weeks

12 weeks

2

Cornua

a

b

c

On pelvic examination the following changes should be noted by the examiner.

1 *Goodell's sign,* softening of the cervix, is present at 5 to 6 weeks.

2 *Piskacek's sign* can be noted at about 6 weeks (a). The uterus is palpated as asymmetric, with softening at the cornua when the ovum has implanted there.

3 *Braun-Fernwald's sign* can be noted at about 6 to 7 weeks (b). One lateral half of the uterus is softer than the other throughout its length, and there may be a groove separating the soft and firm halves.

4 *Ladin's sign,* early softening of the uterus, can be noted at 5 to 6 weeks. A soft spot on the midline of the uterus between the corpus and the cervix occurs.

5 *Hegar's sign* is noted between 6 and 8 weeks (c). The examiner places two fingers of one hand behind the cervix in the posterior vaginal fornix, then compresses the lower part of the corpus anteriorly by retropubic pressure with the other hand. A distinct area of uterine softening is noted between the two structures, the fundus above and the cervix below.

Day 44
Eye retina nerve cells form. Palate of mouth forms. Ear canals form

Day 46
Gonads (ovaries and testes) have differentiated. Nasal passages open to outside. Palate begins to close. Urogenital and rectal passages are separate. The anal membrane, which ruptures during the eighth week to form the anus, appears.

Day 50
The clitoris appears in the female. Ovaries and testes begin to descend.

Day 56
The eyes move from side to front of head.

All facial clefts close. Palate for roof of mouth is forming. Major blood vessels assume their final plan. Stomach moves to its final position.

The *eight-week embryo* is 1¼ inches (30 mm) long, and weighs 1/30 ounce (1 g).

Taste buds form. Hands and feet are well formed. Endocrine glands (thyroid, thymus, and adrenal) are developing. Lungs have lobes and bronchioles. The heart is complete and functioning. Muscles development makes movement possible.

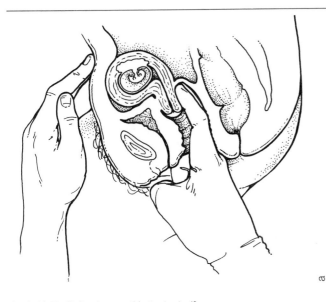

a

6 *McDonald's sign* is noted about 6 weeks. The examiner can easily flex the uterine body and the cervix against one another on bimanual examination (a). This depends on the localized softening responsible for Hegar's sign occurring simultaneously with it.

7 *Chadwick's sign* is noted at about 6 to 8 weeks. The examiner, on inspection, can see the mucous membranes of the vulva, vagina, and cervix take on a bluish-violet hue. This is due to vascular congestion.

Embryo/Fetus (9-12 weeks gestation)

A woman seen for the first time at this stage of pregnancy will show with all the previously described subjective and objective signs.

The major difference at this time is that the examiner can palpate the fundus of the uterus abdominally above the symphysis pubis.

The embryo is now called a *fetus*. The 9-week fetus has a crown to rump length of 1½ inches, and weighs 1/7 ounce.

The examiner palpates the fundus with the client in a supine position. The flat of the fingers and palm are used.

Fingernails, toenails, and hair follicles develop. Irises and eyelids form. When eyelids or palms are touched, they respond by closing, indicating that both nerves and muscles are functioning.

At 12 weeks the fundus is one to two finger breadths above the symphysis pubis (a).

Teeth are beginning to form. The male is distinguished by its penis. The female begins to form a uterus, vagina, and bladder.

The examiner will note that the uterus is no longer pyriform but ovoid by the end of the third month (b). There is symmetrical softening of the entire uterus.

The *10-week fetus* is 2⅝ inches in length, and weighs ¼ ounce.

When assessing the breasts, instruct the client to express colostrum, the precursor of true milk. Periodic expression during pregnancy will prevent clogged milk ducts.

The head is large to accommodate rapid brain growth (1). The palate forms. Thyroid and pancreas are complete. Lungs are complete. The gallbladder is secreting bile. Bones are forming everywhere (2). Blood is beginning to form in the bone marrow. Secondary external sex characteristics are further refined.

The *11-week fetus* is 2½ inches long and weighs 1/3 ounce.

Tooth buds for 20 temporary teeth appear. Vocal cords begin to form. The liver starts to pour bile into the intestines. Islets of Langerhans in the pancreas begin to form insulin.

The *12-week fetus* is 3 inches long and weighs ½ ounce.

Swallowing and sucking reflexes develop further. Digestive glands are complete. Salivary glands form. Motions of breathing and eating, and general body movement become more purposeful.

Third Month

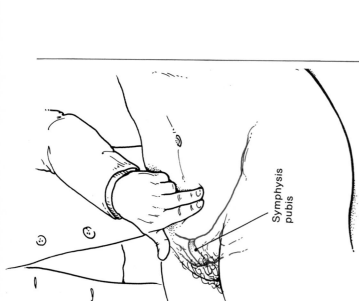

Symphysis pubis

a

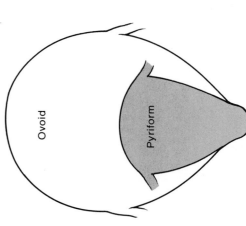

Ovoid

Pyriform

b

Source: J. Dickason and M. Schult, *Maternal and Infant Care*, 2d ed., McGraw-Hill, New York, 1979.

Fetus (13 to 16 weeks gestation).

By the end of the first trimester the fetus has developed all of its major systems.

During the fourth month, the fetus lengthens from 3½ to 6 inches, and its weight increases from 1 to 4 ounces.

The fetal heart is circulating 25 quarts of blood per day. Heart muscles are strong. Lungs are collapsed and inactive.

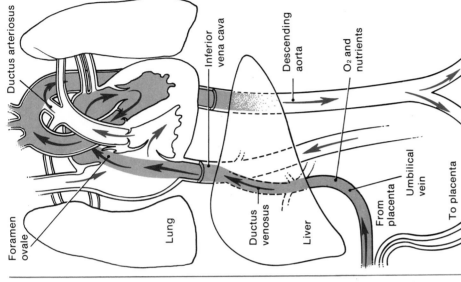

Foramen ovale

Ductus arteriosus

Inferior vena cava

Descending aorta

O_2 and nutrients

Lung

Ductus venosus

Liver

From placenta

Umbilical vein

Umbilical arteries

To placenta

c

Fourth Month

On physical examination the examiner will note:

1 The height of the fundus can be palpated half way between the symphysis and the umbilicus at 16 weeks (a).

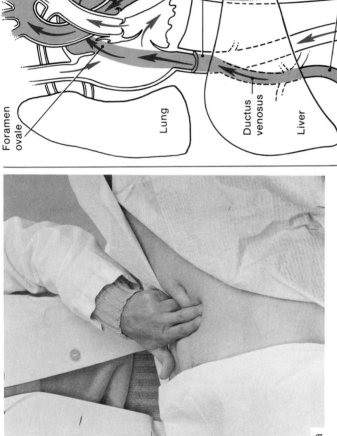

a

b

2 Ballottement of the uterus is possible. Fetal movements are elicited when the anterior vaginal wall and the lower pole of the uterus are tapped sharply upward by two fingers (b). This pushes the fetal body up and it will fall back and be felt as a bump against the fingertip of the examiner.

Pigmentation changes can be noted by the sixteenth week (see skin changes discussed earlier in this chapter).

Fifth Month

Fetus (17 to 20 weeks gestation).

The second trimester is a period of rapid fetal growth, increasing the burden on maternal heart, lungs, and kidneys.

By the end of the fifth month the fetus will measure 8 inches and weigh ½ pound (1).

Vernix caseosa appears. Lanugo develops. Hair can be seen on head, eye-brows, and eyelashes. Pale pink nipples develop over the mammary glands

At 20 weeks the examiner can palpate the fundus at or just below the umbilicus (a).

On auscultation, the uterine bruit will be audible (a rushing sound synchronous with the mother's pulse) and can be heard bilaterally just above the uterus. It is due to increased blood flow to the uterus through the arteries of increased diameter.

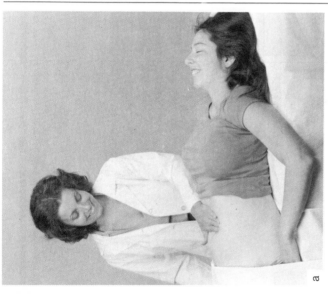

a

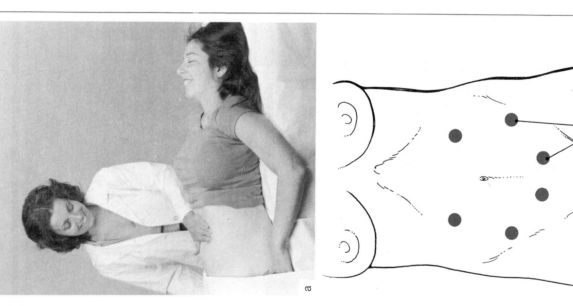

Points of maximum intensity of fetal heartbeat (depends upon position of fetus)

b

Fetal heart sounds are audible on auscultation (b). A rapid tick-tock at a rate of from 120 to 140 beats per minute is the sound of the fetal heart. Fetal heartbeat is a *positive sign of pregnancy.*

The Doppler ultrasound technique may also be used to detect fetal heart tones.

The client should be questioned as to the onset of *quickening*, or presence of fetal movements, which may now be recognized by the woman.

Sixth Month

The examiner can palpate the uterine fundus 1 to 2 fingerbreadths above the umbilicus (a).

Fetus (21 to 24 weeks gestation).

The fetus measures 10 to 12 inches long, and weighs 1 to 1½ pounds.

Hands develop a strong grip. Male testes approach the scrotum. Meconium accumulates in the intestines. Each eye is complete. Eyelids open.

Fat deposits are minimal, and, therefore, skin is wrinkled.

Seventh Month

The examiner can palpate the fundus at a height midway between the umbilicus and the xiphoid (b).

On inspection the examiner notes upward displacement of the diaphragm. Thoracic breathing replaces abdominal breathing.

Auscultation of the fetal heart can be done with a fetascope (c).

Murmurs of maternal heart may be heard on auscultation as cardiac displacement is also occurring in response to the enlarging uterus.

Fetus (25 to 28 weeks gestation).

The fetus measures 12 inches long, and weighs 2 to 3 pounds by 28 weeks (1).

The nervous system can direct breathing and body temperature, but the lungs are still collapsed.

Eyelids reopen. Pupils react to light.

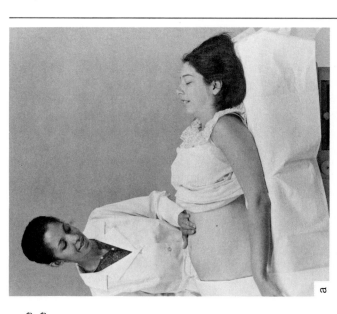

a

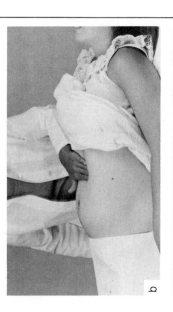

b

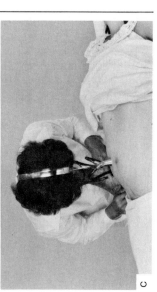

c

Fetus (29 to 32 weeks gestation). The fetus measures 13 inches long, and weighs 3 to 5 pounds.

Rate of weight gain continues. Fat deposits under skin appear.

Fetus (33 to 36 weeks gestation). The fetus measures approximately 13 to 14 inches and weighs 5 to 6 pounds.

Rate of weight gain slows down.

General lanugo is disappearing.

Reflexes which are present include the sucking, rooting, moro, grasp, and stepping reflexes. (See Chap. 5 for reflexes.)

The fetus may assume position for delivery.

Eighth Month

The examiner can palpate the uterine fundus just below the xiphoid and costal margin (a). Fetal heart tones are noted.

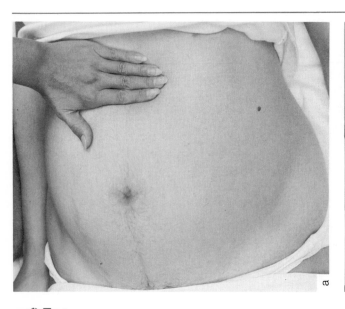

Ninth Month

The examiner can palpate the fundus at the xiphoid and costal margins.

At this time the examiner also palpates the position and lie of the fetus in relation to the mother using *Leopold's maneuvers.*

The first three maneuvers are carried out with the examiner facing the client's head and standing to one side of her as she lies supine on the examining table.

The first maneuver determines what fetal part occupies the fundus.

The examiner palpates the fundal area to ascertain whether it is occupied by a hard, round, mobile head or by an irregular nodular breech (b).

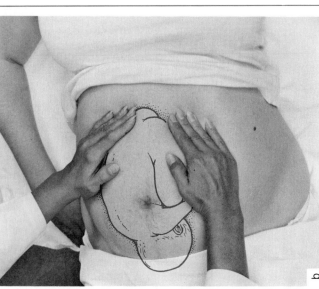

Fetus
Fetal position continues to be evaluated to determine readiness for birthing.

The second maneuver determines which side the fetal back occupies.

Palms of the hands are placed on either side of the abdomen (a). On one side the back feels like a linear bony ridge. On the other side the hands and feet are felt as numerous nodular masses.

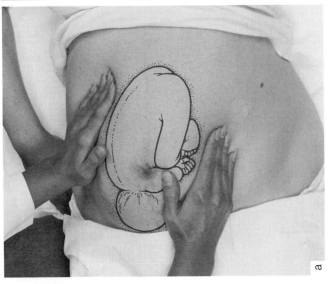

The third maneuver determines what fetal part lies over the pelvic inlet.

A single examining hand is placed just above the symphysis so as to grasp between the thumb and third finger the fetal part that overrides the symphysis (b). If the head is not engaged, it will feel like a round, hard, and smooth object that can easily be displaced or ballotted upward. After engagement, a shoulder is felt as a fixed, knoblike part.

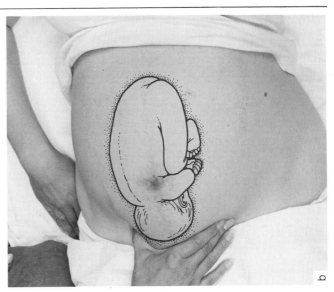

The fourth maneuver determines on which side there is cephalic prominence.

The examiner faces the client's feet and places both hands on either side of the lower pole of the uterus just above the inlet. If the presenting part is floating, this maneuver cannot be done.

When pressure is exerted in the direction of the inlet, one hand can descend further than the other. The part of the fetus that prevents the deep descent of one hand is called the cephalic prominence.

When the head is flexed, the cephalic prominence is on the same side as the hands and feet (a).

When the head is extended, the cephalic prominence is on the same side as the back (b).

Tenth Month

In a primapara, engagement (c) may take place in the 38th week and, therefore, palpation will reveal the fundus below the xiphoid.

A multipara may not engage until the onset of labor.

Leopold's maneuvers are repeated at each weekly examination.

Pelvic examination may be done to evaluate cervical status (effacement and dilatation), to confirm the presenting part, and to establish its station.

The examiner is evaluating the potential for labor beginning, as well as confirming the progress of pregnancy.

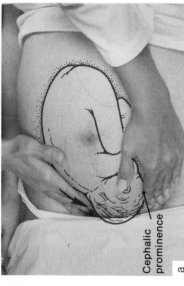

Cephalic prominence

a

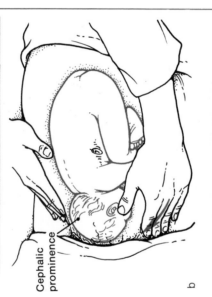

Cephalic prominence

b

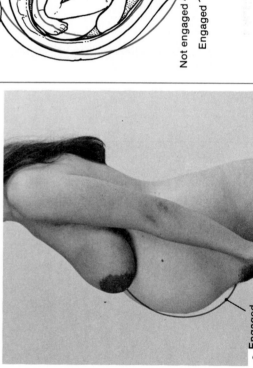

c Engaged

Fetus (37 to 40 weeks gestation)

The fetus now measures 19 to 21 inches long, and weighs 6 to 8 pounds.

Myelination of the brain begins.

More meconium accummulates in the intestines.

Antibodies are acquired from the mother's blood.

Nails grow.

Gums are ridged.

The fetus is less active since there is less space available for movement.

The fetus assumes position for delivery (1).

Testes are in the scrotum.

Labia majora is well developed in the female.

Not engaged

Engaged

1

The gestational period of the fetus is now complete. With the onset of labor the fetus normally progresses through the maternal pelvis, and vaginal delivery of the baby occurs. The full-term baby should be able to successfully complete this transition from intrauterine to extrauterine life (1).

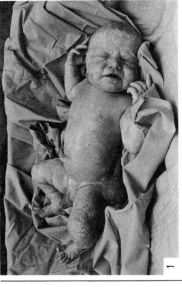

1

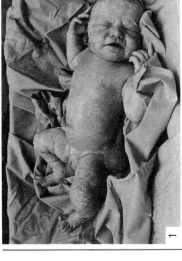

a

The client should be questioned regarding the following subjective symptoms, which may be present at this time:

1 Urinary frequency as the enlarged uterus imposes on the bladder (a)

2 Lightening as the presenting part descends into the pelvis

3 Constipation as the colon is displaced

4 Thoracic breathing

5 A waddling gait as the musculoskeletal system accommodates to the advanced pregnancy

Women will often complain of pelvic heaviness and fatigue as the pregnancy progresses toward term.

When labor begins, this signifies pregnancy is coming to an end.

THE MIDDLE ADULT

**CHAPTER
THIRTEEN**

Mary P. Cadogan

The period of "middle adulthood" is perhaps the most difficult life stage to define chronologically. In contrast to the limits of the spectrum where one is clearly young or old, the middle is more nebulous. Admittedly, few people would have difficulty identifying a person who is "middle aged," but the more difficult task is identification of the beginning and ending of middle adulthood.

Traditionally, the years from 40 to 60 or 65 have been designated as midlife, but this may be changing. Since the mandatory retirement age in the United States increased to 70 years in April 1978, a large number of people will continue "middle-age activities" until age 70. Similarly, some individuals may begin such activities much earlier than age 40, and thus the boundaries continue to blur.

> The age span for middle adulthood is broadly defined between the ages of 40 and 70 years.

On the basis of a current combined average life expectancy of 73.2 years, midlife occurs at age 36.6 years. Future projections suggest a life expectancy of 120 years by the twenty-first century. Although this figure may be exaggerated, the human life cycle is lengthening. A question arises, therefore, as to whether the extra years will be added to the end of the total life span or whether the upper limit of "middle adulthood" will expand to accommodate these added years.

> Currently the average life expectancy is 73.2 years.

Surely factors other than chronological age determine one's place in the life cycle. Acknowledgment of an overlap with young and older adulthood is one way to accommodate the diverse rate of physical, psychological, and developmental changes that occur to individuals in middle adulthood. Emphasis remains, however, on the middle years between the extremes of 30 and 70.

HEALTH HISTORY

For a complete assessment of an individual's level of wellness, all factors which influence health of the middle adult must be thoroughly explored. Such pattern areas as nutrition, developmental status, sexuality, and activity are essential components of the health history in all age groups. The particular importance of investigating each of these functional areas with the middle adult is presented in this chapter.

Establishing a Data Base

As in other age groups, significant changes take place in many areas of any individual's life during the middle years. A comprehensive assessment will help to determine the impact of these changes on the client's present and future state of health.

During midlife many people first become aware that they are growing "old." As the person reaches a stage where the years that have passed are equal to or greater in number than the years remaining, anxiety can increase. Future physical and emotional changes, which are poorly understood but greatly feared by a youth-oriented society, inten-

> It is during the middle years that people first become aware of aging.

sify the problems of the middle years. Through a holistic health history, the nurse will help the client to determine the positive and negative aspects of health, identify fears and concerns about aging, and make the client aware of the need to become actively involved in maintaining and monitoring present and future personal health status.

Client Profile

All data discussed in Chap. 3 are essential for a health history of the middle adult and should be obtained in a similar manner. Of interest is the middle adult's reason for entry into the health care system. Often a client is prompted to accept health care after a traumatic event. For instance, news of a friend or associate having a myocardial infarction or being diagnosed as having a chronic illness may serve as a powerful incentive to seek care.

Refer to Chap. 3 for a discussion of client profile.

These factors require that the nurse not only be sensitive to the concerns of the client, but identify surrounding events that may mimic a client's problems (e.g., chest pain in the absence of a myocardial infarction). Awareness of the concerns of the middle-aged client and increase in one's perception of health may ease the transition through these years.

The middle-aged adult will often seek health care in response to a problem or following the disrupted health state of a peer.

Occupation For a significant percentage of middle adults, work occupies a major portion of time and is a *key* factor influencing one's well-being.

Work occupies much of the middle adult's time.

Definition of the duties and responsibilities of the client's current occupation, the length of time spent in the current position and the number of hours worked weekly, estimation of the level of job satisfaction, and identification of the client's future career goals and plans are all added considerations. Of particular importance in middle age are the risks associated with *sedentary* positions or *repetitive*, timed (assembly-line) jobs.

Health Perception/Health Management

Assessment of the middle-aged client's health state will often reveal a variety of health beliefs and behaviors. Depending on the client's age, health may be viewed as a valued commodity or be something taken for granted. Each person's values and beliefs as related to health are critical to the health practices in which the person engages on a daily basis.

The middle adult should be encouraged to maintain those health practices that enhance the level of wellness. If the individual participates in health habits that could be detrimental to the health state, encouragement should be given to terminate such behaviors. Often this may be difficult to do, especially if the individual has maintained a particular habit (e.g., smoking) for an extended number of years and does not see the value in stopping (refer to discussion of Breslow's health habits in Chap. 1).

For the middle-aged adult, health has a variety of meanings.

For the middle adult, health beliefs are influenced by current trends and attitudes toward health promotion. The younger middle adult may be conscious of changing health practices and pursue them aggressively. Health movements oriented toward physical fitness and optimal wellness may promote a variety of health habits.

Older middle adults exposed to similar information later in life may be influenced to change health practices or be sufficiently comfortable with current health beliefs and resist changing health habits.

Health Habits Clear evidence linking certain health habits with an increased or decreased risk for alteration or disruption of health status appears to be growing. Assessment of these habits, therefore, is an essential component of the health history. During the middle years, special attention should be focused on the following factors:

Smoking. Determine the number of cigarettes smoked per day and the total number of years that the client has smoked, as this is often an established habit by the middle years. Emphasize the harmful effects of smoking to the client and encourage the desire to quit. Identify any previous attempts to quit and assess the reasons for failure.

Assessment of health habits of the middle adult should focus on smoking habits, physical activity, alcohol and food consumption, medications, safety practices, and health promotion behavior.

Physical exercise. Assess the amount and type of physical exercise, and determine whether these are appropriate for the age and health status of the client. Reiterate the need for gradual increase, with warm-up and cooling-down periods before and after activity.

Alcohol consumption. Identify the quantity and type of alcohol ingestion, the use of alcohol as a tension or anxiety reliever, and the relative value of alcohol as a disruptive factor in the client's interpersonal relationships or work. Ascertain any history of "blackouts" as a result of drinking or any previous history of delirium tremens (DT).

Medication use. Identify the use of prescribed drugs (especially estrogen use in women) and tranquilizers as well as nonprescription drugs. During the middle years there is likely to be a high incidence in the use of vitamins, "tonics," and laxatives.

During middle age there is often an increase in the use of vitamins, tonics, and laxatives.

Accident prevention behavior. Determine the use of seat belts, safe driving practices, and alcohol intake during driving; also determine any use or abuse of firearms.

Self-care. Assess the client's awareness of the importance of and ability to perform regular self-examination of breasts, testes, mouth and teeth, pharynx, and skin.

Illness awareness. Determine the client's knowledge of danger signs of potential changes in health that may occur during the middle years, such as signs of impending myocardial infarction and the warning signs of cancer. Also determine the client's or family members' knowledge of cardiopulmonary resuscitation (CPR).

Family History The importance of determining one's family history becomes increasingly significant for the middle adult. This is the stage in life when many inherited diseases have their onset. Indeed, genetic patterns in addition to family health practices are the major etiological factors in most of the leading causes of morbidity and mortality in middle age.

The significance of family history becomes important during middle adulthood since the onset of many inherited diseases occurs at this time.

When obtaining the family history, the following information is most pertinent for middle adults:

1 The age and present state of health of grandparents, parents, siblings, cousins, aunts, and uncles. If a family member is deceased, particular attention should be paid to the cause of death of all family members who died during middle age. Similarly, any increased incidence of certain problems in the family, even those without known genetic links, should be assessed.

Attention should be paid to history surroundings and family members who died during the middle years.

2 Occupations of all family members (or others) with whom the client lived in earlier years should be identified. This is particularly significant if family members were exposed to toxic substances which may have been transferred to the client. The extended latency period of many malignancies related to environmental exposure make this data most important to observe.

Any toxic substances to which family members may have been exposed should be identified.

3 In addition to determining one's risk factors through heredity, the family history is useful in highlighting real or potential stresses for the client. For instance, serious illness of one's spouse would place tremendous physical, psychological, and economic stresses on an individual and would certainly influence one's state of health.

4 Family habits that may positively or negatively influence health such as past and current dietary patterns or unique ways of dealing with health and illness should be carefully analyzed.

Family health habits that have a positive or negative influence on health should be identified.

Life Patterns and Lifestyle

Those patterns that make up the lifestyle of the middle adult are complex. They are often developed over many years and are difficult to change.

Age During the middle years there is an increase in the incidence and prevalence of disease, especially chronic problems. Among these are arthritis, cardiovascular disease and hypertension, diabetes, cancer, obesity, genitourinary disturbances, and problems related to diminished functioning of sensory organs.

In addition, the middle years, often considered to be the most stable period in life, are filled with change. The multiple roles and responsibilities one assumes at this time can be tremendously stressful, yet as these roles are lost, grief and depression frequently occur.

Refer to Roles and Relationship Patterns section discussed later in this chapter.

Heredity While heredity occupies a major role in determination of the risk of an individual for developing disease or disability in middle age, heredity may also have a more subtle influence on one's health state. Parents and grandparents undoubtedly remain role models (either positive or negative) throughout life. Surely one's adaption to new roles will be influenced by the behavior of significant others who have assumed the same roles. For example, one's image of the duties and responsibilities of being a grandparent may be established on the basis of an individual's recollection of his or her own grandparent.

Heredity includes both genetic determination and role models provided by older adults within the family unit.

The pattern and response of a mother to menopause may affect the time of occurrence of her daughter's menopause and her adjustment to the many changes occurring at that time. General response to "being a middle-aged adult" will also reflect familial patterns, including engagement in activities "proper" for middle adults, determination of when one *is* middle-aged, and establishment of future patterns as one observes the lifestyle of parents and other family members as they continue the aging process.

Culture Various cultures define middle age differently. When obtaining a health history, the nurse must carefully examine the influence of ethnic and religious influences on one's adjustment to middle adulthood.

The initial assessment should include information regarding the client's definition of what it actually means to be "middle-aged." For example, in cultures where advancing age is revered and elders are consulted for their advice and wisdom, one looks forward to the prestige and rewards which can be expected in the middle and later years. If, however, one is a part of a culture which idealizes youth and disdains aging, the arrival of the middle years may signal real or imagined doom.

If a culture reveres their elderly, aging is something to anticipate positively.

The nurse should investigate the client's expectations of the implications of changes which occur during the middle years. In some cultures, people firmly believe that the need and capacity for sexual expression and fulfillment disappears with the arrival of menopause. This idea is encouraged within religious groups which hold the view that the sole purpose of sexual activity is procreation.

Ethnicity is another important factor which contributes to one's predisposition to certain middle-age diseases. Awareness of the incidence and prevalence of major diseases among various ethnic groups is a vital component of comprehensive health assessment. In addition to eliciting information on risk factors for certain diseases, it is important to ask clients about any special fears they may have regarding certain diseases which may appear within a particular group. The onset of "cardiac phobia" may occur in middle-aged men in the United States as cardiovascular disease remains the leading cause of death for men during the middle years. Analysis of risk factors and identification of methods for modifying harmful factors may help to allay an individual's particular fears.

The nurse should explore ethnic and other influences which will *enhance* clients' health state. Traditional remedies for "ailments" of middle age should be identified (e.g., herbal treatments for symptoms of menopause). Similarly, an assessment of group supports for middle adults should be included as part of the health history. Religious practices and beliefs as well as other cultural traditions may be a source of stability during some of the crises of the middle years and should be identified.

Any cultural remedies for ailments that accompany middle age (e.g., herbal treatments for menopause) should be explored during the health history.

Growth and Development To people who are not middle-aged, this life stage is regarded as one of extreme stability, to be handled with ease. But those who are middle adults know only too well the psychological impact of the many significant changes that occur during this period.

In order to fully understand and assess the impact of such changes on middle adults, it is helpful to first consider the developmental tasks of midlife.

Erikson[1] has designated the task of middle adults as "generativity versus stagnation." [Refer to Chapters 3 and 14 for further discussion.] Stevenson has expanded this concept and has divided the period of middle adulthood into two "middlescence" phases, each with specific developmental tasks. The "core of the middle years" (Middlescence I) is 30 to 50 years and the "new middle years" (Middlescence II) covers the years 50 to 70.

Erikson has designated the task of middle adult as "generativity versus stagnation."

Stevenson expanded the period of middle adulthood to:

1 Period I (30 to 50 years)— "core of the middle years"
2 Middlescence II (50 to 70)—"new middle years"

Developmental Tasks of Middlescence I Stevenson[2] describes the tasks of this phase as follows:

1 "Developing socioeconomic consolidation." By middle adulthood economic and social patterns are well determined. Roots have been put down and continue to be nurtured during this time. For some people, financial security is attained and may well continue. For others, particularly the unemployed or poor, patterns have been likewise established which become increasingly difficult to change as the years pass.

2 "Evaluating one's occupation or career in light of a personal value system." Career changes are not uncommon in middle age. Ideals toward which one strove in earlier years are reassessed more realistically. Previously determined goals are challenged as younger employees introduce new ideas and which challenge value systems. The awareness of middle age brings to light the question of one's purpose in life and is often accompanied by a decision to "get off the treadmill" and "really live." Social changes, most notably the women's liberation movement, have caused many women to reevaluate their roles. The number of middle-aged women choosing to work outside the home during this period is rapidly increasing.

Stages of Middlescence I include:
1 Developing socioeconomic consolidation
2 Evaluating one's occupation or career in light of personal value system
3 Helping younger persons
4 Enhancing or redeveloping intimacy with spouse or others
5 Developing a few deep friendships
6 Helping aging persons
7 Assuming responsible positions
8 Maintaining or improving the home environment
9 Creative use of leisure time
10 Adjusting to biological and personal life changes

One's purpose in life is brought to light during the middle years.

3 "Helping younger persons (e.g., biologic offspring) to become integrated human beings." As people continue to delay childbearing until the early or middle thirties, this task of actual child rearing that we tend to associate with the period of young adulthood may be extended to the middle years. For the most part, however, this task represents a time for "letting go" of children and for encouraging them to develop ideas and ideals of their own. This task is also expanded to include relationships with young adults who are not biologic offspring. The role of mentor is being increasingly recognized as an important stage in adult development (for both the mentor and the "mentee"). Early middle age is the time when one stops being mentored and begins to mentor. Although this is most commonly considered in terms of occupation or career, social mentorship is a significant application of this concept.

4 "Enhancing or redeveloping intimacy with spouse or most significant other." The activities of young adulthood (active childrearing and career development and advancement) often slow down in the middle years. People then begin to recognize the need to redirect energy toward relationships with the spouse or significant others, which may have been previously neglected or taken for granted. There is increasing awareness of the need to share the excitement and apprehension of a new life stage with a caring, understanding partner. A less subtle message centers around the realization of advancing years and the need to renew and enhance significant relationships "before it's too late."

5 "Developing a few deep friendships." As indicated above, previous demands of family life and career lessen and the focus on self-development increases. Spending time with friends is imperative for expansion of one's horizons, increase of self-esteem, and for combating the loneliness that can occur when activities revolving around a previous lifestyle have ceased.

6 "Helping aging persons (e.g., parents or in-laws) progress through the later years of life." As family size decreases and social mobility increases, helping aging persons becomes increasingly important for middle adults. Financial burdens which may have been shared by several offspring in the past often now become the responsibility of one or two people. Similarly, social relationships with aging parents can be hampered by physical distance. Guilt surrounding the responsibilities and obligations for ensuring the best arrangements for parents is exceedingly common for middle adults. Counseling with all family members is most useful, particularly with a focus on anticipation of needs rather than crisis intervention.[3] The nurse should attempt to identify any anxieties or underlying motivations which may influence decision making or augment guilt. For example, caring for one's aging parents may represent insurance for some middle adults who hope that by "paying their dues" they will be guaranteed similar care during their later years.

7 "Assuming responsible positions in occupational, social and civic activities, organizations, and communities." Middle adults frequently serve as the decision makers of society. This is the stage that the previous years have prepared one for. Emphasis changes from striving *toward* these positions of responsibility to *maintaining* them. Inherent in positions of authority are the stresses of productivity and accountability. Counseling and anticipatory guidance must focus on the need to share the burdens of responsibility and recognize realistic goals and abilities. Assessment of this phase is critical.

8   "Maintaining and improving the home or other forms of property." Physical and financial hardships may weigh heavily on the middle adult who is involved in this task. It may be overlooked by the nurse but can be a major problem for the client. Frequently, ambivalence over whether to sell one's property occurs, and is often overwhelming. Attention should be directed toward helping the client to explore the benefits of all alternatives before reaching a decision.

9   "Using leisure time in satisfying and creative ways." Use of leisure time was discussed previously (Chap. 3) but is reemphasized here as a developmental task on which middle adults will continually work. In the early middle years, the issue may be making time in one's schedule for leisure time. With advancing years, emphasis is changed to deal with increased availability of leisure time. In addition to ensuring satisfaction in the middle years, creative use of leisure time is an imperative aspect of anticipating guidance which should be discussed with middle adults in preparation for the later years.

Refer to Chap. 3 under Exercise Activity Patterns for discussion of leisure time.

10 "Adjusting to biological or personal system changes that occur." Successful adjustment to the multiple changes occurring in middle age is enhanced through understanding of and preparation for these changes. The nurse is responsible for educating the client and, more importantly, for advising the client of all the ways in which health habits and physical and psychological adjustment can enhance one's lifestyle.

All the developmental tasks mentioned above continue to be refined and integrated throughout the later middle years. Stevenson makes this evident through the tasks outlined for the new middle years (age 50 through 70).

Adaptation of the multiple changes occurring during the middle years is eased through understanding and preparation.

Developmental Tasks of Middlescence II[4] Additional tasks associated with the "new middle years" (Middlescence II) include:

1   Maintaining flexible views in occupational, civic, political, religious, and social positions; avoiding rigidity.

2   Keeping current on relevant scientific, political, and cultural changes.

3   Developing mutually supportive (interdependent) relationships with grown offspring and other members of the younger generation.

4   Reevaluating and enhancing the relationship with spouse or significant other or adjusting to their loss.

5   Helping aged parents or other relatives progress through the last stage of life.

6   Deriving satisfaction from increased availability of leisure time.

7   Preparing for retirement and planning another career when feasible.

8   Adjusting self and behavior to signals of accelerated aging processes.

Tasks associated with Middlesence II include keeping current with socioeconomic changes, developing supportive relationships, helping aged parents, and preparing for retirement.

Biological Rhythms *Sleep-Wakefulness Patterns* For the middle adult, gradual changes in the sleep patterns develop in earlier life and continue through middle adulthood. Specifically, total sleep time decreases, with a particular decrease in the amount of Stage IV sleep. The number of sleep arousals increases, and the percentage of time in bed spent awake begins to increase.[5] This will be exaggerated in people who follow previously established sleep patterns after their sleep requirements have decreased.

Because of the multiple changes and stresses in middle age, sleep disturbances are common. However, any sleep aberration should be investigated to exclude the possibility of underlying anxiety or depression which can be reflected by difficulty in falling asleep, early-morning awakening, or alternatively, hypersomnia. Sleeping pills or other aids may be used by middle adults, and such use should be determined during the health history.

Elimination Patterns Bowel patterns may change in middle age. A decrease in frequency of bowel movements may occur as a result of decrease in gastrointestinal motility and a decline in physical activity levels. Increase in the use of laxatives during the middle years may be present and should be assessed by the nurse.

Urinary frequency and nocturia are commonly experienced particularly by late-middle-aged men, as a result of mechanical compression of the urethra from an enlarged prostrate gland. In addition, the use of medications (e.g., diuretics) may alter urinary patterns. These changes may result in increased urinary frequency.

Environment Assessment of safety factors in the home should address the use of such items as smoke detectors and fire extinguishers as well as safety practices, including home fire drills. For middle-aged adults, information about home chores and repairs should be included in the assessment. In this age group, overzealous attempts to undertake strenuous chores may be fatal. Similarly, the use of time- and energy-saving tools and appliances should be discussed with special focus on safety.

Neighborhood In addition to seeking information about his or her living area, details of the condition and safety of the client's neighborhood must be obtained.

The proximity of potential environmental pollutants or other hazards in the area should be identified. Factors such as chemicals and refuse from power plants, oil refineries and metal smelters; the use of pesticides in the area; contaminated water sources; and the amount of automobile traffic and proximity to an airport should be identified. The length of exposure should be isolated as it may impact on the health of the middle-aged client.

The safety of one's neighborhood, including adequacy and availability of police protection and emergency health care assistance, should also be examined. Homicide remains a leading cause of death in middle age, especially with the poor, primarily non-white people, living in urban areas. Violent crimes of rape, burglary, and assault occur in all age groups, and clients should be recognized so that preventive tactics and safety practices can be instituted.

Occupational Hazards Because of the long latency periods of many health problems, middle adulthood is the time when the extended exposure to environmental toxins takes its toll. Past or present exposure to substances such as coal dust, asbestos, vinyl chloride, and plutonium as well as radiation must be assessed. In addition, past and present exposure of other family members to such substances should be determined.

Each client's risk for occupational injuries should be determined.

During the middle years there is a decrease in Stage IV sleep.

Identification of pollutants and safety factors affecting the neighborhood is important when assessing the middle-aged client.

Occupational hazards (e.g., pollutants) as well as easy access to substances (e.g., drugs) may increase the risk of potential occupational risk factors.

Availability of safety provisions and adequate health supervision should be investigated with this age group.

Other less obvious hazards must also be noted. For example, certain health professions are associated with an increased incidence of particular health disorders.[6] Individuals who have occupational access to drugs (e.g., pharmacists, nurses, physicians, and pharmaceutical salespeople) may have increased opportunity for substance abuse.

Nearly every occupation has some hazards, and careful questioning must be done to ascertain an individual's occupational risks.

Economic Patterns The middle years are very often a time of economic security. Usually, children have grown and become financially independent. However, care of aging parents as well as illness or death of one's spouse are examples of financial burdens often encountered in middle adulthood. Additionally, middle age is the time when people must scrimp and save in an attempt to ensure economic stability in the later years. Therefore, this area should be carefully assessed to determine the impact of economic stress on lifestyle.

Community Resources After assessment of one's life patterns, the nurse should be sure that the client is aware of community resources available for various needs. For a middle adult, these needs might include programs for smoking control, weight reduction, and alcoholic treatment programs, as well as educational organizations such as national heart, lung, and cancer associations. Free or low-cost health screening programs should also be identified and access to emergency services clearly established.

Roles and Relationship Patterns

The traditional concept of "the empty nest syndrome" is rapidly being redefined. Largely related to women in the past, this syndrome may now be experienced by men who have assumed a major responsibility for child rearing in the marriage or in the case of single, widowed, or divorced fathers.

Childless couples or working parents who have established social networks outside the family will less likely be affected than will people whose energy and emotions have been entirely devoted to children. For many people, however, middle adulthood becomes a time of overextending themselves into multiple roles.

Understanding one's potentials and limitations becomes easier for both the nurse and the client. Boredom, fatigue, and anxiety may be alleviated merely by adding or eliminating activities or changing activities to maximize time spent on enjoyable activities and minimize time spent on tedious or dreaded activities. (See discussion on Activity Patterns.)

Family Middle adulthood is usually the time when roles within a family are most expansive. It is now that the client may have the potential of being someone's spouse, parent, grandparent or possibly great-grandparent, or uncle or aunt, as well as son or daughter, sibling, niece or nephew, and so on. With each of these roles comes responsibility.

Information should be gathered regarding the quality of relationships with significant family members. Often later middle age is a time of reexamination of the relationship with one's spouse, which becomes significant as children move away from home. Many couples find increased enjoyment in the new privacy. They are now free of parenting

Substance abuse is associated more frequently with persons who have greater access to drugs.

Many middle-aged adults participate in multiple roles during this time.

Many couples find that middle years are a time for increased privacy and self-fulfillment and development of personal interests.

responsibilities and can become involved in developing other areas of interest either individually or together. Those couples who have remained together "for the sake of the children" may now realize that they have little in common and may decide to separate.

Relationships between middle-aged parents and their grown children often change and mature. Similarly, relationships with aging parents are frequently deepened and enriched during one's middle years.

Societal Relationships The influence of the women's liberation movement has drastically influenced the ideas and aspirations of many middle-aged women and men. As a result, previously accepted roles are being challenged. In addition, there are a limited number of new role models available. Therefore, confusion and uncertainty exist for many people. Adults may find themselves dealing with many social changes initiated by other age groups. One notable example is the decision of many young couples to postpone childbearing or to choose not to have children, thus postponing or eliminating the prospect of some middle adults becoming grandparents. The result can be devastating for some and for others, totally acceptable.

This unchartered journey is made alone as breakdown of the extended family and increased mobility of young adults occurs. The potential for social isolation and loneliness as well as increased freedom may result.

Many middle-aged adults experience conflict as society emphasizes the need to meet one's own needs whereas they perceive their role as meeting the needs of others.

Emphasis on "doing one's own thing" is now a predominant theme. Many middle adults may have to be given the "permission" to do so. For individuals who have felt and continue to feel that their major role in life is service to others (children, elderly parents, etc.), focus on meeting one's own needs is often accompanied by guilt.

The nurse is in an excellent position to discuss the impact of social changes on each client's life. Attention to feelings of anxiety, disappointment, or guilt will allow the client to vocalize such feelings and will assist the nurse in identifying useful methods of dealing with these "by-products" of social change.

Identification of social supports such as community groups are useful and necessary. The breakdown of stereotypes and roles will enable clients to realize the potential for full and rewarding middle years.

Self-Perception and Self-Concept Patterns

Adapting to the inevitable changes of aging is not easily accomplished in a society which equates beauty with youth. For people whose sense of self-esteem has been based primarily on physical appearance, the transition to middle adulthood is extremely difficult. This is complicated even more for people whose occupation centers around physical appearance (dancers, models, actors and actresses, etc.), where changes due to aging may mean unemployment.

For adults who have equated self-esteem with physical appearance, middle age may be a difficult period.

During middle adulthood disturbed body self-image may be reflected by a compulsion to retain a youthful appearance through cosmetics, face lifts, hair transplants, hair coloring, or "youthful" hair styles. Additionally, wearing clothing designed for much younger or much older people may also reflect an altered self-image. There is a fine line between maintaining pride in one's appearance and trying to totally conceal the normal changes of aging.

Investigation of one's reactions to ongoing bodily changes is an integral part of the holistic health history. Such practical advice as exercising to increase muscle tone and circulation to the skin can do much to allay fears and help an individual to adapt to the physical changes that normally occur in middle age less stressfully.

Health and Self-Concept Generally, women have fewer health problems than do men during the middle years. Excluding diabetes, which is more common in women than men during this period, most of the other major acute and chronic illnesses show a significantly higher incidence in men. The question of whether women have been biologically or socially protected from certain diseases remains unanswered. Current evidence suggests that as women assume the same occupational and social roles and habits as men, the incidence of certain diseases accelerates. This may be stress-related and associated with leadership positions.

Men and women may respond differently to the actual fact of being middle-aged. In this society where women are considered beautiful when young and slender but unattractive as the changes of age take their toll, it is understandable that many women are disturbed with advancing age. While similar feelings may be true for men, they at least have the approval of society, which considers aging changes in men to be attractive signs of maturity.

Cognitive and Perceptual Patterns

As the adult ages, cognitive patterns may change and grow. This is influenced by life experiences as well as educational preparation.

Educational Preparations The early middle years may be a time when one strives toward satisfying ambitions or competing with younger employees in the job market. Often this involves returning to school to obtain additional credentials. For some people, readjustment to school is difficult. Financial burdens are often heavy, and the strain of combining education with a full-time job is difficult.

As the years progress, educational level as a means to an end becomes less important. However, education may be pursued as an end in itself for self-development or achievement of previously denied aspirations often unrelated to one's career.

Intelligence During the middle years the adult continues to grow intellectually. Life experiences gained through daily contact with occupation, society, friends, and relatives all contribute to the "wisdom of age." Additional knowledge can also be gained through educational pursuit and exploration of personal interests. A person's ability to solve problems expands as available solutions increase.

Sensory Perception The number of functioning neurons begins to decline at about age 25 years. Throughout the succeeding years degenerative changes occur in all the sense organs. Normally, these degenerative changes are gradual. As the individual progresses through the middle years, these changes may become more obvious and can threaten one's self-concept if not discussed and perceived as normal by the client.

Vision Age-associated changes in vision are largely the result of changes in the lens. *Presbyopia* (far-sightedness) occurs in the fourth to fifth decades as a result of decreased flexibility of the lens, causing inability to focus accurately. This change is evidenced by diminished near vision and can occur in people who have never previously had vision problems. Some people find that they need reading glasses for close work, while others must make the switch to bifocals.

Thickening of the lens causes three additional changes: these include diminished visual acuity, lengthening of the time period for visual adjusting from light to dark environment, and decreased peripheral vision.

Yellowing of the lens makes it more difficult for a person to discern certain color intensities, especially the cool colors (blue, green, and violet)

Generally, women are less ill than men during the middle years.

Physical changes of aging may be considered positive for males and less so for females.

Learning continues through the middle years.

Sensory changes may occur gradually during the middle years.

Visual changes associated with aging are often due to changes in the lens.

Thickening of the eye lens results in diminished visual acuity. Increased time is needed to adjust to changes in light, and decreased peripheral vision may also occur.

which are filtered out. Warm colors (yellow, red, and orange) are generally seen more easily.[7]

Hearing Presbycusis (impaired auditory acuity) usually begins during middle age with loss of high-pitched frequencies (above speech frequencies). This is due to progressive degeneration of the sensory hair cells, supporting cells, and the strial vascularis of the cochlea. Therefore, clients may not report any hearing loss in early middle age. However, in later middle age and after, atrophy occurs in the neurons of the cochlea, causing inability to hear middle frequencies (containing most speech sounds) and lower frequencies.[8] Exposure to harmful environmental noise (e.g., occupational noise) will cause an earlier and more pronounced loss of auditory acuity.

Taste There may be a slight decrease in taste sensitivity due to atrophy of the papillae of the lateral edges of the edges of the tongue in persons past the age of 45.[9] This will not become obvious until the later middle years. Frequently, weight loss in this group as well as the elderly can be associated with a loss in one's taste for food. Since each individual's taste perception is unique, changes in one's diet may be needed to respond to those taste perceptions still present.

Sexuality and Reproduction Patterns

Factors influencing sexuality in middle adulthood are numerous. Most pervasive is the myth that sexual needs and desires cease when one makes the transition from "youth" to middle age. However, sexual satisfaction will be affected by such considerations as availability of partners, menopause, reliable and safe contraceptive devices, and information about physical capability and sexual behavior considered "normal" in the middle years.

Simply stated, sexual needs in middle age do not differ significantly from those in earlier years. Variations do occur, however, including the fact that women's interest in and desire for sex often rises after age 35 while men's interest either remains stable or decreases slightly. Of course, this is not a standard, and sexual needs remain very individualized.

During the middle years emphasis on sex for procreation is replaced by emphasis on sex for recreation, thereby changing the focus and purpose of sexual activity. In midlife, sex is often less directed toward performance and more toward intimacy and mutual gratification of personal needs. According to Yeaworth and Friedman,[10] "in mutually satisfying sexual activity, not only can sexual identity be reaffirmed, but also the self-concept can be bolstered by the feeling that one is desired by, attractive to and valued by another."

The middle adult can remain an exciting and creative lover who experiments with new sexual approaches and techniques to maintain or enhance the pleasure and satisfaction of the sexual experiences.

Availability of Partners Loss of one's spouse through death or divorce is not uncommon in the middle years. For several reasons women are found to be without sexual partners more frequently than men. Although both men and women often remarry after divorce, men are much more likely than women to remarry after the death of their spouse. However, during the middle years, the death rate is higher for men than for women.

Social mores also contribute to the problem. Our society generally condones relationships or marriage between older men and young women but frowns on relationships between older women and young men. Dis-

Presbycusis—impaired auditory acuity, begins during middle age.

Refer to sections on the ear and the eye in Chap. 4 for discussion of assessing the structures.

There may be a slight decrease in taste perception during middle age.

Sexual needs do not significantly change during the middle years.

During the middle years the focus of sex is directed less toward sexual performance and more toward intimacy.

Loss of one's spouse is not uncommon during the middle years.

crimination on the basis of physical attractiveness, which is more commonly against women than men, continues in midlife.

Additionally, societal and often personal disapproval prohibits homosexuality as a feasible alternative. However, even among those whose choice is homosexuality, age discrimination may severely limit the availability of partners.[11] Masturbation, too, may be an unacceptable practice for some people. Celibacy, preferred by many, is often considered to be an "abnormal" sexual preference by some.

The problem of lack of suitable sexual partners is one that continues through the later years. Alternatives will have to be found and supported as life expectancy continues to rise; the number of middle-aged and older adults increases; and the need for sexual expression remains constant.

Menopause Menopause occurs in women as a result of a decline in ovarian function and is accompanied by symptoms associated with diminished estrogen (and to a lesser extent progesterone) secretion. Disappearance of the luteal phase is the principal ovarian functional change during this period and is reflected in the menstrual cycle.[12]

According to the National Center for Health Statistics, the average age at menopause is currently approximately 50 years. For several years before this, an irregular bleeding pattern may be observed. Commonly, menstrual periods are spread further apart, with diminished flow and shorter duration. There is an increase in the number of anovulatory cycles. Periods of amenorrhea may persist for a few months and be followed by excessive and prolonged flow. Some women may experience breakthrough bleeding.

In addition, estrogen stimulates many target organs in the body. Decreases in the amount of estrogen production can result in a wide range of symptoms. However, the extent and severity of symptoms will vary greatly among women.

"Hot flashes" are the chief source of distress during menopause and occur in about 65 percent of women.[13] Headaches, palpitations, numbness and tingling of extremities, and cold hands and feet are additional examples of vasomotor changes accompanying decrease in hormonal production.

Emotional instability is frequently described as a characteristic of perimenopausal women. Nervousness, anxiety, and wide mood swings may occur during this time as a result of hormonal fluctuations. In addition, serious consideration must be given to other life events which may be occurring simultaneously, as these may also contribute to the symptoms mentioned above.

Thinning and dryness of the vaginal epithelium results from the lack of estrogenic stimulation. Atrophic vaginitis can predispose women to vaginal burning and itching as well as discomfort during intercourse. The nurse should elicit these symptoms during the history so that appropriate interventions can be instituted to relieve these problems.

In men, the hormone testosterone plateaus between the ages of 40 to 60. After age 60 the levels begin to decline. At about age 70 or later, one can expect symptoms related to testosterone deficiency to occur. These changes can affect sexual performance and may be stressful to the individual.

As a result, men may experience symptoms of urinary frequency, urgency, hesitancy, and nocturia as the prostate gland enlarges. However, other causes for these symptoms should also be investigated.

Behavioral responses can also be altered in the middle-aged male. Often these changes are associated with personal accomplishments and

The average age for menopause is around 50 years.

Menopause has not occurred until menstrual periods have been absent for 1 year.

Physical and emotional changes accompany menopause.

"Hot flashes" are a chief source of distress for women during menopause.

Mood swings and increased anxiety may be observed during menopause.

Hormonal changes in both the male and female may affect sexual performance and satisfaction.

achievement of personal goals. Disappointment in attaining these goals or aspirations held throughout the young adult and early middle adult periods can be a source of stress and can precipitate changes in the individual's health status.

The nurse should be sensitive to this period of one's life and reflect on it during the assessment, especially when discussing self-perception patterns and occupation. Menopause can be a time of great stress for some individuals and a time of great growth for others. Clarification of expected physical and emotional changes, for both the male and female, can help to emphasize the normalcy of this life process and help to ease the transition through this time.

Contraception Since procreation is seldom the desired purpose of intercourse for middle adults, the need to find a safe, reliable, and acceptable contraceptive method becomes an important issue. Choice of any method is dependent primarily on the client's preference for and degree of confidence with the contraceptive. However, the risks and benefits of all methods should be identified to enable the client to make a reasonable and informed decision.

Women over the age of 35 to 40 are strongly cautioned against using oral contraceptives because of the increased incidence of thromboembolism in this group. The risk is increased for women who smoke.[14] Use of the diaphragm, foam, and condoms remains reliable during the middle years. While intrauterine devices (IUDs) can be chosen, their use is controversial. Both tubal ligation and vasectomy are becoming increasingly popular alternatives.

Individuals who oppose the use of contraceptives on religious grounds may have particular difficulty in midlife. Although fertility declines with diminishing ovarian function, conception remains a real possibility. Reliance on the rhythm method becomes more difficult as menstrual irregularities commonly occur. In addition, personal conflicts over the purpose of sexual intercourse (i.e., for recreation, not procreation) can be major stressors for these people. The nurse should be aware of the potential problems that can occur and assist the client in recognizing and handling them. With the increase in middle adult parenting, the use of contraception and pregnancy may be important issues for the persons involved.

Physical Ability Both men and women are able to continue satisfying sexual activities throughout and far beyond middle age. Hormonal and local genital changes occur which may affect enjoyment of intercourse; however, clear understanding of and preparation for these changes will enhance the likelihood of competent and pleasurable sexual function.

Age-related physiological and anatomic changes affecting men begin in the late middle years and continue into subsequent years. These include:

1 A longer time needed to achieve a full erection and to reach a climax

2 Fewer genital spasms experienced and a reduction in both the force and amount of ejaculation

3 Longer intervals between erections

Physical changes may also be seen in postmenopausal women. These include:

1 Decrease in the lubrication and elasticity of the vagina

Menopause should be considered a normal part of the aging process.

Contraception is still a concern during the middle years.

The rhythm method of contraception may have limited effectiveness during menopause because of irregularities in menstrual patterns.

Physical changes in males which can affect sexual performance include delayed erection, fewer erections, and decrease in force and amount of ejaculation.

2 Increase in irritation to tissue of the vagina

3 Spasmodic and painful vagina uterine contractions accompanying orgasm[15]

Highlights

Physical changes in the female which can affect sexual performance include decrease in lubrication of the vaginal wall, tissue irritation, and pain accompanying orgasm.

Physical changes associated with aging in the middle-aged male do not interfere with satisfaction for either himself or his partner. The changes described for women can often be prevented with the use of lubricating jelly or a local estrogen cream. Also, Masters and Johnson[16] have found that continued and regular intercourse helps to keep the vagina youthful, so that women who remain sexually active have vaginas that do not decrease significantly in size, continue to lubricate well, and respond to orgasms with little or no discomfort.

Continued regular intercourse during the middle years can help to reduce physical changes and increase sexual satisfaction.

The nurse must investigate other factors which may influence physical ability. Stanford[17] has identified the following six reasons for a loss of sexual responsiveness in women as well as men during the middle years: (1) boredom, (2) mental or physical fatigue, (3) preoccupation with business interests, (4) overindulgence in food or drink, (5) fear of failure, and (6) physical illness and certain medications. All these factors should also be evaluated when assessing sexual satisfaction.

Stanford identified 6 factors which affect sexual satisfaction: boredom, mental or physical fatigue, preoccupation with business interests, overindulgence in food or drink, fear of failure, and physical illness and certain medications.

One of the strongest predictors of sexual behavior in middle and later years is the pattern of previous sexual activity.[18] "Normal" behavior is determined by the level of a client's satisfaction. Aside from the pioneering works of Kinsey and Masters and Johnson, there are very little data available on actual sexual behavior in middle age.

One recent study[19] examined the occurrence of sexual "dysfunction" in couples who did not seek treatment for their problems. The population was predominantly white, well-educated, middle- to upper-class "happily married" couples with a mean age of 35 for women and 37.4 for men. Although the results of this study cannot be universally applied, they are, nonetheless, enlightening.

The frequency of intercourse reported by these couples was 2 percent never, 8 percent less than once a month, 23 percent once a week, 31 percent two to three times a week, 12 percent four to five times a week, and 1 percent daily.[20]

In addition to some of the physical changes described above, inability to relax, disinterest, too little foreplay, choice of inconvenient time by partner, and too little "tenderness" after intercourse were frequently reported by women. Men, reported attraction to person(s) other than the mate and different sexual practices as issues of importance.

The frequency of sexual dysfunction and difficulties for the most part did not negatively affect either sexual relationships or marriages of those involved.

Among women, masturbation shows very little variation with age. Masturbation rates in males drop with advancing years beyond the teens, but the female rate remains fairly constant, approximating the male level by the forties. In previously married women, masturbation becomes more important with age, relative to other sexual activity.[21]

Sexual assessment and determination of "normal" behavior for the individual involved is most easily done by asking clients the following two questions:

1 Is your sex life satisfactory?

2 If you could change any aspect, what would it be?

It is important also to consider the sexual patterns and behaviors of single middle-aged adults. Assessment can be aided through use of the questions noted above. The important thing is to remember that single

Assessment of the sexual patterns of the single middle-aged adult should not be neglected.

adults are not asexual but have the same needs as anyone else. It is not the place of the nurse to convert clients to certain sexual beliefs, but rather to encourage open discussion of needs and problems with emphasis on the client's choice and comfort.

Further assessment of this pattern area is discussed in Chap. 3 in the section on sexuality and reproductive patterns.

Refer to the section on sexuality and reproductive patterns in Chap. 3 for further discussion of this pattern area.

Nutritional/Metabolic Patterns

Problems most frequently encountered with nutrition of middle adults relate to misconceptions about the need to reduce or alter one's dietary intake. Nutrition patterns begun in earlier years often continue into the middle years, when metabolism and activity have slowed down and when the risk of cardiovascular disease and cancer pose major threats.

Nutritional needs must be adjusted to meet the body's reduced metabolic needs and activity patterns.

As the body's basal metabolic rate (BMR) declines during middle age, feelings of fatigue and diminished energy can occur. These decreases in BMR can also contribute to weight gain in the middle years if caloric intake is not restricted.

As the BMR declines, the client may experience decreased energy, increased fatigue, and potential for weight gain.

The thyroid gland gradually undergoes a reduction in cell size and function from the age of 25 until the eighth decade, when there is stabilization.[22] This, too, contributes to exaggeration of feelings of fatigue and diminished energy and can increase the tendency toward weight gain.

Careful attention must be given to clients' intake of excess calories during the middle years. At least 30 percent of all middle-aged adults are overweight, but the highest incidence is in the 50- to 59-year-old group, where about 60 percent of people are at least 10 percent overweight.[23] For each year after age 25, caloric intake should be reduced by approximately 7.5 percent.[24] Weight loss should be encouraged through a sound, balanced diet. Diet fads promising quick weight loss should be discouraged.

Additionally, nutritional assessment should focus on the intake of cholesterol and saturated fats, sugar, salt, food additives, fiber, and fluids. After recording a typical day's diet, the client should be asked to evaluate the quantity and quality of the food and fluid intake. Identification of nutritional excesses and deficiencies as risk factors for the major life-threatening diseases of middle age must be clearly discussed. Together with the client, dietary modifications can be planned and a reasonable diet established.

A comprehensive evaluation of dietary foods is essential if modifications are to be planned and a diet to optimize health established.

Physical changes involving the ingestion of food are also reported by middle adults. These include difficulty in chewing food because of missing teeth, weakened tooth support, and adjustment to new dentures. Also common are complaints resulting from reduced salivation and decreased secretion of gastric acid. Diminished gastrointestinal motility, combined with a reduction in physical mobility, can also contribute to constipation, as is discussed earlier in this chapter.

It is important for the nurse to consider all the factors that influence the nutrition of the middle-aged adult. Early treatment of dental problems, regulation of mealtimes, and the planning of a well-balanced diet may help to decrease those problems associated with this pattern area.

Refer to the section on nutritional metabolic patterns in Chap. 3 for a list of questions for evaluation of nutritional status.

Coping and Stress Tolerance Patterns

Behavioral assessment of middle adults is a complex and challenging undertaking. Emotional health is dramatically influenced by social changes, handling of "normal," recognizing and adapting to changes in body image, and adjusting to changing sexual feelings and behaviors.

Refer to discussions under Self-Perception and Self-Concept and Sexuality and Reproductive Patterns sections in this chapter when assessing this pattern area.

Each of these areas must be thoroughly examined.

It is important to assess how an individual handles stress and to identify behavioral patterns that predict responses to crisis. Usually, by the middle years individuals have experienced stressors in their lives and can elicit personal responses to each situation.

Stress "Normal" stressors in middle adulthood can result from inability to complete any or all of the developmental tasks outlined for this life stage. This definition is certainly useful in determining the quality of one's coping with the changes of middle adulthood but is enhanced when combined with assessment of additional stressors.

Holmes and Rahe[25] have shown convincing evidence of the detrimental effects of multiple rapid life changes on one's health. Their social readjustment rating scale (Refer to Chapter 1, Table 1-4) can be extremely useful in assessing the amount of change within certain time periods. Since many of the significant changes listed on the tool are likely to occur during the middle years, this tool has an important use in anticipatory guidance of middle adults.

Occupational Stressors In addition to all stressors relating to the quality of the work environment noted above, more obscure but equally detrimental stressors are common and should be identified for each client. Factors such as unreasonable workload (both overload and underload), inadequate preparation for one's current responsibilities, time deadlines, incompetent or inflexible supervisors, and little or no participation on policymaking all add to the stress of one's daily life.

For middle adults, particular focus should be on the issues of job security, inability to achieve desired job status, failure to remain current in one's field, and mandatory retirement. Additional attention should be given to the stressful experiences of the many middle-aged women who reenter the job market after having been away for several years. This becomes significant when the female becomes the "bread winner" following the loss of a spouse.

Finally, one cannot overlook the most devastating occupational stressor of all—unemployment. This is often most detrimental for middle adults with many financial burdens and limited savings.

In addition, plans for retirement should be of concern to the middle adult. Many suggest that attention to one's retirement should begin in the young adult period. Assessment of all these stressors is important in determining one's stress response pattern.

Exercise and Activity Patterns

Extremes of activity may be seen during middle adulthood. For some people, activity may represent an attempt to deny aging. Other individuals consistently work overtime to prove their value as an employee and then spend the evening "out on the town" to demonstrate the ability to maintain a previous "youthful" activity level.

Another variation of overactivity during the middle years results from an attempt to fulfill one's dreams before "it's too late." This pattern is manifest by cramming every day with a month's worth of activities. Often these people take on activities for which they are inadequately instructed and poorly conditioned and are thus at high risk for injury.

For some individuals, middle age is often a time of depression and lethargy resulting from the feeling that one is indeed "over the hill." This will be manifest by inactivity and boredom, with reports of empty days.

Increased stress may result from an inability to complete these developmental tasks as outlined for this age period.

Refer to Table 1-4 for reference to the Holmes and Rahe stress scale.

Occupational stressors, including responsibilities, workload, threat of unemployment, and retirement can intensify stress reactions during the middle years.

Middle-aged adults also report physical changes in terms of being easily fatigued and noting a gradual decline in physical work and exercise capacity.

This is due in part to a decrease in pulmonary vital capacity, accompanied by a decrease in elasticity and compliance of the chest wall. In addition, the arterial oxyhemoglobin saturation is slightly diminished and residual lung volume may increase in the middle years.[26]

Age-related physiological changes in the heart include a loss of elasticity of the aorta, a reduction in cardiac muscle strength, and a decreased cardiac output. After age 20, there is approximately a 0.85 percent annual loss of heart muscle strength.[27] However, cardiac output remains adequate to meet necessary requirements due to atrophy of other tissues and decreased physical demands.

Osteoporosis, which results in decreased skeletal mass and density, may contribute to the "backaches" often occurring in middle adulthood. Symptoms will be worsened by degenerative arthritic changes as well as excess weight which causes undue pressure on the spine. Osteoporosis is also manifest by a decrease in height occurring in the late middle years.

Many years of wear and tear on the joints will also be manifest by aches and pains. Similarly, complaints of decreased strength and "flabby" muscles occur as a result of declining muscle mass. A regular weekly exercise plan, however, will help to maintain muscle strength and to increase physical endurance.

Assessment of an individual's activity pattern should result in a profile of that client's daily activities. Focus should be placed on the amount of time the client spends on pleasurable activities (leisure time) which may be tension-relieving in comparison with the time spent on stress-producing activities. Other critical factors to examine are dramatic changes in activity level and expressed satisfaction or dissatisfaction with the daily activities of one's life.

Summary

The middle years can be a time of growth and change for each individual. Since the process of aging is a normal one, recognition and evaluation of the physical, behavioral, and social changes that accompany this period can create the atmosphere for optimal creativity and enjoyment as one moves toward the next life stage.

REFERENCES

1. Erik Erikson, *Childhood and Society,* 2d ed., Norton, New York, 1963.

2. Joanne Sabol Stevenson, *Issues and Crises during Middlescence,* Appleton-Century-Crofts, New York, 1977, p. 18.

3. Nancy Diekelmann (ed.), *Primary Health Care of the Well Adult,* McGraw-Hill, New York, 1977, p. 93.

4. Stevenson, *Issues and Crises,* p. 25.

5. Anthony Kales (ed.), *Sleep Physiology and Pathology: A Symposium,* Lippincott, Philadelphia, 1969, p. 43.

6. Michael Colligan et al., "Occupational Incidence Rates of Mental Health Disorders," *Human Stress* 34–39 (September 1977).

7. Cary Kart et al., *Aging and Health: Biologic and Social Perspectives,* Addison-Wesley, New York, 1978, p. 61.

8. Austin Chinn (ed.), *Working with Older People—A Guide to Practice,* U.S. Department of Health, Education, and Welfare Publication, No. 1459, July 1971, p. 40.

9. Lois Malasanos et al., *Health Assessment,* Mosby, St. Louis, 1981, p. 630.

10. Rosalee Yeaworth and Joyce Sutkamp Friedman, "Sexuality in Later Life," *Nurs Clin N Am* **10**:565 (September 1975).

Normal physiological changes in the lungs, heart, and skeletal muscular structures can affect an individual's activity tolerance.

Osteoporosis is a structural weakness in bones due to changes within bone tissue (calcification, decreased thickness of the cortex, and enlargement of bone marrow).

Evaluation of an individual's activity pattern should also include use of leisure time.

11. Joseph Harry and William DeVall, "Age and Sexual Culture among Homosexually Oriented Males," *Arch Sex Behav* **7**:199–209 (1978).

12. Langdon Parsons and Sheldon Sommers, *Gynecology,* 2d ed., W. Saunders, Philadelphia, 1978, Chap. 63, pp. 1470–1494.

13. Ibid., p. 1476.

14. Robert Hatcher et al., *Contraceptive Technology,* 9th ed., Hatchford Press, New York, 1978, p. 48.

15. Ibid., p. 48

16. William Masters and Virginia Johnson, *Human Sexual Inadequacy,* Little, Brown, Boston, 1970, p. 342.

17. Dennise Stanford, "All About Sex . . . After Middle Age", *Am J Nurs* **77**:608–611 (April 1977).

18. Eric Pfeiffer and Glen Davis, "Determinants of Sexual Behavior in Middle and Old Age," *J Am Geriatr Soc* **20**:153 (April 1972).

19. Ellen Frank et al., "Frequency of Sexual Dysfunction in 'Normal' Couples," *New Engl J Med* **299**:111–115 (July 20, 1978).

20. Ibid., p. 113.

21. Matilda Riley and Anne Fonner, *Aging and Society,* Russel Sage Foundation, New York, 1968.

22. Chinn, *Working with Older People,* p. 199.

23. Richard Stuart and Barbara Davis, *Slim Chance in a Fat World,* Research Press Company, 1972.

24. Sue Rodwell Williams, *Nutrition and Diet Therapy,* 3d ed., Mosby, St. Louis, 1977, p. 463.

25. Thomas Holmes and Richard Rahe, "The Social Readjustment Rating Scale," *J Psychosom Res* **11**:213–218 (1967).

26. Chinn, *Working with Older People,* p. 117.

27. Kart, *Aging and Health,* p. 120.

BIBLIOGRAPHY

Burcell, R. Clay: "Counselling the Formerly Married," *Clinical Obstetrics and Gynecology* **21**(1):259 (March 1978).

Cadogan, Mary: "Adult Development," in D. Jones (ed.): *Medical-Surgical Nursing,* McGraw-Hill, New York, 1982.

Dosey, M., et al.: "The Climacteric Woman," *Patient Counseling Health Education,* First quarter 1980, 14–21.

Eckhom, Eric: *The Picture of Health: Environmental Sources of Disease,* Norton, New York, 1977.

Fuchs, Estelle: *The Second Season: Life, Love and Sex for Women in the Middle Years,* Anchor Books, New York, 1978.

Genest, Jacques, et al.: *Hypertension—Pathophysiology and Treatment,* McGraw-Hill, New York, 1977.

Haggerty, Robert J.: "Changing Lifestyles to Improve Health," *Preventive Medicine* **6**:276–289 (1977).

Hawkins, J. W.: "A Nursing Model for Delivery of Primary Health Care for Women," ANA Publication G-147 (1980), 22–28.

Haspels, A. A., and H. Muspah: *Psychosomatics in Perimenopause,* University Park Press, Baltimore, 1979.

Levinson, Daniel, et al.: *The Seasons of a Man's Life,* Knopf, New York, 1978.

Lowenthal, Marjorie Fiske, Majda Thurnker, and David Chiriboga: *Four Stages of Life,* Jossey-Bass, San Francisco, 1976.

McGlone, Frank B., and Ella Kick: "Health Habits in Relation to Aging," *J Amer Geriatr Soc* **26** (11):481–488 (November 1978).

Peplau, Hildegard E.: "Mid-Life Crises," *Amer J Nurs* **75**(10):1761–1765 (October 1975).

Pruett, H.: "Stressors in Middle Adulthood," *Family Community Health* **2**(4):53–60 (1980).

Gail Sheehy: *Passages,* Bantam Books, New York, 1977.

PHYSICAL EXAMINATION
APPROACH TO THE EXAMINATION

Preparation of the middle aged client for a physical examination is similar to that described in Chap. 4. Privacy and maintaining a comfortable environment for the client is of particular importance. Providing information about the examination will help the individual feel less threatened by the procedure (a).

The middle adult years herald the onset of age-related physical changes. It is during this period that one begins to notice the signs of "wear and tear" on the body which will become more significant with advanced age.

The rate of physical changes will be influenced by many factors. Past and present health habits and heredity largely determine an individual's rate of physical aging.

THE EXAMINATION
General Appearance

The middle aged client's general appearance varies with each person (b). Frequently, increased weight gain, thinning or loss of hair, changes in hair color, decrease in stature, and diminished agility of body movement will be observed.

Highlights

Refer to Chap. 4 when performing a physical examination of the middle adult.

During the middle years physical changes begin to occur in a variety of body parts.

Increased weight gain in the middle aged client can occur because of a decrease in basal metabolic rate, increased caloric intake, and decreased activity.

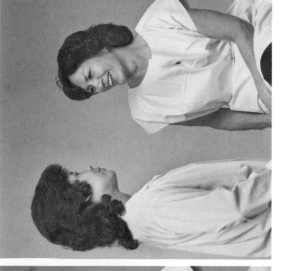

a

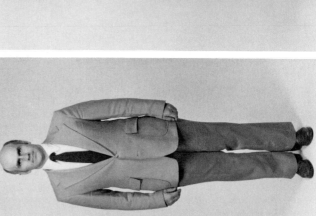

b

Highlights

Measurements of vital signs similar as presented in Chap. 4.

Refer to table A-14 for height and weight measurements of middle aged clients.

During the middle years, thinning of the hair (seen in women) and balding (seen in men) may be a frequent finding when examining the hair.

Heredity can influence the incidence of balding in males.

Graying of hair is a gradual process which usually begins during the 40's.

Table a adapted from Master, A.M., and Lasser, R.P., Blood Pressure Elevation in the Elderly, Lea and Febiger, 1961.

Table a - Average Blood Pressure of Middle Adult

Measurements

Assessment of the vital signs of the middle adult is similar to assessment of the young adult. Temperature range is from 36.7°C (97°F) to 37.6°C (99.6°F); pulse rate from 50 to 100 beats per minute (regular rhythm); respirations 16 to 20 per minute (regular rhythm); and blood pressure 120/80 with individual normal variations influenced by aging (e.g. up to 140/80-90 at age 60-65 [a]).

Head, Hair, and Scalp

Much of the examination of the head, hair, and scalp is similar to the examination described in Chap. 4.

Inspection

Observation of the hair of the middle aged client may show signs of thinning and or balding (b).

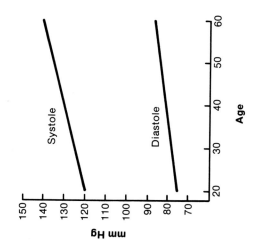

b

Usually these changes begin early in the middle years. Heredity can affect the time of onset. Hair loss results from a reduction in blood flow to the skin and occurs more frequently in male clients.

Graying of the hair is a gradual process. It occurs during the fifth decade in both sexes, but the time of onset can be determined genetically. Changes in hair color result from a decreased number of functioning pigment cells.

Palpation

Palpation of the scalp may reveal increased dryness and scaling. This can be due to a diminished amount of oil in the scalp cells.

Face, Mouth

Inspection

Due to a loss of subcutaneous fat, there is a gradual change in facial features (a). The face may appear coarser and boney. The nose is often more dominant.

The skin may be dry and wrinkled with increasing age due to a reduction of water content and atrophy of sebaceous glands. While drying of the skin is a gradual process, it usually accelerates during the middle half of the middle years. Excessive exposure to sun over the years can intensify this process.

Inspection of the chin will often reveal an increased amount of facial hair. This frequently is seen in postmenopausal women due to a decreased amount of estrogen present in the body.

The examination described in Chap. 4 can be used to inspect the mouth. Particular attention should be paid to the teeth, the lips, the internal mucosa of the oral cavity, and the tongue.

Changes in tooth structure due to bone loss, decay, ineffective dental care, and poor oral hygiene over the years contribute to loss of teeth. Approximately 50 percent of all Americans have lost a varying number if not all their teeth by age 65.

Regardless of the cause, with increasing age many adults have dentures. The fit and condition of these dentures should be noted. When inspecting the oral mucosa the condition of the gums should be inspected. The integrity of gum tissue should be pink, with no bleeding noted upon stimulation (b).

Highlights

Inspection of face may reveal a change in features due to a loss of subcutaneous fat.

Dryness of bodily skin accelerates during the middle years.

Increase in facial hair is often seen on the chin of middle adult females due to diminished amounts of estrogen.

Changes in tooth structure, bone loss, and poor dental hygiene may contribute to loss of teeth or dental caries during the middle years.

a

b

Inspection of the tongue is important when examining the internal oral structures (a). Atrophy of the papillae of the lateral edge of the tongue may begin in later middle years.

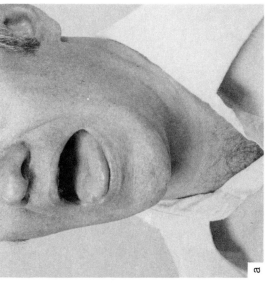

a

Eye

Changes in vision occur during the middle years, even when previous vision has been good. Because of this, individuals over 40 should be encouraged to have an annual eye examination.

Inspection (External Eye)

When inspecting the external eye, no significant changes are normally observed. However, changes in the ocular structures may occur. Tests of *visual acuity* (b) may show diminished readability in visual charts at 35cm (14 inches).

Decrease in visual acuity may be accompanied by a decreased sensitivity to darkness and diminished peripheral vision. These changes occur as the cornea becomes less transparent. As a result, a decreased amount of light is admitted into the eye, affecting sensitivity to light.

Presbyopia (farsightedness) is a common problem in the middle aged client. This change begins to occur during the fourth and fifth decade due to degeneration of the lens. Eyeglasses may be needed for reading and close work.

b

Atrophy of the papillae of the lateral edge of the tongue may be noted in the older middle adult client.

Refer to Chap. 4 under discussion of the mouth.

Eye examination should be part of the annual physical for all middle aged clients.

Refer to Chap. 4 for a complete discussion of the eye examination.

Decrease in visual acuity, diminished sensitivity to darkness, and diminished peripheral vision are changes often seen during the middle years.

Presbyopia (or farsightedness) is a problem often seen in the middle aged client.

Inspection (Internal Eye)

Ophthalmic examination of internal eye structures usually reveals information similar to that described in Chap. 4. As one ages, an increasing number of vessels may be observed.

Within the inner eye structure, the optic disc is normally visible; however, in the presence of increased ocular pressure (e.g. glaucoma) it may be occluded.

Palpation

When testing the *corneal reflexes* (a) a diminished response may be noted. In addition, persons over 40 may begin to experience changes in intraocular pressure. This is *not* a normal occurence. A *Schiotz tonometer* (b) is used to measure a reading of intraocular pressure.

When using a Schiotz tonometer the cornea is anesthetized; the footplate of the tonometer is placed on the cornea. Pressures are recorded in millimeters on a scale above the footplate. Normal readings are below 20 mmHg.

Ears
Inspection

Inspection of the middle adult's external ear is similar to the discussion presented in Chap. 4. With aging, increased dryness and loss of skin turgor of the ear lobe may be observed (c).

Corneal reflex usually diminishes during the middle years.

Persons over 40 should have a tonometry reading done annually.

Diminished auditory acuity, especially for highpitched sounds, is often present in middle aged clients.

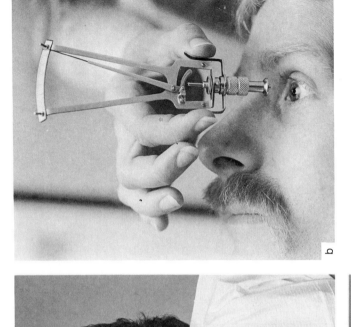

a

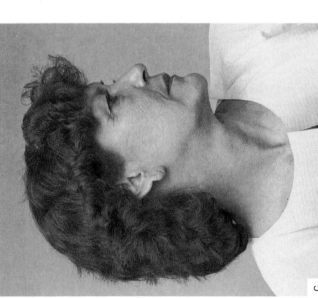

b

c

Highlights

Refer to discussion of the ear in Chap. 4 for an explanation of hearing tests.

Presbycusis is another name for impaired hearing.

Loss of hair cells in the organ of Corti is thought to be a common cause of presbycusis.

Increased amounts of cerumen may contribute to diminished hearing in the middle aged client.

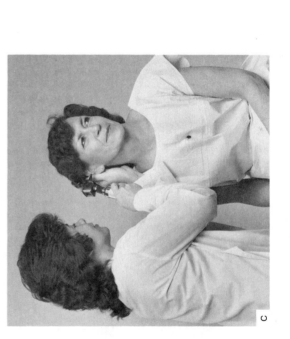

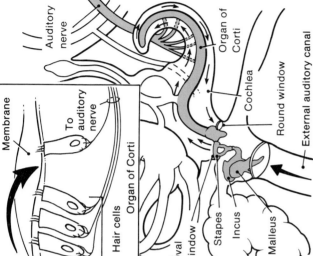

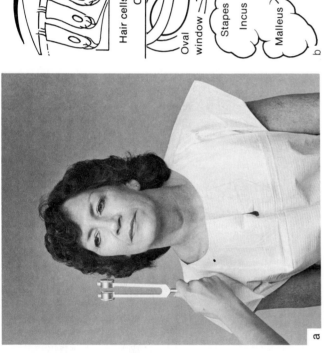

Evaluation of *auditory acuity* (using the Weber, the clock ticking, and the whisper tests) may reveal changes in hearing (a). Diminished auditory acuity may be seen in males, but occurs more frequently in females.

Presbycusis, or impaired hearing, usually affects both ears, though impairment may not be symmetrical. Presbycusis is most frequently the result of changes in the organ of Corti, a structure in the cochlea. Delicate hair cells within this structure are stimulated and in turn transfer stimuli to the auditory nerve (b) which carries the auditory sensations to the brain, where they are perceived as sound. It is believed that the loss of these hair cells in the organ of Corti is the most common cause of presbycusis. The first sounds lost are high-pitched, high-frequency sounds (e.g., a woman's voice).

Examination of the internal ear should reflect findings similar to those described in Chap. 4 (c). For the older middle aged client hearing may be diminished due to an increased amount of cerumen (wax) in the internal ear canal.

Highlights

Breasts

Inspection

Breast adipose tissue begins to atrophy during middle years. This tissue becomes replaced by areolar connective tissue which causes a loss of elasticity. As a result drooping, pendulous breasts may be observed with less rounded contour. With increasing age, breasts become less firm and appear flattened (a).

The examination of the breasts is similar to that described in Chap. 4.

Refer to Chap. 12 for breast changes that occur with pregnancy.

Breast tissue can begin to droop or flatten with age due to a decrease in tissue elasticity.

Palpation

Palpation of breast tissue should continue to be encouraged (self breast examination) during the middle years. Self breast examination should follow the procedure described in Chap. 4.

Self breast examination should be continued during the middle years. (See Chap. 4)

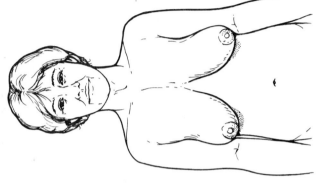

a

Thorax and Lungs

Examination of the lungs is similar to that described in Chap. 4.

Inspection

The shape and contour of the thoracic cavity may change with age and increased roundness of the chest wall may be noted. Changes in weight (gain or loss) can be revealed by inspecting the thoracic cavity.

Kyphosis or *lordosis* of the spine can affect the shape and contour of the thoracic cavity and can contribute to its roundness and posterior protrusion of the spine (b). These changes are exaggerated upon movement (e.g. having the client move forward).

Changes in the shape and contour of the thoracic cavity may contribute to the roundness observed.

Kyphosis: a flexion deformity of the spine.

Lordosis: deformity of lumbar area, extension of the spine.

Refer to Chap. 4 for a complete examination of the lungs.

Palpation

Intercostal spaces of the spine are more easily palpated in thin clients. Increase in weight during the middle years can make this process more difficult.

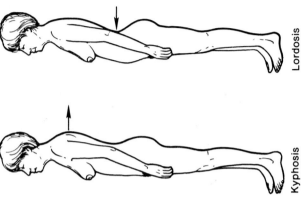

Kyphosis   Lordosis

b

Heart

Examination of the heart is similar to that described in Chap. 4. It should be noted that diminished energy expenditure will affect the amount of oxygen used. This in turn will decrease the amount of blood pumped by the heart. When this occurs, a sudden demand on the heart (e.g. increased exercise) may place stress on the pump, and create changes in pressure and rhythm. Regular, planned exercise or activity is therefore essential during the middle years in order to optimize cardiac function (a).

Increased amounts of calcium and salt deposits can make arteries less elastic. Atherosclerotic deposits can continue to decrease arterial lumen and may affect blood flow (b).

These changes may be progressively occuring during the early years through young adulthood. Manifestation of changes can occur with the stress test (treadmill) used to measure cardiac efficiency; assessment of vital signs including pulse, respiration, and blood pressure; and level of fatigue following exercise.

Abdomen
Inspection

Deposits of fat in suprapubic area can be observed in middle aged women. This change occurs due to a decrease in estrogen levels.

Increased amounts of adipose tissue may also be observed over the abdomen, related to a generalized weight gain (c). The so-called "spare tire" reflects an accumulation of fat in the abdominal area, often seen in the middle aged clients.

Highlights

Refer to Chap. 4 for examination of the heart.

With decreased energy expenditure, there is decreased oxygen used.

Decreased elasticity and size of blood vessel lumen can occur during middle age.

Stress test measures cardiovascular efficiency.

Increased gastric juices may increase complaints of belching.

Refer to Chap. 4, for examination of the abdomen.

Increase in weight may be observed in the abdominal area.

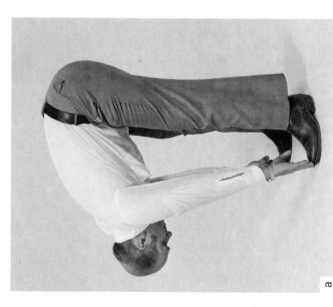

a

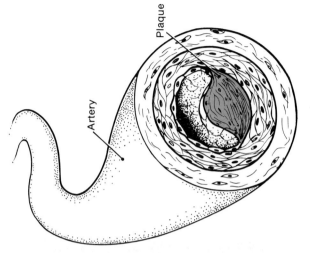

Plaque

Artery

b

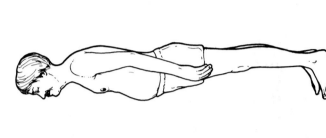

c

Abdomen

Inspection

Abdominal scars may be present if the client has had surgery (e.g. appendectomy or cesarian section). Scars should be described in terms of location, length, and general appearance. *Keloids* may be noted over scars (anywhere on the body) particularly in blacks and those of Asian descent.

Striae (linea albicantes) may be observed on the abdominal surface, particularly if the client has gained and then lost weight. Pregnancy may be the cause of this change.

Striae appears as streaks or atrophic lines on the abdomen that are usually observed after prolonged stretching (a). This stretching causes a disruption in the reticular layer of cutis. Striae initially have a pink or blue hue, later these lines become silver or white.

Palpation

Normally, palpation of the abdomen will reveal findings similar to those described in Chap. 4. Palpation of the liver may reveal an increase in liver span (b). Normally, these changes occur within suggested limits. (Normal liver span is 6 to 12 cm.)

The lower portion of the right kidney may be palpable in thin older middle adults. This occurs because diminished muscle tone and elasticity over the organ make it more accessible to palpation.

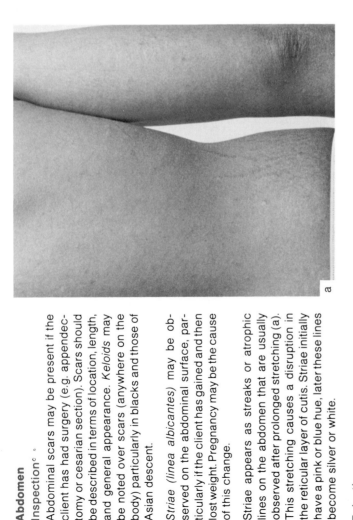

a

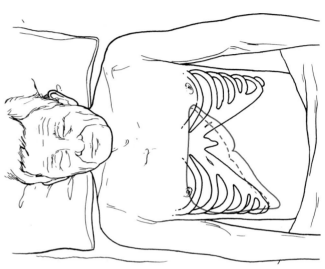

b

Female Genitalia

Inspection

Inspection of the external genitalia in the middle aged client reflect changes that include a gradual reduction of labia and the size of the clitoris; a thinning of the skin around the vulva area and a decreased amount of pubic hair.

These changes are thought to be related to gradual decline in estrogen production and lack of stimulation of target organs previously stimulated by estrogen (a).

Internal Inspection

Vagina Internal gynecological examination of the vaginal canal may reveal increasing dryness, a loss in reddish appearance. The mucosa becomes pale pink; muscle tone may diminish; a decrease in vaginal secretions occurs during this age period.

Cervix Examination of the cervix often reveals tissue shrinkage and retraction of cervical tissue making it appear flush with the vaginal wall. This is frequently due to diminished hormone production.

Palpation

Uterus As the client ages, the uterus becomes smaller and is less firm. These changes occur as the fundal portion of the uterus regresses, as a result of the development of more connective tissue than muscle (c).

Ovaries The ovaries atrophy with age due to diminished hormonal stimulation. They are often not palpable during this time period.

The internal examination, however, is similar to that described in Chapter 4 (b).

Highlights

Inspection of the external genitalia in middle age females reveals the following changes:

1 reduction of the size of the labia
2 decrease in the size of the clitoris
3 thinning of the skin around the vulva
4 decreased pubic hair

Changes in female genitalia occur due to decreased amounts of estrogen.

Vaginal mucosa may become pale and less moist during the middle years.

The cervix may shrink and retract during middle age.

Figure a from Dorothy A. Jones, et. al., Medical-Surgical Nursing, A Conceptural Approach, 1982, p. 65, fig. 4-2. Used with permission of McGraw-Hill Publishing Book Company.

The uterus is smaller and less firm as the client ages.

The ovaries are less palpable in the older middle adult.

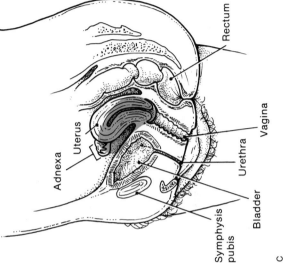

Estrogens excreted in urine, mg/24 h

Puberty

Menopause

Age, yr

a

Vagina

b

Adnexa

Uterus

Symphysis pubis

Bladder

Rectum

Vagina

Urethra

c

Male Genitalia
Inspection

Due to decreased testosterone production, smaller size, less firmness, and elevation of testes are observed.

The prostate gland often is symmetrically enlarged, elastic and rubbery or firm on palpation (a). The median sulcus may be obliterated.

In males over 50, benign prostatic hypertrophy is a common finding. It may occur from a conversion of testosterone to dihydrotestosterone (DHT). The DHT stimulates the prostate gland and accounts for prostatic enlargement over time.

Extremities
Inspection

During the middle years there is a decrease in density and bone mass. Complaints of joint soreness are common, due to weight gain or to continuous wear and tear on bone and joint structures.

There may be shrinkage noted in the client's height due to some compression of the vertebrae column.

Inspection of skin on the extremities should reveal intact structures (b). Pigmentations such as moles should be observed and referred for futher evaluation as needed.

Range of motion activities may also be limited in the middle aged client depending upon the physical fitness and mobility of the joints (c).

Diminished testosterone production in the male can result in decreased size, firmness, and elevation of testes.

Enlargement of the prostate usually begins after age 50.

Compression of vertebrae may result in decrease in height.

The skin of the extremities should be inspected for changes in pigmentation and moles.

Muscle strength and reflexes may be diminished during the middle years.

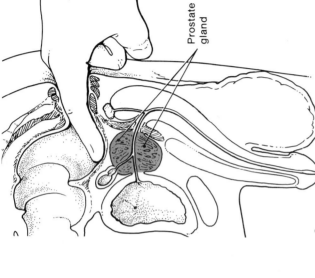

Prostate gland

a

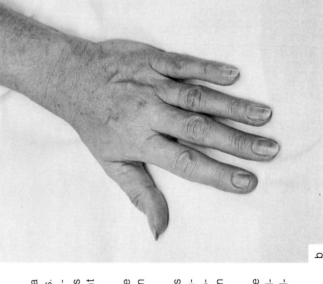

b

c

Regular activity can maintain muscle endurance and peripheral circulation.

Palpation

Muscle strength may be reduced due to diminished muscle tone. Muscles may feel flabby due to the fact that adipose and connective tissue has replaced muscle cells. This may be determined through grip test (a) and muscle strength assessment. The speed of muscle reflexes may also be slowed. However, exercise may help to maintain muscle endurance.

In apparently normal people over age 45, the dorsalis pedis or the posterior tibial pulses may be impalpable (b). Usually this change never occurs in the same foot. Inelasticity or decrease in lumen of peripheral blood vessels may affect palpation of peripheral pulses.

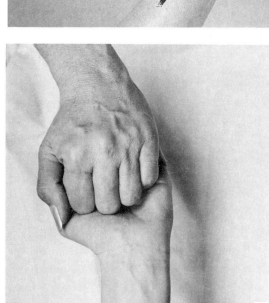

a

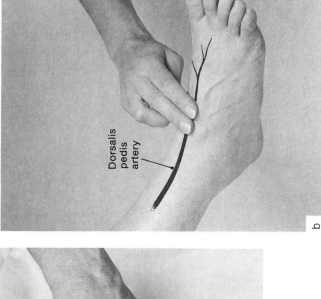

Dorsalis pedis artery

b

AGING*   CHAPTER FOURTEEN

Nancy J. Kehrli and Marian G. Spencer

THE HEALTH HISTORY

Holistic health is a complex state, fluid in nature and influenced by multiple variables. Those committed to the study of aging are still trying to describe healthy aging and to determine what specific factor or combination of factors contribute to healthy older years.

This chapter presents a discussion on healthy aging and considers clinical application of currently available knowledge. From information available it is not always possible to distinguish between age-related changes and pathological changes. Chronological age, that is, the number of years since birth, is not the biopsychosociological age.

The number of years to death, currently being explored, is in the process of testing the *terminal drop hypothesis* and may provide a more accurate indication of one's position in the life-death continuum. Simply stated, the terminal drop hypothesis supports health factors which bring an individual closer to death, related to a decline in intellectual performance.[1] This has implications for explaining the great variability of our older population, for influencing data collection strategies, and for predicting, and thus intervening in, those situations where death may be avoidable. We also know that biological aging occurs at different rates among people and even within different systems and organs within the same person.

Later maturing has been defined in several stages (e.g., "younger old," 55 to 70 years and "older-old," 85 to 100+ years). For purposes of this chapter, 65 to 70+ years will be the age used to describe the older adult.[2]

According to the 1976 U.S. Census, approximately 10.5 percent of the total population of the United States (or more than 22 million persons) were 65 years of age.[3] By the year 1990, the percentage estimate increases to 11.0 percent and to 11.7 percent by the year 2000.[4] This means that over the coming years there will be an increased amount of research into the needs and lifestyle of the elderly. This chapter focuses on changes that normally occur during the life process of the elderly client.

Chapter 14 focuses on healthy aging.

The "terminal drop" theory supports those health factors that bring an individual closer to death as related to a decline in intellectual performance.

Younger old—55 to 70 years; older old—85 to 100+ years.

By the year 2000, 11.7 percent of the population will be older than 65 years of age.

*Physical Assessment edited by Geryln Spollette R.N., M.S.N., Clinical Specialist in Primary Care.

Table 14-1
Percentage of Older Persons in the United States by Age Group in Elderly Population, Years 1900 to 2000

Age	1900	1950	1975	2000
65–74	71	68	62	53
75–84	25	27	30	34
85+	4	5	8	11

Source: National Council on the Aging, *Fact Book on Aging: A Profile of America's Older Population* (Washington, D.C.: NCOA, 1978, p. 7).

Establishing a Data Base

The quality of the initial nurse-client interaction occurs during the health history and influences the amount of data collected and impacts in future nurse-client encounters. As the nurse assesses the client's verbal and nonverbal behavior, the nurse's behavior is also being assessed by the client. Behavioral responses, along with the stoic appearance of many older persons, can be deceptive and should not trigger labels of indifference, apathy, or depression. Rather, it may simply present the older person's struggle with a question of trust.

Behavioral reactions and responses of the elderly can be misleading and must be clarified by the nurse during the interview.

Interviewing principles and techniques discussed in Chap. 3 are also applicable to the aged population. In addition, there are several points to emphasize that are particularly relevant when interviewing the elderly. Consideration should be given to the client's physical comfort. The temperature of the room, lighting, arrangement and type of furniture, and setting all contribute to a client's ease during the interview. Confusion generated by multiple stimuli may be controlled by ensuring freedom from interruptions and turning off radios or television sets (if the interview is conducted in a hospital room) and providing the client with a comfortable chair. The nurse should also be conscious of the older person's ability to hear. Body posture may provide the first clue and should be explored further (see section on cognitive-perceptual patterns).

When interviewing the elderly client, consideration should be given to room temperature, physical environment, and personal comfort.

In addition, the nurse should be sensitive to the older client's level of fatigue. The health professional may find that several short intake sessions are more beneficial than one or two lengthy ones. This means that the health professional must give the older client time and flexibility to initiate the interview where the client feels most comfortable and terminate when the level of fatigue is reached.

The nurse should be sensitive to the client's level of fatigue and divide data collection into several sessions.

The current generation of elders may have had elementary school education or less and may be sensitive or embarrassed about this aspect of their lives, thus adding to their inability to freely express themselves. Furthermore, deafness or memory impairment will slow the history-taking process. Thus the nurse should ask questions in a simple, straightforward manner. If the client appears too ill, confused, or debilitated to answer questions, it may be necessary to obtain pertinent information from a relative or significant other. Use of previous health records may also be necessary.

Deafness, physical limitations, and memory deficit may affect data collection from the elderly client.

Vagueness and lack of specificity of symptoms can further obscure data collection. When this occurs, a careful analysis of symptoms and the obtaining of additional data such as information regarding the level of overall wellness or functional impairment will be necessary for a more accurate interpretation of symptoms.

Vagueness and diminished specificity of factors related to a client's health status may affect the accuracy of data collected during the assessment process.

When interviewing elderly clients of different cultures or ethnic origins, the nurse should be attentive and ask the client to explain or clarify meaning to avoid misinterpretation. It is important not to make value judgments or convey disapproval when confronted with conflicting values and beliefs. Being honest, admitting lack of understanding, and asking the client to repeat, if appropriate, are all important ways to avoid obtaining an inaccurate data base.

One of the most helpful approaches in eliciting information from an older person is to ask open-ended questions which indicate interest in learning about the client as a whole person. Past experiences; expectations, both realized and unrealized; and present concerns can be integrated into the data collection process. This provides older clients an opportunity to start the interaction by stating what is important to them. Giving older clients time to talk will yield information about multiple health patterns that make up the whole individual.

One of the most helpful approaches to use when eliciting data from the elderly client is to ask open-ended questions.

Entry into the Health Care System

The elderly client frequently seeks health care for a perceived or actual dysfunction in health. Therefore, the client may wish to focus on the problem at hand and not a health assessment. It is important to remember that the older person has spent a lifetime interacting with a health care system that has had a medical or disease focus; therefore, they may come to the encounter with preconceived ideas about resource utilization and behavior expectation of the client and the health professional. It is possible to meet clients where they wish to start and at the same time meet the health professional's goal of a holistic health assessment. This may be accomplished by explaining to the client the health professional's interest in the older client's total well-being.

Highlights

Frequently elderly clients seek health care for a perceived or actual health problem.

Elderly clients enter a health care facility with a variety of expectations.

Negative experiences related to health care may hamper an initial nurse-client interaction.

Client Profile

The elderly client is a result of a multiplicity of factors that are influenced by age, sex, genetic inheritance, marriage, place of birth, nationality, and religion. In addition, the functional patterns are examined to reflect a client's total life experience. The client profile provides the nurse with beginning demographic data to initiate the assessment process.

Refer to Chap. 3 under Client Profile for complete discussion of this aspect of assessment.

Health Perception/Health Management

The older person's concept of health is generally a functional one, and their reason for entry into the health care system is usually because of a perceived dysfunction. This means that older people actively engaged in life consider themselves healthy while those whose movement is limited generally respond with statements which indicate they believe they experience a low levels of wellness.

Client's health values also contribute to their health perception. Their particular health belief model (refer to discussion in Chaps. 1 and 3) may contribute to their use of the health care system. For the elderly, to be healthy is considered a gift to be emulated since for many elderly, death and illness seem to be a living part of one's daily existence.

According to Alford, the well older adult is one who participates in life's activities with zest. They have no time to be ill, and enjoy life.[5]

Older persons consider themselves healthy when they actively engage in life processes.

The well older adult has a zest for life.

Current Health Status A person's daily health habits affect the current level of wellness. Older clients are generally interested and concerned about health and may hold very specific views of what has and is influencing their wellness. It may be difficult for the health professional to change lifelong behavior patterns, but older people can change. What constitutes good health habits at a younger age also constitutes good health habits at an older age. Breslow's suggestions for commonsense health practices (e.g., moderate exercise, 7 to 8 hours of sleep per night, no smoking, moderate weight, and moderate alcohol use) are just as appropriate for both young and old adults. [Refer to Chapter 1]

An older client's health habits develop over many years and can be difficult to change.

Refer to Chap. 1 for a complete discussion of Breslow's health habits.

Questions to elicit data

1 What do you think has influenced your health?

2 Do you do anything in particular to maintain your health?

3 Do you use any home remedies when you are not feeling well?

4 Have you ever sought health care from someone other than doctors and nurses?

5 If so, please explain.

Cheraskin and Ringsdorf suggest that expanding an older person's belief system begins with a holistic health assessment which attempts to determine the client's level of wellness.[6] Many feel that the success of holistic health practices for the elderly is determined by a person's perceived locus of control.[7] Allen notes that those elderly who are externally controlled depend on external resources to promote health; those elderly who are internally controlled assume responsibility for their health and are excellent candidates for health programs.[8]

Past Health Status Evaluation of the client's past health status is important. Reference to those areas for consideration can be found in Chap. 3. Those actual or potential health problems can be more easily identified as the client's past health is reviewed. Populations at risk for specific nursing and medical problems can be isolated through evaluation of present and past health records.

Life Patterns and Lifestyles

The lifestyle of the elderly, that is, those life patterns that help to make up part of the life process, are important factors to consider when determining a client's health status. Assessment of a person's age, race, genetic inheritance, cultural influences, growth and development patterns, biological rhythms, and environmental and economic factors, as well as the availability of community resources, contribute in some ways to judgments made about one's lifestyling.

Age The key concept to remember when assessing the elderly client is that biological age is different from chronological age. Aging which is a gradual slowing-down process for each person may be viewed from three levels—molecular, cellular, and organ and organ systems. The health professional is concerned with biological aging at the organ and organ systems level.

Recent life-expectancy projections show that white males reaching age 60 years are likely to live until age 77 and females until age 82. Blacks and other nonwhites reaching age 60 will live until 76 (males) and 81 (females), respectively.[9] In addition, the group of elderly living over age 65 is also increasing and females continue to have a longer life expectancy than do males (refer to Table 14-1).[10]

Race Approximately 15 percent of the elderly U.S. population is foreign born.[11] Racial and ethnic minorities continue to have low visibility on the American health scene. Extreme poverty, language barriers, lifelong educational deprivation, social isolation and stigma, inability to negotiate complex organizational bureaucracy, and maldistribution of health-related services all tend to keep minority members out of the mainstream of the health delivery system. Mistrust and fear of the consequences of medical intervention cause many of these people to seek health care as a last resort.

The foreign-born elderly tend to return to their culture of origin health practices. This is especially noticeable in eating habits and dietary preferences as well as the use of home remedies. They may combine modern treatment modalities with healing potions and rituals that bring about startling results. If it works for them (and why not?), direct questioning about practices used for health maintenance or illness can be enlightening.

The elderly of different ethnic groups tend to live in urban areas. For example, Arizona, New Mexico, Texas, and Colorado have large

Expansion of an older person's belief system begins with a holistic assessment to determine the person's level of wellness.

Successful use of holistic health practices may be affected by an individual's perceived locus of control.

Internally controlled persons respond well to holistic health care.

Evaluation of a client's past health status helps to determine actual or potential nursing and medical problems.

Lifestyle comprises those functional components that affect the elderly client's lifestyle.

Refer to section on Life Patterns and Lifestyles in Chap. 3.

Aging is seen as a slowing-down process for each individual.

The number of males and females living over 65 years of age is steadily increasing.

Females continue to have a longer life expectancy than do males.

Older racial and ethnic minorities have low visibility in terms of health care.

Fifteen percent of the elderly clients in the United States are foreign-born.

Elderly of various ethnic groups tend to live in specific urban areas.

Spanish American populations. California and Hawaii, on the other hand, have large elderly Asian populations.

Heredity Caird and Judge attribute little importance to family history in the elderly as there are few familial disorders of diagnostic value which commonly commence during old age.[12] Family history might reveal availability and suitability of possible sources of caretaking for the elderly client or provide insight into existing social networks.

Those persons who live to become old reflect a combination of factors which might be considered of a holistic nature. Their capacity to cope with stress, genetic endowment, early family life, quality of community life, and health status all combine to influence the stamina and well-being of older adults.

Culture An elderly person's culture may facilitate or impede health and health care. Clients often respond better to a health provider who shares a similar ethnic and cultural background. When client and health provider represent different cultures, care must be taken to avoid miscommunication. Clients may not be familiar with the health values and practices of the larger society. Health professionals may not be sensitive to or understand the client's health beliefs or practices. This lack of sensitivity may result in health care dropouts, disregard for health advisement, and incomplete or inaccurate data.

The health professional can ask questions intended to isolate those cultural factors that influence an individual's health status.

Questions to elicit data

1 Tell me about your cultural background?

2 Is this an important part of your life?

3 How have you been able to carry on your culture's customs and traditions?

4 If this were not possible, in what way were changes made?

Where possible, a detailed account of such practices of folk medicine, self-healing, or religiocultural healing rites should be obtained. The nurse should never overlook the role of the local druggist as a source of self-treatment through the use of over-the-counter drugs. Also, older people often use a lay-referral system; that is, they may discuss common complaints with neighbors or friends and frequently exchange medications or home remedies.

Care must be taken in the choice of terminology. The older person may not have been exposed to the vernacular of the day. For example, the word "client" may be foreign to the elderly person who is used to being called "patient." Also, the older person takes "medicines," not "drugs." Familiarity with the individual's language, cultural customs, and health practices are all needed to determine the quality of one's health.

Growth and Development Aging is currently considered a natural phenomena. Just why it occurs is unknown. There are many proposed theories, a large number of which focus on the coded cellular system of protein manufacture. Organic organisms differ from inorganic organisms in two ways: (1) their ability to reproduce and (2) their ability to use energy taken from the external environment in an organized manner. Both of these processes depend on the cell's ability to synthesize protein. Each living cell has within its nucleus a message in code which gives exact instructions for the synthesis of all protein. Scientists believe that the coded process of protein production is the most likely place for errors to occur. Brocklehurst classifies these proposed changes into two theoretical groups. One school subscribes to the "molecular clock" concept, and the second believes that aging is caused by a deterioration of the protein synthesizing machinery.[13]

In the first theory cellular growth and differentiation is genetically programmed, with genes "turned on" and "turned off" in selected cells by some kind of molecular clock. Theories based on deterioration of the protein synthesizing mechanisms on the other hand, are *primary error theories* and *random error theories*. Most *primary error theories* focus on abnormalities of DNA making RNA and are concerned with the possible ways in which the coded information on DNA could be distorted. Errors may occur in deformation of letters themselves through oxidative changes in the DNA cross-linkages in macromolecules, irreparable breakages in the DNA information strand, and changed capacity of DNA to react with histones which are basic proteins that can cover parts of the codes.

The *autoimmune theory* is a special subtheory based on DNA mutation. It proposes that lymphocytes are capable of somatic mutation and that this will modify their antigenic properties. The result of such a process would be widespread antigen-antibody reaction in different tissues. *Random error theories* occur due to a deletion of one or more code letters, insertion of one or more code letters, or a combination of insertion and deletion.

Aging has also been viewed as a developmental process which allows for the integration of body, mind, and spiritual dimensions. Erikson describes an eighth stage of development for the elderly called "integrity versus despair."[14] The process of integration can be seen as a way of pulling together one's entire life (past, present, and future) into perspective. If well done, it is expected that the individual will experience a sense of completeness and comfort with the life state. Failure to achieve this results in feelings of despair and hopelessness about the present and future.

Peck has added some additional insights into the developmental perspectives on aging. His work suggests that "to successfully adapt to aging one must transcend (rise above) in three areas: roles, bodies and the end of life course."[15] Within this framework, Peck suggests that as one ages, the role of spouse, mother, and occupation may need to be discarded as the person transcends the self to assume a life without attachment to a specific label.

To transcend one's body, Peck emphasizes the need to engage in activity despite physical limitations. *Transcending the end of life course,* on the other hand can be achieved by the recognition of one's personal contribution to society, through awareness of one's continued interaction with the universal life process, and through the experience of spiritual transcendence which suggest preparation for eternal life with God.[16]

Psychosocial Capabilities The impact of many psychosocial factors also affects one's growth and development. Neugarten cautions us against using the biological clock as the sole frame of reference for psychological development in adulthood.[17] She suggests that a social clock may take precedence in understanding personality development from maturity onset to approximately 70 years of age. Each society has norms which are derived from age-expected behaviors. Thus we are provided with timing patterns or a sociological clock which governs our lives. We are aware of these timing patterns and are able to describe ourselves as "early," "late," or "on time."

As a result of the above, we are able to make several generalizations. There are significant differences in the older population which has caused the development of two age categories: the younger old, 55 to 70 years, and the older old, 85 to 100+ years, with age 70 approximately, designating a "middle old" age division. The approach to and response of each age group is different. An example of this may be seen in the orientation each group holds toward age and death. The very elderly are proud of their years and may be more willing to discuss death. The younger elderly are hesitant to share their age and may or may not be willing to discuss death with any degree of comfort. There are changes which are generation-related, specific to that particular cohort, versus age-related, where all aging people in any time period will experience the change. Graying of hair is an example of the latter, while reluctance to give a sexual history is an example of the former. Although older people throughout their lives have experienced and generally adapted to multiple societal changes, their diminished physical, economic, and social resources (family and friends) make them more vulnerable to loss and change. Assessment should focus on the client's concept of life satisfaction with respect to the varied stages and phases of personal development. Older people are more susceptible to chronic and disabling illnesses which once experienced are usually present until death. In 1972, chronic conditions led to mobility problems for 18 percent of those 65 and over.[18] Of this 18 percent, 6 percent had trouble getting around alone, 7 percent needed mechanical assistance, and 5 percent were homebound. However, the majority of elderly persons are functioning independently or optimally with assistive auxiliary services. Only a small number of the elderly are institutionalized.[19] These factors affect one's satisfaction level.

Variations in the aging process may be seen in the ages between 65 and 100+.

The views of the younger old regarding life and life satisfaction may differ considerably from those of the older old.

The majority of older persons are functioning independently or optimally with assistance.

Only a small number of the elderly are in institutions.

Behavioral Development Human behavior is complex, representing the interacting forces of biology, psychology, and sociology. The unity of these forces provide us with a developmental framework which encompasses the whole life cycle from birth to death. The nervous system organizes behavior and regulates the functions of the body; this is the "go power." The human organism undergoes sequential stages of development, growth, and contraction. There are stress and crisis points along the way in the working out of roles and responsibilities in life cycle events. The psychosocial environment shapes personality development. The personality system is unique for each individual. Sex-role identity, age-role identity, and age expectations exert strong influence on the adult personality. (Refer to discussion under Growth and Development section in this chapter.)

Each aged person's personality is different.

It is important to realize that an individual's personality as he or she ages is the result of years of development. Therefore, personality traits will be difficult to change without a personal commitment to do so on the part of the client. Asking the client to describe his or her personality to the nurse may give some insights into unique traits. In addition, eliciting past reactions to particular situations may further clarify these areas.

Changing the behavior and personality traits of the elderly is difficult but possible.

Biological Rhythms The question of breakdown in circadian rhythms in old age was answered in part in a study comparing old and young people. Body temperature, urine flow, heart rate, and potassium excretion were measured. "Of six elderly men, three exhibited dissociation; there was no neat parallel between the peaks and troughs of their four measure functions, . . . Four out of five depressed patients showed dissociation." There is the possibility that dissociation might be indicative of depression among older people. "A dissociation of physiological rhythms

Biological rhythms play an important role in the elderly's life process.

might emanate from many origins—organic illnesses, lack of social pressures and schedules, irregular habits, virus, fever, shock, and emotional stress. All of these may contribute to the increasing load of mental and physical disease that a person suffers as he grows older."[20]

Sleep and Rest Patterns Sleep-wakefulness patterns are altered in the aged. Old people know they no longer sleep deeply. Luce (1971) discusses the influence of circadian rhythms in elderly clients. "The proportion of rapid eye-movement REM sleep in the sleep cycle remains the same throughout life unless a person has suffered brain damage from cardiovascular or other diseases. Some changes in sleep rhythms are an indication of illness within the maturing and aging brain, but others may only mean that the restrictions of society have loosened their hold on the individual who no longer needs to meet daily schedules of job and family."[21]

"Rhythms and social schedule may be very important in treating geriatric disease. It is possible that internal discordance evolves when one's activity and rest schedule are not strong enough to force one to follow an unvarying routine of sleep and wakefulness. The typical insomnia of older people grows worse when there is no routine and they nap all afternoon. A greater knowledge of physiological rhythms might make it easier to time meals and ministrations, to treat them at the pace they need."[22]

Elimination Patterns Elimination patterns are altered in normal aging. The assessment process must differentiate between age-related structural changes in these systems and lifelong bowel habits. Reference to the discussions regarding normal elimination patterns are discussed in Chap. 3.

In the elderly, the biggest constraint related to maintaining normal elimination patterns has to do with nutritional patterns and the use of external sources (e.g., laxatives) to maintain regularity. In the absence of structural problems the elderly should be able to have and maintain elimination with regularity. Reference to nutrition patterns (discussed later in this section) can be made to review those food and water sources that help to maintain proper elimination. Evaluation of the source and frequency of laxatives or enemas must be determined also when assessing this pattern area.

Environmental Factors *Environment* is assessed in relation to the older client's need for resources and safety. Access to family and friends, markets, stores, churches, and health care facilities becomes an important factor to consider when evaluating this component. Questions must be asked regarding the availablity of transportation, fear of physical harm or loss of possessions, the state of repairs in the house or apartment, the length of time the person has lived in the present home or neighborhood, and the amount of money and work required to maintain the home, as these are important pieces of data. Discussions about the convenient location to stores, friends, family, and so on; the safety of the neighborhood; and how the client can get assistance if needed, are added areas to explore.

Approximately 73 percent of the elderly live in urban areas.[23] While the problems associated with urban living (e.g., crime, air pollution, and congestion) are many, they seem to have certain advantages. These include access to transportation, availability of health care facilities, and socialization with other elderly persons. According to Kart et al., the number of elderly living alone has increased during recent years. This has been due primarily to the large number of widows living into their seventies and beyond and the economic changes (e.g., low-income housing for the elderly) that have made living alone possible.[24]

Highlights

Changes in one's "internal clock" can alter behavioral and physical response patterns.

The sleep-wakefulness cycle can be altered in the elderly.

REM sleep remains constant throughout life.

Insomnia in the elderly increases when there is a lack of a daily schedule.

Refer to Chap. 3 under Elimination Patterns section.

Disturbances in elimination patterns of the elderly can often be associated with changes in nutritional patterns.

Most elderly people live in urban areas.

A large number of elderly people are living alone today.

Economics Current economic conditions find everyone including the elderly with decreased purchasing power. However, it is particularly difficult for the elderly who must manage on fixed incomes. Budget cuts appear in all categories from senior citizen recreation to prescription medications. To cope with financial constraints, the older person may regulate medication by decreasing a dosage, taking one pill instead of two per day or by delaying filling empty medication bottles. The health professional's greatest responsibility after assessing the client's ability to manage is to ensure that the client has knowledge of available resources. Help may also be required in obtaining resources.

For many elderly, retirement benefits may be minimal. Therefore, dependence on Social Security may be the major source of income for the client. Originally, Social Security was seen as a supplement to the cost of living for the aged. However, today 90 percent or more of the total income for 1 out of 4 single elderly and 1 out of 12 older couples, Social Security is the main source of income.[25]

Today many individuals continue to work after 65 years of age. Often, this is encouraged by employers who have extended retirement to age 70. This may help the client financially and socially during this time.

It is important to remember that the elderly of today grew up with a strong work ethic and still maintain pride in being able to provide for themselves. Several sessions of explanation, encouragement, and above all tact will be required for the elderly to discuss their economic status.

The economic constraints of the 1980s have seriously affected the elderly person's lifestyle.

Social Security, once regarded as supplemental income for the elderly, is the main financial resource for many people today.

An increasing number of elderly persons continue to work after age 65.

Questions to elicit data

1 Have you been able to manage your present state of living with the costs so high and money so tight?

2 How satisfied are you with your present income?

3 What kinds of things do you not do because of insufficient monies?

In situations where there has been a loss of a spouse, the financial status may worsen for the elderly. The client may need to be put in touch with services that could ease the financial burden.

Community Resources Community resources may influence the older person's quality of life by providing services which range from assistance through advocacy in respect to political action to expanding the older client's community by friendly visiting.

Questions to elicit data

1 Are you a member of any club or social group?

2 Do you receive services from any community group?

3 Do you belong to a senior citizens group (e.g., Association of Retired Persons)?

Over the past few years more services have been provided locally to support the elderly. Community senior citizen centers offer opportunities for socialization, nutrition, health counseling, and screening activities (e.g., blood pressure screening). Services such as "Meals on Wheels" provide nourishment for the elderly in the home. In addition, groups such as the Gray Panthers,[26] SAGE in California,[27] the Activated Senior Citizens program in Virginia,[28] and the Life Enrichment programs for older adults offered by the Gerontology Program at the School of Allied Health in Dallas, Texas,[29] are examples of other community services for

Community resources serving the elderly include:
1 Senior citizen groups
2 Gray Panthers
3 SAGE (California)
4 Association of Retired Persons
5 School and community groups

the elderly. These programs help to promote recognition of the worth of the elderly and help the elderly to reach holistically enriched lives.

Highlights

Many community programs are offered to the elderly through community schools.

Roles and Relationship Patterns

As the individual ages, roles and relationships with family and friends change. This can be a difficult time for the person who sees long-time supports weakening or leaving them entirely. Fear and anxiety can be prompted by the loss of many roles (spouse, mother, teacher, etc.) as well as relationships (wife, sister, children, or friend). Peck (see discussion under Growth and Development section) suggests that the elderly need to refocus and transcend these roles in order to relieve themselves of the loss of such components.

As an individual ages, roles such as spouse, child, brother, sister, mother, and father are often lost.

Fears associated with loss of one's role need to be addressed during the assessment.

Family Relationships Family composition may be determined by asking the client to tell the health professional about the family dynamics.

Family relationships tend to affect the quality of life for the elderly.

Questions to elicit data

1 Who belongs to your family?
2 Who are the members of your family?
3 How frequently do you talk or visit with one another?
4 How close are you to your family (as a whole or to specific individuals)?
5 How close do you live to family members?
   (Refer to Chap. 3 for additional questions).

It is important that personal relationships established with and among family members do not dramatically change as one ages. Those families who have remained close over the years continue to do so. For some, estrangement over the years may remain the same or intensify as family members age. Societal changes have decreased emphasis on the family and the elderly and caused families to separate as a result of increased occupational and personal mobility.

Social mobility and the role of the family in today's society has seriously affected the elderly person's life.

Because of these changes, many elderly live lonely lives. In cultures where the elderly are revered, this loss of family support is less obvious even in the midst of personal and emotional losses.

Societal views of aging and the elderly are frequently stereotyped perceptions of illness, dependence, and loneliness. Unfortunately, older persons as societal members may share in these perceptions. They may become fearful or anxious about the quality of their later years and the influence this will have on their family. The older person who drops cues should be encouraged to discuss these concerns: "What's it like to be an older person today?"

In some cultures the elderly are revered and regarded as those members to be sought out for their wisdom.

Social policies for the elderly have been reflected in terms of particular programs that may improve living conditions for the elderly. These include Social Security benefits, care of the blind, and the Medicare Law of 1965.

The Social Security Act and the Medicare Law (1965) have been social policies established to aid the aged.

Occupation Americans are identified as a "youth-" or "productivity-" oriented society. In fact, the meaning of work is significant in the human life cycle. Work confers status and social position in this society. Chronological age influences the work-productivity cycle of the individual. Since society mandates the standards for life cycle productivity, one's work-productive cycle is time-dependent. Both the entry and the exit points of one's work cycle become a factor of age.

Retirement is a significant time in a person's life.

The occupation role of the individual engaged in a specific work experience ends in retirement (even the homemaker experiences role termination as the children begin to establish independent lives.) Retirement means many things to different people. For some, it means the end of the middle years and the beginning of old age. For others, it is a time of fulfillment and reward, marking the beginning of the leisure years. For others, retirement can mean the loss of social role or status, (a person's work denotes social position), loss of income (which means reduced standard of living), and loss of meaningful relationships through one's loss of social contact; it can also mean increased freedom to complete one's life goals and a time for discovery. According to Kimmel, "Retirement is a major social shift for the individual, but it does not necessarily involve a major psychosocial crisis. It clearly involves a process of anticipation and adjustment. . . . The meaning of retirement for the individual reflects a complex array of social and cultural factors that reflect his unique life situation and also his perception of the social meaning of retirement."[30]

It is important to remember that the current generation of elderly have experienced more societal (economic, technical, and social) changes than any other group of individuals. The interacting forces of ethnicity and sociocultural variations create the diversity which determines how the person has moved through life, time, and space. These activities can influence one's response to retirement.

Many industrial centers are recognizing the wisdom of aging and are retaining elderly workers as consultants or extending the mandatory retirement age. For others, volunteer work in hospital agencies may help to fill increased leisure time. Senior citizen groups may provide a source of socialization for the elderly.

Therefore one's occupation has an influence on economic, biopsychosociological wellbeing, and personal self-worth.

Questions to elicit data

1   What was the meaning of work for you?

2   What does retirement mean to you?

3   Do you participate in volunteer work which allows a continued sense of productivity and, hence, maintenance of a sense of self-worth?

4   What have you done in your life that's been important to you?

5   How satisfied are you with what you've been able to accomplish?

These questions may be utilized to obtain specific information from the elderly about the importance of one's occupation to personal life state.

Self-Perception and Self-Concept Patterns

The elderly client is faced with a multiplicity of physical and emotional changes and, in some instances, impairments which can affect one's self-concept. Adjustment to these changes is related to one's perception of one's own "ego sense" as one has developed throughout life.

For many, feeling good about the self begins when the person looks well. Therefore, attention should be paid to personal appearance. It is important for the elderly to go to the hairdressers and so on and for others to tell them how nice they look.

The elderly person's self-concept can also be affected by the loss of touch. The use of "hugs and kisses" can be therapeutic for many elderly persons, as can massage and reflexology (relaxation). Whatever the contact, "several hours of being 'center stage' by having their bodies . . . 'ooh'd' and 'ah'd' over can be very therapeutic for the elderly."[31]

Reminiscing about one's accomplishments over the years can positively influence one's self-worth. This process can help the client deal with regrets and guilt as well as focus on those events that gave the person joy and happiness. "Reminiscing can be enriching whether done alone, in pairs or groups. It can be redundant . . . and for the listener this repetition may provide insight into the person's life."[32]

Many elderly clients are actively involved in activities with churches, hospitals, and family members (baby-sitting) to maintain a sense of self-worth. These activities should be encouraged, since it is important to consider the impact of these activities in one's life. Being sensitive to the older person's reluctance to expose personal parts of the self, such as feelings, is an important fact for the nurse to remember. An older person's experience with a health care system may vary. Therefore, the client may perceive the relationship between the client's concern and the health professional's as limited. Once a client-health professional's relationship has matured, the client may readily share thoughts and concerns related to the personal needs and perceptions.

It is also important to determine the elderly client's need for privacy and space. For many individuals, living space holds memories and surrounds the person with a sense of the past and present. In addition, this space increases one's sense of independence and personal control over the life situation to whatever degree possible. By retaining this freedom, elderly clients feel they are able to actively participate in their life's direction and thereby improve their self-confidence.[33]

Cognitive and Perceptual Patterns

During the aging process, changes occur in the central nervous system (CNS) as well as in the cardiovascular and other systems. These changes can result in cognitive impairment, memory loss, learning difficulties, and sensory deficits.

Determining the impact of aging on one's cognitive and perceptual functioning is an important part of assessment. Questions presented in Chap. 3 under the Cognitive and Perceptual Patterns section need to be reviewed when collecting data in this area. Care must be taken to recognize limits placed on data collection due to memory and sensory deficits or underreporting of changes in one's health status.

Sensory Perception Although a hearing deficit may not be difficult for the health professional to detect, older people are not always aware that such a deficit exists. Both hearing and vision should control spatial distance of the client and the health professional. With a deficit in either sense, placement of chairs should be closer than normal. In *The Silent Language,* Hall states that personal subject matter for Americans is generally discussed in a soft voice with low volume at a distance of 50 to 90 centimeters (20 to 36 inches).[34] High-frequency hearing is diminished first. Increasing one's volume is a spontaneous response to hearing losses; however, speaking slowly in a low-pitched voice is more effective.[35] Burnside reports that older people respond better when looking at their interviewer, but if there is a hearing deficit, the health professional should sit on the side of the good ear.[36] To determine which is the better ear, the interviewer should ask the client. With a decrease in vision, the health professional should be positioned to provide the client with maximum visibility.

Massage, meditation, and reflexology can help to bring the elderly person in touch with their feelings of self.

Reminiscing about one's accomplishments of the past positively influences the aged person's sense of self-worth.

The elderly may have a difficult time talking about inner feelings.

The elderly clients' need for privacy and personal space is important to assess when evaluating lifestyle.

Changes in the CNS as well as other physiological changes may result in cognitive and perceptual pattern alterations due to normal aging.

Refer to Chap. 3 for a discussion of questions regarding cognitive perceptual patterns.

Visual, auditory, taste, tactile, and temperature changes associated with aging may affect the elderly client's sensory perception.

The sense of touch which gave us our initial contact with the world, may still be a significant tool for communication. It is a highly personal sense which may replace or reinforce verbal messages of empathy, gentleness, and caring to the client. It conveys to the health professional strength, tenseness, temperature, tremulousness, and the need or reluctance to engage in physical contact with another person.

Age-related changes present in the hyothalamus may contribute to altered temperature regulation. This may affect perception of environmental (heat and cold) temperature and affect the client's need for external heat. Room temperature (during the interview and in the home) becomes an important factor to consider during the assessment.

Visual changes (discussed in the physical examination section) can affect an individual's degree of mobility and personal safety. If glasses are used, they should be noted along with the frequency of eye examinations, and changes in vision should be determined.

Education Educational level may contribute to the older person's ability to solve problems [including the ability to find and use resources] and it may also influence income level. It is important to remember that older clients were not subjected to equal educational opportunities nor were opportunities as available to them as they are today. According to the 1970 U.S. Census, the average white elderly person had completed 8.7 years of school and the black elderly, 5.6 years.[37] By 1990 it is expected that 50 percent of the elderly population will be high-school graduates.[38]

Questions to elicit data

1 What was school like when you were a pupil?

2 Was it possible for you to accomplish your educational goals?

3 If not, what deterred you from them?

4 Would you ever consider attending school now to accomplish your goals?

In addition, questions related to how the client best learns are important. Changes in attention span, memory, and sensory alterations may affect learning in the elderly. By recognizing the client's educational background, teaching activities can be planned to optimize personal resources.

Intelligence The questions as to whether intellectual capacity declines, stabilizes, or improves with age necessitates a qualified answer. At present there is no consensus among psychologists as to how intelligence should be defined or operationalized for study. If one determines that intelligence requires long-term memory and use of acquired skills, there may be little change noted for most adults up to age 65 years. If emphasis is placed on the use of acquired skills, an increase in intelligence may be noted since theoretically, competency in acquired skills should increase with age. On the other hand, if intelligence is defined as requiring the ability to respond rapidly and to possess competence with visual-spatial problem solving abilities, there would be a discrepancy between elderly and young age groups. Elias et al. suggest that the more crucial question to ask is what behaviors are significant for adaptation and survival and at what age.[39] For example, does increased competency in acquired skills compensate for lost abilities in visual-spatial problem-solving?

The nurse should be sensitive to potential sensory deficits when collecting data about the elderly client and make adjustments accordingly (e.g., sitting nearer to the client).

Changes in the thermoregulatory system of the elderly client alters perception of the temperature.

Visual examination is an important part of the elderly person's yearly checkup.

The educational level of each elderly client will vary from person to person.

By 1990 it is expected that more than 50 percent of the elderly population will have completed high school.

Intellectual competence of the elderly may be affected by the aging process. However, it is a controversial issue and depends upon the type of learning being discussed (e.g., skills vs. rapid response of the CNS).

Elias et al. also point to several other problems which need to be considered when studying intellectual capacity.[40] (It is important to remember information gleaned from these studies refer to group trends, not individuals.) A very highly educated, healthy older person may show a better test performance level at an old age than may a younger, less educated, and less healthy individual. The problem then becomes one of identifying the significant variable. Is intellectual capacity maintained because of the higher educational level achieved, or do higher educated people continue to use the same cognitive skills that are required in test performance and thus perform well? Intrinsic changes in physiological health such as functional changes of the heart, brain, and other neurological components may influence intellectual performance. Mental health problems such as anxiety and depression also have a profound effect on performance. Factors such as study design, test content, learning orientation of sample, and personality traits may influence outcomes. Longitudinal studies are confronted with a biased sample attrition with those who test poorly dropping out; thus longitudinal studies tend to minimize age deficits. Cross-sectional studies, which emphasize age deficits, are criticized because they compare people born at different times. Behavior modifiers and developmental opportunities may differ for each group. The choice of content and method of scoring may be manipulated to influence test outcomes. Older people may be more susceptible to test anxiety because they have not practiced scholastic skills. They tend to be more cautious and rigid than younger people. These traits may compensate for age-related losses, but they may also influence test efficiency, particularly on those tests which require rapid decision making and versatility.

The above discussion should alert the health professional to be skeptical of definitive statements concerning aging and intelligence and further emphasize the uniqueness of each older person.

Some studies indicate that short-term memory (1 second to 10 minutes) and long-term memory (10 to 20 minutes) may decline with aging.[41] However, recall of events in the distant past are seldom affected. Furthermore, an elderly person's attention span may decrease, particularly if the subject is not interesting to the learner. If the client is in control of the pace, learning sometimes is more successful. This is an important point to remember when planning teaching sessions.

Studies do indicate that short-term memory may decline with aging.

Memories of the distant past are not seriously affected by aging.

The elderly clients seem to be able to retain new information, but at times they experience difficulty finding the right answer on questioning. However, "if the person is provided with 'cues' or recognition tasks, little or no deficit is observed."[42]

The elderly person is able to retain new information but may need assistance in retrieving the data.

Sexuality and Reproductive Patterns

Today's society frequently denies the elderly expression of sexuality because of the many prevailing myths and sterotypes. While it is safe to assume that there is a decline in sexual drive for both males and females, the need for intimacy, that is, touching, embracing, or caressing must be noted. Widowhood and greater longevity decreases the likelihood of a sexual partner for old women, and impotence or poor health decreases the possibility of a sexual partner for old men.

The elderly client can have sexual needs and desires.

According to Masters and Johnson, healthy old couples have the capacity for satisfying sexual relations into the seventies and eighties. They also report

The elderly client can have an effective sexual relationship.

The most important factor in the maintenance of effective sexuality for the aging male is consistency of active sexual expression. When the male is stimulated to high sexual output during his formative years and similar tenor of activity is established for the 31-40 years age range, his middle-aged and involutional years usually are marked by constantly recurring physiologic evidence of maintained sexuality. Certainly it is true for the male geriatric sample that those men currently interested in relatively high levels of sexual expression report similar activity levels from their formative years. It does not appear to matter what manner of sexual expression has been employed as long as high levels of activity were maintained.[43]

In brief, significant sexual capacity and effective sexual performance are not confined to the human female's premenopausal years. Generally, the intensity of physiologic reaction and duration of anatomic response to effective stimulation are reduced. . . . with the advancing years. . . . Regardless of involutional changes in the reproductive organs, the aging human female is fully capable of sexual performance at orgasmic response levels, particularly if she is exposed to regularity of effective sexual stimulation.[44]

Highlights
The frequency of sexual activity engaged in during one's life seems to influence the person's capacity for effective sexual performance as he or she ages.

The elderly male's or female's attempt to express sexuality is more often frowned on by children or caretakers. Persistence in attempting to meet their needs for sexual expression is colored by the term "dirty old man" or "dirty old woman."

Of course, if the person has always been indifferent to sexual expression, it is not likely that he or she will become a highly sexually active person at age 70.

Nutritional Metabolic Patterns

The adequacy of one's nutritional state is an area of importance throughout the life cycle. Therefore, a complete evaluation of this area is important in the elderly client. Nutritional status is influenced by multiple variables, not the least of which is money. Most older people live on a fixed income, which does not increase as costs spiral. In addition to the purchase of food, money can be used in the transportation of foods, such as use of a taxi from the local market, and in the preparation of foods (e.g., homemaking services). The health professional needs to explore the client's access to the market, energy for procuring and preparing food, cooking facilities, food preference, and perceived meaning of food.

It is important to evaluate the nutritional needs of the elderly.

Many factors influence an elderly person's nutritional patterns, including food supply, money, ability to prepare foods, and availability of stores.

Questions to elicit data

1 Was mealtime a time for socialization? Who is available now to share in that experience?

2 How have work eating habits influenced retirement eating patterns?

Information regarding these factors and physical competence such as the mechanical ability to chew and the normal physiological slowing down of metabolism is needed to understand those variables influencing the older client's nutritional status.

In addition, a review of a daily diet should be completed (see Chap. 3 for a complete discussion of nutritional patterns). Starting with breakfast, have the client describe food eaten during the past 24 hours.

Questions to elicit data

1 How do you do your food shopping? What kind of cooking facilities do you have?

2 How has your meal pattern differed since retirement?

Changes in weight may also need to be considered when assessing nutritional patterns. Most elderly people require a balanced diet (carbohydrates, fat, protein, vitamins, minerals, and water). However, within

Weight changes due to over- or under-nutrition are areas that need much exploration when assessing the elderly person's nutrition.

this age group, fewer calories are required because of a decrease in the individual's basal metabolic rate (BMR).

Weight gain can be seen in the aged but tends to decrease after age 70. Often, elderly persons tend to consume a large amount of carbohydrates, often because they are cheaper, easier to prepare, and easy to eat (especially if chewing is a problem). Review of the need for all nutrients, including fresh fruits, fish, vegetables, and whole grain bread should be encouraged (see Table 14-2). When food access is limited because of such things as economic status, inability to prepare specific meals, or altered senses (of taste or smell), the availability of meals through senior citizens centers or groups such as Meals on Wheels should be considered.

While some elderly persons may be *overnourished,* many older clients are *undernourished.* A variety of factors (economic, decreased sensory perception, etc.) already noted tend to contribute to this health problem. Use of some of the strategies noted above may be helpful. Family members may also help by purchasing food, assisting with preparation, or preparing meals.

In addition, adequate hydration should be encouraged. Vitamin supplements may be another source used to achieve adequate nutrition.[45] Maintenance of nutritional patterns not only contributes to a sense of personal well-being, but can optimize other pattern areas (e.g., elimination patterns).

Highlights

Elderly persons tend to eat a large amount of carbohydrates.

The need for a balanced diet is critically important for the elderly client.

Food sources for the elderly are often supplied by community groups (e.g., Meals on Wheels).

In the elderly, nutritional patterns can affect other pattern areas (e.g., elimination patterns).

Table 14-2

Recommended Dietary Allowances for Persons over Age 50[a]

		Men	Women
Weight:	kg	70	55
	lb	154	120
Height:	cm	178	163
	in	70	64
Energy (kcal)[b]		2400	1800
Protein (g)		56	44
Fat-Soluble Vitamins			
Vitamin A (μg RE)[c]		1000	800
Vitamin D (μg)[d]		5	5
Vitamin E (mg α-TE)[e]		10	8
Water-Soluble Vitamins			
Vitamin C (mg)		60	60
Thiamin (mg)		1.2	1.0
Riboflavin (mg)		1.4	1.2
Niacin (mg NE)[f]		16	13
Vitamin B_6 (mg)		2.2	2.0
Folacin (μg)[g]		400	400
Vitamin B_{12} (μg)		3.0	3.0
Minerals			
Calcium (mg)		800	800
Phosphorus (mg)		800	800
Magnesium (mg)		350	300
Iron (mg)		10	10
Zinc (mg)		15	15
Iodine (μg)		150	150

[a] The allowances are intended to provide for individual variations among most normal persons as they live in the United States under usual environmental stresses. Diets should be based on a variety of common foods in order to provide other nutrients for which human requirements have been less well defined.
[b] The energy allowances for the older age group represent mean energy needs, allowing for a 2 percent decrease in basal (resting) metabolic rate per decade and a reduction in activity of 200 kcal/day for men and women between 51 and 75 years, 500 kcal for men over 75 years, and 400 kcal for women over 75 years.
[c] Retinol equivalents. 1 retinol equivalent = 1 μg retinol or 6 μg β-carotene.
[d] As cholecalciferol. 10 μg cholecalciferol = 400 IU of vitamin D.
[e] α-Tocopherol equivalents. 1 mg D-α-tocopherol = 1 α-TE.
[f] 1 NE (niacin equivalent) is equal to 1 mg of niacin or 60 mg of dietary tryptophan.
[g] The folacin allowances refer to dietary sources as determined by *Lactobacillus casei* assay after treatment with enzymes (conjugases) to make polyglutamyl forms of the vitamin available to the test organism.

Exercise and Activity Patterns

Activity level is determined by one's physical and financial resources as well as how one defines role responsibilities and interests. The client can be asked to describe an average day, ability to accomplish tasks with a sustained level of tolerance ("if not, please explain"), how daily responsibilities are met, or what the client does with leisure time; this profile will help determine what the client's activity schedule is.

According to Feldenkrais and Houston, the healthy elderly client should be able to engage in well-planned exercise.[46] "Each exercise should be localized to a specific body part so that for example, the head moves smoothly, fine finger dexterity improves, and gait and equilibrium are more stable."[47]

Activity helps to improve the individual's mobility and personal safety. Techniques such as visual imagery and relaxation are techniques used to help facilitate activity. Walking and hiking, swimming, various aerobic games, and dancing are considered best for the older adult.[48]

From research it appears that "at least 50 percent of the degeneration and decline in the older adults is not due to aging but to disuse atrophy resulting from an increasingly sedentary life style".[49] Therefore, if a plan of exercise is appropriately incorporated into an elderly person's lifestyle, it should improve one's general health status.

Use of leisure time is sometimes an area of difficulty for the elderly client. Access to transportation, physical limitations, or economic constraints all contribute to a decrease in leisure time activities. Since socialization is of great importance to the elderly, leisure time activities also become important for many people.

Today, local and national senior citizen groups provide opportunities for socialization and activities that involve exercise classes, nutritional planning sessions, games, and dancing. In addition many groups plan trips for the elderly which allow for increased use of leisure time. Family activities are additional sources of leisure activity among people who are supportive to the individual's well-being.

Coping Patterns and Stress Tolerance Patterns

Aging is a time of great change for many individuals. How an individual copes with these changes is often a reflection of how the elderly person has dealt with crisis situations throughout his or her life.

Anxiety, depression, and grief responses commonly are seen after the death of a loved one. Fear of being alone, anxiety associated with assumption of unfamiliar responsibilities (e.g., managing money or paying bills), and other emotional responses (e.g., anger and depression) may accompany aging.

Many times, these feeling are new to the elderly individual and require opportunities for verbalization of these reactions to another. Often the nurse becomes the person to assist in this process.

While stress is a normal part of the life process, the manner in which a person copes with and/or adapts to stressful events will in part determine successful aging. In Erikson's grid, maintenance of "ego integrity versus despair" becomes a critical variable in a "productivity-oriented" society. While there are those persons who accept old age with equanimity and dignity, there are persons who become morose and depressed as they begin to experience losses. There are those persons who deny personal aging and engage in behaviors which identify them in the eyes of some as "bent adolescents."

Bromley cites the research findings of Reichard et al. in *Aging and Personality: A Study of Eighty-seven Older Men*. The study describes "five strategies of adjustment in old age."[50] They are as follows:

Highlights

The healthy elderly person can and should engage in activity and exercise.

Exercises that involves multiple body parts are most effective.

Walking, swimming, games, and dancing are good exercises for the elderly adult.

Decline of physical function in the elderly can often be attributed to disuse atrophy.

The use of leisure time needs to be encouraged for the elderly client.

Local and regional services (e.g., senior citizen centers) often provide activities for the elderly person to engage in daily.

An individual copes with the aging process in a way quite similar to the manner in which other life stressors were managed.

Fear, anxiety, depression, and grief are common reactions associated with aging.

Some people accept aging with dignity and others with despair.

Constructiveness. This individual is humorous, tolerant, flexible, and aware of achievements, failings, and prospects. The person has had a happy childhood, suffered relatively little emotional stress in adult life, has had a stable occupational history, is free from financial worries, happily married, and has a life history which shows continuity and development.

Personal satisfaction with achievements, being self-assertive without being aggressive, capable of expressing feelings appropriately, (neither inhibited or uncontrolled) are additional characteristics of this personality. Furthermore, this individual is not prejudiced against minority groups and is tolerant of faults in other people. He or she has accepted the facts of old age, including retirement and eventual death, the prospect of which is dealt with calmly and undespairingly. For this group there is a constructive (future-oriented), optimistic attitude toward life. By being self-sufficient (within the limits set by physical condition and circumstances), this individual influences his or her own future, reflected in self-responsibility and the ability to delay immediate satisfactions in the interests of superior long-term benefits. This person can plan, save, and tolerate temporary deprivations and frustrations.

While retaining a capacity for enjoyment of food and drink, work recreation, and even sexual activity with interests well developed (showing a continuity with the earlier part of his life), the person's sense of self-worth increases. Friendships are close, and feelings of hostility toward others who have been injurious in some way seem to dissipate. This individual's self-esteem is high as he or she looks *back* on life with approval and few regrets and *forward* with anticipation to what is yet to come.

Dependence. Also socially acceptable, this personality tends toward passivity and dependence rather than activity and self-sufficiency. It is basically that of a well-integrated individual who tends to rely on others for material well-being and emotional support. The individual is unambitious, glad to retire and be free of work with its responsibilities and efforts, and derives no enjoyment from such work. This person eats and drinks a little too much, gambles, tends to live beyond personal means, tires easily, and enjoys relaxing in the privacy of the home. In this personality profile the wife is the dominant partner, with the husband giving way to her frequently and without resentment, continuing a pattern of adjustment in relation to women which may have evolved from experiences with a dominant mother. Many individuals of this sort marry late and raise only small families. Their relationships with other people show a mixture of passive tolerance and unwillingness to become involved in relationships which threaten to disturb their security and comfort. They have fairly good insight into their own personal qualities and actions and manage to combine feelings of general satisfaction with the work (they are not disappointed or hostile) with tendencies toward being unrealistic, overoptimistic, and impractical.

Defensiveness. This personality represents a less acceptable mode of adjustment in old age. It could be described as emotionally overcontrolled, habit-bound, conventional, and compulsively active. These individuals usually had a stable occupational history and had been well-adjusted at work. They were actively engaged in social organizations, had planned well in advance to meet the financial problems of old age, and although they worked hard, seemed to move more for extrinsic (defensive) reasons than because they found their

Highlights
Bromley states five personality responses to the aging process:
1 Constructiveness
2 Dependency
3 Defensiveness
4 Hostility
5 Self-hate

The *constructive* person adjusts well to the aging process.

The *dependent* person adjusts well to aging but tends to rely on others for material and emotional support.

The *defensive* person ages less effectively doing what is expected but seeing little value in old age.

work interesting. Individuals are self-sufficient and often refuse help in order to prove to themselves that they were not dependent on others. Usually these individuals express only stereotyped conventional beliefs and feelings and say what is considered normal and socially desirable rather than venturing a personal view. These defensive old people (men in this instance) seem afraid of the threatened dependency and relative inactivity of old age, putting off retirement and keeping a busy schedule of activities which prevents them from facing the facts of old age. They can see few advantages in old age and are envious of young people, even though they are satisfied with their own lives and achievements. They will come to terms with old age only when forced to do so. In the meantime, the prospect of old age and eventual death is ignored and avoided by keeping busy.

Hostility-Anger. These individuals (men in this instance) tend to blame circumstances or other people for their problems. They are aggressive and complaining in their dealings with other people and are both competitive and suspicious. On account of their reduced standard of living and lower income, they regard old age in terms of starvation and poverty. Their views are oversimplified, and they are prejudiced against minority groups. They are habit-bound and inflexible in their attitudes and values and hold unrealistic notions about themselves and the world. Often their suspicions verge on feelings of paranoia, thus encouraging withdrawn modes of adjustment. They envy young people and are hostile toward them. They can see nothing good in old age, are not reconciled with it, and are afraid of death.

Self-hate. Self-hating individuals turn their hostilities on themselves, are critical and contemptuous of the lives they have led, are unambitious, and have no desire to live their lives over again. They have moved steadily downward in terms of socioeconomic standards and are passive, somewhat depressed, and lacking in initiative, unable to make proper financial provision or to accept responsibility. The self-haters are well aware of the facts of aging; they feel that they have had quite enough and are not envious of young people. Their main feelings are those of regret, self-recrimination, and depression. Death appears not to worry them, since they perceive it is a merciful release from a very unsatisfactory existence.

These strategies of adjustment are not intended for use as a grid by which old people can be evaluated, but rather to sensitize the health professional to the shades of gray in the spectrum of psychosocial adjustment in aging.

Diekelmann describes four major developmental tasks with which the health professional may be of help. The *first* task involves "recognizing that aging can be a positive experience."[51] The life history review would be useful in assisting older persons to deal with their own personhood. The *second* task involves "making adjustments and redefining physical and social space." Changing physical capacities and decreased economic resources due to retirement may speed up this aspect of personal adjustment. The *third* task is "to maintain feelings of self-worth, pride and usefulness." Cultivation of new hobbies or interests, seeking different ways for emotional expression and fulfillment, developing an interest in life-long learning activities, volunteer work as a means of helping others less fortunate, acquisition of a set of meaningful recreational interests, can all provide opportunity for self-fulfillment and suc-

The *hostile* personality blames circumstances for problems on other people. They are suspicious, competitive, and habit-bound.

The *self-hating* personality assumes an ineffective mode of responding to the aging process.

Diekelmann describes four major developmental tasks which facilitate the aging process including a positive attitude toward aging, and maintaining self worth.

cessful aging in the postretirement years. The *fourth* developmental task is to "strive toward developing a personal set of goals as one prepares for death." During this stage the older adult increases interest in himself or herself and begins to think about life after death. For some individuals this is a time for increased religious activities or concentration on one's inevitable separation from life and those in it.

In Rossman's discussion of age-related changes he states: "Age changes are often due to a complex of interacting forces, and in some sites, it may be difficult to be sure what are intrinsic and inevitable changes, and what are changes imposed by common or uncommon external forces."[52] His statements are illustrated by the examples of sclerosis and osteoporosis. The processes which produce both of these conditions were once regarded as being an inevitable aging change. Now it is recognized that extrinsic factors such as diet and cigarette smoking influence the development of sclerosis. It may be more accurate to say that with the passage of time, sclerosis occurs in many people in certain societies. Osteoporosis is generally seen in many people as they age; however, it is more severe in women than in men and in whites than in blacks. Its development may be aggravated by low-calcium diets, inactivity, and early menopause, either surgical or otherwise. Excessive secretion of the thyroid, parathyroid, or adrenal gland may produce or aggravate osteoporosis. Hypofunction of the thyroid may increase the development of other sclerosis.

Aging is often due to a complexity of interacting forces and processes.

Summary

If holistic health is the integration of mind, body, and spirit with one's environment, then old people represent living examples of this concept. The elderly are the sum total of the biopsychosocial experiences of living. In spite of the infirmities imposed by normal aging, the zest for life may continue through old age. Old people can emerge with very distinctive personalities. They may possess wisdom and wit and can be charming and endearing. They can suffer accumulated losses and grieve with courage and humor, exemplifying the epitome of inner strengths and capacity for self-healing.

The holistic health assessment in the elderly is critical to the implementation of a nursing plan to optimize a person's level of wellness.

Health is precious at any age. For the old, it tends to be determined in a functional state; that is, old people see themselves as healthy as long as they are able to engage in activities of personal importance. While aging and illness are not synonymous, age-related decrements increase vulnerability and susceptibility to illness. Aging is a unique experience for the individual, influenced by heredity, nutrition, environment, and time.

The human clockworks strike biological, psychological, and sociological hours. We clock in more hours growing old than during any other period in the human life cycle. The inevitability of this time-dependent process results in a decline in efficiency of functioning of the various body systems working together. However, the role of aging varies among individuals.

Assessment of the older adult is an exquisite process. The assessment process demands that the health professional fine-tune his or her detective sensorium as well as cognitive skills to elicit the subtleties and nuances of the aging process at each client encounter.

Review of Body Components

Review of body components discussed in Chap. 3 can be referred to when evaluating the elderly client. Changes peculiar to this population are throughout the functional assessment as well as the physical examination section.

Recording the Holistic Health History

One of the most important characteristics of a communication tool for recording of the elderly client's history is its ability to permit transfer of information from one health facility to another. As the client moves from community to a nursing home and back to the community, pertinent historical and care information needs to be shared. The functional health assessment as presented in Chap. 3 seems to facilitate this process.

A few nations initiate a client's health record at birth, which then becomes the client's or the designated adult's responsibility to keep with health professionals recording at appropriate times. In the United States some gerontologists have begun to provide their clients with copies of their own health records. As our population becomes more sophisticated in health matters and assumes an alliance relationship with the health professional, this may become a more prevalent practice. In the interim, collection of information must continue to be obtained and recorded in a way that permits quick retrieval and easy access. Reference to Chap. 3 (under the section on data recording) may assist the reader in this process.

REFERENCES

1. Elias, Merrill F., Penelope Kelly Elias, and Jeffrey W. Elias: *Basic Process in Adult Developmental Psychology,* Mosby, St. Louis, 1977, p. 222.

2. Futrell, M., et al. (eds.): *Primary Health Care of the Older Adult.* Duxbury Press, Scituate, Mass. 1980, p. 13.

3. U.S. Bureau of the Census: *Demographic Aspects of Aging and the Older Population,* Current Population Reports Special Studies, Series 23, No. 59, U.S. Government Printing Office, Washington, D.C., 1976.

4. Ibid, p. 9.

5. Alford, D.M.: "Expanding Older Persons' Belief Systems" in *Topics in Clinical Nursing,* **1**:1, (January 1982), p. 36.

6. Cheraskin, E., and W. Ringsdorf: *Predictive Medicine—A Study in Strategy,* Keats Publishers, New Caanan, Conn., 1973.

7. Alford, "Expanding Belief Systems," p. 38.

8. Rotter, J.: "Generalized Expectancies for Internal versus External Control of Reinforcement," *Psychological Monographs,* **80**:1 (1966), pp. 1-25.

9. U.S. Department of Health, Education and Welfare: *Health United States, 1975,* Public Health Service, Health Resources Administration, National Center for Statistics, Washington, D.C., 1975.

10. Ibid.

11. Kart, C., E. Metress, et. al.: *Aging and Health: Biological and Social Perspectives,* Addison-Wesley, Menlo Park, Cal. 1978, p. 8.

12. Caird, F. I., and J. T. Judge: *Assessment of the Elderly Patient,* Pitman, London, 1974, p. 19.

13. Brocklehurst, J. C., and T. Hanley: *Geriatric Medicine for Students,* Churchill Livingston, New York, 1976, pp. 4-11.

14. Erikson, E. H.: "Reflections on Dr. Borg's Life Cycle," *Daedolus,* **105**:11 (1976).

15. Futrell, *Primary Health Care,* p. 236.

16. Ibid., p. 237.

17. Neugarten, Bernice, (ed.): *Middle Age and Aging,* University of Chicago Press, Chicago, 1968, p. 142.

18. U.S. Department of Health, Education and Welfare: *Facts about Older Americans 1975,* U.S. Government Printing Office, Washington, D.C., 1975.

19. Alford, D., "Expanding Belief Systems," p. 36.

20. Luce, Gay Gaer: *Body Time,* Bantam Books, New York, 1973, pp. 107-109.

21. Ibid., p. 108.

22. Ibid., p. 109.

23. Atchley, R.: *The Social Forces in Later Life,* 2d ed., Wadsworth, Belmont, Cal. 1977, p. 14.

24. Kart and Metress, *Aging and Health,* p. 18.

25. U.S. Senate: "A Report of the Special Committee on Aging," U.S. Government Printing Office, Washington, D.C., 1976, p. 77.

26. Kuhn, M.: "The Gray Panthers-Networking for New Community," *Dromenon,* **2**:1 (1979), p. 24-25.

27. Luce, G.: "The Coming of Age of Aging", *Dromenon* **2**:1 (1979), p. 3-12.

28. Alford, "Expanding Belief Systems," p. 37.

29. Ibid., p. 38.

30. Kimmel, Douglas C.: *Adulthood and Aging,* John Wiley, New York, 1974, p. 261.

31. Alford, "Expanding Belief systems," p. 40.

32. Futrell, *Primary Health Care,* p. 236.

33. Ibid., p. 263.

34. Hall, Edward T.: *The Silent Language,* Fawcett, Greenwich, Conn., 1969, pp. 163-164.

35. Mezey, Mathy H. (ed.) et al.: "The Health History of the Aged Person," *J Geront Nurs* **3**:47-51 (May-June, 1977).

36. Burnside, Irene Mortenson: *Psychosocial Nursing Care of the Aged,* McGraw-Hill, New York, 1980, p. 8.

37. U.S. Bureau of the Census, *Demographic Aspects.*

38. U.S. Department of Health, Education and Welfare, 1975.

39. Elias, et al., *Basic Process,* p. 72.

40. Ibid., pp. 88-91.

41. Futrell, M. *Primary Health Care,* p. 41.

42. Ibid.

43. Masters, W.H., and V. Johnson: *Human Sexual Response,* Little Brown, Boston, 1966, pp. 262-263.

44. Ibid., p. 238.

45. Futrell, *Primary Health Care,* p. 35.

46. Alford, *"Expanding Belief Systems,"* p. 39.

47. Goldberg, W. and J. Fitzpatrick: "Movement Therapy with the Aged," *Nurs Res* **29**:6 (1980), pp. 339-46.

48. Morse, C., and E. Smith: "Physical Activity Programming for the Aged," in Smith, E., et. al., (ed.): *Exercise and Aging: The Scientific Basis* Enslaw Publishers, Hillside, N.J., 1981, p. 114.

49. Smith, E.: *Exercise and Aging: The Scientific Basis,* Enslaw Publishers, Hillside, N.J., 1981, p. 16.

50. Bromley, D. B.: *The Psychology of Human Aging,* Penguin, Baltimore, 1974, pp. 257-262.

51. Diekelmann, Nancy: *Primary Health Care of the Well Adult,* McGraw-Hill, New York, 1977, pp. 161-166.

52. Rossman, Isadore: "Human Aging Changes" in Burnside, I. M. ed.: *Nursing and the Aged,* McGraw-Hill, New York, 1980, p. 82.

BIBLIOGRAPHY

Adams, George: *Essentials of Pediatric Medicine,* Oxford University Press, New York, 1977, p. 4-11.

Bailey, P.: "Physical Assessment of the Elderly," *Topics in Clinical Nursing,* **3**:1 (April 1981), pp. 15-19.

Bartlett, B. J.: "Normal Changes with Aging," *J Nurs Care,* (Feb. 1980), pp. 19-22.

Bowles, L. T., V. Portnoi, and R. Kenney, "Wear and Fear: Common Biologic Changes of Aging," *Geriatrics,* **36**:4 (April, 1981), pp. 77-83.

Burnside, Irene: *Nursing and the Aged,* McGraw-Hill, New York, 1980.

Busick, S. A.: "Visual Status of the Elderly,"*J Geront Nurs,* **2**:5 (Sept/Oct., 1976), pp. 34-39.

Caird, F. I., and T. G. Judge: *Assessment of the Elderly Patient,* Pitman, London, 1977.

Campbell, E. J., and S. S. Lefrak: "How Aging Affects the Structures and Function of the Respiratory System," *Geriatrics* **33:**6 (June 1978), pp. 68-74.

Densmore, P.: "A Health Education Program for Elderly Residents in the Community," *Nurs Clinics of North Amer,* **14:**4 (Dec. 1979), pp. 585-593.

Forbes, E., and V. Fitzsimons: *The Older Adult: A Process for Wellness,* Mosby, St. Louis, 1981.

Gelun, J. L., and P. Heiple: "Aging," *Health Care of Women: A Nursing Perspective,* Mosby, St. Louis, 1981, pp. 363-394.

Goldman, Ralph: "Decline in Organ Function with Aging" in Rossman, Isadore (ed.): *Clinical Geriatric,* Lippincott, Philadelphia, 1971, p. 30.

Heller, B.: "Hearing Loss and Aural Rehabilitation of the Elderly," *Topics in Clin Nurs* **3:**1 (April 1981), pp. 21-29.

Keeney, A., and V. Keeney: "A Guide to Examining the Aging Eye," *Geriatrics* **35:**2 February 1980), pp. 81+.

Kent, S.: "The Aging Lung; Part I—Loss of Elasticity," *Geriatrics* **33:**2 (February 1978), pp. 124+.

————: "The Aging Lung; Part II," *Geriatrics* **33:**3 (March 1978), pp. 100+.

Malasanos, L., V. Barkanskas, M. Moss, and K. Stollenberg-Allan: *Health Assessment, 2d ed.,* Mosby, St. Louis, 1981.

Morden, P.: "A Self-Help Guide to the Aging Process," *Canadian Nurse* **76:**7 (July/August 1980), pp. 19-26.

Moyer, N. C.: "Health Promotion and the Assessment of Health Habits in the Elderly," *Topics in Clin Nurs* **3:**1 (April 1981), pp. 51-57.

Murray, R., M. Huelskoetter, and D. O'Driscoll: *The Nursing Process in Later Maturity,* Prentice-Hall, Englewood Cliffs, N.J., 1980.

Murray, R., and J. Zentner: *Nursing Assessment and Health Promotion through the Life Span,* Prentice-Hall, Englewood Cliffs, N.J., 1979.

Quinn, J. L., and N. E. Ryan: "Assessment of the Older Adult: A Holistic Approach," *J Geront Nurs* **1:**5 (March/April 1979), pp. 14-18.

Rossman, Isadore (ed.): *Clinical Geriatrics,* Lippincott, Philadelphia, 1971.

Schrock, M. M.: *Holistic Assessment of the Healthy Aged,* Wiley, New York, 1980.

Stokes, S., L. Rauckhorst, and M. Mezey: "Health Assessment—Consideraitons for the Older Individual," *J Geront Nurs* **6:**6 (June 1980), pp. 328-337.

Tichy, A. M., and D. Chong: "When Assessing the Aged Don't Be Fooled by These False Alarms," *RN* **44:**9 (Sept. 1981), pp. 58-62+.

Tichy, A. M., and L. Malasanos: "Physiological Parameters of Aging—Part One," *J Geront Nurs* **5:**2 (January/February 1979), pp. 42-46.

———— and ————: "Physiological Parameters of Aging—Part Two," *J Geront Nurs* **5:**1 (March/April 1979), pp. 38-41.

Waisman, M.: "A Clinical Look at the Aging Skin," *Postgraduate Medicine* **66:** 7, (July 1979), pp. 87-96.

Wright, E. T.: "Identifying and Treating Common Benign Skin Tumors," *Geriatrics* **33:** 6 June 1978), pp. 37+.

Yoselle, H.: "Sexuality in the Later Years," *Topics in Clin Nurs* **3:**1 (April 1981), pp. 59-70.

PHYSICAL EXAMINATION

Contributed by Geralyn Spollett, R.N., C., M.S.N.

In general, the physical examination of the older adult closely follows the format discussed in Chap. 4. Normal differences in the examination of the elderly client are emphasized in the discussion which follows. The reader will be referred to Chap. 4 for a more complete discussion of specific examination components.

General Appearance

The client's face and thorax have a bony, angular appearance. The ears and nose appear disproportionately large in relation to other structures. The client's arms are long and the neck and trunk are shortened.

The loss of subcutaneous fat and the redistribution of adipose tissue from extremities, hips and abdomen account for some of the changes of the elderly client's physique (a).

Gait The elderly client's gait may be affected by aging (b). The toes point out and the steps are short. An adaptive gait, involving a widened base for increased stability, is noted. This gait compensates for a loss of sensitivity in those mechanisms controlling posture, antigravity support, and balance.

As a result of loss of subcutaneous fat and redistribution of adipose tissue, the client's general appearance changes with aging.

The client's gait widens at the base with aging. This adaptive mechanism helps control the client's posture and balance.

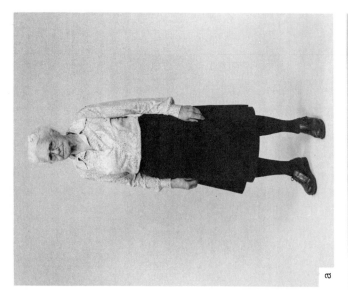

a

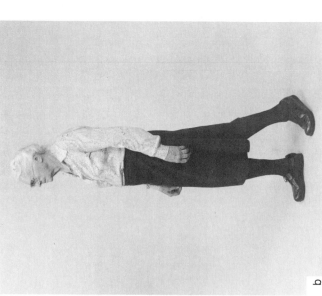

b

Measurements

Height A rounded, kyphotic posture is often seen in the elderly adult, as is a decrease in height [approximately 1/2 to 2 inches (6 to 10 cm)]. This change in posture is more pronounced in women and black males. *Senile kyphosis* commonly occurs in the thoracic region of the spine in women (a). Dehydration and shrinkage of the fibroelastic discs between the vertebrae account for these changes. As the disc becomes calcified the changes are fixed.

The loss of height in the elderly contributes the long, thin, gangly look of the extremities. Arm span, is proportionately greater in relation to present height. Reduction in shoulder width and size is noted in women. Right flexion at hips and knees can be observed.

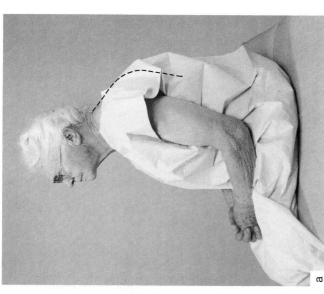

a

Weight There is a general decrease in weight in the elderly adult, especially in elderly men. Women's weight tends to increase from age 50 to 70 and decrease after age 70 (b).

Temperature In the elderly client a change in temperature may not accurately reflect the client's state of health. The changes that are noted may occur as a result of changes in the client's temperature regulatory mechanism, a decrease in sweat gland activity, as well as changes in certain neurosensory mechanisms. These alterations can result in hyper- and hypothermia in the elderly client.

The client's height decreases with aging from 1/2 to 2 inches.

Senile kyphosis is commonly seen in elderly females in the thoracic region.

There is generally a weight loss in elderly men.

Women tend to have a weight gain between the ages of 50 and 70 and a decrease in weight thereafter.

Normal alterations in thermoregulatory mechanisms that accompany the aging process may cause changes in the elderly client's temperature.

Table b adapted from a table by Master, A.M., et al.: *J.A.M.A.* 172: 658, 1960.

Table b - Mean Change in Weight With Age

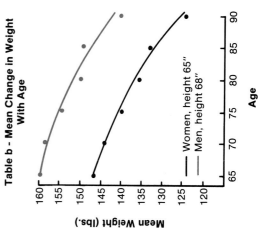

Mean Weight (lbs.) vs Age

— Women, height 65"
— Men, height 68"

b

Highlights

The pulse in the elderly is usually palpated easily.

Changes in the pulse rate may be caused by physical and structural alteration of the blood vessels (e.g., rigidity of the arterial wall).

Refer to discussion in Chap. 4 for location of various pulse sites.

Because of a decrease in maximum breathing capacity and inspiratory volume, respiratory rates in the elderly may increase.

Increased peripheral resistance caused by arterial and atherosclerotic changes can alter blood pressure.

With aging, vascular changes as well as changes in general physical health status may cause variations in the average blood pressure range.

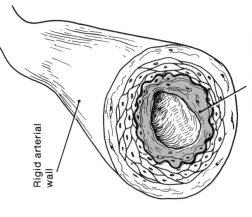

Rigid arterial wall

Fatty deposits in thickened intima

c

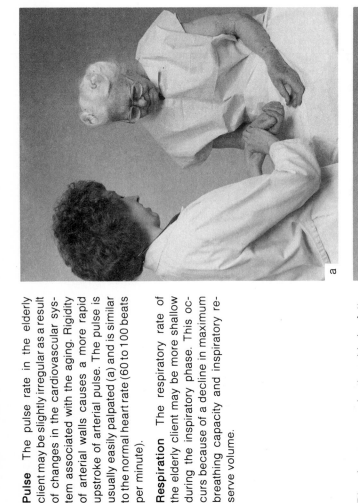

a

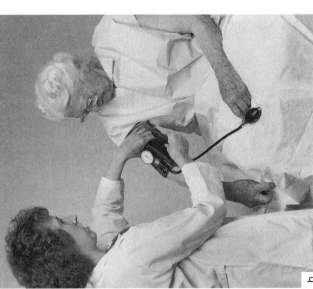

b

Pulse The pulse rate in the elderly client may be slightly irregular as a result of changes in the cardiovascular system associated with the aging. Rigidity of arterial walls causes a more rapid upstroke of arterial pulse. The pulse is usually easily palpated (a) and is similar to the normal heart rate (60 to 100 beats per minute).

Respiration The respiratory rate of the elderly client may be more shallow during the inspiratory phase. This occurs because of a decline in maximum breathing capacity and inspiratory reserve volume.

Blood pressure In the elderly, fatty deposits in the arteries can cause an increased rigidity of arterial walls, circulatory insufficiency, and increased peripheral resistance (c). Reduced cardiac output can affect systolic and diastolic pressures.

A rise in systolic pressure can lead to a widened pulse pressure. There is disagreement in the literature regarding the average normal range of blood pressure in the elderly, but changes (increase) may occur in both the systolic and/or diastolic readings as a result of the physiologic alterations noted above.

Blood pressure reading is measured similar to the procedure described in Chap. 4 (b).

Head

Inspection

The size and shape of an older adult's head may appear changed because of alterations in hair distribution and texture (a). Men with maternal hereditary balding trait exhibit a receding hairline between the ages of 20 and 30. Subsequent loss of vertex hair occurs randomly. There is no pattern of balding in men without hereditary balding or in women.

During aging, there is a decrease in hair follicle production. Hair color changes to gray or yellowish gray. As a result of a decrease in melanin and secretion of sebaceous oil, the scalp may appear dry and flaky.

Palpation

Hair texture is often coarse to the touch and lacks luster, there may also be a decrease in curling. The changes are caused by diminished oil secretion in the elderly.

Face

Inspection

The elderly person's skin may appear dry, thin, wrinkled, and inelastic (b). Wrinkles are particularly evident on the face and neck, and forehead. Nasolabial lines are also accentuated and multiple wrinkles can be seen radiating out from the mouth.

The skin changes seem to be caused by a decrease in collagen and elastic fibers, slowed keratin formation, diminished sebum production, a diminished number of sweat glands, and a decrease in subcutaneous fat.

Facial features appear prominent and angular. An increased amount of facial hair may be observed. This is more noticeable in women, especially in the area of the chin.

Men with hereditary balding traits, bald early in adulthood. Refer to Chap. 13.

Women are less affected by significant hair loss with aging.

As the individual ages, hair normally turns gray or yellowish gray and the scalp may appear dry and flaky.

Decreased pigmentation and sebaceous secretions affect hair color and texture and cause scalp dryness.

A decrease in the number of sweat glands causes the skin of older persons to lose elasticity and become dried.

Facial hair may increase with age, especially in females.

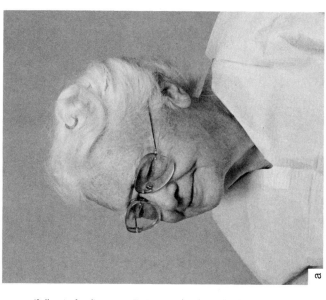

a

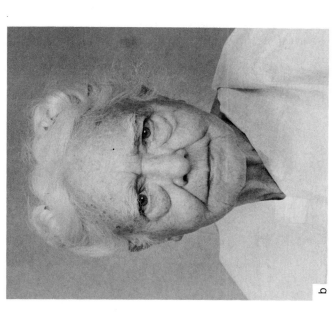

b

Highlights

Liver spots (**lentigines**), skin tags (**acrohordons**), and **ichthyosis** (dry, "fish-scale" lesions) may be noted aound the head, neck, and face region of the elderly person.

Lentigines (liver spots), **acrohordons** (skin tags), **ichthyosis** (dry, "fish-scale" lesions), and **senile telangiectasis** (small reddish areas on the skin caused by enlargment and dilation of capillaries) are commonly found in the head and neck region of the elderly individual.

Spotty pigmentation may be present (a) and skin in whites appears more white with age. The whiteness is accentuated by loss of skin ruddiness. Because of the fragility of the blood vessels, ecchymoses resulting from relatively trivial trauma, may be apparent.

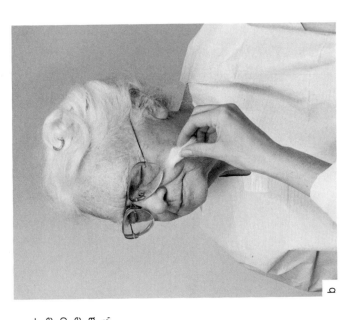

a

b

As a result of a decrease in the number of sensory receptors, dermatomes, and neurons, the elderly exhibit diminished sensitivity to tactile stimulation.

Palpation
There is a general dulling of facial sensation and hence diminished response to palpation. Decreased responses to temperature, pain, and light touch are noted (b). This is usually the result of a loss in the number of sensory receptors, dermatomes, and neurons.

Highlights

In the elderly, the eyebrows may lose hair. A decrease in orbital fat can cause the eyes to have a sunken appearance.

Loss of elasticity in orbital tissue may cause **pseudoptosis**, a laxness of the upper lid.

Pinqueculae, thickened areas of the bulbar conjunctiva may be observed.

For a discussion of visual acuity, visual fields, and pupil response refer to Chap. 4.

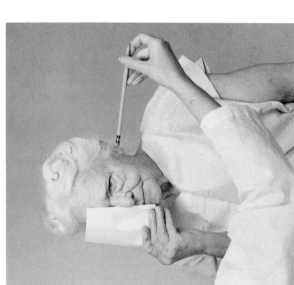

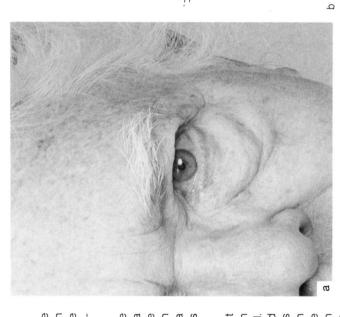

Sagging lower eyelid

Eyes
Inspection

The decrease in hair follicles in the elderly client can result in a loss of hair in the outer one-half to one-third of the eyebrow. The remaining hair of the eyebrow is more coarse.

Periorbital puffiness present during the middle years decreases with age and a diminished fatty tissue around the eye can be observed. These changes can give a dark appearance to the area around the eye socket, making the eyes appear sunken (a).

The lids become lax, which may result in a *pseudoptosis* of the upper lid and an *eversion* or *entroversion* of the lower lid. Decrease in orbital fat and generalized atrophy of the elastic and fibrous tissues account for these changes. Relaxation of the lower lid tissue can be severe enough to cause the lid to fall away from the eye, causing impaired function of the lacrimal glands (b).

Development of *pinqueculae* (thickened areas of the bulbar conjunctiva at the nasal side of the eye) may also be seen on the temporal side.

Eye tests are used to assess visual function (c). Generally they demonstrate a decrease in visual acuity and visual fields and a delayed adaptive pupil response to dark. (Refer to the discussion of the examination of the eye in, Chap. 4.)

Alterations in specific eye structures (iris, vitreous humor, retina, and choroid areas) also occur. They result in changes such as a decreased tolerance to glare and an increase in the minimal threshold of light perception.

The pupils often become small and show a slowed reflex response (a). This has been attributed to the effects of aging on the parasympathetic tone which alters function in the muscles of accommodation.

With age, pupils show a slowed reflex response.

A decrease in the pupil's ability to accommodate may result in *presbyopia*. Loss of lens elasticity and sclerosis contribute to the severity of this problem. In addition, visual-spatial perception may be altered and discrimination of objects may be less accurate as aging progresses.

Presbyopia, a loss of visual accommodation or a recession of near point, may occur with aging.

Ophthalmic examination of the internal eye may reveal a pale fundus, with veins and arteries noted in an approximate 1:1 ratio.

Internal eye examination may reveal a pale fundus and a 1:1 ratio of arteries to veins.

Ears

Inspection

Inspection of the external ear usually reveals elongation of the earlobes (b). This condition is due to loss of subcutaneous fat. Dry skin may also surround the ear canals.

In the elderly client, the earlobes often appear elongated as a result of loss of subcutaneous fat.

Otoscopic examination of the internal ear will reveal changes in the tympanic membrane. Loss of elasticity of the membrane may be reflected by the thickened appearance of the membrane and a diminished cone of light (c). Varying amounts of wax may be present in the external canal, and may account for hearing loss in the elderly.

Otoscopic examination of the ear may reveal a thickened tympanic membrane with a diminished cone reflex.

Changes in the organ of hearing and related structures may diminish sound perception and/or transmission, resulting in hearing loss.

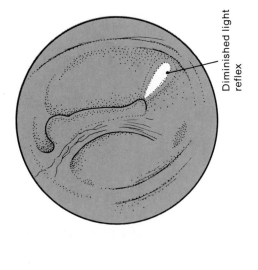

Diminished light reflex

c

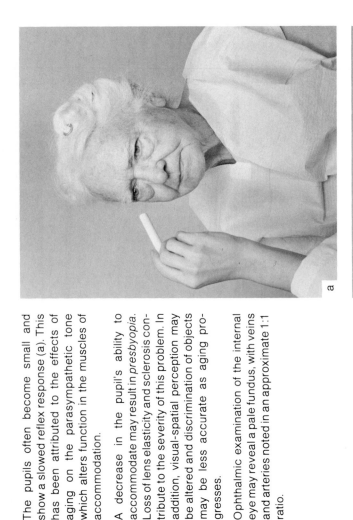

a

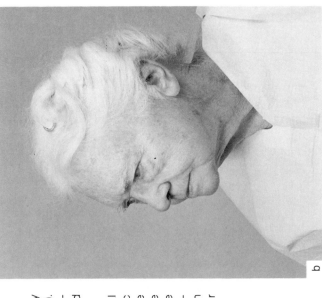

b

Hearing loss in the elderly occurs because of

1—Degeneration of the corti
2—Loss of neurons in cochlea
3—Atrophy of stria vascularis
4—Impaired elasticity
5—Otosclerosis of the ossicular chain.

Increased nasal hair may be observed.

Sinuses are more easily illuminated during examination of elderly client.

The sense of smell may diminish with age.

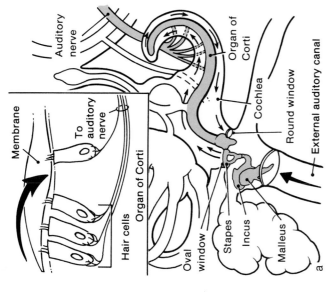

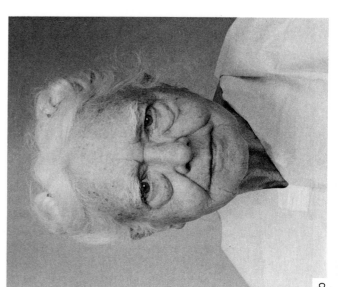

Additional changes which may account for hearing loss in the elderly client include:

Degeneration of organ of Corti (a) (loss of hair cells), can alter a person's sensitivity to high tones

Loss of neurons in cochlea (ganglion cells) and temporal cortex occurs which can affect sound perception

Impaired elasticity affects vibration of the basilar membrane and may interfere with sound localization

Otosclerosis of ossicular chain in middle ear and/or excessive wax accumulation, can develop and may lead to impaired transmission of sound

Atrophy of stria vascularis (impaired endolymph production), may impair air reflex postural control

Nose and Sinuses
Inspection

As a result of the decrease in fat tissue, the nose is often a prominent facial feature of the elderly client (b). Increased nasal hair may also be observed during examination of the internal nasal canal.

The sinuses often illuminate more easily in the elderly, as a result of the lack of sebaceous fat in the cheeks.

Highlights

As the individual ages, there is a relaxation of facial musculature.

A decrease in salivary gland secretion may become apparent during aging.

Varicosities of the sublingual mucosal vessels may be seen.

Tooth loss, loose teeth, and recession of the gingiva may be observed during the oral examination of the elderly client.

Tooth loss is often the result of loss of bone structure. (**Osteoporosis**).

Mouth

Inspection

A general relaxation of facial musculature causes the appearance of the elderly client to change. A loss of vermilion is apparent at the border of the lips. If the mouth is edentulous, the space between chin and nose lessens, with a pulling inward of the lips.

Inspection of the oral cavity will reveal several changes (a). A decrease in salivary gland secretion occurs, and saliva becomes more alkaline. Oral mucosal vessels may become engorged, with varicosities apparent. Atrophy of the papillae of the lateral edges of the tongue may be seen.

Further examination of the teeth (b) and gums may reveal missing teeth, flattened and worn tooth surfaces, recession of gingiva, and lessening of tooth structure and support. Because of this, the teeth may move easily on palpation. The enamel is worn, and yellowish dentin is visible.

As a result of the exposure of the teeth to extremes of temperature over the individual's life, vertical cracks in the enamel of the incisors may be present. Changes in the tooth structure can cause the teeth to have a glassy appearance in transmitted light.

Tooth loss generally occurs as a result of inflammatory bone absorption around the teeth in a condition known as **osteoporosis**. Osteoporosis is caused by an increase in enamel and dentin with a decrease in the size of the pulp chamber; migration apically of supporting structures of the teeth; an increase in the amount of cementum as a result of continuous apposition; and an increased area of sclerosis in root dentin (c).

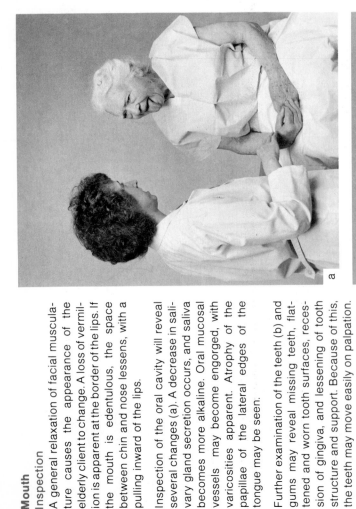

a

b

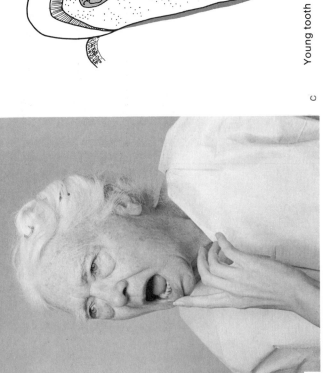

Abrasion

Dental decay

Decrease in size of pulp chamber

Increased cementum

Young tooth

Old tooth

c

The elderly adult often describes changes in taste sensation and a lessened sensitivity to food perception. Normal neuronal degenerative changes that accompany aging may result in diminished cough and swallowing reflexes.

Neck

Inspection

There is a shortening of the neck with age, as well as increased wrinkling of the skin of the neck. The elasticity of the platysma muscle is lost, producing neck folds and forming two curvilinear parallel lines extending from the clavicles up toward the chin (**upper dorsal scoliosis**) (a). Tracheal deviation due to muscular atrophy and loss of fat tissue may also be evident.

A slackening of the vocal folds, along with atrophy and loss of elasticity in laryngeal muscles and cartilages, may cause a change in voice pitch. The examiner may note a reduction in power and range of the voice and a rise in pitch.

The arteries of the neck may become more prominent, rigid, and tortuous. This can occur due to structural changes that result in splitting and fragmentation. When increasing quantities of calcium are present, the problem is called **elastic calcinosis** (c).

In small muscular arteries, intimal thickening narrows the lumen and reduces blood supply to the various organs. The aorta and great muscular arteries dilate, lengthen, and become less elastic. Pulsation of the carotid arteries may become more obvious, and venous pressure may become elevated.

Palpation

Palpation of the carotid arteries may reveal a pulse rate and rhythm similar to that found in Chap. 4 (b).

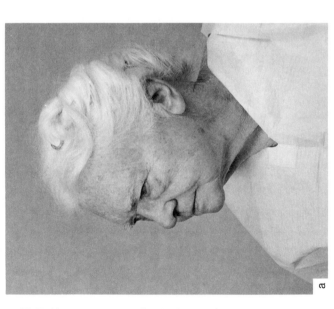

a

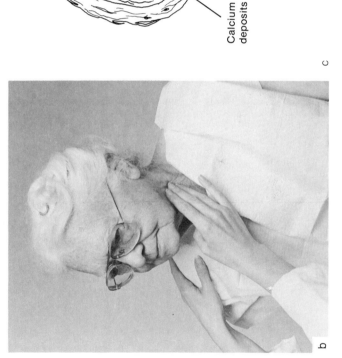

b

Elastic fibers

Calcium deposits

c

Diminishing taste perception often accompanies the aging process.

Diminished cough and swallowing reflexes may be present in the elderly.

There may be a shortening of the neck with increased skin wrinkling in elderly client.

Tracheal deviation due to muscle atrophy may accompany the aging process.

Increased elasticity of the laryngeal muscles and slackening of the vocal cords may cause the voice of the elderly client to become high-pitched and to lose power.

Changes in elasticity of arteries associated with increased quantities of calcium are called **elastic calcinosis.**

Refer to the discussion of the neck in Chap. 4 for a description of assessment of normal arterial and venous pressure.

Palpation of the carotid arteries of the adult client should be done with extreme caution; avoiding excessive pressure over the carotid vessels.

The thyroid gland does not change in size but may be more nodular when palpated. This may be due to increased fibrous tissue.

Chest and Lungs

Inspection

In the elderly, skeletal-muscular changes such as osteoporosis, calcification of costal cartilages, and weakness of intercostal and accessory muscles of respiration may affect the anatomical structure of the chest wall and alter landmarks. **Kyphosis,** which partially contributes to an increased anterior-posterior diameter, may alter the older client's posture (a). Reduced mobility of ribs and overall chest excursion may also be observed.

The older adult may exhibit a decrease in the force of expiration resulting from a loss of elastic recoil of thoracic musculature. This is compensated by an increase in lung fibrosis and loss of flexibility in the chest wall. There is little clinical manifestation of these changes unless the condition is stressed by illness. In addition, a reduction in vital capacity and an increase in residual volume may be present. Reduction in maximum breathing capacity, forced vital capacity, and inspiratory reserve are also apparent.

Diminished muscle tone and sensitivity to stimuli may weaken the coughing response. In addition, drying and a-trophy of the epithelium, sclerosis of the bronchi and supporting tissue, an increase in the size of the alveoli, and rigidity of the lungs are normal changes that affect the respiratory mechanism in the elderly (b).

Highlights

Refer to the discussion of examination of the neck in Chap. 4 for a complete coverage of the thyroid examination.

Skeletal-muscular changes normally affecting the elderly may alter thoracic landmarks.

For a complete discussion of thoracic landmarks, refer to examination of the thorax in Chap. 4.

Kyphosis is an exaggeration of the normal posterior curve of the spine.

A decrease in force of expiration, with little clinical manifestation, may accompany normal aging.

Structural changes, diminished muscle tone, and a decreased sensitivity to stimuli may weaken the coughing response.

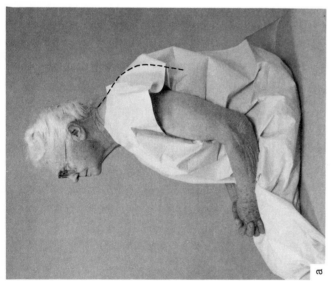

a

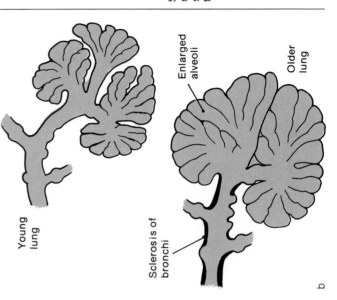

Young lung

Enlarged alveoli

Sclerosis of bronchi

Older lung

b

Palpation and auscultation of the lungs should reflect findings similar to those described in Chap. 4 where the examination of normal breath sounds is discussed.

Gynecomastia is an enlargement of breast tissue in males, and may be more apparent in the elderly male client.

Female breast may become pendulous and flattened with aging. Decreased fullness is a result of loss of subcutaneous fat.

Palpation of breasts should reveal findings similar to those described in Chap. 4 in the discussion of the breast examination.

Palpation and Auscultation

Normally, aging does not alter the quality of breath sounds assessed during palpation and auscultation (a). When kyphosis is present, breath sounds may seem distant. Skeletal-muscular changes causing weakness of the intercostal musculature may cause respiratory excursion to be diminished.

Breast

Inspection

In the male, slight breast enlargement, known as **gynecomastia,** may occur as a result of testosterone deficiency.

In the female, a flattening of breast tissue as a result of changes in muscle structure and hormonal deficits may cause the breasts to become pendulous (b). The terminal ducts will appear more prominent, and a decrease in breast fullness is a result of the loss of subcutaneous fat will be observed. Changes in breast tissue during aging are influenced by the client's overall breast size and hence vary from individual to individual.

Palpation

Palpation of the breast in the elderly client follows the procedures described in Chap. 4. Retracted nipples can be easily inverted with gentle pressure. There should be no discharge evident when palpating the nipple in either males or females.

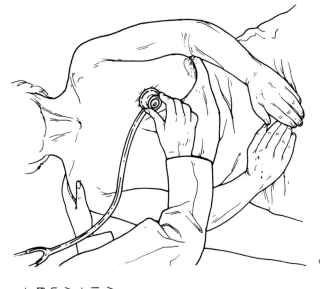

a

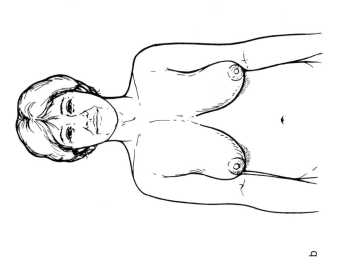

b

Heart

Changes in the heart are the result of decreased efficiency in converting nutrients into mechanical energy and a decline in enzymes needed to maintain strength of contraction. In the elderly client there is less effective mobilization of the catecholamines necessary to maintain the speed and force of contractions. The heart is less able to use oxygen, which decreases cardiac power in the presence of increased energy demands.

Inspection

Electrocardiographic changes show a decrease in the amplitude of the QRS complex and a lengthening of PR, QRS, and QT intervals (a). In addition, skin color as well as peripheral circulation can be observed to evaluate systemic circulation.

Diminished heart size may be the result of diminished work requirements. Atrial atrophy and decreased aortic elasticity may lead to difficulty in filling and emptying the heart. An increase in subpericardial fat may result in myocardial fibrosis, deposits of lipofuscin (brown pigment), and amyloidosis (excessive deposits of starchlike material).

Palpation

Palpation of the heart rate follows procedures described in Chap. 4. After stress, the heart rate in the elderly client usually returns to a predemand state more slowly. A downward dislocation of the cardiac apex may make it difficult to isolate the apical pulse (b). Senile kyphosis may alter usual chest landmarks and add to this problem.

Highlights

Refer to Chap. 4 for a complete discussion of the examination of the heart.

The ability of the aging heart to effectively mobilize catecholamines under stress is diminished.

EKG changes in the elderly client reflect a decreased QRS amplitude and a lengthening of the PR, QRS, and QT intervals. Refer to Chap. 4 for a discussion of normal EKG findings.

The apex of the heart is often dislocated downward, which may affect isolation of the apical pulse.

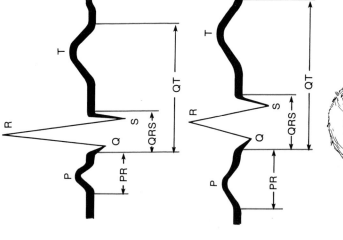

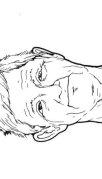

a

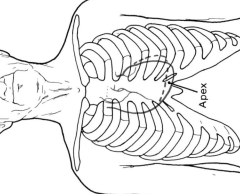

Apex

b

Auscultation

Auscultation of the heart in the elderly individual should produce findings similar to those discussed in Chap. 4. In addition, systolic murmur (aortic or mitral) may be present, without being an indication of cardiovascular complications (a). This change may be the result of calcification, sclerosis, and fibrosis which are present in elderly and can cause an increase in valvular rigidity, impeding complete closure of the valves.

Abdomen
Inspection

The general appearance of the elderly client's abdomen varies from individual to individual. There may be an increased amount of tissue and a protuberance of the abdomen itself. Muscular wasting and loss of fibroconnective tissue can occur. Adipose tissue is redistributed to abdomen and hips. The abdominal wall is thinner and less taut. Slow undulations (peristalsis) are often more visible as a result.

Stress incontinence may be observed by the examiner during the inspection of the perineal floor (valsalva maneuver). A decrease in muscle tone of ureters, bladder, and urethra often accounts for this problem in the elderly. Other changes in the elderly are weakening of the perineal musculature, a slowing of inhibitory neural impulses, and diminished time span between signal for urination and elimination.

a

An early systolic murmur (S₄) may be present in the elderly client in the absence of cardiovascular complications.

The abdomen of the elderly client may exhibit muscle wasting.

With aging, the abdominal wall becomes thinner and less taut, making peristalsis more visible.

Atrophic changes in the stomach mucosa may affect digestion.

Inspection of the perineal floor in the elderly client may reveal stress incontinence. Weakened musculature and slowed inhibitory responses may account for release of urine during the valsalva maneuver. See vaginal examination.

The abdominal wall feels soft to the touch.

The elderly client may have diminished perception of pain in the abdominal wall.

Changes in the structure of the diaphragm lower the position of the liver and make it more palpable.

There is a decrease in kidney mass with aging.

Bladder capacity may decrease by as much as 50 percent as the client ages.

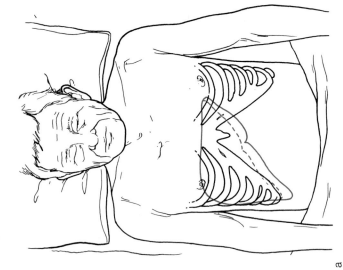

a

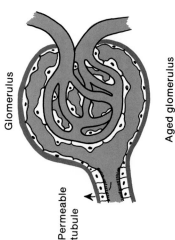

Glomerulus

Permeable tubule

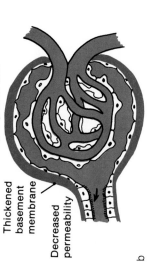

Aged glomerulus

Thickened basement membrane

Decreased permeability

b

Palpation

The abdominal wall feels soft on palpation. Organs are palpated more easily. A decrease in the number and sensitivity of abdominal wall sensory receptors can lead to a dulled sensitivity to pain (pinprick).

The *liver* increases in size with age, making it easier to palpate (a). Changes in chest and diaphragm structure lower the position of the liver, which helps account for its increased palpability. Functional capabilities should be within normal limits. (See the discussion in Chap. 4 of the examination of the liver.)

As the client ages, there is a decrease in *kidney* mass, which makes the kidneys less palpable. Internally, thickening of the basement membrane of Bowman's capsule (b) and impaired permeability may affect excretion and reabsorption. Atrophy of the connecting tubules may also be present.

Auscultation

Auscultation of the abdominal cavity will reveal normal variations as outlined in the discussion of the abdomen in Chap. 4.

There is a decrease in esophageal mobility, and this may result in "popping" sounds heard when auscultating the stomach area. In the elderly, atrophic changes in the mucosa and musculature may be present. A decrease in secretion of digestive enzymes may result in an increase in hypoacidity and achlorhydria.

The *bladder* is palpable when full. As the aging process progresses there may be a decrease in bladder capacity of as much as 50 percent.

Male Genitalia

Inspection

Inspection will reveal a decreased amount of pubic hair, with graying. The penis decreases in size, and the client experiences fewer sustained erections. The testes decrease in size and hang lower (a). The scrotal rugae diminish, and vasocongestion of the scrotum during excitement or stimulation lessens. Loss of perineal subcutaneous fat, diminished cellular metabolic activity, and a decrease in testosterone levels contribute to these changes.

Palpation

On palpation, the testes are hard and firm, and the penis is normally flaccid when unstimulated. The prostate is enlarged, but it remains smooth and symmetrical.

Female Genitalia

External Inspection

Pubic hair in the elderly female becomes thin, sparse, and brittle. The fat pad over the mons pubis atrophies with age, and appears reduced in size. In inspecting the vulva, the examiner will note a thinning of the epidermis which makes the labia majora and minora seem flatter. The clitoral size begins to decrease after age 60, and the clitoral hood will appear atrophied.

Relaxation of the sacral ligaments along with diminished muscle support can cause a dropping of the usual anteroflexed position of the uterus (b).

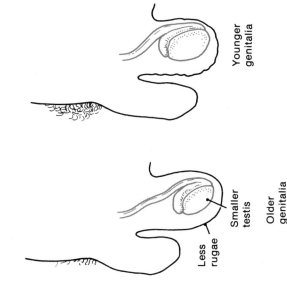

Younger genitalia

Smaller testis

Older genitalia

Less rugae

a

Rectum

Uterus

Adnexa

Vagina

Urethra

Bladder

Symphysis pubis

b

Highlights

The testes and penis decrease in size in the elderly male.

There is a decrease in the production of spermatozoa with aging.

The prostrate is enlarged, but smooth and symmetrical, in the elderly male.

Clitoral size decreases after age 60.

Inspection of the perineal floor may reveal uterovaginal prolapse, rectocele, or ceptocele of varying degrees of intensity when the client is asked to bear down. Further evaluation is needed.

Internal Inspection

As the client ages, the vaginal barrel becomes shorter, narrower, and less elastic. Without sexual activity, the vagina can atrophy to one-half its former length and width (a). During inspection, of the internal genitalia the following changes are observed. The vaginal walls can lose rugal folds. Thinning of the epithelium can cause the canal to appear pale and may make the client susceptible to bleeding in the canal.

There is a decrease in lubrication, which can make the vaginal canal susceptible to irritation and pain during intercourse and discomfort during examination. An increase in submucosal connective tissue, which replaces muscular tissue, accounts for some of the changes described above. The cervix shrinks, becomes pale, and has a thick glistening epithelium.

The cells of the reproductive tract are estrogen-dependent and the changes noted in the female genitalia stem from a decrease in estrogen production (b) rather than from the process of aging per se. Decreases in estrogen also alter the pH of vaginal secretions and can affect the tissue integrity of the vaginal wall.

Highlights

Without sexual activity, the vagina can atrophy to one-half its former length and width.

Thinning of the vaginal epithelium gives a pale appearance to the canal and can easily predispose the area to bleeding.

Changes in female genitalia stem from a decrease in estrogen production rather than aging per se.

The pH of vaginal secretions becomes more alkaline with age.

Figure b adapted from Dorothy A. Jones, et al., Medical-Surgical Nursing, A Conceptual Approach, McGraw-Hill, 1978, fig. 3-2, p. 51. Used with permission of McGraw-Hill Book Company.

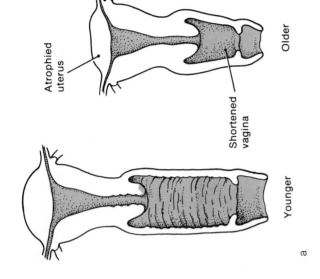

Atrophied uterus

Shortened vagina

Younger

Older

a

Estrogens excreted in urine, mg/24 h

Puberty

Menopause

Age, yr

b

Palpation

The ovaries become progressively smaller with age and are nonpalpable after menopause. Follicular activity is rare in women past the age of 50. Gradual replacement of the follicles by fibroblasts and connective tissue is responsible for this diminished activity. As aging progresses, the fallopian tubes become increasingly atrophied until eventually they are nonpalpable. (See the discussion of the gynecologic examination in Chap. 4.)

After menopause, there is a marked decrease in size and weight of the uterus (a) which may become nonpalpable upon examination. The reduction in the size of the uterus is caused by progressive decrease in the thickness of the myometrium and a decrease in estrogen levels.

The ovarian stroma can still synthesize androgens and, to a lesser degree, estrogens. Ovulation can occur sporadically up to and sometimes after menopause. Phases of sexual response are present but are less intense. Physiologic response to stimulation slows and, once achieved, is shorter in duration.

Rectum and Anus

Physical examination of rectoanal area (b) should demonstrate findings similar to those described in the discussion of the recto-anal examination in Chap. 4. Decreased sphincter control and relaxation of the perineal musculature may be observed when the client is asked to bear down.

Highlights

The ovaries in the elderly client are often nonpalpable.

Follicular activity is rare in the female over 50.

Fallopian tubes become nonpalpable as the individual ages.

The size of the uterus can decrease as much as 50 percent with aging.

Ovulation can occur sporadically up to and sometimes after menopause.

The phases of sexual response are present but are usually less intense as the individual ages.

The rectal examination of the elderly client produces results similar to those described in Chap. 4 in the discussion of the rectal examination.

A decrease in rectal sphincter control may be observed in the elderly client.

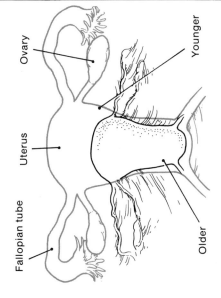

Ovary

Uterus

Fallopian tube

Younger

Older

a

Sacrum

Coccyx

Levator ani muscle

Rectal valves

Rectal ampulla

Pectinate line

b

Lengthening of the skin and decreased skin turgor may accompany aging.

As the individual ages, muscles
may lose strength and bulk.

A slowing of most muscle reflexes
will often accompany aging.

Hand-grip strength will be more
pronounced on the client's dominant side.

Decreased joint mobility can affect the elderly person's ability to
perform range-of-motion activities
(refer to Chap. 4).

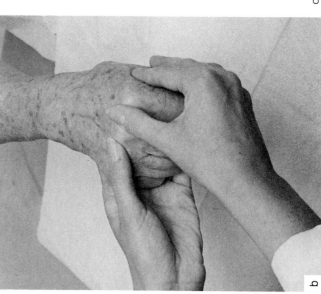

Roughened
cartilagenous
surfaces

Thickened
subchondral
bone

c

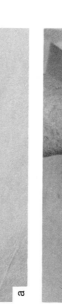

a

b

Upper Extremities

Inspection

The nails on the hands and feet appear
thickened, and there is noticeable vertical ridging. The skin of the upper extremities appears elongated, and a "tenting"
of the skin and a decrease in skin turgor
is noted in the hands. Changes in skin
pigmentation may result in appearance
of "brown spots" (a).

A loss of subcutaneous fat and elastic
fibers, along with a decrease in connective tissue, makes the muscle mass of
the biceps and triceps more clearly
defined.

Palpation

Measurement of the muscle areas of the
arm will reveal a decrease in muscle
size that is usually correlated with a
decrease in muscle bulk. These changes occur in the elderly because of disuse and atrophy, which affect both the
number and size of muscle fibers.

Palpation of the biceps and triceps will
usually reveal a slowing of reflexes,
although in some cases these reflexes
become hyperactive. Handgrip strength
may be more pronounced on the dominant side.

Palpation of the joint may reveal stiffness and crepitation upon movement
(b). Degenerative joint changes in both
upper and lower extremities frequently
accompany the aging process (c).
Rough cartilaginous surfaces together
with some thickening of the periarticular
surfaces contribute to the problem. The
extent of such change will vary with
each individual.

Movement and general range of motion
(of upper and lower extremities) should
follow the description offered in Chap. 4
in the discussion of the extremities.

Lower Extremities

Inspection

Hair loss due to decreased hair follicle production may be noted. Lipofuscin ("wear and tear" pigment) may be noted on the skin. Toenails are thick and hard.

A decrease in bone growth, and an increase in hip and knee flexion is noted.

Palpation

As a result of a decrease in peripheral circulation, the skin is cooler to the touch. A decrease in sensory appreciation of pain, touch, temperature, and peripheral vibrations, as well as a decrease in proprioceptivity, can be noted during the examination.

There is a decrease in speed and intensity of neuronal reflexes (a), especially the ankle jerk, as a result of cellular degeneration and the death of neurons.

Range of movement can be affected by the following observable age-related changes:

Muscular weakness, joint stiffness, and impaired central mechanisms for sensory-motor performance

Atrophy of bones

Loss of resilience and elasticity in ligaments, cartilage, and particular tissues

Degeneration, erosion, and calcification in cartilage and capsule

These changes result in:

Less precision in fine movements and in rapid alternating movements

Irregular timing of action—loss of smooth flow of one action into another

Slowing down to await outcome of one action before planning the next

A reduction in confidence in ability to perform activities reliably

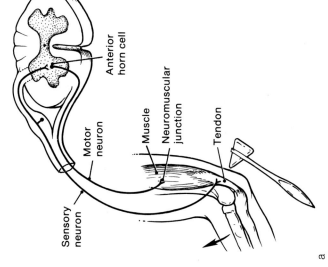

Sensory neuron

Motor neuron

Anterior horn cell

Muscle

Neuromuscular junction

Tendon

a

The skin of the legs may be cool to the touch.

A decrease in peripheral sensory responses may accompany aging.

A slowing of the ankle-jerk reflex is frequently present in the elderly.

In the older individual, muscular weakness, joint stiffness, and impaired sensory-motor performance may result in limitation of movement.

Loss of mobility of the extremities may result in:

Decrease in fine movements

Slowed reactions

Decreased self-confidence

Increased difficulty in completing certain tasks

Table A-1
Normal Laboratory Values

BODY FLUIDS AND OTHER MASS DATA

Body fluid, total volume: 56% (in obese) to 70% (lean) of body weight
    Intracellular: 30 to 40% of body weight
    Extracellular: 23 to 25% of body weight
Blood:
    Total volume:
        Male: 69 ml/kg body weight
        Female: 65 ml/kg body weight
    Plasma volume:
        Male: 39 ml/kg body weight
        Female: 40 ml/kg body weight
    Red blood cell volume:
        Males: 30 ml/kg body weight (1.15–1.21 liters per m^2 body surface area)
        Females: 25 ml/kg body weight

$$meq/liter = \frac{mg/100\ ml \times 10 \times valence}{atomic\ weight}$$

$$mg/100\ ml = \frac{meq/liter \times atomic\ weight}{10 \times valance}$$

TABLE A-1
Atomic weights of elements commonly encountered in clinical medicine

Calcium	40.08	Magnesium	24.32
Carbon	12.01	Nitrogen	14.008
Chlorine	35.46	Oxygen	16.00
Copper	63.54	Phosphorus	30.98
Hydrogen	1.008	Potassium	39.100
Iodine	126.91	Sodium	22.997
Iron	55.85	Sulfur	32.07

CEREBROSPINAL FLUID

Cells: 5/mm³, all lymphocytes
Pressure, initial (horizontal position): 70–200 mm water
Colloidal gold test: Not more than one to two in first few tubes
Creatinine: 0.4–1.5 mg/100 ml
Glucose*: 44–100 ml/100 ml
pH*: 7.35–7.70
Protein:
    Lumbar: 14–45 mg/100 ml; gamma-globulin. <10% of total
    Cisternal: 10–20 mg/100 ml
    Ventricular: 1–15 mg/100 ml

CHEMICAL CONSTITUENTS OF BLOOD†
(See also under Function Tests, especially Metabolic and Endocrine)

Acetone, serum: 0.3–2.0 mg/100 ml
Albumin, serum: 3.5–5.5 g/100 ml
Aldolase: 0–8 IU/liter
Alpha-amino nitrogen, plasma: 3.0–5.5 mg/100 ml
Ammonia, whole blood, venous: 30–70 μg/100 ml
Amylase, serum (Somogyi): 60–180 units/100 ml; 0.8–3.2 IU/liter

* Since cerebrospinal fluid concentrations are equilibrium values, measurement of blood plasma obtained at the same time is recommended.

† IU = International units.

Arterial blood gases:
    HCO_3^-: 21–28 meq/liter
    P_{CO_2}: 35–45 mmHg
    pH: 7.38–7.44
    P_{O_2}: 80–100 mmHg
Ascorbic acid, serum: 0.4–1.0 mg/100 ml
    Leukocytes: 25–40 mg/100 ml
Barbiturates, serum: 0
    "Potentially fatal" level (Schreiner) phenobarbital: Approx. 8 mg/100 ml
    Most short-acting barbiturates: 3.5 mg/100 ml
Base, total, serum: 145–155 meq/liter
Bilirubin, total, serum (Mallory-Evelyn): 0.3–1.0 mg/100 ml
    Direct, serum: 0.1–0.3 mg/100 ml
    Indirect, serum: 0.2–0.7 mg/100 ml
Bromides, serum: 0
    Toxic levels: Above 17 meq/liter; 150 mg/100 ml
Bromsulphalein, BSP (5 mg/kg body weight, IV): 5% or less retention after 45 min
Calcium, ionized: 2.3–2.8 meq/liter; 4.5–5.6 mg/100 ml
Calcium, serum: 4.5–5.5 meq/liter; 9–11 mg/100 ml
Carbon dioxide-combining power, serum (sea level): 21–28 meq/liter; 50–65 vol%
Carbon dioxide content, plasma (at sea level): 21–30 meq/liter; 50–70 vol%
Carbon dioxide tension, arterial blood (sea level): 35–45 mmHg
Carbon monoxide content, blood: Symptoms with over 20% saturation of hemoglobin
Carotenoids, serum: 50–300 μg/100 ml
Ceruloplasmin, serum: 27–37 mg/100 ml
Chlorides, serum (as Cl): 98–106 meq/liter
Cholesterol:
    Total, serum (Man-Peters method): 180–240 mg/100 ml
    Esters, serum: 100–180 mg/100 ml
Cholesterol ester fraction of total cholesterol, serum: 68–72%
Complement, serum, total hemolytic (CH_{50}): 150–250 units/ml
Copper, serum (means ± 1 SD): 114 ± 14 μg/100 ml
Corticosteroids, plasma (Porter-Silber) (mean ± 1 SD): 13 ± 6 μg/100 ml at 8:00 A.M.
Cortisol (competitive protein binding): 5–20 μg/100 ml at 8:00 A.M.
Creatine phosphokinase, serum:
    Females: 5–25 U/ml
    Males: 5–35 U/ml
Creatinine, serum: 1–1.5 mg/100 ml
Dilantin, plasma:
    Therapeutic level, 10–20 μg/ml
    Toxic level, > 30 μg/ml
Ethanol, blood:
    Mild to moderate intoxication: 80–200 mg/100 ml
    Marked intoxication: 250–400 mg/100 ml
    Severe intoxication: Above 400 mg/100 ml
Fatty acids, serum: 380–465 mg/100 ml
Fibrinogen, plasma: 160–415 mg/100 ml
Folic acid, serum: 6–15 ng/ml
Gastrin, serum: 40–150 pg/ml
Globulins, serum: 2.0–3.0 g/100 ml
Glucose (fasting):
    Blood (Nelson-Somogyi): 60–90 mg/100 ml
    Plasma: 75–105 mg
Hemoglobin, blood (sea level):
    Males: 14–18 g/100 ml
    Female: 12–16 g/100 ml

Immunoglobulins, serum:
  IgA: 90–325 mg/100 ml
  IgG: 800–1.500 mg/100 ml
  IgM: 45–150 mg/100 ml
Iron, serum:
  Males and females (mean ± 1 SD): 107 ± 31 μg/100 ml
Iron-binding capacity, serum (mean ± 1 SD): 305 ± 32 μg/100 ml
  Saturation: 20–45%
Ketones, total: 0.5–1.5 mg/100 ml
Lactic acid, blood: 0.6–1.8 meq/liter
Lactic dehydrogenase, serum:
  200–450 units/ml (Wrobleski)
  60–100 units/ml (Wacker)
  25–100 IU/liter
Lead, serum: < 20 μg/100 ml
Lipase, serum (Cherry-Crandall): 1.5 ml N/20 NaOH (upper limit of normal). (However, values above 1.0 should be regarded with suspicion.)
Lipids, total, serum: 500–600 mg/100 ml
Lipids, triglyceride, serum: 50–150 mg/100 ml
Magnesium, serum: 1.5–2.5 meq/liter; 2–3 mg/100 ml
Nitrogen, nonprotein, serum: 15–35 mg/100 ml
5'-Nucleotidase, serum: 0.3–2.6 Bodansky units/100 ml
Nutrients, various: See Table 81-3
Osmolality, serum: 280–300 mOsm/kg serum water
Oxygen content:
  Arterial blood (sea level): 17–21 vol%
  Venous blood, arm (sea level): 10–16 vol%
Oxygen percent saturation (sea level):
  Arterial blood: 97%
  Venous blood, arm: 60–85%
Oxygen tension, blood: 80–100 mmHg
pH blood: 7.38–7.44
Phosphatase, acid, serum:
  Bessey-Lowry method: 0.10–0.63 unit
  Bodansky method: 0.5–2.0 units
  Fishman-Lerner (tartrate sensitive): <0.6 unit/100 ml (up to 0.15/100 ml)
  Gutman method: 0.5–2.0 units
  International units: 0.2–1.8
  King-Armstrong method: 1.0–5.0 units
  Shinowara method: 0.0–1.1 units
Phosphatase, alkaline, serum:
  Bessey-Lowry method: 0.8–2.3 units (3.4–9)*
  Bodansky method: 2.0–4.5 units (3.0–13.0)*
  Gutman method: 3.0–10.0 units
  International units: 21–91 U/liter at 37°C incubation
  King-Armstrong method: 5.0–13.0 units (10.0–20.0)*
  Shinowara method: 2.2–8.6 units
Phospholipids, serum: 150–250 mg/100 ml (as lecithin)
Phosphorus, inorganic, serum: 1–1.5 meq/liter; 3–4.5 mg/100 ml
Potassium, serum: 3.5–5.0 meq/liter
Proteins, total, serum: 5.5–8.0 g/100 ml
Protein fractions, serum:
  Albumin: 3.5–5.5 g/100 ml (50–60%)
  Globulin: 2.0–3.5 g/100 ml (40–50%)
    α₁: 0.2–0.4 g/100 ml (4.2–7.2%)
    α₂: 0.5–0.9 g/100 ml (6.8–12%)
    β: 0.6–1.1 g/100 ml (9.3–15%)
    γ: 0.7–1.7 g/100 ml (13–23%)
Pyruvic acid, serum: 0–0.11 meq/liter

Salicylate, plasma: 0
  Therapeutic range: 20–25 mg/100 ml
  Toxic range: over 30 mg/100 ml
Sodium, serum: 136–145 meq/liter
Steroids: See under Function Tests: Metabolic and Endocrine
Transaminase, serum glutamic oxalacetic (SGOT): 10–40 Karmen units/ml; 6–18 IU/liter
Transaminase, serum glutamic pyruvic (SGPT): 10–40 Karmen units/ml; 3–26 IU/liter
Urea nitrogen, whole blood: 10–20 mg/100ml
Uric acid, serum:
  Males: 2.5–8.0 mg/ml
  Females: 1.5–6.0 mg/ml
Vitamin A, serum: 50–100 μg/100/ml
Vitamin B₁₂, serum: 200–600 pg/ml
Zinc, serum: 120 ± 20 μg/100 ml

FUNCTION TESTS
Circulation

Cardiac output (Fick): 2.5–3.6 liters/m²/min
Circulation time: Arm to lung, ether: 4–8 s
  Arm to tongue:
    Calcium gluconate: 12–18 s
    Decholin: 10–16 s
    Saccharin: 9–16 s
Ejection fraction:
  Stroke volume/end-diastolic volume (SV/EDV), normal range: 0.55–0.78; A₁: 0.67
Left ventricular work:
  Stoke work index: 30–110 g-m/m²
  Left ventricular minute work index: 1.8–6.6 kg-m/m²/min
Pressure, intracardiac and intraarterial:
  Aorta: systole: 100–140 mmHG
    Diastole: 60–90 mmHg
  Atrium: Left (mean): 2–12 mmHg
    Right (mean): 0–5 mmHg
  Pulmonary artery: Systole: 12–28 mmHg
    Diastole: 3–13 mmHg
    Wedge (mean): 3–13 mmHg
  Ventricle, left: Systole: 120 mmHg
    Diastole: 2–12 mmHg
  Ventricle, right: Systole: 25 mmHg
    Diastole: 0–5 mmHg
  Venous (antecubital): 70–140 mmH₂O
Systemic vascular resistance: 770–1,500 dynes-sec-cm⁻⁵
Pulmonary vascular resistance: 100–250 dynes-sec-cm⁻⁵
Systolic time intervals (see Table A-2)

TABLE A-2
Systolic time intervals in normal individuals (in ms)

Regression equation		SD of index
QS₂ (M) =	−2.1 HR + 546	14
QS₂ (F) =	−2.0 HR + 549	14
PEP (M) =	−0.4 HR + 131	13
PEP (F) =	−0.4 HR + 133	11
LVET (M) =	−1.7 HR + 413	10
LVET (F) =	−1.6 HR + 418	10

QS_2 = total electromechanical systole, PEP = preejection phase, $LVET$ = left ventricular ejection time, HR = heart rate, M = male, F = female, SD = standard deviation of the systolic time interval index.
(From AM Weissler, CL Garrard, Mod Concepts Cardiovasc Dis 40:1, 1971)

Values in parentheses are those found in children.

Gastrointestinal
(See also Stool)

Absorption tests:

D-Xylose absorption test: After an overnight fast, 25 g xylose is given in aqueous solution by mouth. Urine collected for the following 5 h should contain 5–8 g (or >20% of ingested dose). Serum xylose should be 25–40 mg/100 ml 1 h after the oral dose.

Vitamin A absorption test: A fasting blood specimen is obtained and 200,000 units vitamin A in oil given by mouth. Serum vitamin A levels should rise to twice fasting level in 3 to 5 h.

Gastric juice:

Volume: 24 h. 2–3 liters; nocturnal, 600–700 ml; basal, fasting, 30–70 ml/h

Reaction: as pH, 1.6–1.8; titratable acidity of fasting juice, 15–35 meq/h

Acid output:

Basal: Females 2.0 ± 1.8 meq/h
Males 3.0 ± 2.0 meq/h

Maximal (after subcutaneous histamine acid phosphate 0.04 mg/kg, preceded by 50 mg Phenergan, or Histalog 1.7 mg/kg):

Females 16 ± 5 meq/h
Males 23 ± 5 meq/h

Basal acid output/maximal acid output ratio: 0.6 or less

Tubeless gastric analysis with azure A dye: Acid present if more than 0.6 mg dye is excreted in urine over a 2-h period. (CAUTION: A negative test is meaningless and requires performance of the ordinary test with a gastric tube.)

Metabolic and endocrine

Adrenal-pituitary function tests (see Chap. 93)

Adrenal steroid values, including cortisol, aldosterone, ketosteroids, renin, and angiotensin (see Table 93-1)

Corticotropin (ACTH) response tests (see Table 93-4)

Insulin tolerance test: Blood glucose usually falls to 50% of fasting level in 20–30 min and returns to normal levels in 90–120 min after IV administration of 0.1 unit crystalline insulin per kg body weight

Metyrapone test (see page 532)

Basal metabolic rate: −15 to +15% of mean standard

Catecholamines, urinary excretion (24 h):

Free catecholamines, epinephrine, and norepinephrine: Less than 100 μg

Metanephrine, normetanephrine: Less than 1.3 mg

VMA: Less than 8 mg/24 h

Estrogens, gonadotropins, and progesterone:

Estrogens, urinary (Brown method):

Females (postpubertal, premenopausal):
Estrone: 5–20; estradiol: 2–10; estriol: 5–30 μg/24 h

Females (postmenopausal):
Estrone: 0.3–2.4; estradiol: 0–14; estriol: 2.2–7.5 μg/24 h

Males and prepubertal females:
Estrone: 0–15; estradiol: 0–5; estriol: 0–10 μg/24 h

Gonadotropins (radioimmunoassay):

Females (postpubertal, premenopausal, except at ovulation):
FSH: 10–30; LH: 10–25 mIU/ml

Ovulatory surge:
FSH: 25–35; LH: 35–100 mIU/ml

Females (postmenopausal):
FSH: 40–150; LH: 30–100 mIU/ml

Males (postpubertal):
FSH: 10–30; LH: 10–25 mIU/ml

Males and females (prepubertal):
FSH: 2–10; LH: 2–10 mIU/ml

Progesterone (radioimmunoassay):

Females (preovulatory): 0.2–2.0 μm/ml

Females (postovulatory): 2.0–20.0 μm/ml

Males, prepubertal and postmenopausal females: 0.2 μm/ml

Glucose tolerance test, oral: 100 g glucose or 1.75 g glucose/kg body weight. Blood sugar not more than 160 mg/100 ml "true glucose" (Somogyi-Nelson) after 1/2 h; return to normal by 2 h; sugar not present in any urine specimen.

Hyperparathyroidism, tests for (see pages 2017–2018)

Pancreatic islet cell function tests (see pages 559–560)

Plasma and urine steroids

	Plasma	Urine
Cortisol	9–24 μg/100 ml (8 A.M.)	2–10 mg/24 h (Porter-Silbert) 5–23 mg/24 h (ketogenic)
Free cortisol		7–25 mg/24 h (male) 4–15 mg/24 h (female)
Testosterone	0.3–1.0 μg/100 ml (male) 0.01–0.1 μg/100 ml (female)	47–156 μg/24 h (male) 0–15 μg/24 h (female)
Aldosterone		2–10 μg/24 h

Renin test (see page 530)

Thyroid function tests:

Iodine, protein-bound: 4–8 μg/100 ml

Iodine radioactive uptake: Range 5–45% in 24 h (range and mean vary widely in specific geographic areas owing to variations in iodine intake)

Resin T_3 uptake: 25–35% (expressed as ratio to normal: 0.82–1.17)

Thyroxine (competitive protein binding): 4–11 μg/100 ml (radioimmunoassay): 5–12 μg/100 ml

Thyroxine, free concentration (dialysis or ultrafiltration): 2.4 ng/100 ml (values vary among laboratories)

Triiodothyronine (radioimmunoassay): 80–160 ng/100 ml

TSH (radioimmunoassay): 0–6 μU/ml (upper limit normal varies among laboratories)

T_3 suppression test: Measure thyroid radioiodine uptake before and after 10 days of T_3 (100 μg/day p.o.). Uptake should decrease to half of original value or into subnormal range.

Pulmonary

TABLE A-3
Normal spirometric values for seated subjects

Age	Men	Women
FORCED EXPIRATORY VOLUME IN 1 S (FEV_1), LITERS		
20–39	3.11–4.64	2.16–3.65
40–59	2.45–3.98	1.60–3.09
60–70	2.09–3.32	1.30–2.53

FEV₁/VITAL CAPACITY (FEV%)

20–39	77	82
40–59	70	77
60–70	66	74

MAXIMAL MIDEXPIRATORY FLOW (MMEF $_{25-75\%}$)LITERS/S

20–39	3.8	3.4
40–59	2.8	2.2
60–70	2.2	1.6

Arterial blood gas measurements in normal subjects (at sea level):
P_{CO_2} in mmHg: 38 (± 2.9 SD) seated; no change with age
P_{O_2} in mmHg: seated. $104.2 - 0.27 \times$ age in years; supine, $103.5 - 0.42 \times$ age in years

TABLE A-4
Prediction formulas* for lung volumes and spirometric tests in seated subjects

	Age, to nearest year (A)	Height, m (H)	Weight, kg (W)	Constant (C)	Residual standard deviation (RSD)
MEN					
TLC, liters		+6.92	−0.017	−4.30	0.67
VC, liters	−0.020	+4.81		−2.81	0.50
FRC, liters	+0.015	+5.30	−0.037	−3.89	0.56
FRC/TLC, %	+0.18		−0.12	+52.3	6.8
FEV₁, liters	−0.033	+3.44		−1.00	0.50
FEV%	−0.37			+91.8	7.2
MMEF$_{25-75\%}$	−0.0523			+5.85	1.00
WOMEN					
TLC, liters	−0.015	+6.71		−5.77	0.48
VC, liters	−0.022	+4.04		−2.35	0.40
FRC, liters		+5.13	−0.028	−4.50	0.41
FRC/TLC, %	+0.16		−0.08	+45.2	4.7
FEV₁, liters	−0.028	+2.67		−0.54	0.36
FEV%	−0.26			+92.1	5.4
MMEF$_{25-75\%}$	−0.0579			+5.63	0.71

* Answer = (A × age) + (H × height) + (W × weight) + C ± 2 RSD. Example: The normal value and lower limit for the FEV₁ are sought in a man, age forty years, height 1.77 m, and weight 76 kg. The following equation gives the normal value:
FEV₁ = (−0.033 × 40) + (3.44 × 1.77) + (−1.00) = 3.77 liters
The lower limit of normal: 3.77 − 2 × 0.50 = 2.77 liters
Only 2.5% of a normal population will fall below this value (2 SD below the mean).
Key: FRC, functional residual capacity; FEV₁, forced expiratory volume in l s; FEV%, FEV₁ expressed as percent of nonforced expiratory VC; MMEF $_{25-75\%}$, mean flow rate during the middle half of the forced expiratory vital capacity.
SOURCE: Birath et al. Acta Med Scand 173:193, 1963; Grimby, Soderholm, Acta Med Scand 173:199, 1963.

Renal

Clearances (corrected to 1.73 m² body surface area):
 Measures of glomerular filtration rate:
  Inulin clearance (C_1):
   Males: 124 ± 25.8 ml/min
   Females: 119 ± 12.8 ml/min
  Endogenous creatinine: 91–130 ml/min
  Urea: 60–100 ml/min
 Measures of effective renal plasma flow and tubular function:
  Para-aminohippuric acid (C_{PAH}):
   Males: 654 ± 163 ml/min
   Females: 594 ± 102 ml/min
  Tubular maximum for PAH, males and females:
   77.2 mg/min

 Diodrast: 600–800 ml/min: 20–30% excretion in 15 min
Concentration and dilution test:
 Specific gravity of urine:
  After 12 h fluid restriction: 1.025 or more
  After 12 h deliberate water intake: 1.003 or less
Phenolsulfonphthalein:
 After intravenous injection:
  Excretion in urine in 15 min: 25% or more
  Excretion in urine in 2 h: 55–75%
 After intramuscular injection:
  Excretion in urine in 2 h: 55–75%
Protein excretion, urine: <150 mg/24 h
 Males: 0–60 mg/24 h
 Females: 0–90 mg/24 h
Specific gravity, maximal range: 1.002–1.028
Tubular reabsorption phosphorus:
 79–94% of filtered load

HEMATOLOGIC EXAMINATIONS
(See also Chemical Constituents of Blood)

Bone marrow
(See Table A-7)

Erythrocytes and hemoglobin
(See also Table A-5)

Carboxyhemoglobin:
 Nonsmoker: 0–2.3%
 Smoker: 2.1–4.2%
Fragility, osmotic:
 Slight hemolysis: 0.45–0.39%
 Complete hemolysis: 0.33–0.30%
Haptoglobin, serum: 128 ± 25 mg/100 ml
Hemochromogens plasma: 3–5 mg/100 ml
Hemoglobin, fetal: <2% of fetal
"Life span":
 Normal survival: 120 days
 Chromium, half-life (T½): 28 days
Methemoglobin: Up to 1.7% of total
Plasma iron turnover rate: 20–42 mg/24 h (0.47 mg/kg)
Protoporphyrin, free erythocyte (EP):
 16–36 μg/100 ml RBCs
Reticulocytes: 0.5–2.0% of red blood cells
Sedimentation rate:
 Westergren: <15 mm/1 h
 Wintrobe: Males: 0–9 mm/1 h
  Females: 0–20 mm/1 h

Leukocytes

TABLE A-6
Normal values

	Percent	Average	Minimum	Maximum
Total number, per mm³		7,000	4,300	10,000
Neutrophils:				
Juvenile and band	0–21	520	100	2,100
Segmented	25–62	3,000	1,100	6,050
Eosinophils	3–8	150	0	700
Basophils	0.6–1.8	30	0	150
Lymphocytes	20–53	2,500	1,500	4,000
Monocytes	2.4–11.8	430	200	950

TABLE A-5
Normal values at various ages

| Age | Red blood cell count, millions/mm³ | Hemoglobin, g/100 ml | Vol.packed RBC, ml/100 ml | Corpuscular values* | | | | |
				MCV, fl	MCH, pg	MCHC, g/100 ml	MCD, μm
Days 1–13	5.1 ± 1.0†	19.5 ± 5.0†	54.0 ± 10.0†	106–98	38–33	36–34	8.6
Days 14–60	4.7 ± 0.9	14.0 ± 3.3	42.0 ± 7.0	90	30	33	8.1
3 mon–10 yr	4.5 ± 0.7	12.2 ± 2.3	36.0 ± 5.0	80	27	34	7.7
11–15 yr	4.8	13.4	39.0	82	28	34	
Adults:							
Females	4.8 ± 0.6	14.0 ± 2.0	42.0 ± 5.0	90 ± 7	29 ± 2	34 ± 2	7.5 ± 0.3
Males	5.4 ± 0.9	16.0 ± 2.0	47.0 ± 5.0	90 ± 7	29 ± 2	34 ± 2	7.5 ± 0.3

Note: MCV = mean corpuscular volume, MCH = mean corpuscular hemoglobin, MCHC = mean corpuscular hemoglobin concentration, MCD = mean corpuscular diameter, (Wintrobe et al: Clinical Hematology, 7th ed. Philadelphia, Lea & Febiger, 1974).
* *fl = cu μm; pg = μμχ*
† *The range of values represents almost the extremes of observed variations (93 percent or more) at sea level. The blood values of healthy persons should fall well within these figures.*

Platelets and coagulation

Bleeding time (Ivy method. 5-mm wound), 1–9 min; Duke method, 1–4 min
Clot retraction:
  Qualitative: Apparent in 60 min, complete in <24 h, usually <6 h
Coagulation time (Lee-White):
  Majority and range (glass tubes): 9–15 min, 2–19 min
  Majority and range (siliconized tubes): both 20–60 min
Prothrombin time (Quick's one stage): Comparable to normal control (with most thromboplastins, 11–16 s)
Partial thromboplastin time (PTT) (Nye-Brinkhous method): Comparable to normal control. With standard technique, 68–82 s; activated, 32–46 s
Plasma thrombin time: 13–17 s
Platelets, per mm³, Brecher-Cronkite method: 290,000 (150,000–400,000)
Whole-clot lysis: >24 h

Schilling test

Excretion in urine of orally administered radioactive vitamin B_{12} following "flushing" parenteral injection of B_{12}: 7–40%

STOOL

Bulk:
  Wet weight: <197.5 g/day (mean 115 ± 41)
  Dry weight: <66.4 g/day (mean 34 ± 16)
Coproporphyrin: 400–1,000 μg/24 h
Fat, on diet containing at least 50 g fat: <7.0 g/day when measured on a 3-day (or longer) collection (mean 4.0 ± 1.5)
  As percent of dry weight: <30.4 (mean 13.3 ± 8.07)
  Coefficient of fat absorption: >93%
Fatty acid:
  Free: 1–10% of dry matter
  Combined as soap: 0.5–12% of dry matter

TABLE A-7
Differential nucleated cell counts of bone marrow

	Normal mean %*		Range†	AGL	CGL	CLL	Multiple myeloma	Hemolytic anemia
Myeloid	56.7							
Neutrophilic series		53.6						
Myeloblast		0.9	0.2– 1.5	↑ ↑ ↑	↑			
Promyelocyte		3.3	2.1– 4.1		↑			
Myelocyte		12.7	8.2–15.7		↑			
Metamyelocyte		15.9	9.6–24.6		↑			
Band		12.4	9.5–15.3		↑			
Segmented								
Eosinophilic series		3.1	1.2– 5.3		↑			
Basophilic series		< 0.1	0 – 0.2		↑			
Erythroid	25.6							
Pronormoblasts		0.6	0.2– 1.3					↑ ↑
Basophilic normoblasts		1.4	0.5– 2.4					↑ ↑
Polychromatophilic normoblasts		21.6	17.9–29.2					↑ ↑
Orthochromatic normoblasts		2.0	0.4– 4.6					↑ ↑
Megakaryocytes	<0.1							
Lymphoreticular	17.8							
Lymphocytes		16.2	11.1–23.2			↑ ↑ ↑		
Plasma cells		1.3	0.4– 3.9				↑ ↑ ↑	
Reticulum cells		0.3	0– 0.9					

* *Taken from Wintrobe et al: Clinical Hematology, 7th ed., Philadelphia: Lea & Febiger, 1974*
† *Range observed in 12 healthy men.*
Abbreviations: AGL = acute granulocytic leukemia, CGL = chronic granulocytic leukemia, CLL = chronic lymphocytic leukemia

Nitrogen: <1.7 g/day (mean 1.4 ± 0.2)
Protein content: minimal
Urobilinogen: 40–280 mg/24 h
Water: Approximately 65%

URINE
(See also Function Tests: Metabolic and Endocrine)

Acidity, titratable: 20–40 meq/24 h
α-Amino nitrogen: 0.4–1.0 g/24 h
Ammonia: 30–50 meq/24 h
Amylase (Somogyi): 35–260 units/h
Calcium, 10 meq or 200 mg calcium diet:
  <7.5 meq/24 h or <150 mg/24 h
Catecholamines: Less than 100 μg/24 h
Copper: 0–25 μg/24 h

Coproporphyrins (types I and III): 100–300 μg/24h
Creatine, as creatinine:
  Adult males: <50 mg/24 h
  Adult females: <100 mg/24 h
Creatinine: 1.0–1.6 g/24 h
Glucose, true (oxidase method): 50–300 mg/24 h
5-Hydroxyindoleacetic acid (5HIAA): 2–9 mg/24 h
Ketones, total (mean ± 1 SD): 50.5∓30.7 mg/24 h
Lactic dehydrogenase: 560–2.050 units/8 h urine
Lead: <0.08 μg/ml or <120 μg/24 h
Protein: <50 mg/24 h
Porphobilinogen: 0 μg/24 h
Potassium: 25–100 meq/24 h (varies with intake)
Sodium: 100–260 meq/24 h (varies with intake)
Urobilinogen: 1–3.5 mg/24 h
Vanillylmandelic acid (VMA): 0.7–6.8 mg/24 h
D-Xylose excretion: 5–8 g/5 after oral dose of 25 g

SOURCE: G W Thorne et al: *Harrison's Principles of Internal Medicine*, 8th ed., McGraw-Hill, New York, 1977

Table A-2
Major Tracts (Pathways) of the Spinal Cord

Tract	Spinal Cord Location	Site of Origin	Site of Termination	Function
Ascending tracts				
Fasciculus gracilis (T7 and below) Fasciculus cuneatus (T6 and above)	Posterior white columns	Spinal ganglions on the same side of the cord	Medulla	Touch, two-point discrimination. position sense (kinesthesia), motion, weight perception, vibration sense
Spinocerebellar posterior	Lateral white columns	Neuromuscular receptors on the same side of the cord	Cerebellum	Unconscious proprioception (muscle sense)
Spinocerebellar anterior	Lateral white columns	Neuromuscular receptors on the same *and* opposite sides of the cord	Cerebellum	Coordination of posture and limb movement
Spinothalamic lateral	Lateral white columns	Cell bodies in the posterior horn on the opposite side of the cord	Thalamus	Pain and temperature sensation on the opposite sides of the body
Spinothalamic anterior	Anterior white columns	Cell bodies in the posterior horn on the opposite side of the cord	Thalamus	Touch and pressure on the opposite sides of the body
Descending tracts				
Pyramidal Lateral Corticospinal	Lateral white columns	Voluntary motor areas of the cerebral cortex (fibers cross in the medulla)	Anterior gray or anterolateral columns in the spinal cord	Voluntary movement especially of the arms and legs
Anterior corticospinal	Anterior or ventral columns	Voluntary motor areas of the cerebral cortex (uncrossed fibers)	Anterior gray or anterolateral columns in the spinal cord	Voluntary movement of the trunk muscles
Extrapyramidal Rubrospinal	Lateral white columns	Red nucleus of the midbrain (fibers cross immediately)	Anterior gray or anterolateral columns in the spinal cord	Muscle tone and coordination. posture
Vestibulospinal	Anterior or ventral columns	Vestibular nuclei in the medulla	Anterior gray or anterolateral columns in the spinal cord	Equilibrium and posture

Table A-3
Cranial Nerves

Number and Name	Type of Nerve	Site of Origin	Site of Termination	Function
I Olfactory	Sensory (afferent)	Sensory receptors in the nasal mucosa	Olfactory bulb in the brain	Smell
II Optic	Sensory (afferent)	Sensory cells in the retina	Occipital lobe of the cerebrum	Vision and associated reflexes
III Oculomotor	Motor (efferent)	Gray matter in the midbrain	Levator palpebrae, superior, medial, and inferior rectus, and inferior oblique muscles	Movement of the eyeball, pupillary constriction and accommodation
IV Trochlear	Motor (efferent)	Gray matter in the midbrain	Superior oblique muscles	Movement of the eyeball
V Trigeminal	Sensory (afferent)	Ophthalmic branch: Eye, lacrimal gland, nose, forehead	Sensory: Midpons, below the fourth ventricle	General sensations from the anterior surface of the face, mouth, nose, and tongue
	Sensory (afferent)	Maxillary branch: Teeth and gums of the upper jaw, upper lip, cheek	Motor: Muscles of mastication	Mastication, swallowing; movement of the soft palate, auditory tube, ear ossicles, and tympanic membrane.
	Mixed	Manidibular branch: Sensory from teeth and gums of lower jaw, chin, lower lip, tongue. Motor from the midpons		
VI Abducent	Motor (efferent)	Lower pons beneath fourth ventricle	Lateral rectus muscle	Movement of the eyeball
VII Facial	Motor (efferent)	Lower pons	Muscles of face and forehead; parasympathetic fibers to lacrimal, submandibular, and sublingual glands	Facial expression; lacrimation, salivation, and vasodilatation
	Sensory (afferent)	Anterior two-thirds of tongue, external ear, and facial glands	Genticulate ganglion in temporal bone	Taste: sensation from external ear and glands
VIII Vestibulocochlear	Sensory (afferent)	Cochlear branch: Sensory receptors in cochlea	Temporal lobe of the cerebrum	Hearing
		Vestibular branch: Sensory receptors in the semicircular canals and vestibule	Cerebellum	Equilibrium
IX Glossopharyngeal	Motor (efferent)	Medulla	Muscles of the pharynx, parotid gland via parasympathetic fibers	Swallowing movements, vasodilatation, and salivation
	Sensory (afferent)	Tonsils, mucous membrane of the pharynx, external ear and posterior one-third of the tongue, pressoreceptors and chemoreceptors in the cortoid body.	Medulla	Taste, general sensation to the posterior tongue, tonsils, and upper pharynx; cardiovascular and respiratory effects from receptors in the carotid sinus and carotid body.

Table A-3 Cranial Nerves (continued)

Number and Name	Type of Nerve	Site of Origin	Site of Termination	Function
X Vagus	Sensory (afferent)	Mucous membrane lining respiratory and digestive tracts	Medulla	Taste and general sensation from larynx, neck, thorax, and abdomen
	Motor (efferent)	Medulla	Muscles of pharynx and larynx	Swallowing, movement of pharynx and larynx
			Parasympathetic fibers to thoracic and abdominal viscera	Inhibitory fibers to the heart; secretion of gastric glands and pancreas; vasodilator fibers to abdominal viscera
XI Accessory	Motor	Cranial portion: Medulla	Pharyngeal and laryngeal muscles	Movement of the soft palate, pharynx, and larynx
		Spinal portion: Upper cervical region of the spinal cord	Sternocleidomastoid and trapezius muscles	Shoulder and head movement
XII Hypoglossal	Motor	Medulla	Muscles of the tongue	Speaking and swallowing, tongue movement

Table A-4
Fahrenheit and Celsius Equivalents: Body Temperature Range

F°	C°	F°	C°	F°	C°	F°	C°	F°	C°
94.0	34.44	97.0	36.11	100.0	37.78	103.0	39.44	106.0	41.11
94.2	34.56	97.2	36.22	100.2	37.89	103.2	39.56	106.2	41.22
94.4	34.67	97.4	36.33	100.4	38.00	103.4	39.67	106.4	41.33
94.6	34.78	97.6	36.44	100.6	38.11	103.6	39.78	106.6	41.44
94.8	34.89	97.8	36.56	100.8	38.22	103.8	39.89	106.8	41.56
95.0	35.00	98.0	36.67	101.0	38.33	104.0	40.00	107.0	41.67
95.2	35.11	98.2	36.78	101.2	38.44	104.2	40.11	107.2	41.78
95.4	35.22	98.4	36.89	101.4	38.56	104.4	40.22	107.4	41.89
95.6	35.33	98.6	37.00	101.6	38.67	104.6	40.33	107.6	42.00
95.8	35.44	98.8	37.11	101.8	38.78	104.8	40.44	107.8	42.11
96.0	35.56	99.0	37.22	102.0	38.89	105.0	40.56	108.0	42.22
96.2	35.67	99.2	37.33	102.2	39.00	105.2	40.67		
96.4	35.78	99.4	37.44	102.4	39.11	105.4	40.78		
96.6	35.89	99.6	37.56	102.6	39.22	105.6	40.89		
96.8	36.00	99.8	37.67	102.8	39.33	105.8	41.00		

Table A-5
Celsius and Fahrenheit Equivalents: Body Temperature Range

C°	F°	C°	F°	C°	F°	C°	F°	C°	F°
34.0	93.20	35.5	95.90	37.0	98.60	38.5	101.30	40.0	104.00
34.1	93.38	35.6	96.08	37.1	98.78	38.6	101.48	40.1	104.18
34.2	93.56	35.7	96.26	37.2	98.96	38.7	101.66	40.2	104.36
34.3	93.74	35.8	96.44	37.3	99.14	38.8	101.84	40.3	104.54
34.4	93.92	35.9	96.62	37.4	99.32	38.9	102.02	40.4	104.72
34.5	94.10	36.0	96.80	37.5	99.50	39.0	102.20	40.5	104.90
34.6	94.28	36.1	96.98	37.6	99.68	39.1	102.38	40.6	105.08
34.7	94.46	36.2	97.16	37.7	99.86	39.2	102.56	40.7	105.26
34.8	94.64	36.3	97.34	37.8	100.04	39.3	102.74	40.8	105.44
34.9	94.82	36.4	97.52	37.9	100.22	39.4	102.92	40.9	105.62
35.0	95.0	36.5	97.70	38.0	100.40	39.5	103.10	41.0	105.80
35.1	95.18	36.6	97.88	38.1	100.58	39.6	103.28		
35.2	95.36	36.7	98.06	38.2	100.76	39.7	103.46		
35.3	95.54	36.8	98.24	38.3	100.94	39.8	103.64		
35.4	95.72	36.9	98.42	38.4	101.12	39.9	103.82		

Table A-6
Fahrenheit and Celsius Equivalents

Fahrenheit to Celsius: $(F - 32) \times 5/9 = C$ or $C = \dfrac{F - 32}{1.8}$

F°	C°	F°	C°	F°	C°	F°	C°	F°	C°
−40	−40.0	11	−11.67	62	16.67	113	45.0	164	73.33
−39	−39.44	12	−11.11	63	17.22	114	45.56	165	73.89
−38	−38.89	13	−10.56	64	17.78	115	46.11	166	74.44
−37	−38.33	14	−10.0	65	18.33	116	46.67	167	75.0
−36	−37.78	15	−9.44	66	18.89	117	47.22	168	75.56
−35	−37.22	16	−8.89	67	19.44	118	47.78	169	76.11
−34	−36.67	17	−8.33	68	20.0	119	48.33	170	76.67
−33	−36.11	18	−7.78	69	20.56	120	48.89	171	77.22
−32	−35.56	19	−7.22	70	21.11	121	49.44	172	77.78
−31	−35.0	20	−6.67	71	21.67	122	50.0	173	78.33
−30	−34.44	21	−6.11	72	22.22	123	50.56	174	78.89
−29	−33.89	22	−5.56	73	22.78	124	51.11	175	79.44
−28	−33.33	23	−5.0	74	23.33	125	51.67	176	80.0
−27	−32.78	24	−4.44	75	23.89	126	52.22	177	80.56
−26	−32.22	25	−3.89	76	24.44	127	52.78	178	81.11
−25	−31.67	26	−3.33	77	25.0	128	53.33	179	81.67
−24	−31.11	27	−2.78	78	25.56	129	53.89	180	82.22
−23	−30.56	28	−2.22	79	26.11	130	54.44	181	82.78
−22	−30.0	29	−1.67	80	26.67	131	55.0	182	83.33
−21	−29.44	30	−1.11	81	27.22	132	55.56	183	83.89
−20	−28.89	31	−0.56	82	27.78	133	56.11	184	84.44
−19	−28.33	32	0.0	83	28.33	134	56.67	185	85.0
−18	−27.78	33	0.56	84	28.89	135	57.22	186	85.56
−17	−27.22	34	1.11	85	29.44	136	57.78	187	86.11
−16	−26.67	35	1.67	86	30.0	137	58.33	188	86.67
−15	−26.11	36	2.22	87	30.56	138	58.89	189	87.22
−14	−25.56	37	2.78	88	31.11	139	59.44	190	87.78
−13	−25.0	38	3.33	89	31.67	140	60.0	191	88.33
−12	−24.44	39	3.89	90	32.22	141	60.56	192	88.89
−11	−23.89	40	4.44	91	32.78	142	61.11	193	89.44
−10	−23.33	41	5.0	92	33.33	143	61.67	194	90.0
−9	−22.78	42	5.56	93	33.89	144	62.22	195	90.56
−8	−22.22	43	6.11	94	34.44	145	62.78	196	91.11
−7	−21.67	44	6.67	95	35.0	146	63.33	197	91.67
−6	−21.11	45	7.22	96	35.56	147	63.89	198	92.22
−5	−20.56	46	7.78	97	36.11	148	64.44	199	92.78
−4	−20.0	47	8.33	98	36.67	149	65.0	200	93.33
−3	−19.44	48	8.89	99	37.22	150	65.56	201	93.89
−2	−18.89	49	9.44	100	37.78	151	66.11	202	94.44
−1	−18.33	50	10.0	101	38.33	152	66.67	203	95.0
0	−17.78	51	10.56	102	38.89	153	67.22	204	95.56
1	−17.22	52	11.11	103	39.44	154	67.78	205	96.11
2	−16.67	53	11.67	104	40.0	155	68.33	206	96.67
3	−16.11	54	12.22	105	40.56	156	68.89	207	97.22
4	−15.56	55	12.78	106	41.11	157	69.44	208	97.78
5	−15.0	56	13.33	107	41.67	158	70.0	209	98.33
6	−14.44	57	13.89	108	42.22	159	70.56	210	98.89
7	−13.89	58	14.44	109	42.78	160	71.11	211	99.44
8	−13.33	59	15.0	110	43.33	161	71.67	212	100.0
9	−12.78	60	15.56	111	43.89	162	72.22		
10	−12.22	61	16.11	112	44.44	163	72.78		

Table A-7
Celsius and Fahrenheit Equivalents

Celsius to Fahrenheit: 9/5 C + 32 = F or F = (C × 1.8) + 32

C°	F°	C°	F°	C°	F°	C°	F°	C°	F°
-50	-58.0	-19	-2.2	12	53.6	43	109.4	74	165.2
-49	-56.2	-18	-0.4	13	55.4	44	111.2	75	157.0
-48	-54.4	-17	1.4	14	57.2	45	113.0	76	168.8
-47	-52.6	-16	3.2	15	59.0	46	114.8	77	170.6
-46	-50.8	-15	5.0	16	60.8	47	116.6	78	172.4
-45	-49.0	-14	6.8	17	62.6	48	118.4	79	174.2
-44	-47.2	-13	8.6	18	64.4	49	120.2	80	176.0
-43	-45.4	-12	10.4	19	66.2	50	122.0	81	177.8
-42	-43.6	-11	12.2	20	68.0	51	123.8	82	179.6
-41	-41.8	-10	14.0	21	69.8	52	125.6	83	181.4
-40	-40.0	-9	15.8	22	71.6	53	127.4	84	183.2
-39	-38.2	-8	17.6	23	73.4	54	129.2	85	185.0
-38	-36.4	-7	19.4	24	75.2	55	131.0	86	186.8
-37	-34.6	-6	21.2	25	77.0	56	132.8	87	188.6
-36	-32.8	-5	23.0	26	78.8	57	134.6	88	190.4
-35	-31.0	-4	24.8	27	80.6	58	136.4	89	192.2
-34	-29.2	-3	26.6	28	82.4	59	138.2	90	194.0
-33	-27.4	-2	28.4	29	84.2	60	140.0	91	195.8
-32	-25.6	-1	30.2	30	86.0	61	141.8	92	197.6
-31	-23.8	0	32.0	31	87.8	62	143.6	93	199.4
-30	-22.0	1	33.8	32	89.6	63	145.4	94	201.2
-29	-20.2	2	35.6	33	91.4	64	147.2	95	203.0
-28	-18.4	3	37.4	34	93.2	65	149.0	96	204.8
-27	-16.6	4	39.2	35	95.0	66	150.8	97	206.6
-26	-14.8	5	41.0	36	96.8	67	152.6	98	208.4
-25	-13.0	6	42.8	37	98.6	68	154.4	99	210.2
-24	-11.2	7	44.6	38	100.4	69	156.2	100	212.0
-23	-9.4	8	46.4	39	102.2	70	158.0		
-22	-7.6	9	48.2	40	104.0	71	159.8		
-21	-5.8	10	50.0	41	105.8	72	161.6		
-20	-4.0	11	51.8	42	107.6	73	163.4		

Table A-8

List of Nursing Diagnoses Accepted for Clinical Testing by the North American Nursing Diagnosis Association, April 1982

*Activity Intolerance
 Airway Clearance Ineffective
*Anxiety
 Bowel Elimination, Alterations in: Constipation
 Bowel Elimination, Alterations in: Diarrhea
 Bowel Elimination, Alterations in: Incontinence
 Breathing Patterns, Ineffective
 Cardiac Output, Alterations in: Decreased
 Comfort, Alterations in: Pain
 Communication, Impaired Verbal
 Coping, Ineffective Individual
 Coping, Ineffective Family: Compromised
 Coping, Ineffective Family: Disabling
 Coping, Family: Potential for Growth
 Diversional Activity, Deficit
*Family Process, Alteration in
 Fear
 Fluid Volume Deficit, Actual
 Fluid Volume Deficit, Potential
*Fluid Volume, Alterations in: Excess
 Gas Exchange, Impaired
 Grieving, Anticipatory
 Grieving, Dysfunctional
*Health Maintenance, Alterations in
 Home Maintenance Management, Impaired
 Injury, Potential for
 Knowledge Deficit (specify)
 Mobility, Impaired Physical
 Non-compliance (specify)
 Nutrition, Alterations in: Less Than Body Requirements
 Nutrition, Alterations in: More Than Body Requirements
 Nutrition, Alterations in: Potential For More Than Body Requirements
*Oral Mucous Membranes, Alterations in
 Parenting, Alterations in: Actual
 Parenting, Alterations in: Potential
*Powerlessness
 Rape-Trauma Syndrome
 Self-Care Deficit (specify level: Feeding, Bathing/hygiene, Dressing/grooming, Toileting)
 Self-concept, Disturbance in
 Sensory Perceptual Alterations
 Sexual Dysfunction
 Skin Integrity, Impairment of: Actual
 Skin Integrity, Impairment of: Potential
 Sleep Pattern Disturbance
*Social Isolation
 Spiritual Distress (Distress of the Human Spirit)
 Thought Processes, Alterations in
 Tissue Perfusion, Alteration in
 Urinary Elimination, Alteration in Patterns
 Violence, Potential for

*New diagnoses accepted by the Fifth National Conference on Classification of Nursing Diagnosis. See Table A-9.

Table A-9 New Diagnoses Accepted for Clinical Testing by the Fifth National Conference on Classification of Nursing Diagnosis

ACTIVITY INTOLERANCE

Etiology: bedrest/immobility, generalized weakness, sedentary lifestyle, imbalance between oxygen supply and demand
Defining characteristics (* critical defining characteristics):

*1 verbal report of fatigue or weakness

2 abnormal heart rate or blood pressure response to activity

3 exertional discomfort or dyspnea

4 electrocardiographic changes reflecting arrythmias or ischemia

ANXIETY

Definition: a vague, uneasy feeling the source of which is often nonspecific or unknown to the individual.
Etiology: unconscious conflict about essential values and goals of life; threat to self concept; threat of death; threat to or change in health status; threat to or change in socioeconomic status; threat to or change in role functioning; threat to or change in environment; threat to or change in interaction patterns; situational/maturational crises; interpersonal transmission/contagion unmet needs
Defining characteristics (* critical defining characteristics):

I. *Subjective*
1. increased tension

2. apprehension

3. painful and persistent increased helplessness

4. uncertainty

5. fearful

6. scared

7. regretful

8. overexcited

9. rattled

10. distressed

11. jittery

12. feelings of inadequacy

13. shakiness

14. fear of unspecific consequences

15. expressed concerns re change in life events

16. worried

17. anxious

II. *Objective*
*1. sympathetic stimulation—cardiovascular excitation, superficial vasoconstriction, pupil dilation

2. restlessness

3. insomnia

4. glancing about

5. poor eye contact

6. trembling/hand tremors

7. extraneous movement (foot shuffling, hand/arm movements)

8. facial tension

9. voice quivering

10. focus "self"

11. increased wariness

12. increased perspiration

FAMILY PROCESSES, ALTERATION IN

Etiology: situation transition and/or crisis; development transition and/or crisis
Defining characteristics:

1. family system unable to meet physical needs for its members

2. family system unable to meet emotional needs of its members

3. family system unable to meet spiritual needs of its members
4. parents do not demonstrate respect for each other's views on child-rearing practices
5. inability to express or accept wide range of feelings
6. inability to express or accept feelings of members
7. family unable to meet security needs of its members
8. inability to accept or receive help appropriately
9. family does not demonstrate respect for individuality and autonomy of its members
10. inability of the family members to relate to each other for mutual growth and maturation
11. family uninvolved in community activities
12. rigidity in function and roles
13. family inability to adapt to change or deal with traumatic experience constructively
14. family fails to accomplish current or past developmental task
15. unhealthy family decision-making process
16. failure to send and receive clear messages
17. inappropriate boundary maintenance
18. inappropriate or poorly communicated family rules, rituals, symbols
19. unexamined family myths
20. inappropriate level and direction of energy

FLUID VOLUME, ALTERATION IN: EXCESS

Etiology: comprised regulatory mechanism; excess fluid intake; excess sodium intake
Defining characteristics:

1. edema
2. effusion
3. anasarca
4. weight gain
5. SOB, orthopnea
6. intake greater than output
7. S_3 heart sound
8. pulmonary congestion: chest x ray
9. abnormal breath sounds: crackles (rales)
10. change in respiratory pattern
11. change in mental status
12. decreased hemoglobin and hematocrit
13. blood pressure changes
14. central venous pressure changes
15. pulmonary artery pressure changes
16. jugular vein distention
17. positive hepatojugular reflex
18. ollguria
19. specific gravity changes
20. azotemia
21. altered electrolytes
22. restlessness and anxiety

HEALTH MAINTENANCE ALTERATION

Definition: inability to identify, manage and/or seek out help to maintain health
Etiology: lack of, or significant alteration in, communication skills (written, verbal and/or gestural); lack of ability to make deliberate and thoughtful judgments; perceptual/cognitive impairment complete or partial lack of gross and/or fine motor skills; ineffective individual coping, dysfunctional grieving; unachieved developmental tasks; ineffective family coping: disabling spiritual; lack of material resources
Defining characteristics:

1. demonstrated lack of knowledge regarding basic health practices
2. demonstrated lack of adaptive behaviors to internal/external environmental changes

3. reported or observed inability to take responsibility for meeting basic health practices in any or all functional pattern areas

4. history of lack of health seeking behavior

5. expressed client interest in improving health behaviors

6. reported or observed lack of equipment, financial and/or other resources

7. reported or observed impairment of personal support system

ORAL MUCUS MEMBRANE, ALTERATIONS IN

Etiology: pathological condition—oral cavity radiation to head and/or neck dehydration; chemical trauma (e.g., acidic foods, drugs, noxious agents, alcohol); mechanical trauma (e.g., ill-fitting dentures, braces, tubes); endotracheal/nasogastric, surgery-oral cavity; NPO—greater than 24 hours; ineffective oral hygiene; mouth breathing; malnutrition; infections; lack of or decreased salivation; medication

Defining characteristics:

1. oral pain/discomfort

2. coated tongue

3. xeroxtomia (dry mouth)

4. stomatitis

5. oral lesions or ulcers

6. lack of or decreased salivation

7. leukoplakia

8. edema

9. hyperemia

10. oral plaque

11. desquamation

12. vesicles

13. hemorrhagic gingivitis

14. carious teeth

15. halitosis

POWERLESSNESS

Definition: the perception of the individual that one's own action will not significantly affect an outcome. Powerlessness is a perceived lack of control over a current situation or immediate happening.

Etiology: health care environment; interpersonal interaction; illness related regime; life style of helplessness

Defining characteristics:

I. *Severe*
  1 verbal expressions of having no control or influence over situation
  2 verbal expressions of having no control or influence over outcome
  3 verbal expressions of having no control over self-care
  4 depression over physical deterioration which occurs despite patient compliance with regimes
  5 apathy

II. *Moderate*
  1 nonparticipation in care or decision making when opportunities are provided
  2 expressions of dissatisfaction and frustration over inability to perform previous tasks and/or activities
  3 does not monitor progress
  4 expression of doubt regarding role performance
  5 reluctance to express true feelings fearing alienation from care givers
  6 passivity
  7 inability to seek information regarding care
  8 dependence on others that may result in irritability, resentment, anger, and guilt
  9 does not defend self-care practices when challenged

III. *Low-Passivity*
  1 expressions of uncertainty about fluctuating energy levels

SOCIAL ISOLATION

Definition: Condition of aloneness experienced by the individual and perceived as imposed by others and as a negative or threatened state.

Etiology: factors contributing to the absence of satisfying personal relationships (e.g.: 1. delay in accomplishing developmental tasks; 2. immature interests; 3. alterations in physical appearance; 4. alterations in mental status; 5. unaccepted social behavior; 6. unaccepted social values; 7. altered state of wellness; 8. inadequate personal resources; 9. inability to engage in satisfying personal relationships)

Defining characteristics (* critical defining characteristics):

I. *Objective*
   1 absence of supportive significant others: family, friends, group
   2 sad, dull, affect
   3 inappropriate or immature interests and activities for developmental age or stage
   4 uncommunicative, withdrawn, no eye contact
   5 preoccupation with own thoughts, repetitive, meaningless actions
   6 projects hostility in voice, behavior
   7 seeks to be alone, or exists in a subculture
   8 evidence of physical or mental handicap or altered state of wellness
   9 shows behavior unaccepted by dominant cultural group

II. *Subjective*
   1 expresses feelings of aloneness imposed by others
   2 expresses feelings of rejection
   3 experiences feelings of difference from others
   4 inadequacy in or absence of significant purpose in life
   5 inability to meet expectations of others
   6 insecurity in public
   7 expresses values acceptable to the subculture but unacceptable to the dominant cultural group
   8 expresses interests inappropriate to the developmental age or stage

Table A-10
Approximation of Frame Size

Men		Women	
Height in 1″ heels	Elbow breadth	Height in 1″ heels	Elbow breadth
5′2″–5′3″	$2\frac{1}{2}″-2\frac{7}{8}″$	4′10″–4′11″	$2\frac{1}{4}″-2\frac{1}{2}″$
5′4″–5′7″	$2\frac{5}{8}″-2\frac{7}{8}″$	5′0″–5′3″	$2\frac{1}{4}″-2\frac{1}{2}″$
5′8″–5′11″	$2\frac{3}{4}″-3″$	5′4″–5′7″	$2\frac{3}{8}″-2\frac{5}{8}″$
6′0″–6′3″	$2\frac{3}{4}″-3\frac{1}{8}″$	5′8″–5′11″	$2\frac{3}{8}″-2\frac{5}{8}″$
6′4″	$2\frac{7}{8}″-3\frac{1}{4}″$	6′0″	$2\frac{1}{2}″-2\frac{3}{4}″$

Extend your arm and bend the forearm upward at a 90 degree angle. Keep fingers straight and turn the inside of your wrist toward your body. If you have a caliper, use it to measure the space between the two prominent bones on *either side* of your elbow. Without a caliper, place thumb and index finger of your other hand on these two bones. Measure the space between your fingers against a ruler or tape measure. Compare it with these tables that list elbow measurements for *medium-framed* men and women. Measurements lower than those listed indicate you have a small frame. Higher measurements indicate a large frame.

Source: Metropolitan Life Insurance Company, Health and Safety Education Division, 1983.

Table A-11
Height and Weight Tables

Men					Women				
Height Feet	Inches	Small frame	Medium frame	Large frame	Height Feet	Inches	Small frame	Medium frame	Large frame
5	2	128–134	131–141	138–150	4	10	102–111	109–121	118–131
5	3	130–136	133–143	140–153	4	11	103–113	111–123	120–134
5	4	132–138	135–145	142–156	5	0	104–115	113–126	122–137
5	5	134–140	137–148	144–160	5	1	106–118	115–129	125–140
5	6	136–142	139–151	146–164	5	2	108–121	118–132	128–143
5	7	138–145	142–154	149–168	5	3	111–124	121–135	131–147
5	8	140–148	145–157	152–172	5	4	114–127	124–138	134–151
5	9	142–151	148–160	155–176	5	5	117–130	127–141	137–155
5	10	144–154	151–163	158–180	5	6	120–133	130–144	140–159
5	11	146–157	154–166	161–184	5	7	123–136	133–147	143–163
6	0	149–160	157–170	164–188	5	8	126–139	136–150	146–167
6	1	152–164	160–174	168–192	5	9	129–142	139–153	149–170
6	2	155–168	164–178	172–197	5	10	132–145	142–156	152–173
6	3	158–172	167–182	176–202	5	11	135–148	145–159	155–176
6	4	162–176	171–187	181–207	6	0	138–151	148–162	158–179

Weights at ages 25–59 based on lowest mortality. Weight in pounds according to frame (in indoor clothing weighing 5 lbs. for men and 3 lbs. for women; shoes with 1″ heels).

Source of basic data: 1979 Build Study, Society of Actuaries and Association of Life Insurance Medical Directors of America, 1980.

Source: Metropolitan Life Insurance Company Health and Safety Education Division, 1983.

Table A-12
Recommended Daily Dietary Allowance,[a] Revised 1980

		Weight (kg) (lb.)	Height (cm) (in)	Protein (g)	Fat-Soluble Vitamins Vitamin A (μg R.E.)[b]	Vitamin D (μg)[c]	Vitamin E (mg α T.E.)[d]	Water-Soluble Vitamins Vitamin C (mg)	Thiamin (mg)	Riboflavin (mg)	Niacin (mg N.E.)[e]	Vitamin B6 (mg)	Folacin[f] (μg)	Vitamin B12 (μg)	Minerals Calcium (mg)	Phosphorus (mg)	Magnesium (mg)	Iron (mg)	Zinc (mg)	Iodine (μg)
Infants																				
	birth–6 mo	6 13	60 24	kg × 2.2	420	10	3	35	0.3	0.4	6	0.3	30	0.5[g]	360	240	50	10	3	40
	6 mo–1 year	9 20	71 28	kg × 2.0	400	10	4	35	0.5	0.6	8	0.6	45	1.5	540	360	70	15	5	50
Children																				
	1–3	13 29	90 35	23	400	10	5	45	0.7	0.8	9	0.9	100	2.0	800	800	150	15	10	70
	4–6	20 44	112 44	30	500	10	6	45	0.9	1.0	11	1.3	200	2.5	800	800	200	10	10	90
	7–10	28 62	132 52	34	700	10	7	45	1.2	1.4	16	1.6	300	3.0	800	800	250	10	10	120
Males																				
	11–14	45 99	157 62	45	1000	10	8	50	1.4	1.6	18	1.8	400	3.0	1200	1200	350	18	15	150
	15–18	66 145	176 69	56	1000	10	10	60	1.4	1.7	18	2.0	400	3.0	1200	1200	400	18	15	150
	19–22	70 154	177 70	56	1000	7.5	10	60	1.5	1.7	19	2.2	400	3.0	800	800	350	10	15	150
	23–50	70 154	178 70	56	1000	5	10	60	1.4	1.6	18	2.2	400	3.0	800	800	350	10	15	150
	51+	70 154	178 70	56	1000	5	10	60	1.2	1.4	16	2.2	400	3.0	800	800	350	10	15	150
Females																				
	11–14	46 101	157 62	46	800	10	8	50	1.1	1.3	15	1.8	400	3.0	1200	1200	300	18	15	150
	15–18	55 120	163 64	46	800	10	8	60	1.1	1.3	14	2.0	400	3.0	1200	1200	300	18	15	150
	19–22	55 120	163 64	44	800	7.5	8	60	1.1	1.3	14	2.0	400	3.0	800	800	300	18	15	150
	23–50	55 120	163 64	44	800	5	8	60	1.0	1.2	13	2.0	400	3.0	800	800	300	18	15	150
	51+	55 120	163 64	44	800	5	8	60	1.0	1.2	13	2.0	400	3.0	800	800	300	10	15	150
Pregnant				+30	+200	+5	+2	+20	+0.4	+0.3	+2	+0.6	+400	+1.0	+400	+400	+150	h	+5	+25
Lactating				+20	+400	+5	+3	+40	+0.5	+0.5	+5	+0.5	+100	+1.0	+400	+400	+150	h	+10	+50

[a]The allowances are intended to provide for individual variations among most normal persons as they live in the United States under usual environmental stresses. Diets should be based on a variety of common foods in order to provide other nutrients for which human requirements have been less well defined. See heights, weights, and recommended intake.

[b]1 Retinol equivalent = 1 μg retinol or 6 μg carotene.

[c]As cholecalciferol, 10 μg cholecalciferol = 400 I.U. vitamin D.

[d]1 mg d-α-tocopherol = 1 α T.E. See text for variation in allowances and calculation of vitamin E activity of the diet as α-tocopherol equivalents.

[e]1 N.E. (niacin equivalent) is equal to 1 mg of niacin or 60 mg of dietary tryptophan.

[f]The folacin allowances refer to dietary sources as determined by *Lactobacillus casei* assay after treatment with enzymes ("conjugases") to make polyglutamyl forms of the vitamin available to the test organism.

[g]The RDA for vitamin B12 in infants is based on average concentration of the vitamin in human milk. The allowances after weaning are based on energy intake (as recommended by the American Academy of Pediatrics) and consideration of other factors such as intestinal absorption.

[h]The increased requirement during pregnancy cannot be met by the iron content of habitual American diets nor by the existing iron stores of many women; therefore the use of 30–60 mg of supplemental iron is recommended. Iron needs during lactation are not substantially different from those of nonpregnant women, but continued supplementation of the mother for 2 to 3 months after parturition is advisable in order to replenish stores depleted by pregnancy.

Source: Food and Nutrition Board, National Academy of Sciences–National Research Council, Washington, D.C.

Table A-13
Recommended Dietary Allowances of Selected Vitamins and Minerals[a] Revised 1980

	Vitamins			Trace Elements[b]						Electrolytes		
	Vitamin K (µg)	Biotin (µg)	Pantothenic Acid (mg)	Copper (mg)	Manganese (mg)	Fluoride (mg)	Chromium (mg)	Selenium (mg)	Molybdenum (mg)	Sodium (mg)	Potassium (mg)	Chloride (mg)
Infants												
birth–6 mo	12	35	2	0.5–0.7	0.5–0.7	0.1–0.5	0.01–0.04	0.01–0.04	0.03–0.06	115–350	350–925	275–700
6 mo–1 year	10–20	50	3	0.7–1.0	0.7–1.0	0.2–1.0	0.02–0.06	0.02–0.06	0.04–0.08	250–750	425–1275	400–1200
Children												
1–3	15–30	65	3	1.0–1.5	1.0–1.5	0.5–1.5	0.02–0.08	0.02–0.08	0.05–0.1	325–975	550–1650	500–1500
4–6	20–40	85	3–4	1.5–2.0	1.5–2.0	1.0–2.5	0.03–0.12	0.03–0.12	0.06–0.15	450–1350	775–2325	700–2100
7–10	30–60	120	4–5	2.0–2.5	2.0–3.0	1.5–2.5	0.05–0.2	0.05–0.2	0.1–0.3	600–1800	1000–3000	925–2775
Adolescents												
11+	50–100	100–200	4–7	2.0–3.0	2.5–5.0	1.5–2.5	0.05–0.2	0.05–0.2	0.15–0.5	900–2700	1525–4575	1400–4200
Adults	70–140	100–200	4–7	2.0–3.0	2.5–5.0	1.5–4.0	0.05–0.2	0.05–0.2	0.15–0.5	1100–3300	1875–5625	1700–5100

[a]Because there is less information on which to base allowances, these figures are not given in the main table of the RDA and are provided here in the form of ranges of recommended intakes.
[b]Since the toxic levels for many trace elements may be only several times usual intakes, the upper levels for the trace elements given in this table should not be habitually exceeded.
Source: Food and Nutrition Board, National Academy of Sciences–National Research Council, Washington, D.C.

Table A-14
Mean Heights and Weights and Recommended Energy Intake[a]

	Weight		Height		Energy Needs (with range)	
	(kg)	(lb)	(cm)	(in)	(kcal)	(MJ)
Infants						
birth–6 mo	6	13	60	24	kg × 115 (95–145)	kg × .48
6 mo–1 year	9	20	71	28	kg × 105 (80–135)	kg × .44
Children						
1–3	13	29	90	35	1300 (900–1800)	5.5
4–6	20	44	112	44	1700 (1300–2300)	7.1
7–10	28	62	132	52	2400 (1650–3300)	10.1
Males						
11–14	45	99	157	62	2700 (2000–3700)	11.3
15–18	66	145	176	69	2800 (2100–3900)	11.8
19–22	70	154	177	70	2900 (2500–3300)	12.2
23–50	70	154	178	70	2700 (2300–3100)	11.3
51–75	70	154	178	70	2400 (2000–2800)	10.1
76+	70	154	178	70	2050 (1650–2450)	8.6
Females						
11–14	46	101	157	62	2200 (1500–3000)	9.2
15–18	55	120	163	64	2100 (1200–3000)	8.8
19–22	55	120	163	64	2100 (1700–2500)	8.8
23–50	55	120	163	64	2000 (1600–2400)	8.4
51–75	55	120	163	64	1800 (1400–2200)	7.6
76+	55	120	163	64	1600 (1200–2000)	6.7
Pregnancy					+300	
Lactation					+500	

[a]The data in this table have been assembled from the observed median heights and weights of children, together with desirable weights for adults for the mean heights of men (70 in) and women (64 in) between the ages of 18 and 34 years as surveyed in the U.S. population (HEW/NCHS data).

Energy allowances for children through age 18 are based on median energy intakes of children of these ages followed in longitudinal growth studies. The values in parentheses are 10th and 90th percentiles of energy intake to indicate the range of energy consumption among children of these ages.

Energy allowances for the young adults are for men and women doing light work. The allowances for the two older groups represent mean energy needs over these age spans, allowing for a 2% decrease in basal (resting) metabolic rate per decade and a reduction in activity of 200 kcal/day for men and women between 51 and 75 years, 500 kcal for men over 75 years and 400 kcal for women over 75. The customary range of daily energy output is shown for adults in parentheses, and is based on a variation in energy needs of ±400 kcal at any one age, emphasizing the wide range of energy intakes appropriate for any group of people.

Table A-15
Basic Four Food Groups with Nutrient Pattern and Recommended Quantity

Group	Nutrients	Quantity	Comments
Milk	Calcium Protein Phosphorus Riboflavin	*Servings:* Three or more for children, four or more for teenagers, two or more for adults *Serving size equals:* 　8 oz milk or yogurt 　1 oz cheese 　1½ cup cottage cheese, ice cream, or custard	Butter is not included in this group as it is a fat and does not contain other essential nutrients.
Meat	Protein B vitamins Iron	*Servings:* Two or more *Serving size equals:* 　3 oz meat, poultry, or fish 　2 eggs 　2 tbsp peanut butter 　½ cup lentils or beans	Legumes, nuts, and soy extenders can be substituted for meat although the protein has a lower biological value than meat has. These foods can be combined with animal or grain products to increase protein quality.
Vegetable and fruit	Vitamin A Vitamin C Carbohydrate (fiber) Iron	*Servings:* Four or more *Serving size equals:* 　½ cup vegetable or fruit 　4 oz citrus juice 　1 medium size fruit 　½ cup dark green or yellow vegetables	One serving daily should be vitamin C—rich (e.g., citrus fruits). Vitamin A—rich foods (e.g., leafy green and yellow vegetables) should be consumed 3–4 times/wk.
Grain	Carbohydrate (fiber) B vitamins Iron	*Servings:* Four or more *Serving size equals:* 　1 slice bread 　½ cup cereal	Whole grain and enriched products are recommended grain foods.

Source: R. B. Howard and N. H. Herbold, *Nutrition in Clinical Care,* McGraw-Hill, New York, 1978.

DENVER ASSESSMENT TESTS APPENDIX B

THE DENVER EYE SCREENING TEST (DEST)

The Denver Eye Screening Test is made up of four parts. These are:

1. Vision Test
   a. "E" Test
   b. Picture Card Test
   c. Fixation Test
2. Question
3. Cover Test
4. Pupillary Light Reflex Test

For children from 6 to 30 months of age, the examiner tests the child for (1) fixation (ability to follow a moving light source or spinning toy), (2) squinting (observation of the child's eyes or report by parent), and (3) strabismus (report by parent and performance on the cover and pupillary light reflex tests).

For children from age $2\frac{1}{2}$ to 2 years 11 months, or for children who are untestable with the letter E test, picture cards (or Allen cards) are used. Pictures include familiar objects such as a tree, car, house, stuffed bear, telephone, and birthday cake. The child must identify objects at a close range and at 15 feet.

For children 3 years and older, visual acuity is tested by using a single card containing the letter E. This test is more accurate than the picture card test. At a distance of 15 feet the child must identify the different directions the arms of the small E point as the examiner changes the position of the E.

Refer to the DEST manual/workbook for a detailed description of each part included in testing (William K. Frankenburg, Arnold D. Goldstein, and John Barker, University of Colorado Medical Center, 1973).

DENVER EYE SCREENING TEST

Name
Hospital No.
Ward
Address

	1ST SCREENING: DATE — Right Eye			Left Eye			RESCREENING: DATE — Right Eye			Left Eye		
Vision Tests	Normal	Abnormal	Untestable	Normal	Abnormal	Untestable	Normal	Abnormal	Untestable	Normal	Abnormal	Untestable
1. "E" (3 years and above—3 to 5 trials)	3P	3F	U	3P	3F	U	3P	3F	U	3P	3F	U
2. Picture Card (2 1/2 – 2 11/12 yrs.—3 to 5 trials)	3P	3F	U	3P	3F	U	3P	3F	U	3P	3F	U
3. Fixation (6 months – 2 5/12 years)	P	F	U	P	F	U	P	F	U	P	F	U
4. Squinting		yes			yes			yes			yes	

	1ST SCREENING: DATE			RESCREENING: DATE		
Tests for Non-Straight Eyes	Normal	Abnormal	Untestable	Normal	Abnormal	Untestable
1. Do your child's eyes turn in or out, or are they ever not straight?	NO	YES	U	NO	YES	U
2. Cover Test	P	F	U	P	F	U
3. Pupillary Light Reflex	P	F	U	P	F	U

Total Test Rating (Both Eyes) — 1ST SCREENING: Normal / Abnormal / Untestable — RESCREENING: Normal / Abnormal / Untestable

Normal (passed vision test plus no squint, plus passed 2/3 tests for non-straight eyes)

Abnormal (abnormal on any vision test, squinting or 2 of 3 procedures for non-straight eyes)

Untestable (untestable on any vision test or untestable on 2/3 tests for non-straight eyes)

Future Rescreening Appointment for Total Test Rating (Abnormal or Untestable)

Date:

Date:

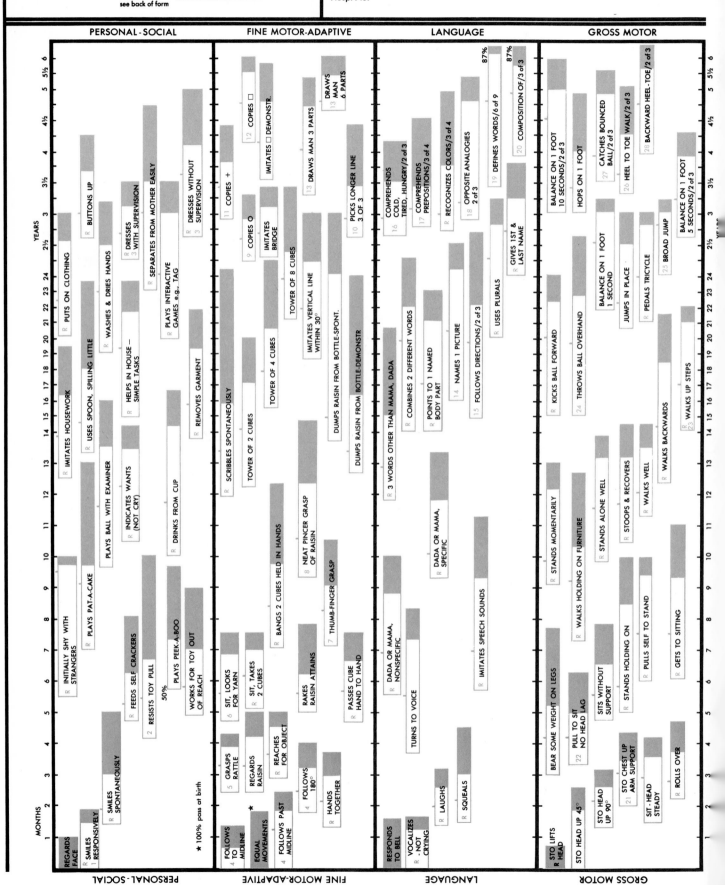

DENVER DEVELOPMENTAL SCREENING TEST

STO.=STOMACH
SIT=SITTING

PERCENT OF CHILDREN PASSING

25 50 75 90

May pass by report →
Footnote No. →
see back of form

Date

Name

Birthdate

Hosp. No.

PERSONAL-SOCIAL   FINE MOTOR-ADAPTIVE   LANGUAGE   GROSS MOTOR

1. Try to get child to smile by smiling, talking or waving to him. Do not touch him.
2. When child is playing with toy, pull it away from him. Pass if he resists.
3. Child does not have to be able to tie shoes or button in the back.
4. Move yarn slowly in an arc from one side to the other, about 6" above child's face.
   Pass if eyes follow 90° to midline. (Past midline; 180°)
5. Pass if child grasps rattle when it is touched to the backs or tips of fingers.
6. Pass if child continues to look where yarn disappeared or tries to see where it went. Yarn
   should be dropped quickly from sight from tester's hand without arm movement.
7. Pass if child picks up raisin with any part of thumb and a finger.
8. Pass if child picks up raisin with the ends of thumb and index finger using an over hand
   approach.

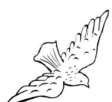 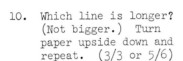 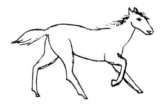 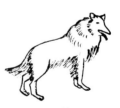

9. Pass any en-
   closed form.
   Fail continuous
   round motions.

10. Which line is longer?
    (Not bigger.) Turn
    paper upside down and
    repeat. (3/3 or 5/6)

11. Pass any
    crossing
    lines.

12. Have child copy
    first. If failed,
    demonstrate

When giving items 9, 11 and 12, do not name the forms. Do not demonstrate 9 and 11.

13. When scoring, each pair (2 arms, 2 legs, etc.) counts as one part.
14. Point to picture and have child name it. (No credit is given for sounds only.)

 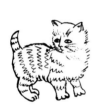 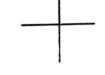 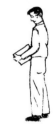

15. Tell child to: Give block to Mommie; put block on table; put block on floor. Pass 2 of 3.
    (Do not help child by pointing, moving head or eyes.)
16. Ask child: What do you do when you are cold? ..hungry? ..tired? Pass 2 of 3.
17. Tell child to: Put block on table; under table; in front of chair, behind chair.
    Pass 3 of 4. (Do not help child by pointing, moving head or eyes.)
18. Ask child: If fire is hot, ice is ?; Mother is a woman, Dad is a ?; a horse is big, a
    mouse is ?. Pass 2 of 3.
19. Ask child: What is a ball? ..lake? ..desk? ..house? ..banana? ..curtain? ..ceiling?
    ..hedge? ..pavement? Pass if defined in terms of use, shape, what it is made of or general
    category (such as banana is fruit, not just yellow). Pass 6 of 9.
20. Ask child: What is a spoon made of? ..a shoe made of? ..a door made of? (No other objects
    may be substituted.) Pass 3 of 3.
21. When placed on stomach, child lifts chest off table with support of forearms and/or hands.
22. When child is on back, grasp his hands and pull him to sitting. Pass if head does not hang back.
23. Child may use wall or rail only, not person. May not crawl.
24. Child must throw ball overhand 3 feet to within arm's reach of tester.
25. Child must perform standing broad jump over width of test sheet. (8-1/2 inches)
26. Tell child to walk forward, ⚬⚬⚬⚬⚬→ heel within 1 inch of toe.
    Tester may demonstrate. Child must walk 4 consecutive steps, 2 out of 3 trials.
27. Bounce ball to child who should stand 3 feet away from tester. Child must catch ball with
    hands, not arms, 2 out of 3 trials.
28. Tell child to walk backward, ←⚬⚬⚬⚬⚬ toe within 1 inch of heel.
    Tester may demonstrate. Child must walk 4 consecutive steps, 2 out of 3 trials.

DATE AND BEHAVIORAL OBSERVATIONS (how child feels at time of test, relation to tester, attention
span, verbal behavior, self-confidence, etc,):

THE DENVER ARTICULATION SCREENING EXAM*

Screening tests and procedures are intended to serve as tools which can be applied readily and economically to large population groups to ferret out the individual who has a high probability of harboring the disease or dysfunction.

The Denver Articulation Screening Exam (DASE) was designed to meet the above criteria and to: (1) reliably detect disorders in preschool children aged 2½ to 6 years, (2) be useful and acceptable to speech pathologists, and (3) be readily understandable so as to gain wide use among other child workers (doctors, nurses, teachers and paraprofessionals, who may not be well versed in articulation development. The DASE is designed to reliably discriminate between significant developmental delay and normal variations in the acquisition of speech sounds, and to detect common abnormal conditions such as hyponasality, hypernasality, lateral lisp, and tongue thrust. It was hoped that by including norms for articulation development of economically disadvantaged children, incorrect referrals among this population due to dialect, regional pronunciation, or foreign language background would be minimized.

Administration of the DASE

Tell the child to say some words after you. "If I say *car*, then you say *car*." Give the child several examples to ensure understanding. Start with the first word, '*table*"; have the child repeat all 22 words after you. The examiner will score the child's pronunciation of the underlined *sounds or blends* in each word. A perfect raw score is *30 correctly articulated* sound elements.

For purposes of scoring the DASE, a child is considered to be the closest previous age shown on the percentile rank chart. For example, a child 3 years, 11 months of age is considered 3.5 years when scoring the DASE.

To determine test results, match the raw score (number of correct sounds) line with the column denoting child's age. Where the line and column meet, child's percentile rank is given. Percentiles above heavy line are abnormal. Percentiles below heavy line are normal.

Rate the child's spontaneous speech in terms of intelligibility: (1) easy to understand, (2) understandable half the time, (3) not understandable, or (4) cannot evaluate (if the child does not speak in sentences or phrases during the interview). Score intelligibility as follows:

2½ years	NORMAL: "Easy" or understandable half the time	ABNORMAL: Not understandable
3 years and older	NORMAL: Easy to understand	ABNORMAL: Understandable half the time; not understandable

Rate the child's total test result as follows:

1. *Normal* = Normal on DASE *and* intelligibility.
2. *Abnormal* = Abnormal on DASE *and/or* intelligibility.

In case of abnormal screening results, rescreening with DASE within two weeks would further decrease the chance of incorrect referral.

*Amelia F. Drumwright

DENVER ARTICULATION SCREENING EXAM
for children 2 1/2 to 6 years of age

Instructions: Have child repeat each word after you. Circle the underlined sounds that he pronounces correctly. Total correct sounds is the Raw Score. Use charts on reverse side to score results.

NAME

HOSP. NO.

ADDRESS

Date: _____ Child's Age: _____ Examiner: _____ Raw Score: _____

Percentile: _____ Intelligibility: _____ Result: _____

1. table	6. zipper	11. sock	16. wagon	21. leaf
2. shirt	7. grapes	12. vacuum	17. gum	22. carrot
3. door	8. flag	13. yarn	18. house	
4. trunk	9. thumb	14. mother	19. pencil	
5. jumping	10. toothbrush	15. twinkle	20. fish	

Intelligibility: (circle one)   1. Easy to understand   3. Not understandable
                                2. Understandable 1/2   4. Can't evaluate
                                   the time.

Comments:

Date: _____ Child's Age: _____ Examiner: _____ Raw Score _____

Percentile: _____ Intelligibility: _____ Result: _____

1. table	6. zipper	11. sock	16. wagon	21. leaf
2. shirt	7. grapes	12. vacuum	17. gum	22. carrot
3. door	8. flag	13. yarn	18. house	
4. trunk	9. thumb	14. mother	19. pencil	
5. jumping	10. toothbrush	15. twinkle	20. fish	

Intelligibility: (circle one)   1. Easy to understand   3. Not understandable
                                2. Understandable 1/2   4. Can't evaluate
                                   the time.

Comments:

Date: _____ Child's Age: _____ Examiner: _____ Raw Score_____

Percentile: _____ Intelligibility: _____ Result: _____

1. table	6. zipper	11. sock	16. wagon	21. leaf
2. shirt	7. grapes	12. vacuum	17. gum	22. carrot
3. door	8. flag	13. yarn	18. house	
4. trunk	9. thumb	14. mother	19. pencil	
5. jumping	10. toothbrush	15. twinkle	20. fish	

Intelligibility: (circle one)   1. Easy to understand   3. Not understandable
                                2. Understandable 1/2   4. Can't evaluate
                                   the time.

Comments:

To score DASE words: Note Raw Score for child's performance. Match raw score line (extreme left of chart) with column representing child's age (to the closest *previous* age group). Where raw score line and age column meet number in that square denotes percentile rank of child's performance when compared to other children that age. Percentiles above heavy line are ABNORMAL percentiles, below heavy line are NORMAL.

PERCENTILE RANK

Raw Score	2.5 yr.	3.0	3.5	4.0	4.5	5.0	5.5	6 years
2	1							
3	2							
4	5							
5	9							
6	16							
7	23							
8	31	2						
9	37	4	1					
10	42	6	2					
11	48	7	4					
12	54	9	6	1	1			
13	58	12	9	2	3	1	1	
14	62	17	11	5	4	2	2	
15	68	23	15	9	5	3	2	
16	75	31	19	12	5	4	3	
17	79	38	25	15	6	6	4	
18	83	46	31	19	8	7	4	
19	86	51	38	24	10	9	5	1
20	89	58	45	30	12	11	7	3
21	92	65	52	36	15	15	9	4
22	94	72	58	43	18	19	12	5
23	96	77	63	50	22	24	15	7
24	97	82	70	58	29	29	20	15
25	99	87	78	66	36	34	26	17
26	99	91	84	75	46	43	34	24
27		94	89	82	57	54	44	34
28		96	94	88	70	68	59	47
29		98	98	94	84	84	77	68
30		100	100	100	100	100	100	100

To Score intelligibility

	NORMAL	ABNORMAL
2 1/2 years	Understandable 1/2 the time, or, "easy"	Not Understandable
3 years and older	Easy to understand	Understandable 1/2 time Not understandable

Test Result: 1. NORMAL on Dase and Intelligibility = NORMAL
2. ABNORMAL on Dase and/or Intelligibility = ABNORMAL

* If abnormal on initial screening rescreen within 2 weeks. If abnormal again child should be referred for complete speech evaluation.

CLIENT PROFILE/BIOGRAPHICAL DATA

Date 6-1-84

Name Mr. James S. ———

Address 221 York St., Denver, Colorado 80262

Sex Male Age 37 Birthdate: 10-8-46

Place of Birth: Detroit, Michigan

Race: White Nationality: Irish-American

Marital Status: Married

Religion: Catholic

Occupation: Attorney

Employer's Address: 1600 Lincoln St., Suite 50, Denver, Colorado 80115

Social Security Number: 001-02-0003

Source of Referral: Self; reliable informant

Reason for Referral: Pre-employment physical

HEALTH/HEALTH MANAGEMENT PERCEPTION

Client states, "My health is very important to me. I usually try to have a physical check-up at least every few years, but I don't see a doctor unless I think it is necessary. It's important that I have some say in how I am treated by health care providers, and I've been satisfied with care so far."

Current Health Status/Health Habits

Client states, "I feel like I'm in good health, physically and mentally."

Exercises regularly; denies use of any type of drugs, unless prescribed. Personal hygiene appears good—well groomed.

Past Health Status

Birth history:

Exact details unknown. States he is not aware of any complications.

Growth and development:

Previous records from 7 to 16 years of age indicate height was between the 60th and 75th percentiles, and weight consistently at the 60th to 65th percentiles. All developmental milestones were completed within normal limits according to pediatric records.

Common childhood illnesses:

Positive history for measles, mumps, and chickenpox prior to 10 years; cannot recall ever having had rubella, diphtheria, pertussis, or tetanus. Recalls a problem with streptococcal infections between 11 and 13 years of age; ". . . a lot of sore throats." Denies history of rheumatic fever.

Immunizations:

Recalls being immunized; types and dates of immunizations noted on previous records.

Previous hospitalizations:

1. Age 12 (1958), St. Joseph's Hospital, Denver; length of stay unknown; tonsillectomy with no complications.
2. Age 19 (1965), St. Joseph's Hospital, Denver; 3 week stay; fractured left femur due to basketball accident; casted for 11 weeks; resolved.
3. Age 30 (1976), St. Joseph's Hospital, Denver; 6 week stay; fractured T 10 vertebra secondary to a roller coaster ride; traction, bedrest and narcotics; resolved.

Accidents or injuries:

1965 and 1976, see above. Some limitation of activity due to fx T 10—minimal running and contact sports recommended to client by physician (Dr. Patrick King).

Allergies or allergic reactions:

Pollen allergies since age 7 (1953); presently uses decongestants prn. No known allergies to drugs or foods.

Family history:

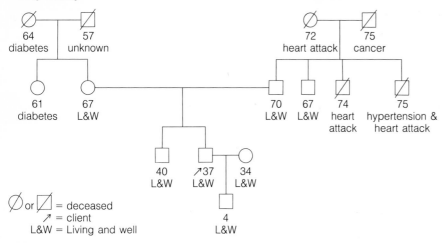

⊘ or ▧	= deceased
↗	= client
L&W	= Living and well

LIFE PATTERNS/LIFESTYLES

Age:
"I'm not really concerned about growing old. My parents are both healthy and that makes me feel good. Retirement is so far off, I don't think about it."

Race:
Client does not consider this to be a significant factor for his health.

Heredity:
Client is most concerned with paternal family history of heart disease; has fears of heart problems and, thus, tries to follow health habits that will decrease risk factors (diet, exercise, no smoking).

Culture:
Strong Irish-Catholic background; remembers a happy childhood and maintains a close relationship with parents who live in town. Wife is Presbyterian, but they have no religious conflicts. Client states, "I think my lifestyles and habits are certainly influenced by my cultural background."

Growth and Development:
No physical or cognitive deficits known. Socially, client gets along well with his wife of 7 years; has many friends. Encounters stress almost weekly in his job; has never sought professional counseling and deals with stress through exercise, sports, and self-hypnosis. Feels he is emotionally stable.

Behavioral development:
History unknown for childhood. Client states that his mother told him that he was always a well-behaved and cooperative child. Describes his behavior using the following terms: trusting, motivated, responsible, ethical and loving, sometimes stubborn and cynical.

Biological rhythms:
Sleep-rest: "I'm a night person, and usually retire by 11 or 12 at night and awaken by 7 or 8 A.M. Occasionally I have to change my pattern and am forced to arise earlier. This leaves me tired most of the day, unless I nap. I feel my best after 10 A.M. Sometimes I use self-hypnosis to fall asleep."
Elimination: Urinates approximately 8 times per day; defecates every 2 or 3 days. No history of problems.
Nutrition: Eats breakfast approximately 4 times per week; daily lunch and dinner; snacks at night. Largest meal is about 6:30 P.M.
Activity: Runs 5 miles at least 4 times per week; lifts weights 3 times per week if schedule allows; swims occasionally.
Vital signs: No current record of peaks and troughs.

Environmental factors:
Enjoys winter and summer sports, so weather not a concern. Most aware of air pollution at work (smoke) and when driving (auto); tries to avoid overexposure. He does not use a sunscreen unless reminded by wife.

Economics:
Annual income over $35,000. Wife works part-time. Has a good health insurance policy, and carries disability insurance also. No major outstanding bills, but only has a small savings for emergencies. Client states he feels financially secure, but is concerned about inflation.

Community resources:
Sought information on contraceptives from Planned Parenthood while in college. No other usage noted.

ROLES AND RELATIONSHIP PATTERNS
Identifies major roles as husband, father, and professional (attorney).

Family life:
Wife, son, and parents are most significant. Spends as much time with family as his job allows. States wife is very supportive and understanding of his professional commitment. Stress does occur when he's consistently busy with work day and night for more than 2 or 3 weeks.

Occupation:
Happy with career and position, although would like to make more money. Periodically gets burned out, but seems to be able to cope with wife's support. Stress is the greatest health hazard in his job; sometimes takes an extra day off for relief.

Societal relationships:
Believes he has attained desirable social status with regard to family and occupation. Maintains numerous relationships in the community, ie., business, political and peer groups within his profession. A member of the Colorado Bar Association. Feels comfortable taking time off from work or business when ill.

SELF PERCEPTION AND SELF-CONCEPT PATTERNS
Client appears very self-confident. States he most often is satisfied with himself, but would like to achieve a stronger reputation as "a really good trial attorney."

CONCEPTUAL AND PERCEPTUAL PATTERNS

Sensory Perception
Vision is corrected with contact lenses worn during waking hours; began wearing glasses at age 11; exact correction unknown.
Acute hearing; does not recall any history of ear infections as a child. Keen sense of taste and smell; enjoys a wide variety of foods. Good sense of touch, but has experienced numbness and tingling in toes of right foot within past 5 months; most uncomfortable after sitting for long periods. States he has high pain tolerance.

Education:
Highest degree is J.D. Enjoyed college and law school and attained high grades. Participates in continuing education; values education and definitely wants his son to be well educated.

Intelligence:
Client articulates well; above average intelligence apparent based on educational achievements. Social behavior and mannerisms appropriate during this encounter.

SEXUALITY AND REPRODUCTIVE PATTERNS
Feels good about his masculinity and enjoys his sexual relationship with his wife; they plan on 2 more children. No history of venereal disease, impotence, or other sexual problems. Does not routinely perform self-examination of genitalia.

NUTRITIONAL/METABOLIC PATTERNS
24 hour recall:
breakfast—orange juice, cereal and milk
lunch—hamburger and bun, fries, cola, and ice cream
snacks—granola bar and 2 oranges
dinner—chicken, baked potato with margarine, green salad, corn, and milk
snack—popcorn and cake, soda
Diet adequate with exception of vegetables; could increase protein intake. No food intolerances and eats a variety of foods. Drinks alcohol in moderation and only on weekends.

EXERCISE AND ACTIVITY PATTERNS
Regular exercise by running 5 miles at least 4 times per week and lifting weights 3 times per week. Does yardwork at home. Family outings at least one weekend a month (hiking, skiing, etc.). Understands cardiovascular benefits of exercise, and feels increased alertness and stamina with exercise.

COPING PATTERNS AND STRESS TOLERANCE PATTERNS
Experiences the most stress in job-related situations. Copes through exercise and use of self-hypnosis, which promote relaxation. Gains emotional support from wife and close friends. Thinks some stress is healthy, as long as it doesn't incapacitate him emotionally and psychologically. Has never sought professional counseling for stress. No significant losses or crises during the past year.

PHYSICAL GROWTH CHARTS APPENDIX D

The physical growth charts in this appendix have been adapted from National Center for Health Statistics growth charts, 1976 *(Monthly Vital Statistics Report* 25:3, Supp. HRA 76-1120). Data are from The Fels Research Institute, Yellow Springs, Ohio.

Reproduced with the kind permission of Ross Laboratories, Columbus, Ohio, a division of Abbot Laboratories. Copyright 1976 by Ross Laboratories.

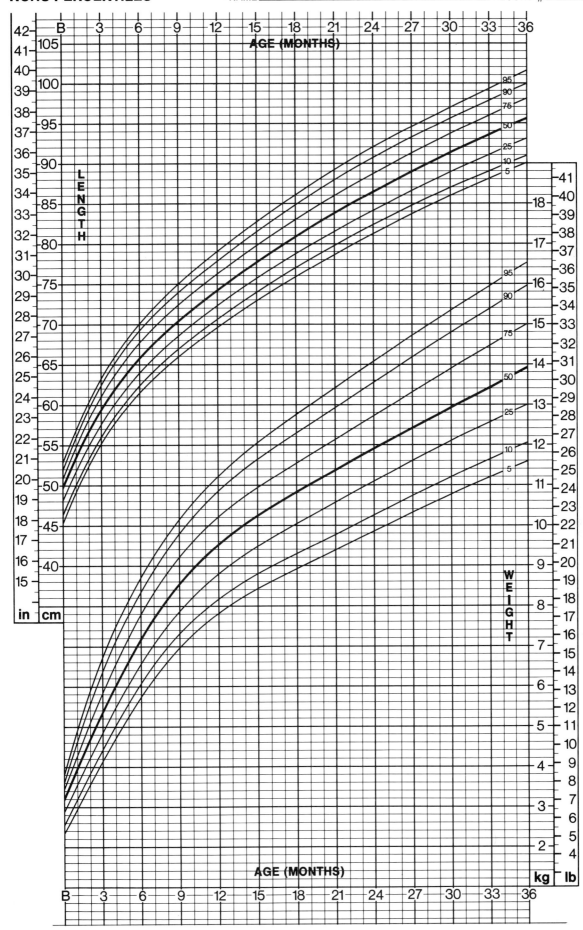

GIRLS: BIRTH TO 36 MONTHS
PHYSICAL GROWTH
NCHS PERCENTILES*

NAME _____ RECORD # _____

AGE (MONTHS)

LENGTH

WEIGHT

AGE (MONTHS)

GIRLS: BIRTH TO 36 MONTHS
PHYSICAL GROWTH
NCHS PERCENTILES*

NAME _____ RECORD # _____

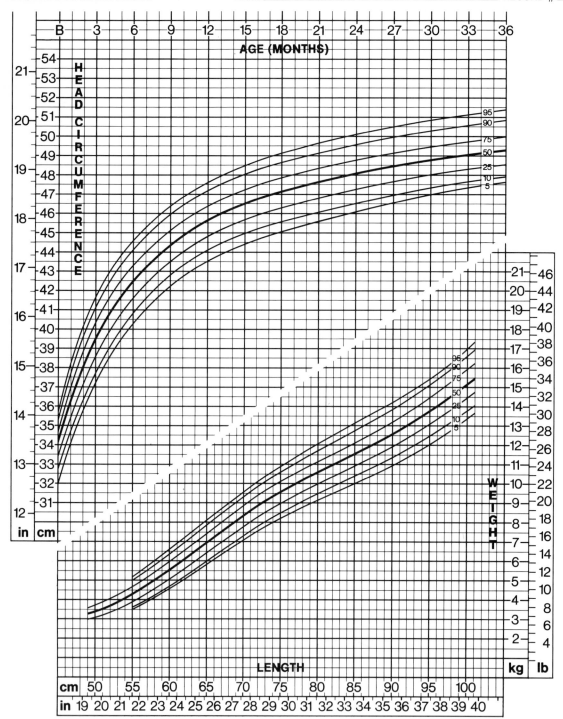

DATE	AGE	LENGTH	WEIGHT	HEAD C.
	BIRTH			

DATE	AGE	LENGTH	WEIGHT	HEAD C.

NAME _____   RECORD # _____

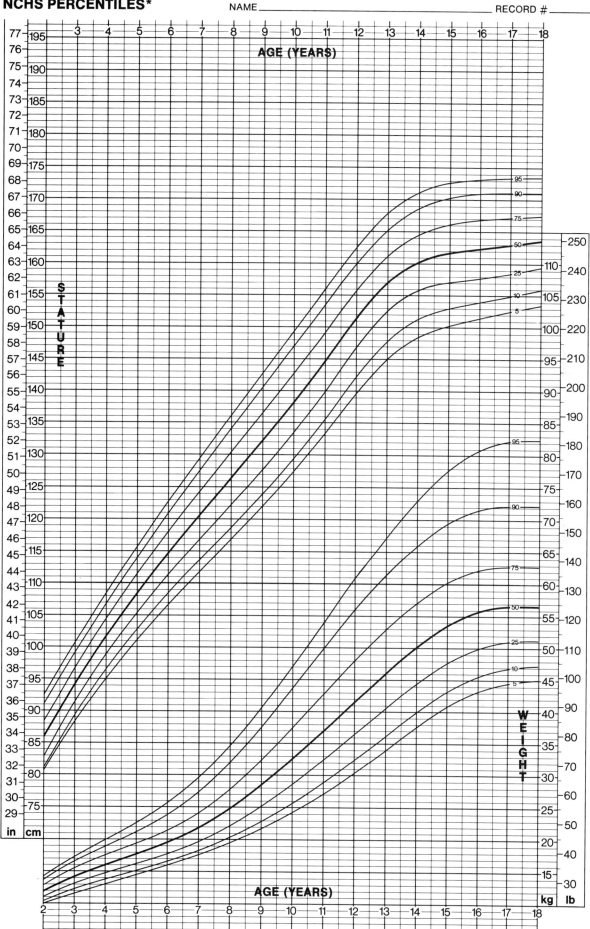

GIRLS: PREPUBESCENT
PHYSICAL GROWTH
NCHS PERCENTILES*

NAME _____ RECORD # _____

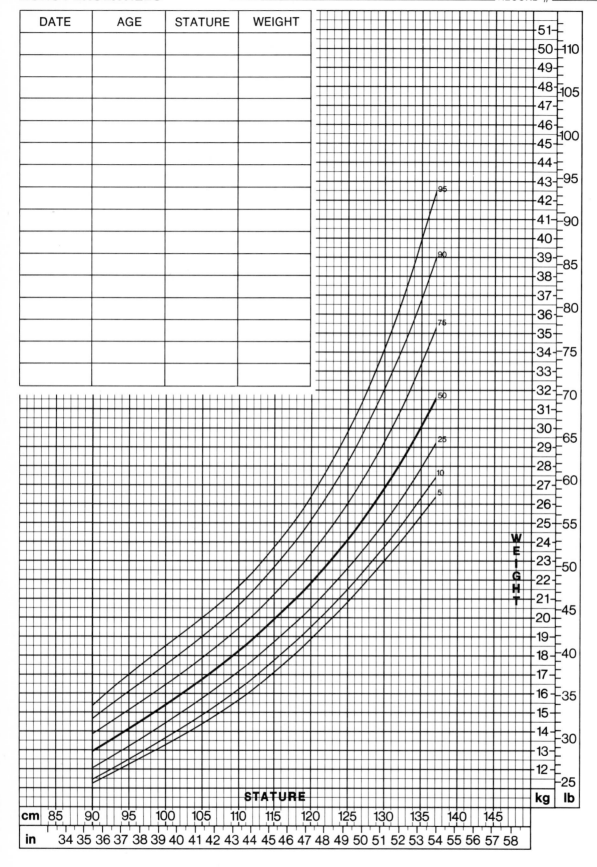

DATE	AGE	STATURE	WEIGHT

STATURE

WEIGHT

cm 85 90 95 100 105 110 115 120 125 130 135 140 145

in 34 35 36 37 38 39 40 41 42 43 44 45 46 47 48 49 50 51 52 53 54 55 56 57 58

kg lb

NAME _____ RECORD # _____

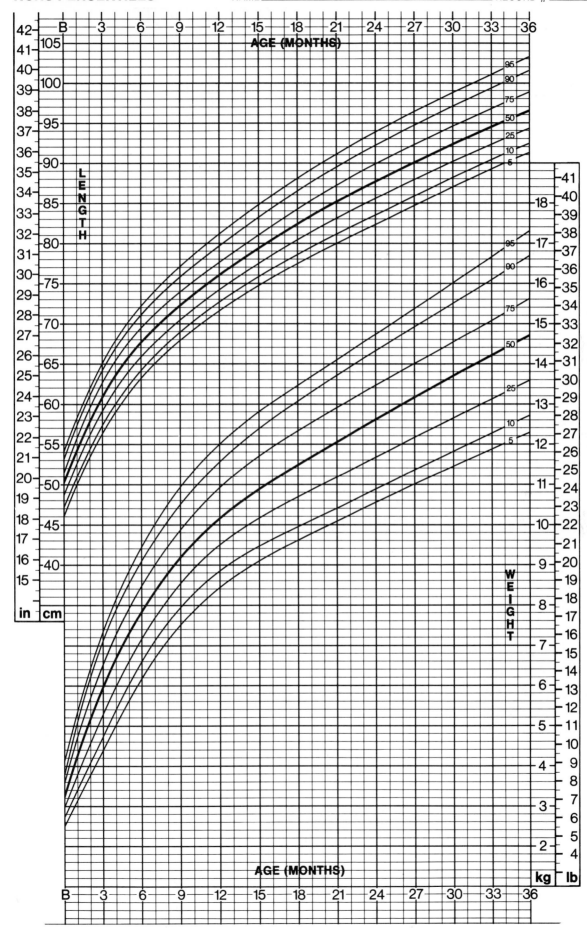

BOYS: BIRTH TO 36 MONTHS
PHYSICAL GROWTH
NCHS PERCENTILES*

NAME _____   RECORD # _____

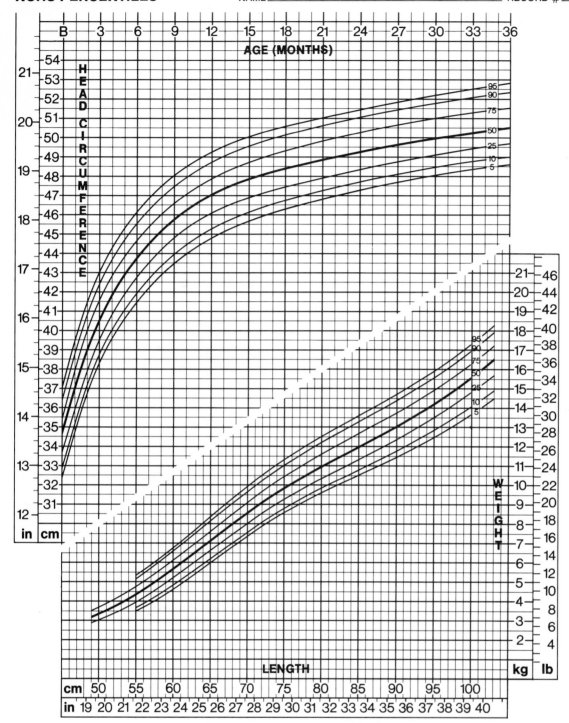

DATE	AGE	LENGTH	WEIGHT	HEAD C.
	BIRTH			

DATE	AGE	LENGTH	WEIGHT	HEAD C.

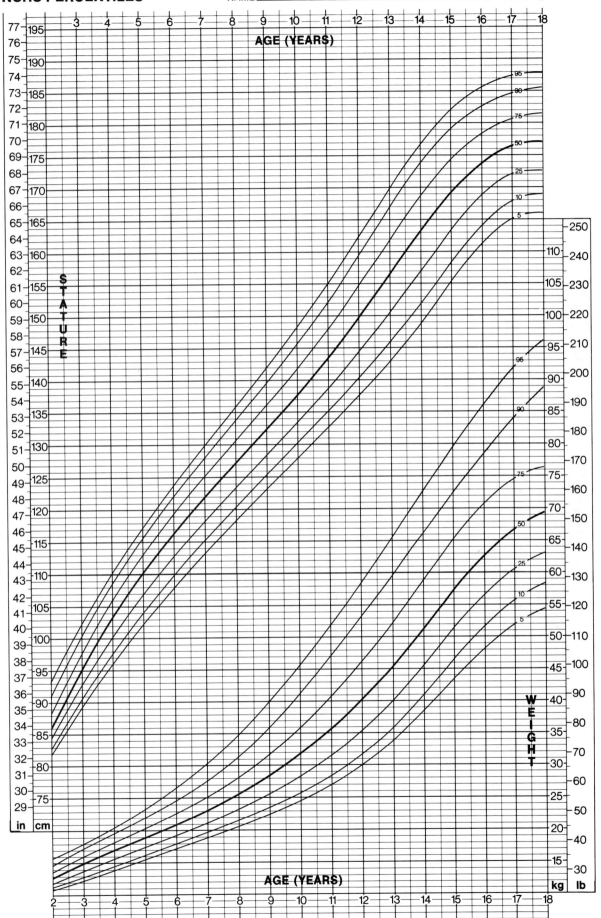

BOYS: PREPUBESCENT
PHYSICAL GROWTH
NCHS PERCENTILES*

NAME _____ RECORD # _____

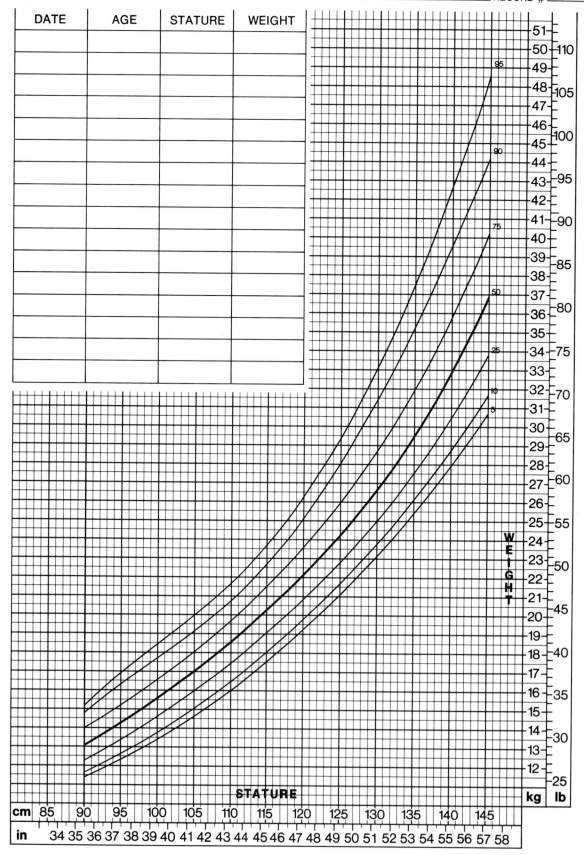

DATE	AGE	STATURE	WEIGHT

AUTHOR AND TITLE INDEX

Page numbers in *italic* indicate illustrations or tables.

Abbey, H., 686
Abdellah, Faye, 17
Abernethy, M., 686
Ackerman, Nathan, 54–56
Adler, Alfred, *645*
Adolescence (G. S. Hall), 617
Alford, Delores, 759
American Academy of Pediatrics, 351, 365, 408, *431,* 439, 441, 565
American Journal of Clinical Nutrition, 145
American Journal of Health Planning, 415
American Journal of Maternal-Child Nursing, 428
American Journal of Nursing, 297
American Nurses' Association, 14, 15, 669, 679
Amundson, Mary Jane, 37–42, 45–49
Annual Review of Psychiatry, 637
Anthony, E., 427
Ardell, Don, 3–4

Baer, Donald, 47–48
Bangai, Andrew, 686
Barker, John, *820–821*
Barnard, Martha, *515, 568*
Barness, Lewis, *439*
Battle, Constance, 358
Bell, Norman, 54
Bernard, Claude, 2
Berry, Keith, 517
Bibring, Grete, 681
Bientema, David, 371
Bijou, Sidney, 47–48
Bindelglass, P. M., 570–571
Binder, F. Z., 578
Birch, Herbert, 32
Blatman, Saul, *568*
Blood Pressure Elevation in the Elderly (A. Master and R. Lasser), 745
Bowlby, John, 426, 477
Brasel, JoAnne, *439*
Brazelton, T. Berry, 357
Breslow, Lester, 11–12, 759
Brocklehurst, J. C., 762
Bromley, D. B., 773, 774
Broussard, Elsie, 429
Brown, Jeanne B., 428
Brozek, J., 145
Brunell, Philip, *568*
Buesch, B., 661
Butler, J. E., 578
Butler, Julius, *691*
Butler, N. R., 686

Caird, F. I., 761
Caldwell, Bettye, *423,* 483, 484–485, 525, *526–528*
Cannon, Walter, 1, 2
Carey, W., 429
Centers for Disease Control, U.S. Department of Health, Education and Welfare, 145
Chard, Marilyn, *515, 568*
Cheraskin, E., 760
Chess, Stella, 32, 428
Child Development (Mary Tudor), 37–42, 45–49, *590*
Child and Family (M. Smith et al.), 589
Child Health Maintenance (P. Chinn and C. Leitch), *550*
Children Are Different: Developmental Physiology (T. Johnson), *523, 543*
Chinn, Peggy, *550*
Cohen, Michael, 570
Comprehensive Pediatric Nursing (G. Scipien et al.), *517, 568*
Comstock, G. W., 686
Confucius, 4
Cumming, Elaine, 43

Danaher, K., 11
Davies, D. P., 686
Davis, R., 524
Décarie, Thérèse, *436*

Dement, W., 430
Descartes, René, 6
Detection of Developmental Problems in Children (M. Krajicek and A. Tearney), *423, 516*
Developmental Psychology Today (R. Schell), *645*
Dialogues in Infant Nutrition: A Foundation for Lasting Health, 438, 439
Diekelmann, Nancy, 775–776
Dimensions of a New Identity (Erik Erikson), 51
Doll, Edgar, 517
Drumm, John, 686
Drumwright, Amelia, *824–826*
Dubos, René, 2
Dubowitz, Lillie, 404–407
Dubowitz, Victor, 404–407
Dunbar, Claire, *24, 162, 166, 252, 289–291, 306, 316, 632, 705, 753, 796*
Dunn, Halpert, 1, 2
Dunn, Lloyd, 517

Eating Right for You (Carlton Fredricks), 21
Ego and the Mechanisms of Defense, The (Anna Freud), 61
Elias, Jeffrey, 769, 770
Elias, Merrill, 769, 770
Elias, Penelope, 769, 770
Eliopoulos, Charlotte, 43–44
Ellwood, P. C., 686
Engle, George, 2, 8, 58, 59, *64*
Erikson, Erik, 36–37, 50–51, 61, 98, 426, 467, 476–477, 569, 617, *645,* 648, 649, 729, 762, 773

Fact Book on Aging: A Profile of America's Older Population (National Council on the Aging), 757
Fenichel, Otto, 58
Fink, Donald, 415
Food and Nutrition Board, National Academy of Sciences–National Research Council, *817, 818*
Food, Nutrition, and Diet Therapy (M. V. Krause and L. K. Mahan), *536*
Fraiberg, Selma, 477–478
Frank, Lawrence, 413
Frankenburg, William, *820–823*
Fredricks, Carlton, 21
Freud, Anna, 52–53, 61
Freud, Sigmund, 34–36, 58, 60, 61, 98, 426, 534, *645*
Friedman, Joyce, 736
Friedman, Stanford, *586*
Frisancho, A., 145
Fromm, Erich, *645*

Garrick, J. C., 580
Gerontological Nursing (Charlotte Eliopoulos), 43–44
Gessell, Arnold, 37–38, 617
Ghiselli, E., 661
Goldberg, Cissie, 404–407
Goldstein, Arnold, *820–821*
Goldstein, H., 686
Goldstein, K., 51
Goodenough, Florence, 517
Goodman, Julie, 589
Gordon, Marjorie, 16, 17, 22, *23*
Graham, Sylvester, 7
Gray, O. P., 686
Greenacre, Phyllis, 427
Growth at Adolescence (James Tanner), *624, 625, 633*

Hahnemann, Samuel, 6
Hall, Edward, 78–79, 768
Hall, G. Stanley, 617
Handel, George, 55
Hanley, T., 762
Hanson, S., 524
Harper, John, 413, *415*
Harris, D. B., 517
Hassenein, R., 524
Hastings, A. C., *11*

Havighurst, Robert, 43–44, 617
Hayes-Bautista, David, 8
Healing Mind, The (Irving Oyle), 8
Health for the Whole Person (A. C. Hastings), *11*
Heider, Fritz, 48–49
Heisler, Alice, 582
Hellbrügge, Theodor, 360
Henderson, Virginia, 14, 17
Henry, William, 43
Herbold, Nancie, *819*
Hess, Robert, 55
Hester, Nancy, 524
Hettler, B., 3
Hippocrates, 5
Hoekelman, Robert, *568*
Hofmann, F. G., 615
Holism and Evolution (J. C. Smuts), 3
Holmes, Thomas, 110, 741
Howard, Rosanne, *819*
Howe, Jeanne, *515, 568*
Howell, M., 435

Intelligence and Affectivity in Early Childhood (T. Décarie), *436*
International Symposium on Infant and Child Feeding, 438
Introduction to Physical Anthropology, An (M. F. A. Montagu), 145
Issues in Comprehensive Pediatric Nursing, 565

Jahoda, Marie, 65
Jarvis, Linda, 565
Jirovec, Mary, *24, 162, 166, 252, 289–291, 306, 316, 632, 705, 753, 796*
Johnson, Dorothy, 14, 17
Johnson, T., *523, 543*
Johnson, Virginia, 691, 739, 770–771
Jones, Dorothy, *24, 162, 166, 252, 289–291, 306, 316, 632, 705, 753, 796*
Jones, K., 685, *686*
Journal of the American Medical Association, 781
Journal of Obstetric, Gynecologic, and Neonatal Nursing, 684
Judge, J. T., 761

Kart, C., 764
Keniston, K., 658
Kenneth, John, 358
Kierkegaard, Søren, 427
Kimmel, Douglas, 767
Kinlein, Lucille, 638
Kinsey, Alfred, 739
Klaus, Marshall, 358
Kmetz, Rose, *415*
Knowles, John, 18
Koestler, Arthur, 3
Kohlberg, Lawrence, 42–43
Krajicek, Marilyn, *423, 516*
Krause, M. V., *536*
Kugelmass, I. Newton, 614

Laborivie, G., 661
Lancet, 686
Lao-Tzu, 4
Lasser, R. P., *745*
Lederer, Henry, 75
Leitch, Cynthia, *550*
Levine, Myra, 13
Lewin, Kurt, 38–39
Lipton, Rose, 433
Lovell, K., 40
Luce, Gay, 764

McBroom, W. H., 91
McFarland, Margaret, 413

McKay, R. J., *448, 454*
Magic Years, The (Selma Fraiberg), 477–478
Mahan, L. K., *536*
Mahler, Margaret, 426–428
Maslow, Abraham, 681
Master, A. M., *745, 781*
Masters, William, 691, 739, 770–771
Mead, George, 50
Meade Johnson Company, *372–375, 382, 398, 401, 465, 822–823*
Medical-Surgical Nursing: A Conceptual Approach (D. Jones et al.), *24, 162, 166, 252, 289–291, 306, 316, 632, 705, 753, 796*
Metress, E., 764
Metropolitan Life Insurance Company, *107, 140, 815, 816*
Meyer, M. B., 686
Mind as Healer, Mind as Slayer, (K. Pelletier), 22
Mischel, Walter, *645*
Mitchell, P., 14
Montagu, M. F. A., 145
Moore, K. L., *684*
Murphy, John, 686
Muzio, J., 430

Nahigian, Eileen, *515*
National Center for Health Statistics, *587,* 611, 626, 669, 737, *827–834*
National Council on the Aging, *757*
Neugarten, Bernice, 44–45, 653, 762
New England Journal of Medicine, 691
New Guide to Health (Samuel Thomson), 7
Nightingale, Florence, 13
North American Nursing Diagnosis Association, *811*
Notes on Nursing (F. Nightingale), 13
Nursing Diagnosis: Process and Application (M. Gordon), *16, 23*
Nutrition in Clinical Care (R. Howard and N. Herbold), *819*
Nutrition in Infancy and Childhood (P. Pipes), *490*

Orem, Dorothea, 14
Orlando, Ida, 14
Ouellette, E. M., 685–686
Owen, George, *438*
Owens, E., 685–686
Oyle, Irving, 8

Parmalee, Arthur, 358
Parsons, Talcott, 75

Pasternack, Sarah, 589
Pasteur, Louis, 6
Pediatrics, 351, 588
Pelletier, Kenneth, 9, 22
Persaud, T. V. N., *684*
Phillips, D. C., 3
Phillips, Patricia, *515, 568*
Piaget, Jean, 39–42, 61, 98, 364, 436, 487–488, 532, 533, 569, 574, 608, 617
Pipes, Peggy, *490*
Polgar, Promadhat, *628*
Prazar, Gregory, 569
Prechtl, Heinz, 371
Principles of Pediatrics (R. Hoekelman et al.), *568*
Problems in Child Behavior and Development (M. Senn and A. Solnit), *424–425*
Provence, Sally, 433
Psychology of Careers, The (D. E. Super), *649*
Pulmonary Function Testing in Children: Techniques and Standards (P. Polgar), *628*

Rahe, R. H., 110, 741
Ramsey, Nancy, 589
Recommended Dietary Allowance (National Research Council), *692*
Report of the Committee on Infectious Diseases (American Academy of Pediatrics), *431*
Ribble, Margaret, 419
Riesteard, Melcahy, 686
Ringquist, Mary Ann, 681
Ringsdorf, W., *760*
Roberts, Pamela, *423, 516*
Robson, Kenneth, 358
Roffwarg, H., 430
Rogers, Carl, 72
Rogers, Martha E., 13–14
Rosett, H. L., 685–686
Ross, E. M., 686
Ross Laboratories, *827–834*
Rossman, Isadore, 776
Roy, Callista, 2, 14, 17
Roy, Claude, *438, 439*
Rubin, Reva, 358, 680

Sarles, Richard, 582
Sarnesu, Edith, *415*
Saruer, Roy, *415*
Schell, Robert, *645*
Scipien, Gladys, *515, 568*
Sears, Robert, 45–47
Seidel, Henry, *568*

Selye, Hans, 63, 64
Senn, Milton, *424–425*
Shah, F. K., 686
Shaie, W., 661
Silent Language, The (Edward Hall), 768
Smith, D., 685, *686*
Smith, Marjorie, 589
Smuts, Jan C., 3
Solberg, Don, *691*
Solnit, Albert, *424–425*
Stanford, Dennise, 739
Steele, J. L., 91
Stevenson, Joanne, 729–731
Sullivan, Harry Stack, *645*
Super, D. E., *649*
Switzer, David, 58

Tanner, James, *624, 625, 633*
Task Force on Blood Pressure Control in Children, *588*
Tearney, Alice, *423, 516*
Ten-State Nutrition Survey (Center for Disease Control), 145
Thomas, Alexander, 32, 428
Thomson, Samuel, 6–7
Toffler, Alvin, 56, 57, 63
Tom, Cheryl, 99
Travis, John, 1, 3
Tudor, Mary, 37–42, 45–49, *590*

United States Department of Health, Education and Welfare, 145, *587,* 611, 626, 669, 737, *827–834*
University of California at Los Angeles (UCLA), 11–12

Vaughn, Victor, *448, 454*
Vogel, Ezra, 54

Wagner, Nathaniel, *691*
Weed, Lawrence, 112
Wegman, M., *351*
Weidenbach, Ernestine, 14, 31
Weiner, L., 685–686
Wellness Workbook (John Travis), *10*
Williams, Cicely, 437
Williamson, J. D., 11
World Health Organization (WHO), 1, 2, 351
Wright, Fanny, 6

Yeaworth, Rosalee, 736

SUBJECT INDEX

Page numbers in *italic* indicate illustrations or tables.

Abdomen, 265–279
  of adolescent, 630
  of infant, 458–459
  of middle adult, 751–752
  of neonate, 388–392
  of older adult, 793–794
  in pregnancy, 703–704
    month by month changes in, 711–723
  of preschooler, 547–548
  of school-aged child, 594
  of toddler, 505
Abducens nerve (cranial nerve VI), 170, 172, *807*
  of preschooler, 551
Abuse:
  of alcohol and other substances (*see* Drugs, use and
    abuse of)
  of child, 434, 472
Accessory nerve (cranial nerve XI), 214, *808*
Accidents (*see* Safety)
Acne, 152, 618, 627
Acrocyanosis, 370, 372, 402
Activity (*see* Exercise and activity pattern)
Adaptation as positive response to loss, 57
Adaptation model of health (C. Roy), 2, 14, 17
Adolescent(s), 597–636
  abdomen of, 630
  age differences among, 601–604
  alcohol and (*see* drug use and abuse by, *below*)
  anxiety of, 60, 61, 614
  behavioral development of, 603–604, 609, 617–618
  biological rhythms of, 604–605
  blood pressure of, 624
  body image of, 610, 612, 619, 623
  breasts of, 618, 629, *633*
  chest of, 619, 628
  client profile and biographical data about, 599
  cognitive and perceptual pattern of, 41, 607–608, 617
  community resources for, 605–606
  coping and stress tolerance pattern of, 613–616
  diagnostic laboratory tests for, 636
  drug use and abuse by, 612, 614–616
  ears of, 628
  elimination pattern of, 604
  environment of, 604–605
  exercise and activity pattern of, 613
  extremities of, 630–631
  eyes of, 628
  face of, 627
  family history of, 600
  family life of, 606
  finances of, 605
  general appearance of, 618–619, 624
  genitals of, 619, *633*, 634–636
  growth and development of, 603–604
    developmental tasks in, 601, 607, 612, 617
      according to Erikson, 36–37, 617, 649
    physical size increments in, 579, 587, 594, 625,
      829–830, 833–834
    theories about, 35–37, 41–43, 50–51, 617
  hair of, 618
    pubic, 594, *633*, 634, *636*
  head of, 627–628
  health education for, 601, 620
  health habits of, 600
    (*See also* drug use and abuse by, *above*)
  health history of, 597–622
  health status and health perception pattern of,
    599–600
  hearing of, 628
  heart of, 619, 629, 631
  height of, 625–626
    growth spurt in, 579, 587, 594, 625
  hormones of, 625–626, 632–633
  independence of, 617–618
  legal status of, 598–599
  life pattern and lifestyle of, 600–606
  lungs of, 628
  moodiness of, 618
  morality and ethics of, 42–43, 614–615
  mouth of, 627
  neck of, 627–629

Adolescent(s) (*Cont.*):
  nose of, 627
  nursing approach to, 597–599, 623
  nutrition pattern of, 107, 612–613
  occupation of, 605–607
  parent of: role of, in health history or physical
    examination, 598
    as parent, 434, 611–612
  peer group and, 602–603, 618
  physical examination of, 623–636
    role of parent in health history or, 598
  pregnancy of, 611–612
  rectum of, 619, 630
  review of body components of, 618
  role and relationship pattern of, 602–603, 606–607,
    617–619
  school and, 607–608
  self-perception and self-concept pattern of, 50–51,
    616–618
    (*See also* body image of, *above*)
  sexual maturity rating of (Tanner stages), *629, 633,
    634, 636*
  sexuality and reproductive pattern of, 52–54,
    609–612
  skin of, 618, 627
  sleep and wakefulness pattern of, 604
  teeth of, 627, 636
  thorax of, 619, 628
  vision of, 628
  weight of, 625–626, *829–830, 833–834*
    growth spurt in, 579, 587, 594, 625
Aerobics, 664
Age:
  biological versus chronological, in older adult, 760
  differences in and changes accompanying: among
    adolescents, 601–604
    among infants, 419, *421*
    among neonates, 355, 403–409
    among older adults, 760, 763
    among school-aged children, 565–566
  gestational: classification of neonate by weight and,
    409
    estimation of, 403–408
  as health factor, 18–19
    for adolescent, 601–604
    for middle adult, 728
    for neonate, 355, 409
    in pregnancy, 676–677
    for preschooler, 513
    for toddler, 472
    for young adult, 642
Age of Reason, 5–6
Aged (*see* Older adult)
Aging, theories of, 43–45, 761–762
Alcohol:
  effects of, in pregnancy, 685–686
  use and abuse of (*see* Drugs, use and abuse of)
Alienation and family, 56, 57
Allergy:
  to food: in infancy, 438–439
  health history about, 94–95
Allopathy, 6
Ambivalence:
  toward pregnancy, 679
  of toddler, 476, 479
Amniocentesis, 683
Ankles, 326, 340
Anoscope, 137
Anus, 301, 304
  of adolescent, 619
  of infant, 461
  of neonate, 394
  of older adult, 797
  of pregnant client, 709
  of preschooler, 548
  of toddler, 506
Anxiety:
  of adolescent, 60, 61, 614
  defense mechanisms and, 61–62
  definition of, 59
  family as aid in, 55, 56

Anxiety (*Cont.*):
  and grief, 58–59
  of infant, 59–61, 427, 428, 440
    management of, 62–65
    normal, 59–61
  positive aspects of, 56, 59, 62, 63, 681
  in pregnancy, 680–681, 693
  of preschooler, 60, 61
  of school-aged child, 60, 61
    with school phobia, 582–583
  about separation: of infant, 440
    of toddler, 60, 428, 477, 479, 491
  about strangers, 60, 427, 428, 469
  of toddler, 60, 61
    about separation, 60, 428, 477, 479, 491
    about strangers, 469
  (*See also* Coping and stress tolerance pattern)
Aorta, abdominal pulsations of, 269, 270, 278
Apgar score of neonate, 402
Appearance, assessment of, 138–140
Arms (*see* Extremities, upper)
Arteries:
  of lower extremities, 315, 332–333
  of neck, 216, 220
    of neonate, 384
    of preschooler, 556
  of upper extremities, 313, 332
  [*See also* Pulse(s)]
Asceticism, 53, 61
Asia, influences of, on holism, 4–5
Assessment:
  as component of nursing process, 16–22
  equipment for, 129–137, 308
  functional patterns and, *16*, 17–22
  in problem-oriented record (POR), 112–113
  (*See also* Health history; Physical examination)
Athletics:
  and nutritional needs, 612–613
  safety in, 580–581
Attachment between parent and neonate or infant, 56,
  98, 357–358, 429, 431
Auditory nerve (cranial nerve VIII), 184, 187, *807*
Auscultation as physical examination technique,
  127–128
  (*See also* Bowel sounds; Heart sounds; Lung sounds)
Autism, infant developmental stage of, 426
Autogenic training, 25
Autonomy versus shame and doubt, 36, 467

Back (*see* Spine; Thorax)
Balance, assessment of, 178, 187–188, 312–313
Barlow's test for infant hip dislocation, 464, 465
Bartholin's glands, 283, 284
Basic four food groups, 107, 108, *819*
Bayley Mental Scales, *423*
Bedwetting, 570–571
Behavior, observation of, during physical examination,
  139
Behavioral development, 31–68
  of adolescent, 603–604, 609, 617–618
  family as influence on, 54–57
    in infancy, 429
  of infant, 424–429
    states of consciousness in, 429–430
    temperament in, 32
  of middle adult, 729–731
  of neonate, 357–358
    states of consciousness in, 371
    temperament in, 32
  of older adult, 763
  in pregnancy, 679–682
  of preschooler, 518–521
  principles of, 31–32
  of school-aged child, 567–570
  theories of, 34–49
    of adolescent, 35–37, 41–43, 50–51, 617, 649
    of infant and newborn, 34, 36, 39–40, 46, 426
    of middle adult, 37, 649, 729
    of older adult, 37, 43–45, 761–762, 773
    in pregnancy, 358, 681

Behavioral development, theories of (*Cont.*):
  of preschooler, 35, 36, 40, 42, 46–47, 532–533
  of school-aged child, 35, 36, 41, 42, 47, 569
  of toddler, 34–36, 40, 46–47, 467
  of young adult, 37, 648–649, 663
  of toddler, 475–479
  of young adult, 648–650
Behavioral Developmental Profile (Marshalltown), *423*
Behavioral states of neonate and infant, 371, 429–430
Behavioral systems model (D. Johnson), 14, 17
Behaviorism, 45–48
Beliefs (*see* Values and beliefs)
Bell's palsy, 376
Bimanual examination, 288–291, 306
  in pregnancy, 703, 705
Bing test of hearing, 186
Biofeedback, 25
Biological data (*see* Client profile and biographical data)
Biological rhythms, *16,* 17–19, 98–99
  of adolescent, 604–605
  of female client, 682
  of infant, 99, 429–433
  of middle adult, 732
  of neonate, 99, 358–360
  of older adult, 763–764
  and pregnancy, 682
  of preschooler, 99, 521–524
  of school-aged child, 99, 570–571
  of toddler, 99, 479–481
  of young adult, 650–651
Birth, 723
  alternative settings for, 688
  fetal position before, 720–722
  health history about, 93
    of infant, 417–419
    of neonate, 354–355
    of toddler, 471
  natural, 690
  physical examination of neonate at time of, 402–412
  psychological, Mahler's theory of, 426–428
Birth defects, causes of, 418, 673, 674, 683–687
Birth rate, 669
Birthmarks, 152
  of infant, spontaneous disappearance of, 448
  of neonate, 372–373
  of preschooler, 542, 543
Bladder:
  of infant, 459
  of neonate, 390, 392
  of older adult, 794
  pelvic examination and, 280, 281, 287
  in pregnancy, 704
  of preschooler, 538
  of school-aged child, 594
Blood pressure, 130, 142–144
  of adolescent, 624
  alternative methods of measuring, 412, 432, 497
  cuff size for measuring: of adult, 143
    of preschooler, 524, 543
    of toddler, 497
  of infant, 432, 447, 456
  of middle adult, 745, 751
  of neonate, 360, 412
  normal values of: for adolescent, 624
    for infant, 432
    for middle adult, 745
    for neonate, 360, 412
    for older adult, 782
    in pregnancy, 682, 702, 710
    for preschooler, *523, 543*
    for school-aged child, *588*
    for toddler, 497
  of older adult, 782
  in pregnancy, 682, 702, 710
  of preschooler, *523,* 524, 543
  of school-aged child, 583, 587, 588
  of toddler, 497
Blood tests:
  for adolescent, 636
  normal laboratory values for, *801–802, 804–805*
  in pregnancy, 702
  for preschooler, *538, 558*
  for toddler, 507
Body build, frame size approximation of, *815*
Body components, review of, 110–111
  of adolescent, 618
  of infant, 440–441
  of neonate, 367
  of older adult, 776–777
  of pregnant client, 693–694
  of preschooler, 537–538
  of school-aged child, 583
  of toddler, 492
  of young adult, 665
Body image, 50–51
  of adolescent, 610, 619, 623

Body image, of adolescent (*Cont.*):
  in pregnancy, 612
  of infant, 426
  of middle adult, 734, 740
  in pregnancy, 612, 689–690, 693
  of toddler, 478
Body language:
  in children, 78–79
  in health history interview, 74–75, 77–79, 97
Bonding (*see* Attachment)
Bone age and sexual maturity, 595, 636
Bones of extremities, 309–310
Bottle-feeding, 438–439
  and caries, 422
  for neonate, 366
  stools of infants who receive, 391, 431
Bowel, 269–271
  of infant, 459
  of neonate, 389, 391, 392
  of older adult, 793, 794
  of preschooler, 547, 548
  of school-aged child, 594
  (*See also* Rectum)
Bowel elimination (*see* Elimination pattern; Stool)
Bowel sounds, 270
  of infant, 459
  of neonate, 389
  of older adult, 794
  of preschooler, 548
Boyd Developmental Progress Scale, *423*
Braun-Fernwald's sign of pregnancy, 714
Brazelton Neonatal Assessment Scale, 357
Breast-feeding, 438
  advantages of, 365
  community resources to assist with, 687
  preparation of, for breast-feeding, 702
  stools of infants who receive, 391, 431
Breasts, 259–263
  of adolescent, 619, 629, *633*
  of infant, 458
  of male, 261, 264, 791
  of middle adult, 750
  of neonate, 388
    in gestational age estimation, 403
  of older adult, 791
  in pregnancy, 698, 702, 713
    preparation of for breast-feeding, 702
  of preschooler, 546
  of school-aged child, 593
  self-examination of, 727
  and sexual maturity rating of adolescent, 629, *633*
  of toddler, 505
Breath sounds, 248–249
  of infant, 455–456
  of neonate, 386, 411
  of older adult, 791
  of preschooler, 546
  of toddler, 504
Breathing (*see* Respiration)
Bursa, 317, 334, 336, 337

Calipers, skinfold, 134, 144–145
Cattell Infant Intelligence Test, *423*
Cerebellum, 341, 557
Cerebrospinal fluid, laboratory values for, *801*
Cervix, 135–136, 285–288
  culture or smear of, 286, 287
  of middle adult, 753
  of older adult, 796
  during pregnancy, 286, 704, 705
Chadwick's sign of pregnancy, 286, 704, 715
Change:
  as loss, 57–58
  need for, 63
  reactions to, 57–65
Chart (*see* Record, client)
Cheeks, 197, 208
Chest (*see* Thorax)
Chest circumference:
  of infant, 447, 454
    norms for, *454*
  of neonate, 410
  of toddler, 504
Child abuse, 434, 472
Childhood illnesses, 93
  (*See also* Immunization)
China, influence of, on holism, 4–5
Circulation, fetal, 386, 387
Clavicle, 231
  lymph nodes near, 222, 223
  of neonate, 384, 385
  of preschooler, 544
Client:
  mental set of, 73–74
  as participant in own care, 10, 25–27, 69, 84
    as preschooler, 509–510, 541
    as school-aged child, 560

Client (*Cont.*):
  role of, young adult development into, 638, *639*
  versus traditional word, *patient,* 26–27, 69
Client profile and biographical data, 89–91
  of adolescent, 599
  of infant, 417
  of middle adult, 726
  of neonate, 353
  of older adult, 759
  in pregnancy, 671–672
  of preschooler, 511
  of school-aged child, 560–563
  of toddler, 469–470
  of young adult, 639–640
Clitoris, 283
  of adolescent, 636
  of infant, 460
  of middle adult, 753
  of neonate, 393
  of older adult, 795
  of preschooler, 548
Cochlea, 184, 186
  of neonate, 380
  of older adult, 787
Cognitive and perceptual pattern, *16,* 17, 21, 39–42, 104–105, 341–346
  of adolescent, 41, 607–608, 617
  of infant, 39–40, *423,* 435–437
  of middle adult, 735–736
  of neonate, 39–40, 363–364
  of old adult, 768–770, 784, 799
  of pregnant client, 690–691
  of preschooler, 40–41, *423,* 515, 516, 531–534
  of school-aged child, 41, 567, *568,* 574–578
  of toddler, 40, *423,* 486–489, *516,* 517, *568*
  of young adult, 660–661
  (*See also* Hearing; Intelligence; Language; Memory; Smell, sense of; Taste, sense of; Touch, sense of; Vision)
Collaboration in nurse-client relationship, 84, 415–416
Color blindness, tests for, 577
Communication, 70–86
  with child or adolescent, 70, 71, 73, 92
  congruence in, 72, 84
  contract for, 75–76
  with deaf, blind, or mute client, 77
  factors affecting, 76–77
  impediments to, 85–86
  with older adult, 71, 73
  techniques for, 79–85, 416
  verbal and nonverbal, 74–79, 83, 84
  of adolescent, 598
Community resources, 101
  for adolescent, 605–606
  health facilities available as, 19–20
  for infant, 433–434
  for middle adult, 733
  for neonate, 361–362
  for older adult, 765–766
  for pregnant client, 687–688
  for preschooler, 525
  for school-aged child, 572
  for toddler, 483
  for young adult, 639, 653
Confidentiality:
  of adolescent health history record, 598–599
  in nurse-client relationship, 72
  with child or adolescent, 92
Conscience (*see* Morality)
Conservation of wholeness, principles of (M. Levine), 13
Consumer of health care, role of, 638, *639*
Continuity theory of aging (B. Neugarten), 44–45
Contraception:
  and gestational age, 675
  teaching and counseling about, 612, 619, 622, 674, 738
  pelvic examination as part of, 280
Contract between client and nurse, 24
  for communication, 75–76
Coordination of body movement, 312, 341–343, 347, 557, *806*
Coping and stress tolerance pattern, *16,* 17, 22, 57–65, 109–110
  of adolescent, 613–616
  family as factor in, 55, 56
  of infant, 440
  of middle adult, 740–741
  and neonate, 366–367
  of older adult, 773–776
  in pregnancy, 680–681, 693
  of preschooler, 537
  of school-aged child, 581–583
  of toddler, 491–492
  of young adult, 665
Cover-uncover test of eye muscles, 170, 172, 500
Cranial nerve I (olfactory nerve), 193, *807*
  of toddler, 499

Cranial nerve II (optic nerve), 166, 167, *807*
Cranial nerve III (oculomotor nerve), 170, 172, *807*
Cranial nerve IV (trochlear nerve), 170, 172, *807*
  of preschooler, 551
Cranial nerve V (trigeminal nerve), 156–159, 162, 177, *807*
  of toddler, 499
Cranial nerve VI (abducens nerve), 170, 172, *807*
  of preschooler, 551
Cranial nerve VII (facial nerve), 153–154, 199, 207,, *807*
  birth injury to, 376
  of toddler, 499
Cranial nerve VIII (auditory nerve), 184, 187, *807*
Cranial nerve IX (glossopharyngeal nerve), 206, 207, 210, 222, *807*
Cranial nerve X (vagus nerve), 210, *808*
Cranial nerve XI (accessory nerve), 214, *808*
Cranial nerve XII (hypoglossal nerve), 206–207, *808*
Cranial nerves, location and function of, *807–808*
Cricoid cartilage, 215–216, 226
Cremasteric muscle, 297
  reflex contraction of, in infant, 461
  in neonate, 394
Crying:
  of infant, 430
    types of, 428
  of neonate, 366, 367, 371, 382, 430
Culture, 97
  of adolescent, 601–602
  and communication, 76
  of infant, 420
  of middle adult, 728–729
  of neonate, 356
  of older adult, 760–761
  of pregnant client, 677–678
  of preschooler, 514
  of school-aged child, 566–567
  of toddler, 473
  of young adult, 643

DASE (Denver Articulation Screening Examination), 489, *516*, 517, *824–826*
Data:
  objective: physical examination as, 111
    in problem-oriented record (POR), 112–113
  recording of, 88, 111–113
  subjective: health history as, 111
    in problem-oriented record (POR), 112–113
Data base (*see* Health history; Physical examination)
Data collection (*see* Health history; Physical examination)
Day care, environment of, 482, 487, 524, 532
DDST (*see* Denver Developmental Screening Test)
Death:
  older adult attitudes about, 763
  preschooler concept of, 519
  school-aged child reaction to, 581–582
  of spouse of middle adult, 736
Defense mechanisms, 56, 59, 61–62
  list of, *62*
  pathology in, 62
  in pregnancy, 680–681
  and sexuality, 53
Denver Articulation Screening Examination (DASE), 489, *516*, 517, *824–826*
Denver Developmental Screening Test (DDST), 19, 98, *822–823*
  for infant, *423*, 435
  for preschooler, *516*, 517, 533
  for school-aged child, 567, *568*, 576
  for toddler, 474–475, 488, 489
Denver Eye Screening Test (DEST), *423*, 500, *516*, 517, *820–821*
Depression in older adult, 763
DEST (Denver Eye Screening Test), *423*, 500, *516*, 517, *820–821*
Development:
  tests of, 423–424, *516*, 517, 567, *568*, *820–834*
    (*See also* Intelligence testing; *names of particular tests*)
  (*See also* Behavioral development; Developmental tasks; Growth and Development)
Developmental tasks:
  of adolescent, 601, 607, 612, 617
    according to Erikson, 36–37, 617, 649
  of infant, *424–425*
    according to Erikson, 36, 426
  of middle adult, 729–731
    according to Erikson, 37, 649, 729
  of neonate, *424–425*
    according to Erikson, 36, 426
  of older adult, 775–776
    according to Erikson, 37, 762
  of parents of neonate and infant, *424–425*
  pregnancy as, 681–682

Developmental tasks (*Cont.*):
  of preschooler, 509, 513, 529
    according to Erikson, 36
  of school-aged child, according to Erikson, 36
  of toddler, according to Erikson, 36, 467
  of young adult, 648–650
    according to Erikson, 37, 648–649, 663
Developmental Test of Visual-Motor Integration (VMI), *516*, 517, 567, *568*
Diagnoses, nursing (*see* Nursing diagnoses)
Diagnostic tests:
  for adolescent, 636
  normal laboratory values for, *539, 801–806*
  as nursing assessment component, 16
  in pregnancy, 702, 705
  for preschooler, *538, 539, 558*
  for toddler, 507
Diaper rash, 460
Diet (*see* Nutrition pattern)
Differentiation, infant developmental attainment of, 426–427
Discipline of preschooler, 520–521, *527*, 529
Disease:
  causes of: in holistic view, 3, 9
    in nineteenth-century theory, 6
  client awareness of danger signs of, 727
  familial, 94–96
  health as absence of, 1–2, 11–12
  holistic view of, 11
    as "dis-ease," 4
  sex differences in patterns of, 735
Disengagement theory of aging (E. Cumming and W. Henry), 43
Distance, interpersonal, 78–79
Disuse phenomenon, 21
Divorce:
  of middle adult, 736
  of young adult, 655–656
Doll's-eye test:
  of infant, 451
  of neonate, 378
Drugs:
  medicinal and over-the-counter: in middle adulthood, 727
  older adult finances and, 765
  in pregnancy, 673, 674, *684*, 685
  in young adulthood, 651
  use and abuse of, 92
    by adolescent, 612, 614–616
    by middle adult, 727, 733
    by pregnant client, *684*, 685
    by young adult, 651, 665
Dubowitz method of estimating gestational age, 404–407

Eardrum, 182, 183
  of infant, 451
  of neonate, 380
  of preschooler, 552, 553
  of toddler, 501
  of older adult, 786
Ears, 131, 134, 178–188
  of adolescent, 628
  of infant, 451–452
  of neonate, 379–380
    in gestational age estimation, 403
  of older adult, 786–787
  position of, 152, 179, 379
  in pregnancy, 700
  of preschooler, 552–554
  of school-aged child, 591
  of toddler, 492, 501
  wax in: of middle adult, 749
    of older adult, 786
    of preschooler, 553
    removal of, 553
  (*See also* Hearing)
Ecology, 13
Economic status (*see* Finances)
Ecosystem, 13
Education, 104, 105
  of adolescent, 607–608
  of infant and caretakers, 435–436
  of middle adult, 737
  of neonate and caretakers, 363–364
  of older adult, 769
  of pregnant client, 690
  of preschooler, 524, 531–532
    (*See also* Day care, environment of)
  of school-aged child, 575–576
    (*See also* School)
  for toddler, 486–487
  of young adult, 660
  (*See also* Health education; Sex education)
Ego:
  and defense mechanisms, 61–62

Ego (*Cont.*):
  in Erikson's theory, 36
  in Freud's theory, 35, 36
  functions of, 36
Ego integrity versus despair, 37, 762, 773
Elbow, 321, 334–335
  muscles and nerves of, 330
Electra complex, 35–36, 534
Elimination pattern, *16*, 17, 18, 98–99
  of adolescent, 604
  of infant, 431
  of middle adult, 732, 737
  of neonate, 359, 391
  of older adult, 764, 793, 794
  in pregnancy, 704, 709, 713, 723
  of preschooler, 522–523
  of school-aged child, 570–571
  of toddler, 480–481
  of young adult, 651
Embryo:
  environment of, 683
  growth and development of, 711–716
Empathy in nurse-client relationship, 72
Employee, health examination of, 88–89
Enuresis, 570–571
Environment, 19, 97, 100
  of adolescent, 604–605
  behaviorist viewpoint on, 47–48
  holistic viewpoint on, 3
  home, 19, 89–90, 100
    tool for assessing (see Home Observation for Measurement of the Environment)
  of infant, 433
  intrauterine, 683
  of middle adult, 732
  of neonate, 360–361
  Nightingale on, 13
  occupational, 19, 91, 102–103, 727, 732–733
    for pregnant client, 689
  of older adult, 764
  of pregnant client, 683–687, 689
  of preschooler, 524–525, *526–528,* 532
  school, 19, 103
    (*See also* Day care, environment of)
  of school-aged child, 571
  of toddler, 481–482, *484–485*, 487
    for play, 486–487, 490–491
  of young adult, 651–652
Epididymus, 296–297
Ethics (*see* Morality)
Ethnicity:
  and communication, 76
  definition of, 18
Eustachian tube, 182
Evaluation:
  as component of nursing process, 17, 26
  in problem-oriented record (POR), 112
Examining room, equipment of, 129
Exercise and activity pattern, *16*, 17, 21, 108–109
  of adolescent, 613
  of infant, 440
  of middle adult, 727, 741–742
  of neonate, 366, 371
  of older adult, 763, 773
  in pregnancy, 693
  of preschooler, 536–537
  of school-aged child, 580–581
  of toddler, 490–491
  of young adult, 664–665
Extremities, 308–349
  of adolescent, 630–631
  bones of, 309–310
  of infant, 461–465
  lower, 310, 314–316, 325–327
    arteries of, 315, 332–333
    muscles and nerves of, 316, 331, 337, 339–340
    reflexes of, 349
  of middle adult, 754–755
  of neonate, 395–400
    of gestational age estimate, 404–407
  of older adult, 798–799
  in pregnancy, 709–710
  of preschooler, 557
  of school-aged child, 591
  of toddler, 492, 506–507
  upper, 310, 313–314, 320–324
    arteries of, 313, 332
    muscles and nerves of, 330, 334, 338
    reflexes of, 348
  (*See also* Joints)
Eyebrows, 151, 161
  of older adult, 785
Eyelashes, 161
Eyelids, 161
  inversion of, 163
Eyes, 132–133, 151, 160–177
  of adolescent, 628
  of infant, 450–451

Eyes (Cont.):
  of middle adult, 747–748
  muscles of, 170–173, 450, 500, 551
  of neonate, 377–378
  of older adult, 785–786
  in pregnancy, 699
  of preschooler, 551
  of school-aged child, 591
  of toddler, 492, 500
  (See also Vision)

Face, 150–160
  of adolescent, 627
  of infant, 449
  of middle adult, 746
  of neonate, 376
  of old adult, 783–784
  in pregnancy, 698, 699
  of preschooler, 549, 550
  of school-aged child, 589
  of toddler, 497, 499
Facial nerve (cranial nerve VII), 153–154, 199, 207, 807
  birth injury to, 376
  in toddler, 499
Fallopian tubes, 285–290
  of older adult, 797
  in pregnancy, 706
Family:
  alternative forms of, 57
  and child development, 37, 46–47, 53–57, 429, 563
  functions or tasks of, 20, 54–56
  future of, 56–57
  and mental health, 55–56
  as social system, 54–57
Family history, 94–97
  of adolescent, 600
  of infant, 419–420
  of middle adult, 727–728
  of neonate, 355
  of older adult, 761
  of pregnant client, 676
  of preschooler, 512, 514
  of school-aged child, 562, 565
  of toddler, 472
  of young adult, 642
Family life, 102
  of adolescent, 606
  of infant, 433–435
  of middle adult, 733–734
  of neonate, 362
  of older adult, 766
  in pregnancy, 688–689
  of preschooler, 525–529
  of school-aged child, 572–573
  of toddler, 483
Fantasies of toddler, 477–479
Fatigue:
  of middle adult, 742
  of older adult, 758
  during pregnancy, 689, 693
Fears of toddler, 477–479
Feces, tests of:
  for blood, 307
  normal laboratory values for, 805–806
Feet, 327, 338, 340
  of infant, 423, 462, 463
  of neonate, 395, 398, 399
    in gestational age estimation, 403
  of toddler, 506–507
Femoral canals, 295, 298
Fetal alcohol syndrome, 685–686
Fetoscope, 137, 719
Fetus:
  circulation of, 386, 387
  environment of, 683
  growth and development of, 716–723
  position of, before birth, 720–722
Field theory (K. Lewin), 38–39
Fifth National Conference Group on the Classification of Nursing Diagnosis (1982), 22, 23
Finances, 101
  of adolescent, 605
  of infant, 433
  of middle adult, 729, 733
  of neonate, 361
  of older adult, 765
    and medications, 765
    and nutrition, 771
  of pregnant client, 687, 693
  of preschooler, 525
  of school-aged child, 571–572
  of toddler, 473–474, 483
  of young adult, 652–653
Fingers, 323–324
  muscles and nerves of, 330, 339

Fingers (Cont.):
  of neonate, 395, 397
  (See also Hands; Nails)
First National Conference on the Classification of Nursing Diagnosis (1970), 17
Fontanels:
  of infant, 448, 449
  of neonate, 374–375
  of toddler, 499
Food groups, basic four, 107, 108, 819
Food intake record, 108
Forceps, facial marks from delivery by, 375, 376
Forehead, 151
Formula, infant, 438–439
Frame size, method of approximating, 815
Function tests, laboratory values for:
  circulatory, 802
    gastrointestinal, 803
    metabolic and endocrine, 803
    pulmonary, 803–804
    renal, 804
Functional patterns:
  definitions of, 18–22
  health history format for, 87
  and nursing assessment, 16, 17–22
  and problem-oriented record (POR), 113

Gait, 139, 312, 343
  of older adult, 780
  in pregnancy, 697, 709
  of preschooler, 557
  of toddler, 506–507
Gallbladder, 277
General adaptation syndrome (H. Selye), 63–65
Generativity versus stagnation, 37, 649, 729
Genetic counseling, 95, 642–643
Genetics, 94–97
  (See also Heredity)
Genitals, 280–299, 304, 307
  of adolescent, 619, 633, 634–646
  female, 280–291
  of infant, 460–461
  male, 292–299, 304, 307
  of middle adult, 753–754
  of neonate, 393–394
  of older adult, 795–797
  of pregnant client, 704–708, 711–723
  of preschooler, 548–549
  of school-aged child, 594–595
  of toddler, 506
Germ theory of disease causation, 6
Glaucoma, 137, 162, 748
Glossopharyngeal nerve (cranial nerve IX), 206, 207, 210, 222, 807
Goals:
  client role in establishment of, 84
  as component of nursing process, 16–17, 24–26
  in problem-oriented record (POR), 112
Goniometer, 137
Goodell's sign of pregnancy, 714
Goodenough-Harris Drawing Test, 516, 517, 567, 568
Greece, influence of, on holism, 5
Grief, 57–59, 63–64
  of preschooler, 519–520
  of school-aged child, 581–582
  stages of, 58–59, 64
Growth charts for children to 18 years, 827–834
Growth and development, 18–19, 93, 97–98
  of adolescents, 603–604
    developmental tasks in, 601, 607, 612, 617
      according to Erikson, 36–37, 617, 649
    physical size increments in, 579, 587, 594, 625, 829–830, 833–834
    theories about, 35–37, 41–43, 50–51, 617
    (See also sexual maturation in, below)
  of embryo and fetus, 711–723
  of infant, 413–414, 415, 420–429
    anticipatory guidance about, 414, 420, 422, 428, 441
    developmental tasks in, 424–425
      according to Erikson, 36, 426
    physical size increments in, 447, 827–828, 831–832
    theories about, 34, 36, 40, 46, 426
  of middle adult, 37, 729–731
    developmental tasks in, 37, 649, 729–731
    theories about, 37
  of neonate, 355–358
    anticipatory guidance about, 369
    developmental tasks in, 424–425
      according to Erikson, 36, 426
    physical size increrments in, 410, 827–828, 831–832
  of older adult, 761–763
    developmental tasks in, 775–776
      according to Erikson, 37, 762

Growth and development, of older adult (Cont.):
    theories about, 43–45, 761–762
  in pregnancy, 678–682
  of preschooler, 515–521
    developmental tasks in, 509, 513, 529
      according to Erikson, 36
    physical size increment in, 515
    theories about, 35, 40–42
  of school-aged child, 567–570
    developmental task in, 36
    physical size increment in, 587, 829–830, 833–834
    theories about, 35, 41, 42, 47
    sexual maturation in (Tanner stages): and athletics, 581
    of breasts, 593, 629, 633
    of genitals, 594, 633, 634, 646
    laboratory tests related to, 636
  of toddler, 474–475
    developmental tasks in, 36, 467
    physical size increment in, 474, 829–830, 833–834
    theories about, 34–36, 40, 46–47, 467
  of young adult, 643–650
    developmental tasks in, 37, 648–650, 663
    theories of, 37
Guaiac test for fecal blood, 307
Gum stimulator in physical examination, 136, 201, 204, 205
Gums, 136, 201, 203–205
  of infant, 453
  of neonate, 381–382
  of older adult, 788
  in pregnancy, 700
Gynecomastia, 264, 791

Hair, 149
  of adolescent, 618
    (See also pubic, below)
  axillary, 231
  chest, 231
  facial, 153, 699
  of infant, 448
  lower extremity, 316, 799
  of middle adult, 745, 753
  of neonate, 376
    in gestational age estimation, 403
  of older adult, 783, 795, 799
  in pregnancy, 699
  of preschooler, 549
  pubic, 594, 795
    of female, 282, 753, 795
    of male, 292, 795
    and sexual maturity rating of adolescent, 633, 634, 636
  of school-aged child, 589, 594
  of toddler, 499
  upper extremity, 314
Hammer, reflex, 135, 347–349
Hands, 313–314, 322–324, 339
  (See also Fingers; Thumbs; Wrists)
Hardy-Rand-Rittler color blindness test, 577
Head, 146–210
  of adolescent, 627–628
  of infant, 448–453
    circumference of, 447, 448, 828, 832
  of middle adult, 745–749
  of neonate, 374–383
    circumference of, 410, 828, 832
  of older adult, 783–789
  of pregnant client, 699–700
  of preschooler, 549–555
    circumference of, 550, 828, 832
  of school-aged child, 589–591
  of toddler, 492, 499
    circumference of, 499, 828, 832
Health:
  definition of, 1–4, 51
    by client, 91
    by Hippocrates, 5
  factors affecting, 13
  holistic (see Holistic health)
  mental (see Mental health)
Health care:
  facilities for, 19–20
  models for delivery of, 8–12
    holistic, 9–12
    medical, 8–9
  motives for seeking, 70, 88–89
    in adolescence, 599
    in older adulthood, 759
    in school-aged period, 560
    in young adulthood, 639
Health education:
  for adolescent, 601, 620
  about contraception, 280, 612, 619, 662, 674, 738
  during health history 83, 85, 86, 638

Health education (*Cont.*):
in pregnancy, 674, 683, 686–687, 690–691
of school children, 560, 563
(*See also* Sex education)
Health habits:
of adolescent, 600
(*See also* Adolescent, drug use and abuse by)
of infant, 417
and life expectancy, 11–12
of middle adult, 726–727
of older adult, 759
of pregnant client, 673–674
of preschooler, 511–512
of toddler, 470–471
of young adult, 640–641, 652
Health history, 69–116
accuracy of, 70–71
of adolescent, 597–622
about biological rhythms, 98–99
(*See also particular age groups*)
about birth, 93
of infant, 417–419
of neonate, 354–355
of previous children of pregnant client, 675
of toddler, 471
about cognitive and perceptual pattern, 104–105
(*See also particular age groups*)
communication in, 70–86
with child or adolescent client, 70, 71, 73, 92
impediments to, 85–86
with older adult, 71, 73
techniques for, 79–85
verbal and nonverbal language in, 74–79, 83, 84
of adolescent, 598
components of, 89–111
about coping and stress tolerance pattern, *16, 17,* 22,
57–65, 109–110
(*See also particular age groups*)
about culture, 97
about elimination pattern, *16, 17,* 18, 98–99
(*See also particular age groups*)
about environment, 19, 97, 100
about exercise and activity pattern, *16, 17,* 21,
108–109
(*See also particular age groups*)
format for, 86–113
functional patterns in, *87*
functions of, 69, 87
about growth and development, 18–19, 93, 97–98
health education during, 83, 85, 86, 836
about health status and health perception pattern, *16,*
17, 18, 91–96
(*See also particular age groups*)
of infant, 414–444
data tool for, *415*
interview techniques for, 79–85
introductions in, 77
about life pattern and lifestyle, *16,* 17–20, 96–101
(*See also particular age groups*)
mental set and, 73–74
of middle adult, 725–743
of neonate, 352–367
and nursing diagnosis, 87, 111
as nursing process component, 16
about nutrition pattern, 106–108
(*See also particular age groups*)
observations during, 77
about occupation, 91, 102–103
of older adult, 71, 73, 757–779
in pregnancy, 354–355, 417, 670–696
of preschooler, 509–540
record of, 88, 111–113
confidentiality of, 598–599
of older adult, 777
of pregnant client, 671
of toddler, 469
about role and relationship pattern, *16,* 17, 20,
101–104
(*See also particular age groups*)
of school-aged child, 559–584
about self-perception and self-concept pattern, *16,* 17,
21, 50–51, 104
(*See also particular age groups*)
setting for, 72–73
about sexuality and reproductive pattern, *16,* 17,
20–21, 106
(*See also particular age groups*)
about sleep and wakefulness pattern, *16,* 17, 18,
98–99
time required for, 70
timing of, 73
of toddler, 467–494
of young adult, 637–666
Health status and health perception pattern, *16,* 17, 18,
91–96
of adolescent, 599–600
of infant, 417

Health status and health perception pattern (*Cont.*):
of middle adult, 726–728
of neonate, 353
of older adult, 759–760
of pregnant client, 672–676
of preschooler, 511–512
of school-aged child, 563
of toddler, 470–472
of young adult, 640–642
Health teaching (*see* Health education)
Hearing, 21, 104, 134, 184–187
of adolescent, 628
of infant, *421, 422,* 435, 452
of middle adult, 736, 749
of neonate, 363
of older adult, 768, 786–787
in pregnancy, 690
of preschooler, 517, 531
of school-aged child, 564, 577–578, 591
of toddler, 486
Weber test of, 186, 578, 749
Heart, 250–258
of adolescent, 619, 629, 631
of infant, 456–457
of middle adolescent, 751
of neonate, 386–387
of older adult, 792–793
in pregnancy, 702
of preschooler, 544–545
of school-aged child, 593
of toddler, 492, 505
Heart rate:
of infant, 447
of middle adult, 745, 751
of neonate, 360, 387, 411
of older adult, 782, 792
in pregnancy, 682
of preschooler, 523–524, 543
of school-aged child, 583, 587, 588
of toddler, 497
Heart sounds, 250, 252–258
of adolescent, 619
of infant, 457
of neonate, 387
of older adult, 258, 793
in pregnancy, 257, 702
of preschooler, 545
respiratory effect on, 256
of school-aged child, 593
of toddler, 505
Hegar's sign of pregnancy, 714
Height, 138, 140
of adolescent, 625–626, *829–830, 833–834*
growth spurt in, 579, 587, 594, 625
of infant (length), 447, *827–828, 831–832*
of middle adult, 754
recommended weight for, *107, 140, 816, 819*
of neonate (length), 410, *827–828, 831–832*
norms of: for adults, *107, 140, 816*
for children to 18 years, *827–834*
of older adult, 781
of preschooler, 515–516, 543, *829–830,*
833–834
of school-aged child, 568, 583, 587, *829–830,*
833–834
of toddler, 474, 498, *827–828, 831–832*
weight recommended for, *107, 140, 816, 819*
Hemangioma, 152
Hematology, laboratory values for, *801–802,*
804–805
Hemorrhoids, 302
in pregnancy, 709
Heredity, 96–97
of adolescent, 601
of infant, 419–420
of middle adult, 727–728
of neonate, 355–356
of older adult, 761
of pregnant client, 676, 677
of preschooler, 514
of school-aged child, 566
of toddler, 473
of young adult, 642–643
Hernia, 295, 298–299
umbilical, 458, 505, 547
Hips, 325, 336, 339
of neonate and infant, 396, 464–465
Hirschberg test of eye muscles, 170, 171, 500, 551
History (*see* Health history)
Holistic health, 1–30
consumer role in, 26–27
health history interview in, 69, 74, 75
history of, 3–7
and nursing, 12–17, 25–27
principles of, 3, 9–12
Home:
environment of, 19, 89–90, 100

Home, environment of (*Cont.*):
tool for assessment of (*see* Home Observation for
Measurement of the Environment)
Home Observation for Measurement of the
Environment (HOME), *423,* 482, *484–485,* 525,
526–528
Homeopathy, 6
Homeostasis, 1, 2
Homosexuality, 659, 737
Hormones:
in adolescence, 625–626, 632–633
at menopause, 737, 753, 754
Hygienic movement in history of holistic health, 7
Hyoid bone, 214
Hyperactivity of school-aged child, 578
Hypoglossal nerve (cranial nerve XII), 206–207, *808*

Id, 35
Identity (*see* Self-perception and self-concept pattern)
Identity versus role confusion, 36–37, 617, 649
Illness (*see* Disease)
Imaginary playmate, 537
Immunization, 93
of infant, 431–432
of pregnant client, 683
of preschooler, 523
schedule for, *431*
of child not immunized in infancy, 565
of school-aged child, 564–565
of toddler, 472, 481
Income (*see* Finances)
Incus, 182, 183
Independence:
of adolescent, 617–618
of preschooler, 531
of young adult, 644–645
Industry versus inferiority, 36
Infant, 413–465
abdomen of, 458–459
age factors in health of, 419, *421*
anxiety of, 59–61, 440
behavioral development of, 424–429
states of consciousness in, 429–430
temperament in, 32–33
behavioral states of, 429–430
biological rhythms of, 99, 429–433
blood pressure of, 432, 447, 456
chest of, 454–458
client profile and biographical data of, 417
cognitive and perceptual pattern of, 39–40,
435–437
community resources for, 433–434
coping and stress tolerance pattern of, 440
crying of, 430
types of, 428
ears of, 451–452
elimination pattern of, 431
environment of, 433
exercise and activity pattern of, 440
extremities of, 461–465
eyes of, 450–451
face of, 449
family history of, 419–420
family life of, 433–435
finances of, 433
general appearance of, *421,* 447–448
genitals of, 460–461
growth and development of, 413–414, *415,* 420–429
anticipatory guidance about, 414, 420, 422, 428,
441
developmental tasks in, *424–425*
according to Erikson, 36, 426
physical size increments in, 447, *827–828,*
831–832
theories about, 34, 36, 40, 46, 426
hair of, 448
head of, 448–453
circumference of, 447, 448, *828, 832*
health care schedule for, 414, *415*
health habits of, 417
health history of, 414–444
data tool for, *415*
health status and health perception pattern of, 417
hearing of, *421, 422,* 435, 452
heart of, 456–457
heart rate of, 447
height (length) of, 447, *827–828, 831–832*
hips of, 464–465
immunization of, 431–432
language of, *421, 422,* 436
length of, 447, *827–828, 831–832*
life pattern and lifestyle of, 419–429
low birth weight, 351, 409
lungs of, 455–456
mental health of, *424–425*
mortality rates of, 351, 355, 409, 439

Infant (*Cont.*):
mouth of, 453
nails of, 448
neck of, 454
nose of, 452
nursing approach to, 414–416, 445–446
nutrition pattern of, 107, *415*, 437–440
oropharynx of, 453, 454
parent of: attitude of, toward birth and baby,
418–419, 428–429
developmental tasks of, *424–425*
mental health of, *424–425*
occupation of, 434, 435
role of, in child health history or physical
examination, 413–414, 437, 445
single, 435
physical examination of, 437, 445–465
parent role in health history of, 413–414, 437, 445
premature, definition of, 351
respiration of, 432, 447, 452, 454–456
restraints for, 446
review of body components of, 440–441
role and relationship pattern of, 434–435
safety of, 422–423
screening tests and tools for, 423–424
separation-individuation of, 426–428, 430
sexuality and reproduction pattern of, 52–53, 437
skin of, 447–448, 460
sleep and wakefulness pattern of, 426–427, 429–431
spine of, 465
states of arousal (consciousness) of, 429–430
stimulation of, 430–431, 433, 440
teeth of, 420, *421*, 453
bottle-feeding and, 422
temperament of, 32–33, 428–429
temperature of, 431
thorax of, 454–458
vision of, 435
developmental changes in, 420, *421*, 450
testing of, *422, 423*, 451
weight of, 447, *827–828, 831–832*
Inguinal canals, 295, 298–299
Inguinal rings:
of infant, 460
of neonate, 394
of preschooler, 549
Initiative versus guilt, 36, 513, 529
Inspection as physical examination technique, 119
Integrity versus despair, 37, 762, 773
Intellectualization, 53, 61
Intelligence (*see* Cognitive and perceptual pattern)
Intelligence testing, 105
of adolescent, *568*, 608
of infant, *423, 568*
of middle adult, *568*, 769–770
of older adult, *568*, 770
of preschooler, *423, 516*, 533–534, *568*
of school-aged child, 567, *568*
of toddler, *423*, 488, *516*, 517, *568*
of young adult, *568*, 661
Interdependence of young adult, 644–646
International Society for the Study of Biological
Rhythms, 650
Intervention:
as component of nursing process, 17, 25
in holistic nursing, 25
Interview (*see* Health history, communication in)
Intimacy versus isolation, 37, 648–649, 663
Ishihara color blindness test, 577

Japan, influences of, on holism, 4
Jaundice, in pregnancy, 703
Jaw, 198
Job (*see* Occupation)
Joints, 311, 316–327, 334–337
of middle adult, 754
of neonate, 396
of older adult, 798
Jugular veins, 216–219

Kidneys, 279
of infant, 459
laboratory values for tests of, *804*
of middle adult, 752
of neonate, 390, 392
of older adult, 794
in pregnancy, 703
of preschooler, 547
of school-aged child, 594
(*See also* Elimination pattern; Urinalysis; Urinary
tract infection)
Kiesselbach's plexus of the nose, 192
Knees, 326, 336–337
of preschooler, 557
Korotkoff sound, 143
Kyphosis of older adult, 781, 790–792

Labia majora, 282
of adolescent, 636
of infant, 460
of middle adult, 753
of neonate, 393
of older adult, 795
of preschooler, 548
Labia minora, 283
of adolescent, 636
of infant, 460
of middle adult, 753
of neonate, 393
of older adult, 795
of preschooler, 548
Laboratory tests (*see* Diagnostic tests)
Ladin's sign of pregnancy, 714
Language, 21, 138, 139
of infant, *421, 422*, 436
of nurse, 76
of preschooler, *515*, 517, 531, 533
of school-aged child, 567, *568*, 575
of toddler, 474, 488–489, 501
verbal and nonverbal, 74–79, 83, 84
(*See also* Denver Articulation Screening
Examination; Denver Developmental Screening
Test; Peabody Picture Vocabulary Test)
Law about rights of minors, 598–599
Laxatives, 727, 764
Lead poisoning, testing for, 507
Learning disabilities, 576–578
Legs (*see* Extremities, lower)
Leisure time, use of, 109, 665, 773
Leopold's maneuvers for assessing fetal position,
720–722
Life expectancy, 11–12, 760
Life pattern and lifestyle, *16*, 17–20, 96–101
of adolescent, 600–606
of infant, 419–429
of middle adult, 728–733
of neonate, 355–361
nontraditional or alternative, 640–641, 658–659,
661–662
of older adult, 760–766
of pregnant client, 676–679, 682
of preschooler, 513
of school-aged child, 565–567
of toddler, 472–483
of young adult, 640–653
nontraditional, 640–641, 658–659, 661–662
Lips, 199–200
Liver, 272, 276
of infant, 459
of middle adult, 752
of neonate, 390, 391
of older adult, 794
in pregnancy, 703
of preschooler, 547
of toddler, 505
Locus of control, 641, 760
Loneliness, 56, 90
Loss:
behavioral reaction to, 57–65
change as, 57–58
definition of, 57
theories about, 58–59
Low birth weight infant, definition of, 351
Lungs, 238–249
of adolescent, 628
of infant, 455–456
of middle adult, 750
of neonate, 385–386, 411
of older adult, 790–791
in pregnancy, 701
of preschooler, 538, 545–546
of school-aged child, 593
of toddler, 504
Lying of school-aged child, 569–570
Lymph nodes:
axillary, 262
breast, 262
cervical, 222–224
of neonate, 384
in pregnancy, 699
of preschooler, 556
of school-aged child, 592
facial, 156
inguinal, 299
postauricular, of preschooler, 554

McDonald's rule for estimating duration of pregnancy,
403, 715
Magical thinking of toddler, 478
Malleus, 182, 183
Mandible, 198
of neonate, 382
Marital status, 90
of pregnant client, 672

Marriage:
of middle adult, 733–734
of young adult, 654–655, 658–659, 664
Masseter muscle, 156–157
Mastoid process, 178–180
Masturbation:
by child, 60, 534
by middle adult, 737, 739
Maturation:
Gesell's theory of, 37–38, 617
pregnancy as crisis of, 682
sexual, rating scale for (Tanner stages):
and athletics, 581
of breasts, 593, *629, 633*
of genitals, 594, *633, 634, 636*
laboratory tests related to, 636
Maturity:
and child rearing, 656–657
of young adult, 644–648
Meconium, 359, 391, 394
Medical record (*see* Record, client)
Medication (*see* Drugs)
Meditation, 25, 768
Memory, 21
of older adult, 770
of school-aged child, 574
Menarche, 579, 594, 610, 619, 632
breast development with, 593
Menopause, 737–738
male, 737–738
physical changes after, 282, 286, 737–738, 796–797
Menstruation, 98–99
in adolescence, 610–611, 632
disorders of, 99, 611
history of, of pregnant client, 674–675, 682
pelvic examination during, 280
Mental health:
definition of, 65
family role in, 55–56
of infant, *424–425*, 429
of middle adult, 740
of neonate, *424–425*
of older adult, 773–775
of parents of neonate and infant, *424–425*
Mental status, 139
Mentor, 650, 730
Metabolic rhythms (*see* Blood pressure; Heart rate;
Respiration; Temperature)
Middle adult, 725–755
abdomen of, 751–752
age of, as health factor, 728
behavioral development of, 729–731
biological rhythms of, 732
blood pressure of, 745, 751
body image of, 740, 743
chest of, 750–751
client profile and biographical date of, 726
cognitive and perceptual pattern of, 735–736
community resources for, 733
coping and stress tolerance pattern of, 740–741
definition of, 725
drug use and abuse by, 727, 733
elimination pattern of, 732, 737
environment of, 732
exercise and activity pattern of, 741–742
extremities of, 754–755
eyes of, 747–748
face of, 746
family history of, 727–728
family life of, 733–734
finances of, 729, 733
general appearance of, 744
genitals of, 753–754
growth and development of, 37, 729–731
developmental tasks in, 37, 649, 729–731
theories about, 37
hair of, 745, 753
head of, 745–749
health habits of, 726–727
health history of, 725–743
health status and health perception pattern of,
726–728
hearing of, 736, 749
heart of, 751
heart rate of, 745, 751
height of, 754
weight recommended for, *107, 140, 816, 819*
life pattern and lifestyle of, 728–733
lungs of, 750
menopause in, 737–738
male, 737–738
physical changes following, 282, 286, 737–738, 797
mouth of, 746
nursing approach to, 744
nutrition pattern of, 740
occupation of, 726, 727, 729, 741
hazards of, 732–733
physical examination of, 744–755

Middle adult (*Cont.*):
  respiration of, 745, 751
  role and relationship pattern of, 733–734
  self-perception and self-concept pattern of, 734–735, 740
  sense of taste of, 736
  sexual and reproductive pattern of, 728–729, 736–740
    sexual dysfunction in, 739
  skin of, 746, 748, 752, 754
  sleep and wakefulness pattern of, 732
  spine of, 750
  teeth of, 746
  temperature of, 745
  thorax of, 750–751
  vision of, 735–736, 747
Middle ages, influence of, on holism, 5
Middlescence, 729–731
Minors, legal rights of, 598–599
Models, conceptual:
  of health care, 9–12
  of nurse-client relationship, 415–416
"Molecular clock" theory of aging, 762
Money (*see* Finances)
Morality:
  of adolescent, 42–43, 614–615
  of preschooler, 35–36, 42, 534
  of school-aged child, 35–36, 569–570
  of young adult, 658, 659
Mortality rates of newborns and infants, 351, 355, 409, 433
Motor pathways, 312, 347, *806*
Motor skills:
  of preschooler, *515,* 516, 531, 536–537, 557
  of school-aged child, 657
  of toddler, 471, 474–475, 490–491
Mourning, 57–59
  (*See also* Grief)
Mouth, 136, 152, 197–210
  of adolescent, 627
  of infant, 453
  of middle adult, 746
  of neonate, 381–383
  of older adult, 788–789
  in pregnancy, 700
  of preschooler, 555
  of school-aged child, 590
  self-examination of, 727
  of toddler, 502–503
Muscle mass, 329
Muscles, 328–331, 340
  of eye, 170–173, 450, 500, 551
  of face, 156–158, 197, 199
  of lower extremity, 316, 331, 337, 339–340
  of neck, 212–214, 221
  of upper extremities, 330, 338

Naegele's rule for calculating length of pregnancy, 403
Nailbiting, 582
Nails, 313, 316, 333
  of infant, 448
  of older adult, 798, 799
Naïve theory of behavior (F. Heider), 48–49
Narcissism in infancy, 426, 428
Neck, 211–229
  of adolescent, 627–629
  arteries of, 216, 220
    of neonate, 384
    of preschooler, 556
  of infant, 454
  lymph nodes of, 222–224
    of neonate, 384
    in pregnancy, 699
    of preschooler, 556
    of school-aged child, 592
  muscles of, 212–214, 221
    of neonate, 383–384
  of older adult, 789–790
  in pregnancy, 699, 701
  of preschooler, 556
  of school-aged child, 592
  of toddler, 502–503
  veins of, 216–219
    of adolescent, 629
    of neonate, 384
    of preschooler, 556
Negativism of toddler, 476–477, 479
Neonatal Perception Index (E. Broussard), 429
Neonate, 351–412
  abdomen of, 388–392
  of adolescent mother, 611–612
  age of, gestational and chronological, 355, 403–409
  Apgar scoring of, 402
  attachment behavior of, 357–358
  behavioral development of, 357–358
    states of consciousness in, 371

Neonate, behavioral development of (*Cont.*):
    temperament in, 32
  behavioral states of, 371
  biological rhythms of, 99, 358–360
  birth history of, 354–355
  blood pressure of, 360, 412
  chest of, 385–388, 410
  classification of, by birth weight and gestational age, 409
  client profile and biographical data of, 353
  cognitive and perceptual pattern of, 39–40, 363–364
  community resources for, 361–362
  coping and stress tolerance pattern of, 366–367
  crying of, 366, 367, 371, 382, 430
  definition of, 351
  ears of, 379–380
    in gestational age estimation, 403
  elimination pattern of, 359, 391
  environment of, 360–361
  exercise and activity pattern of, 366, 371
  extremities of, 395–400
    in gestational age estimation, 404–407
  eyes of, 377–378
  face of, 376
  family history of, 355
  family life of, 362
  finances of, 361
  general appearance of, 370
  genitals of, 393–394
  gestational age estimation of, 403–408
  growth and development of, 355–358
    anticipatory guidance about, 369
    developmental tasks in, *424–425*
      according to Erikson, 36, *426*
    physical size increments in, 410, 827–828,. 831–832
  head of, 374–383
    circumference of, 410, *828, 832*
  health history of, 352–376
  health status and health perception pattern of, 353
  hearing of, 363
  heart of, 386–387
  heart rate of, 360, 387, 411
  height (length) of, 410, 827–828, 831–832
  hips of, 396
  length of, 410, 827–828, 831–832
  life pattern and lifestyle of, 355–361
  low birth weight, 351, 409
  lungs of, 385–386, 411
  mental health of, *424–425*
  mortality rates of, 351, 355, 409
  mouth of, 381–383
  neck of, 383–384
  nose of, 380, 385, 411
  nursing approach to, 369–370
  nutrition pattern of, 365–366
  parent of: attitude of, toward birth and baby, 418–419, 428–429
    developmental tasks of, *424–425*
    mental health of, *424–425*
    occupation of, 362
    role of, in child health history or physical examination, 352–353, 369
  physical examination of, 369–412
    at birth, 402–412
    parent role in health history or, 352–353, 369
    schedule for, 369
  reflexes of, 379, 383, 384, 392, 394, 397–401
  respiration of, 360, 385–386, 411
  review of body components of, 367
  role and relationship pattern of, 362
  sexuality and reproduction pattern in, 52–53, 364–365
  skin of, 372–373
    color of, 370, 372, 386, 395, 402
  sleep and wakefulness pattern of, 358–359, 371
  spine of, 397
  states of arousal (consciousness) of, 371
  teeth of, 381
  temperature of, 359–360, 412
  thorax of, 385–388, 410
  vision of, 363
  weight of, 408–410, 827–828, 831–832
Nerves:
  cranial (*see* Cranial nerves)
  of lower extremities, 331
  of upper extremities, 330, 334
Nevi (*see* Birthmarks)
Nipples, 261, 263, 264
  of infant, 458
  of neonate, 388
  of older adult, 791
  in pregnancy, 698, 702, 713
  of preschooler, 546
Nocturnal seminal emissions, 594, 611, 632
Nose, 133, 152, 189–196
  of adolescent, 627
  of infant, 452

Nose (*Cont.*):
  of neonate, 380, 385, 411
  of older adult, 787
  in pregnancy, 700
  of preschooler, 554
  of school-aged child, 590
  of toddler, 502
Nosebleed in pregnancy, 700
Nurse:
  mental set of, 73–74
  sensory stimuli transmitted by, 79
  values and beliefs of, 73–74
Nurse-client relationship:
  collaboration in, 84, 415–416
  factors influencing, 70–74
  Szasz model of, 415–416
Nursing diagnoses, 17, 22–24
  as component of nursing process, 16
  definition of, 22
  functions of, 23
  health history as basis for, 87, 111
  list of accepted, 22, *23, 811–815*
  and problem list, 22
  in problem-oriented record (POR), 112
Nursing history (*see* Health history)
Nursing practice:
  definition of, 14–15
  standards of, 15
    for pregnant client, 669, 679
Nursing process:
  components of, 15–26
  and health assessment, 111
  and holistic health, 12–17
Nursing theory, 13–15
Nutrition pattern, *16,* 17, 21, 106–108
  of adolescent, 107, 612–613
  basic four food groups in, 107, 108, *819*
  of infant, 107, *415,* 437–440
  of middle adult, 740, *772*
  of neonate, 365–366
  of older adult, 771–772, *776*
  in pregnancy, 107, 692–693
  of preschooler, 518, 535–536
  recommended daily dietary allowances in, 21, 107, 108, *817*
    for calories, for height and weight, *819*
    for persons over 50 years, *772*
    for pregnancy and lactation, *692*
    for selected vitamins and minerals, *818*
  of school-aged child, 579–580
  skinfold thickness as indicator of, 134, 144–145, 626, 636
  of toddler, 489–490
  of young adult, 663–664
  (*See also* Obesity; Weight)

Obesity:
  cultural variations in, 678
  and gynecomastia in adolescence, 619
  of infant, 365, 438, 439
  of middle adult, 740
  of preschooler, 535–536
  of school-age male, 594
Object permanence, 436–437, 487
Occupation, 91, 102–103
  of adolescent, 605–607
  hazards of, 19, 91, 102–103, 727, 732–733
    for pregnant client, 689
  of middle adult, 726, 727, 729, 741
    hazards of, 732–733
  of older adult, 765–767
  of parent of infant, 434, 435
  of parent of neonate, 362
  of parent of preschooler, 529–530
  of parent of toddler, 483
  of pregnant client, 672, 689
  of young adult, 649–650, 657–658
Oculomotor nerve (cranial nerve III), 170, 172, *807*
Oedipal complex, 35–36, 534
Older adult, 757–799
  abdomen of, 793–794
  age differences and subgroups of, 760, 763
  attitude of, toward death, 763
  behavioral development of, 763
  biological rhythms of, 763–764
  blood pressure of, 782
  chest of, 790–793
  client profile and biographical data of, 759
  cognitive and perceptual pattern of, 768–770, 784, 799
  community resources for, 765–766
  constructiveness as adjustment strategy of, 774
  coping and stress tolerance pattern of, 773–776
  defensiveness as adjustment strategy of, 774–775
  definition of, 757
  dependence as adjustment strategy of, 774
  depression of, and biological rhythms, 763

Older adult (*Cont.*):
  ears of, 786–787
  elimination pattern of, 764, 793, 794
  environment of, 764
  exercise and activity pattern of, 763, 773
  extremities of, 798–799
  eyes of, 785–786
  face of, 783–784
  family history of, 761
  family life of, 766
  finances of, 765
    and medications, 765
    and nutrition, 771
  general appearance of, 780, 781
  genitals of, 795–797
  growth and development of, 761–763
    developmental tasks in, 775–776
      according to Erikson, 37, 762, 773
    theories about, 43–45, 761–762
  head of, 783–789
  health habits of, 759, 776
  health history of, 71, 73, 757–779
  health status and health perception pattern of,
    759–760
  hearing of, 768, 786–787
  heart of, 792–793
  heart rate of, 782, 792
  height of, 781
  hostility-anger as adjustment strategy of, 775
  joints of, 798
  life pattern and lifestyle of, 760–766
  lungs of, 790–791
  medication dosage and finances of, 765
  mouth of, 788–789
  neck of, 789–790
  nose and sinus of, 787
  nursing approach to, 758
  nutrition pattern of, 771–772, 776
  occupation of, 765–767
  personality types of, 773–775
  physical examination of, 780–799
  rectum of, 797
  reminiscing by, 768
  respiration of, 782, 790–791
  review of body components of, 776–777
  role and relationship pattern of, 766–767
  self-hate as adjustment strategy of, 775
  self-perception and self-concept pattern of, 767–768,
    775
  sense of touch of, 767–769, 784, 799
  sexuality and reproduction pattern of, 770–771, 796,
    797
  skin of, 783, 784, 798
  sleep and wakefulness pattern of, 764
  spine of, 781, 789–792
  teeth and gums of, 788
  temperature of, 769, 781
  terminal drop hypothesis about, 757
  thorax of, 790–793
  vision of, 768, 769, 785, 786
  weight of, 781
Olfactory nerve (cranial nerve I), 193, *807*
  of toddler, 499
Ophthalmoscope, 132–133, 174–176
  and middle adult, 748
  and neonate, 378
  and older adult, 786
  and pregnant client, 699
  and preschooler, 551
  and school-aged child, 586
  and toddler, 500
Optic nerve (cranial nerve II), 166, 167, *807*
Orem's self-care agency model, 14
Orient, influences of, on holism, 4–5
Oropharynx, 208–209
  of infant, 453, 454
  of neonate, 381–383
  in pregnancy, 701
  of preschooler, 538, 556
  self-examination of, 727
  of toddler, 502–503
Ortolani's maneuver for infant hip assessment, 396, 464
Osteoporosis, 742, 776, 790
  dental, 788
Otoscope, 131, 179, 181–182, 191
  and infant, 451
  and neonate, 380
  and preschooler, 552–553
  and school-aged child, 586
  and toddler, 501
Ovaries, 285, 290–291
  of adolescent, 636
  of middle adult, 753
  of older adult, 797
  in pregnancy, 706

Pain, 21, 97, 104
  health as freedom from, 1–3

Pain (*Cont.*):
  perception of, 341, 344, 346
Palate, 208–210
  of infant, 453
  of neonate, 383
Palpation as physical examination technique, 120–122
Pancreas, 277
Papanicolaou test, 287
  in pregnancy, 674, 705
Parent:
  adolescent as, 434, 611–612
  of adolescent, role of, in health history or physical
    examination of adolescent, 598
  of infant: attitude of, toward birth and baby, 418–419,
    428–429
    developmental tasks of, *424–425*
    mental health of, *424–425*
    occupation of, 434, 435
    role of, in child health history or physical
      examination, 413–414, 437, 445
  of neonate: attitude of, toward birth and baby,
    418–419, 428–429
    developmental tasks of, *424–425*
    mental health of, *424–425*
    occupation of, 362
    role of, in health history or physical examination of
      child, 352–353, 369
  middle adult as, 733–734
  nurse relationship with, 415–416
  of preschooler: occupation of, 529–530
    role of, in child health history or physical
      examination, 541
    sex education needs of, 534
  role of, in health history or physical examination: of
    adolescent, 598
    of infant, 413–414, 437, 445
    of neonate, 352–353, 369
    of preschooler, 541
    of school-aged child, 585
    of toddler, 491, 495–496
  of school-aged child: role of, in health history or
    physical examination of child, 585
  single, 572
  single, 657
    of infant, 435
    of school-aged child, 572
  young adult as, 656–657
Patient (*see* Client)
Patterns (*see* Functional patterns)
PDQ (Prescreening Developmental Questionnaire), 423,
  516
Peabody Picture Vocabulary Test, 489, *516*, 567, *568*,
  576
Peers:
  of adolescent, 602–603, 618
  of preschooler, 531
  of school-aged child, 569, 572, 574
Pelvic examination (*see* Genitals)
Pelvimeter, 137
Pelvis, bony, diameters of, 706–708
Penis, 292–295
  of adolescent, 619, *633*, 634
  of infant, 460
  of neonate, 393
  of older adult, 795
  of preschooler, 549
  of school-aged child, 594
  and sexual maturity rating of adolescent, *633*, 634
  of toddler, 506
Percussion as physical examination technique,
  123–126
Pharynx (*see* Oropharynx)
Physical examination, 117–349
  of adolescent, 623–636
  annual, 88–89
  as component of nursing process, 16
  equipment for, 129–137, 308
  general appearance in, 138–145
  of infant, 445–465
    parent role in health history or, 413–414, 437,
    445
  measurements taken in, 140–145
  of middle adult, 744–755
  of neonate, 369–412
    at birth, 402–412
    schedule for, 369
  of older adult, 780–799
  in pregnancy, 697–723
    schedule for, 697
  of preschooler, 541–558
    parent role in health history or, 541
  report to client about, 349
  of school-aged child, 585–596
    parent role in health history or, 585
  techniques for, 119–128
  of toddler, 495–507
    parent role in health history or, 491
Pilonidal area, 302

Piskacek's sign of pregnancy, 714
Plan in problem-oriented record (POR), 112–113
Planning as component of nursing process, 24
Play, 36
  of preschooler, 513, 519, 536–537
  of toddler, 486–487, 490–491
Point of maximum impulse (PMI), 251
Poisoning:
  of infant, 422
  of preschooler, 524–525
  of toddler, 472, 481–482
Posture, 138
Practicing as step in separation-individuation of infant,
  427–428
Pregnancy, 669–723
  abdomen in, 703–704
    month by month changes in, 711–723
  during adolescence, 611–612
  age as health factor in, 676–677
  alcohol and, 685–686
  anemia in, 702
  anxiety during, 680–681, 693
  attitude toward, 672, 682
    of client's family, 689
  behavioral development in, 679–682
  biological rhythms associated with, 682
  blood pressure in, 682, 702, 710
  blood volume in, 709, 710
  body image in, 612, 689–690, 693
  breasts in, 698, 702, 713
    preparation of, for breast-feeding, 702
  chest in, 701–702
  client profile and biographical data in, 671–672
  client record in, 671
  cognitive and perceptual pattern in, 690–691
  community resources helpful in, 687–688
  coping and stress tolerance pattern in, 680–681,
    693
    as crisis, 682
    as developmental task, 681–682
  diagnosis of, 280, 286, 711–715, 718
  diagnostic laboratory tests performed during, 702,
    705
  drug use in, 673, 674, *684*, 685
  ears in, 700
  edema in, 710
  elimination pattern during, 704, 709, 713, 723
  environmental influences on, 683–687, 689
  exercise and activity pattern in, 693
  extremities in, 709–710
  eyes in, 699
  face in, 698, 699
  family history in, 676
  family life in, 688–689
  fatigue during, 689, 693
  finances in, 687, 693
  general appearance in, 697–698
  genitals in, 704–708, 711–723
  goiter of, 701
  growth and development in, 678–682
  hair during, 699
  head of client during, 699–700
  health habits during, 673–674
    (*See also* Pregnancy, smoking and)
  health history during, 354–355, 417, 670–696
  health status and health perception pattern during,
    672–676
  health teaching in, 674, 683, 686–687, 690–691
  hearing in, 690
  heart in, 702
  heart rate in, 682
  life pattern and lifestyle in, 676–679, 682
  lungs in, 701
  mouth in, 700
  neck in, 699, 701
  nose in, 700
  nursing approach to client in, 670–671, 697
  nutrition pattern in, 107, 692–693
  occupation during, 672, 689
  pelvic measurement in, 706–708
  physical changes during each month and trimester of,
    680, 711–723
  physical examination in, 697–723
    schedule for, 697
  radiation and, 687
  rectum in, 708, 709
  respiration in, 682, 700, 701
  review of body components in, 693–694
  role and relationship pattern in, 688–689
  self-perception and self-concept pattern during,
    689–690
  sexuality and reproductive pattern during,
    691–692
  skin in, 698, 699, 703, 713, 717
  smoking and, 686–687
  spine in, 709
  temperature in, 682
  thorax in, 701–702

Pregnancy (*Cont.*):
  values and beliefs in, 677
  vision in, 690
  (*See also* Birth defects)
Prematurity, definition of, 351
Preschool (*see* Day care, environment of)
Preschooler, 509–558
  abdomen of, 547–548
  age of, as health factor, 513
  anxiety of, 60, 61
  behavioral development of, 518–521
  biological rhythms of, 99, 521–524
  bladder of, 538
  blood pressure of, *523, 524, 543*
  chest of, 544–547
  client profile and biographical data of, 511
  cognitive and perceptual pattern of, 40–41, *423, 515,
    516,* 531–534
  community resources for, 525
  concept of, about death, 519
  coping and stress tolerance pattern of, 537
  diagnostic laboratory tests for, *538, 539, 558*
  discipline for, 520–521, *527,* 529
  ears of, 552–554
  education of, 524, 531–532
  elimination pattern of, 522–523
  environment of, 524–525, *526–528,* 532
  exercise and activity pattern of, 536–537
  extremities of, 557
  eyes of, 551
  face of, 549, 550
  family history of, 512, 514
  family life of, 525–529
  finances of, 525
  general appearance of, 542–543
  genitals of, 548–549
  grief and mourning of, 519–520
  growth and development of, 515–521
    developmental tasks in, 509, 513, 529
      according to Erikson, 36
    physical size increment in, 515
    theories about, 35, 40–42
  hair of, 549
  head of, 549–555
    circumference of, 550, *828, 832*
  health habits of, 511–512
  health history of, 509–540
  health status and health perception pattern of,
    511–512
  hearing of, 517, 531
  heart of, 544–545
  heart rate of, 523–524, 543
  height of, 515–516, 543, *829–830, 833–834*
  immunization of, 523
  language of, *515,* 517, 531, 533
  life pattern and lifestyle of, 513
  lungs of, 538, 545–546
  morality and ethics of, 35–36, 42
  motor skills of, *515,* 516, 531, 536–537, 557
  mouth of, 555
  neck of, 556
  nose and sinus of, 554
  nurse approach to, 73, 509–510, 541–542
  nutrition pattern of, 518, 535–536
  oropharynx of, 538, 556
  parent of: occupation of, 529–530
    role of, in child health history or physical
      examination, 541
    sex education needs of, 534
  as participant in health care, 509–510, 541
  peers of, 531
  physical examination of, 541–558
    parent role in, 541
  play of, 513, 519, 536–537
  rectum of, 548
  reflexes of, 551, 557
  respirations of, *523,* 524, 543, 545
  restraints for, 552
  review of body components of, 537–538
  ritualism of, 537
  role and relationship pattern of, 525–530
  safety of, 513, 524–525
  self-care skills of, 511–512, 518–519, 536–537
  self-perception and self-concept pattern of, 530–531
  sexuality and reproduction pattern of, 53, 534–535
  skin of, 542–543
  sleep and wakefulness pattern of, 518, 521–522
  spine of, 549
  stimulation for, 524, 525, *526–528*
  teeth of, 511, 555
  temperature of, 523
  thorax of, 544–547
  toilet training of, 512, 518, 537
  vior, 509, 517, 531
  weight of, 515, 543, *829–830, 833–834*
Prescreening Developmental Questionnaire (PDQ), 423,
  516
Primary Mental Abilities Test, 661

Problem list:
  as component of nursing process, 16, 22
  in problem-oriented record (POR), 112
Problem-oriented record (POR), 112–113
  and functional pattern problems, 113
Proprioception, 188, 312, 341–343, 346, 799
Prostate gland, 300, 317
  of middle adult, 732, 737, 754
  of older adult, 795
Protein synthesis theory of aging, 762
Psychological birth, Mahler's theory of, 426–428
Pterygoid muscles, 156, 158
Pulse(s), 138, 141
  of abdomen, 269, 270, 278
  aortic, 269, 270, 278
  apical: of older adult, 792
    of preschooler, 524, 544
    of toddler, 505
  brachial, 332
    of infant, 456
    of neonate, 387, 396
    of preschooler, 544
    of toddler, 505
  carotid, 220, 227–229
    of neonate, 363
    older adult, 789
    of preschooler, 524, 544
    of toddler, 505
  dorsalis pedis, 333
    of infant, 456
    of middle adult, 755
    of neonate, 387
  femoral, 333
    of infant, 456
    of neonate, 387, 396
    of preschooler, 524, 544
    of toddler, 505
  grading scale for, 332
  jugular, 216–219, 228
  popliteal, 332
  posterior tibial, 333
    of middle adult, 755
  radial, 332
  temporal, 155
  venous, 216–219, 228
  (*See also* Heart Rate)
Pulse pressure, definition of, 142
Pupil of eye, 172–173

Race:
  and communication, 76
  dental development and, 590
  effects of, on health, 18, 90, 96
    of adolescent, 601
    of infant, *351,* 419
    of neonate, *351,* 355
    of older adult, 760–761
    in pregnancy, 677
    of preschooler, 513–514
    of school-aged child, 566
    of toddler, 473
  infant mortality rates and, *351*
Radiation in pregnancy, 687
Range of motion, 139, 311, 318–327
  aging and, 311
  of lower extremity, 325–327
  of neonate, 396
  of spine, 214, 319
  of upper extremity, 320–324
Rapprochement in separation-individuation, 428
Readiness:
  as developmental characteristic, 31–32
  for school, 575–576
Reassessment as component of nursing process, 26
Recommended daily dietary allowances (RDA), 21, 107,
  108, *817*
  of calories, for height and weight, *819*
  for persons over 50 years, *772*
  in pregnancy and lactation, *692*
  of selected vitamins and minerals, *818*
Record:
  client, 88, 111–113
    confidentiality of, 598–599
    of older adult, 777
    of pregnant woman, 671
    sharing of, with client, 441
    of toddler, 469
  problem-oriented (POR), 112–113
    and functional pattern problems, 113
Rectum:
  of adolescent, 619, 630
  of female adult, 280, 285, 287, 291, 305–306
    positioning for examination of, 301
  of infant, 461
  of male adult, 305–307
  of neonate, 394
  of older adult, 797

Rectum (*Cont.*):
  in pregnancy, 708, 709
  of preschooler, 548
  of school-aged child, 595
  of toddler, 506
  (*See also* Anus)
Reflex, 135, 347–349
  abdominal, 274, 392, 459
  achilles, 349, 397, 464, 799
  anal (gluteal), 394, 461
  arm recoil, 398
  Babinski, 399, 463, 557
  Bauer's (crawling), 399
  biceps, 348, 397, 464
  blink, 379
  brachioradialis, 348, 397
  corneal, 159, 177
  cremasteric, 394, 461
  crossed extension, 399
  fencing (tonic neck), 384, 461
  finger and thumb, 348
  gag, 210
  Galant's, 401, 465
  gluteal (anal), 394, 461
  hyperactivity of, in pregnancy, 710
  magnet, 398
  maxillary, 159
  Moro, 379, 397
  palmar grasp, 397, 463
  patellar, 349, 397, 464, 557
  placing, 462
  plantar, 398, 463
  protective turning, 401
  pupillary (light), 450, 551
  red, 175, 450, 551
  rooting, 383, 453
  sucking, 383, 453
  stepping, 462
  tonic neck (fencing), 384, 461
  triceps, 348
  withdrawal, 398
Reflex hammer, 135, 347–349
Relaxation, 25
Religion:
  effects of, on health, 90–91, 677
  of older adult, 762
  in young adulthood, 659
Reminiscing by older adult, 768
Renal function tests, laboratory values, for, *804*
Reproduction (*see* Sexuality and reproductive
  pattern)
Resources (*see* Community resources)
Respiration, 142, 238–242, 247–249
  abdominal movement in, 269
  and heart sounds, 256
  of infant, 432, 447, 452, 454–456
  of middle adult, 745, 751
  of neonate, 360, 385–386, 411
  of older adult, 782, 790–791
  in pregnancy, 682, 700, 701
  of preschooler, *523,* 524, 543, 545
  of school-aged child, 583, 587, 588
  sex differences in, 269
  of toddler, 497
  (*See also* Lungs)
Restraints:
  for infant, 446
  for preschooler, 552
  for toddler, 495, 501–503
Retina, 165–166, 174–176
Retirement:
  and older adult, 765, 767
  plans for, of middle adult, 741
Review of systems (*see* Body components, review of)
Rhythms (*see* Biological rhythms)
Ribs, 233, 236, 237, 239
  of infant, 455
  of preschooler, 544
Rinne test of hearing, 134, 186, 578
Ritualism:
  of preschooler, 537
  of toddler, 476, 479
Role and relationship pattern, *16,* 17, 20, 97,
  101–104
  of adolescent, 602–603, 606–607, 617–619
  changes in, 51–52
  development of, 51–52
  of infant, 434–435
  of middle adult, 733–734
  of neonate, 362
  of older adult, 766–767
  in pregnancy, 688–689
  of preschooler, 525–530
  of school-aged child, 572–573
  of toddler, 483–486
  of young adult, 653–659
  (*See also* Family life)
Role strain, 75, 76

Romberg test of balance and proprioception, 188, 312, 342, 343
Rubella and pregnancy, 673, 684

Safety:
  for infant, 422–423
  for middle adult, 727, 732
  for preschooler, 513, 524–525
  for toddler, 472, 481–482
  (See also Environment)
Salivary glands, 207, 208
Scalp, 148–149
  of middle adult, 745
  of neonate, 376
  of preschooler, 550
Scapulae, 237
School, 19, 103
  adjustment to entering, 568–569
  adolescent and, 607–608
  health examination before, 88–89
  performance in, 576–578
  readiness for, 575–576
School-aged child, 559–596
  abdomen of, 594
  adjustment of, to school, 568–569
  age characteristics of, 565–566
  anxiety of, 60, 61
    in school phobia, 582–583
  behavioral development of, 567–570
  biological rhythms of, 99, 570–571
  blood pressure of, 583, 587, 588
  chest of, 592–593
  client profile and biographical data of, 560–563
  cognitive and perceptual pattern of, 41, 567, 574–578
  community resources for, 572
  coping and stress tolerance pattern of, 581–583
  ears of, 591
  elimination pattern of, 570–571
  environment of, 571
  exercise and activity pattern of, 580–581
  extremities of, 595–596
  eyes of, 591
  face of, 589
  family history of, 562, 565
  family life of, 572–573
  finances of, 571–572
  general appearance of, 587
  genitals of, 594–595
  growth and development of, 567–570
    developmental task in, 36
    physical size increment in, 587, 829–830, 833–834
    theories about, 35, 41, 42, 47
  hair of, 589, 594
  head of, 589–591
  health history of, 559–584
  health status and health perception pattern of, 563
  health teaching of, 560, 563
  hearing of, 564, 577–578, 591
  heart of, 593
  heart rate of, 583, 587, 588
  height of, 568, 583, 587, 829–830, 833–834
  immunization of, 564–565
  language of, 567, 568, 575
  life pattern and lifestyle of, 565–567
  lungs of, 593
  morality and ethics of, 35–36, 569–570
  motor skills of, 567
  mouth of, 590
  neck of, 592
  nose of, 590
  nurse approach to, 559–560, 585–586
  nutrition pattern of, 579–580
  parent of: role of, in health history or physical examination of child, 585
    single, 572
  as participant in own care, 560
  peer relationships of, 569, 572, 574
  physical examination of, 585–596
    parent role in health history or, 585
  rectum of, 595
  respiration of, 583, 587, 588
  review of body components of, 583
  role and relationship pattern of, 572–573
  screening tests for, 563–564, 577, 578, 592
    developmental, 568
  self-perception and self-concept pattern of, 596, 573, 574, 576, 580
  sexuality and reproductive pattern of, 53, 578–579, 581, 593, 594
  sleep and wakefulness pattern of, 570
  spine of, scoliosis screening of, 592, 596
  teeth of, 580, 590
  temperature of, 583, 587, 588
  thorax of, 592–593
  values and beliefs of, 563, 569–570
  vision of, 564, 577, 591
  weight of, 568, 583, 587, 829–830, 833–834

School health care, 560
School phobia, 582–583
Schwaback test of hearing, 187
Science of unitary man (M. Rogers), 13–14
Scoliosis:
  screening school-aged child for, 592, 596
  of older adult, 789
    (See also Kyphosis)
Scrotum, 294, 296–297, 299
  of adolescent, 634
  of neonate, 393, 394
    in gestational age estimation, 403
  of older adult, 795
"Security blanket" (transition object), 427
Self-breast examination (SBE), 259, 593, 674, 727, 750
Self-care agency model of health care (D. Orem), 14
Self-care skills of preschooler, 511–512, 518–519, 536–537
Self-examination as preventive health practice, 727
Self-perception and self-concept pattern, 16, 17, 21, 50–51, 104
  of adolescent, 50–51, 616–618
  and emotional development, 98
  of middle adult, 734–735, 740
  in mourning, 58
  of older adult, 767–768, 775
  during pregnancy, 689–690
  of preschooler, 530–531
  of school-aged child, 569, 573, 574, 576, 580
  and sexuality, 106
  of toddler, 486
  of young adult, 659–660
Semicircular canals, 184
Separation anxiety:
  of infant, 440
  of toddler, 60, 428, 447, 479, 491
Separation-individuation, Mahler's theory of, 426–428
Set:
  mental, in health history, 73–74
Sex, curiosity about, 489, 534, 579, 610, 620
Sex education:
  for child and adolescent, 535, 579, 594, 610, 611
  for parent, 534
  (See also Health education)
Sexual maturation, 593, 594
  laboratory tests related to, 636
  Tanner classification of, 629, 633, 634, 636
Sexuality and reproductive pattern, 16, 17, 20–21, 53–54, 106
  of adolescent, 52–54, 609–612
    (See also physical development in, below)
  and emotional stability, 98
  of infant, 52–53, 437
  of middle adult, 728–729, 736–740
  of neonate, 52–53, 364–365
  of older adult, 770–771, 796, 797
  physical development in: athletics and, 581
    breasts and, 593, 629, 633
    genitals and, 594, 633, 634, 636
    laboratory tests related to, 636
  in pregnancy, 691–692
  of preschooler, 53, 534–535
  of school-aged child, 53, 578–579, 581, 593, 594
  sexual dysfunction in, 739
  of toddler, 53, 489
  of young adult, 52–54, 661–663
Shoes for infant, 423, 462
Shoulders, 320, 330, 334, 338
Sick role, 75, 638
Sight (see Vision)
Signs and symptoms:
  definition of, 91
  in SOAP format, 112–113
Sinuses, paranasal, 194–196
  of adolescent, 627
  of neonate, 381
  of older adult, 787
  of school-aged child, 590
Skeleton of extremities, 309–310
Skene's ducts, 283, 284, 394
Skin, 138, 251, 268, 333
  of adolescent, 618, 627
  of infant, 447–448, 460
  of middle adolescent, 746, 748, 752, 754
  of neonate, 372–373
    color of, 370, 372, 386, 395, 402
  of older adult, 783, 784, 798
  in pregnancy, 698, 699, 703, 713, 717
  of preschooler, 542, 543
  self-examination of, 727
  of toddler, 498
  (See also Acne; Birthmarks)
Skinfold, measurement of, 134, 144–145, 626, 636
Sleep and wakefulness pattern, 16, 17, 18, 98–99
  of adolescent, 604
  of infant, 426–427, 429–431

Sleep and wakefulness pattern (Cont.):
  of middle adult, 732
  of neonate, 358–359, 371
  of older adult, 764
  of preschooler, 518, 521–522
  rapid eye movement (REM) sleep in, 764
    of infant, 430
    of neonate, 358
    of preschooler, 521
    of young adult, 651
  of school-aged child, 570
  sleeping medications and, 651
  of toddler, 479–480
  of young adult, 650–651
Slosson Intelligence Test (SIT), 516, 567, 568
Smell, sense of, 21, 104, 105
  of adolescent, 627
  of infant, 435
  of older adult, 787
  in pregnancy, 690
  of preschooler, 531
  of toddler, 486
Smoking, 92
  by adolescent, 600
  and infant health, 354, 417
  by middle adult, 727
    and contraceptive pills, 738
  and physical changes of older adult, 776
  in pregnancy, 686–687
  by young adult, 652
Snellen eye chart, 79, 167–168, 517, 551, 577
SOAP format, 112–113
"Social clock" theory of aging, 762
Social learning theory (R. Sears), 45–48
Speculum:
  nasal, 133, 191–193
  vaginal, 135–136, 285–287, 704
Speech (see Language)
Sphygmomanometer, 130, 142–143
  cuff size of: for adult, 143
    for preschooler, 524, 543
    for toddler, 497
Spinal cord, major tracts (pathways) of, 806
Spinal fluid, laboratory values for, 801
Spine, 233, 311, 319
  cervical, 214
    of older adult, 789
  of infant, 465
  of middle adult, 750
  of neonate, 397
  of older adult, 781, 789–792
  in pregnancy, 709
  of preschooler, 549
  of school-age child, scoliosis screening for, 592, 596
  thoracic, 232–233
    of older adult, 781, 790–792
  of toddler, 507
Spleen, 273, 277
  of infant, 459
  of neonate, 390, 391
  in pregnancy, 703
  of preschooler, 547
  of toddler, 505
Sports:
  and nutritional needs, 612–613
  safety in, 580–581
Stanford Binet Intelligence Test, 488, 533, 661
Stapes, 182, 183
Stature, 138–140
Stealing by school-aged child, 569, 582
Step test for endurance, 631
States of arousal (consciousness) of newborn and infant, 371, 429–430
Sternocleidomastoid muscle, 212–214, 221, 240, 330, 592
Stethoscope, 127–128, 130, 586
  in abdominal assessment, 269–270
  in heart assessment, 253–258
  in lung assessment, 247–249
Stimulation:
  of infant, 430–431, 433, 440
  of neonate, 363–364
  of preschooler, 524, 525, 526–528
Stimulus-response theory, 45–48
Stomach, 273
  of neonate, 390, 391
Stool, tests of:
  for blood, 307
    normal laboratory values for, 805–806
  (See also Elimination pattern; Meconium)
Strabismus:
  of infant, 450
  of preschooler, 551
  tests for, 170–172, 500
Stranger anxiety, 60, 427, 428, 469
Stress (see Coping and stress tolerance pattern)
Striae, 268, 751

Stuttering of preschooler, 517
Superego, 35–36
  of preschooler, 534
  of school-aged child, 569
  (*See also* Morality)
Swallowing, 216, 225, 226
Symbiosis, infant developmental stage of, 426
Symptoms:
  definition of, 91
  in SOAP format, 112–113
System:
  open: client as, 25
Systems, review of (*see* Body components, review of)
Szasz model of nurse-client relationship, 415–416

Tanner stages of sexual maturation:
  and athletics, 581
  of breasts, 593, *629, 633*
  of genitals, 594, *633, 634, 636*
  laboratory tests related to, 636
Taoism, influence of, on holism, 4
Taste, sense of, 21, 104, 105, 207
  of infant, 435
  of middle adult, 736
  of older adult, 789
  in pregnancy, 690
  of preschooler, 531
  of toddler, 486
Teaching (*see* Health education; Sex education)
Teeth, 138, 201–205
  of adolescent, 627, 636
  of infant, 420, *421*, 453
    bottle-feeding and, 422
  of middle adult, 746
  of neonate, 381
  of older adult, 788
  of preschooler, 511, 555
  of school-aged child, 580, 590
  self-examination of, 727
  stains of, 201
  of toddler, 481, 503
Temper tantrums, 478–479
Temperament of neonate and infant, 32–33, 428–429
Temperature, 138, 141
  Celsius-Fahrenheit conversion of, 141, *808–810*
  of infant, 431
  of middle adult, 745
  of neonate, 359–360, 412
  of older adult, 769, 781
  and ovulation, 682
  of pregnant client, 682
  of preschooler, 523
  of school-aged child, 583, 587, 588
  teething and, 481
  of toddler, 481, 497
Temporal muscles, 156, 157
Teratogens, 418, 673, 674, 683–687
Terminal drop hypothesis about aging, 757
Territoriality, 78–79
Testes, 296
  of adolescent, 594, *633*, 634
  of infant, 460, 461
  migration of, 297
  of middle adult, 754
  of neonate, 394
    in gestational age estimation, 403
  of older adult, 795
  of preschooler, 549
  of school-aged child, 594, 595
  self-examination of, 727
  of toddler, 506
Thorax, 230–263
  of adolescent, 619, 628
  of infant, 454–458
  of middle adult, 750–751
  of neonate, 385–388, 410
  of older adult, 790–793
  in pregnancy, 701–702
  of preschooler, 544–547
  of school-aged child, 592–593
  of toddler, 504–505
Thorpe Developmental Inventory, 517
Throat (*see* Neck; Oropharynx)
Thumbs, 324, 330
Thumb-sucking, 520
Thyroid cartilage, 215–216, 225–226
Thyroid gland, 215–216, 225–226
  enlargement of, in pregnancy, 701
  of middle adult, 740
  of neonate, 384
  of older adult, 790
  of preschooler, 556
Toddler, 467–507
  abdomen of, 505
  age of, as health factor, 472
  ambivalence of, 476, 479

Toddler (*Cont.*):
  anxiety of, 60, 61
    about separation, 60, 428, 477, 479, 491
    about strangers, 469
  bedtime resistance of, 478
  behavioral development of, 475–479
  biological rhythms of, 99, 479–481
  blood pressure of, 497
  body image of, 478
  chest of, 504–505
  client profile and biographical data of, 469–470
  cognitive and perceptual pattern of, 40, *423*,
    486–489, *516*, 517, *568*
  community resources for, 483
  coping and stress tolerance pattern of, 491–492
  day-care environment of, 482, 487
  diagnostic laboratory tests for, 507
  ears of, 492, 501
  education for, 486–487
  elimination pattern of, 480–481
  environment of, 481–482, *484–485*, 487
  exercise and activity pattern of, 490–491
  extremities of, 492, 506–507
  eyes of, 492, 500
  face of, 497, 499
  family history of, 472
  family life of, 483
  fears and fantasies of, 477–479
  finances of, 473–474, 483
  general appearance of, 497–498
  genitals of, 506
  growth and development of, 474–475
    developmental tasks in, 36, 467
    physical size increment in, 474, *829–830, 833–834*
    theories about, 34–36, 40, 46–47, 467
  head of, 492, 499
    circumference of, 499, *828, 832*
  health habits of, 470–471
  health history of, 467–494
  health status and health perception pattern of,
    470–472
  hearing of, 486
  heart of, 492, 505
  heart rate of, 497
  height of, 474, 498, *827–828, 831–832*
  immunization of, 472, 481
  language development of, 474, 488–489, 501
  life pattern and lifestyle of, 472–483
  lungs of, 504
  magical thinking of, 478
  motor skills of, 471, 474–475, 490–491
  mouth of, 502–503
  neck of, 502–503
  negativism of, 476–477, 479
  nose and sinus of, 502
  nurse approach to, 73, 468, 495–496
  nutritional pattern of, 489–490
  parent of: attitude of, toward child, 468, 469,
    475–477, 491
    occupation of, 483
    role of, in health history or physical exam of child,
    491
  physical examination of, 495–507
    parent role in health history or, 491
  play of, 486–487, 490–491
  rectum of, 506
  reflexes of, 507
  respiration of, 497
  restraints for, 495, 501–503
  review of body components of, 492
  ritualism of, 476, 479
  role and relationship pattern of, 483–486
  safety of, 472, 481–482
  self-perception and self-concept pattern of, 486
  separation-individuation of, 428
  sexuality and reproductive pattern of, 53, 489
  skin of, 498
  sleep and wakefulness pattern of, 479–480
  spine of, 507
  stranger anxiety of, 469
  teeth of, 503
  teething and fever of, 481
  temper tantrums of, 478–479
  temperature of, 481, 497
  thorax of, 504–505
  toilet training of, 474, 480–481
  vision of, 486, 500
  weight of, 474, 498, *829–830, 833–834*
Toes, 327, 395
Toilet training:
  and enuresis, 571
  Freudian views on, 34–35
  of preschooler, 512, 518, 537
  of toddler, 474, 480–481
Tongue, 205–208
  of middle adult, 747
  of neonate, 382
Tonometer, 137, 162, 748

Tonsils, 208, 210
  of infant, 453
  of toddler, 503
Touch:
  client responses to, 78
    older adult, 767–769
  sense of, 21, 104, 105, 341, 344–346
    of infant, 435
    of neonate, 363
    of older adult, 767–769, 784, 799
    in pregnancy, 690
    of preschooler, 531
    of toddler, 486
  therapeutic, 25
Trachea, 215–216, 235, 240
  of adolescent, 628
  of infant, 454
  of neonate, 384
  of older adult, 789
  of preschooler, 556
Transition objects, 427
Trapezius muscle, 212–214, 221, 240, 330
Trigeminal nerve (cranial nerve V), 156–159, 162, 177,
    807
  of toddler, 499
Trochlear nerve (cranial nerve IV), 170, 172, *807*
  of preschooler, 551
Trunk, 311, 319
Trust in nurse-client relationship, 71, 83, 85, 86
Trust versus mistrust, 36, 426
Tuberculosis, screening for:
  of infant, 432
  of school-aged child, 564
  of toddler, 472, 481, 507
Tuning fork, 185, 186
Tympanic membrane (*see* Eardrum)

Umbilicus, 268
  of infant, 458
  of neonate, 389
  of preschooler, 547
  of toddler, 505
Urethra, 283, 292
  of infant, 460
  of neonate, 393
  of preschooler, 548
Urinalysis, *539, 806*
  for preschooler, *538*, 558
  for toddler, 507
Urinary tract infection:
  in pregnancy, 704
  of preschooler, 558
  of school-age child, 570
Urination (*see* Elimination pattern)
Uterus, 285, 288–289
  of adolescent, 636
  of middle adult, 753
  of older adult, 795, 797
  in pregnancy, 703–706
    monthly changes in, 711–723

Vagina, 135–136, 283–287
  of adolescent, 636
  culture or smear of, 286
  of infant, 460
  of middle adult, 737, 738, 753
  of neonate, 393
  of older adult, 796
  in pregnancy, 704
  of preschooler, 548
Vagus nerve (cranial nerve X), 210, *808*
Values and beliefs, *16*, 17, 18, 51, 97
  of nurse, 73–74
  of older adult, 762
  of pregnant client, 677
  of school-aged child, 563, 569–570
  (*See also* Religion)
Veins:
  of lower extremities, 315
  of neck, 216–219
    of adolescent, 629
    of neonate, 384
    of preschooler, 556
  of upper extremities, 314
Venous pressure of older adult, 789
Venous pulse, 216–219, 228
Verbal Language Development Scale (VLDS), *568*
Vertebrae (*see* Spine)
Vestibulocochlear nerve (cranial nerve VIII) (*see*
    Auditory nerve)
Vietnam war as influence on health, 662–663
Vineland Social Maturity Scale, 489, 517
Viruses, effects of, on pregnancy, 683–685
Vision, 21, 104, 166–173
  of adolescent, 628

Vision (*Cont.*):
Denver Eye Screening Test (DEST) of, *423, 500, 516, 517, 820–821*
Hardy-Rand-Rittler test of, 577
of infant, 435
developmental changes in, 420, *421*, 450
testing of, *422, 423,* 451
Ishihara test of, 577
of middle adult, 735–736, 747
of neonate, 363
of older adult, 768, 769, 785, 786
in pregnancy, 690
of preschooler, 509, 517, 531
of school-aged child, 564, 577, 591
Snellen tests of, 79, 167–168, *517,* 551, 577
of toddler, 486, 500
Visualization, 25
Vital signs (*see* Blood pressure; Heart rate; Respiration; Temperature)
Vitamins:
recommended daily dietary allowances for, *818*
supplemental: for infant, 440
for older adult, 772
for toddler, 490
VLDS (Verbal Language Developmental Scale), 568
VMI (Developmental Test of Visual-Motor Integration), *516,* 517, 567, *568*
Voice and chest fremitus, 243–245

Walking of infant, 427–428
(*See also* Gait)
Weaning:
and preschooler, 512
readiness for, 422, 427
Weber test of hearing, 186, 578, 749

Wechsler Intelligence Scale for Children, 488, 533
Weight, 138, 140
in adolescence, 625–626, *829–830, 833–834*
at birth, 408
classification by gestational age and, 351, 409
of children to 18 years, *827–834*
and height, caloric requirements for, *819*
of infant, 447, *827–828, 831–832*
of neonate, 408–410, *827–828, 831–832*
of older adult, 781
of preschooler, 515, 543, *829–830, 833–834*
recommended for height, *107, 140, 816, 819*
of school-aged child, *568,* 583, 587, *829–830, 833–834*
of toddler, 474, 498, *829–830, 833–834*
Wellness, 1–4
Wholeness, Levine's principles of conservation of, 13
Wholism (*see* Holism)
Wide Range Achievement Test (WRAT), 567, *568*
Women:
biological rhythms of, 682
recommended daily dietary allowances for, *692*
Work (*see* Occupation)
Worms, testing toddler for, 507
Wrists, 322, 335, 339
muscles and nerves of, 330, 339

Ying and yang, 5, 25
Young adult, 637–668
age of, as health factor, 642
biological rhythms of, 650–651
client profile and biographical data of, 639–640
cognitive and perceptual pattern of, 660–661
community resources for, 639, 653

Young adult (*Cont.*):
coping and stress tolerance pattern of, 665
definition of, 637
divorce of, 655–656
drug use and abuse by, 651, 665
elimination pattern of, 651
environmental influences on health of, 651–652
exercise and activity pattern of, 664–665
family history of, 642
finances of, 652–653
generativity versus stagnation of, 649
growth and development of, 643–650
developmental tasks in, 37, 648–650, 663
theories of, 37
health habits of, 640–641, 652
health history of, 637–666
health risks of, 641
health status and health perception pattern of, 640–642
intimacy versus isolation of, 648–649, 663
life pattern and lifestyle of, 640–653
nontraditional, 640–641, 658–659, 661–662
marriage of, 654–655, 658–659, 664
maturity of, 644–648
morality and ethics of, 658, 659
nutritional pattern of, 663–664
occupation of, 649–650, 657–658
as parent, 656–657
review of body components of, 665
role acquisition of, as client, 638, *639*
role and relationship pattern of, 653–659
self-perception and self-concept pattern of, 659–660
sexuality and reproduction pattern of, 52–54, 661–663
sleep and wakefulness pattern of, 650–651